Stressed out by the complicated details of Pharmacology?
Cut through the confusion with

The Student Resource CD-ROM to Accompany Focus on Nursing Pharmacology 4th Edition

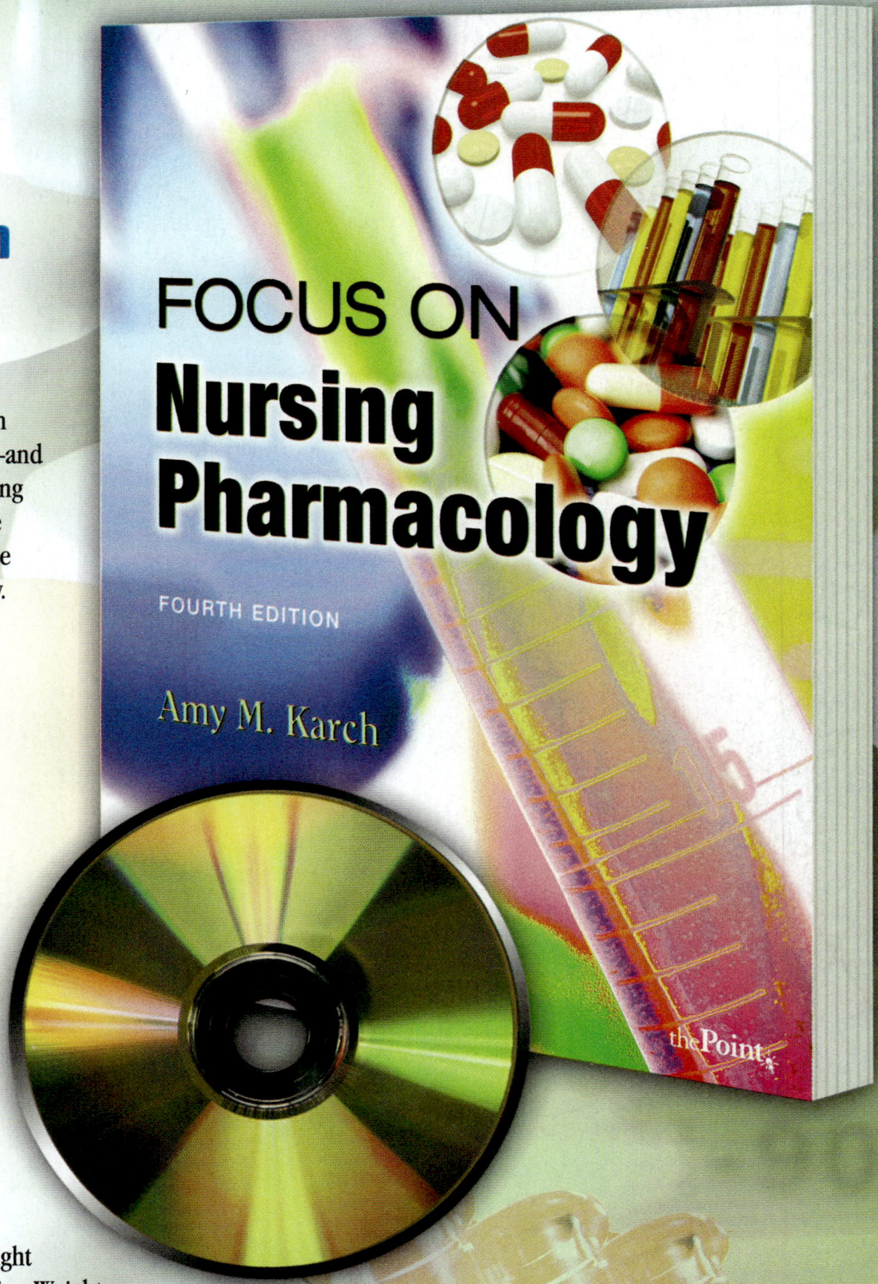

Your Student Resource CD-ROM features awesome tools to help you learn!

Studying and understanding nursing pharmacology can seem overwhelming, but this clearly organized, streamlined text—and its amazing bound-in CD-ROM—breaks down the intimidating complexities into small, easy-to-learn steps, zeroes in on the need-to-know specifics, and moves smoothly from the simple to the more difficult, building your knowledge along the way.

Dynamic audio and video on the CD-ROM includes:

- NCLEX Alternate Item Format Tutorial
- Monographs of 100 most commonly prescribed drugs
- Concepts in Action™ Animations covering:
  - Absorption
  - Drug Binding
  - Intramuscular Injection
  - Distribution
  - Excretion
  - Intravenous Injection
  - And More!
- Watch and Learn™ Medication Administration Videos on:
  - Preparing Unit Dose-Packaged Medications
  - Administering Oral Medications
  - Administering Subcutaneous and Intramuscular Injections
  - IV Medication by Piggyback Infusion
  - And More!
- Dosage Calculation Quizzes including:
  - Solving for Dose
  - Solving for Dosing Rate
  - Comprehensive Review
  - Solving for Dose Using Weight
  - Solving for Dosing Rate Using Weight
- Spanish-English Audio Glossary

...and much, much more!

FOCUS ON
Nursing Pharmacology
FOURTH EDITION
Amy M. Karch
thePoint

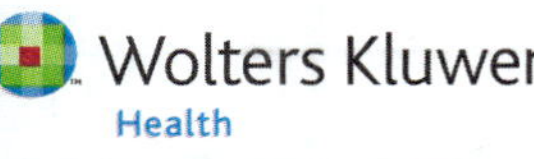

Lippincott Williams & Wilkins

Check it out today!

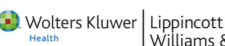

FOCUS ON Nursing Pharmacology

FOURTH EDITION

Amy M. Karch, RN, MS
Associate Professor of Clinical Nursing
University of Rochester School of Nursing
Rochester, New York

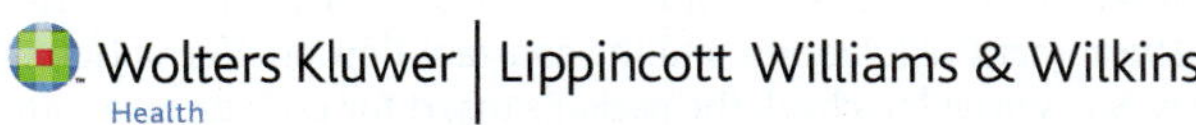

Philadelphia • Baltimore • New York • London
Buenos Aires • Hong Kong • Sydney • Tokyo

Acquisitions Editor: Margaret Zuccarini
Senior Managing Editor: Helen Kogut
Managing Editor: Michelle Clarke
Senior Managing Editor, Production: Erika Kors
Senior Production Manager: Helen Ewan
Design Coordinator: Holly Reid McLaughlin
Indexer: Ellen Brennan
Compositor: Circle Graphics
Printer: R. R. Donnelley—Willard

The author and the publisher have endeavored to ensure that Web sites listed in the text were active prior to publication. However, due to the Internet's evolving nature, Web addresses may have changed or sites may have ceased to exist since publication.

9 8 7 6 5 4 3 2

Library of Congress Cataloging-in-Publication Data

Karch, Amy Morrison, 1949-
Focus on nursing pharmacology / Amy M. Karch. — 4th ed.
p. ; cm.
Includes bibliographical references and index.
ISBN-13: 978-0-7817-9047-5 (alk. paper)
ISBN-10: 0-7817-9047-6 (alk. paper)
1. Pharmacology. 2. Nursing. I. Title.
[DNLM: 1. Pharmaceutical Preparations—Nurses' Instruction. 2. Drug Therapy—Nurses' Instruction. 3. Pharmacology—Nurses' Instruction. QV 4 K183f 2007]
RM300.K37 2007
615'.1—dc22
2006029012

Care has been taken to confirm the accuracy of the information presented and to describe generally accepted practices. However, the authors, editors, and publisher are not responsible for errors or omissions or for any consequences from application of the information in this book and make no warranty, express or implied, with respect to the contents of the publication.

The authors, editors and publisher have exerted every effort to ensure that drug selection and dosage set forth in this text are in accordance with current recommendations and practice at the time of publication. However, in view of ongoing research, changes in government regulations, and the constant flow of information relating to drug therapy and drug reactions, the reader is urged to check the package insert for each drug for any change in indications and dosage and for added warnings and precautions. This is particularly important when the recommended agent is a new or infrequently employed drug.

Some drugs and medical devices presented in this publication have Food and Drug Administration (FDA) clearance for limited use in restricted research settings. It is the responsibility of the health care provider to ascertain the FDA status of each drug or device planned for use in clinical practice.

Dedicated to my many students, past and present, who have taught me how to teach and kept me inspired and enthusiastic about the wonders of learning; to the hard-working nursing faculty across the country who are tirelessly striving to educate new nurses . . . and to my family, who have been my support, my inspiration, and my sunshine.

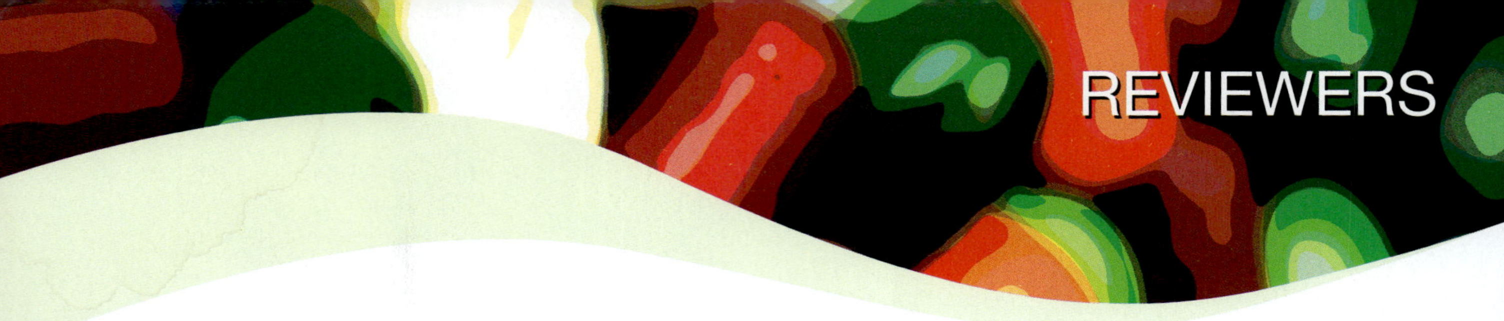

REVIEWERS

Joanne Bonesteel, RN, MSN
Nursing Faculty
Excelsior College
Albany, New York

Gina S. Brown, RN, PhD
Chair and Professor
Columbia Union College
Edyth T. James Department of Nursing
Takoma Park, Maryland

Susan Buchholz, RN, BSN, MSN
Associate Professor of Nursing
Georgia Perimeter College
Lawrenceville, Georgia

Barbara M. Carranti, RN, MS, CNS
Instructor—Nursing
LeMoyne College
Syracuse, New York

Cynthia L. Dakin, RN, PhD
Assistant Professor
Northeastern University School of Nursing
Boston, Massachusetts

Loretta B. Delargy, RN, MSN
Assistant Professor
North Georgia College and State University
Dahlonega, Georgia

Carol Fanutti, RN, EdD, MSN,
Director of Nursing
Trocaire College
Buffalo, New York

Mary-Margaret Finney, RN, MSN
Assistant Professor, Department of Nursing
North Georgia College and State University
Dahlonega, Georgia

Charlene Beach Gagliardi, BS, RN, MSN
Instructor
Mount Saint Mary's College
Los Angeles, California

Nancy B. Hartel, RN, MS
Nursing Faculty
St. Joseph's College of Nursing at St. Joseph's Hospital
Syracuse, New York

Annette Hutcherson, RN, MN, EdD
Professor of Nursing
Polk Community College
Winter Haven, Florida

Jodie Lane, RN, MSN
Nursing Faculty NSC and Critical Care Educator
Summerlin Medical Center
Nevada State College
Henderson, Nevada

Cynthia L. Lapp, BS, RN
Practical Nursing Instructor
Jefferson–Lewis BOCES
Lowville, New York

Rhonda Lawes, RN, MN
Instructor
University of Oklahoma College of Nursing
Tulsa, Oklahoma

A. Renee Leasure, RN, PhD, CCRN, CNS
Associate Professor and Deputy Director, Evidence Based Practice Center Oklahoma
University of Oklahoma College of Nursing
Oklahoma City, Oklahoma

Barbara Lee-Learned, RN, MSN
Nursing Faculty
Technical College of the Lowcountry
Beaufort, South Carolina

Colleen Ley, RN, BSN, MSN
AD Instructor
Madison Area Technical College
Watertown, Wisconsin

Linda McIntosh Liptok, RN, BMus, MSN, APRN, BC
Assistant Professor
Kent State University, Tuscarawas
New Philadelphia, Ohio

Robin D. Lockhart, RN, MSN
Assistant Professor of Nursing
Midwestern State University
Wichita Falls, Texas

Angela Phillips-Lowe, RN, EdD
Associate Professor of Nursing
Mount Carmel College of Nursing
Columbus, Ohio

Janet Massoglia, BSN, MSN
Instructor
Delta College
University Center, Michigan

Dorothy Mathers, RN, MSN
Associate Professor
Pennsylvania College of Technology
Pittsburgh, Pennsylvania

Jeffrey C. McManemy
Associate Professor
University Center, Missouri
St. Louis Community College at Florissant Valley
St. Louis, Missouri

Cathy Michalenko, RN, MN, GNC(c)
Instructor
Red Deer College
Red Deer, Alberta, Canada

Patricia J. Neafsey, RD, PhD
Professor
University of Connecticut
Storrs, Connecticut

Winifred A. Olmstead, BSN, MSN
Nursing Faculty
St. Joseph's College of Nursing at St. Joseph's Hospital
Syracuse, New York

Nola Ormrod, RN, MSN
Nursing Director
Centralia College
Centralia, Washington

Eva Ann Pihlgren, BSN, MN
Professor of Nursing
Antelope Valley College
Lancaster, California

Susan L. Piva, RN, MSN, BSN
Associate Professor of Nursing
Brevard Community College
Cocoa, Florida

Loretta G. Quigley, RN, MS
Associate Dean
St. Joseph's College of Nursing at St. Joseph's Hospital
Syracuse, New York

Luanne G. Richardson
Assistant Professor
Duquesne University
Pittsburgh, Pennsylvania

Patricia Roper, RN, MSN
Professor of Nursing
Columbus State Community College
Columbus, Ohio

Carol A. Sheldon, RN, MS, CEN
Nursing Faculty
St Joseph's College of Nursing at St. Joseph's Hospital Health Center
Syracuse, New York

Thomas J. Smith
Faculty–BSN Program
Nicholls State University
Thibodaux, Louisiana

Fran Soukup
Faculty
Madison Area Technical College
Reedsburg, Wisconsin

Martha A. Spies, RN, PhD
Professor
Deaconess College of Nursing
St. Louis, Missouri

Carol A. Storm, MSN, APRN, BC
Director
B. M. Spurr School of Practical Nursing
Glen Dale, West Virginia

Scott Carter Thigpen, RN, MSN, CCRN, CEN
Assistant Professor of Nursing
South Georgia College, Division of Nursing
Douglas, Georgia

Dina L. Wilson, RN, MN
Professor, Nursing
Johnson County Community College
Overland Park, Kansas

Regina L. Wright, RN, MSN, CEN
Clinical Assistant Professor
Drexel University
Philadelphia, Pennsylvania

Carolyn Johnson Wyss, RN, MSN
Associate Professor of Nursing, Technology Coordinator
Walters State Community College
Morristown, Tennessee

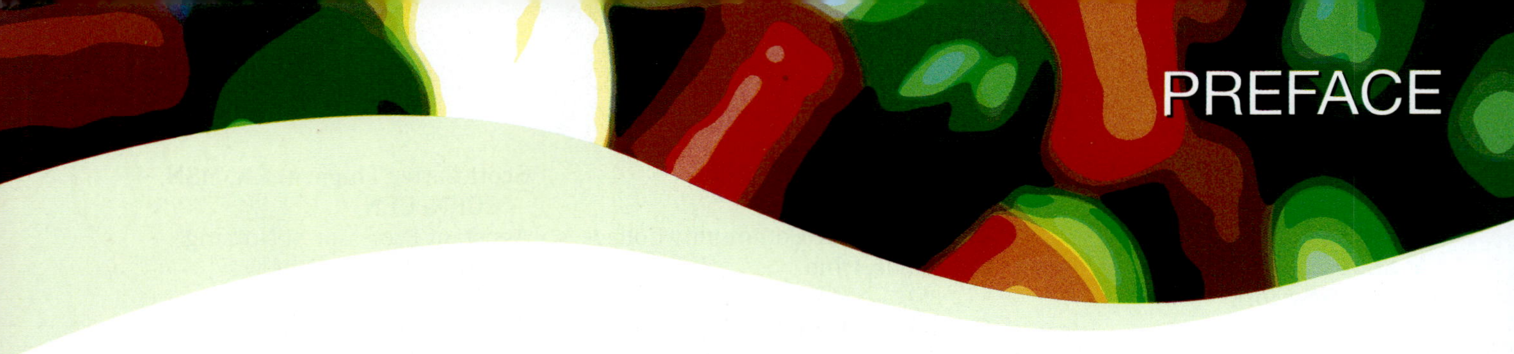

PREFACE

Pharmacology is a difficult course to teach in a standard nursing curriculum, whether it be a diploma, associate, baccalaureate, or graduate program. Teachers are difficult to find, and time and money often dictate that the invaluable content of such a course be incorporated into other courses. As a result, the content is often lost. At the same time, changes in medical care delivery—more outpatient and home care, shorter hospital stays, and more self-care—have resulted in additional legal and professional responsibilities for nurses, making them more responsible for the safe and effective delivery of drug therapy.

Pharmacology should not be such a formidable obstacle in the nursing curriculum. The study of drug therapy incorporates physiology, pathophysiology, chemistry, and nursing fundamentals—subjects that are already taught in most schools. A textbook that approaches pharmacology as an understandable, teachable, and learnable subject would greatly facilitate the incorporation of this subject into nursing curricula. Yet many nursing pharmacology texts are large and burdensome, mainly because they have needed to cover not only the basic pharmacology but also the particulars included in each area considered.

The fourth edition of *Focus on Nursing Pharmacology* is based on the premise that students first need to have a solid and clearly focused concept of the principles of drug therapy before they can easily grasp the myriad details associated with individual drugs.

Armed with a fundamental knowledge of pharmacology, the student can appreciate and use the specific details that are so readily available in the many annually updated and published nursing drug guides, such as *Lippincott's Nursing Drug Guide.*

With this goal in mind, *Focus on Nursing Pharmacology* provides a concise, user-friendly, and uncluttered text for the modern student. This difficult subject is presented in a streamlined, understandable, teachable, and learnable manner. Because this book is designed to be used in conjunction with a handbook of current drug information it remains streamlined. This fourth edition of *Focus on Nursing Pharmacology* continues to emphasize "need-to-know" concepts.

The text reviews and integrates previously learned knowledge of physiology, chemistry, and nursing fundamentals into chapters focused on helping students conceptualize what is important to know about each group of drugs. Illustrations, side bars and tables sum up concepts to enhance learning. Special features further focus student learning on clinical application, critical thinking, patient safety, lifespan issues related to drug therapy, evidence-based practice, patient teaching, and case-study–based critical thinking exercises that incorporate nursing process principles. The text incorporates study materials that conclude each chapter. *Check Your Understanding* provides both new- and old-format NCLEX-style review questions as well as study guide review questions to help the student master the material and prepare for the national licensing exam.

Focus on Teaching/ Learning Activities

thePoint

ThePoint (http://thepoint.lww.com/), a trademark of Wolters Kluwer Health, is a web-based course and content management system that provides every resource instructors and students need in one easy-to-use site. ThePoint . . . where teaching, learning, and technology click!

Student Resources

Students can visit thePoint to access supplemental multimedia resources to enhance their learning experience, check the course syllabus, download content, upload assignments, and join an online study group. ThePoint offers a variety of free student resources, including Watch and Learn video clips, Practice and Learn activities, NCLEX-Style Student Review Questions, an Alternate-Format NCLEX Tutorial, and a Spanish-English Audioglossary. It also has free journal articles related to topics discussed in the Focus on Patient Safety boxes from the book. Also, included are **WATCH & LEARN** videos on preventing medication errors and **CONCEPTS** in action **ANIMATION** 3-D animated depictions of pharmacology concepts. In addition, an online course is available that includes interactive activities.

Instructor Resources

Advanced technology and superior content combine at thePoint to allow instructors to design and deliver online and offline courses, maintain grades and class rosters, and communicate with students. In addition to housing the material from the Instructor's Resource CD-ROM, thePoint also provides additional resources, including pre-lecture quizzes, guided lecture notes, topics for discussion, and assignments.

Organization

Focus on Nursing Pharmacology is organized following a "simple to complex" approach, much like the syllabus for a basic nursing pharmacology course. Because students learn best "from the bottom up," the text is divided into distinct parts.

Part I begins with an overview of basic nursing pharmacology, including such new challenges as bioterrorism, street drugs, herbal therapies, and the information overload; each of the other parts begins with a review of the physiology of the system affected by the specific drugs being discussed. This review refreshes the information for the student and provides a quick and easy reference when reading about drug actions.

Part II of the text introduces the drug classes, starting with the chemotherapeutic agents—both antimicrobial and antineoplastic drugs. Because the effectiveness of these drugs depends on their interference with the most basic element of body physiology—the cell—students can easily understand the pharmacology of this class. Mastering the pharmacotherapeutic effects of this drug class helps establish a firm grasp of the basic principles taught in Part I. Once the easiest pharmacologic concepts are understood, the student is prepared to move on to the more challenging physiologic and pharmacologic concepts.

Part III focuses on drugs affecting the immune system, because recent knowledge about the immune system has made it the cornerstone of modern therapy. All of the immune system drugs act in ways that the immune system would itself act if it were able. Recent immunologic research has contributed to a much greater understanding of this system, making it important to position information about drugs affecting this system close to the beginning of the text, instead of at the end as has been the custom.

Parts IV and **V** of the text address drugs that affect the nervous system, the basic functioning system of the body. Following the nervous system, and closely linked with it in **Part VI**, is the endocrine system. The sequence of these parts introduces students to the concept of control, teaches them about the interrelatedness of these two systems, and prepares them for understanding many aspects of shared physiologic function and the inevitable linking of the two systems into one: the neuroendocrine system.

Parts VII, VIII and **IX** discuss drugs affecting the reproductive, cardiovascular, and renal systems, respectively. The sequencing of cardiovascular and renal drugs is logical because most of the augmenting cardiovascular drugs (such as diuretics) affect the renal system.

Part X covers drugs that act on the respiratory system, which provides the link between the left and right ventricles of the heart.

Part XI addresses drugs acting on the gastrointestinal system. The gastrointestinal system stands on its own; it does not share any actions with any other system.

Text Features

The features in this text are skillfully designed to support the text discussion, encouraging the student to look at the whole patient and to focus on the essential information that is important to learn about each drug class. Important features in the fourth edition focus on incorporating basic nursing skills, patient safety, critical thinking, and application of the material learned to the clinical scenario, helping the student to understand the pharmacology material.

Special Elements and Learning Aids

Each chapter opens with a list of learning objectives for that chapter, helping the student to understand what the key learning points will be. A list of featured drugs and key terms is also found on the opening chapter page. *Focus Points* appear periodically throughout each chapter to summarize important concepts. The text of each chapter ends with a bulleted list of *Points to Remember,* which summarizes important concepts. This is followed by a series of review exercises, *Check Your Understanding,* which includes NCLEX-style questions in the new format to focus student learning on the seminal information presented in the chapter.

- In the *Nursing Considerations* section of each chapter, *italics* highlight the *rationale* for each nursing intervention, helping the student to apply the information in a clinical situation. Elsewhere in the text, the rationale is consistently provided for therapeutic drug actions, contraindications and adverse effects. In the *Drug List* at the beginning of each chapter, a special icon appears next to the drug that is considered the prototype drug of each class. In each chapter, *Pharmacokinetic Tables* spotlight the pharmacokinetic information for each prototype drug. A *Glossary* found in the back of the book, defines all of the key terms listed in each chapter.
- *Drugs in Focus* are summary tables that clearly identify the drugs within a class, highlighting them by generic and trade names, usual dosage, and indications. A special icon appears in these tables next to each drug that is considered to be the prototype for its specific class.
- *Web Links* alert the student to electronic sources of drug information and sources of drug therapy information for specific diseases.
- *Focus on Clinical Skills* points to accurate drug administration practices and the salient and sometimes life-

preserving nursing interventions for a specific drug or drug therapy.

- *Focus on the Evidence* boxes compile information based on research to identify the best nursing practices associated with specific drug therapy.
- *Herbal and Alternative Therapies* displays highlight known interactions with specific herbs or alternative therapies that could affect the actions of the drugs being discussed.
- *Focus on Patient Safety* points alert the student to potentially serious drug–drug interactions, name confusions to watch for, common dosing errors associated with specific drugs, and reported unsafe drug practices.
- *Focus on Calculations* reviews are designed to help the student hone calculation and measurement skills while learning about the drugs for which dosages might need to be calculated.
- *Drug Therapy Across the Lifespan* tables concisely summarize points to consider when using the drugs of each class with children, adults, and older adults.
- Similarly, where appropriate, discussion of *gender and cultural considerations* encourages the student to think about cultural awareness and to consider the patient as a unique individual with a special set of characteristics that not only influence variations in drug effectiveness but could influence a patient's perspective on drug therapy.
- *Critical Thinking Scenarios* tie each chapter's content together by presenting clinical *scenarios* about a patient using a particular drug from the class being discussed. Included in the case study are hints to guide critical thinking about the case and a discussion of *drug- and nondrug-related nursing considerations* for that particular patient and situation. Most importantly, the case study provides a *plan of nursing care* specifically developed for that patient and specifically based on the nursing process. The care plan is followed by a checklist of *patient teaching points* designed for the patient presented in the case study. This approach helps the student to see how assessment and the collected data are applied in the clinical situation.
- *Check Your Understanding* sections present NCLEX-style questions, including alternate format questions, to help the student prepare for that exam. Other questions and activities in this section are designed to help students test their knowledge of the information that has been learned in the chapter.

To the Student Using This Text

As you begin your study of pharmacology, don't be overwhelmed or confused by all of the details. The study of drugs fits perfectly into your study of the human body—anatomy, physiology, chemistry, nutrition, psychology, and sociology. Approach the study of pharmacology from the perspective of putting all of the pieces together; this can be not only fun but challenging! Work to understand the concepts and all of the details will fall into place, be easy to remember, and apply to the clinical situation. This understanding will help you in creating the picture of the whole patient as you are learning to provide comprehensive nursing care. This text is designed to help you accomplish all of this in a simple and concise manner. Good luck!

Amy M. Karch, RN, MS

How To Use *Focus on Nursing Pharmacology, 4e*

The fourth edition of *Focus on Nursing Pharmacology* offers an abundance of learning tools to help you focus on what you need to know to administer, monitor, and teach patients about safe and effective drug therapy.

The **Drug List** at the beginning of each chapter contains featured drugs that appear throughout the chapter. An icon appears next to prototype drugs found in the list.

ALPHA- AND BETA-ADRENERGIC BLOCKING AGENTS
amiodarone
bretylium
carvedilol
guanadrel
guanethidine
P labetalol

ALPHA-ADRENERGIC BLOCKING AGENTS
P phentolamine

ALPHA$_1$-SELECTIVE ADRENERGIC BLOCKING AGENTS
alfuzosin
P doxazosin
prazosin
tamsulosin
terazosin

BETA-ADRENERGIC BLOCKING AGENTS
carteolol
nadolol
penbutolol
pindolol
P propranolol
sotalol
timolol

BETA$_1$-SELECTIVE ADRENERGIC BLOCKING AGENTS
acebutolol
P atenolol
betaxolol
bisoprolol
esmolol
metoprolol

LEARNING OBJECTIVES

Upon completion of this chapter, you will be able to:

1. Describe the sites of action of the various anti-inflammatory agents.
2. Describe the therapeutic actions, indications, pharamacokinetics, contraindications, most common adverse reactions, and important drug–drug interactions associated with each class of anti-inflammatory agents: salicylates, nonsteroidal anti-inflammatory drugs, and miscellaneous agents.
3. Discuss the use of anti-inflammatory drugs across the lifespan.
4. Compare and contrast the prototype drugs for each class of anti-inflammatory drugs with the other drugs in that class.
5. Outline the nursing considerations and teaching needs for patients receiving each class of anti-inflammatory agents.

Learning Objectives let students know what they're going to learn in each and every chapter.

BOX 10.2 **DRUG THERAPY ACROSS THE LIFESPAN**

Antivirals

CHILDREN

Children are very sensitive to the effects of most antiviral drugs, and more severe reactions can be expected when these drugs are used in children.

Many of these drugs do not have proven safety and efficacy in children, and extreme caution should be used.

Most of the drugs for prevention and treatment of influenza virus infections can be used, in smaller doses, for children.

Acyclovir is the drug of choice for children with herpes virus or cytomegalovirus infections.

The drugs used in the treatment of AIDS are frequently used in children, even when no scientific data are available, because of the seriousness of the disease. Dosage should be lowered according to body weight, and children must be monitored very closely for adverse effects on kidneys, bone marrow, and liver.

ADULTS

Adults need to know that these drugs are specific for the treatment of viral infections. The use of antibiotics to treat such infections can lead to the development of resistant strains and superinfections that can cause more problems.

Patients with HIV infection who are taking antiviral medications need to be taught that these drugs do not cure the disease, that opportunistic infections can still occur, and that precautions to prevent transmission of the disease need to be taken.

Pregnant women, for the most part, should not use these drugs unless the benefit clearly outweighs the potential risk to the fetus or neonate. Women of childbearing age should be advised to use barrier contraceptives if any of these drugs are used. Zidovudine has been safely used in pregnant women.

The Centers for Disease Control and Prevention advises that women with HIV infection should not breast-feed, to protect the neonate from the virus.

OLDER ADULTS

Older patients may be more susceptible to the adverse effects associated with these drugs; they should be monitored closely.

Patients with hepatic dysfunction are at increased risk for worsening hepatic problems and toxic effects of those drugs that are metabolized in the liver. Drugs that are excreted unchanged in the urine can be especially toxic to patients who have renal dysfunction. If hepatic or renal dysfunction is expected (extreme age, alcohol abuse, use of other hepatotoxic or nephrotoxic drugs), the dosage may need to be lowered and the patient should be monitored more frequently.

Drug Therapy Across the Lifespan boxes summarize the important differences in drug effects in children, adults, and older adults.

Table 26.5 DRUGS IN FOCUS

Antimigraine Triptans

Drug Name	Dosage/Route	Usual Indications
almotriptan (*Axert*)	6.25–12.5 mg PO at onset of aura or symptoms	Acute migraines in adults
eletriptan (*Relpax*)	20–40 mg PO; may repeat in 2 h if needed; do not exceed 80 mg/day	Acute migraines in adults
frovatriptan (*Frova*)	2.5 mg PO as a single dose at first sign of headache; may repeat in 2 h; do not exceed three doses in 24 h	Acute migraines in adults
naratriptan (*Amerge*)	1–2.5 mg PO with fluid; may repeat in 4 h if needed	Acute migraines in adults
rizatriptan (*Maxalt; Maxalt MLT*)	5–10 mg PO; may repeat in 2 h; do not exceed 30 mg/day	Acute migraines in adults; orally disintegrating tablet may be useful with difficulty swallowing
P sumatriptan (*Imitrex*)	50–100 mg PO at first sign of headache, may repeat in 2 h, do not exceed 200 mg/day; *or* 6 mg Sub-Q; *or* 5, 10, *or* 20 mg by nasal spray in one nostril, may repeat in 2 h, do not exceed 40 mg/day	Acute migraines, cluster headaches in adults
zolmitriptan (*Zomig, Zomig ZMT*)	2.5 mg PO; may repeat in 2 h; do not exceed 10 mg/day	Acute migraines in adults

Drugs in Focus tables provide a quick guide to drug dosages, routes, and usual indications.

Focus Points boxes summarize important content and concepts throughout the chapters.

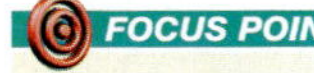

FOCUS POINTS

- Selective adrenergic blocking agents have specific affinity for alpha- or beta-receptors or for specific alpha$_1$-, beta$_1$-, or beta$_2$-receptor sites. Nonspecific alpha-adrenergic blocking agents are used to treat pheochromocytoma, a tumor of the adrenal medulla. A reflex tachycardia commonly occurs when the blood pressure falls.
- Alpha$_1$-selective adrenergic blocking agents decrease blood pressure by blocking the postsynaptic alpha$_1$-receptor sites, decreasing vascular tone, and a promoting vasodilation.

BOX 16.3 FOCUS ON **CLINICAL SKILLS**

Rheumatoid Arthritis

Pathophysiology

Rheumatoid arthritis is a chronic, systemic disease that affects people of all ages. It is considered to be an autoimmune disease. Patients with rheumatoid arthritis have high levels of rheumatoid factor (RF), an antibody to immunoglobulin G (IgG). RF interacts with circulating IgG to form immune complexes, which tend to deposit in the synovial fluid of joints as well as in the eye and other small vessels. The formation of the immune complex activates complement and precipitates an inflammatory reaction. During the immune reaction, lysosomal enzymes are released that destroy the tissues surrounding the joint. This destruction of normal tissue causes a further inflammatory reaction, and a cycle of destruction and inflammation ensues. Over time, the joint becomes severely damaged and the synovial space fills with scar tissue.

Effects of Disease

The patient with rheumatoid arthritis is in chronic pain, related to the release of the chemicals involved in the inflammatory process and the pressure of the swelling tissues in the joint capsule. At this time there is no cure for rheumatoid arthritis. Treatment is aimed at relieving the signs and symptoms of inflammation and delaying the progressive damage to the joints. The patient with this disease will progressively lose the use of the joint, which affects mobility as well as the ability to carry on the activities of daily living. Depression is not an uncommon side effect to this disease.

Clinical Skills

Specific nursing interventions can help to alleviate some of the signs and symptoms of rheumatoid arthritis and help the patient to cope with the disease. These interventions include physical therapy; range-of-motion exercises; application of hot and cold packs to the joints; weight-bearing exercises; spacing activities throughout the day to make the most of energy and movement reserves; and assistance devices for normal daily activities (e.g. big handles on utensils and pens to help patients do things for themselves when they cannot grasp small handles). Thorough teaching about drug regimens can also help prevent adverse effects and increase compliance.

Patients may have to progress through a series of drugs as various agents lose their effectiveness. Aspirin, NSAIDs, gold therapy, and more potent antiarthritis drugs may all be used at one time or another. The patient with rheumatoid arthritis will profit from a relationship with a consistent, reliable health care provider who listens, offers support, and has knowledge of new drugs and treatments to improve the quality of life. Many community support and information groups are available as resources to patients—and to health care providers who work with these patients. For a listing of available resources in your area, contact the Arthritis Foundation: **http://www.arthritis.org**.

Focus on Clinical Skills provide accurate drug administration practices and nursing interventions for a specific drug or drug therapy.

Prototype Summaries inform the student about the indications, actions, pharmacokinetics, half-life, and adverse effects of the most typical drug in a drug class.

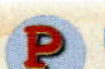

Prototype Summary: Phenelzine

Indications: Treatment of patients with depression who are unresponsive to other antidepressive therapy or in whom other antidepressive therapy is contraindicated

Actions: Irreversibly inhibits MAO, allowing norepinephrine, serotonin, and dopamine to accumulate in the synaptic cleft; this accumulation is thought to be responsible for the clinical effects

Pharmacokinetics:

Route	Onset	Duration
Oral	Slow	48–96 h

$T_{1/2}$: Unknown, metabolized in the liver, excreted in the urine

Adverse effects: Dizziness, vertigo, headache, overactivity, hyperreflexia, tremors, mania, weakness, drowsiness, fatigue, sweating, orthostatic hypotension, constipation, diarrhea, dry mouth, edema, anorexia, potential for hypertensive crisis

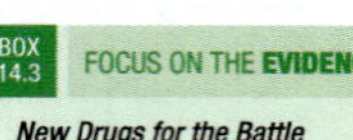

BOX 14.3 FOCUS ON THE **EVIDENCE**

New Drugs for the Battle Against Cancer

Arsenic trioxide *(Trisenox)*, known as a poison in forensic medicine, has been approved for the induction and remission of promyelocytic leukemia (PML) in patients whose disease is refractory to conventional therapy and whose leukemia is characterized by t(15:17) translocation of PML/RAR-alpha gene expression. It is given intravenously at a rate of 0.15 mg/kg/day until bone marrow remission occurs and then 0.15 mg/kg/day starting 3 to 6 wk after induction. The patient needs to be screened carefully for toxic reactions.

Other drugs are under development that target specific areas of the human genome. In the future, antineoplastic drugs may be able to target abnormal cells and not affect the healthy cells. This could relieve the suffering of many patients undergoing cancer chemotherapy.

Several familiar drugs are being studied for their ability to block angiogenesis. By blocking the development of new blood vessels to feed the tumor, the growing cells in the tumor will lack nutrition and oxygen and will not be able to survive. Celecoxib (*Celebrex*), an anti-inflammatory drug, is being studied in various cancer combination drug trials for this effect. Some low-molecular-weight heparins, such as dalterparin (*Fragmin*), are also being studied for this effect.

Focus on the Evidence boxes help students identify the best nursing practices associated with specific drug therapies.

Nursing Considerations contain the rationale for each nursing intervention, helping the student to apply the information in a clinical situation.

Nursing Considerations for Patients Receiving Alpha-Adrenergic Blocking Agents

Assessment: History and Examination

Screen for the following conditions, *which could be cautions or contraindications to the use of the drug:* any known allergies to these drugs; presence of any cardiovascular diseases, *which may be contraindications to the use of these drugs;* and pregnancy or lactation, *which require caution for drug use.* Include screening *for baseline status and for any potential adverse effects:* assess orientation, affect, and reflexes to monitor for CNS changes related to drug therapy; blood pressure, pulse, ECG, peripheral perfusion, and cardiac output; and urine output.

Nursing Diagnoses

The patient receiving an alpha-adrenergic blocking agent may also have the following nursing diagnoses related to drug therapy:

- Risk for Injury related to CNS, CV effects of drug
- Decreased Cardiac Output related to blood pressure changes, arrhythmias, vasodilation
- Deficient Knowledge regarding drug therapy

Implementation With Rationale

- Monitor heart rate and blood pressure very carefully *in order to arrange to discontinue the drug if adverse reactions are severe;* provide supportive management if needed.
- Inject phentolamine directly into the area of extravasation of epinephrine or dopamine *to prevent local cell death.*
- Arrange for supportive care and comfort measures, such as rest, environmental control, and other measures, *to decrease CNS irritation;* provide headache medication *to alleviate patient discomfort;* arrange safety measures if CNS effects or orthostatic hypotension occur *to prevent patient injury.*
- Provide thorough patient teaching, including dosage, potential adverse effects, measures to avoid adverse effects, and warning signs of problems, *to enhance patient knowledge about drug therapy and to promote compliance.*
- Offer support and encouragement *to help the patient deal with the drug regimen.*

Evaluation

- Monitor patient response to the drug (improvement in signs and symptoms of pheochromocytoma, improvement in tissue condition after extravasation).
- Monitor for adverse effects (orthostatic hypotension, arrhythmias, CNS effects).
- Evaluate the effectiveness of the teaching plan (patient can name drug, dosage, adverse effects to watch for, specific measures to avoid adverse effects).
- Monitor the effectiveness of comfort measures and compliance to the regimen.

FOCUS ON **PATIENT SAFETY**

There have been several reports of name confusion between trade names, particularly *Lamisil* (terbinafine) the antifungal agent, and *Lamictal* (lamotrigine), an antiepileptic agent. Patients who needed Lamictal have been given the potentially toxic antifungal agent *Lamisil* with the result being seizures. Conversely, patients expecting to be treated for a serious systemic fungal infection received the antiepileptic preparation *Lamictal* and experienced CNS effects related to the drug. The Food and Drug Administration (FDA) has asked the manufacturers of these drugs to change the labels to bring attention to the differences. All health care providers should be especially cautious when using either one of the drugs and should alert the patient to the potential for errors and encourage the patient to be vigilant and to ask questions.

Focus on Patient Safety material alerts student to potentially serious drug–drug interactions, drug name confusions, and common dosing errors.

BOX 21.4 HERBAL AND ALTERNATIVE THERAPIES

Patients being treated with SSRIs are at an increased risk of developing a severe reaction, including serotonin syndrome, as well as an increased sensitivity to light if they are also taking St. John's wort. Because this herbal therapy is often used to self-treat depression, it is important to forewarn any patient who is taking an SSRI not to combine it with taking St. John's wort.

Also caution patients that there is an increased risk of seizures if evening primrose is used with antidepressants, and patients should be cautioned against this combination. Interactions have also been reported when antidepressants are combined with ginkgo, ginseng, and valerian. Patients should be cautioned against using these herbs while taking antidepressants.

Herbal and Alternative Therapies are highlighted so students are aware of how these alternative therapies can interact with traditional medications.

BOX 20.2 FOCUS ON CALCULATIONS

Your 3-year-old patient, weighing 25 kg, is prescribed chloral hydrate as a hypnotic at bedtime. The order reads: 50 mg/kg/day PO at bedtime. The drug comes in a syrup form as 500 mg/5 mL. How much syrup would you give as the bedtime dose?

First, figure out what the correct dose would be:

50 mg/kg × 25 kg = 1250 mg

Set up the equation using available form = prescribed dose:

500 mg/5 mL = 1250 mg/dose

Then, cross-multiply:

500 mg (dose) = 6250 mg (mL)
dose = 6250 mg (mL)/500 mg
dose = 12.5 mL

Because this is a child, it is good practice to ask another nurse to calculate the correct dosage and then compare your work, so you can double-check the accuracy of your calculations.

Focus on Calculations are designed to help the student practice and refine math skills.

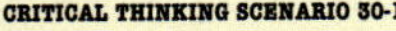
CRITICAL THINKING SCENARIO 30-1

Adrenergic Agonist Toxicity

The Situation

M.C. is a 26-year-old man who has recently moved to the northeastern United States from New Mexico. He has been suffering from sinusitis, runny nose, and cold-like symptoms for 2 weeks. He appears at an outpatient clinic with complaints of headache, "jitters," inability to sleep, loss of appetite, and a feeling of impending doom. He states that he feels "on edge" and has not been productive in his job as a watch repairman and jewelry maker. According to his history, M.C. has been treated with several different drugs for nocturnal enuresis, a persisting childhood problem. Only ephedrine, which he has been taking for 2 years, has been successful. He has no other significant health problems. He denies any side effects from the use of ephedrine but does admit to self-medicating his nagging cold with over-the-counter (OTC) preparations—a nasal spray used four times a day and a combination decongestant–pain reliever. A physical examination reveals a pulse of 104, BP 154/86, R 16. The patient appears flushed and slightly diaphoretic.

Critical Thinking

What are the important nursing implications for M.C.? *Think about the problems that confront a patient in a new area seeking health care for the first time.*

What could be causing the problems that M.C. presents with? *The diagnosis of ephedrine overdose was eventually made based on the patient history of OTC drug use and the presenting signs and symptoms.*

Keeping in mind that this diagnosis means M.C. has an overstimulated sympathetic stress reaction; what other physical problems can be anticipated? *Overwhelming feelings of anxiety and stress are influencing M.C.'s response to work and health care.*

Given this fact, how may the nurse best deal with explaining the problem and how it could have happened—without making the patient feel uninformed or that the practice of his former health care provider is being questioned?

What treatment should be planned and what teaching points should be covered for M.C.?

Discussion

The first step in caring for M.C. is establishing a trusting relationship to help alleviate some of the anxiety he is feeling. Being in a new state and seeking health care in a new setting can be very stressful for patients under normal circumstances. In M.C.'s case, the sympathomimetic effects of the drugs that he has been taking make him feel even more anxious and jittery.

A careful patient history will help determine whether there are any underlying medical problems that could be exacerbated by these drug effects. A review of M.C.'s nocturnal enuresis and the treatments that have been tried will enhance understanding of his former health care and suggest possible implications for further study. This questioning will also reassure M.C. that he is an important member of the health team and that the information he has to offer is valued.

A careful review of the OTC drugs that M.C. has been using will be informative for the patient as well as for the health care providers who have not actually checked OTC drugs for those specific ingredients, but combining them to ease signs and symptoms often results in toxic levels and symptoms of overdose. M.C. will need a full teaching program about the effects of his ephedrine and which OTC drugs to avoid. The treatment for his current problems involves withdrawal of the OTC drugs; when these drug levels fall, the signs and symptoms will disappear. M.C. may also wish to avoid nicotine and caffeine, because these stimulants could increase his "jitters."

To build trust and ensure that the underlying cause of the problem was drug toxicity, M.C. should receive written patient instructions that highlight warning signs to report, including chest pain, palpitations, and difficulty voiding. He also should be given the health care provider's telephone number with instructions to call the next day and report on his health status. Finally, specimens of nasal discharge should be cultured and antibiotic treatment prescribed, if appropriate.

Nursing Care Guide for M.C.: Adrenergic Agonist Toxicity

Assessment: History and Examination

Assess the patient's history of drug allergies, cardiovascular dysfunction, pheochromocytoma, narrow-angle glaucoma, prostatic hypertrophy, thyroid disease, or diabetes, as well as concurrent use of MAOIs, tricyclic antidepressants, reserpine, ephedrine, or urinary alkalinizers. Focus the physical examination on the following:

CV: Blood pressure, pulse rate, peripheral perfusion, and ECG

called an adrenergic agonist (or a sympathomimetic drug). Ephedrine acts by mimicking the effects of the sympathetic nervous system, which is the part of your nervous system that is responsible for your response to fear or danger (this is called the "fight-or-flight"

- ☐ Tell any health care provider who takes care of you that you are taking this drug.
- ☐ Keep this drug and all medication out of the reach of children. And do not share this drug with other people.

Critical Thinking Scenarios appear at the end of each chapter and encourage students to imagine a true-to-life patient situation, to develop and follow through on a nursing plan of care, and to create a checklist of teaching points related to a specific drug therapy.

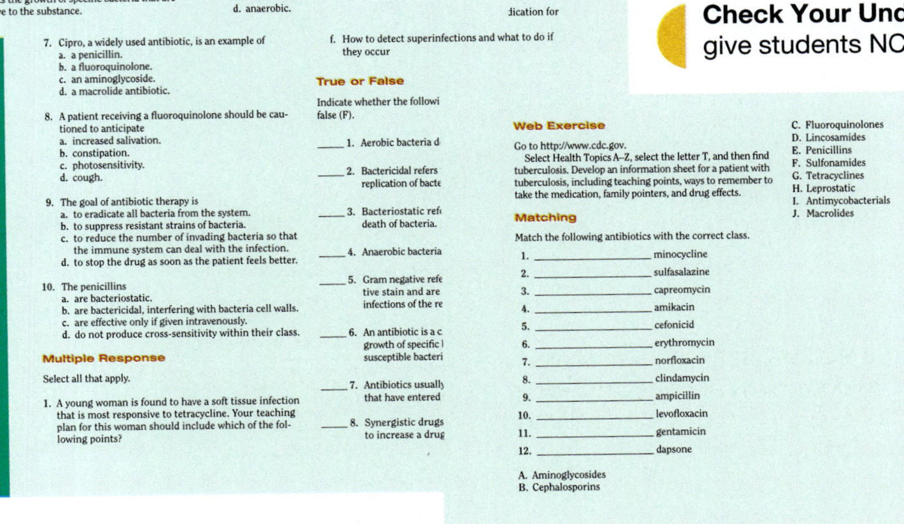
CHECK YOUR UNDERSTANDING

Answers to the questions in this chapter may be found in the Answer Key in the back of the book.

Multiple Choice

Select the best answer to the following.

1. A bacteriostatic substance is one that
   a. directly kills any bacteria it comes in contact with.
   b. directly kills any bacteria that are sensitive to the substance.
   c. prevents the growth of any bacteria.
   d. prevents the growth of specific bacteria that are sensitive to the substance.
2. Gram-negative bacteria
   a. are mostly found in the respiratory tract.
   b. are mostly associated with soft tissue infections.
   c. are mostly found in the GI and GU tracts.
   d. accept a positive stain when tested.
3. Antibiotics that are used together to increase their effectiveness and limit the associated adverse effects are said to be
   a. broad spectrum.
   b. synergistic.
   c. bactericidal.
   d. anaerobic.

7. Cipro, a widely used antibiotic, is an example of
   a. a penicillin.
   b. a fluoroquinolone.
   c. an aminoglycoside.
   d. a macrolide antibiotic.
8. A patient receiving a fluoroquinolone should be cautioned to anticipate
   a. increased salivation.
   b. constipation.
   c. photosensitivity.
   d. cough.
9. The goal of antibiotic therapy is
   a. to eradicate all bacteria from the system.
   b. to suppress resistant strains of bacteria.
   c. to reduce the number of invading bacteria so that the immune system can deal with the infection.
   d. to stop the drug as soon as the patient feels better.
10. The penicillins
   a. are bacteriostatic.
   b. are bactericidal, interfering with bacteria cell walls.
   c. are effective only if given intravenously.
   d. do not produce cross-sensitivity within their class.

Multiple Response

Select all that apply.

1. A young woman is found to have a soft tissue infection that is most responsive to tetracycline. Your teaching plan for this woman should include which of the following points?

f. How to detect superinfections and what to do if they occur

True or False

Indicate whether the followi false (F).

____ 1. Aerobic bacteria d

____ 2. Bactericidal refers replication of bacte

____ 3. Bacteriostatic ref death of bacteria.

____ 4. Anaerobic bacteria

____ 5. Gram negative refe tive stain and are infections of the re

____ 6. An antibiotic is a c growth of specific susceptible bacteri

____ 7. Antibiotics usually that have entered

____ 8. Synergistic drugs to increase a drug

Web Exercise

Go to http://www.cdc.gov.

Select Health Topics A–Z, select the letter T, and then find tuberculosis. Develop an information sheet for a patient with tuberculosis, including teaching points, ways to remember to take the medication, family pointers, and drug effects.

Matching

Match the following antibiotics with the correct class.

1. ____________ minocycline
2. ____________ sulfasalazine
3. ____________ capreomycin
4. ____________ amikacin
5. ____________ cefonicid
6. ____________ erythromycin
7. ____________ norfloxacin
8. ____________ clindamycin
9. ____________ ampicillin
10. ____________ levofloxacin
11. ____________ gentamicin
12. ____________ dapsone

A. Aminoglycosides
B. Cephalosporins
C. Fluoroquinolones
D. Lincosamides
E. Penicillins
F. Sulfonamides
G. Tetracyclines
H. Leprostatic
I. Antimycobacterials
J. Macrolides

Check Your Understanding sections give students NCLEX-style questions.

ACKNOWLEDGMENTS

I would like to thank the various people who have worked so hard to make this book a reality: especially the many students and colleagues who have, for so long, pushed for a pharmacology book that was straightforward and user-friendly and who have taken the time to make suggestions to improve each edition. Thanks also to Charlotte Torres, Rita D'Aoust and Carolanne Bianchi, fellow "boatmates" with vision tempered by reality; my acquisitions editor at Lippincott Williams & Wilkins, Margaret Zuccarini, who had the vision and the drive to see this project through and who has become a mentor and a friend; my managing editor, Michelle Clarke, and senior managing editor, Helen Kogut, who stepped in and pulled it all together to make deadlines and yet kept an upbeat spirit and smile when one was needed; Erika Kors, production managing editor and Holly McLaughlin, designer, whose careful attention to detail and artistic expression are apparent throughout the book; to Tim, Jyoti, Mark, Tracey, Cortney, Bryan and Kathryn, who continue to thrive and grow and have become the wonderful, supportive people in my life; to little Vikas Fred who has returned the sunshine and hope to our lives and lastly to Duncan and Brodie, whose happily wagging tails never fail to bring smiles and help to keep everything in perspective.

CONTENTS

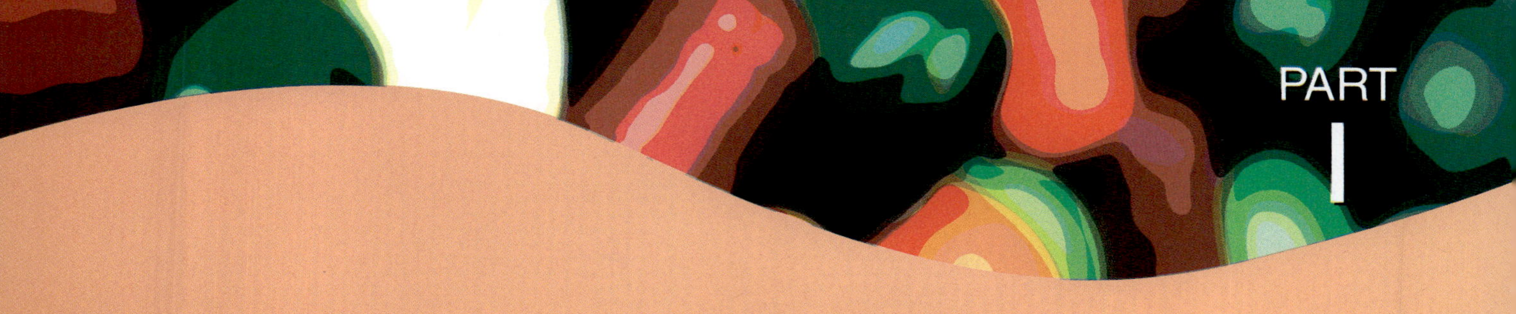

PART I

Introduction to Nursing Pharmacology

CHAPTER

1

Introduction to Drugs

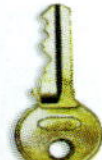

KEY TERMS

adverse effects

brand name

chemical name

drugs

Food and Drug Administration (FDA)

generic drugs

generic name

genetic engineering

orphan drugs

over-the-counter (OTC) drugs

pharmacology

pharmacotherapeutics

phase I study

phase II study

phase III study

phase IV study

preclinical trials

teratogenic

LEARNING OBJECTIVES

Upon completion of this chapter, you will be able to:

1. Define the word pharmacology.
2. Outline the steps involved in developing and approving a new drug in the United States.
3. Describe the federal controls on drugs that have abuse potential.
4. Differentiate between generic and brand name drugs, over-the-counter drugs, and prescription drugs.
5. Explain the benefits and risks associated with the use of over-the-counter drugs.

The human body works through a complicated series of chemical reactions and processes. **Drugs** are chemicals that are introduced into the body to cause some sort of change. When drugs are administered, the body begins a sequence of processes designed to handle the new chemicals. These processes, which involve breaking down and eliminating the drugs, in turn affect the body's complex series of chemical reactions.

For many reasons, understanding how drugs act on the body to cause changes and applying that knowledge in the clinical setting are important aspects of nursing practice. For instance, patients today often follow complicated drug regimens and receive potentially toxic drugs. Many also manage their own care at home. The nurse is in a unique position regarding drug therapy because nursing responsibilities include the following:

- Administering drugs
- Assessing drug effects
- Intervening to make the drug regimen more tolerable
- Providing patient teaching about drugs and the drug regimen
- Monitoring the overall patient care plan to prevent medication errors

Knowing how drugs work makes these tasks easier to handle, thus enhancing drug therapy.

This text is designed to provide the pharmacological basis for understanding drug therapy. The physiology of a body system and the related actions of many drugs on that system are presented in a way that allows clear understanding of how drugs work and what to anticipate when giving a particular type of drug. Thousands of drugs are available for use, and it is impossible to memorize all of the individual differences among drugs in a class.

This text addresses *general* drug information. The nurse can refer to *Lippincott's Nursing Drug Guide* (*LNDG*), or to another drug guide, to obtain the *specific* details required for safe and effective drug administration. Drug details change constantly, and the practicing nurse should rely on an up-to-date and comprehensive drug guide in the clinical setting.

A nursing care guide in each chapter of *Focus on Nursing Pharmacology* serves as a model for developing nursing care guides for any drugs being administered (Table 1.1). The various sections of each drug monograph in *LNDG* also can be used to develop other care guides or teaching plans. See Figure 1.1 for an example of a drug monograph. The CD-ROM found at the back of this book contains patient teaching guides for all of the drugs found in *LNDG*. The nurse can use this text as a resource for basic concepts of pharmacology and a nursing drug guide as an easy-to-use reference in the clinical setting.

Understanding how to read a drug label is essential. Drug labels have specific features that identify the drug, and it is important to become familiar with each aspect of a drug label (Figure 1.2).

Pharmacology

Pharmacology is the study of the biological effects of chemicals. In clinical practice, health care providers focus on how chemicals act on living organisms. Nurses deal with **pharmacotherapeutics**, or clinical pharmacology, the branch of pharmacology that uses drugs to treat, prevent, and diagnose disease. Clinical pharmacology addresses two key concerns: the drug's effects on the body, and the body's response to the drug.

Because a drug can have many effects, the nurse must know which ones may occur when a particular drug is administered. Some drug effects are therapeutic, or helpful, but others are undesirable or potentially dangerous. These negative effects are called **adverse effects**. (See Chapter 3 for a detailed discussion of adverse effects.)

Sources and Evaluation of Drugs

Drugs are available from varied sources, both natural and synthetic. The drugs listed in this book have been through rigorous testing and are approved for sale to the public, either with or without a prescription from a health care provider.

Sources of Drugs

Chemicals that might prove useful as drugs can come from many natural sources, such as plants, animals, or inorganic compounds, or they may be developed synthetically. To become a drug, a chemical must have a demonstrated therapeutic value or efficacy without severe toxicity or damaging properties.

Plants

Plants and plant parts have been used as medicines since prehistoric times. Even today, plants are an important source of chemicals that are developed into drugs. For example, digitalis products used to treat cardiac disorders and various opiates used for sedation are still derived from plants. Table 1.2 provides examples of drugs derived from plant sources.

Drugs also may be processed using a synthetic version of the active chemical found in a plant. An example of this type of drug is dronabinol (*Marinol*), which contains the active ingredient delta-9-tetrahydrocannabinol found in marijuana. It helps prevent nausea and vomiting in cancer patients but does not have all of the adverse effects that occur when the marijuana leaf is smoked. Marijuana leaf is a controlled substance with high abuse potential and has no legal or accepted medical use. The synthetic version of the active ingredient allows for an accepted form to achieve the desired therapeutic effect in cancer patients.

Sometimes a drug effect occurs from ingestion of a plant-derived food. For instance, the body converts natural licorice

Table 1.1 Sample Nursing Care Plan From *Lippincott's Nursing Drug Guide* for a Patient Receiving Oral Linezolid

Assessment	Nursing Diagnosis	Implementation	Evaluation
History (contraindications/cautions) Hypertension Hyperthyroidism Blood dyscrasias Hepatic dysfunction Pheochromocytoma Phenylketonuria Carcinoid syndrome Pregnancy Lactation Known allergy to: linezolid **Medication History** (possible drug–drug interactions) Pseudoephedrine SSRIs MAOIs Antiplatelet drugs **Diet History** (possible drug–food interactions) Foods high in tyramine **Physical Assessment** (screen for contraindications and to establish a baseline for evaluating effects and adverse effects) Local: Culture site of infection CNS: Affect, reflexes, orientation CV: P, BP, peripheral perfusion GI: Bowel sounds, liver evaluation Skin: Color, lesions Hematologic: CBC with differential, liver function tests	Potential for imbalanced nutrition, less than body requirements, related to GI effects Potential for pain related to GI effects, headache Ineffective tissue perfusion related to bone marrow effects Deficient knowledge related to drug therapy	Safe and appropriate administration of drug: Culture infection site to ensure appropriate use of drug Provision of safety and comfort measures: • Monitor BP periodically • Monitor platelet counts before and periodically during therapy • Alleviation of GI upset • Ready access to bathroom facilities • Nutritional consult • Safety provisions if dizziness and CNS effects occur • Avoidance of tyramine-rich foods Patient teaching regarding: Drug Side effects to anticipate Warnings Reactions to report Support and encouragement to cope with disease, high cost of therapy, and side effects Provision of emergency and life-support measures in cases of acute hypersensitivity	Monitor for therapeutic effects of drug: resolution of infection. If resolution does not occur, reculture site. Monitor for adverse effects of drug: • GI upset—nausea, vomiting, diarrhea • Liver function changes • Pseudomembranous colitis • Blood dyscrasias—changes in platelet counts • Fever • Rash • Sweating • Photosensitivity • Acute hypersensitivity reactions Evaluate effectiveness of patient teaching program: patient can name drug, dose of drug, use of drug, adverse effects to expect, reactions to report Evaluate effectiveness of comfort and safety measures Monitor for drug–drug, drug–food interactions as appropriate Evaluate effectiveness of life-support measures if needed

From Karch, A.M. (2006). *2007 Lippincott's nursing drug guide.* Philadelphia: Lippincott Williams & Wilkins.

to a false aldosterone, resulting in fluid retention and hypokalemia or low serum potassium levels if large amounts of licorice are eaten. However, people seldom think of licorice as a drug.

Finally, plants have become the main component of the growing alternative therapy movement. Chapter 6 discusses the alternative therapy movement and its impact on today's drug regimens.

Animal Products

Animal products are used to replace human chemicals that are not produced because of disease or genetic problems. Until recently, insulin for treating diabetes was obtained exclusively from the pancreas of cows and pigs. Now **genetic engineering**—the process of altering DNA—permits scientists to produce human insulin by altering *Escherichia coli* bacteria, making insulin a better product without some of the impurities that come with animal products.

Thyroid drugs and growth hormone preparations also may be obtained from animal thyroid and hypothalamus tissues. But many of these preparations are now created synthetically, and the synthetic preparations are considered to be purer and safer than preparations derived from animals.

Inorganic Compounds

Salts of various elements can have therapeutic effects in the human body. Aluminum, fluoride, iron, and even gold are used to treat various conditions. The effects of these elements

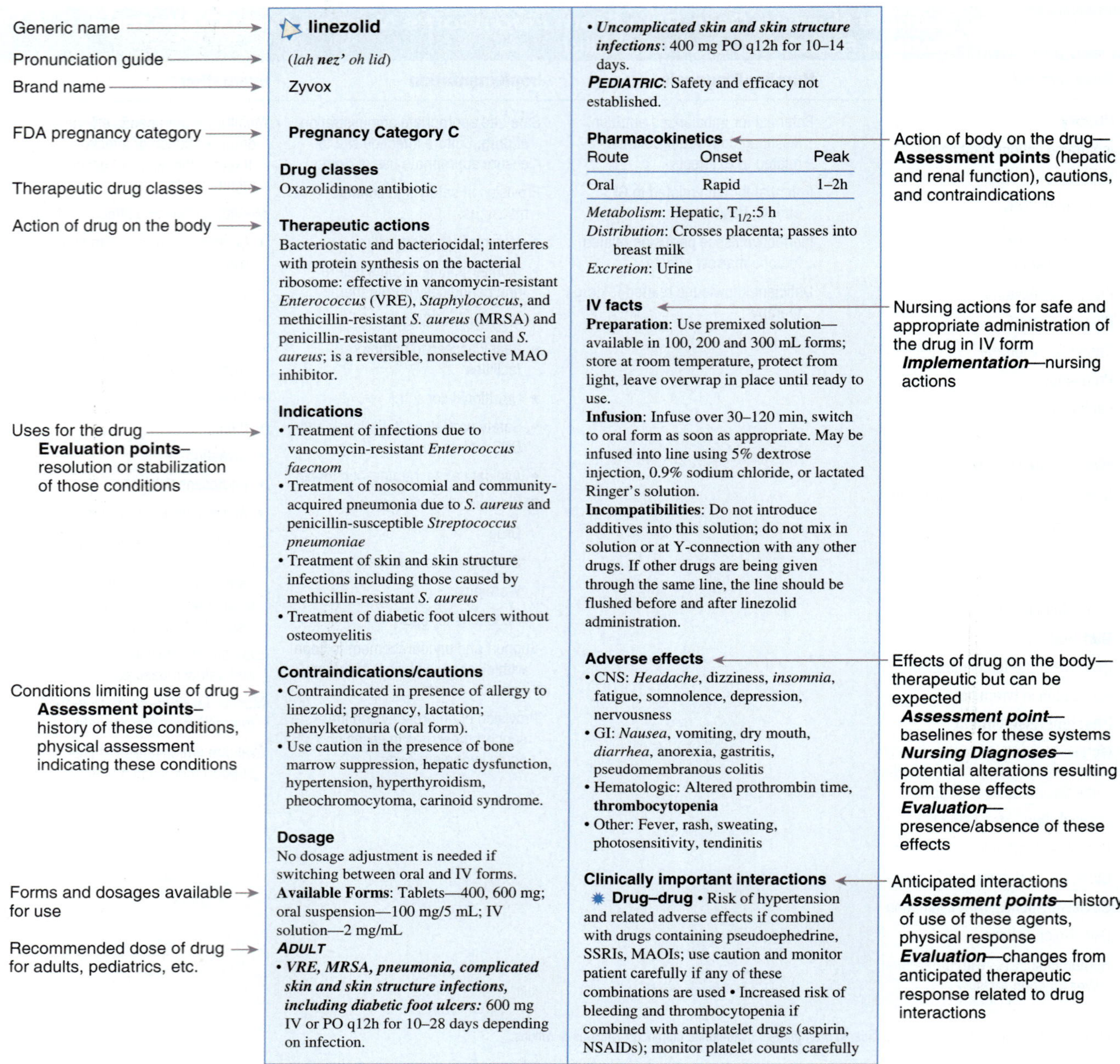

linezolid

(lah nez' oh lid)

Zyvox

Pregnancy Category C

Drug classes
Oxazolidinone antibiotic

Therapeutic actions
Bacteriostatic and bacteriocidal; interferes with protein synthesis on the bacterial ribosome: effective in vancomycin-resistant *Enterococcus* (VRE), *Staphylococcus*, and methicillin-resistant *S. aureus* (MRSA) and penicillin-resistant pneumococci and *S. aureus*; is a reversible, nonselective MAO inhibitor.

Indications
- Treatment of infections due to vancomycin-resistant *Enterococcus faecnom*
- Treatment of nosocomial and community-acquired pneumonia due to *S. aureus* and penicillin-susceptible *Streptococcus pneumoniae*
- Treatment of skin and skin structure infections including those caused by methicillin-resistant *S. aureus*
- Treatment of diabetic foot ulcers without osteomyelitis

Contraindications/cautions
- Contraindicated in presence of allergy to linezolid; pregnancy, lactation; phenylketonuria (oral form).
- Use caution in the presence of bone marrow suppression, hepatic dysfunction, hypertension, hyperthyroidism, pheochromocytoma, carinoid syndrome.

Dosage
No dosage adjustment is needed if switching between oral and IV forms.
Available Forms: Tablets—400, 600 mg; oral suspension—100 mg/5 mL; IV solution—2 mg/mL
ADULT
- ***VRE, MRSA, pneumonia, complicated skin and skin structure infections, including diabetic foot ulcers:*** 600 mg IV or PO q12h for 10–28 days depending on infection.
- ***Uncomplicated skin and skin structure infections***: 400 mg PO q12h for 10–14 days.

PEDIATRIC: Safety and efficacy not established.

Pharmacokinetics

Route	Onset	Peak
Oral	Rapid	1–2h

Metabolism: Hepatic, $T_{1/2}$:5 h
Distribution: Crosses placenta; passes into breast milk
Excretion: Urine

IV facts
Preparation: Use premixed solution—available in 100, 200 and 300 mL forms; store at room temperature, protect from light, leave overwrap in place until ready to use.
Infusion: Infuse over 30–120 min, switch to oral form as soon as appropriate. May be infused into line using 5% dextrose injection, 0.9% sodium chloride, or lactated Ringer's solution.
Incompatibilities: Do not introduce additives into this solution; do not mix in solution or at Y-connection with any other drugs. If other drugs are being given through the same line, the line should be flushed before and after linezolid administration.

Adverse effects
- CNS: *Headache*, dizziness, *insomnia*, fatigue, somnolence, depression, nervousness
- GI: *Nausea*, vomiting, dry mouth, *diarrhea*, anorexia, gastritis, pseudomembranous colitis
- Hematologic: Altered prothrombin time, **thrombocytopenia**
- Other: Fever, rash, sweating, photosensitivity, tendinitis

Clinically important interactions
Drug–drug • Risk of hypertension and related adverse effects if combined with drugs containing pseudoephedrine, SSRIs, MAOIs; use caution and monitor patient carefully if any of these combinations are used • Increased risk of bleeding and thrombocytopenia if combined with antiplatelet drugs (aspirin, NSAIDs); monitor platelet counts carefully

FIGURE 1.1 Example of a drug monograph from *Lippincott's Nursing Drug Guide.*

usually were discovered accidentally when a cause–effect relationship was observed. Table 1.3 shows examples of some elements used for their therapeutic benefit.

Synthetic Sources

Today, many drugs are developed synthetically after chemicals in plants, animals, or the environment have been screened for signs of therapeutic activity. Scientists use genetic engineering to alter bacteria to produce chemicals that are therapeutic and effective. Other technical advances allow scientists to alter a chemical with proven therapeutic effectiveness to make it better. Sometimes, a small change in a chemical's structure can make that chemical more useful as a drug—more potent, more stable, less toxic. These technological advances have led to the development of groups of similar drugs, all of which are derived from an original prototype, but each of which has slightly different properties, making a particular drug more desirable in a specific situation. Throughout this book, the icon P will be used to designate those drugs of a class that are considered the prototype of the class. For example, the cephalosporins are a group of antibiotics

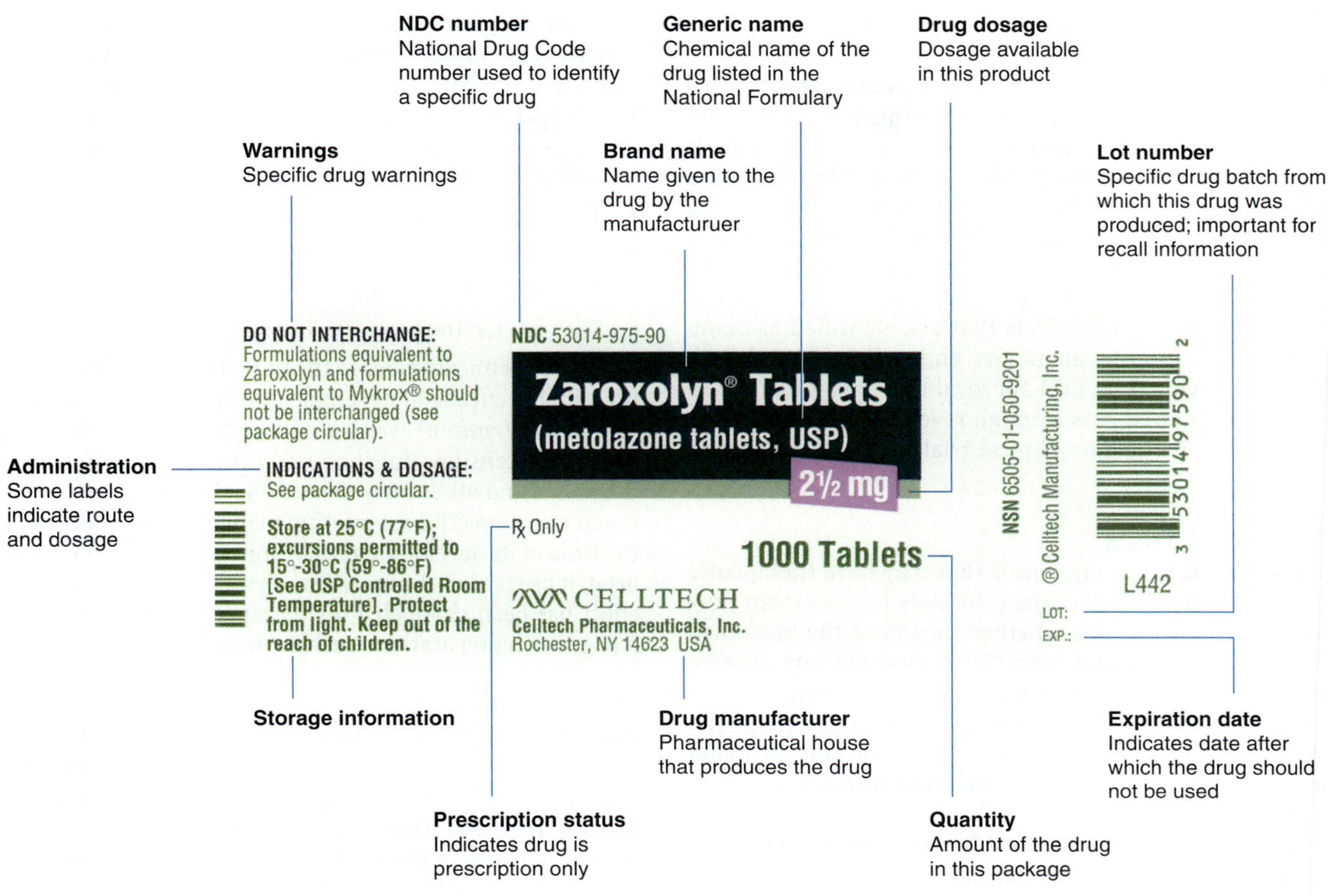

(Courtesy of CellTech Pharmaceuticals)

FIGURE 1.2 Reading a drug label (sample drug label courtesy of Celltech Pharmaceuticals, Rochester, NY).

derived from the same chemical structure. Alterations in the chemical rings or attachments to that structure make it possible for some of these drugs to be absorbed orally, whereas others must be given parenterally. Some of these drugs cause severe toxic effects (e.g., renal toxicity), but others do not.

Table 1.2 Focus on Drugs Derived From Plants

Plant	Product
Ricinus communis	Seed Oil Castor oil (*Neolid*)
Digitalis purpurea (foxglove plant)	Leaves Dried leaves Digitalis leaf
Papaver somniferum (poppy plant)	Unripe capsule Juice Opium (paregoric) Morphine (*Roxanol*) Codeine Papaverine (*Pavabid*)

FOCUS POINTS

- Clinical pharmacology is the study of drugs used to treat, diagnose, or prevent a disease.
- Drugs are chemicals that are introduced into the body and affect the body's chemical processes.
- Drugs can come from plants, foods, salts, animals, or synthetic sources.

Table 1.3 Focus on Elements Used for Their Therapeutic Effects

Element	Therapeutic Use
Aluminum	Antacid to decrease gastric acidity Management of hyperphosphatemia Prevention of the formation of phosphate urinary stones
Fluoride	Prevention of dental cavities Prevention of osteoporosis
Gold	Treatment of rheumatoid arthritis
Iron	Treatment of iron deficiency anemia

Drug Evaluation

After a chemical that might have therapeutic value is identified, it must undergo a series of scientific tests to evaluate its actual therapeutic and toxic effects. This process is tightly controlled by the **Food and Drug Administration (FDA)**, an agency of the U.S. Department of Health and Human Services that regulates the development and sale of drugs. FDA-regulated tests are designed to ensure the safety and reliability of any drug approved in this country. For every 100,000 chemicals that are identified as being potential drugs, only about five end up being marketed. Before receiving final FDA approval to be marketed to the public, drugs must pass through several stages of development. These include preclinical trials and phase I, II, and III studies.

Preclinical Trials

In **preclinical trials**, chemicals that may have therapeutic value are tested on laboratory animals for two main purposes: (1) to determine whether they have the presumed effects in living tissue, and (2) to evaluate any adverse effects. Animal testing is important because unique biological differences can cause very different reactions to the chemical. These differences can be found only in living organisms, so computer-generated models alone are often inadequate.

At the end of the preclinical trials, some chemicals are discarded for the following reasons:

- The chemical lacks therapeutic activity when used with living animals.
- The chemical is too toxic to living animals to be worth the risk of developing into drugs.
- The chemical is highly **teratogenic** (causing adverse effects to the fetus).
- The safety margins are so small that the chemical would not be useful in the clinical setting.

Some chemicals, however, are found to have therapeutic effects and reasonable safety margins. This means that the chemicals are therapeutic at doses that are reasonably different from doses that cause toxic effects. Such chemicals will pass the preclinical trials and advance to phase I studies.

Phase I Studies

Phase I studies use human volunteers to test the drugs. These studies are more tightly controlled than preclinical trials and are performed by specially trained clinical investigators. The volunteers are fully informed of possible risks and may be paid for their participation. Usually, the volunteers are healthy, young men. Women are not good candidates for phase I studies because the chemicals may exert unknown and harmful effects on a woman's ova, and too much risk is involved in taking a drug that might destroy or alter the ova. Men produce sperm daily, so there is less potential for complete destruction or alteration of the sperm.

Some chemicals are therapeutic in other animals but have no effects in humans. Investigators in phase I studies scrutinize the drugs being tested for effects in humans. They also look for adverse effects and toxicity. At the end of phase I studies, many chemicals are dropped from the process for the following reasons:

- They lack therapeutic effect in humans.
- They cause unacceptable adverse effects.
- They are highly teratogenic.
- They are too toxic.

Some chemicals move to the next stage of testing despite undesirable effects. For example, the antihypertensive drug minoxidil (*Loniten*) was found to effectively treat malignant hypertension, but it caused unusual hair growth on the palms and other body areas. However, because it was so much more effective for treating malignant hypertension at the time of its development than any other antihypertensive drug, it proceeded to phase II studies. (Now, its hair-growing effect has been channeled for therapeutic use into various hair-growth preparations such as *Rogaine*.)

Phase II Studies

Phase II studies allow clinical investigators to try the drug in patients who have the disease that the drug is meant to treat. Patients are told about the possible benefits of the drug and are invited to participate in the study. Those who consent to participate are fully informed about possible risks and are monitored very closely, often at no charge to them, to evaluate the drug's effects. Usually, phase II studies are performed at various sites across the country—in hospitals, clinics, and doctors' offices—and are monitored by representatives of the pharmaceutical company studying the drug. At the end of phase II studies, a drug may be removed from further investigation for the following reasons:

- It is less effective than anticipated.
- It is too toxic when used with patients.
- It produces unacceptable adverse effects.
- It has a low benefit-to-risk ratio, meaning that the therapeutic benefit it provides does not outweigh the risk of potential adverse effects that it causes.
- It is no more effective than other drugs already on the market, making the cost of continued research and production less attractive to the drug company.

A drug that continues to show promise as a therapeutic agent receives additional scrutiny in phase III studies.

Phase III Studies

Phase III studies involve use of the drug in a vast clinical market. Prescribers are informed of all the known reactions to the drug and precautions required for its safe use. Prescribers observe patients very closely, monitoring them for any adverse effects. Sometimes, prescribers ask patients to keep journals and record any symptoms they experience. Prescribers then evaluate the reported effects to determine whether they are caused by the disease or by the drug. This information is collected by the drug company that is developing the drug and is shared with the FDA. When a drug is used widely, totally unexpected responses may occur. A drug that produces unacceptable adverse effects or unforeseen reactions is usually removed from further study by the drug company. In some cases, the FDA may have to request that a drug be removed from the market.

Food and Drug Administration Approval

Drugs that finish phase III studies are evaluated by the FDA, which relies on committees of experts familiar with the specialty area in which the drugs will be used. Only those drugs that receive FDA committee approval may be marketed. Figure 1.3 recaps the various phases of drug development discussed.

The entire drug development and approval process can take 5 to 6 years, resulting in a so-called drug lag in the United States. In some instances, a drug that is available in another country may not become available here for years. The FDA regards public safety as primary in drug approval, so the process remains strict; however, it can be accelerated in certain instances involving the treatment of deadly diseases. For example, some drugs (including delavirdine [*Rescriptor*] and efavirenz [*Sustiva*]) that were thought to offer a benefit to patients with acquired immune deficiency syndrome (AIDS), a potentially fatal immune disorder, were pushed through because of the progressive nature of AIDS and the lack of a cure. All literature associated with these drugs indicates that long-term effects and other information about the drug may not yet be known.

In addition to the drug lag issue, there also are concerns about the high cost of drug approval. In 2004, *Fortune* magazine did a study that found the estimated cost of taking a chemical from discovery to marketing as a drug was about $802 million. Because of this kind of financial investment, pharmaceutical companies are unwilling to risk approval of a drug that might cause serious problems and prompt lawsuits.

Continual Evaluation

An approved drug is given a **brand name** (trade name) by the pharmaceutical company that developed it. The **generic name** of a drug is the original designation that the drug was given when the drug company applied for the approval process. **Chemical names** are names that reflect the chemical structure of a drug. Some drugs are known by all three names. It can be confusing to study drugs when so many different names are used for the same compound. In this text, the generic and chemical names always appear in straight print, and the brand name is italicized (e.g., minoxidil [*Rogaine*]). See Box 1.1 for examples of drug names.

After a drug is approved for marketing, it enters a phase of continual evaluation or **phase IV study**. Prescribers are obligated to report to the FDA any untoward or unexpected adverse effects associated with drugs they are using, and the FDA continually evaluates this information. Some drugs cause unexpected effects that are not seen until wide distribution occurs. Sometimes, those effects are therapeutic. For example, patients taking the antiparkinsonism drug amantadine (*Symmetrel*) were found to have fewer cases of influenza

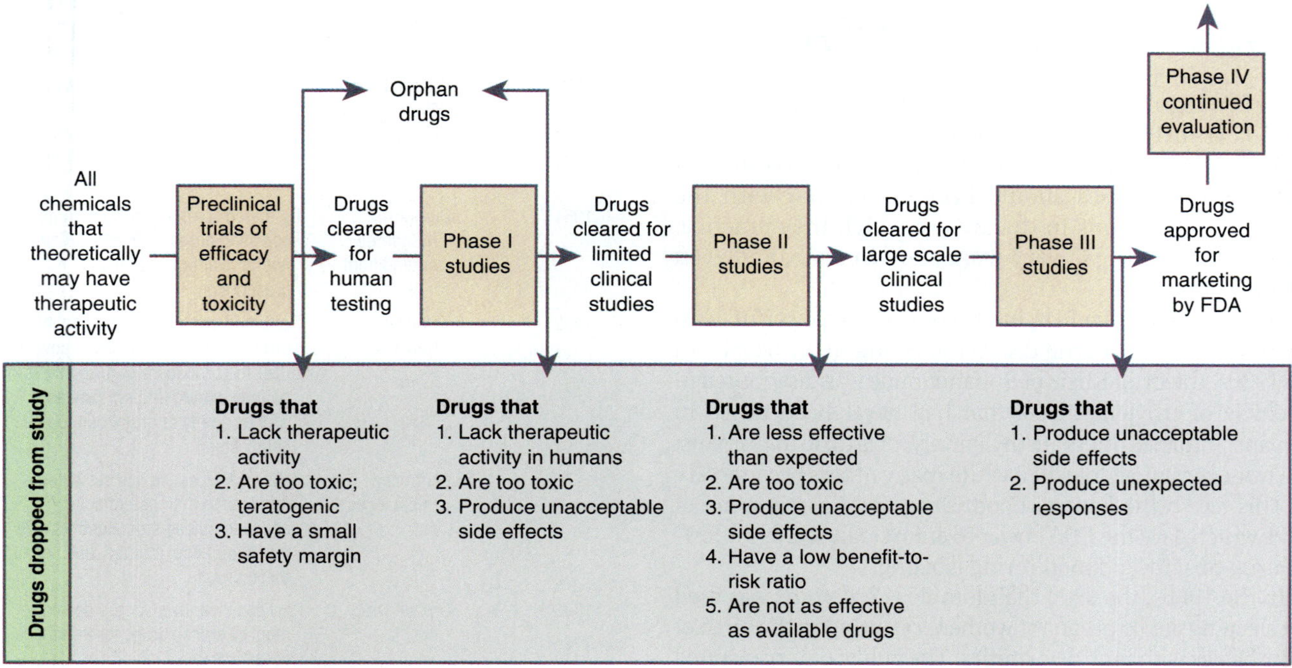

FIGURE 1.3 Phases of drug development.

BOX 1.1 Focus on Generic, Chemical, and Brand Names of Drugs

levothyroxine sodium	←	**generic name**	→	colfosceril palmitate
L-thyroxine, T_4	←	**chemical name**	→	dipalmitoylphosphatidylcholine
Eltroxin, Levothroid, Synthroid	←	**brand names**	→	*Exosurf Neonatal*

than other patients, leading to the discovery that amantadine is an effective antiviral agent.

In other instances, the unexpected effects are dangerous. In 1998, the antihypertensive drug mibefradil (*Posicor*) was removed from the market not long after its release because patients taking it were found to have more cardiac morbidity. In 1997, the diet drug dexfenfluramine (*Redux*) was removed from the market only months after its release because patients taking it developed serious heart problems. These problems were not seen in any of the premarket studies.

FOCUS POINTS

- The FDA carefully regulates the testing and approval of all drugs in this country.
- To be approved for marketing, a drug must pass through animal testing, testing on healthy humans, select testing on people with the disease being treated, and then broad testing on people with the disease being treated.

Legal Regulation of Drugs

The FDA regulates the development and sale of drugs. Local laws further regulate the distribution and administration of drugs. In most cases, the strictest law is the one that prevails. Nurses should become familiar with the rules and regulations in the area in which they practice. These regulations can vary from state to state, and even within a state.

Over the years, the FDA has become more powerful, usually in response to a drug disaster affecting many people. In the 1930s, the drug Elixir of Sulfanilamide was distributed in a vehicle of ethylene glycol that had never been tested in humans. It turned out that ethylene glycol is toxic to humans, and hundreds of people died while many others became very ill. This led to the Federal Food, Drug and Cosmetic Act of 1938, which gave the FDA power to enforce standards for testing drug toxicity and monitoring labeling.

In the 1960s, the drug thalidomide (*Thalomid*) was used as a sleeping aid by pregnant women, resulting in the birth of many babies with limb deformities. The public outcry resulted in the Kefauver-Harris Act of 1962, which gave the FDA regulatory control over the testing and evaluating of drugs and set standards for efficacy and safety.

Other laws have given the FDA control over monitoring of potentially addictive drugs and responsibility for monitoring, to some extent, the sale of drugs that are available without prescription. Table 1.4 provides a summary of these laws.

Pregnancy Categories

As part of the standards for testing and safety, the FDA requires that each new drug be assigned to a pregnancy category (Box 1.2). The categories indicate a drug's potential or actual teratogenic effects, thus offering guidelines for use of that particular drug in pregnancy. Research into the development of the human fetus, especially the nervous system,

Table 1.4 Focus on Federal Legislation Affecting the Clinical Use of Drugs

Year Enacted	Law	Impact
1906	Pure Food and Drug Act	Prevented the marketing of adulterated drugs; required labeling to eliminate false or misleading claims
1938	Federal Food, Drug and Cosmetic Act	Mandated tests for drug toxicity and provided means for recall of drugs; established procedures for introducing new drugs; gave FDA the power of enforcement
1951	Durham-Humphrey Amendment	Tightened control of certain drugs; specified drugs to be labeled "may not be distributed without a prescription"
1962	Kefauver-Harris Act	Tightened control over the quality of drugs; gave FDA regulatory power over the procedure of drug investigations; stated that efficacy as well as safety of drugs had to be established
1970	Controlled Substances Act	Defined drug abuse and classified drugs as to their potential for abuse; provided strict controls over the distribution, storage, and use of these drugs
1983	Orphan Drug Act	Provided incentives for the development of orphan drugs for treatment of rare diseases

BOX 1.2 FDA Pregnancy Categories

The Food and Drug Administration (FDA) has established five categories to indicate the potential for a systemically absorbed drug to cause birth defects. The key differentiation among the categories rests on the degree (reliability) of documentation and the risk-benefit ratio.

Category A: Adequate studies in pregnant women have not demonstrated a risk to the fetus in the first trimester of pregnancy, and there is no evidence of risk in later trimesters.

Category B: Animal studies have not demonstrated a risk to the fetus but there are no adequate studies in pregnant women, *or* animal studies have shown an adverse effect, but adequate studies in pregnant women have not demonstrated a risk to the fetus during the first trimester of pregnancy, and there is no evidence of risk in later trimesters.

Category C: Animal studies have shown an adverse effect on the fetus but there are no adequate studies in humans; the benefits from the use of the drug in pregnant women may be acceptable despite its potential risks, *or* there are no animal reproduction studies and no adequate studies in humans.

Category D: There is evidence of human fetal risk, but the potential benefits from the use of the drug in pregnant women may be acceptable despite its potential risks.

Category X: Studies in animals or humans demonstrate fetal abnormalities or adverse reaction; reports indicate evidence of fetal risk. The risk of use in a pregnant woman clearly outweighs any possible benefit.

Regardless of the designated Pregnancy Category or presumed safety, *no* drug should be administered during pregnancy unless it is clearly needed.

BOX 1.3 DEA Schedules of Controlled Substances

The Controlled Substances Act of 1970 regulates the manufacturing, distribution, and dispensing of drugs that are known to have abuse potential. The Drug Enforcement Agency (DEA) is responsible for the enforcement of these regulations. The controlled drugs are divided into five DEA schedules based on their potential for abuse and physical and psychological dependence.

Schedule I *(C-I):* High abuse potential and no accepted medical use (heroin, marijuana, LSD)

Schedule II *(C-II):* High abuse potential with severe dependence liability (narcotics, amphetamines, and barbiturates)

Schedule III *(C-III):* Less abuse potential than schedule II drugs and moderate dependence liability (nonbarbiturate sedatives, nonamphetamine stimulants, limited amounts of certain narcotics)

Schedule IV *(C-IV):* Less abuse potential than schedule III and limited dependence liability (some sedatives, antianxiety agents, and non-narcotic analgesics)

Schedule V *(C-V):* Limited abuse potential. Primarily small amounts of narcotics (codeine) used as antitussives or antidiarrheals. Under federal law, limited quantities of certain schedule V drugs may be purchased without a prescription directly from a pharmacist. The purchaser must be at least 18 years of age and must furnish suitable identification. All such transactions must be recorded by the dispensing pharmacist.

Prescribing physicians and dispensing pharmacists must be registered with the DEA, which also provides forms for the transfer of Schedule I and II substances and establishes criteria for the inventory and prescribing of controlled substances. State and local laws are often more stringent than federal law. In any given situation, the more stringent law applies.

has led many health care providers to recommend that no drug should be used during pregnancy because of potential effects on the developing fetus. In cases in which a drug is needed, it is recommended that the drug of choice be one for which the benefit outweighs the potential risk.

Controlled Substances

The Controlled Substances Act of 1970 established categories for ranking of the abuse potential of various drugs. This same act gave control over the coding of drugs and the enforcement of these codes to the FDA and the Drug Enforcement Agency (DEA), a part of the U.S. Department of Justice. The FDA studies the drugs and determines their abuse potential; the DEA enforces their control. Drugs with abuse potential are called *controlled substances.* Box 1.3 contains descriptions of each category, or schedule.

The prescription, distribution, storage, and use of these drugs is closely monitored by the DEA in an attempt to decrease substance abuse of prescribed medications. Each prescriber has a DEA number, which allows the DEA to monitor prescription patterns and possible abuse. A nurse should be familiar with not only the DEA guidelines for controlled substances, but also the local policies and procedures, which might be even more rigorous.

Generic Drugs

When a drug receives approval for marketing from the FDA, the drug formula is given a time-limited patent, in much the same way as an invention is patented. The length of time for which the patent is good depends on the type of chemical involved. When the patent runs out on a brand-name drug, the drug can be produced by other manufacturers. **Generic drugs** are chemicals that are produced by companies that just manufacture drugs. Because they do not have the research, the advertising, or, sometimes, the quality control departments that pharmaceutical companies have, they can produce the generic drugs more cheaply. In the past, some quality-control problems were found with generic products. For example, the binders used in a generic drug might not be the same as those used in the brand-name product; as a result, the way the body breaks down and uses the drug may differ. In that case, the bioavailability of the drug is different from that of the brand-name product.

Many states require that a drug be dispensed in the generic form if one is available. This requirement helps keep down the cost of drugs and health care. Some prescribers, however, specify that a drug prescription be "dispensed as written" (DAW); that is, that the brand-name product be used. By doing so, the prescriber ensures the quality control and bioavailability expected with that drug. These elements may be most important in drugs that have narrow safety margins, such as digoxin (*Lanoxin*), a heart drug, and warfarin (*Coumadin*), an anticoagulant. The initial cost may be higher, but some prescribers believe that, in the long run, the cost to the patient will be less.

Orphan Drugs

Orphan drugs are drugs that have been discovered but are not financially viable and therefore have not been "adopted" by any drug company. Orphan drugs may be useful in treating a rare disease, or they may have potentially dangerous adverse effects. Orphan drugs are often abandoned after preclinical trials or phase I studies. The Orphan Drug Act of 1983 provided tremendous financial incentives to drug companies to adopt these drugs and develop them. These incentives help the drug company put the drug through the rest of the testing process, even though the market for the drug in the long run may be very small (as in the case of a drug to treat a rare neurological disease that affects only a small number of people). Some drugs in this book have orphan drug uses listed.

Over-the-Counter Drugs

Over-the-counter (OTC) drugs are products that are available without prescription for self-treatment of a variety of complaints. Some of these agents were approved as prescription drugs but later were found to be very safe and useful for patients without the need of a prescription. Some were not rigorously screened and tested by the current drug evaluation protocols because they were developed and marketed before the current laws were put into effect. Many of these drugs were "grandfathered" into use because they had been used for so long. The FDA is currently testing the effectiveness of many of these products and, in time, will evaluate all of them. Although OTC drugs have been found to be safe when taken as directed, nurses should consider several problems related to OTC drug use:

- Taking these drugs could mask the signs and symptoms of underlying disease, making diagnosis difficult.
- Taking these drugs with prescription medications could result in drug interactions and interfere with drug therapy.
- Not taking these drugs as directed could result in serious overdoses.

Many patients do not consider OTC drugs to be medications and therefore do not report their use. Nurses should always include specific questions about OTC drug use when taking a drug history and should provide information in all drug-teaching protocols about avoiding OTC use while taking prescription drugs.

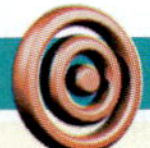

FOCUS POINTS

- Generic drugs are no longer protected by patent and can be produced by companies other than the one that developed it.
- Over-the-counter (OTC) drugs are deemed safe when used as directed and are available without a prescription.
- Orphan drugs are drugs that have been discovered but that are not financially viable because they have a limited market or a narrow margin of safety. These drugs have then been adopted for development by a drug company in exchange for tax incentives.

Sources of Drug Information

The fields of pharmacology and drug therapy change so quickly that it is important to have access to sources of information about drug doses, therapeutic and adverse effects, and nursing-related implications. Textbooks provide valuable background and basic information to help in the understanding of pharmacology, but in clinical practice it is important to have access to up-to-the-minute information. Several sources of drug information are readily available.

Package Inserts

All drugs come with a package insert prepared by the manufacturer according to strict FDA regulations. The package insert contains all of the chemical and study information that led to the drug's approval. Package inserts sometimes are difficult to understand and are almost always in very small print, making them difficult to read.

Reference Books

The *Physician's Drug Reference* (*PDR*) is a compilation of the package insert information from drugs used in this country, along with some drug advertising. This information is heavily cross-referenced. The book may be difficult to use.

Drug Facts and Comparisons provides a wide range of drug information, including comparisons of drug costs, patient information sections, and preparation and administration guidelines. This book is organized by drug class and can be more user friendly than the *PDR*. It is very large and very expensive.

AMA Drug Evaluations contains detailed monographs in an unbiased format and includes many new drugs and drugs still in the research stage.

Lippincott's Nursing Drug Guide (*LNDG*) has drug monographs organized alphabetically and includes nursing implications and patient teaching points.

Journals

Medical Letter is a monthly review of new drugs, drug classes, and specific treatment protocols. *American Journal of Nursing* offers information on new drugs, drug errors, and nursing implications.

Internet Information

Box 1.4 lists some informative Internet sites for obtaining drug information, patient information, or therapeutic information related to specific disease states. Many patients now use the Internet as a source of medical information and advice. It is a good idea for the nurse to become familiar with what is available on the Internet and what patients may be referencing.

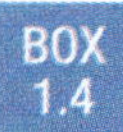

BOX 1.4 **Focus on Internet Information**

Ways to get started and to evaluate sites with drug information on the Internet

Good Places to Begin (Search Tools and Places to Browse)

Alta Vista:
http://www.altavista.com

Cliniweb:
http://www.ohsu.edu/cliniweb

Hardin Meta Directory of Internet Health Sources:
http://www.lib.uiowa.edu/hardin/md/index.html

MetaCrawler:
http://www.metacrawler.com

Yahoo Search:
http://www.yahoo.com

Learning More About the Internet

Learn the Net:
http://learnthenet.com

To find an Internet service provider (ISP):
http://www.thelist.com

Evaluating web sites:
http://hitiweb.mitretek.org/docs/policy.html

Government Sites

Agency for Health Care Research and Quality (AHRQ):
http://www.ahcpr.gov

CancerNet (National Cancer Institute):
http://www.cancer.gov

Centers for Disease Control:
http://www.cdc.gov

Drug Formulary:
http://www.intmed.mcw.edu/drug.html

Food and Drug Administration:
http://www.fda.gov

Healthfinder:
http://www.healthfinder.gov

National Institutes of Health:
http://www.nih.gov

National Institute for Occupational Safety and Health:
http://www.cdc.gov/niosh

National Library of Medicine:
http://www.nlm.nih.gov

Office of Disease Prevention and Health Promotion:
http://www.odphp.osophs.dhhs.gov

Nursing and Health Care Sites

American Diabetes Association:
http://www.diabetes.org

American Nurses Association:
http://www.ana.org

Cumulative Index to Nursing and Allied Health Literature:
http://www.cinahl.com

International Council of Nurses:
http://www.icn.ch

Joint Commission on Accreditation of Healthcare Organizations:
http://www.jcaho.org

Journal of American Medical Association:
http://www.jama.ama-assn.org

Lippincott's Nursing Center:
http://www.nursingcenter.com

Mayo Health Oasis:
http://www.mayohealth.org

Medscape:
http://www.medscape.com

Merck & Co. (search the Merck Manual):
http://www.merck.com

New England Journal of Medicine:
http://www.nejm.org

Nurse Practitioner resources:
http://nurseweb.ucsf.edu/www/arwwebpg.htm

RxList:
http://www.rxlist.com

Points to Remember

- Drugs are chemicals that are introduced into the body to bring about some sort of change.
- Drugs can come from many sources: plants, animals, inorganic elements, and synthetic preparations.
- The FDA regulates the development and marketing of drugs to ensure safety and efficacy.
- Preclinical trials involve testing of potential drugs on laboratory animals to determine their therapeutic and adverse effects.
- Phase I studies test potential drugs on healthy human subjects.
- Phase II studies test potential drugs on patients who have the disease the drugs are designed to treat.
- Phase III studies test drugs in the clinical setting to determine any unanticipated effects or lack of effectiveness.
- FDA pregnancy categories indicate the potential or actual teratogenic effects of a drug.
- DEA controlled substance categories indicate the abuse potential and associated regulation of a drug.
- Generic drugs are sold under their chemical names, not brand names; they may be cheaper but are not necessarily as safe as brand-name drugs.
- Orphan drugs are chemicals that have been discovered to have some therapeutic effect but that are not financially advantageous to develop into drugs.
- OTC drugs are available without prescription for the self-treatment of various complaints.

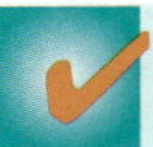

CHECK YOUR UNDERSTANDING

Answers to the questions in this chapter may be found in the Answer Key in the back of the book.

Multiple Choice

Select the best answer to the following.

1. Clinical pharmacology is the study of
   a. the biological effects of chemicals.
   b. drugs used to treat, prevent, or diagnose disease.
   c. plant components that can be used as medicines.
   d. binders and other vehicles for delivering medication.

2. Phase I drug studies involve
   a. the use of laboratory animals to test chemicals.
   b. patients with the disease the drug is designed to treat.
   c. mass marketing surveys of drug effects in large numbers of people.
   d. healthy human volunteers who are often paid for their participation.

3. The generic name of a drug is
   a. the name assigned to the drug by the pharmaceutical company developing it.
   b. the chemical name of the drug based on its chemical structure.
   c. the original name assigned to the drug at the beginning of the evaluation process.
   d. often used in advertising campaigns.

4. An orphan drug is a drug that
   a. has failed to go through the approval process.
   b. is available in a foreign country but not in this country.
   c. has been discovered but is not financially viable and therefore has not been "adopted" by any drug company.
   d. is available without a prescription.

5. The FDA pregnancy categories
   a. indicate a drug's potential or actual teratogenic effects, offering guidelines for use of a particular drug in pregnancy.
   b. are used for research purposes only.
   c. list drugs that are more likely to have addicting properties.
   d. are tightly regulated by the DEA.

6. The storing, prescribing, and distributing of controlled substances—drugs that are more apt to be addictive—are monitored by
   a. the FDA.
   b. the Department of Commerce.
   c. the FBI.
   d. the DEA.

7. Healthy young women are not usually involved in Phase I studies of drugs because
   a. male bodies are more predictable and responsive to chemicals.
   b. females are more apt to suffer problems with ova, which are formed before birth and not formed in later years.
   c. males can tolerate the unknown adverse effects of many drugs better than females.
   d. there are no standards to use to evaluate the female response.

8. A patient has been taking fluoxetine (*Prozac*) for several years, but when picking up the prescription this month, found that the tablets looked different and became concerned. The nurse, checking with the pharmacist, found that fluoxetine had just become available in the generic form and the prescription had been filled with the generic product. The nurse should tell the patient
   a. that the new tablet may not work and the patient should carefully monitor response.
   b. that generic drugs are available without a prescription because they are very safe.
   c. that the law requires that prescriptions be filled with the generic form if one is available to cut down the cost of medications.
   d. that the pharmacist filled the prescription with the wrong drug and it should be returned to the pharmacy for a refund.

Multiple Response

Select all that apply.

1. When teaching a patient about over-the-counter (OTC) drugs, which points should the nurse include?
   a. These drugs are very safe and can be used freely to relieve your complaints.
   b. These compounds are called drugs, but they aren't really drugs and don't need to be reported to your health care provider.
   c. Some of these drugs were once prescription drugs, but are now thought to be safe when used as directed.
   d. Reading the label of these drugs is very important; the active ingredient is very prominent; you should always check the ingredient name.
   e. It is important to read the label to see what the recommended dose of the drug is; some of these drugs can cause serious problems if too much of the drug is taken.
   f. It is important to report the use of any OTC drug to your physician, because many of them can interact with drugs that might be prescribed for you.

2. A patient asks what generic drugs are and if he should be using them to treat his infection. Which of the following statements should be included in the nurse's explanation?
   a. A generic drug is a drug that is sold by the name of the ingredient, not by brand name.
   b. Generic drugs are always the best drugs to use because they are never any different from the familiar brand names.
   c. Generic drugs are not available until the patent expires on a specific drug.
   d. Generic drugs are usually cheaper than the well-known brand names and some insurance companies require that you receive a generic drug if one is available.
   e. Generic drugs are forms of a drug that are available over the counter and do not require a prescription.
   f. Your physician may want you to have the brand name of a drug, not the generic form, and DAW, or "dispense as written," will be on your prescription.
   g. Generic drugs are less likely to cause adverse effects than brand-name drugs.

Web Exercise

Go to the FDA home page on the Internet (www.fda.gov). Click on "Drugs" in the column on the left hand side of the page. This will take you to the CDER home page (Center for Drug Evaluation and Research). The left hand column contains news items about new drug releases. Select a drug that has been recently released. Click on Drugs @fda on the right side of the page. This will take you to a page with a keyboard. Select the letter that represents the first letter in the brand name of the new drug. Drugs beginning with that letter will appear; scroll down the page to find the drug that you selected. Click on that name. This will take you to that drug's page. Identify the brand name, generic name, and therapeutic class of the drug. Click on label information to get specific information regarding the therapeutic use, adverse effects, and dosage of the drug. Try to find the manufacturer's home page for this drug. (This can be done by entering the generic name of the drug into a search.) Compare the information available on that site with the FDA information. Return to the FDA site and try this search for another drug.

Matching

Match the word with the appropriate definition.

1. ________________ genetic engineering
2. ________________ Food and Drug Administration (FDA)
3. ________________ pharmacology
4. ________________ phase I study
5. ________________ over-the-counter (OTC) drugs
6. ________________ preclinical study
7. ________________ teratogenic
8. ________________ pharmacotherapeutics
9. ________________ generic drugs
10. ________________ drugs

A. The study of the actions of chemicals on living organisms
B. Drugs sold by their chemical names, not brand-name products

C. Having adverse effects on the fetus
D. Chemicals that are introduced into the body to bring about some sort of change
E. A drug that is available without a prescription
F. Federal agency responsible for the regulation and enforcement of drug evaluation and distribution policies
G. Process of altering deoxyribonucleic acid (DNA) to produce a chemical to be used as a drug
H. Pilot study of a potential drug conducted with a small number of selected, healthy human volunteers
I. Initial trial of a chemical believed to have therapeutic potential; uses laboratory animals, not human subjects
J. Clinical pharmacology, the branch of pharmacology that deals with drugs

Bibliography and References

Anderson, P. O. (2000). *Handbook of critical drug data* (9th ed.). Hamilton, IL: Drug Intelligence.

Cardinale, V. (1998). Consumers looking for more answers, clearer directions. *Drug Topics Supplement, 142*(11), 23a.

Fitzgerald, M. (1994). Pharmacological highlights: Principles of pharmacokinetics. *Journal of the American Academy of Nursing Practice, 6*(12), 581.

Food and Drug Administration. (1994). FDA launches MEDWATCH program: Monitoring adverse drug reactions. *NP News, 2,* 1, 4.

Gilman, A., Hardman, J. G., & Limbird, L. E. (Eds.). (2006). *Goodman and Gilman's the pharmacological basis of therapeutics* (11th ed.). New York: McGraw-Hill.

The medical letter on drugs and therapeutics. (2006). New Rochelle, NY: Medical Letter.

CHAPTER

2

Drugs and the Body

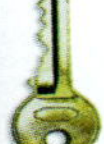

KEY TERMS

absorption
active transport
biotransformation
chemotherapeutic agents
critical concentration
distribution
excretion
first-pass effect
half-life
passive diffusion
pharmacodynamics
pharmacogenomics
pharmacokinetics
placebo effect
receptor sites
selective toxicity

LEARNING OBJECTIVES

Upon completion of this chapter, you will be able to:

1. Describe how body cells respond to the presence of drugs that are capable of altering their function.
2. Outline the process of dynamic equilibrium that determines the actual concentration of a drug in the body.
3. Explain the meaning of half-life of a drug and calculate the half-life of given drugs.
4. List six factors that can influence the actual effectiveness of drugs in the body.
5. Define drug–drug, drug–alternative therapy, drug–food, and drug–laboratory test interactions.

To understand what happens when a drug is administered, the nurse must understand **pharmacodynamics**, or how the drug affects the body, and **pharmacokinetics**, or how the body acts on the drug. These processes form the basis for the guidelines that have been established regarding drug administration—for example, why certain agents are given intramuscularly (IM) and not intravenously (IV), why some drugs are taken with food and others are not, and the standard dose that should be used to achieve the desired effect. Knowing the basic principles of pharmacodynamics and pharmacokinetics helps the nurse to anticipate therapeutic and adverse drug effects and to intervene in ways that ensure the most effective drug regimen for the patient.

Pharmacodynamics

Pharmacodynamics is the science dealing with interactions between the chemical components of living systems and the foreign chemicals, including drugs, that enter those systems. All living organisms function by a series of complicated, continual chemical reactions. When a new chemical enters the system, multiple changes in and interferences with cell functioning may occur. To avoid such problems, drug development works to provide the most effective and least toxic chemicals for therapeutic use.

Drug Actions

Drugs usually work in one of four ways:

1. To replace or act as substitutes for missing chemicals.
2. To increase or stimulate certain cellular activities.
3. To depress or slow cellular activities.
4. To interfere with the functioning of foreign cells, such as invading microorganisms or neoplasms. (Drugs that act in this way are called **chemotherapeutic agents**.)

Drugs can act in several different ways to achieve these results.

Receptor Sites

Many drugs are thought to act at specific areas on cell membranes called **receptor sites**. The receptor sites react with certain chemicals to cause an effect within the cell. In many situations, nearby enzymes break down the reacting chemicals and open the receptor site for further stimulation.

To better understand this process, think of how a key works in a lock. The specific chemical (the key) approaches a cell membrane and finds a perfect fit (the lock) at a receptor site (Figure 2.1). The interaction between the chemical and the receptor site affects enzyme systems within the cell. The activated enzyme systems then produce certain effects, such as increased or decreased cellular activity, changes in cell membrane permeability, or alterations in cellular metabolism.

Some drugs interact directly with receptor sites to cause the same activity that natural chemicals would cause at that site. These drugs are called *agonists* (see Figure 2.1). For example, insulin reacts with specific insulin receptor sites to change cell membrane permeability, thus promoting the movement of glucose into the cell.

Other drugs act to prevent the breakdown of natural chemicals that are stimulating the receptor site. For example, monoamine oxidase (MAO) inhibitors block the breakdown of norepinephrine by the enzyme MAO. (Normally, MAO breaks down norepinephrine, removes it from the receptor site, and recycles the components to form new norepinephrine.) The blocking action of MAO inhibitors allows norepinephrine to stay on the receptor site, stimulating the cell longer and leading to prolonged norepinephrine effects. Those effects can be therapeutic (e.g., relieving depression) or adverse (e.g., increasing heart rate and blood pressure). Selective serotonin reuptake inhibitors (SSRIs) work similarly to MAO inhibitors in that they also exert a blocking action. Specifically, they block removal of serotonin from receptor sites. This action leads to prolonged stimulation of certain brain cells, which is thought to provide relief from depression.

Some drugs react with receptor sites to block normal stimulation, producing no effect. For example, curare (a drug used on the tips of spears in the Amazon to paralyze prey and cause death) occupies receptor sites for acetylcholine, which is necessary for muscle contraction and movement. Curare prevents muscle stimulation, causing paralysis. Curare is said to be a *competitive antagonist* of acetylcholine (see Figure 2.1).

Still other drugs react with specific receptor sites on a cell and, by reacting there, prevent the reaction of another chemical with a different receptor site on that cell. Such drugs are called *noncompetitive antagonists* (see Figure 2.1). For some drugs, the actual mechanisms of action are unknown. But speculation exists that many drugs use receptor site mechanisms to bring about their effects.

Drug–Enzyme Interactions

Drugs also can cause their effects by interfering with the enzyme systems that act as catalysts for various chemical reactions. Enzyme systems work in a cascade effect, with one enzyme activating another and eventually causing a cellular reaction. If a single step in one of the many enzyme systems is blocked, normal cell function is disrupted. Acetazolamide (*Diamox*) is a diuretic that blocks the enzyme carbonic anhydrase, which subsequently causes alterations in the hydrogen ion and water exchange system in the kidney, as well as the eye.

Selective Toxicity

Ideally, all chemotherapeutic agents would act only on enzyme systems that are essential for the life of a pathogen or neoplastic cell and would not affect healthy cells. The

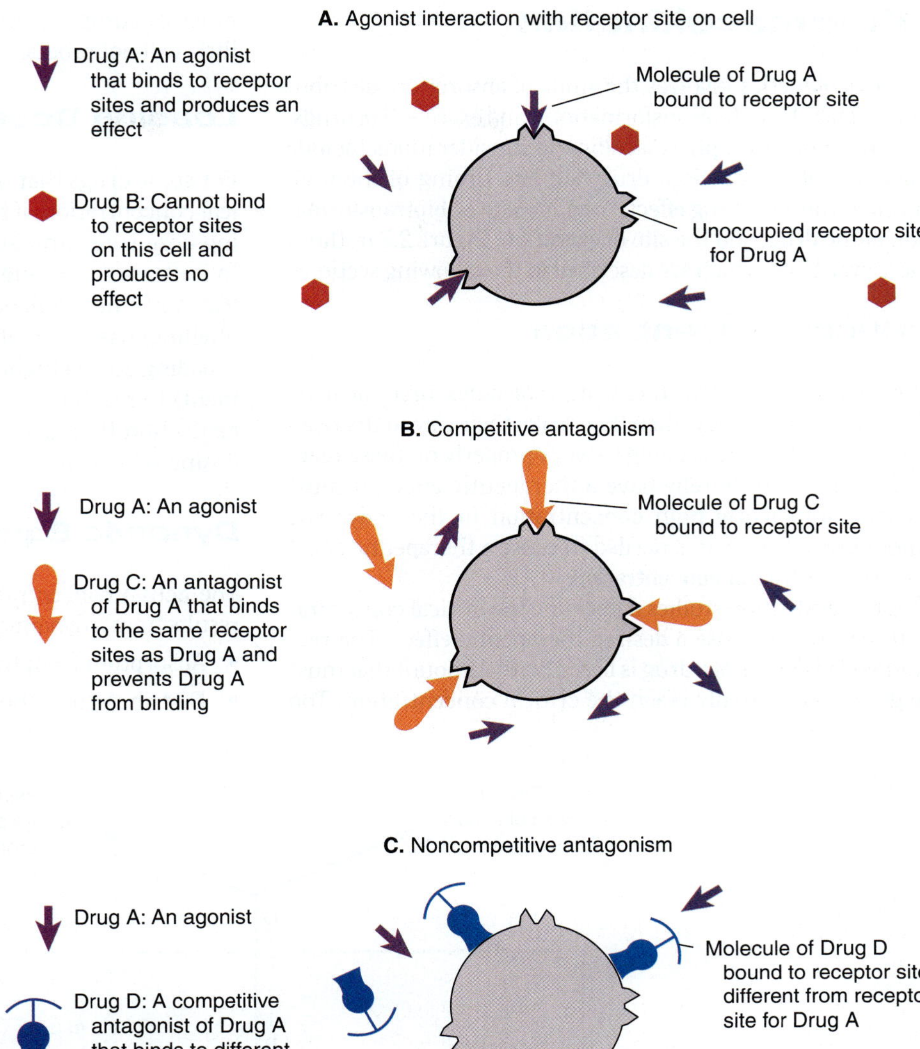

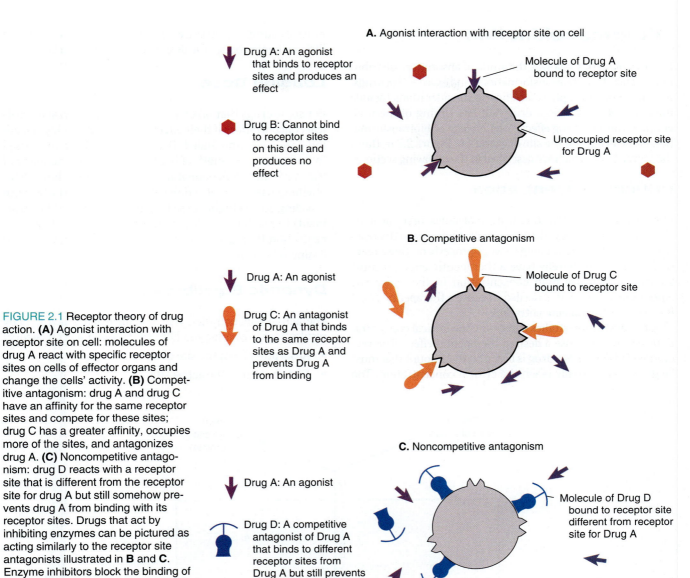

FIGURE 2.1 Receptor theory of drug action. **(A)** Agonist interaction with receptor site on cell: molecules of drug A react with specific receptor sites on cells of effector organs and change the cells' activity. **(B)** Competitive antagonism: drug A and drug C have an affinity for the same receptor sites and compete for these sites; drug C has a greater affinity, occupies more of the sites, and antagonizes drug A. **(C)** Noncompetitive antagonism: drug D reacts with a receptor site that is different from the receptor site for drug A but still somehow prevents drug A from binding with its receptor sites. Drugs that act by inhibiting enzymes can be pictured as acting similarly to the receptor site antagonists illustrated in **B** and **C**. Enzyme inhibitors block the binding of molecules of normal substrate to active sites on the enzyme.

ability of a drug to attack only those systems found in foreign cells is known as selective toxicity. Penicillin, an antibiotic used to treat bacterial infections, has **selective toxicity**. It affects an enzyme system unique to bacteria, causing bacterial cell death without disrupting normal human cell functioning.

Unfortunately, most other chemotherapeutic agents also destroy normal human cells, causing many of the adverse effects associated with antipathogen and antineoplastic chemotherapy. Cells that reproduce, or are replaced, rapidly (e.g., bone marrow cells, gastrointestinal [GI] cells, hair follicles) are more easily affected by these agents. Consequently, the goal of many chemotherapeutic regimens is to deliver a dose that will be toxic to the invading cells yet cause the least amount of toxicity to the host.

FOCUS POINTS

- Pharmacodynamics is the process by which a drug works on the body.
- Drugs may work by replacing a missing body chemical, by stimulating or depressing cellular activity, or by interfering with the functioning of foreign cells.
- Drugs are thought to work by reacting with specific receptor sites or by interacting with enzyme systems in the body.

Pharmacokinetics

Pharmacokinetics involves the study of absorption, distribution, metabolism (biotransformation), and excretion of drugs. In clinical practice, pharmacokinetic considerations include the onset of drug action, drug half-life, timing of the peak effect, duration of drug effects, metabolism or biotransformation of the drug, and the site of excretion. Figure 2.2 outlines these processes, which are described in the following sections.

Critical Concentration

After a drug is administered, its molecules first must be absorbed into the body; then they make their way to the reactive tissues. If a drug is going to work properly on these reactive tissues, and thereby have a therapeutic effect, it must attain a sufficiently high concentration in the body. The amount of a drug that is needed to cause a therapeutic effect is called the **critical concentration.**

Drug evaluation studies determine the critical concentration required to cause a desired therapeutic effect. The recommended dosage of a drug is based on the amount that must be given to eventually reach the critical concentration. Too much of a drug will produce toxic (poisonous) effects, and too little will not produce the desired therapeutic effects.

Loading Dose

For some drugs that take a prolonged period to reach a critical concentration, if their effects are needed quickly, a loading dose is recommended. Digoxin (*Lanoxin*), a drug used to increase the strength of heart contractions, and many of the xanthine bronchodilators (e.g., aminophylline, theophylline) used to treat asthma attacks are often started with a loading dose (a higher dose than that usually used for treatment) to reach the critical concentration. The critical concentration then is maintained by using the recommended dosing schedule.

Dynamic Equilibrium

The actual concentration that a drug reaches in the body results from a dynamic equilibrium involving several factors:

- Absorption from the site of entry
- Distribution to the active site

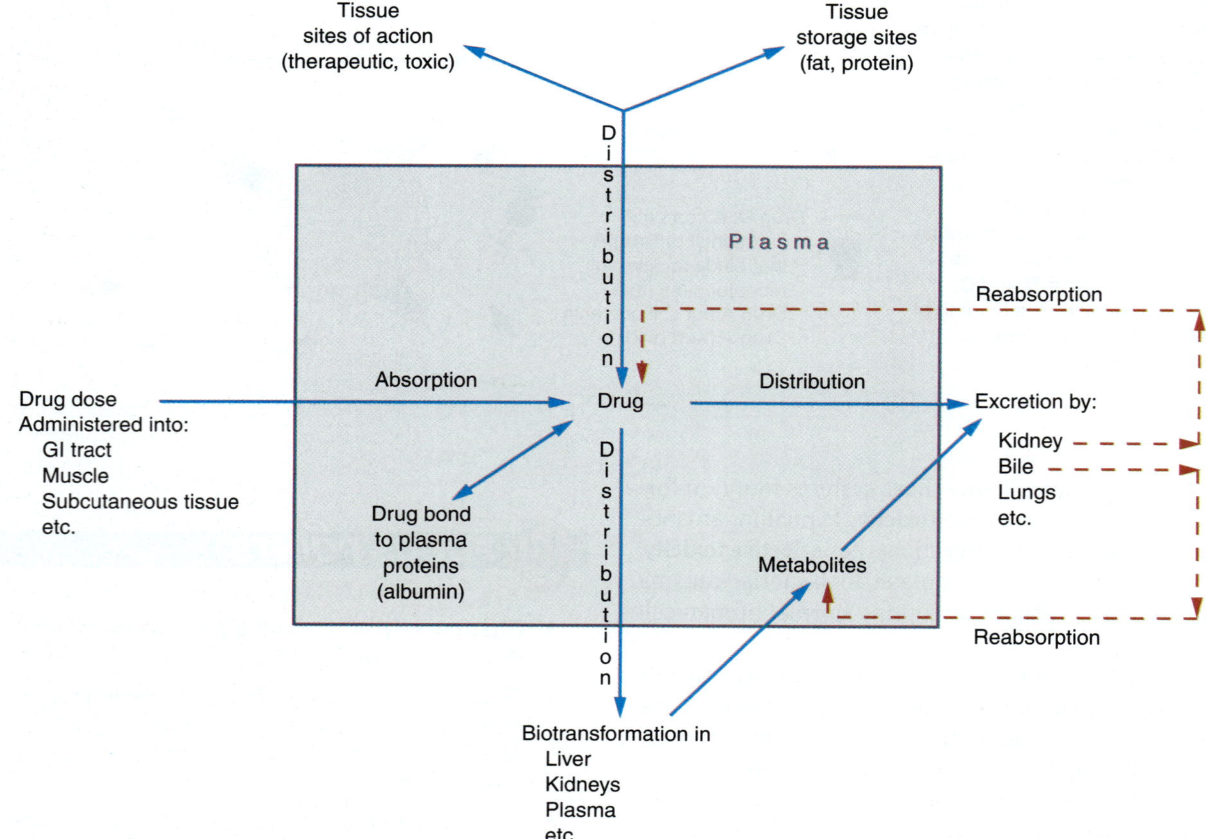

FIGURE 2.2 The processes by which a drug is handled by the body. *Dashed lines* indicate that some portion of a drug and its metabolites may be reabsorbed from the excretory organs. The dynamic equilibrium of pharmacokinetics is shown.

- Biotransformation (metabolism) in the liver
- Excretion from the body

These factors are key elements in determining the amount of drug needed (dose) and the frequency of dose repetition (scheduling) required to achieve the critical concentration for the desired length of time. When administering a drug, the nurse needs to consider the phases of pharmacokinetics so that the drug regimen can be made as effective as possible.

Absorption

In order to reach reactive tissues, a drug must first make its way into the circulating fluids of the body. **Absorption** refers to what happens to a drug from the time it is introduced to the body until it reaches the circulating fluids and tissues. Drugs can be absorbed from many different areas in the body: through the GI tract either orally or rectally, through mucous membranes, through the skin, through the lung, or through muscle or subcutaneous tissues (see Figure 2.2).

Drugs can be absorbed into cells through various processes, which include passive diffusion, active transport, and filtration. **Passive diffusion** is the major process through which drugs are absorbed into the body. Passive diffusion occurs across a concentration gradient. When there is a greater concentration of drug on one side of a cell membrane, the drug will move through the membrane to the area of lower concentration. This process does not require any cellular energy. It occurs more quickly if the drug molecule is small, is soluble in water and in lipids (cell membranes are made of lipids and proteins—see Chapter 7), and has no electrical charge that could repel it from the cell membrane.

Unlike passive diffusion, **active transport** is a process that uses energy to actively move a molecule across a cell membrane. The molecule may be large, or it may be moving against a concentration gradient. This process is not very important in the absorption of drugs, but it is often involved in drug excretion in the kidney.

Filtration is another process the body commonly uses in drug excretion. Filtration involves movement through pores in the cell membrane, either down a concentration gradient or as a result of the pull of plasma proteins (when pushed by hydrostatic, blood, or osmotic pressure).

CONCEPTS in action ANIMATION

Administration

The oral route is the most frequently used drug administration route in clinical practice. Oral administration is not invasive, and as a rule, oral administration is less expensive than drug administration by other routes. It is also the safest way to deliver drugs. Patients can easily continue their drug regimen at home when they are taking oral medications.

Oral administration subjects the drug to a number of barriers aimed at destroying ingested foreign chemicals. The acidic environment of the stomach is one of the first barriers to foreign chemicals. The acid breaks down many compounds and inactivates others. This fact is taken into account by pharmaceutical companies when preparing capsules or tablets of drugs. The binders that are used often are designed to break down in a certain acidity and release the active drug to be absorbed.

When food is present, stomach acidity is higher and the stomach empties more slowly, thus exposing the drug to the acidic environment for a longer period. Certain foods that increase stomach acidity, such as milk products, alcohol, and protein, also speed the breakdown of many drugs. Other foods may chemically bind drugs or block their absorption. To decrease the effects of this acid barrier and the direct effects of certain foods, oral drugs ideally should be given 1 hour before or 2 hours after a meal.

Some drugs that cannot survive in sufficient quantity when given orally need to be injected directly into the body. Drugs that are injected intravenously (IV) reach their full strength at the time of injection, avoiding initial breakdown. These drugs are more likely to cause toxic effects because the margin for error in dosage is much smaller. Drugs that are injected intramuscularly (IM) are absorbed directly into the capillaries in the muscle and sent into circulation. This takes time because the drug must be picked up by the capillary and taken into the veins. Because men have more vascular muscles than women do, IM drugs in men reach a peak level faster than in women. Subcutaneous injections deposit the drug just under the skin, where it is slowly absorbed into circulation. Timing of absorption varies with subcutaneous injection, depending on the fat content of the injection site and the state of local circulation. Table 2.1 outlines the various factors that affect drug absorption.

First-Pass Effect

Drugs that are taken orally are usually absorbed from the small intestine directly into the portal venous system (the blood vessels that flow through the liver on their way back to the heart). Aspirin and alcohol are two drugs that are known to be absorbed from the lower end of the stomach. The portal veins deliver these absorbed molecules into the liver, which immediately transforms most of the chemicals delivered to it by a series of liver enzymes. These enzymes break the drug into metabolites, some of which are active and cause effects in the body and some of which are deactivated and can be readily excreted from the body. As a result, a large percentage of the oral dose is destroyed at this point and never reaches the tissues. This phenomenon is known as the **first-pass effect**. The recommended dose for oral drugs can be considerably higher than the recommended dose for parenteral drugs, taking the first-pass effect into account.

Injected drugs and drugs absorbed from sites other than the GI tract undergo a similar biotransformation when they pass through the liver. Because some of the active drug already has had a chance to reach the reactive tissues before reaching the liver, the injected drug is more effective at a lower dose than the oral equivalent.

Table 2.1 Factors That Affect Absorption of Drugs

Route	Factors Affecting Absorption
IV (intravenous)	None: direct entry into the venous system
IM (intramuscular)	Perfusion or blood flow to the muscle Fat content of the muscle Temperature of the muscle: cold causes vasoconstriction and decreases absorption; heat causes vasodilation and increases absorption
Sub-Q (subcutaneous)	Perfusion or blood flow to the tissue Fat content of the tissue Temperature of the tissue: cold causes vasoconstriction and decreases absorption; heat causes vasodilation and increases absorption
PO (oral)	Acidity of stomach Length of time in stomach Blood flow to gastrointestinal tract Presence of interacting foods or drugs
PR (rectal)	Perfusion or blood flow to the rectum Lesions in the rectum Length of time retained for absorption
Mucous membranes (sublingual, buccal)	Perfusion or blood flow to the area Integrity of the mucous membranes Presence of food or smoking Length of time retained in area
Topical (skin)	Perfusion or blood flow to the area Integrity of skin
Inhalation	Perfusion or blood flow to the area Integrity of lung lining Ability to administer drug properly

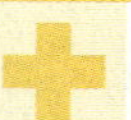

FOCUS ON PATIENT SAFETY

The liver is very important in metabolizing drugs in the body, and the kidneys are responsible for a large part of the excretion of drugs from the body. Therefore, it is a good idea to get into the habit of always checking a patient's liver and renal functions before a patient starts a drug regimen. If the liver is not functioning properly, the drug may not be metabolized correctly and may reach toxic levels in the body. If the kidneys are not functioning properly, the drug may not be excreted properly and could accumulate in the body. Dosage adjustment should be considered if a patient has problems with either the liver or the kidneys.

Distribution

The portion of the drug that gets through the first-pass effect is delivered to the circulatory system for transport throughout the body. **Distribution** involves the movement of a drug to the body's tissues (see Figure 2.2). As with absorption, factors that can affect distribution include the drug's lipid solubility and ionization and the perfusion of the reactive tissue.

For example, tissue perfusion is a factor in treating a diabetic patient who has a lower leg infection and needs antibiotics to destroy the bacteria in the area. In this case, systemic drugs may not be effective because part of the disease process involves changes in the vasculature and decreased blood flow to some areas, particularly the lower limbs. If there is not adequate blood flow to the area, little antibiotic can be delivered to the tissues and little antibiotic effect will be seen.

In the same way, patients in a cold environment may have constricted blood vessels (vasoconstriction) in the extremities, which would prevent blood flow to those areas. The circulating blood would be unable to deliver drugs to those areas, and the patient would receive little therapeutic effect from drugs intended to react with those tissues.

Many drugs are bound to proteins and are not lipid soluble. These drugs cannot be distributed to the central nervous system (CNS) because of the effective blood–brain barrier (see later discussion), which is highly selective in allowing lipid-soluble substances to pass into the CNS.

CONCEPTS in action ANIMATION

Protein Binding

Most drugs are bound to some extent to proteins in the blood to be carried into circulation. The protein–drug complex is relatively large and cannot enter into capillaries and then into tissues to react. The drug must be freed from the protein's binding site at the tissues.

Some drugs are tightly bound and are released very slowly. These drugs have a very long duration of action because they are not freed to be broken down or excreted and therefore are very slowly released into the reactive tissue. Some drugs are loosely bound; they tend to act quickly and to be excreted quickly. Some drugs compete with each other for protein binding sites, altering effectiveness or causing toxicity when the two drugs are given together.

CONCEPTS in action ANIMATION

Blood–Brain Barrier

The blood–brain barrier is a protective system of cellular activity that keeps many things (e.g., foreign invaders, poisons) away from the CNS. Drugs that are highly lipid soluble are more likely to pass through the blood–brain barrier and reach the CNS. Drugs that are not lipid soluble are not able to pass the blood–brain barrier. This is clinically significant in treating a brain infection with antibiotics. Almost all antibiotics are not lipid soluble and cannot cross the blood–brain barrier. Effective antibiotic treatment can occur only when the infection is bad enough to alter the blood–brain barrier and allow antibiotics to cross.

Although many drugs can cause adverse CNS effects, these are often the result of indirect drug effects and not the actual reaction of the drug with CNS tissue. For example, alterations in glucose levels and electrolyte changes can interfere with nerve functioning and produce CNS effects.

Placenta and Breast Milk

Many drugs readily pass through the placenta and affect the developing fetus in pregnant women. As stated earlier, it is best not to administer any drugs to pregnant women because of the possible risk to the fetus. Drugs should be given only when the benefit clearly outweighs any risk. Many other drugs are secreted into breast milk and therefore have the potential to affect the neonate. Because of this possibility, the nurse must always check the ability of a drug to pass into breast milk when giving a drug to a breast-feeding mother.

Biotransformation (Metabolism)

The body is well prepared to deal with a myriad of foreign chemicals. Enzymes in the liver, in many cells, in the lining of the GI tract, and even circulating in the body detoxify foreign chemicals to protect the fragile homeostasis that keeps the body functioning (see Figure 2.2). Almost all of the chemical reactions that the body uses to convert drugs and other chemicals into nontoxic substances are based on a few processes that work to make the chemical less active and more easily excreted from the body.

Liver Enzyme Systems

The liver is the single most important site of drug metabolism or **biotransformation**, the process by which drugs are changed into new, less active chemicals. Think of the liver as a sewage treatment plant. Everything that is absorbed from the GI tract first enters the liver to be "treated." The liver detoxifies many chemicals and uses others to produce needed enzymes and structures.

The hepatic cells' intracellular structures are lined with enzymes, which are packed together in what is called the *hepatic microsomal system.* Because orally administered drugs enter the liver first, the enzyme systems immediately work on the absorbed drug to biotransform it. As explained earlier, this first-pass effect is responsible for neutralizing most of the drugs that are taken. Phase I biotransformation involves oxidation, reduction, or hydrolysis of the drug via the cytochrome P450 system of enzymes. These enzymes are found in most cells but are especially abundant in the liver. Phase II biotransformation usually involves a conjugation reaction that makes the drug less polar and more readily excreted by the kidneys.

The presence of a chemical that is metabolized by a particular enzyme system often increases the activity of that enzyme system. This process is referred to as *enzyme induction.* Only a few basic enzyme systems are responsible for metabolizing most of the chemicals that pass through the liver. Increased activity in an enzyme system speeds the metabolism of the drug that caused the enzyme induction, as well as any other drug that is metabolized via that same enzyme system. This explains why some drugs cannot be taken together effectively: The presence of one drug speeds the metabolism of others, preventing them from reaching their therapeutic levels. Some drugs inhibit an enzyme system, making it less effective. As a consequence, any drug that is metabolized by that system will not be broken down for excretion, and the blood levels of that drug will increase, often to toxic levels. These actions also explain why liver disease is often a contraindication or a reason to use caution when administering certain drugs. If the liver is not functioning effectively, the drug will not be metabolized as it should be, and toxic levels could develop rather quickly. Table 2.2 gives some examples of drugs that induce or inhibit the cytochrome P450 system.

Excretion

Excretion is the removal of a drug from the body. The skin, saliva, lungs, bile, and feces are some of the routes used to excrete drugs. The kidneys, however, play the most important role in drug excretion (see Figure 2.2). Drugs that have been made water soluble in the liver are often readily excreted from the kidney by *glomerular filtration*—the passage of water and water-soluble components from the plasma into the renal tubule.

Other drugs are secreted or reabsorbed through the renal tubule by active transport systems. The acidity of the urine can play an important part in the excretions. The active transport systems that move the drug into the tubule often do so by exchanging it for acid or bicarbonate molecules. This is an important concept to remember when trying to clear a drug rapidly from the system or trying to understand why a drug is being given at the usual dose but is reaching toxic levels in the system. It is important to consider the patient's kidney function and urine acidity before administering a drug. Kidney dysfunction can lead to toxic levels of a drug in the body because the drug cannot be excreted. Figure 2.3 outlines the pharmacokinetic processes that are undergone by a drug administered orally.

CONCEPTS in action ANIMATION

Half-Life

The **half-life** of a drug is the time it takes for the amount of drug in the body to decrease to one-half of the peak level it previously achieved. For instance, if a patient takes 20 mg of a drug with a half-life of 2 hours, 10 mg of the drug will remain

Table 2.2 Examples of Drugs That Alter the Effects of the Cytochrome P450 Enzyme System in the Liver

Drugs That Induce or Increase Activity	Drugs That Inhibit or Decrease Activity
Nicotine (cigarette smoking)	Ketoconazole (*Nizoral*)
Alcohol (drinking)	Mexiletine (*Mexitil*)
Glucocorticoids (*Cortone*, others)	Quinidine (*generic*)

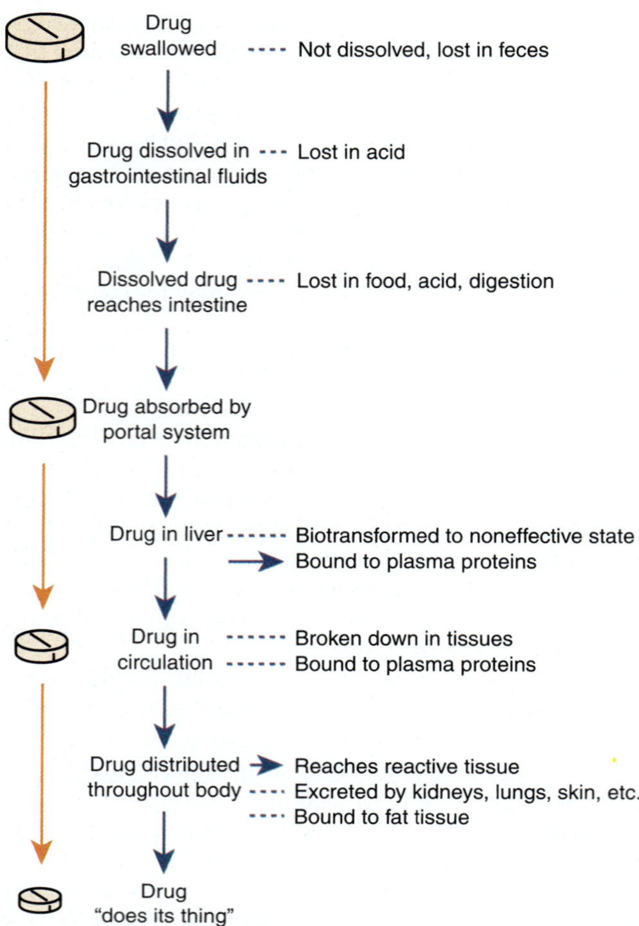

FIGURE 2.3 Pharmacokinetics affect the amount of a drug that reaches reactive tissues. Very little of an oral dose of a drug actually reaches reactive sites.

2 hours after administration. Two hours later, 5 mg will be left (one-half of the previous level); in 2 more hours, only 2.5 mg will remain. This information is important in determining the appropriate timing for a drug dose or determining the duration of a drug's effect on the body. (See Box 2.1.)

The absorption rate, the distribution to the tissues, the speed of biotransformation, and how fast a drug is excreted are all taken into consideration when determining the half-life of the drug. The half-life that is indicated in any drug monograph is the half-life for a healthy person. Using this information, the half-life of a drug for a patient with kidney or liver dysfunction (which could prolong the biotransformation and the time required for excretion of a drug) can be estimated and changes made in the dosage schedule by the prescriber.

The timing of drug administration is important to achieve the most effective drug therapy. Nurses can use their knowledge of drug half-life to explain the importance of following a schedule of drug administration in the hospital or at home. Figure 2.4 shows the effects of drug administration on the critical concentration of a drug.

BOX 2.1 FOCUS ON **CALCULATIONS**

Determining the Impact of Half-Life on Drug Levels

A patient is taking a drug that has a half-life of 12 hours. You are trying to determine when a 50-mg dose of the drug will be gone from the body:

- In 12 hours, half of the 50 mg (25 mg) would be in the body.
- In another 12 hours (24 hours), half of 25 mg (12.5 mg) would remain in the body.
- After 36 hours, half of 12.5 mg (6.25 mg) would remain.
- After 48 hours, half of 6.25 mg (3.125 mg) would remain.
- After 60 hours, half of 3.125 (1.56 mg) would remain.
- After 72 hours, half of 1.56 (0.78 mg) would remain.
- After 84 hours, half of 0.78 (0.39 mg) would remain.
- Twelve more hours (for a total of 96 hours) would reduce the drug amount to 0.195 mg.
- Finally, 12 more hours (108 hours) would reduce the amount of the drug in the body to 0.097 mg, which would be quite negligible.
- Therefore, it would take 4½ to 5 days to clear the drug from the body.

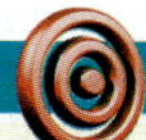

FOCUS POINTS

- Pharmacokinetics is the study of how the body deals with a drug.
- The concentration of a drug in the body is determined by the balance of absorption, metabolism, distribution, and excretion of the drug.
- In determining the dosage, route, and appropriate timing of a drug dose, the pharmacokinetics of that drug have to be considered.

Factors Influencing Drug Effects

When administering a drug to a patient, the nurse must be aware that the human factor has a tremendous influence on what actually happens to a drug when it enters the body. No two people react in exactly the same way to any given drug. Even though textbooks and drug guides explain the pharmacodynamics and pharmacokinetics of a drug, it must be remembered that such information usually is based on studies of healthy, adult males. Things may be very different in the clinical setting. Consequently, before administering any drug, the nurse must consider a number of factors. These are discussed in detail in the following sections and summarized in Box 2.2.

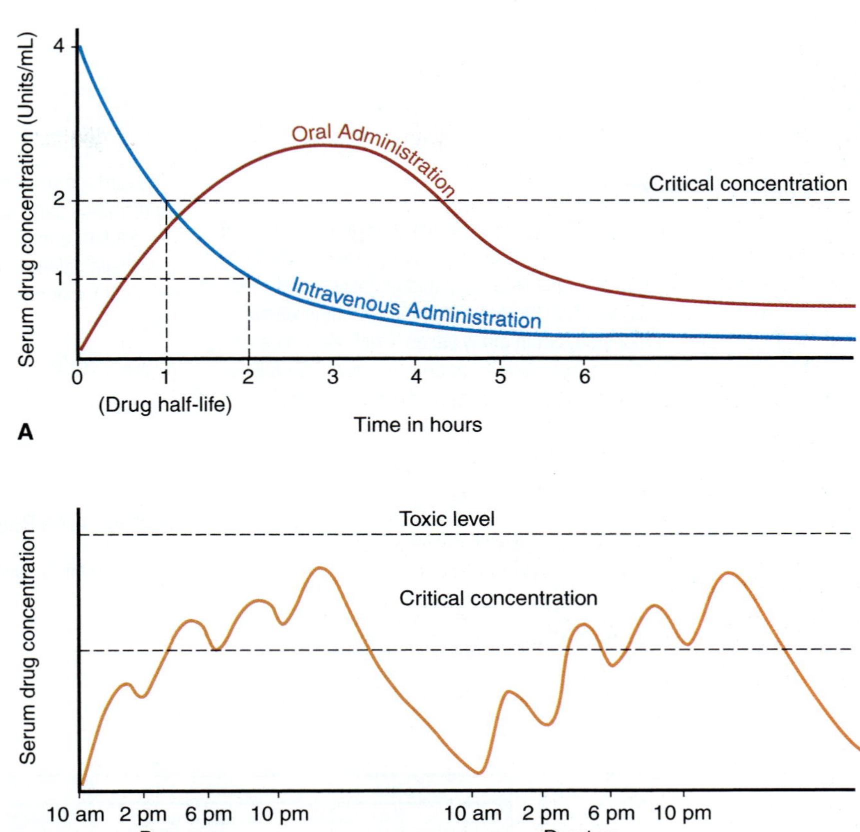

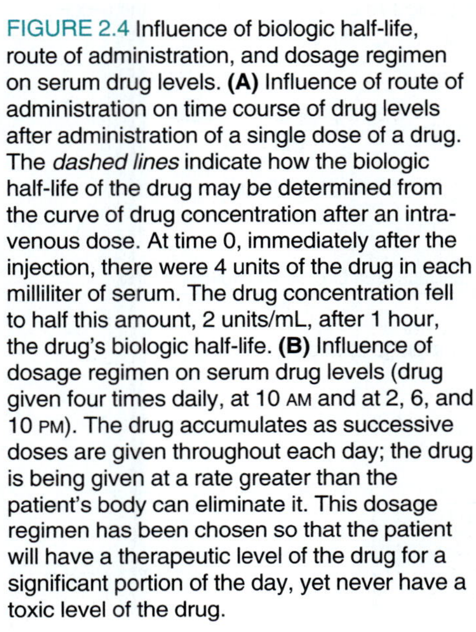
FIGURE 2.4 Influence of biologic half-life, route of administration, and dosage regimen on serum drug levels. **(A)** Influence of route of administration on time course of drug levels after administration of a single dose of a drug. The *dashed lines* indicate how the biologic half-life of the drug may be determined from the curve of drug concentration after an intravenous dose. At time 0, immediately after the injection, there were 4 units of the drug in each milliliter of serum. The drug concentration fell to half this amount, 2 units/mL, after 1 hour, the drug's biologic half-life. **(B)** Influence of dosage regimen on serum drug levels (drug given four times daily, at 10 AM and at 2, 6, and 10 PM). The drug accumulates as successive doses are given throughout each day; the drug is being given at a rate greater than the patient's body can eliminate it. This dosage regimen has been chosen so that the patient will have a therapeutic level of the drug for a significant portion of the day, yet never have a toxic level of the drug.

BOX 2.2 Factors Affecting the Body's Response to a Drug

Weight

Age

Gender

Physiological factors—diurnal rhythm, electrolyte balance, acid–base balance, hydration

Pathological factors—disease, hepatic dysfunction, renal dysfunction, gastrointestinal dysfunction, vascular disorders, low blood pressure

Genetic factors

Immunological factors—allergy

Psychological factors—placebo effect, health beliefs, compliance

Environmental factors—temperature, light, noise

Drug tolerance

Cumulation effects

Weight

The recommended dosage of a drug is based on drug evaluation studies and is targeted at a 150-pound person. People who are much heavier than that may require larger doses to get a therapeutic effect from a drug because they have increased tissues to perfuse and increased receptor sites in some reactive tissue. People who are much lighter than the norm may require smaller doses of a drug. Toxic effects may occur at the recommended dosage if the person is very small.

Age

Age is a factor primarily in children and older adults. Children metabolize many drugs differently than adults do, and they have immature systems for handling drugs. Many drugs come with recommended pediatric dosages, and others can be converted to pediatric dosages using one of several conversion formulas (Box 2.3).

Older adults undergo many physical changes that are a part of the aging process. Their bodies may respond very differently in all aspects of pharmacokinetics—less effective absorption, less efficient distribution because of fewer plasma proteins and less efficient perfusion, altered biotransformation or metabolism of drugs because of liver changes with age,

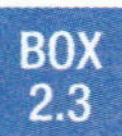

BOX 2.3 Formulas for Calculating Dosages

Pediatric Dosages

Children often require different doses of drugs than adults because children's bodies often handle drugs very differently from adults' bodies. The "standard" drug dosages listed in package inserts and references such as the PDR refer to the adult dosage. In some cases, a pediatric dosage is suggested, but in many cases it will need to be calculated based on the child's age, weight, or body surface. The following are some standard formulae for calculating the pediatric dose.

Fried's Rule

$$\text{infant's dose } (<1 \text{ year}) = \frac{\text{infant's age (in months)}}{150 \text{ months}} \times \text{average adult dose}$$

Young's Rule

$$\text{child's dose } (1\text{–}12 \text{ years}) = \frac{\text{child's age (in years)}}{\text{child's age (in years)} + 12} \times \text{average adult dose}$$

The surface area of a child is determined using a nomogram which determines surface area based on height and weight measurements.

Pediatric dosage calculations should be checked by two persons. Many institutions have procedures for double checking the dosage calculation of those drugs (e.g., digoxin) used most frequently in the pediatric area.

Clark's Rule

$$\text{child's dose} = \frac{\text{weight of child (in pounds)}}{150} \times \text{average adult dose}$$

Surface Area Rule

$$\text{child's dose} = \frac{\text{surface area of child (in square meters)}}{1.73} \times \text{average adult dose}$$

Nomogram for estimating surface area of infants and young children. To determine the surface area of the patient, draw a straight line between the point representing the height on the left vertical scale and the point representing the weight on the right vertical scale. The point at which this line intersects the middle vertical scale represents the patient's surface area in square meters.

and less effective excretion owing to less efficient kidneys. Many drugs now come with recommended geriatric dosages. Other drugs may also need decreased dosages in the elderly.

When administering drugs to a patient at either end of the age spectrum, the nurse should monitor closely for desired effects. If the effects are not what would normally be expected, a dosage adjustment should be considered.

Gender

Physiological differences between men and women can influence a drug's effect. When giving IM injections, for example, it is important to remember that men have more vascular muscles, so the effects of the drug will be seen sooner in men than in women.

Women have more fat cells than men do, so drugs that deposit in fat may be slowly released and cause effects for a prolonged period. For example, gas anesthetics have an affinity for depositing in fat and can cause drowsiness and sedation sometimes weeks after surgery. Women who are given any drug should always be questioned about the possibility of pregnancy because, as stated previously, the use of drugs in pregnant women is not recommended unless the benefit clearly outweighs the potential risk to the fetus.

Physiological Factors

Physiological differences such as diurnal rhythm of the nervous and endocrine systems, acid–base balance, hydration, and electrolyte balance can affect the way that a drug works on the body and the way that the body handles the drug. If a drug does not produce the desired effect, review the patient's acid–base and electrolyte profiles and the timing of the drug.

Pathological Factors

Drugs are usually used to treat disease or pathology. However, the disease that the drug is intended to treat can change the functioning of the chemical reactions within the body and thus change the response to the drug.

Other pathological conditions can change the basic pharmacokinetics of a drug. For example, GI disorders can affect the absorption of many oral drugs. Vascular diseases and low blood pressure alter the distribution of a drug, preventing it from being delivered to the reactive tissue and rendering it nontherapeutic. Liver or kidney diseases affect the way that a drug is biotransformed and excreted and can lead to toxic reactions when the usual dose is given.

Genetic Factors

Genetic differences can sometimes explain patients' varied responses to a given drug. Some people lack certain enzyme systems necessary for metabolizing a drug, whereas others have overactive enzyme systems and break down drugs very quickly. Still others have differing metabolisms or slightly different enzymatic makeups that alter their chemical reactions and the effects of a given drug. Predictable differences in the pharmacokinetics and pharmacodynamic effects of drugs can be anticipated with people of particular cultural backgrounds because of their genetic makeup. **Pharmacogenomics** is a new area of study that explores the unique differences in response to drugs that each individual possesses, based on genetic makeup. The mapping of the human genome has accelerated research in this area. It is thought that in the future, medical care and drug regimens could be personally designed, based on the person's own unique genetic makeup. Trastuzumab (*Herceptin*) (see Chapter 17, Immune Modulators) is a drug that was developed to treat breast cancer when the tumor expresses human epidermal growth factor receptor 2—a genetic defect seen in some tumors. The drug has no effect on tumors that do not express that genetic defect. This drug was developed as a personalized or targeted medicine, based on genetic factors. Such differences are highlighted throughout this book.

Immunological Factors

People can develop an allergy to a drug. After exposure to its proteins, a person can develop antibodies to a drug; with future exposure to the same drug, that person may experience a full-blown allergic reaction. Sensitivity to a drug can range from dermatological effects to anaphylaxis, shock, and death. (Drug allergies are discussed in detail in Chapter 3.)

Psychological Factors

The patient's attitude about a drug has been shown to have a real effect on how that drug works. A drug is more likely to be effective if the patient thinks it will work than if the patient believes it will not work. This is called the **placebo effect.**

The patient's personality also influences compliance with the drug regimen. Some people who believe that they can influence their health actively seek health care and willingly follow a prescribed regimen. These people usually trust the medical system and believe that their efforts will be positive. Other people do not trust the medical system; they may believe that they have no control over their own health and may be unwilling to comply with any prescribed therapy. Knowing a patient's health-seeking history and feelings about health care is important in planning an educational program that will work for that particular patient. It is also important to know this information when arranging for necessary follow-up procedures and evaluations.

As the caregiver most often involved in drug administration, the nurse is in a position to influence the patient's attitude about drug effectiveness. Frequently, the nurse's positive attitude, combined with additional comfort measures, can improve the patient's response to a medication.

Environmental Factors

The environment can affect the success of drug therapy. Some drug effects are helped by a quiet, cool, nonstimulating environment. For example, sedating drugs are given to help a patient relax or to decrease tension. Cutting down on external stimuli to decrease tension and stimulation will help the drug be more effective. Other drug effects may be influenced by temperature. For example, antihypertensives that are working well during cold, winter months may become too effective in warmer environments, when natural vasodilation to release heat tends to lower the blood pressure. If a patient's response to a medication is not as expected, the nurse might look for changes in environmental conditions.

Tolerance

Some drugs become tolerated by the body over time. Tolerance may come about because of increased biotransformation of the drug, increased resistance to its effects, or other pharmacokinetic factors. Drugs that are tolerated no longer cause the same reaction, and they need to be taken in increasingly larger doses to achieve a therapeutic effect. An example of this type of drug is morphine, an opiate used for pain relief. The longer morphine is taken, the more tolerant the body becomes to the drug, so that larger and larger doses are needed to relieve pain. Clinically, this situation can be avoided by giving the drug in smaller doses or in combination with other drugs that may also relieve pain. Cross-tolerance, or resistance to drugs within the same class, may also occur in some situations.

Cumulation

If a drug is taken in successive doses at intervals that are shorter than recommended, or if the body is not able to eliminate a drug properly, the drug can accumulate in the body, leading to toxic levels and adverse effects. This can be avoided by following the drug regimen precisely. In reality, with many people managing their own therapy at home, strict compliance with a drug regimen seldom occurs. Some people take all of their medications first thing in the morning, so that they won't forget to take the pills later in the day. Others realize that they forgot a dose and then take two to make up for it. Many interruptions of everyday life can interfere with strict adherence to a drug regimen. If a drug is causing serious adverse effects, review the drug regimen with the patient to find out how the drug is being taken, and then educate the patient appropriately.

Drug–Drug or Drug–Alternative Therapy Interactions

When two or more drugs are taken together, there is a possibility that the drugs will interact with each other to cause unanticipated effects in the body. Alternative therapies, such as herbal products, act as drugs in the body and can cause these same interactions. Usually this is an increase or decrease in the desired therapeutic effect of one or all of the drugs or an increase in adverse effects.

Clinically significant drug–drug interactions occur with drugs that have small margins of safety. If there is very little difference between a therapeutic dose and a toxic dose of the drug, interference with the drug's pharmacokinetics or pharmacodynamics can produce serious problems. For example, drug–drug interactions can occur in the following situations:

- *At the site of absorption:* One drug prevents or accelerates absorption of the other drug. For example, the antibiotic tetracycline is not absorbed from the GI tract if calcium or calcium products (milk) are present in the stomach.
- *During distribution:* One drug competes for the protein binding site of another drug, so the second drug cannot be transported to the reactive tissue. For example, aspirin competes with the drug methotrexate (*Rheumatrex*) for protein binding sites. Because aspirin is more competitive for the sites, the methotrexate is bumped off, resulting in increased release of methotrexate and increased toxicity to the tissues.
- *During biotransformation:* One drug stimulates or blocks the metabolism of the other drug. For example, warfarin (*Coumadin*), an oral anticoagulant, is biotransformed more quickly if it is taken at the same time as barbiturates, rifampin, or many other drugs. Because the warfarin is biotransformed to an inactive state more quickly, higher doses will be needed to achieve the desired effect.
- *During excretion:* One drug competes for excretion with the other drug, leading to accumulation and toxic effects of one of the drugs. For example, digoxin (*Lanoxin*) and quinidine (generic) are both excreted from the same sites in the kidney. If they are given together, the quinidine is more competitive for these sites and is excreted, resulting in increased serum levels of digoxin, which cannot be excreted.
- *At the site of action:* One drug may be an antagonist of the other drug or may cause effects that oppose those of the other drug, leading to no therapeutic effect. This is seen, for example, when an antihypertensive drug is taken with an allergy drug that also increases blood pressure. The effects on blood pressure are negated, and there is a loss of the antihypertensive effectiveness of the drug.

Whenever two or more drugs are being given together, the nurse should first consult a drug guide for a listing of clinically significant drug–drug interactions. Sometimes problems can be avoided by staggering the administration of the drugs or adjusting their dosages.

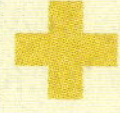

FOCUS ON PATIENT SAFETY

Check the monograph of any drug that is being given to monitor for clinically important drug–drug interactions.

Drug–Food Interactions

Certain foods can interact with drugs in much the same way that drugs can interact with each other. For the most part, this interaction occurs when the drug and the food are in direct contact in the stomach. Some foods increase acid production, speeding the breakdown of the drug molecule and preventing absorption and distribution of the drug. Some foods chemically react with certain drugs and prevent their absorption into the body. The antibiotic tetracycline cannot be taken with iron products for this reason. Tetracycline also binds with calcium to some extent and should not be taken with foods or other drugs containing calcium.

As stated earlier, oral drugs are best taken on an empty stomach. If the patient cannot tolerate the drug on an empty stomach, the food selected to be taken with the drug should be something that is known not to interact with it. Drug monographs usually list important drug–food interactions and give guidelines to avoid problems and optimize the drug's therapeutic effects.

Drug–Laboratory Test Interactions

As explained previously, the body works through a series of chemical reactions. Because of this, administration of a particular drug may alter results of tests that are done on various chemical levels or reactions as part of a diagnostic study. This drug–laboratory test interaction is caused by the drug being given and not necessarily by a change in the body's responses or actions. It is important to keep these interactions in mind when evaluating a patient's diagnostic tests. If one test result is off and does not fit in with the clinical picture or other test results, consider the possibility of a drug–laboratory test interference. For example, dalteparin (*Fragmin*), a low-molecular-weight heparin used to prevent deep vein thrombosis after abdominal surgery, may cause increased levels of the liver enzymes aspartate aminotransferase (AST) and alanine aminotransferase (ALT) with no injury to liver cells or hepatitis.

Achieving the Optimal Therapeutic Effect

As overwhelming as all of this information may seem, most patients can follow a drug regimen to achieve optimal therapeutic effects without serious adverse effects. Avoiding problems is the best way to treat adverse or ineffective drug effects. The nurse should incorporate basic history and physical assessment factors into any care plan, so that obvious problems can be spotted and handled promptly. If a drug just does not do what it is expected to do, the nurse should further examine the factors that are known to influence drug effects (see Box 2.2). Frequently, the drug regimen can be modified to deal with that influence. Rarely is it necessary to completely stop a needed drug regimen because of adverse or intolerable effects. And in many cases, the nurse is the caregiver in the best position to assess problems early.

Points to Remember

- Pharmacodynamics is the study of the way that drugs affect the body.
- Most drugs work by replacing natural chemicals, by stimulating normal cell activity, or by depressing normal cell activity.
- Chemotherapeutic agents work by interfering with normal cell functioning, causing cell death. The most desirable chemotherapeutic agents are those with selective toxicity to foreign cells and foreign cell activities.
- Drugs frequently act at specific receptor sites on cell membranes to stimulate enzyme systems within the cell and to alter the cell's activities.
- Pharmacokinetics, the study of the way the body deals with drugs, includes absorption, distribution, biotransformation, and excretion of drugs.
- The goal of established dosing schedules is to achieve a critical concentration of the drug in the body. This critical concentration is the amount of the drug necessary to achieve the drug's therapeutic effects.
- Arriving at a critical concentration involves a dynamic equilibrium among the processes of drug absorption, distribution, metabolism or biotransformation, and excretion.
- Absorption involves moving a drug into the body for circulation. Oral drugs are absorbed from the small intestine, undergo many changes, and are affected by many things in the process. IV drugs are injected directly into the circulation and do not need additional absorption.
- Drugs are distributed to various tissues throughout the body depending on their solubility and ionization. Most drugs are bound to plasma proteins for transport to reactive tissues.
- Drugs are metabolized or biotransformed into less toxic chemicals by various enzyme systems in the body. The liver is the primary site of drug metabolism or biotransformation. The liver uses the cytochrome P450 enzyme system to alter the drug and start its biotransformation.
- The first-pass effect is the breakdown of oral drugs in the liver immediately after absorption. Drugs given by other routes often reach reactive tissues before passing through the liver for biotransformation.
- Drug excretion is removal of the drug from the body. This occurs mainly through the kidneys.
- The half-life of a drug is the period of time it takes for an amount of drug in the body to decrease to one-half of the peak level it previously achieved. The half-life is affected by all aspects of pharmacokinetics. Knowing the half-life of a drug helps in predicting dosing schedules and duration of effects.
- The actual effects of a drug are determined by the pharmacokinetics, the pharmacodynamics, and many human factors that can change the drug's effectiveness.
- To provide the safest and most effective drug therapy, the nurse must consider all of the interacting aspects that influence drug concentration and effectiveness.

CHECK YOUR UNDERSTANDING

Answers to the questions in this chapter may be found in the Answer Key in the back of the book.

Multiple Choice

Select the best answer to the following.

1. Chemotherapeutic agents are drugs that
   a. are used only to treat cancers.
   b. replace normal body chemicals that are missing because of disease.
   c. interfere with the functioning of foreign cells, such as invading microorganisms or neoplasms.
   d. stimulate a cell's normal functioning.

2. Receptor sites
   a. are a normal part of enzyme substrates.
   b. are protein areas on cell membranes that react with specific chemicals to cause an effect within the cell.
   c. can usually be stimulated by many different chemicals.
   d. are responsible for all drug effects in the body.

3. Selective toxicity is
   a. the ability of a drug to seek out a specific bacterial species or microorganism.
   b. the ability of a drug to cause only specific adverse effects.
   c. the ability of a drug to cause fetal damage.
   d. the ability of a drug to attack only those systems found in foreign or abnormal cells.

4. The absorption of a drug taken orally can be affected by
   a. the blood flow to muscle beds.
   b. the acidity of the gastric juices, often influenced by the presence of food.
   c. the weight and age of the patient.
   d. the temperature of the peripheral environment.

5. Much of the biotransformation that occurs when a drug is taken occurs as part of
   a. the protein binding effect of the drug.
   b. the functioning of the renal system.
   c. the first-pass effect through the liver.
   d. the distribution of the drug to the reactive tissues.

6. The half-life of a drug
   a. is determined by a balance of all of the factors working on that drug—absorption, distribution, biotransformation, and excretion.
   b. is a constant factor for all drugs taken by a patient.
   c. is influenced by the fat distribution of the patient.
   d. can be calculated with the use of a body surface nomogram.

7. Jack B. has Parkinson's disease that has been controlled for several years with levodopa. After he begins a health food regimen with lots of vitamin B_6, his tremors return, and he develops a rapid heart rate, hypertension, and anxiety. The nurse investigating the problem discovers that vitamin B_6 can speed the conversion of levodopa to dopamine in the periphery, leading to these problems. The nurse would consider this problem:
   a. a drug–laboratory test interaction.
   b. a drug–drug interaction.
   c. a cumulation effect.
   d. a sensitivity reaction.

Multiple Response

Select all that apply.

1. When reviewing a drug to be given, the nurse notes that the drug is excreted in the urine. What points should be included in the nurse's assessment of the patient?
   a. The patient's liver function tests
   b. The patient's bladder tone
   c. The patient's renal function tests
   d. The patient's fluid intake
   e. Other drugs the patient might be taking that could affect the kidney
   f. The patient's intake and output for the day

2. When considering the pharmacokinetics of a drug, what points would the nurse take into consideration?
   a. How the drug will be absorbed
   b. The way the drug affects the body
   c. Receptor site activation and suppression
   d. How the drug will be excreted
   e. How the drug will be metabolized or biotransformed
   f. The half-life of the drug

3. Drug–drug interactions are important considerations in clinical practice. When evaluating a patient for potential drug–drug interactions, what will the nurse be considering?
   a. Bizarre drug effects on the body
   b. The need to adjust drug dosage or timing of administration to ensure effective drug therapy because of the actions of one drug on the other
   c. The need for more drugs in the drug regimen to balance the effects of the drugs being given
   d. A new therapeutic effect not encountered with either drug alone

e. Increased adverse effects because of the action of both drugs in the body
f. The use of herbal or alternative therapies, which could act to affect the pharmacokinetics or pharmacodynamics of the drugs being given

Word Scramble

Unscramble the following letters to form words related to pharmacotherapeutics.

1. tsrmafaomrtnioibo ____________________
2. sittriobnudi ____________________
3. cobplea ____________________
4. xncoriete ____________________
5. msacciotkeinprha ____________________
6. ptoercersstie ____________________
7. llffiahe ____________________
8. tchietruaepmeoch ____________________

Fill in the Blanks

1. ____________________ describes how drugs affect the body.
2. ____________________ describes how the body acts on drugs.
3. Drugs that interfere with the functioning of foreign cells, such as invading microorganisms or neoplasms, are called ____________________.
4. The amount of a drug that is needed to cause a therapeutic effect is called the ____________________.
5. The dynamic equilibrium that must be considered when administering a drug considers four main factors: ____________________, ____________________, ____________________, and ____________________.
6. Drugs taken orally are absorbed from the GI tract and delivered directly to the liver for metabolism. This phenomenon is called the ____________________.
7. The presence of a chemical that is metabolized by a particular enzyme system often increases the activity of that enzyme system. This process is referred to as ____________________.
8. The ____________________ of a drug is the time it takes for the amount of drug in the body to decrease to one-half of the peak level it previously achieved.

Bibliography and References

Batt, A. M., et al. (1994). Drug metabolizing enzymes related to laboratory medicine: Cytochrome P-450 and UDP glucuronosyltransferases. *Clinica Chimica Acta, 226,* 171–190.

DeMaagd, G. (1995). High-risk drugs in the elderly population. *Geriatric Nursing, 16*(5), 198–207.

Edwards, J. (1997). Guarding against adverse drug events. *American Journal of Nursing, 97*(5), 26–31.

Gilman, A., Hardman, J. G., & Limbird, L. E. (Eds.). (2006). *Goodman and Gilman's the pharmacological basis of therapeutics* (11th ed.). New York: McGraw-Hill.

Kelly, J. (1995). Pharmacodynamics and drug therapy. *Professional Nursing, 10*(12), 792–796.

The medical letter on drugs and therapeutics. (2006). New Rochelle, NY: Medical Letter.

O'Mahoney, M. S., & Woodhouse, K. W. (1994). Age, environmental factors and drug metabolism. *Pharmacology and Therapeutics, 61,* 279–287.

Pirmohamed, M., et al. (1996). The role of active metabolites in drug toxicity. *Drug Safety, 11,* 114–144.

Wetterberg, L. (1994). Light and biological rhythms. *Journal of Internal Medicine, 235,* 5–19.

Wissmann, J. (1996). Strategies for teaching critical thinking in pharmacology. *Nurse Educator, 21,* 42–46.

CHAPTER 3

Toxic Effects of Drugs

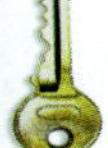

KEY TERMS

blood dyscrasia

dermatological reactions

drug allergy

hypersensitivity

poisoning

stomatitis

superinfections

LEARNING OBJECTIVES

Upon completion of this chapter, you will be able to:

1. Define the term adverse drug reaction and explain the clinical significance of this reaction.
2. List four types of allergic responses to drug therapy.
3. Discuss five common examples of drug-induced tissue damage.
4. Define the term poison.
5. Outline the important factors that should be considered in the application of the nursing process to selected situations of drug poisoning.

All drugs are potentially dangerous. Even though chemicals are carefully screened and tested in animals and in people before they are released as drugs, drug products often cause unexpected or unacceptable reactions when they are given. Drugs are chemicals, and the human body operates by a vast series of chemical reactions. Consequently, many effects can be seen when just one chemical factor is altered. Today's potent and amazing drugs can cause a great variety of reactions, many of which are more severe than ever seen before.

Adverse Effects

Adverse effects are undesired effects that may be unpleasant or even dangerous. They can occur for many reasons, including the following:

- The drug may have other effects on the body besides the therapeutic effect.
- The patient is sensitive to the drug being given.
- The drug's action on the body causes other responses that are undesirable or unpleasant.
- The patient is taking too much or too little of the drug, leading to adverse effects.

The nurse, as the caregiver who most frequently administers medications, must be constantly alert for signs of drug reactions of various types. Patients and their families need to be taught what to look for when patients are taking drugs at home. Some adverse effects can be countered with specific comfort measures or precautions. Knowing that these effects may occur and what actions can be taken to prevent or cope with them may be the most critical factor in helping the patient to comply with drug therapy (Box 3.1). Adverse drug effects can be of several types: primary actions, secondary actions, and hypersensitivity reactions.

BOX 3.1 Safety and the Nursing Process

Before administering any drug to a patient, it is important to review the contraindications and cautions associated with that drug, as well as the anticipated adverse effects of the drug. This information will direct your assessment of the patient, helping you to focus on particular signs and symptoms that would alert you to contraindications or to proceed cautiously, and to establish a baseline for that patient so that you will be able to identify adverse effects that occur. When teaching the patient about a drug, you should list the adverse effects that should be anticipated, along with the appropriate actions that the patient can take to alleviate any discomfort associated with these effects. Being alert to adverse effects—what to assess and how to intervene appropriately—can increase the effectiveness of a drug regimen, provide for patient safety, and improve patient compliance.

Primary Actions

One of the most common occurrences in drug therapy is the development of adverse effects from simple overdosage. In such cases, the patient suffers from effects that are merely an extension of the desired effect. For example, an anticoagulant may act so effectively that the patient experiences excessive and spontaneous bleeding. This type of adverse effect can be avoided by monitoring the patient carefully and adjusting the prescribed dose to fit that particular patient's needs.

In the same way, a patient taking an antihypertensive drug may become dizzy, weak, or faint when taking the "recommended dose" but will be able to adjust to the drug therapy with a reduced dose. These effects can be caused by individual response to the drug, high or low body weight, age, or underlying pathology that alters the effects of the drug.

Secondary Actions

Drugs can produce a wide variety of effects in addition to the desired pharmacological effect. Sometimes the drug dose can be adjusted so that the desired effect is achieved without producing undesired secondary reactions. But sometimes this is not possible, and the adverse effects are almost inevitable. In such cases, the patient needs to be informed that these effects may occur and counseled about ways to cope with the undesired effects. For example, many antihistamines are very effective in drying up secretions and helping breathing, but they also cause drowsiness. The patient who is taking antihistamines needs to know that driving a car or operating power tools or machinery should be avoided because the drowsiness could pose a serious problem.

Hypersensitivity

Some patients are excessively responsive to either the primary or the secondary effects of a drug. This is known as **hypersensitivity**, and it may result from a pathological or underlying condition. For example, many drugs are excreted through the kidneys; a patient who has kidney problems may not be able to excrete the drug and may accumulate the drug in the body, causing toxic effects.

Hypersensitivity also can occur if a patient has an underlying condition that makes the drug's effects especially unpleasant or dangerous. For example, a patient with an enlarged prostate who takes an anticholinergic drug may develop urinary retention or even bladder paralysis when the drug's effects block the urinary sphincters. This patient needs to be taught to empty the bladder before taking the drug. A reduced dosage also may be required to avoid potentially serious effects on the urinary system.

Drug Allergy

A **drug allergy** occurs when the body forms antibodies to a particular drug, causing an immune response when the person is re-exposed to the drug. A patient cannot be allergic to a drug that has never been taken, although patients can have cross-allergies to drugs within the same drug class as one formerly taken. Many people state that they have a drug allergy because of the effects of a drug. For example, one patient stated that she was allergic to the diuretic furosemide (*Lasix*). On further questioning, the nurse discovered that the patient was "allergic" to the drug because it made her urinate frequently—the desired drug effect, but one that the patient thought was a reaction to the drug. Patients who state that they have a drug "allergy" should be further questioned as to the nature of the allergy. Many patients do not receive needed treatment because the response to the drug is not understood.

Drug allergies fall into four main classifications: anaphylactic reactions, cytotoxic reactions, serum sickness, and delayed reactions (Table 3.1). The nurse, as the primary caregiver involved in administering drugs, must constantly assess for potential drug allergies and must be prepared to intervene appropriately.

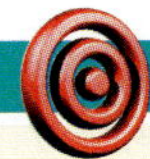

Focus Points

- All drugs have effects other than the desired therapeutic effect.
- Primary actions of the drug can be extensions of the desired effect.
- Secondary actions of the drug are effects that the drug causes in the body that are not related to the therapeutic effect.
- Hypersensitivity reactions to a drug are individual reactions that may be caused by increased sensitivity to the drug's therapeutic or adverse effects, or by drug allergy.

Drug-Induced Tissue and Organ Damage

Drugs can act directly or indirectly to cause many types of adverse effects in various tissues, structures, and organs (Figure 3.1). These drug effects account for many of the

Table 3.1 Focus on the Nursing Process: Types of Drug Allergies

Allergy Type	Assessment	Interventions
Anaphylactic Reaction This allergy involves an antibody that reacts with specific sites in the body to cause the release of chemicals, including histamine, that produce immediate reactions (mucous membrane swelling and constricting bronchi) that can lead to respiratory distress and even respiratory arrest.	Hives, rash, difficulty breathing, increased BP, dilated pupils, diaphoresis, "panic" feeling, increased heart rate, respiratory arrest	Administer epinephrine, 0.3 mL of a 1;1000 solution, Sub-Q for adults or 0.01 mg/kg of 1;1000 Sub-Q for pediatric patients. Massage the site to speed absorption rate. Repeat the dose every 15–20 minutes, as appropriate. Notify the prescriber and/or primary caregiver and discontinue the drug. Be aware that prevention is the best treatment. Counsel patients with known allergies to wear Medic-Alert identification and, if appropriate, to carry an emergency epinephrine kit.
Cytotoxic Reaction This allergy involves antibodies that circulate in the blood and attack antigens (the drug) on cell sites, causing death of that cell. This reaction is not immediate, but may be seen over a few days.	Complete blood count showing damage to blood-forming cells (decreased hematocrit, white blood cell count, and platelets); liver function tests show elevated liver enzymes; renal function test shows decreased renal function	Notify the prescriber and/or primary caregiver and discontinue the drug. Support the patient to prevent infection and conserve energy until the allergic response is over.
Serum Sickness Reaction This allergy involves antibodies that circulate in the blood and cause damage to various tissues by depositing in blood vessels. This reaction may occur up to a week or more after exposure to the drug.	Itchy rash, high fever, swollen lymph nodes, swollen and painful joints, edema of the face and limbs	Notify the prescriber and/or primary caregiver and discontinue the drug. Provide comfort measures to help the patient cope with the signs and symptoms (cool environment, skin care, positioning, ice to joints, administer antipyretics or anti-inflammatory agents, as appropriate).
Delayed Allergic Reaction This reaction occurs several hours after exposure and involves antibodies that are bound to specific white blood cells.	Rash, hives, swollen joints (similar to the reaction to poison ivy)	Notify the prescriber and/or primary caregiver and discontinue drug. Provide skin care and comfort measures that may include anti-histamines or topical corticosteroids.

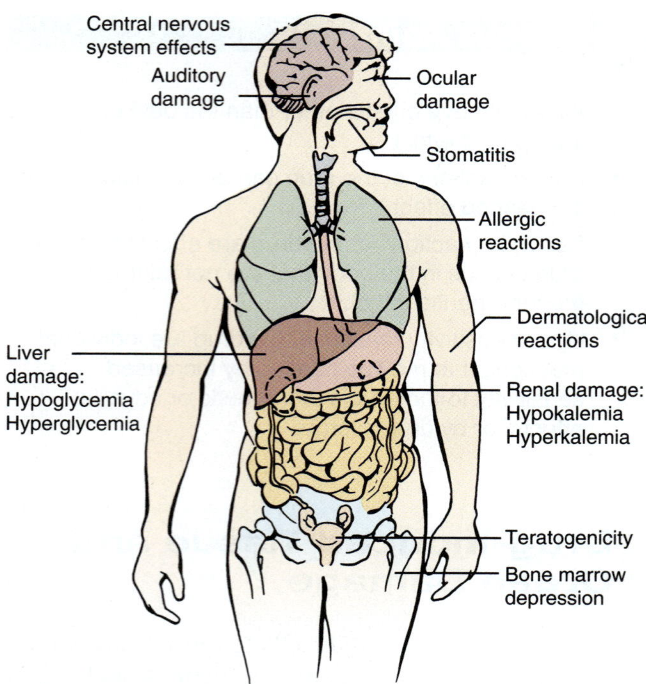

FIGURE 3.1 Variety of adverse effects and toxicities associated with drug use.

cautions that are noted before drug administration begins. The possible occurrence of these effects also accounts for the fact that the use of some drugs is contraindicated in patients with a particular history or underlying pathology. The specific contraindications and cautions for the administration of a given drug are noted with each drug type discussed in this book and in the individual monographs of various drug guides. These effects occur frequently enough that the nurse should be knowledgeable about the presentation of the drug-induced damage and about appropriate interventions that should be used if they occur.

Dermatological Reactions

Dermatological reactions are adverse reactions involving the skin. These can range from a simple rash to potentially fatal exfoliative dermatitis. Many adverse reactions involve the skin because many drugs can deposit there or cause direct irritation to the tissue.

Rashes, Hives

Procainamide (*Pronestyl*) is a drug used to treat cardiac arrhythmias. It causes a characteristic skin rash in many patients.

Assessment

Hives, rashes, and other dermatological lesions may be seen. Severe reactions may include exfoliative dermatitis, which is characterized by rash and scaling, fever, enlarged lymph nodes, enlarged liver, and the potentially fatal erythema multiforme exudativum (Stevens–Johnson syndrome), which is characterized by dark red papules appearing on the extremities with no pain or itching, often in rings or disk-shaped patches.

Interventions

In mild cases, or when the benefit of the drug outweighs the discomfort of the skin lesion, provide frequent skin care; instruct the patient to avoid rubbing, tight or rough clothing, and harsh soaps or perfumed lotions; and administer antihistamines, as appropriate. In severe cases, discontinue the drug and notify the prescriber and/or primary caregiver. Be aware that, in addition to these interventions, topical corticosteroids, antihistamines, and emollients are frequently used.

Stomatitis

Stomatitis, or inflammation of the mucous membranes, can occur because of a direct toxic reaction to the drug or because the drug deposits in the end capillaries in the mucous membranes, leading to inflammation. Fluorouracil (*Adrucil*), an antineoplastic agent, causes mouth sores or stomatitis in most of the patients who take it.

Assessment

Symptoms can include swollen gums, inflamed gums (gingivitis), and swollen and red tongue (glossitis). Other symptoms include difficulty swallowing, bad breath, and pain in the mouth and throat.

Interventions

Provide frequent mouth care with a nonirritating solution. Offer nutrition evaluation and development of a tolerated diet, which usually involves frequent, small meals. If necessary, arrange for a dental consultation. Note that antifungal agents and/or local anesthetics are sometimes used.

Superinfections

One of the body's protective mechanisms is the wide variety of bacteria that live within or on the surface of the body. This bacterial growth is called the *normal flora*. The normal flora protect the body from invasion by other bacteria, viruses, fungi, and so on. Several kinds of drugs (especially antibiotics) destroy the normal flora, leading to the development of **superinfections** or infections caused by the usually controlled organisms.

Assessment

Symptoms can include fever, diarrhea, black or hairy tongue, inflamed and swollen tongue (glossitis), mucous membrane lesions, and vaginal discharge with or without itching.

Interventions

Provide supportive measures (frequent mouth care, skin care, access to bathroom facilities, small and frequent meals).

Administer antifungal therapy as appropriate. In severe cases, discontinue the drug responsible for the superinfection.

Blood Dyscrasia

Blood dyscrasia is bone marrow suppression caused by drug effects. This occurs when drugs that can cause cell death (e.g., antineoplastics, antibiotics) are used. Bone marrow cells multiply rapidly; they are said to be rapidly turning over. Because they go through cell division and multiply so often, they are highly susceptible to any agent that disrupts cell function.

Assessment

Symptoms include fever, chills, sore throat, weakness, back pain, dark urine, decreased hematocrit (anemia), low platelet count (thrombocytopenia), low white blood cell count (leukopenia), and a reduction of all cellular elements of the complete blood count (pancytopenia).

Interventions

Monitor blood counts. Provide supportive measures (rest, protection from exposure to infections, protection from injury, avoidance of activities that might result in injury or bleeding). In severe cases, discontinue the drug or stop administration until the bone marrow recovers to a safe level.

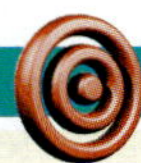

Focus Points

- Adverse drug effects can include skin irritation ranging from rashes and hives to potentially fatal Stevens–Johnson syndrome.
- Superinfections, or infection caused by normal flora bacteria; blood dyscrasias caused by bone marrow suppression of the blood-forming cells; and stomatitis or mucous membrane eruptions are common adverse drug effects.

Toxicity

Liver Injury

Oral drugs are absorbed and passed directly into the liver in the first-pass effect. This exposes the liver cells to the full impact of the drug before it is broken down for circulation throughout the body. Most drugs are metabolized in the liver, so any metabolites that are irritating or toxic will also affect liver integrity.

Assessment

Symptoms may include fever, malaise, nausea, vomiting, jaundice, change in color of urine or stools, abdominal pain or colic, elevated liver enzymes (e.g., aspartate aminotransferase [AST], alanine aminotransferase [ALT]), alterations in bilirubin levels, and changes in clotting factors (e.g., partial thromboplastin time).

Interventions

Discontinue the drug and notify the prescriber and/or primary caregiver. Offer supportive measures (small, frequent meals; skin care; cool environment; rest periods).

Renal Injury

The glomerulus in the kidney has a very small capillary network that filters the blood into the renal tubule. Some drug molecules are just the right size to get plugged into the capillary network, causing acute inflammation and severe renal problems. Some drugs are excreted from the kidney unchanged; they have the potential to directly irritate the renal tubule and alter normal absorption and secretion processes. Gentamicin (*Garamycin*), a potent antibiotic, is frequently associated with renal toxicity.

Assessment

Elevated blood urea nitrogen (BUN), elevated creatinine concentration, decreased hematocrit, electrolyte imbalances, fatigue, malaise, edema, irritability, and skin rash may be seen.

Interventions

Notify the prescriber and/or primary caregiver and discontinue the drug as needed. Offer supportive measures (e.g., positioning, diet and fluid restrictions, skin care, electrolyte therapy, rest periods, controlled environment). In severe cases, be aware that dialysis may be required for survival.

Poisoning

Poisoning occurs when an overdose of a drug damages multiple body systems, leading to the potential for fatal reactions. Assessment parameters vary with the particular drug. Treatment of drug poisoning also varies, depending on the drug. Throughout this book, specific antidotes or treatments to poisoning are identified, if known. Emergency and life support measures often are needed in severe cases.

Alterations in Glucose Metabolism

Hypoglycemia

Some drugs affect metabolism and the use of glucose, causing a low serum blood glucose concentration, or hypoglycemia. Glipizide (*Glucotrol*) and glyburide (*DiaBeta*) are antidiabetic agents that have the desired action of lowering the blood glucose level, but which can lower blood glucose too far, causing hypoglycemia.

Assessment

Symptoms may include fatigue; drowsiness; hunger; anxiety; headache; cold, clammy skin; shaking and lack of coordination (tremulousness); increased heart rate; increased blood pressure; numbness and tingling of the mouth, tongue, and/or lips; confusion; and rapid and shallow respirations. In severe cases, seizures and/or coma may occur.

Interventions

Restore glucose, intravenously (IV) or orally if possible. Provide supportive measures (e.g., skin care, environmental control of light and temperature, rest). Institute safety measures to prevent injury or falls. Offer reassurance to help the patient cope with the experience.

Hyperglycemia

Some drugs stimulate the breakdown of glycogen or alter metabolism in such a way as to cause high serum glucose levels, or hyperglycemia. Ephedrine (generic), a drug used as a bronchodilator and anti-asthma drug and to relieve nasal congestion, can break down stored glycogen and cause an elevation of blood glucose by its effects on the sympathetic nervous system.

Assessment

Fatigue, increased urination (polyuria), increased thirst (polydipsia), deep respirations (Kussmaul's respirations), restlessness, increased hunger (polyphagia), nausea, hot or flushed skin, and fruity odor to breath may be observed.

Interventions

Administer insulin therapy to decrease blood glucose as appropriate. Provide support to help the patient deal with signs and symptoms (e.g., access to bathroom facilities, controlled environment, reassurance, mouth care).

Electrolyte Imbalances

Hypokalemia

Some drugs affecting the kidney can cause low serum potassium levels (hypokalemia) by altering the renal exchange system. For example, loop diuretics function by causing the loss of potassium as well as sodium and water. Potassium is essential for the normal functioning of nerves and muscles.

Assessment

Symptoms include a serum potassium concentration ($[K^+]$) lower than 3.5 mEq/L, weakness, numbness and tingling in the extremities, muscle cramps, nausea, vomiting, diarrhea, decreased bowel sounds, irregular pulse, weak pulse, orthostatic hypotension, and disorientation. In severe cases, paralytic ileus (absent bowel sounds, abdominal distention, and acute abdomen) may occur.

Interventions

Replace serum potassium and carefully monitor serum levels and patient response. Provide supportive therapy (e.g., safety precautions to prevent injury or falls, orientation of the patient, comfort measures for pain and discomfort).

Hyperkalemia

Some drugs that affect the kidney, such as the potassium-sparing diuretics, can lead to potassium retention and a resultant increase in serum potassium levels (hyperkalemia). Other drugs that cause cell death or injury, such as many antineoplastic agents, also can cause the cells to release potassium, leading to hyperkalemia.

Assessment

Symptoms include a serum potassium level higher than 5.0 mEq/L, weakness, muscle cramps, diarrhea, numbness and tingling, slow heart rate, low blood pressure, decreased urine output, and difficulty breathing.

Interventions

Institute measures to decrease the serum potassium concentration, including use of sodium polystyrene sulfonate. Offer supportive measures to cope with discomfort. Institute safety measures to prevent injury or falls. Monitor cardiac effects and be prepared for cardiac emergency. In severe cases, be aware that dialysis may be needed.

Sensory Effects

Ocular Toxicity

The blood vessels in the retina are very tiny and are called "end arteries"; that is, they stop and do not interconnect with other arteries feeding the same cells. Some drugs are deposited into these tiny arteries, causing inflammation and tissue damage. Chloroquine (*Aralen*), a drug used to treat some rheumatoid diseases, can cause retinal damage and even blindness.

Assessment

Blurring of vision, color vision changes, corneal damage, and blindness may be observed.

Interventions

Monitor the patient's vision carefully when the patient is receiving known oculotoxic drugs. Consult with the prescriber and/or primary caregiver and discontinue the drug as appropriate. Provide supportive measures, especially if vision loss is not reversible. Monitor lighting and exposure to sunlight.

Auditory Damage

Tiny vessels and nerves in the eighth cranial nerve are easily irritated and damaged by certain drugs. The macrolide antibiotics can cause severe auditory nerve damage. Aspirin, one of the most commonly used drugs, is often linked to auditory ringing and eighth cranial nerve effects.

Assessment

Dizziness, ringing in the ears (tinnitus), loss of balance, and loss of hearing may be observed.

Interventions

Monitor the patient's perceptual losses or changes. Provide protective measures to prevent falling or injury. Consult with the prescriber to decrease dose or discontinue the drug. Provide supportive measures to cope with drug effects.

Neurologic Effects

General Central Nervous System Effects

Although the brain is fairly well protected from many drug effects by the blood–brain barrier, some drugs do affect neurologic functioning, either directly or by altering electrolyte or glucose levels. Beta-blockers, used to treat hypertension, angina, and many other conditions, can cause feelings of anxiety, insomnia, and nightmares.

Assessment

Symptoms may include confusion, delirium, insomnia, drowsiness, hyperreflexia or hyporeflexia, bizarre dreams, and hallucinations.

Interventions

Provide safety measures to prevent injury. Caution the patient to avoid dangerous situations such as driving a car or operating dangerous machinery. Orient the patient and provide support. Consult with the prescriber to decrease drug dose or discontinue the drug.

Atropine-like (Anticholinergic) Effects

Some drugs block the effects of the parasympathetic nervous system by directly or indirectly blocking cholinergic receptors. Atropine, a drug used to treat Parkinson's disease to dry up secretions before surgery, and for many other indications, is the prototype anticholinergic drug. Many cold remedies and antihistamines also cause anticholinergic effects.

Assessment

Dry mouth, altered taste perception, dysphagia, heartburn, constipation, bloating, paralytic ileus, urinary hesitancy and retention, impotence, blurred vision, cycloplegia, photophobia, headache, mental confusion, nasal congestion, palpitations, decreased sweating, and dry skin may be seen.

Interventions

Provide sugarless lozenges and mouth care to help mouth dryness. Arrange for bowel program as appropriate. Have the patient void before taking the drug, to aid voiding. Provide safety measures if vision changes occur. Arrange for medication for headache and nasal congestion as appropriate. Advise the patient to avoid hot environments and to take protective measures to prevent falling and to prevent dehydration, which may be caused by exposure to heat owing to decreased sweating.

Parkinson-like Syndrome

Drugs that directly or indirectly affect dopamine levels in the brain can cause a syndrome that resembles Parkinson's disease. Many of the antipsychotic and neuroleptic drugs can cause this effect. In most cases, the effects go away when the drug is withdrawn.

Assessment

Lack of activity, akinesia, muscular tremors, drooling, changes in gait, rigidity, extreme restlessness or "jitters" (akathisia), or spasms (dyskinesia) may be observed.

Interventions

Discontinue the drug, if necessary. Know that treatment with anticholinergics or antiparkinson drugs may be recommended if the benefit of the drug outweighs the discomfort of its adverse effects. Provide small, frequent meals if swallowing becomes difficult. Provide safety measures if ambulation becomes a problem.

Neuroleptic Malignant Syndrome

General anesthetics and other drugs that have direct central nervous system effects can cause neuroleptic malignant syndrome, a generalized syndrome that includes high fever.

Assessment

Extrapyramidal symptoms, hyperthermia, autonomic disturbances, and fever may be observed.

Interventions

Discontinue the drug, if necessary. Know that treatment with anticholinergics or antiparkinson drugs may be required. Provide supportive care to lower the body temperature. Institute safety precautions as needed.

Teratogenicity

Many drugs that reach the developing fetus or embryo can cause death or congenital defects, which can include skeletal and limb abnormalities, CNS alterations, heart defects, and the like. The exact effects of a drug on the fetus may not be known. In some cases, a predictable syndrome occurs when a drug is given to a pregnant woman. In any situation, a pregnant woman who is given a drug should be advised of the possible effects on the baby. Before a drug is administered to a pregnant patient, the actual benefits should be weighed against the potential risks. All pregnant women should be advised not to self-medicate during the pregnancy.

Interventions

Provide emotional and physical support for dealing with fetal death or birth defects.

Box 3.2 summarizes all of the adverse effects that have been described throughout this chapter.

Points to Remember

- No drug does only what is desired of it. All drugs have adverse effects associated with them.
- Adverse drug effects can range from allergic reactions to tissue and cellular damage. The nurse, as the health care provider most associated with drug administration, needs

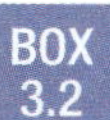

BOX 3.2 Summary of Adverse Drug Effects

- Extension of primary action
- Occurrence of secondary action
- Allergic reactions
  - Anaphylactic reactions
  - Cytotoxic reactions
  - Serum sickness reactions
  - Delayed allergic reactions
- Tissue and organ damage
  - Dermatological reactions
  - Stomatitis
  - Superinfections
  - Blood dyscrasia
- Toxicity
  - Liver injury
  - Renal injury
  - Poisoning
- Alterations in glucose metabolism
  - Hypoglycemia
  - Hyperglycemia
- Electrolyte imbalances
  - Hypokalemia
  - Hyperkalemia
- Sensory effects
  - Ocular toxicity
  - Auditory damage
- Neurological effects
  - General CNS effects
  - Atropine-like (cholinergic) effects
  - Parkinson-like syndrome
  - Neuroleptic malignant syndrome (NMS)
- Teratogenicity

to assess each situation for potential adverse effects and intervene appropriately to minimize those effects.

- Adverse effects can be extensions of the primary action of a drug or secondary effects that are not necessarily desirable but are unavoidable.
- Allergic reactions can occur when a person makes antibodies to a drug or drug protein. If the person is exposed to that drug another time, an immune response may occur. Allergic reactions can be of various types. The exact response should be noted to avoid future confusion in patient care.
- Tissue damage can include skin problems, mucous membrane inflammation, blood dyscrasia, super-infections, liver toxicity, hypoglycemia or hyperglycemia, renal toxicity, electrolyte disturbances, various central nervous system problems (ocular toxicity, auditory damage, atropine-like effects, Parkinson-like syndrome, neuroleptic malignant syndrome), teratogenicity, and overdose poisoning.

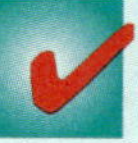

CHECK YOUR UNDERSTANDING

Answers to the questions in this chapter may be found in the Answer Key in the back of the book.

Multiple Choice

Select the best answer to the following.

1. An example of a drug allergy is
   a. dry mouth occurring with use of an antihistamine.
   b. increased urination occurring with use of a thiazide diuretic.
   c. hives and difficulty breathing after an injection of penicillin.
   d. skin rash associated with procainamide use.

2. A patient taking glyburide (an antidiabetic drug) has his morning dose and then does not have a chance to eat for several hours. An adverse effect that might be expected from this would be
   a. teratogenic effects.
   b. a skin rash.
   c. anticholinergic effects.
   d. hypoglycemia.

3. A patient with a severe infection is given gentamicin, the only antibiotic shown to be effective in culture and sensitivity tests. A few hours after the drug is started IV, the patient becomes very restless and develops edema. Blood tests reveal abnormal electrolytes and elevated BUN. This reaction was most likely caused by
   a. an anaphylactic reaction.
   b. renal toxicity associated with gentamicin.
   c. superinfection related to the antibiotic.
   d. hypoglycemia.

4. Patients receiving antineoplastic drugs that disrupt cell function often have adverse effects involving cells that turn over rapidly in the body. These cells include
   a. ovarian cells.
   b. liver cells.
   c. cardiac cells.
   d. bone marrow cells.

5. A woman has had repeated bouts of bronchitis throughout the fall and has been taking antibiotics. She calls the clinic with complaints of vaginal pain and itching. When she is seen, it is discovered that she has developed a yeast infection. You would explain to her that
   a. her bronchitis has moved to the vaginal area.
   b. the antibiotics kill bacteria, and bacteria normally live on your skin to protect you from various environmental organisms, including the yeast causing this infection. This is called a superinfection, and is commonly seen with some antibiotic use.

c. she probably has developed a sexually transmitted disease related to her lifestyle.
d. she will need to take even more antibiotics to treat this new infection.

6. Knowing that a patient is taking a loop diuretic and is at risk for developing hypokalemia, the nurse would assess the patient for
   a. hypertension, headache, and cold and clammy skin.
   b. decreased urinary output and yellowing of the sclera.
   c. weak pulse, low blood pressure, and muscle cramping.
   d. diarrhea and flatulence.

Multiple Response

Select all that apply.

1. A patient is taking a drug that is known to be toxic to the liver. The patient is being discharged to home. What teaching points related to liver toxicity of the drug should the nurse teach the patient to report to the physician?
   a. Fever; changes in the color of urine
   b. Changes in the color of stool; malaise
   c. Rapid, deep respirations; increased sweating
   d. Dizziness; drowsiness; dry mouth
   e. Rash, black or hairy tongue; white spots in the mouth or throat
   f. Yellowing of the skin or the whites of the eyes

2. Pregnant women should be advised of the potential risk to the fetus any time they take a drug during pregnancy. What fetal problems can be related to drug exposure in utero?
   a. Fetal death
   b. Nervous system disruption
   c. Skeletal and limb abnormalities
   d. Cardiac defects
   e. Low-set ears
   f. Deafness

3. A client is experiencing a reaction to the penicillin injection that the nurse administered approximately one-half hour ago. The nurse is concerned that it might be an anaphylactic reaction. What signs and symptoms would validate her suspicion?
   a. Rapid heart rate
   b. Diaphoresis
   c. Constricted pupils
   d. Hypotension
   e. Rash
   f. Client report of a panic feeling

4. A client is experiencing a serum sickness reaction to a recent rubella vaccination. Which of the following interventions would be appropriate when caring for this client?
   a. Administration of epinephrine
   b. Cool environment
   c. Positioning to provide comfort
   d. Ice to joints as needed
   e. Administration of anti-inflammatory agents
   f. Administration of topical corticosteroids

Matching

Match the adverse drug effect with the appropriate intervention.

1. ______________________ hypoglycemia
2. ______________________ hyperglycemia
3. ______________________ hypokalemia
4. ______________________ superinfection
5. ______________________ cholinergic effects
6. ______________________ Parkinson-like effects

A. Replace serum potassium and carefully monitor serum levels; provide supportive therapy (safety precautions to prevent injury or falls, orient patient, comfort measures for pain and discomfort).
B. Provide sugarless lozenges, mouth care to help mouth dryness. Arrange for bowel program; have the patient void before taking the drug; provide safety measures if vision changes occur.
C. Administer insulin therapy to decrease blood glucose as appropriate; provide support to help the patient deal with signs and symptoms (access to bathroom facilities, controlled environment, reassurance, mouth care).
D. Discontinue the drug, if necessary; treat with anticholinergics or antiparkinson drugs if recommended and if the benefit outweighs the discomfort of adverse effects; provide small, frequent meals if swallowing becomes difficult; provide safety measures.
E. Restore glucose intravenously (IV) or orally (PO), if possible; provide supportive measures (skin care, environmental control of light and temperature, rest). Institute safety measures to prevent injury or falls.
F. Provide supportive measures (frequent mouth care, skin care, access to bathroom facilities, small and frequent meals); administer antifungal therapy as appropriate.

Fill in the Blanks

1. Renal injury is a frequent adverse effect associated with ______________________________.

2. Glipizide and glyburide, antidiabetic agents, may cause ____________________, and the patient should be monitored for cool and clammy skin, rapid heart rate, increased blood pressure, and rapid and shallow respirations.

3. Retinal damage and even blindness have been associated with the antirheumatoid agent ____________________.

4. Dizziness, ringing in the ears, loss of balance, and impaired hearing can occur with aspirin therapy and are referred to as ____________________.

5. A common adverse effect associated with chemotherapy is ____________________, which can lead to increased bleeding, increased risk of infection, and fatigue.

6. Patients should be advised to avoid driving or operating machinery, and other safety precautions should be taken if the patient has central nervous system (CNS) effects such as ____________________.

Bibliography and References

Barditch-Crovo, P. (1995). Adverse reactions to therapy for HIV infections. *Emergency Medical Clinics of North America, 13,* 133–146.

Brody, T. M., et al. (1994). *Human pharmacology: Molecular to clinical* (2nd ed.). St. Louis: C. V. Mosby.

Drug facts and comparisons. (2006). St. Louis: Facts and Comparisons.

Food and Drug Administration. (1994). FDA launches MEDWATCH program: Monitoring adverse drug reactions. *NP News, 2,* 1, 4.

Gilman, A., Hardman, J. G., & Limbird, L. E. (Eds.). (2006). *Goodman and Gilman's the pharmacological basis of therapeutics* (11th ed.). New York: McGraw-Hill.

Karch, A. M. (2006). *2007 Lippincott's nursing drug guide.* Philadelphia: Lippincott Williams & Wilkins.

The medical letter on drugs and therapeutics. (2006). New Rochelle, NY: Medical Letter.

CHAPTER 4

Nursing Management

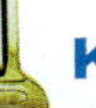

KEY TERMS

assessment
evaluation
intervention
nursing
nursing diagnosis
nursing process

LEARNING OBJECTIVES

Upon completion of this chapter, you will be able to:

1. List the responsibilities of the nurse in drug therapy.
2. Explain what is involved in each step of the nursing process as it relates to drug therapy.
3. Describe key points that must be incorporated into the assessment of a patient receiving drug therapy.
4. Describe the essential elements of a medication order.
5. Outline the important points that must be assessed and considered before administering a drug, combining knowledge about the drug with knowledge of the patient and the environment.

The delivery of medical care today is in a constant state of change and sometimes crisis. The population is aging, resulting in more chronic disease and more complex care issues. The population also is transient, resulting in unstable support systems and fewer at-home care providers and helpers. At the same time, medicine is undergoing a technological boom, including greater use of computed tomography (CT) scans, nuclear magnetic resonance imaging (MRI) scans, experimental drugs, and so on. Patients are being discharged earlier from acute care facilities, or they are not being admitted at all for procedures that used to be treated in-hospital with follow-up support and monitoring provided. Patients also are becoming more responsible for their own care and for adhering to complicated medical regimens at home.

Nursing: Art and Science

Nursing is a unique and complex science as well as a nurturing and caring art. In the traditional sense, nursing has been viewed as ministering to and soothing the sick. In the current state of medical changes, nursing also has become increasingly technical and scientific. Nurses have had to assume increasing responsibilities that involve not only nurturing and caring, but also assessing, diagnosing, and intervening with patients to treat, to prevent, and to educate in order to help patients cope with various health states.

The nurse deals with the whole person, including physical, emotional, intellectual, social, and spiritual aspects. The nurse needs to consider how a person responds to treatment, disease, and the changes in lifestyle that may be required. The nurse is the key health care provider who is in a position to assess the whole patient, to administer therapy as well as medications, to teach the patient how best to cope with the therapy so as to ensure the most favorable outcome, and to evaluate the effectiveness of the therapy. Being able to do this requires broad knowledge in the basic sciences (anatomy, physiology, nutrition, chemistry, pharmacology), the social sciences (sociology, psychology), education, and many other disciplines.

The Nursing Process

Although not all nursing theorists completely agree on the process that defines the practice of nursing, most do include certain key elements in the **nursing process**. These elements are the basic components of the decision-making or problem-solving process:

- **Assessment** (gathering information)
- **Nursing diagnosis** (analyzing the information gathered to arrive at some conclusions)
- **Interventions** (actions undertaken to meet the patient's needs, such as administration of drugs, education, and comfort measures)
- **Evaluation** (determining the effects of the interventions that were performed)

In general, the nursing process provides an effective method for handling all of the scientific and technical information, as well as the unique emotional, social, and physical factors that each patient brings to a given situation. With respect to drug therapy, use of the nursing process ensures that the patient receives the best, most efficient, scientifically based, holistic care. Box 4.1 outlines the steps of the nursing process, which are discussed in detail in the following paragraphs.

Assessment

The first step of the nursing process is the systematic, organized collection of data about the patient. Because the nurse is responsible for holistic care, these data must include information about physical, intellectual, emotional, social, and environmental factors. These data provide the nurse with the facts needed to plan educational and discharge programs, arrange for appropriate consultations, and monitor the physical response to treatment or to disease.

In clinical practice, the process of assessment never ends. The patient is not in a steady state, but rather a dynamic state, adjusting to physical, emotional, and environmental influences. Each nurse develops a unique approach to the organization of the assessment, an approach that is functional and useful in the clinical setting and that makes sense to that nurse and in the particular clinical situation.

Drug therapy is a complex and important part of health care, and the principles of drug therapy should be incorporated into every patient assessment plan. The particular information that is needed varies with each drug, but the concepts involved are similar. Two key areas that need to be assessed are the patient's history (past illnesses and the current problem) and his or her physical status.

History

The patient's past experiences and illnesses can influence a drug's effect.

Chronic Conditions

Certain conditions (e.g., renal disease, heart disease, diabetes, chronic lung disease) may be contraindications to the use of a drug. Or these conditions may require that caution be used when administering a certain drug or that the drug dosage be adjusted.

Drug Use

Prescription drugs, over-the-counter (OTC) drugs, street drugs, alcohol, nicotine, alternative therapies, and caffeine may have an impact on a drug's effect. Patients often neglect to mention OTC drugs or alternative therapies, not considering them to be actual drugs or not willing to admit their use to the health care provider. Patients should be asked specifically about OTC drug or alternative therapy use. Patients also

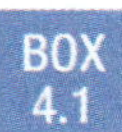

BOX 4.1 The Steps of the Nursing Process

Nursing Process

↓

Assessment

Past history
- Chronic conditions
- Drug use
- Allergies
- Level of education
- Level of understanding of disease and therapy
- Social supports
- Financial supports
- Pattern of health care

Physical assessment
- Weight
- Age
- Physical parameters related to the disease state or known drug effects

↓

Nursing Diagnosis

↓

Interventions

Proper drug administration
- Drug
- Storage
- Route
- Dosage
- Preparation
- Timing
- Recording

Comfort measures
- Placebo effect
- Managing side effects
- Lifestyle adjustments

Patient/family education

↓

Evaluation

Assessment
Nursing diagnosis
Interventions
Evaluation

The continual, dynamic nature of the nursing process.

might forget to mention prescription drugs that they take all the time, for instance oral contraceptives, because it is just routine and they don't think about it. It is a good idea to specifically ask about all types of medications that the patient might use.

Allergies

Past exposure to a drug or other allergens can provoke a future reaction or provide a caution for the use of a drug, food, or animal product. It is important to describe the particular allergic reaction when noting a drug allergy. In some cases, the reaction is not an allergic response but an actual drug effect.

Level of Education

This information helps the nurse determine the level of explanation required and provides a basis for developing patient education programs.

Level of Understanding of Disease and Therapy

This information also helps the development of educational information.

Social Supports

Patients are being discharged earlier than ever before, and often they need help at home with care and drug therapy. A key aspect of discharge planning involves determining what support, if any, is available to the patient at home. In many situations, it also involves referral to appropriate community resources.

Financial Supports

The high cost of health care in general, and of medications in particular, should be considered when initiating drug therapy. In some situations, a less expensive drug might be considered in place of a very expensive drug. Because of financial constraints, a patient may not follow through with a prescribed drug regimen. In such cases, the nurse may refer the patient to appropriate resources that might offer financial assistance.

Pattern of Health Care

Knowing how a patient seeks health care gives the nurse valuable information to include in the educational plan. Does this patient routinely seek follow-up care, or does he or she wait for emergency situations? Does the patient tend to self-treat many complaints, or is every problem brought to a health care provider?

Physical Assessment

Weight

A patient's weight helps determine whether the recommended drug dosage is appropriate. Because the recommended dosage typically is based on a 150-pound adult male, patients who are much lighter or much heavier need a dosage adjustment.

Age

Patients at the extremes of the age spectrum—children and older adults—often require dosage adjustments based on the functional level of the liver and kidneys and the responsiveness of other organs.

Physical Parameters Related to Disease or Drug Effects

Assessing these factors before drug therapy begins provides a baseline level to which future assessments can be compared to determine the effects of drug therapy. The specific parameters that need to be assessed depend on the disease process being treated and on the expected therapeutic and adverse effects of the drug therapy. For example, if a patient is being treated for chronic pulmonary disease, the respiratory status and reserve need to be assessed, especially if a drug is being given that has known effects on the respiratory tract. In contrast, a thorough respiratory evaluation would not be warranted in a patient with no known pulmonary disease who is taking a drug with no known effects on the respiratory system. Because the nurse has the greatest direct and continual contact with the patient, the nurse has the best opportunity to detect minute changes that ultimately determine the course of drug therapy—therapeutic success or discontinuation because of adverse or unacceptable responses.

NOTE: Review the monographs in a drug guide or handbook for specific parameters to be assessed in relation to the particular drug being discussed. This assessment provides not only the baseline information needed before giving that drug, but also the data required to evaluate the effects of that drug on the patient. This information should supplement the overall nursing assessment of the patient, which includes social, intellectual, financial, environmental, and other physical data.

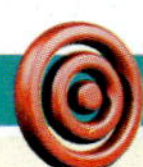

FOCUS POINTS

- Nurses use the nursing process to provide a framework for organizing the information that is needed to provide safe and effective patient care.
- The nursing process involves assessment, nursing diagnosis, interventions, and evaluation.
- The steps of the nursing process are constantly being repeated to meet the ever-changing needs of the patient.

Nursing Diagnosis

Once data have been collected, the nurse must organize and analyze that information to arrive at a nursing diagnosis. A nursing diagnosis is simply a statement of the patient's status from a nursing perspective. This statement directs appropriate nursing interventions. A nursing diagnosis shows actual or potential alterations in patient function based on the assessment of the clinical situation. Because drug therapy is only a small part of the overall patient situation, nursing diagnoses that are related to drug therapy must be incorporated into a total picture of the patient.

In the nursing considerations sections of this book, the nursing diagnoses listed are those that reflect potential alteration of function based only on the particular drug's actions (i.e., therapeutic and adverse effects). No consideration is given to environmental or disease-related problems. These diagnoses, culled from the North American Nursing Diagnosis Association (NANDA) list of accepted nursing diagnoses, are only a part of the overall nursing diagnoses related to the patient's situation. See Box 4.2 for a list of the accepted NANDA nursing diagnoses.

Interventions (Implementation)

The assessment and diagnosis of the patient situation direct the implementation of specific nursing interventions. Three types of interventions are frequently involved in drug therapy: drug administration, provision of comfort measures, and patient/family education.

WATCH & LEARN

Proper Drug Administration

There are seven points to consider in the safe and effective administration of a drug:

1. *Drug:* Know that it is standard nursing practice to ensure that the drug being administered is the correct dose and the correct drug, and that it is being given at the correct time and to the correct patient.
2. *Storage:* Be aware that some drugs require specific storage environments (e.g., refrigeration, protection from light).
3. *Route:* Determine the best route of administration; this is frequently established by the formulation of the drug. Nurses can often have an impact in modifying the route to arrive at the most efficient, comfortable method for the patient based on the patient's specific situation. When establishing the prescribed route, check the proper method of administering a drug by that route.

   CONCEPTS in action ANIMATION
4. *Dosage:* Calculate the drug dosage appropriately, based on the available drug form, the patient's body weight or surface area, or the patient's kidney function.
5. *Preparation:* Know the specific preparation required before administering any drug. For example, oral drugs may need to be shaken or crushed; parenteral drugs may need to be reconstituted or diluted with specific solutions; and topical drugs may require specific handling, such as the use of gloves during administration or shaving of a body area before application.
6. *Timing:* Recognize that the administration of one drug may require coordination with the administration of other drugs, foods, or physical parameters. As the caregiver

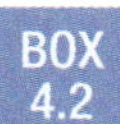

BOX 4.2

NANDA-Approved Nursing Diagnoses

The North American Nursing Diagnosis Association (NANDA) endorsed its first nursing diagnosis taxonomic structure, NANDA Taxonomy I, in 1986. This taxonomy has been revised and updated several times. The new Taxonomy II has a code structure that is compliant with recommendations from the National Library of Medicine concerning health care terminology codes. The taxonomy that appears here represents the currently accepted classification system for nursing diagnosis (2005).

Imbalanced nutrition: More than body requirements
Imbalanced nutrition: Less than body requirements
Risk for imbalanced nutrition: More than body requirements
Risk for infection
Risk for imbalanced body temperature
Hypothermia
Hyperthermia
Ineffective thermoregulation
Autonomic dysreflexia
Risk for autonomic dysreflexia
Constipation
Perceived constipation
Diarrhea
Bowel incontinence
Risk for constipation
Impaired urinary elimination
Stress urinary incontinence
Reflex urinary incontinence
Urge urinary incontinence
Functional urinary incontinence
Total urinary incontinence
Risk for urge urinary incontinence
Urinary retention
Decreased intracranial adaptive capacity
Disturbed energy field
Impaired verbal communication
Impaired social interaction
Social isolation
Risk for loneliness
Ineffective role performance
Impaired parenting
Risk for impaired parenting
Risk for impaired parent/infant/child attachment
Sexual dysfunction
Interrupted family processes
Caregiver role strain
Risk for caregiver role strain
Dysfunctional family processes: Alcoholism
Parental role conflict
Ineffective sexuality patterns
Spiritual distress
Risk for spiritual distress
Readiness for enhanced spiritual well-being
Ineffective coping
Impaired adjustment
Defensive coping
Ineffective denial
Disabled family coping
Compromised family coping
Readiness for enhanced family coping
Readiness for enhanced community coping
Ineffective community coping
Ineffective therapeutic regimen management
Noncompliance (specify)
Ineffective family therapeutic regimen management
Ineffective community therapeutic regimen management
Disorganized infant behavior
Readiness for enhanced organized infant behavior
Disturbed body image
Chronic low self-esteem
Situational low self-esteem
Disturbed personal identity
Disturbed sensory perception (specify: visual, auditory, kinesthetic, gustatory, tactile, olfactory)
Unilateral neglect
Hopelessness
Powerlessness
Deficient knowledge (specify)
Impaired environmental interpretation syndrome
Acute confusion
Chronic confusion
Disturbed thought processes
Impaired memory
Acute pain
Chronic pain
Nausea
Dysfunctional grieving
Anticipatory grieving
Chronic sorrow
Risk for other-directed violence
Risk for self-mutilation
Risk for self-directed violence
Posttrauma syndrome
Rape-trauma syndrome
Rape-trauma syndrome: Compound reaction
Rape-trauma syndrome: Silent reaction
Risk for posttrauma syndrome
Anxiety
Death anxiety
Ineffective tissue perfusion (specify type: renal, cerebral, cardiopulmonary, gastrointestinal, peripheral)
Risk for imbalanced fluid volume
Excess fluid volume
Deficient fluid volume
Risk for deficient fluid volume
Decreased cardiac output
Impaired gas exchange
Ineffective airway clearance
Ineffective breathing pattern
Impaired spontaneous ventilation
Dysfunctional ventilatory weaning response
Risk for injury

(continued)

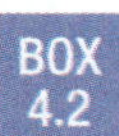

BOX 4.2 NANDA-Approved Nursing Diagnoses *(Continued)*

Risk for suffocation
Risk for poisoning
Risk for trauma
Risk for aspiration
Risk for disuse syndrome
Latex allergy response
Risk for latex allergy response
Ineffective protection
Impaired tissue integrity
Impaired oral mucous membrane
Impaired skin integrity
Risk for impaired skin integrity
Impaired dentition
Effective therapeutic regimen management
Decisional conflict (specify)
Health-seeking behaviors (specify)
Impaired physical mobility
Risk for peripheral neurovascular dysfunction
Risk for perioperative-positioning injury
Impaired walking
Impaired wheelchair mobility
Impaired transfer ability
Impaired bed mobility
Activity intolerance
Fatigue
Risk for activity intolerance
Disturbed sleep pattern
Sleep deprivation
Deficient diversional activity
Impaired home maintenance
Ineffective health maintenance
Delayed surgical recovery
Adult failure to thrive
Feeding self-care deficit
Impaired swallowing
Ineffective breast-feeding
Interrupted breast-feeding
Effective breast-feeding
Ineffective infant feeding pattern
Bathing or hygiene self-care deficit
Dressing or grooming self-care deficit
Toileting self-care deficit
Delayed growth and development
Risk for delayed development
Risk for disproportionate growth
Relocation stress syndrome
Risk for disorganized infant behavior
Fear
Risk for relocation stress syndrome
Risk for suicide
Self-mutilation
Risk for powerlessness
Risk for situational low self-esteem
Wandering
Risk for falls
Risk for sudden infant death syndrome
Readiness for enhanced communication
Readiness for enhanced coping
Readiness for enhanced family processes
Readiness for enhanced fluid balance
Readiness for enhanced knowledge (specify)
Readiness for enhanced management of therapeutic regimen
Readiness for enhanced nutrition
Readiness for enhanced parenting
Readiness for enhanced sleep
Readiness for enhanced urinary elimination
Readiness for enhanced self-concept

most frequently involved in administering drugs, the nurse must be aware of and juggle all of these factors, as well as educate the patient to do this on his or her own.

7. *Recording:* After assessing the patient, making the appropriate nursing diagnoses, and delivering the correct drug, by the correct route, in the correct dose, and at the correct time, the nurse should document that information in accordance with the local requirements for recording medication administration. Box 4.3 summarizes points to consider for proper drug administration.

Comfort Measures

Nurses are in a unique position to help the patient cope with the effects of drug therapy.

Placebo Effect

The anticipation that a drug will be helpful (placebo effect) has proved to have tremendous impact on the actual success of drug therapy. Therefore, the nurse's attitude and support can be a critical part of drug therapy; a back rub, a kind word, and a positive approach may be as beneficial as the drug itself.

Managing Adverse Effects

Interventions can be directed at decreasing the impact of the anticipated adverse effects of a drug and promoting patient safety. Such interventions include environmental control

BOX 4.3 Focus on Proper Drug Administration

Correct drug and patient
Correct storage of drug
Correct and most effective route
Correct dosage
Correct preparation
Correct timing
Correct recording of administration

(e.g., temperature, light), safety measures (e.g., avoiding driving, avoiding the sun, using side rails), and physical comfort (e.g., skin care, laxatives, frequent meals).

Lifestyle Adjustment

Some drug effects require that a patient change his or her lifestyle to cope effectively. For example, patients taking diuretics may have to rearrange their day so as to be near toilet facilities when the drug works. Patients taking monoamine oxidase inhibitors (MAOIs) must adjust their diet to prevent serious adverse effects from interaction of the drug with certain foods. In some cases the change in lifestyle that is needed can have a tremendous impact on the patient and can affect coping and compliance with any medical regimen.

NOTE: Special points regarding drug administration and related comfort measures are noted with each drug class discussed in this book. Refer to the individual drug monographs in a drug guide or handbook for more detailed interventions regarding a specific drug.

Patient and Family Education

With patients becoming increasingly responsible for their own care, it is essential that they have all of the information necessary to ensure safe and effective drug therapy at home. In fact, many states now require that patients be given written information. Key elements that should be included in any drug education program are the following:

1. *Name, dose, and action of drug:* Many patients see more than one health care provider; knowing this information is crucial to ensuring safe and effective drug therapy and avoiding drug–drug interactions.
2. *Timing of administration:* Teach patients when to take the drug with respect to frequency, other drugs, and meals.
3. *Special storage and preparation instructions:* Some drugs require particular handling procedures; inform patients how to carry out these requirements.
4. *Specific OTC drugs or alternative therapies to avoid:* Many patients do not consider OTC drugs or herbal or alternative therapies to be actual drugs and may inadvertently take them along with their prescribed medications, causing unwanted or even dangerous drug–drug interactions. Prevent these situations by explaining which drugs or therapies should be avoided.
5. *Special comfort or safety measures:* Teach patients how to cope with anticipated adverse effects to ease anxiety and avoid noncompliance with drug therapy. Also educate patients about the importance of follow-up tests or evaluation.
6. *Safety measures:* Instruct all patients to keep drugs out of the reach of children. Remind all patients to inform any health care provider they see about the drugs they are taking; this can prevent drug–drug interactions and misdiagnoses based on drug effects.
7. *Specific points about drug toxicity:* Give patients a list of warning signs of drug toxicity. Advise patients to notify their health care provider if any of these effects occur.
8. *Specific warnings about drug discontinuation:* Some drugs with a small margin of safety and drugs with particular systemic effects cannot be stopped abruptly without dangerous effects. Alert patients who are taking these drugs to this problem and encourage them to call their health care provider immediately if they cannot take their medication for any reason (e.g., illness, financial constraints). Box 4.4 summarizes points to consider in patient/family education.

NOTE: Refer to the CD-ROM in the front of this book for teaching guides that can be used for patients in the actual clinical setting.

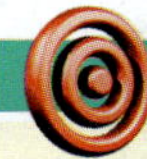

FOCUS POINTS

- Nursing diagnoses are made using the information gathered during the assessment phase of the nursing process. A nursing diagnosis states the actual or potential response of a patient to a clinical situation.
- Interventions include safe and effective drug administration, provisions of comfort measures to help the patient cope with the therapeutic or adverse effects of a drug, and patient and family education to ensure safe and effective drug therapy.

Evaluation

Evaluation is part of the continual process of patient care that leads to changes in assessment, diagnosis, and intervention. The patient is continually evaluated for therapeutic response, the occurrence of adverse drug effects, and the occurrence of drug–drug, drug–food, drug–alternative therapy, or drug–laboratory test interactions. The efficacy of the nursing interventions and the education program must be evaluated. In some situations, the nurse evaluates the patient simply by reapplying the beginning steps of the nursing process and analyzing for change. In some cases of drug therapy, specific therapeutic drug levels also need to be evaluated.

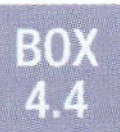

BOX 4.4 Focus on Patient/Family Education

Name, dose, and action of drug
Timing of administration
Special storage and preparation information
Special over-the-counter drugs and herbal or alternative therapies to avoid
Special comfort measures
Safety measures that need to be observed
Specific points about drug toxicity
Specific warnings to report to health care provider

Points to Remember

- Nursing is a complex art and science that provides for nurturing and care of the sick as well as prevention and education services.
- The nursing process is a problem-solving one, involving assessment, nursing diagnosis, interventions, and evaluation. It is an ongoing, dynamic process that provides safe and efficient care.
- Nursing assessment must include information on the history of past illnesses and the current complaint, as well as a physical examination; this provides a database of baseline information to ensure safe administration of a drug and to evaluate the drug's effectiveness and adverse effects.
- Nursing diagnoses use the data gathered during the assessment to determine actual or potential problems that require specific nursing interventions.
- Nursing interventions should include proper administration of a drug; comfort measures to help the patient cope with the drug effects; and patient and family education regarding the drug effects, ways to avoid adverse effects, warning signs to report, and any other specific information about the drug that will facilitate patient compliance.
- Evaluation is a continual process that assesses the situation and leads to new diagnoses or interventions as the patient reacts to the drug therapy.
- A nursing care guide and patient education materials can be prepared for each drug being given, using information about a drug's therapeutic effects, adverse effects, and special considerations.

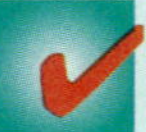

CHECK YOUR UNDERSTANDING

Answers to the questions in this chapter may be found in the Answer Key in the back of the book.

Multiple Choice

Select the best answer to the following.

1. A patient reports to you that she has a drug allergy. In exploring the allergic reaction with the patient, the following might indicate an allergic response:
   a. increased urination.
   b. dry mouth.
   c. rash.
   d. drowsiness.

2. It is important to obtain a medical history from a patient before beginning drug therapy because
   a. many medical conditions alter the pharmacokinetics and pharmacodynamics of a drug.
   b. it is part of the nursing protocol.
   c. a baseline is needed for evaluating drug effects.
   d. it is the first step in the nursing process.

3. A nursing diagnosis
   a. directs medical care.
   b. helps the patient become more compliant.
   c. shows actual or potential alteration in patient function.
   d. determines insurance reimbursement in most cases.

4. A patient receiving an antihistamine complains of dry mouth and nose. An appropriate comfort measure for this patient would be
   a. use of a humidifier and an increase in fluid consumption.
   b. voiding before taking the drug.
   c. avoiding exposure to the sun.
   d. a back rub.

5. When establishing the nursing interventions appropriate for a given patient
   a. the patient should not be actively involved.
   b. the family or other support systems should not be consulted.
   c. teaching is important only if the patient seems compliant.
   d. an evaluation of all of the data accumulated should be incorporated to achieve an effective care plan.

6. The evaluation step of the nursing process
   a. is often not necessary.
   b. is important only in the acute setting.
   c. is a continual process that redirects nursing interventions as needed.
   d. includes making nursing diagnoses.

7. A client has been through a teaching format for digoxin (generic), a drug used to increase the effectiveness of the heart's contractions. Which of the following statements would indicate that the teaching was effective?
   a. "I need to take my pulse every morning before I take my pill."
   b. "Sometimes I forget my pills, but I usually make up the missed ones once I remember."

c. "This pill might help my hay fever."
d. "I don't remember the name of it, but it is the white one."

Multiple Response

Select all that apply.

1. A client is being started on a laxative regimen. Before beginning the regimen, the nurse would perform which of the following assessments?
   a. Liver function test
   b. Abdominal examination
   c. Skin color and lesion evaluation
   d. Lung auscultation
   e. 24-hour urine
   f. Cardiac assessment

2. The nursing care of a patient receiving drug therapy should include measures to decrease the anticipated adverse effects of the drug. Which of the following measures would a nurse consider to decrease adverse effects?
   a. A positive approach
   b. Environmental temperature control
   c. Safety measures
   d. Skin care
   e. Refrigeration of the drug
   f. Involvement of the family

3. A nurse is preparing to administer a drug to a client for the first time. What questions should the nurse consider before actually administering the drug?
   a. Is this the right patient?
   b. Is this the right drug?
   c. Is there a generic drug available?
   d. Is this the right route for this patient?
   e. Is this the right dose, as ordered?
   f. Did I record this properly?

Complete the List

List the seven points to consider in the safe and effective administration of a drug.

1. ______________________________
2. ______________________________
3. ______________________________
4. ______________________________
5. ______________________________
6. ______________________________
7. ______________________________

Fill in the Blanks

1. The first step of the nursing process, which involves the systematic, organized collection of data about the patient, is called ______________.

2. The continual process that assesses the situation and leads to new diagnoses or interventions as the patient reacts to the drug therapy is called ______________.

3. ______________ use the data gathered during the assessment to determine actual or potential problems that require specific nursing interventions.

4. Inadvertent drug–drug interactions may occur when a patient does not report use of ______________ or ______________ when given a prescription drug.

5. Patients should always be told the name, action, and ______________ of each drug being taken.

6. A drug is known to cause dizziness. An important safety warning for the patient taking that drug would be ______________.

Bibliography and References

Bickley, L. (2005). *Bates' guide to physical examination and history taking* (9th ed.). Philadelphia: Lippincott Williams & Wilkins.

Buchanan, L. M. (1994). Therapeutic nursing intervention knowledge development and outcome measures for advanced practice. *Nursing and Health Care, 15*(4), 190–195.

Carpenito, L. J. (2005). *Handbook of nursing diagnoses* (11th ed.). Philadelphia: Lippincott Williams & Wilkins.

Carpenito, L. J. (2005). *Nursing care plans and documentation* (4th ed.). Philadelphia: Lippincott Williams & Wilkins.

Carpenito, L. J. (2005). *Nursing diagnosis: Application in clinical practice* (11th ed.). Philadelphia: Lippincott Williams & Wilkins.

Cohen, M. (1994). Medication errors . . . misprinted doses: FDA precautions. *Nursing, 94*(3), 14.

McCloskey, J., & Bulechek, G. (Eds.). (2000). *Nursing interventions classification* (3rd ed.). St. Louis: C. V. Mosby.

Redman, B. (1997). *The practice of patient education* (8th ed.). St. Louis: Mosby-Year Book.

CHAPTER 5

Dosage Calculations

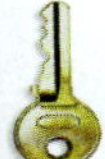

KEY TERMS

apothecary system
Clark's Rule
conversion
Fried's Rule
metric system
ratio and proportion
Young's Rule

LEARNING OBJECTIVES

Upon completion of this chapter, you will be able to:

1. Describe four measuring systems that can be used in drug therapy.
2. Convert between measuring systems when given drug orders and available forms of the drugs.
3. Calculate the correct dose of a drug when given examples of drug orders and available forms of the drugs ordered.
4. Discuss why children require different dosages of drugs than adults.
5. Explain the calculations used to determine a safe pediatric dose of a drug.

To determine the correct dose of a particular drug for a patient, one should take into consideration the patient's sex, weight, age, and physical condition, as well as the other drugs that the patient is taking. Frequently, the dose that is needed for a patient is not the dose that is available, and it is necessary to convert the dosage form available into the prescribed dosage. Doing the necessary mathematical calculations to determine what should be given is the responsibility of the prescriber who orders the drug, the pharmacist who dispenses the drug, and the nurse who administers the drug. This provides for a good set of checks on the dosage being given before the patient actually receives the drug. In many institutions, drugs arrive at the patient care area in unit-dose form, prepackaged for each individual patient. The nurse who will administer the drug may come to rely on the prepackaged unit-dose that is sent from the pharmacy and may not even recalculate or recheck the dose to match the order that was written. But mistakes still happen, and the nurse, as the person who is administering the drug, is legally and professionally responsible for any error that might occur. It is necessary for practicing nurses to know how to convert drug orders into available forms of a drug to ensure that the right patient is getting the right dose of a drug.

Measuring Systems

At least four different systems are currently used in drug preparation and delivery: the metric system, the apothecary system, the household system, and the avoirdupois system. With the growing number of drugs available and increasing awareness of medication errors that occur in daily practice, efforts have been made to decrease the dependence on so many different systems. In 1995, the United States Pharmacopeia Convention established standards requiring that all prescriptions, regardless of the system that was used in the drug dosage, include the metric measure for quantity and strength of drug. It was also established that drugs may be dispensed only in the metric form. Prescribers are not totally converted to this new standard, however, so the nurse must be able to convert what is ordered into the available form to ensure patient safety. It is important to be able to perform **conversions** within each system of measure and between systems of measure.

Metric System

The **metric system** is the most widely used system of measure. It is based on the decimal system, so all units are determined as multiples of 10. This system is used worldwide and makes the sharing of knowledge and research information possible. The metric system uses the gram as the basic unit of solid measure and the liter as the basic unit of liquid measure. Table 5.1 lists the standard units of the metric system.

Apothecary System

The **apothecary system** is a very old system of measure that was specifically developed for use by apothecaries or pharmacists. The apothecary system uses the minim as the basic unit of liquid measure and the grain as the basic unit of solid measure. This system is much harder to use than the metric system and is rarely seen in most clinical settings. Occasionally a prescriber will write an order in this system and the dosage will have to be converted to an available form. An interesting feature of this system is that it uses Roman numerals placed after the unit of measure to denote amount. For example, 15 grains would be written "gr xv." Table 5.1 lists the standard units of the apothecary system.

Household System

The household system is the measuring system that is found in recipe books. Many people are familiar with the teaspoon

Table 5.1 Comparing Basic Units of Measure by Measuring Systems

System	Solid Measure	Liquid Measure
Metric	gram (g) 1 milligram (mg) = 0.001 g 1 microgram (mcg) = 0.000001 g 1 kilogram (kg) = 1000 g	liter (L) 1 milliliter (mL) = 0.001 L 1 mL = 1 cubic centimeter = 1 cc
Apothecary	grain (gr) 60 gr = 1 dram (dr) 8 dr = 1 ounce (oz)	minim (min) 60 min = 1 fluidram (f dr) 8 f dr = 1 fluidounce (f oz)
Household	pound (lb) 1 lb = 16 ounces (oz)	pint (pt) 2 pt = 1 quart (qt) 4 qt = 1 gallon (gal) 16 oz = 1 pt = 2 cups (c) 32 tablespoons (tbsp) = 1 pt 3 teaspoons (tsp) = 1 tbsp 60 drops (gtt) = 1 tsp

and the cup as units of measure. This system uses the teaspoon as the basic unit of fluid measure and the pound as the basic unit of solid measure. Although efforts have been made in recent years to standardize these measuring devices, wide variations have been noted in the capacity of some of these units. Patients need to be advised that flatware teaspoons and drinking cups vary tremendously in the volume that they contain. A flatware teaspoon could hold up to two measuring teaspoons of quantity. When a patient is using a liquid medication at home, it is important to clarify that the measures indicated in the instructions refer to a standardized measuring device. Table 5.1 lists the standard units of the household system.

Avoirdupois System

The avoirdupois system is another older system that was very popular when pharmacists routinely had to compound medications on their own. This system uses ounces and grains, but they measure differently than those of the apothecary and household systems. The avoirdupois system is seldom used by prescribers but may be used for bulk medications that come directly from the manufacturer.

Other Systems

Some drugs are measured in units other than those already discussed. These measures may reflect chemical activity or biological equivalence. One of these measures is the unit. A unit usually reflects the biological activity of the drug in 1 mL of solution. The unit is unique for the drug it measures; a unit of heparin would not be comparable to a unit of insulin. Milliequivalents (mEq) are used to measure electrolytes (e.g., potassium, sodium, calcium, fluoride). The milliequivalent refers to the ionic activity of the drug in question; the order is usually written for a number of milliequivalents instead of a volume of drug. International units (IU) are sometimes used to measure certain vitamins or enzymes. These are also unique to each drug and cannot be converted to another measuring form.

Converting Between Systems

The simplest way to convert measurements from one system to another is to set up a **ratio and proportion** equation. The ratio containing two known equivalent amounts is placed on one side of an equation, and the ratio containing the amount you wish to convert and its unknown equivalent is placed on the other side. To do this, it is necessary to first check a table of conversions to determine the equivalent measure in the two systems you are using. Table 5.2 presents some accepted conversions between systems of measurement. It is a good idea to post a conversion guide in the medication room or on the medication cart for easy access. When conversions are used frequently, it is easy to remember them. When conversions are not used frequently, it is best to look them up.

Table 5.2 Commonly Accepted Conversions Between Systems of Measurement

Metric System	Apothecary System	Household System
Solid Measure		
1 kg		2.2 lb
454 g		1.0 lb
1 g = 1000 mg	15 gr (gr xv)	
60 mg	1 gr (gr i)	
30 mg	½ gr (gr ss)	
Liquid Measure		
1 L = 1000 mL		about 1 qt
240 mL	8 f oz (f oz viii)	1 c
30 mL	1 f oz (f oz i)	2 tbsp
15–16 mL	4 f dr (f dr iv)	1 tbsp = 3 tsp
8 mL	2 f dr (f dr ii)	2 tsp
4–5 mL	1 f dr (f dr i)	1 tsp = 60 gtt
1 mL	15–16 min (min xv or min xvi)	
0.06 mL	1 min (min i)	

Try the following conversion using Table 5.2. Convert 6 f oz (apothecary system) to the metric system of measure. According to Table 5.2, 1 f oz is equivalent to 30 mL. Use this information to set up a ratio:

$$\frac{1 \text{ f oz}}{30 \text{ mL}} = \frac{6 \text{ f oz}}{\text{X}}$$

The known ratio—1 f oz (apothecary system) is equivalent to 30 mL (metric system)—is on one side of the equation. The other side of the equation contains 6 f oz, the amount (apothecary system) that you want to convert, and its unknown (metric system) equivalent, X. Because the fluid ounce measurement is in the numerator (top number) on the left side of the equation, it must also be in the numerator on the right side of the equation. This equation would read as follows: One fluid ounce is to thirty milliliters as six fluid ounces is to how many milliliters?

The first step in the conversion is to cross-multiply (multiply the numerator from one side of the equation by the denominator from the other side, and vice versa):

$$\frac{1 \text{ f oz}}{30 \text{ mL}} = \frac{6 \text{ f oz}}{\text{X}}$$

$$1 \text{ f oz}(\times \text{X}) = 6 \text{ f oz} \times 30 \text{ mL}$$

This could also be written

$$(1 \text{ f oz})(X) = (6 \text{ f oz})(30 \text{ mL})$$

After multiplying the numbers, you have

$$1 \text{ (f oz)}X = 180 \text{ (f oz)(mL)}$$

Next, rearrange the terms to let the unknown quantity stand alone on one side of the equation:

$$X = \frac{180 \text{ (mL)(f oz)}}{1 \text{ f oz}}$$

Whenever possible, cancel out numbers as well as units of measure. In this example, canceling out leaves

$$X = 180 \text{ mL}$$

By canceling out, you are left with the appropriate amount and unit of measure. The answer to the problem is that 6 f oz is equivalent to 180 mL.

Try another conversion. Convert 32 gr (apothecary system) to its equivalent in the metric system, expressing the answer in milligrams. First, find the conversion on Table 5.2: 1 gr is equal to 60 mg. Set up the ratio:

$$\frac{1 \text{ gr}}{60 \text{ mg}} = \frac{32 \text{ gr}}{X}$$

Cross-multiply:

$$(1 \text{ gr})(X) = (32 \text{ gr})(60 \text{ mg})$$

$$1\text{(gr)}X = 1920 \text{ (gr)(mg)}$$

Rearrange:

$$X = \frac{1920 \text{ (gr)(mg)}}{1 \text{ gr}}$$

Finally, cancel out units and numbers:

$$X = 1920 \text{ mg}$$

Therefore, 32 gr is equivalent to 1920 mg.

Calculating Dosage

As mentioned earlier, because there are several systems of measurement available that might be used when ordering a drug and because drugs are made available only in certain forms or dosages, it may be necessary to calculate what the patient should be receiving when interpreting a drug order.

Oral Drugs

Frequently, tablets or capsules for oral administration are not available in the exact dose that has been ordered. In these situations, the nurse who is administering the drug must calculate the number of tablets or capsules that should be given to make up the ordered dose. The easiest way to determine this is once again to set up a ratio and proportion equation. The ratio containing the two known equivalent amounts is put on one side of the equation, and the ratio containing the unknown value is put on the other side. The known equivalent is the amount of drug available in one tablet or capsule; the unknown is the number of tablets or capsules that are needed for the prescribed dose:

$$\frac{\text{amount of drug available}}{\text{one tablet or capsule}} = \frac{\text{amount of drug prescribed}}{\text{number of tablets or capsules to give}}$$

The phrase "amount of drug" serves as the unit, so this information must be in the numerator of each ratio.

Try this example: An order is written for 10 grains of aspirin (gr x, aspirin). The tablets that are available each contain 5 grains. How many tablets should be given? First, set up the equation:

$$\frac{5 \text{ gr}}{1 \text{ tablet}} = \frac{10 \text{ gr}}{X}$$

Cross-multiply the ratio:

$$5 \text{ (gr)}X = 10 \text{ (gr)(tablet)}$$

Rearrange and cancel units and numbers:

$$X = \frac{10 \text{ (gr)(tablet)}}{5 \text{ (gr)}}$$

$$X = 2 \text{ tablets}$$

Try another example: An order is written for 0.05 g *Aldactone* to be given orally (PO). The *Aldactone* is available in 25-mg tablets. How many tablets would you have to give? First, you will need to convert the grams to milligrams.

$$\frac{1 \text{ g}}{1000 \text{ mg}} = \frac{0.05 \text{ g}}{X}$$

Cross-multiply:

$$1 \text{ (g)}X = (0.05 \times 1000)\text{(g)(mg)}$$

Simplify:

$$X = \frac{50 \text{ (g)(mg)}}{1\text{(g)}}$$

$$X = 50 \text{ mg}$$

The order has been converted to the same measurement as the available tablets. Now solve for the number of tablets that you will need, letting X be the desired dose.

$$\frac{25 \text{ mg}}{1 \text{ tablet}} = \frac{50 \text{ mg}}{X}$$

$$25 \text{ (mg)}X = (50 \times 1)\text{(mg)(tablet)}$$

$$X = \frac{50 \text{ (mg)(tablet)}}{25 \text{ (mg)}}$$

$$X = 2 \text{ tablets}$$

Sometimes the desired dose will be a fraction of a tablet or capsule, ½ or ¼. Some tablets come with score markings that allow them to be cut. Pill cutters are readily available in most pharmacies to help patients cut tablets appropriately. One must use caution when advising a patient to cut a tablet. Many tablets today come in a matrix system that allows for slow and steady release of the active drug. These drugs cannot be cut, crushed, or chewed. A drug reference should always be consulted before cutting a tablet. However, as a quick reference, any tablet that is designated as having delayed or sustained release may very well be one that cannot be cut. Capsules can be very difficult to divide precisely, and some of them also come with warnings that they cannot be cut, crushed, or chewed. If the only way to deliver the correct dose to a patient is by cutting one of these preparations, a different drug or a different approach to treating the patient should be tried.

Other oral drugs come in liquid preparations. Many of the drugs used in pediatrics and for adults who might have difficulty swallowing a pill or tablet are prepared in a liquid form. Some drugs that do not come in a standard liquid form can be prepared as a liquid by the pharmacist. If the patient is not able to swallow a tablet or capsule, check for other available forms and consult with the pharmacist about the possibility of preparing the drug in a liquid as a suspension or a solution. The same principle used to determine the number of tablets needed to arrive at a prescribed dose can be used to determine the volume of liquid that will be required to administer the prescribed dose. The ratio on the left of the equation shows the known equivalents, and the ratio on the right side contains the unknown. The phrase "amount of drug" must appear in the numerator of both ratios, and the volume to administer is the unknown (X).

$$\frac{\text{amount of drug available}}{\text{volume available}} = \frac{\text{amount of drug prescribed}}{\text{volume to administer}}$$

Try this example: An order has been written for 250 mg sulfisoxazole. The bottle states that the solution contains 125 mg/5 mL. How much of the liquid should you give?

$$\frac{125\text{ mg}}{5\text{ mL}} = \frac{250\text{ mg}}{\text{X}}$$

Cross-multiply:

$$125\ (\text{mg})\text{X} = (250 \times 5)(\text{mg})(\text{mL})$$

Simplify:

$$\text{X} = \frac{1250\ (\text{mg})(\text{mL})}{125\text{ mg}}$$

So the desired dose is

$$\text{X} = 10\text{ mL}$$

Even if you are working in an institution that provides unit-dose medications, practice your calculation skills occasionally to make sure that you can figure out the dose of a drug to give. Power can be lost, computers can go down, and the ability to determine conversions is a skill that anyone who administers drugs should have in reserve. Periodically throughout this text you will find a "Focus on Calculations" box to help you refresh your dosage calculation skills as they apply to the drugs being discussed.

Parenteral Drugs

All drugs administered parenterally must be administered in liquid form. The person administering the drug needs to calculate the volume of the liquid that must be given to administer the prescribed dose. The same formula can be used for this determination that was used for determining the dose of an oral liquid drug:

$$\frac{\text{amount of drug available}}{\text{volume available}} = \frac{\text{amount of drug prescribed}}{\text{volume to administer}}$$

Try this example: An order has been written for 75 mg meperidine to be given intramuscularly (IM). The vial states that it contains meperidine, 1.0 mL = 50.0 mg. Set up the equation just as before:

$$\frac{50\text{ mg}}{1\text{ mL}} = \frac{75\text{ mg}}{\text{X}}$$

$$50\ (\text{mg})\text{X} = (75 \times 1)(\text{mg})(\text{mL})$$

$$\text{X} = \frac{75\ (\text{mg})(\text{mL})}{50\ (\text{mg})}$$

$$\text{X} = 1.5\text{ mL}$$

Intravenous Solutions

Intravenous (IV) solutions are used to deliver a prescribed amount of fluid, electrolytes, vitamins, nutrients, or drugs directly into the bloodstream. Although most institutions now use electronically monitored delivery systems, it is still important to be able to determine the amount of an IV solution that should be given using standard calculations. Most IV delivery systems come with a standard control called a microdrip, by which each milliliter delivered contains 60 drops. Macrodrip systems, which deliver 15 drops/mL, are also available; they are usually used when a large volume must be delivered quickly. In giving IV drugs, the microdrip system is most commonly encountered. Check the packaging of the IV tubing if you have any doubts or are unfamiliar with the packaging. The ratio that is used to determine how many drops of fluid to administer per minute is the following:

$$\text{drops/minute} = \frac{\text{mL of solution prescribed per hour} \times \text{drops delivered per mL}}{60\text{ minutes/1 hour}}$$

That is, the number of drops per minute, or the rate that you will set by adjusting the valve on the IV tubing, is equal to the amount of solution that has been prescribed per hour times the number of drops delivered per milliliter (mL) divided by 60 minutes in an hour.

Try this example: An order has been written for a patient to receive 400 mL of 5% dextrose in water (D5W) over a period of 4 hours in a standard microdrip system (i.e., 60 drops/mL). Calculate the correct setting (drops per minute).

$$X = \frac{400\ \text{mL}/4\ \text{h} \times 60\ \text{drops/mL}}{60\ \text{min/h}}$$

Simplify:

$$X = \frac{100\ \text{mL/h} \times 60\ \text{drops/mL}}{60\ \text{min/h}}$$

$$X = \frac{6000\ \text{drops/h}}{60\ \text{min/h}}$$

Therefore,

$$X = 100\ \text{drops/min}$$

Now calculate the same order for an IV set that delivers 15 drops/mL:

$$X = \frac{400\ \text{mL}/4\ \text{h} \times 15\ \text{drops/mL}}{60\ \text{min/h}}$$

$$X = \frac{100\ \text{mL/h} \times 15\ \text{drops/mL}}{60\ \text{min/h}}$$

$$X = \frac{1500\ \text{drops/h}}{60\ \text{min/h}}$$

$$X = 25\ \text{drops/min}$$

If a patient has an order to be given an IV drug, the same principle can be used to calculate the speed of the delivery. For example, an order is written for a patient to receive 50 mL of an antibiotic over 30 minutes. The IV set used dispenses 60 drops/mL, which allows greater control. Calculate how fast the delivery should be.

$$X = \frac{50\ \text{mL}/0.5\ \text{h} \times 60\ \text{drops/mL}}{60\ \text{min/h}}$$

$$X = \frac{100\ \text{mL/h} \times 60\ \text{drops/mL}}{60\ \text{min/h}}$$

$$X = \frac{6000\ \text{drops/h}}{60\ \text{min/h}}$$

$$X = 100\ \text{drops/min}$$

Pediatric Considerations

For most drugs, children require dosages different from those given to adults. The "standard" drug dosage that is listed on package inserts and in many references refers to the dose that has been found to be most effective in the adult male. An adult's body handles drugs differently and may respond to drugs differently than a child's. A child's body may handle a drug differently in all areas of pharmacokinetics—absorption, distribution, metabolism, and excretion. The responses of the child's organs to the effects of the drug also may vary because of the immaturity of the organs. Most of the time a child requires a smaller dose of a drug to achieve the comparable critical concentration. On rare occasions, a child may require a higher dose of a drug. For ethical reasons, drug research per se is not done on children. Over time, however, enough information can be accumulated from experience with the drug to have a recommended pediatric dosage. The drug guide that you have selected to use in the clinical setting will have the pediatric dose listed if this information is available. Sometimes there is no recommended dosage but a particular drug is needed for a child. In these situations, established formulas can be used to estimate the appropriate dosage. These methods of determining a pediatric dose take into consideration the child's age, weight, or body surface.

Fried's Rule applies to a child younger than 1 year of age. The rule assumes that an adult dose would be appropriate for a child who is 12.5 years (150 months) old. Fried's Rule states

$$\text{child's dose}\ (\text{age} < 1\ \text{year}) = \frac{\text{infant's age (in months)}}{150\ \text{months}} \times \text{average adult dose}$$

Young's Rule, which applies to children 1 to 12 years of age, states

$$\text{child's dose}\ (\text{age 1–12 years}) = \frac{\text{child's age (in years)}}{\text{child's age (in years)} + 12} \times \text{average adult dose}$$

Clark's Rule uses the child's weight to calculate the appropriate dose and assumes that the adult dose is based on a 150-lb person. It states

$$\text{child's dose} = \frac{\text{weight of child (in pounds)}}{150\ \text{pounds} \times \text{average adult dose}}$$

The child's surface area may also be used to determine the approximate dosage that should be used. To do this, the child's surface area is determined with the use of a nomogram (Figure 5.1). The height and weight of the child are taken into consideration in this chart. The following formula is then used:

$$\text{child's dose} = \frac{\text{surface area in square meters}}{1.73 \times \text{average adult dose}}$$

For example, a 3-year-old child weighing 30 lb is to receive a therapeutic dose of aspirin. The average adult dose is 5 gr, and the dose to be given is the unknown (X). The calculation may be made from the child's age, by Young's Rule:

$$X = \frac{3\ \text{y}}{3 + 12\ \text{y}} \times 5\ \text{gr}$$

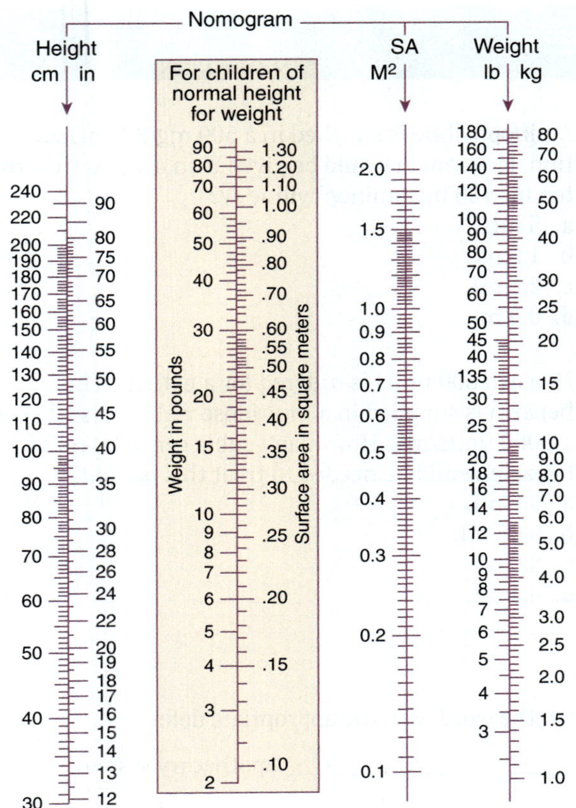

FIGURE 5.1 The West nomogram for calculating body surface area (BSA). Draw a straight line connecting the child's height (left scale) to the child's weight (right scale). The BSA value, which is calculated in square meters, is found at the point where the line intersects the SA column. The formula for estimating a child's dose is: Child's BSA (in m^2) × adult dose ÷ 1.73. Normal values are shown in the box.

$$X = \frac{15\ (y)(gr)}{15\ y}$$

$$X = 1\ gr$$

Alternately, the calculation could be based on the child's weight, using Clark's Rule:

$$X = \frac{30\ lb}{150\ lb} \times 5\ gr$$

$$X = \frac{150\ (gr)(lb)}{150\ lb}$$

$$X = 1\ gr$$

With small children, even a tiny dosage error can be critical. When working in pediatrics, it is important to become familiar with at least one of these methods of determining the drug dose to use. Many institutions require that two nurses check critical pediatric dosages. This is a good practice when working with small children. Box 5.1 summarizes the pediatric conversion formulas.

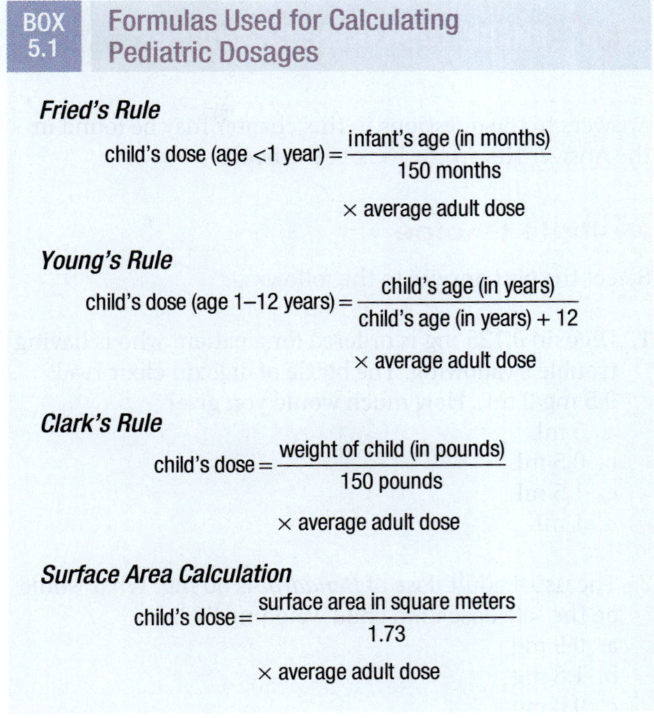
BOX 5.1 Formulas Used for Calculating Pediatric Dosages

Fried's Rule

$$\text{child's dose (age} < 1 \text{ year)} = \frac{\text{infant's age (in months)}}{150 \text{ months}} \times \text{average adult dose}$$

Young's Rule

$$\text{child's dose (age 1–12 years)} = \frac{\text{child's age (in years)}}{\text{child's age (in years)} + 12} \times \text{average adult dose}$$

Clark's Rule

$$\text{child's dose} = \frac{\text{weight of child (in pounds)}}{150 \text{ pounds}} \times \text{average adult dose}$$

Surface Area Calculation

$$\text{child's dose} = \frac{\text{surface area in square meters}}{1.73} \times \text{average adult dose}$$

Points to Remember

- At least four different systems are currently used in drug preparation and delivery. These are the metric system, the apothecary system, the household system, and the avoirdupois system.
- The metric system is the most widely used system of measure. The United States Pharmacopeia Convention established standards requiring that all prescriptions, regardless of the system that was used in the drug dosage, include the metric measure for quantity and strength of drug. All drugs are dispensed in the metric system.
- It is important to know how to convert dosages from one system to another. The method of ratio and proportion, which uses basic principles of algebra to find an unknown, is the easiest method of converting doses within and between systems.
- Children require dosages of most drugs different from those of adults because of the way their bodies handle drugs and the way that drugs affect their tissues and organs.
- Standard formulas can be used to determine the approximate dose that should be given to a child when the average adult dose is known. These include Fried's Rule (which considers age less than 1 year), Clark's Rule (which considers the child's weight), Young's Rule (which considers weight and age greater than 1 year), and the surface area rule, which requires the use of a nomogram to determine body surface area.

CHECK YOUR UNDERSTANDING

Answers to the questions in this chapter may be found in the Answer Key in the back of the book.

Multiple Choice

Select the best answer to the following.

1. Digoxin 0.125 mg is ordered for a patient who is having trouble swallowing. The bottle of digoxin elixir reads 0.5 mg/2 mL. How much would you give?
   a. 5 mL
   b. 0.5 mL
   c. 1.5 mL
   d. 1 mL

2. The usual adult dose of *Benadryl* is 50 mg. What would be the safe dose for a child weighing 27 lb?
   a. 0.9 mg
   b. 1.8 mg
   c. 9.0 mg
   d. 18 mg

3. An order is written for 700 mg ampicillin PO. The drug is supplied in liquid form as 1 g/3.5 mL. How much of the liquid should be given?
   a. 5 mL
   b. 2.5 mL
   c. 6.2 mL
   d. 2.45 mL

4. An order is written for 1000 mL of normal saline to be administered IV over 10 hours. The drop factor on the IV tubing states 15 drops/mL. What is the IV flow rate?
   a. 50 mL/h at 50 drops/min
   b. 100 mL/h at 25 drops/min
   c. 100 mL/h at 100 drops/min
   d. 100 mL/h at 15 drops/min

5. The average adult dose of meperidine is 75 mg. What dose would be appropriate for a 10-month-old infant?
   a. 50 mg
   b. 5 mg
   c. 25 mg
   d. 0.5 mg

6. A patient needs to take 0.75 g tetracycline PO. The drug comes in 250-mg tablets. How many tablets should the patient take?
   a. 2 tablets
   b. 3 tablets
   c. 4 tablets
   d. 30 tablets

7. Aminophylline is supplied in a 500 mg/2.5 mL solution. How much would be given if an order were written for 100 mg aminophylline IV?
   a. 5 mL
   b. 1.5 mL
   c. 2.5 mL
   d. 0.5 mL

8. Heparin 800 units is ordered for a patient. The heparin is supplied in a multidose vial that is labeled 10,000 units/mL. How many cubic centimeters of heparin would be needed to treat this patient?
   a. 0.8 mL
   b. 0.08 mL
   c. 8.0 mL
   d. 0.4 mL

Matching

Match the word with the appropriate definition.

1. ________________________ apothecary system
2. ________________________ Fried's Rule
3. ________________________ metric system
4. ________________________ Young's Rule
5. ________________________ household system
6. ________________________ Clark's Rule

A. A method of conversion from adult dose to pediatric dose that assumes that an adult dose would be appropriate for a child who is 12.5 years of age.
B. A method of conversion from adult dose to pediatric dose based on the child's weight.
C. A method of conversion from adult dose to pediatric dose for children 1 to 12 years of age.
D. A system of measure using teaspoons and cups.
E. A system of measure based on the minim and the grain and originally developed for use by pharmacists.
F. A system of measure based on the decimal system and using the gram and liter.

Complete the Following Problems

1. Change to equivalents within the system:
   a. 100 mg = ______ g
   b. 1500 g = ______ kg
   c. 0.1 L = ______ mL
   d. 500 mL = ______ L

2. Convert to units in the metric system:
   a. 150 gr = ______ g
   b. ¼ gr = ______ mg
   c. 45 min = ______ mL
   d. 2 qt = ______ L

3. Convert to units in the household system:
   a. 5 mL = ______ tsp
   b. 30 mL = ______ tbsp

4. Convert the weights in the following problems:
   a. A patient weighs 170 lb. What is the patient's weight in kilograms?
      170 lb = ______ kg
   b. A patient weighs 3200 g. What is the patient's weight in pounds?
      3200 g = ______ lb

5. Robitussin cough syrup 225 mg PO is ordered. The bottle reads: 600 mg in 1 ounce. How much cough syrup should be given? ______ mL.

6. A postoperative order is written for ¼ gr codeine q4h as needed (PRN) for pain. Each dose given will contain how many milligrams of codeine? ________ mg.

7. Ordered: 6.5 mg. Available: 10 mg/mL.
   Proper dose: ______ mL.

8. Ordered: 0.35 mg. Available: 1.2 mg/2 mL.
   Proper dose: ______ mL.

9. Ordered: 80 mg. Available: 50 mg/mL.
   Proper dose: ______ mL.

10. Ordered: 150,000 units. Available: 400,000 units/5 mL.
    Proper dose: ______ mL.

Bibliography and References

Broussard, M. C., & Pire, S. (1996). Medication problems in the elderly: A home healthcare nurse's perspective. *Home Healthcare Nurse, 14,* 441–443.

Craig, G. (2001). *Clinical calculations made easy.* Philadelphia: Lippincott Williams & Wilkins.

Dosage calculations made incredibly easy. (2001). Ambler, PA: Springhouse Corporation.

Gilman, A. G., Hardman, J. G., & Limbird, L. E. (Eds.). (2006). *Goodman and Gilman's the pharmacological basis of therapeutics* (11th ed.). New York: McGraw-Hill.

Lee, M. (1996). Drugs and the elderly: Do you know the risks? *American Journal of Nursing, 96*(7), 25–32.

Morrison, G. (1996). Drug dosing in the intensive care unit: The patient with renal failure. In J. M. Rippe, R. S. Irwin, & M. P. Fink, *Intensive care medicine* (3rd ed.). Boston: Little, Brown.

CHAPTER
6

Drug Therapy in the 21st Century

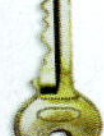

KEY TERMS

alternative therapies
biological weapons
cost comparisons
Internet
off-label uses
self-care
street drugs

LEARNING OBJECTIVES

Upon completion of this chapter, you will be able to:

1. Discuss the impact of the media, the Internet, and direct-to-consumer advertising on drug sales and prescriptions.
2. Explain the growing use of over-the-counter drugs and the impact it has on safe medical care.
3. Discuss the lack of controls on herbal or alternative therapies and the impact it has on safe drug therapy.
4. Define the off-label use of a drug.
5. Describe measures being taken to protect the public in cases of bioterrorism.

The dawn of the 21st century arrived with myriad new considerations and pressures in the health care industry. For the first time, consumers have access to medical and pharmacological information from many sources. Consumers are taking steps to demand specific treatments and considerations. Alternative therapies are being offered and advertised at a record pace, and this is causing people to rethink their approach to medical care and the medical system. At the same time, financial pressures have led to early discharge of patients from health care facilities and to provision of outpatient care for patients who, in the past, would have been hospitalized and monitored closely. Health care providers are being pushed to make decisions about patient care and prescriptions based on finances in addition to medical judgment. The events of 9/11 and the increased threat of terrorism have led to serious concerns about dealing with exposure to biological or chemical weapons. Illicit drug use is at an all-time high, bringing increased health risks and safety concerns. The nurse is caught in the middle of all of this change. Patients are demanding information, but may not understand it when they get it. Patient teaching and home care provisions are vital to the success of any health regimen. The nurse is frequently in the best position to listen, teach, and explain some of this confusing information to the patient and to facilitate the care of the patient in the health system.

Consumer Awareness

Access to information has become so broad in the past decade that consumers are often overwhelmed with details, facts, and choices that affect their health care. Gone is the era when the health care provider was seen as omniscient and always right. The patient now comes into the health care system burdened with the influence of advertising, the Internet, and a growing alternative therapy industry. Many patients no longer calmly accept whatever medication is selected for them. They often come with requests and demands, and they partake of a complex array of over-the-counter (OTC) and alternative medicines that further complicate the safety and efficacy of standard drug therapy.

Media Influence

The past 10 years have seen an explosion of drug advertising in the mass media. It became legal to advertise prescription drugs directly to the public in the 1990s, and it is now impossible to watch television, listen to the radio, or flip through a magazine without encountering numerous drug advertisements.

Federal guidelines determine what can be said in an advertisement, but in some cases this further confuses the issue for many consumers. If a drug advertisement states what the drug is used for, it must also state contraindications, adverse effects, and precautions. Because, in many cases, listing the possible adverse effects is not a good selling point, many advertisements are pure business ploys intended to interest consumers in the drug and to have them request it from their health care providers (even if they don't know what the drug is used for). It is not unusual to see a smiling, healthy-looking person romping through a field of beautiful flowers on a sunny day with a cute baby or puppy in tow. The ad might simply state how wonderful it is to be outside on a day like today—contact your health care provider if you, too, would like to take drug X. Numerous calls to caregivers each day are requests for this drug that makes you feel young, happy, and energetic. Although most people now know what the erectile dysfunction drug *Viagra* is used for, some of the ads for this drug simply show a happy older couple smiling and dancing the night away and then encourage viewers to ask their health care providers about *Viagra*. What older person wouldn't want a drug that makes you feel so happy and energetic?

Parenting magazines, which are often found in pediatricians' offices, are full of advertisements for antibiotics and asthma medications. These ads picture smiling, cute children and encourage readers to check with their pediatricians about the use of these drugs. If the drug's indication is mentioned, the second page of the ad may well have the United States Food and Drug Administration (FDA)-approved drug insert printed out, in extremely tiny print and in full medical lingo. Most readers have trouble reading the words on these required pages. Even if the words are legible, they frequently don't have any meaning for the reader. The pediatrician or nurse may spend a great deal of time explaining why a particular drug is not indicated for a particular child and may actually experience resistance on the part of the parent who wants the drug for his or her child. As the marketing power for prescription drugs continues to grow, the health care provider must be constantly aware of what patients are seeing, what the ads are promising, and the real data behind the indications and contraindications for these "hot" drugs. It is a continuing challenge to stay up to date and knowledgeable about drug therapy.

The media also look for headlines in current medical research or reports. It is not unusual for the media to take a headline or research title and make news. Sometimes the interpretation of the medical report is not accurate, and this can influence a patient's response to suggested therapy or provide a whole new set of demands or requests for the health care provider. Many of the standard talk shows include a medical segment that presents just a tiny bit of information, frequently out of context, which opens a whole new area of interest for the viewer. Some health care providers have learned to deal with the "disease of the week" as seen on these shows; others can be unprepared to deal with what was presented and may lose credibility with the patient.

The Internet

The **Internet** and World Wide Web are now readily accessible to most consumers. People who do not have Internet access at home will find it readily available at the local library, at work, or even in computer centers that allow community access. The information available over the Internet is completely overwhelming to most people. A person can spend hours looking up information on a drug—including pharmaceutical company information sites, chat rooms with other people who are taking the drug, online pharmacies, lists of government regulations, and research reports about the drug and its effectiveness. Many people do not know how to evaluate the information that they can access. Is it accurate or anecdotal? Patients often come into the health care system with pages of information downloaded from the Internet that they think pertains to their particular situation. The nurse or physician can spend a tremendous amount of time deciphering and interpreting the information and explaining it to the patient. Some tips that might be helpful in determining the usefulness or accuracy of information found on the Internet are in Box 6.1.

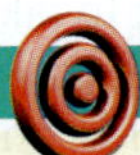

FOCUS POINTS

- An overwhelming amount of readily accessible information is available to consumers. This information has changed the way that people approach the health care system.
- Consumer advertising of prescription drugs, mass media health reports and suggestions, and the Internet influence some patients to request certain treatments, to question therapy, and to challenge the health care provider.

Over-the-Counter Drugs

OTC medications have allowed people to take care of simple medical problems without seeking advice from their health care providers. OTC drugs have been deemed to be safe when used as directed. Many of them were "grandfathered in" as drugs when stringent testing and evaluation systems became law and have not been tested or evaluated to the extent that new drugs are today. Aspirin, one of the nonprescription standbys for many years, falls into this category. Slowly, the FDA is looking at all of these drugs to determine effectiveness and safety. Other OTC drugs are former prescription drugs that have been tested and found to be safe for use by the general public, when they are used as directed. Each year several prescription drugs are reviewed for possible OTC status. In 2004, lovastatin, an antihyperlipidemic drug, was considered for OTC status. The FDA eventually decided that the public would have a hard time self-prescribing this drug because high lipid levels can be determined only with a blood test and present no signs and symptoms, so the drug's OTC status was not approved. Some well-known approved OTC drugs are cimetidine (*Tagamet*), to decrease gastric upset and heartburn; various vaginal antifungal medications for treating yeast infections; and omeprazole and famotidine, two other drugs for dealing with heartburn.

The availability of OTC drugs gives patients freedom for **self-care**, but there are some drawbacks to the use of OTC drugs that should be considered. The use of OTC drugs can mask the signs and symptoms of an underlying problem, making it difficult to arrive at an accurate diagnosis if the condition persists. These drugs are safe when used as directed, but many times the directions are not followed or even read. The idea that "If one makes me feel better, two will make me feel really good" is not always safe in the use of these drugs. Many people are not aware of which drugs are contained in these preparations and can inadvertently overdose when taking one preparation for each symptom they have. Table 6.1 gives an example of the ingredients that are found in some common cold and allergy preparations. Patients who take doses of different preparations to cover their various symptoms could easily wind up with an unintended overdose or toxic reaction.

Many OTC drugs interact with prescription drugs, with possibly serious effects for the patient. Many patients do not consider OTC drugs to be "real" drugs and do not mention their use when reporting a drug history to the health care provider. Every patient drug teaching session should include information on which particular OTC drugs must be avoided

BOX 6.1 Evaluating Internet Sites

Address Identification

- *.com:* commercial, advertising, selling, business site
- *.edu:* education site: school system, university, college
- *.gov:* government site
- *.net:* part of a linked network system, may include any of the above
- *.org:* sponsored by an organization, including professional, charitable, and educational groups

Site Evaluation

- Navigation—Is the site easy to access and navigate or confusing?
- Contributors—Who prepared the site? Is it reviewed? Is it purely commercial? What are the qualifications of the person(s) maintaining the site? Is there a mechanism for feedback or interaction with the site?
- Dates—Is the site updated frequently? When was the site last updated?
- Accuracy/reliability—Is the information supported by other sites? Is the information accurate and in agreement with other sources you have reviewed? Does the site list other links that are reasonable and reliable?

Table 6.1 Ingredients Found in Some Common Cold and Flu OTC Preparations*

Drug Name	Ingredients	Use
Vicks Formula 44 Cough & Decongestant	Pseudoephedrine, dextromethorphan	Cough, stuffy nose
Vicks 44D Cough & Head Congestion	Pseudoephedrine, dextromethorphan	Cough, sinus pressure
Vicks 44M Cold, Flu & Cough	Pseudoephedrine, chlorpheniramine, dextromethorphan	Cough, aches, stuffy head, flu
Vicks NyQuil LiquiCaps	Pseudoephedrine, doxylamine, dextromethorphan	Cough, aches, need to sleep, stuffy head
Thera-Flu Non-Drowsy Formula	Pseudoephedrine, dextromethorphan	Stuffy head, need to stay awake, cough, aches

*Safety Precautions: A patient could take one preparation for cough, a second to cover sinus pressure, a third to cover the aches and pains, and a fourth to stay awake or fall asleep—when the total amounts of the drugs contained in these products is calculated, a serious overdose of pseudoephedrine or dextromethorphan could easily occur.

or advice to check with the health care provider before taking any other medications or over-the-counter products. When taking a drug history, it is important to specifically ask whether the patient is taking any OTC drugs or any other medications. Serious adverse or toxic effects can be avoided if this information is known.

Alternative Therapies and Herbal Medicine

Another aspect of the increasing self-care movement is the rapidly growing alternative or herbal therapies market. Herbal or **alternative therapies** are found in ancient records and have often been the basis for discovery of an active ingredient that is later developed into a regulated medication (see Box 6.2). Today, alternative therapies can also include nondrug measures, such as imaging and relaxation.

Currently, these products are not controlled or tested by the FDA; they are considered to be dietary supplements, and therefore the advertising surrounding these products is not as restricted or as accurate as it would be with classic drugs.

BOX 6.2 HERBAL AND ALTERNATIVE THERAPIES

Many natural substances are used by the public for self-treatment of many complaints. These substances, derived from folklore of various cultures, often have ingredients that have been identified and have known therapeutic activities. Some of these substances have unknown mechanisms of action, but over the years have been reliably used to relieve specific symptoms. There is an element of the placebo effect in using some of these substances. The power of believing that something will work and that there is some control over the problem is often very beneficial in achieving relief from pain or suffering. Some of these substances contain as-yet-unidentified ingredients, which, when discovered, may prove very useful in the modern field of pharmacology. Because these products are not regulated or monitored, there is always a possibility of toxic effects. Some of these products may contain ingredients that interact with prescription drugs. A history of use of these alternative therapies may explain unexpected reactions to some drugs. See Appendix I for an extensive listing of alternative and complementary therapies.

Consumers are urged to use the "natural" approach to medical care and to self-treat with a wide variety of products. Numerous Internet sites point out all of the natural treatments that can be used to cure various disorders. Television ads and magazine spreads push the use of these products in place of prescribed medications. Many people who want to gain control of their medical care or who do not want to take "drugs" for their diabetes, depression, or fatigue are drawn to these products. The Dietary Supplement Health and Education Act of 1994, updated in 2000, states that herbal products, vitamins and minerals, and amino acids are classified as dietary supplements and are not required to go through premarketing testing. The advertising that is permitted for these products does not allow direct claims to cure, treat, diagnose, or prevent a specific disease but does allow for nondisease claims such as "for muscle enhancement," "for hot flashes," or "for memory loss." Appendix E lists common alternative therapies and their suggested uses.

Several issues are of concern to the health care provider when a patient elects to self-treat with alternative therapies. The active ingredients in these products have not been tested by the FDA; when test results are available, often the tests were for only a very small number of people with no reproducible results. When a patient decides to take bilberry to control diabetes, for example, the reaction that will occur is not really known. In some patients, the blood glucose level might decrease; in others, it might increase. The incidental ingredients in many of these products are unknown. Because many of these products are produced directly from plants or from a natural state, the fertilizer used for the plant, the time of the year when the plant was harvested, and the other ingredients that are compounded with the product have a direct effect on its efficacy. Saw palmetto, an herb that has been used successfully to alleviate the symptoms of benign prostatic hypertrophy, is available in a wide variety of preparations from different manufacturers. A random sampling of these products performed in 2000 revealed that the contents of the identified active ingredient varied from 20% to 400% of the recommended dose (*Medical Letter,* Feb. 2001; 1097). It is difficult to guide patients to the correct product with such a wide range of variability.

Patients often do not mention the use of alternative therapies to the health care provider. Some patients believe that the health care provider will disapprove of the use of these products and do not want to discuss it; others believe that these are just natural products and do not need to be mentioned. With the increasing use of these products, however, several drug interactions that can cause serious complications for patients taking prescription medication have been reported to the FDA. Diabetic patients who decide to use juniper berries, ginseng, garlic, fenugreek, coriander, dandelion root, or celery to "maintain their blood glucose level" may run into serious problems with hypoglycemia when they also use their prescription antidiabetic drugs. If the patient does not report the use of these alternative therapies to the health care provider, extensive medical tests and dosage adjustments might be done to no avail.

St. John's wort, a highly advertised and popular alternative therapy, has been found to interact with oral contraceptives, digoxin (a heart medication), the selective serotonin reuptake inhibitors (used for depression), theophylline (a drug used to treat lung disease), various antineoplastic drugs used to treat cancer, and the antivirals used to treat acquired immune deficiency syndrome (AIDS). Patients using St. John's wort for the symptoms of depression who are also taking *Prozac* (fluoxetine) for depression may experience serious side effects and toxic reactions. If the health care provider is not told about the use of St. John's wort, treatment of the toxicity can become very complicated.

Asking patients specifically about the use of any herbal or alternative therapies should become a routine part of any health history. If a patient presents with an unexpected reaction to a medication, ask the patient about any herbal or natural remedies he or she may be using. If a patient reports the use of an unusual or difficult-to-find remedy, try looking it up on the Internet at http://nccam.nih.gov, a site with generalized information about complementary and alternative medicines.

FOCUS POINTS

- OTC (over-the-counter) drugs are drugs that have been deemed safe when used as directed and that do not require a prescription or advice from a health care provider.
- OTC drugs can mask the signs and symptoms of disease, can interact with prescription drugs, and can be taken in greater than the recommended dose, leading to toxicity.
- Herbal or alternative therapies are considered to be dietary supplements and are not tightly regulated by the FDA.
- Herbal therapies can produce unexpected effects and toxic reactions, can interact with prescription drugs, and can contain various unknown ingredients that alter their effectiveness and toxicity.

Off-Label Uses

When a drug is approved by the FDA, the therapeutic indications for which the drug is approved are stated. Once a drug becomes available, it is sometimes used for indications that are not approved. This is called **off-label use** of the drug. It is commonly done for groups of patients for which there is little premarketing testing, particularly pediatric and geriatric groups. With the ethical issues involved in testing drugs on children, the use of particular drugs in children often occurs by trial and error when the drug is released with adult indications. Dosing calculations and nomograms become very important in determining the approximate dose that should be used for a child.

Drugs used to treat various psychiatric problems are often not approved for that use. The fact that little is really known about the way the brain works and what happens when the chemicals in the brain are altered has led to a polypharmacy approach in psychiatry—mixing and juggling drugs until the effect that is wanted is achieved. That same combination might not work in another patient with the same diagnosis because of brain and chemical differences in that patient. The nurse needs to be cognizant of off-label uses of drugs. The liability issues surrounding many of these uses are very fuzzy, and the nurse should be clear about the intended use, why the drug is being tried, and its potential for problems. The off-label use of drugs is widespread and often leads to discovery of a new use for a drug. If the use makes no sense to you, however, question it before you administer the drug.

Health Care Crisis

The cost of medical care and drugs has skyrocketed in the past few years. This is partly due to the demand to have the best possible, most up-to-date, and safest care and drug therapies. The research and equipment requirements to meet these demands are huge. At the same time, the rising cost of health insurance to pay for all of this is a major complaint for employers and consumers. As a result, health maintenance organizations (HMOs) have surged in popularity. These groups run the medical care system like a business, with the financial aspects of business becoming the overriding concern; decisions are often made by nonmedical personnel with a keen eye on the bottom line. Patients are being discharged from hospitals far earlier than ever before, as a cost-saving move, and many are not even admitted to hospitals for surgical or invasive procedures that used to require several days of hospitalization and monitoring. As a result, there is less monitoring of the patient, and more responsibility for care falls on the patient or the patient's significant others. Teaching the patient about self-care, drug therapies, and what to expect is even more crucial now. The nurse is the one who most often is responsible for this teaching.

Health Maintenance Organizations and Regulations

HMOs maintain a centralized control system to provide patients with their medical care within a budget. In many communities, the HMO provides a centralized building with participating physicians and services housed in one area. Consumers are often provided with all of their health care at this facility, and find the HMO insurance cost less expensive than traditional medical insurance. The tradeoff is often a loss of choice. The health care providers in the organization are the only ones who can be consulted. The HMO may regulate access to emergency facilities, types and timing of tests allowed, and procedures covered. Accessibility to prescription drugs is also controlled. The formulary for each HMO differs. Sometimes only generic products are covered, and newer drugs must be paid for by the patient; in other instances, a tier system exists and the patient may urge the provider to choose a drug from a lower tier, at a lower cost. Many health care providers believe that their ability to make decisions is limited by such regulations and that decisions are often made by nonmedical personnel at the other end of a telephone, who have no contact with the patient. The regulatory power of HMOs is being challenged in various court cases and through legislation, and may change dramatically in the coming years.

Cost Considerations

Despite the insurance coverage a patient may have for prescription medications, it is often necessary for the health care provider to choose a drug therapy based on the costs of the drugs available. With more and more of the population reaching retirement age and depending on a fixed income, costs are a real issue. Sometimes this may mean not selecting a first-choice drug but settling for a drug that should be effective. Patients who take antibiotics must be reminded to take the full course and not to stop the drug when they feel better, saving the remaining pills for the next time they feel sick, hoping to avoid the costs of another health care visit and a new prescription. This practice has contributed to the problem of resistant bacteria, which is becoming more dangerous all the time.

Patients also need to be advised not to split tablets in half unless specifically advised to do so. Some drugs can be split, and it is cheaper to order the larger size and have the patient cut the tablet. Some patients think that by cutting the drug in half they will have coverage for twice the time allowed by the prescription and will not be as dependent on the drug. With the new matrix delivery systems used for many medications, however, splitting the drug can cause it to become toxic or ineffective. Patients should be specifically alerted to avoid cutting drugs when it could be dangerous, especially if they are being advised to cut other tablets to be economical. The cost of treating the toxic reactions may far exceed the cost of the original drug.

Generic drug availability in many cases reduces the cost of a drug. Generic drugs are preparations that are off patent and therefore can be sold by their generic name, without the cost associated with brand name products. Generic drugs are tested for bioequivalence with the brand-name product, and resulting information is available to prescribers. When a drug has a small margin of safety (a small difference between the therapeutic and the toxic dose), a prescriber may feel more comfortable ordering the drug by brand name, to ensure that the dosage and binders are what the prescriber expects. When "DAW" (dispense as written) is on a prescription, the prescription is filled with the brand-name drug—such as *Lanoxin* instead of digoxin, or *Coumadin* instead of warfarin. In some situations the generic drug is not less expensive than the brand-name drug, so using only generic drugs does not guarantee that the patient is getting the least expensive preparation. Many pharmacies post the costs of commonly used drugs, and patients may do **cost comparisons** and request that a different drug be prescribed. The nurse is often the person who is in the middle of this issue and must be able to explain the reason for the drug choice or request that the prescriber consider an alternative treatment.

Table 6.2 presents an example of a cost comparison of some beta-blockers commonly used to treat hypertension. When deciding which drug to use, the patient or nurse may need to consider the range of costs. *Drug Facts and Comparisons* (2006) provides a cost comparison of drugs in each class, and *The Medical Letter* (2006) provides cost comparisons of drugs that are reviewed in each issue.

Table 6.2 Generic or Trade-Name Drugs? What Do They Cost?

Drug Name	Dosage (mg)	Cost of a 30-Day Supply
Acebutolol (generic) *Sectral*	200–1200	$21.30 $37.50
Atenolol (generic) *Tenormin*	25–100	$8.70 $32.40
Betaxolol (generic) *Kerlone*	5–40	$24.60 $28.80
bisoprolol (generic) *Zebeta*	5–20	$36.30 $37.80
carvedilol *Coreg*	12.5–50	$92.40
metoprolol (generic) *Lopressor*	50–200	$7.80 $21.90
nadolol (generic) *Corgard*	20–240	$18.30 $41.40
propranolol (generic) *Inderal*	40–240	$8.40 $21.60
timolol (generic) *Blocadren*	10–40	$16.20 $31.80

Note: This table shows general prescription drug prices in the earliest years of the 21st century for beta-blockers used to treat hypertension. It is presented to illustrate the wide price range between generic and trade-name drugs

In the past few years, with the cost of drugs becoming a political as well as a social issue, many people have begun ordering drugs on the Internet, often from other countries. These drugs are often cheaper, do not require the patient to see a health care provider (many of these sites simply have customers fill out a questionnaire that is reviewed by a doctor), and are delivered right to the patient's door. The FDA has begun checking these drugs as they arrive in this country and have found many discrepancies between what was ordered and what is in the product, as well as problems in the storage of these products. Some foreign brand names are the same as brand names in this country, but are associated with different generic drugs. The FDA has issued many warnings to consumers about the risk of taking some of these drugs without medical supervision, reminding consumers that they are not protected by U.S. laws or regulations when they purchase drugs from other countries. The FDA web site, www.fda.gov, contains important information and guidelines for people who elect to use the Internet to get cheaper drugs.

Home Care

The home care industry is one of the most rapidly growing offshoots of the changes in costs and medical care delivery. Patients go home directly from surgery with the responsibility for changing dressings, assessing wounds, and monitoring their own recovery. Patients are being discharged from hospitals because the hospital days allowed for a particular diagnosis have run out. These patients may be responsible for their own monitoring, rehabilitation, and drug regimens. At the same time, the population is aging and may be less accepting of all of this responsibility. Home health aides, visiting nurses, and home care programs are taking over some of the responsibilities that used to be handled in the hospital.

The responsibility of meeting the tremendous increase in teaching needs of patients frequently resides with the nurse. Patients need to know exactly what medications they are taking (generic and brand names), the dose of each medication, and what each is supposed to do. They also need to know what they can do to alleviate some of the adverse effects that are expected with each drug (e.g., small meals if gastrointestinal upset is common, use of a humidifier if secretions will be dried and make breathing difficult); which OTC drugs or alternative therapies they need to avoid while taking their prescribed drugs; and what to watch for that would indicate a need to call the health care provider. With patients who are taking many drugs at the same time, this information should be provided in writing, in language that is clear and understandable. Many pharmacies provide written information with each drug that is dispensed, but trying to organize these sheets of information into a usable and understandable form is difficult for many patients. The nurse is often the one who needs to sort this out and organize, simplify, and make sense of the provided information. The cost of dealing with toxic or adverse effects is often much higher, in the long run, than the cost of the time spent teaching and explaining things to the patient.

The projections for trends in health care indicate even greater expansion of the home health care system, with hospitals being used for only the most critically ill patients. The role of the nurse in this home health system is crucial—as teacher, assessor, diagnostician, and patient advocate.

Emergency Preparedness

The events of 9/11 brought a change in the sense of security and safety that generally prevailed in this country. Now there are terrorist alerts, long lines for security at airports, and increased inspection of bags and carryalls at sporting events and theme parks. One of the potential threats that is being addressed by the Centers for Disease Control and Prevention (CDC) and the Office of Homeland Security is the risk of exposure to biological and chemical weapons. Chemical weapons have been encountered in the wars in the Middle East as well as in terrorist attacks in Japan, and guidelines have been established for dealing with this exposure (Table 6.3). The threat of exposure to **biological weapons**, so-called germ warfare, is somewhat theoretical, but very real as seen in the anthrax mail scares in Washington, D.C., Pennsylvania, and New York. The CDC has worked diligently to establish guidelines for treating possible exposure to biological weapons (see Table 6.3). Education of health care providers and the public is one of the central points in coping effectively with any biological assault. The CDC posts regularly updated information on signs and symptoms of infection by various biological agents; guidelines for management of patients who are exposed and those who are actually infected; and ongoing research into detection, diagnosis, prevention, and management of diseases associated with biological agents. The nurse is often called upon to answer questions, reassure the public, offer educational programs, and serve on emergency preparedness committees. Go to www.cdc.gov and click on Emergency Preparedness to keep up to date and informed about these issues.

Drug Abuse

Illicit drug use in this country is a growing problem. Professional athletes are cited almost daily for abusing anabolic steroids. Hollywood stars are often part of the drug scene, using **street drugs**—nonprescription drugs with no known therapeutic use—to enhance their moods and increase pleasure. Alcohol and nicotine are two commonly abused drugs that cause serious problems for the abuser, but which are often not seen as drug addiction issues. Parents are often very concerned that their children will use street drugs. The "everyone is doing it" argument is hard to counter when today's heroes are thought to be heavily involved. Some people abuse and become addicted to prescription drugs following an injury, when confronted with chronic pain, when their occupation puts them in contact with readily available drugs, or when someone else in the home is using

Table 6.3 Recommended Treatments for Biological/Chemical Weapons Exposure

Biological/Chemical Agent	Suggested Treatment
Anthrax (*Bacillus anthracis*) Cutaneous anthrax	Adult: 500 mg ciprofloxacin PO b.i.d. for 60 days *or* 100 mg doxycycline PO b.i.d. for 60 days Pediatric: 10–15 mg/kg ciprofloxacin PO q12h for 60 days *or* >8 yr and >45 kg: 100 mg doxycycline PO q12h >8 yr and ≤45 kg: 2.2 mg/kg doxycycline PO q12h ≤8 yr: 2.2 mg/kg doxycycline PO q12h for 60 days
Inhalational anthrax	Adult: 400 mg ciprofloxacin IV q12h, then 500 mg ciprofloxacin PO b.i.d. for a total of 60 days *or* 100 mg doxycycline IV q12h, then 100 mg doxycycline PO b.i.d. for a total of 60 days Pediatric: 10–15 mg/kg ciprofloxacin IV q12h, then 10–15 mg/kg PO q12h for a total of 60 days *or* >8 yr and >45 kg: 100 mg doxycycline IV then PO q12h >8 yr and ≤45 kg: 2.2 mg/kg doxycycline IV then PO q12h ≤8 yr: 2.2 mg/kg doxycycline PO q12h for a total of 60 days Switch from IV to PO form is based on patient response. If patient is not responding to ciprofloxacin or doxycycline, one or two additional antimicrobials can be added to the drug regimen, including rifampin, vancomycin, penicillin, ampicillin, chloramphenicol, imipenem, clindamycin, and clarithromycin.
Botulism (*Clostridium botulinum toxin*)	Supportive therapy, antitoxin administered early, available from the CDC
Brucellosis (*Brucella* species)	Adult: 100 mg/day doxycycline PO with 600 mg/day rifampin PO for 6 wk Pediatric: 2.2 mg/day doxycycline PO with 10 mg/kg rifampin PO for 6 wk
Cholera (*Vibrio cholerae*)	Replacement of fluids and electrolytes, IV if necessary
Escherichia coli	Recovery usually occurs in 5–10 days; replace fluids
Hemorrhagic fevers Ebola virus Marburg virus Lassa fever Arenaviruses	Supportive therapy; fresh frozen plasma and judicious use of heparin to control DIC Ribavirin: 30 mg/kg IV followed by 15 mg/kg IV q6h for 4 days, then 7.5 mg/kg IV q8h for 6 days
Nerve gas (sarin, organophosphates)	Adult: atropine 2–4 mg IM and 2-PAM Cl 600 mg IM Severe symptoms: atropine 6 mg IM and 2-PAM Cl 1800 mg IM Pediatric: 0–2 yr: atropine 0.05 mg/kg IM and 2-PAM Cl 15 mg/kg IM Severe symptoms: atropine 0.1 mg/kg IM and 2-PAM Cl 25 mg/kg IM 2–10 yr: atropine 1 mg IM and 2-PAM Cl 15 mg/kg IM Severe symptoms: atropine 2 mg IM and 2-PAM Cl 25 mg/kg IM >10 yr: atropine 2 mg IM and 2-PAM Cl 15 mg/kg IM Severe symptoms: atropine 4 mg IM and 2-PAM Cl 25 mg/kg IM Geriatric: atropine 1 mg IM and 2-PAM Cl 10 mg/kg IM Severe symptoms: atropine 2–4 mg IM and 2-PAM Cl 25 mg/kg IM Repeat atropine (2 mg IM) at 5- to 10-min intervals until secretions have diminished and breathing is comfortable or airway resistance has returned to near normal. Assisted ventilation should be started after administration of antidotes for severe exposures.
Plague (*Yersinia pestis*)	Adults: 100 mg doxycycline PO b.i.d. *or* 500 mg ciprofloxacin PO b.i.d. Pediatric: >45 kg: adult dose of doxycycline <45 kg: 2.2 mg/kg doxycycline PO b.i.d. *or* 20 mg/kg ciprofloxacin PO b.i.d. Treatment of acute plague may include 15 mg/kg streptomycin IM b.i.d. or 2.5 mg/kg gentamicin IM or IV t.i.d.; 15 mg/kg chloramphenicol IV q.i.d. is also useful.
Q fever (*Coxiella burnetii*)	Adults: 100 mg doxycycline PO b.i.d. for 15–21 days Pediatric: >45 kg: adult dose of doxycycline <45 kg: 2.2 mg/kg doxycycline PO b.i.d. for 15–21 days
Ricin poisoning	No antidote exists; the most important factor is then getting the ricin off or out of the body as quickly as possible; medical supportive therapy
Salmonellosis (*Salmonella* species)	Rehydration, support Severe cases: 500 mg ampicillin PO q6h (adults and children >20 kg), or 100 mg/kg/day ampicillin PO (if <20 kg) *or* ciprofloxacin 500 mg PO b.i.d. (adults), or 20 mg/kg PO b.i.d. (children)
Shigellosis (*Shigella*)	Adult: 500 mg ampicillin PO q6h *or* 500 mg ciprofloxacin PO b.i.d. *or Septra/Bactrim* 160 mg trimethoprim/800 mg sulfamethoxazole PO q12h for 5 days Pediatric: <20 kg: 100 mg/kg/day ampicillin PO *or* 20 mg/kg ciprofloxacin PO b.i.d. *or Septra/Bactrim* 160 mg trimethoprim/800 mg sulfamethoxazole in divided doses of 8–10 mg/kg/day PO for 5 days

Table 6.3 Recommended Treatments for Biological/Chemical Weapons Exposure *(Continued)*

Biological/Chemical Agent	Suggested Treatment
Smallpox (*Variola major*)	No treatment available; active immunization possible
Tularemia (*Francisella tularensis*)	Adult: 1 g streptomycin IM b.i.d. *or* 5 mg/kg gentamicin IM or IV once daily If these cannot be used, one of the following: 100 mg doxycycline IV b.i.d. 15 mg/kg chloramphenicol IV q.i.d. 400 mg ciprofloxacin IV b.i.d. Pediatric: 15 mg/kg streptomycin IM b.i.d. *or* 2.5 mg/kg gentamicin IM or IV t.i.d. If these cannot be used, one of the following: 100 mg doxycycline IV b.i.d. (≥45 kg) 2.2 mg/kg doxycycline IV b.i.d. (<45 kg) 15 mg/kg chloramphenicol IV q.i.d. 15 mg/kg ciprofloxacin IV b.i.d.
Typhoid fever (*Salmonella typhi*)	Adult: 500 mg ampicillin PO q6h *or* 500 mg ciprofloxacin PO b.i.d. *or Septra/Bactrim* 160 mg trimethoprim/800 mg sulfamethoxazole PO q12h for 5 days Pediatric <20 kg: 100 mg/kg/day ampicillin PO *or* 20 mg/kg ciprofloxacin PO b.i.d. *or Septra/Bactrim* 160 mg trimethoprim/800 mg sulfamethoxazole in divided doses of 8–10 mg/kg/day PO for 5 days

CDC, Centers for Disease Control and Prevention; DIC, disseminated intravascular coagulation.
The table provides recommended treatments for exposure to biological or chemical weapons. For complete information on presenting signs and symptoms, diagnoses, and current research in this area, go to www.cdc.gov and click on Emergency Preparedness. (Adapted from Karch, A. M. (2006). *2007 Lippincott's nursing drug guide*. Philadelphia: Lippincott Williams & Wilkins.)

a prescription drug. Many of the drugs used illicitly are addictive and can change a person's entire life, with drug-seeking behavior becoming a major factor. Researchers have identified actual changes in the brain and neurotransmitter patterns of people who abuse and become addicted to such drugs. Trying to reverse these changes and return the person to a nonaddicted state is a physiological as well as a psychological challenge. The use of these drugs can have severe consequences on health, can mask underlying signs and symptoms of medical problems, and can interact with other medications that the user may need (Table 6.4).

Being informed about the drugs available in the community, the current trends among teenagers or young adults, and the community resources available to help patients can help parents and health care professionals deal with this drug culture problem. Education, for the public and for health care professionals, is crucial to providing a defense against drug abuse and helps them recognize the problem and deal with it when it occurs. The National Institutes of Health has a division called the National Institute on Drug Abuse. Go to www.nida.nih.gov to find educational programs for teens, parents, and health care professionals; the latest information on the hottest fads in illicit drugs; research on dealing with drug abuse problems; and links to sites for identifying unknown drugs, community resources, and laws.

Points to Remember

- Drugs in the 21st century pose new challenges for patients and health care providers, including information overload, demands for specific treatments, increased access to self-care systems, and financial pressures to provide cost-effective care.
- The mass media bombard consumers with medical reviews, research updates, and advertising for prescription drugs. If the use of a drug is stated, the adverse effects and cautions also must be stated. If the use is not stated, the drug advertisement is free to use any images and suggestions to sell the drug.
- Increasing access to the Internet and World Wide Web has increased consumer access to drug information, advertising, and even purchasing without a mediator of this information. Determining the reliability of an Internet site is a challenge for the consumer and the health care provider.
- OTC drugs and herbal and alternative therapies allow patients to make medical decisions and self-treat many common signs and symptoms. Problems arise when they are used inappropriately, when they interact with prescription drugs, or when they mask signs and symptoms, making diagnosis difficult.
- The health care crisis in this country has led to the emergence of HMOs and tight regulations on medical therapy and drug therapy alternatives. The choice of a drug to be used may be determined by the HMO formulary or by cost comparison with other drugs in the same or a similar class. Cost comparison is a major consideration in the use of many drugs.
- Off-label uses of drugs occur when a drug has been released and is available for use. The use of a drug for an indication that is not approved by the FDA occurs commonly in pediatric and in psychiatric medicine, where testing is limited or made ineffective by individual differences.
- Home care is one of the most rapidly growing areas of medical care. Patients are increasingly more responsible

Table 6.4 Street Drugs Frequently Abused and the Potential Health Consequences of These Drugs

Drug	Street Names	Class	Health Consequences
Amphetamines	Uppers, whites, dexies	Stimulant	Hypertension, tachycardia, insomnia, restlessness
Amyl nitrate	Boppers, pearls	Stimulant	Tachycardia, restlessness, hypotension, vertigo
Anabolic steroids	Roids, muscle	Steroid	Hypertension, hyperlipidemia, acne, cancer, cardiomyopathy
Barbiturates	Downers, reds	Depressant	Bradycardia, hypotension, laryngospasm, ataxia, impaired thinking
Benzodiazepines	M&Ms, Uncle Milty	Depressant	Confusion, fatigue, impaired memory, impaired coordination
Cannabis	Pot, grass, weed, THC	Mixed CNS	Drowsiness, elation, dizziness, memory lapse, hallucinations
Cocaine	Snow, blow, crack	Stimulant	Tachycardia, hypertension, hallucinations, confused thinking
Fentanyl	Jackpot, China white	Opioid	Sedation, arrhythmias, shock, cardiac arrest, decreased respirations, constipation
Gamma hydroxybutyrate	GHB, fantasy, liquid X, liquid E, "date rape" drug	Depressant	Memory loss, hypotension, somnolence
Heroin	Brown sugar, joy, crank, fairy dust	Opioid	Sedation, arrhythmias, shock, cardiac arrest, decreased respirations, constipation
Ketamine	Super acid, special K	Depressant	Paralysis, loss of sensation, disorientation, psychic changes
LSD	Acid, sunshine, blotter acid	Hallucinogen	Hallucinations, hypotension, changes in thinking, loss of social control
MDA	Ecstasy, b-bombs, go, Scooby snacks	Hallucinogen	Hallucinations, psychic change, loss of memory, hypotension, cardiac arrest
Methamphetamine	Crystal, glass, speed, crystal meth	Stimulant	Hypertension, tachycardia, restlessness, changes in thinking
Methylphenidate	Ritalin	Stimulant	Agitation, tachycardia, hypertension, hyperreflexia, fever
Morphine	Mort, miss emma	Opioid	Sedation, arrhythmias, shock, cardiac arrest, decreased respirations, constipation
OxyContin	Oxy, Oxycotton, Oxy 80s, hillbilly heroin, poor man's heroin	Opioid	Sedation, arrhythmias, shock, cardiac arrest, decreased respirations, constipation
PCP	Angel dust, zombie	Hallucinogen	Acute psychosis, CHF, death, seizures, memory loss
Peyote	Button, mesc	Hallucinogen	Acute psychosis, tremor, altered perception, death

CHF, congestive heart failure; CNS, central nervous system; LSD, lysergic acid diethylamide; MDA, methylendioxyamphetamine; PCP, phencyclidine; THC, tetrahydrocannabinol.

for managing their own medical regimens from home with dependence on home health providers and teaching and support from knowledgeable nurses.

- Emergency preparedness in the post-9/11 era includes awareness of risks associated with biological or chemical weapon exposure and medical management for the victims.
- Illicit drug use can lead to dependence on the drug and physiological changes, causing health problems and changing the body's response to traditional drugs.

CHECK YOUR UNDERSTANDING

Answers to the questions in this chapter may be found in the Answer Key in the back of the book.

Multiple Choice

Select the best answer to the following.

1. Drugs can be advertised in the mass media only if
   a. the FDA indication is clearly stated.
   b. the actual use is never stated.
   c. adverse effects and precautions are stated if the use is stated.
   d. all adverse effects are clearly stated.

2. Herbal treatments and alternative therapies
   a. are considered drugs and regulated by the FDA.
   b. are considered dietary supplements and are not regulated by the FDA.
   c. have no restrictions on claims and advertising.
   d. contain no drugs, only natural substances.

3. OTC drugs are drugs that are
   a. deemed to be safe when used as directed.
   b. harmless to the public.
   c. too old to be tested.
   d. cheaper to use than prescription drugs.

4. The home health care industry is booming because
   a. there is a shortage of hospital beds.
   b. patients feel safer at home and prefer to be cared for at home.
   c. patients are going home sooner and becoming responsible for their own care sooner than in the past.
   d. the nursing shortage makes it difficult to care for patients in hospitals.

5. The cost of drug therapy is a major consideration in most areas because
   a. generic drugs are always cheaper.
   b. the high cost of drugs combined with more fixed-income consumers puts constraints on drug use.
   c. pharmacies usually carry only one drug from each class.
   d. patients like to shop around and get the best drug for their money.

6. An off-label use of a drug means that the drug:
   a. was found without a label and its actual contents are not known.
   b. has been found to be safe when used as directed and no restrictions are needed.
   c. is being used for an indication not listed in the approved indications noted by the FDA.
   d. has expired, but is still found to be useful when used as directed.

Multiple Response

Select all that apply.

1. When taking a health history, the nurse should include specific questions about the use of OTC drugs and alternative therapies. This is an important aspect of the health history because
   a. many insurance policies cover these drugs.
   b. patients should be reprimanded about the use of these products.
   c. patients often do not consider them to be drugs and do not report their use.
   d. patients should never use these products when taking prescription drugs.
   e. these products can mask or alter presenting signs and symptoms.
   f. many of these products interact with traditional prescription drugs.

2. A nurse is caring for a patient who has been diagnosed with type 2 diabetes. The patient has reported that he frequently uses herbal remedies. Before administering any antidiabetic medications, the nurse should caution the patient about the use of which of the following herbal therapies?
   a. Glucosamine
   b. Ginseng
   c. St. John's wort
   d. Juniper berries
   e. Garlic
   f. Kava

Matching

Match the following Internet addresses with the appropriate classification:

1. ______________ www.fda.gov
2. ______________ www.amhrt.org
3. ______________ www.pain.com
4. ______________ www.anesthesia.net
5. ______________ www.geocities.com
6. ______________ www.healthy.net
7. ______________ www.healthtouch.com
8. ______________ www.nih.gov

9. ______________ www.brockport.edu
10. ______________ www.monroecc.edu

A. A commercial site that includes advertising, sales, and business
B. An educational site from a school, college, or university
C. A government-sponsored site
D. An official organization site
E. Part of a linked, interconnected network

Definitions

Define the following terms.

1. self-care ______________

____

2. Internet ______________

____

3. over-the-counter (OTC) drugs ______________

____

4. alternative therapies ______________

____

5. off-label uses ______________

____

6. cost comparisons ______________

____

Bibliography and References

Anderson, P. O. (2000). *Handbook of critical drug data* (9th ed.). Hamilton, IL: Drug Intelligence.

Cardinale, V. (1998). Consumers looking for more answers, clearer directions. *Drug Topics Supplement,* 142(11), 23a.

DerMarderosian, A. (Ed.). (2006). *The review of natural products.* St. Louis: Facts and Comparisons.

Drug facts and comparisons. (2006). St. Louis: Facts and Comparisons.

Gilman, A. G., Hardman, J. G., & Limbird, L. E. (Eds.). (2006). *Goodman and Gilman's the pharmacological basis of therapeutics* (11th ed.). New York: McGraw-Hill.

Karch, A. M. (2006). *2007 Lippincott's nursing drug guide.* Philadelphia: Lippincott Williams & Wilkins.

The medical letter on drugs and therapeutics. (2006). New Rochelle, NY: Medical Letter.

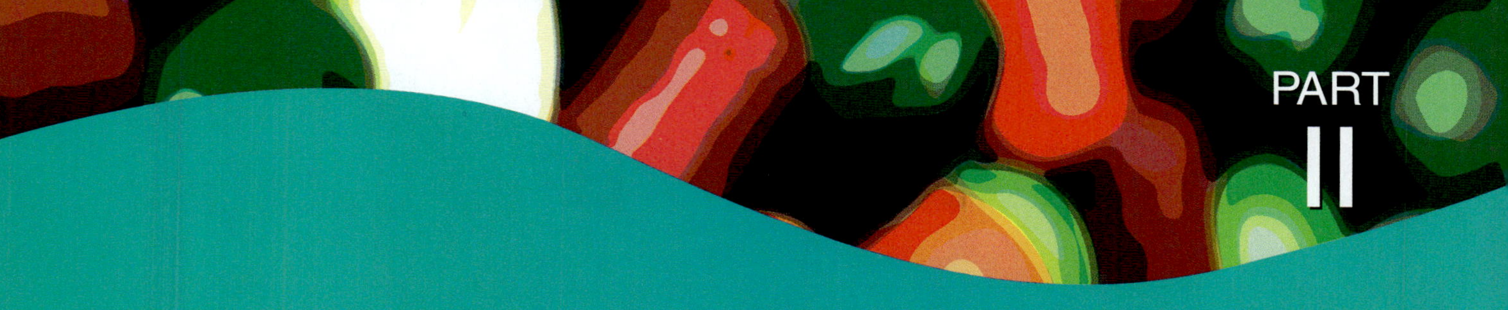

Chemotherapeutic Agents

CHAPTER 7

Introduction to Cell Physiology

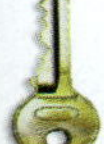

KEY TERMS

cell cycle
cell membrane
cytoplasm
diffusion
endocytosis
exocytosis
histocompatibility antigens
lipoprotein
lysosomes
mitochondria
nucleus
organelles
osmosis
ribosomes

LEARNING OBJECTIVES

Upon completion of this chapter, you will be able to:

1. Identify the parts of the human cell.
2. Describe the role of each organelle found within the cell cytoplasm.
3. Explain the unique properties of the cell membrane.
4. Describe three processes used by the cell to move things across the cell membrane.
5. Outline the cell cycle, including the activities going on within the cell in each phase.

Chemotherapeutic drugs are agents that affect cells (1) by altering cellular function or disrupting cellular integrity, causing cell death, or (2) by preventing cellular reproduction, eventually leading to cell death. To understand the actions and the adverse effects caused by chemotherapeutic agents, it is important to understand the basic functioning of the cell.

Chemotherapeutic drugs are used to destroy both organisms that invade the body (bacteria, viruses, parasites, protozoa, fungi) and abnormal cells within the body (neoplasms, cancers). By keeping in mind the various properties of the cell and cell processes, nurses may help determine interventions that increase the therapeutic effectiveness of a drug and limit the undesired adverse effects.

The Cell

The cell is the basic structural unit of the body. The cells that make up living organisms, which are arranged into tissues and organs, all have the same basic structure. Each cell has a nucleus, a cell membrane, and cytoplasm, which contains a variety of organelles (Figure 7.1).

Cell Nucleus

The **nucleus** of a cell contains all of the genetic material that is necessary for cell reproduction and for regulation of cellular production of proteins. Each cell is "programmed" by the genes for the production of specific proteins that allow the cell to carry out its function, maintain cell homeostasis or stability, and promote cell division. The nucleus is encapsulated in its own membrane and remains distinct from the rest of the cytoplasm. A small spherical mass, called the nucleolus, is located within the nucleus. Within this mass are dense fibers and proteins that will eventually become **ribosomes**, the sites of protein synthesis within the cell.

The nucleus also contains genes, or sequences of DNA, that control basic cell functions and allow for cell division. Genes are responsible for the formation of messenger RNA and transcription RNA, which are involved in production of the proteins unique to the cell. The DNA necessary for cell division is found on long strains called chromatin. These structures line up and enlarge during the process of cell division.

Cell Membrane

The cell is surrounded by a thin barrier called the **cell membrane**, which separates the intracellular fluid from the extracellular fluid. The membrane is essential for cellular integrity, and is equipped with many mechanisms for maintaining cell homeostasis.

Lipoproteins

The cell membrane, which consists of lipids and proteins, is a **lipoprotein** structure. The two components are arranged in a freely moving double layer. The membrane is largely composed of lipids—phospholipids, glycolipids, and choles-

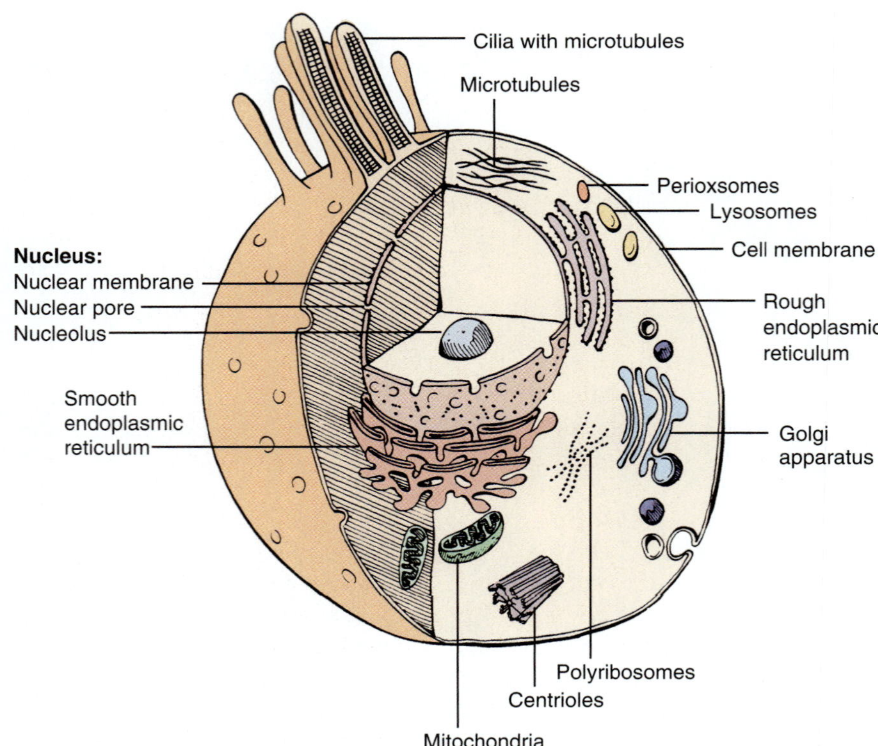

FIGURE 7.1 General structure of a cell and the location of its organelles.

terol. The phospholipids, which are bipolar in nature, line up with their polar regions pointing toward the interior or exterior of the cell and their nonpolar region lying within the cell membrane. The polar regions mix well with water, and the nonpolar region repels water. These properties allow the membrane to act as a barrier, keeping the cytoplasm within the cell and regulating what can enter the cell (Figure 7.2). The freely moving nature of the membrane allows it to adjust to the changing shape of the cell.

Receptor Sites

Embedded in the lipoprotein membrane are a series of peripheral proteins with several functions. As discussed in Chapter 2, one type of protein located on the cell membrane is known as a receptor site. This protein reacts with specific chemicals outside the cell to stimulate a reaction within a cell. For example, the receptor site for insulin reacts with the hormone insulin to cause activation of adenosine triphosphate (ATP) within the cell. This reaction alters the cell's permeability to glucose. Receptor sites are very important in the functioning of neurons, muscle cells, endocrine glands, and other cell types, and they play a very important role in clinical pharmacology.

Identifying Markers

Other surface proteins are surface antigens, or genetically determined identifying markers. These proteins provide the **histocompatibility antigens** or human leukocyte antigens (HLAs) that the body uses to identify a cell as a self-cell (i.e., a cell belonging to that individual). The body's immune system recognizes these proteins and acts to protect self-cells and to destroy non–self-cells. When an organ is transplanted from one person to another, a great effort is made to match as many histocompatibility antigens as possible to reduce the chance that the "new" body will reject the transplanted organ.

Histocompatibility antigens can be changed in several ways: by cell injury, with viral invasion of a cell, with age, and so on. If the markers are altered, the body's immune system reacts to the change and can ignore it, allowing neoplasms to grow and develop. The immune system may also attack the cell, leading to many of the problems associated with autoimmune disorders and chronic inflammatory conditions.

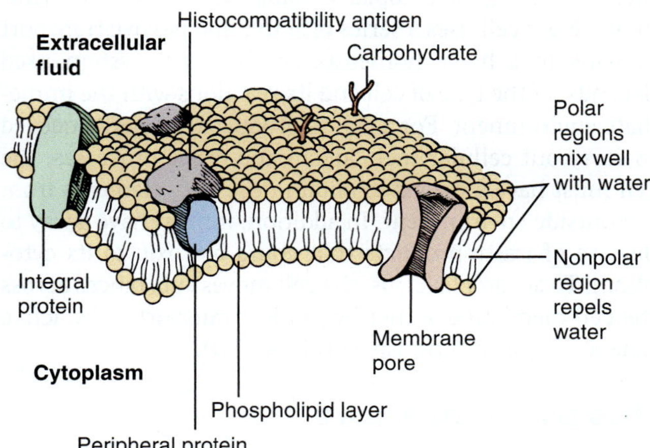

FIGURE 7.2 Structure of the lipid bilayer of the cell membrane.

Channels

Channels or pores within the cell membrane are made by proteins in the cell wall that allow the passage of small substances in or out of the cell. Specific channels have been identified for sodium, potassium, calcium, chloride, bicarbonate, and water, and other channels may also exist. Some drugs are designed to affect certain channels specifically. For example, calcium channel blockers prevent the movement of calcium into a cell through calcium channels.

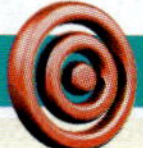

FOCUS POINTS

- The cell is the basic structure of living things.
- Cells are composed of a nucleus and cytoplasm surrounded by a phospholipid cell membrane.
- The cell membrane features specific receptor sites that allow interaction with various chemicals, histocompatibility proteins that allow for self-identification, and channels or pores that allow for the passage of substances into and out of the cell.

Cytoplasm

The cell **cytoplasm** lies within the cell membrane. This complex area, which contains many **organelles** (structures with specific functions), is the site of activities of cellular metabolism and special cellular functions. The organelles within the cytoplasm include the mitochondria, the endoplasmic reticulum, free ribosomes, the Golgi apparatus, and the lysosomes.

Mitochondria

The **mitochondria** are rod-shaped power plants within each cell that produce energy in the form of ATP, which allows the cell to function. Mitochondria are plentiful in very active cells such as muscle cells and are relatively scarce in inactive cells such as bone cells. Mitochondria, which can reproduce when a cell is very active, are always very abundant in cells that consume energy. For example, cardiac muscle cells, which must work continually to keep the heart contracting, contain a great number of mitochondria. Milk-producing cells in breast tissue, which are normally quite dormant, contain very few mitochondria. If a woman is lactating, however, the mitochondria become more abundant to meet the demands of the milk-producing cells. The mitochondria can take carbohydrates, fats, and proteins from the cytoplasm and make ATP via the Krebs cycle, which depends on oxygen. Cells use the ATP to maintain homeostasis, produce proteins, and carry out specific functions. If oxygen is not available, lactic acid builds up as a byproduct of cellular respiration. Lactic acid leaves the cell and is transported to the liver for conversion to glycogen and carbon dioxide.

Endoplasmic Reticulum

Much of the cytoplasm of a cell is made up of a fine network of interconnected channels known as cisternae, which form the endoplasmic reticulum. The undulating surface of the endoplasmic reticulum provides a large surface for chemical reactions within the cell. Many granules that contain enzymes and ribosomes, which produce protein, are scattered over the surface of the endoplasmic reticulum. Production of proteins, nonproteins, hormones, and other substances takes place there. The breakdown of many toxic substances may also occur in these channels.

Free Ribosomes

Other ribosomes that are not bound to the surface of the endoplasmic reticulum exist throughout the cytoplasm. These free-floating ribosomes produce proteins that are important to the structure of the cell and some of the enzymes that are necessary for cellular activity.

Golgi Apparatus

The Golgi apparatus is a series of flattened sacs that may be part of the endoplasmic reticulum. These structures prepare hormones or other substances for secretion by processing them and packaging them in vesicles to be moved to the cell membrane for excretion from the cell. In addition, the Golgi apparatus may produce lysosomes and store other synthesized proteins and enzymes until they are needed.

Lysosomes

Lysosomes are membrane-covered organelles that contain specific digestive enzymes that can break down proteins, nucleic acids, carbohydrates, and lipids. These organelles form a membrane around any substance that needs to be digested and secrete the digestive enzymes directly into the isolated area, protecting the rest of the cytoplasm from injury. The lysosomes are responsible for digesting worn or damaged sections of a cell, which they accomplish by encapsulating the area and self-digesting it. If a cell dies and the membrane ruptures, the release of lysosomes causes the cell to self-destruct.

This phenomenon can be seen with old lettuce in the refrigerator. The side of the lettuce head that has been "lying down" for a prolonged period becomes brown and wet as the lettuce cells die and self-digest when their lysosomes are released. If the lettuce is not used, the released lysosomes begin to digest any healthy lettuce that remains, with eventual destruction of the entire head. Lysosomes are important in ecology. Dead trees, animals, and other organisms self-digest and disappear.

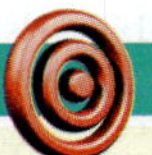

FOCUS POINTS

- The cytoplasm of the cell contains various organelles that are important for cellular function.
- The mitochondria produce energy for the cell; the endoplasmic reticulum contains ribosomes that produce proteins; the Golgi apparatus packages proteins; and lysosomes contain protein-dissolving enzymes that are important for digestion and the recycling of nature.

Cell Properties

Cells have certain properties that allow them to survive. **Endocytosis** involves incorporation of material into the cell. Pinocytosis, a form of endocytosis, refers to the engulfing of specific substances that have reacted with a receptor site on the cell membrane. This process allows cells to absorb nutrients, enzymes, and other materials. Phagocytosis is a similar process; it allows the cell, usually a neutrophil or macrophage, to engulf a bacterium or a foreign protein and destroy it within the cell by secreting digestive enzymes into the area. **Exocytosis** is the opposite of endocytosis. This property allows a cell to move a substance to the cell membrane and then secrete the substance outside the cell. Hormones, neurotransmitters, enzymes, and other substances that are produced within a cell are excreted into the body by this process (Figure 7.3).

Homeostasis

The main goal of a cell is to maintain homeostasis, which means keeping the cytoplasm stable within the cell membrane. Each cell uses a series of active and passive transport systems to achieve homeostasis; the exact system used depends on the type of cell and its reactions with the immediate environment. For a cell to produce the energy needed to carry out cellular metabolism and other processes, the cell must have a means to obtain necessary elements from the outside environment. In addition, it must have a way to dispose of waste products that could be toxic to its cytoplasm. To accomplish this, the cell moves substances across the cell membrane, either by passive transport or by active (energy-requiring) transport (Figure 7.4).

Passive Transport

Passive transport happens without the expenditure of energy and can occur across any semipermeable membrane. There

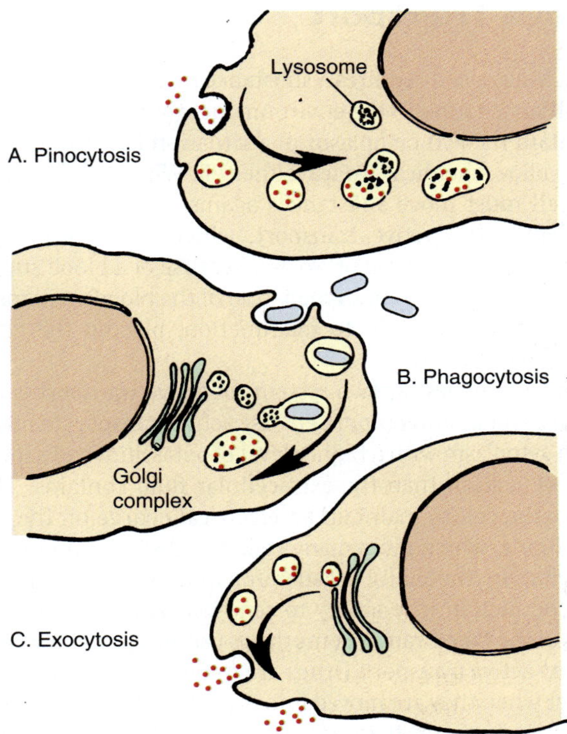

FIGURE 7.3 Schematic representation of endocytosis and exocytosis. Pinocytosis **(A)** is the movement of nutrients and needed substances into the cell through specific receptors on the cell surface. Phagocytosis **(B)** involves the destruction of engulfed proteins or bacteria. Exocytosis **(C)** is the movement of substances (waste products, hormones, neurotransmitters) out of the cell.

are essentially three types of passive transport: diffusion, osmosis, and facilitated diffusion.

Diffusion

Diffusion is the movement of a substance from a region of higher concentration to a region of lower concentration. The difference between the concentrations of the substance in the two regions is called the *concentration gradient* of the substance; usually, the greater the concentration gradient, the faster the substance moves. Movement into and out of a cell is regulated by the cell membrane. Some substances move through channels or pores in the cell membrane. Small substances and materials with no ionic charge move most freely through the channels. Substances with a negative charge move more freely than substances with a positive charge. Substances that move into and out of a cell by diffusion include sodium, potassium, calcium, carbonate, oxygen, bicarbonate, and water.

When a cell is very active and is using energy and oxygen, the concentration of oxygen within the cell decreases. The concentration of oxygen outside the cell remains relatively high, so oxygen moves across the cell membrane (down the concentration gradient) to supply needed oxygen to the inside of the cell. Cells use this process to maintain homeostasis during many activities that occur in the life of a cell.

Osmosis

Osmosis, a special form of diffusion, is the movement of water across a semipermeable membrane from an area that is low in dissolved solutes to one that is high in dissolved

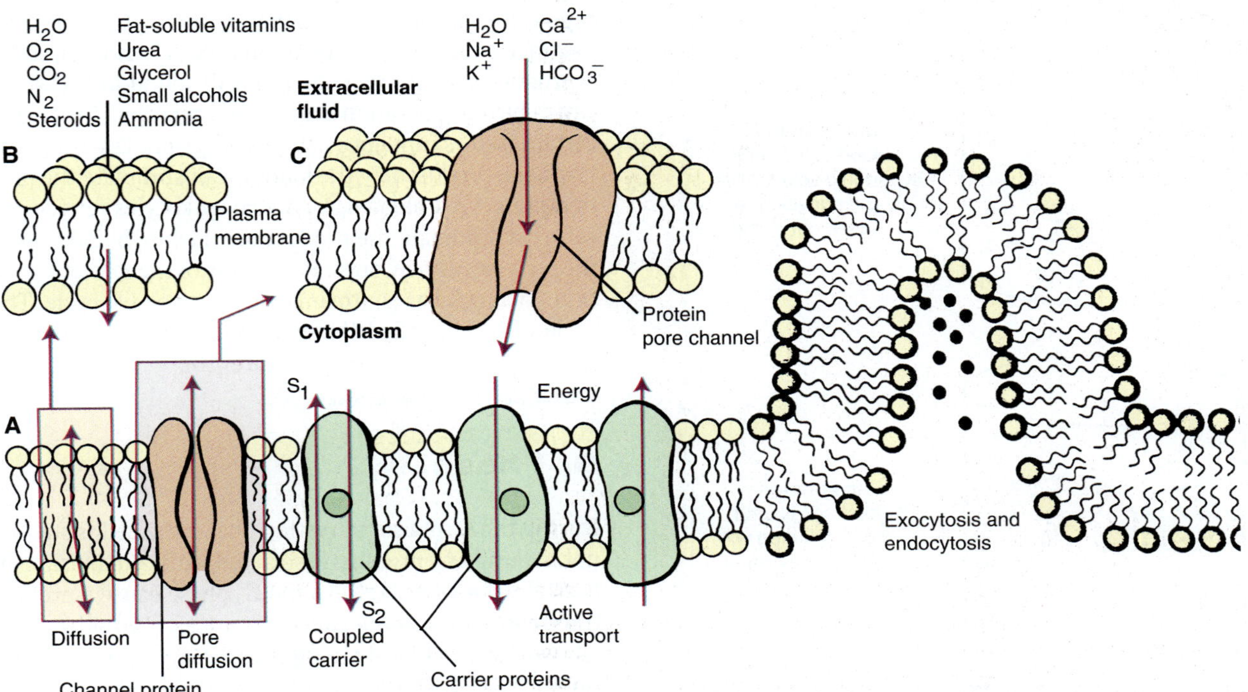

FIGURE 7.4 Schematic representation of transport across a cell membrane **(A)**, which includes *diffusion* through the cell membrane **(B)** and *pore diffusion* through a protein channel **(C)**.

solutes. The water is attempting to equalize the dilution of the solutes. This diffusion of water across a cell membrane from an area of high concentration (of water) to an area of low concentration creates pressure on the cell membrane, called *osmotic pressure.* The greater the concentration of solutes in the solution to which the water is flowing, the higher the osmotic pressure.

A fluid that contains the same concentration of solutes as human plasma is called an *isotonic* solution. A fluid that contains a higher concentration of solutes than human plasma is a *hypertonic* solution, and it draws water from cells. A fluid that contains a lower concentration of solutes than human plasma is *hypotonic;* it loses water to cells. If a human red blood cell, which has a cytoplasm that is isotonic with human plasma, is placed into a hypertonic solution, it shrinks and shrivels because the water inside the cell diffuses out of the cell into the solution. If the same cell is placed into a hypotonic solution, the cell swells and bursts because water moves from the solution into the cell (Figure 7.5).

Facilitated Diffusion

Sometimes a substance cannot move freely on its own in or out of a cell. Such a substance may attach to another molecule, called a carrier, to be diffused. This form of diffusion, known as *facilitated diffusion,* does not require energy, just the presence of the carrier. Carriers may be hormones, enzymes, or proteins. Because the carrier required for facilitated diffusion is usually present in a finite amount, this type of diffusion is limited.

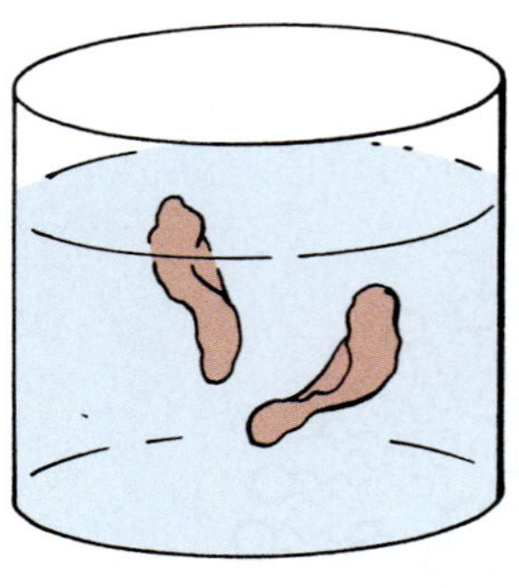

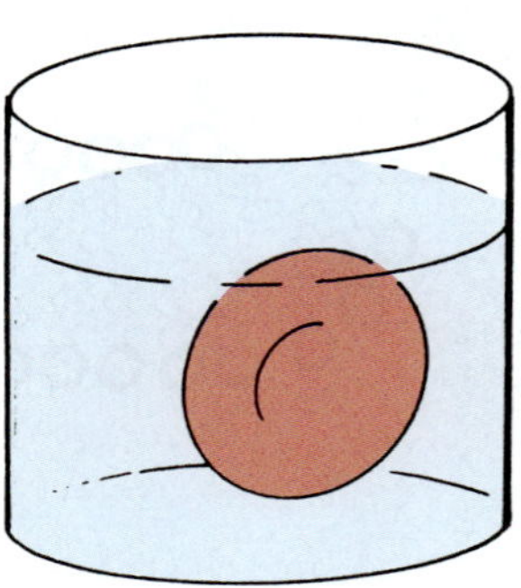
Hypotonic solution
A red blood cell placed in hypotonic solution will swell and burst as water moves into the cell.

FIGURE 7.5 Red blood cell response to hypertonic and hypotonic solutions.

Active Transport

Sometimes a cell requires a substance in greater concentration than is found in the environment around it or needs to maintain its own cytoplasm in a situation that would normally allow chemicals to leave the cell. When this happens, the cell must move substances against the concentration gradient using active transport, which requires energy. When a cell is deprived of oxygen because of a blood supply problem or insufficient oxygenation of the blood, systems of active transport begin to malfunction, placing the cell's integrity in jeopardy.

One of the best known systems of active transport is the sodium–potassium pump. Cells use active transport to maintain a cytoplasm with a higher level of potassium and a lower level of sodium than the extracellular fluid contains. This allows the cell to maintain an electrical charge on the cell membrane, which gives many cells the electrical properties of excitation (the ability to generate a movement of electrons) and conduction (the ability to send this stimulus to other areas of the membrane). Some drugs use energy to move into cells by active transport. Drugs are frequently bonded with a carrier when they are moved into the cell. Cells in the kidney use active transport to excrete drugs from the body as well as to maintain electrolyte and acid–base balances.

Cell Cycle

Most cells have the ability to reproduce themselves through the process of mitosis. The genetic makeup of a particular cell determines the rate at which that cell can multiply. Some cells reproduce very quickly (e.g., the cells lining the gastrointestinal tract, which have a generation time of 72 hours), and some reproduce very slowly (e.g., the cells found in breast tissue, which have a generation time of a few months). In some cases, certain factors influence cell reproduction. Erythropoietin, a hormone produced by the kidney, can stimulate the production of new red blood cells. Active leukocytes release chemicals that stimulate the production of white blood cells when the body needs new ones. Regardless of the rate of reproduction, each cell has approximately the same life cycle. The life cycle of a cell, called the **cell cycle**, consists of four active phases and a resting phase (Figure 7.6).

CONCEPTS in action **ANIMATION**

G_0 Phase

During the G_0 phase, or resting phase, the cell is stable. It is not making any proteins associated with cell division and is basically dormant. Cells in the G_0 phase cause a problem in the treatment of some cancers. Cancer chemotherapy usually works on active, dividing cells, leaving resting cells fairly untouched. When the resting cells are stimulated to become active and regenerate, the cancer can return, which is why

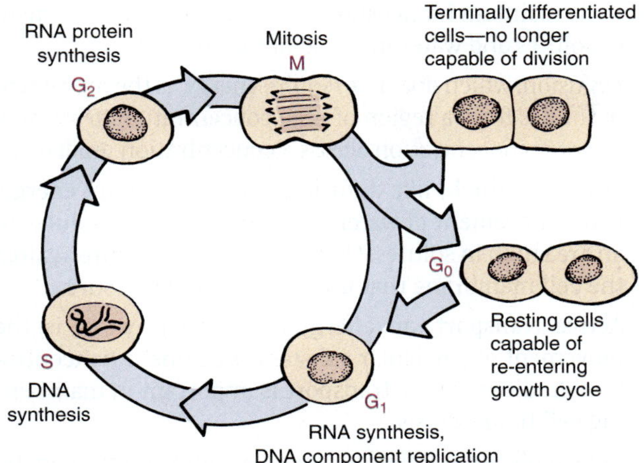

FIGURE 7.6 Diagram of the cell cycle, showing G_0, G_1, S, G_2, and M phases.

cancer chemotherapeutic regimens are complicated and extended over time, and why a 5-year cancer-free period is usually the basic guide for considering a cancer to be cured.

G_1 Phase

When a cell is stimulated to emerge from its resting phase, it enters what is called the G_1 phase, which lasts from the time of stimulation from the resting phase until the formation of DNA. During this period, the cell synthesizes the substances that are needed for DNA formation. The cell is actively collecting materials to make these substances and producing the building blocks for DNA.

S Phase

The next phase, called the S phase, involves the actual synthesis of DNA, which is an energy-consuming activity. The cell remains in this phase until the amount of cellular DNA has doubled.

G_2 Phase

After the cellular DNA has doubled in preparation for replication, the G_2 phase begins. During this phase, the cell produces all the substances that are required for the manufacture of the mitotic spindles.

M Phase

After the cell has produced all the substances necessary for the formation of a new cell, or daughter cell, it undergoes cell division. This occurs during the M phase of the cell cycle. During this phase, the cell splits to form two identical daughter cells, a process called mitosis.

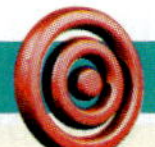

FOCUS POINTS

- All cells progress through a cell cycle, which allows them to reproduce.
- Each cell goes through a resting phase (G_0); a gathering phase (G_1), when the components needed for cell division are collected by the cell; a synthesizing phase (S), when DNA and other components are produced; a final gathering phase (G_2), when the last substances needed for division are collected and produced; and the M phase, when actual cell division occurs, producing two identical daughter cells.

Clinical Significance of Cell Physiology

Knowledge of the basic structure and function of the cell may help in understanding the therapeutic and toxic effects of the various classes of chemotherapeutic agents. Drugs may alter the cell membrane, causing the cell to rupture and die. Or they may deprive the cell of certain nutrients, altering the proteins that the cell produces and interfering with normal cell functioning and cell division. Because most chemotherapeutic agents do not possess complete selective toxicity, they also affect the normal cells of patients to some extent.

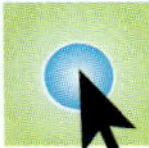

WEB LINKS

Students may want to consult the following Internet sources:

http://www.historyoftheuniverse.com/cell.html Information on cell physiology, theories of cell formation, and ongoing cellular research.

http://www.life.uiuc.edu/plantbio/cell Information on cell structure, properties, and division.

Points to Remember

- The cell is the basic structural unit of all living organisms.
- The cell is composed of a nucleus, which contains genetic material and controls the production of proteins by the cell; a cytoplasm, which contains various organelles important to cell function; and a cell membrane, which separates the inside of the cell from the outside environment.
- The cell membrane functions as a fluid barrier made of lipids and proteins. The arrangement of the lipoprotein membrane controls what enters and leaves the cell.
- Proteins on the cell membrane surface can act either as receptor sites for specific substances or as histocompatibility markers that identify the cell as a self-cell.

- Channels or pores in the cell membrane allow for easier movement of specific substances needed by the cell for normal functioning.
- Mitochondria are rod-shaped organelles that produce energy in the form of ATP for use by cells.
- Ribosomes are sites of protein production within the cell cytoplasm. The specific proteins produced by a cell are determined by the genetic material within the cell nucleus.
- The Golgi apparatus packages particular substances for removal from the cell (e.g., neurotransmitters, hormones).
- Lysosomes are packets of digestive enzymes located in the cell cytoplasm. These enzymes are responsible for destroying injured or nonfunctioning parts of the cell and for cellular disintegration when the cell dies.
- Endocytosis is the process of moving substances into a cell by extending the cell membrane around the substance and engulfing it. Pinocytosis refers to the engulfing of necessary materials, and phagocytosis refers to the engulfing and destroying of bacteria or other proteins by white blood cells.
- Exocytosis is the process of removing substances from a cell by moving them toward the cell membrane and then changing the cell membrane to allow passage of the substance out of the cell.
- Cells maintain homeostasis by regulating the movement of solutes and water into and out of the cell.
- Diffusion, which does not require energy, is the movement of solutes from a region of high concentration to a region of lower concentration across a concentration gradient.
- Osmosis, which, like diffusion, does not require energy, is the movement of water from an area low in solutes to an area high in solutes. Osmosis exerts a pressure against the cell membrane that is called osmotic pressure.
- Active transport, an energy-requiring process, is the movement of particular substances against a concentration gradient. Active transport is important in maintaining cell homeostasis.
- Cells replicate at differing rates depending on the genetic programming of the cell. All cells go through a life cycle consisting of the following phases: G_0, the resting phase; G_1, which involves the production of proteins for DNA synthesis; S, which involves the synthesis of DNA; G_2, which involves manufacture of the materials needed for mitotic spindle production; and M, the mitotic phase, in which the cell splits to form two identical daughter cells.
- Chemotherapeutic drugs act on cells to cause cell death or alteration. All properties of the drug that affect cells should be considered when administering a chemotherapeutic agent.

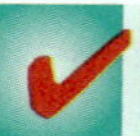

CHECK YOUR UNDERSTANDING

Answers to the questions in this chapter may be found in the Answer Key in the back of the book.

Multiple Choice

Select the best answer to the following.

1. The basic unit of human structure is
   a. the mitochondria.
   b. the nucleus.
   c. the nucleolus.
   d. the cell.

2. The cell membrane is composed of
   a. a phospholipid structure.
   b. channels of protein.
   c. a cholesterol-based membrane.
   d. Golgi apparati.

3. The saying, "One rotten apple can spoil the whole barrel," refers to the cell-degrading properties of
   a. calcium channels.
   b. lysosomes.
   c. histocompatibility receptors.
   d. nuclear spindles.

4. The ribosomes are important sites for
   a. digestion of nutrients.
   b. excretion of waste products.
   c. production of proteins.
   d. hormone receptors.

5. A human cell placed in salty sea water will
   a. burst from water entering the cell.
   b. shrivel and die from water leaving the cell.
   c. not be affected in any way.
   d. break apart from the salt effect.

6. The sodium–potassium pump maintains a negative charge on the cell membrane by
   a. osmosis.
   b. diffusion.
   c. active transport.
   d. facilitated diffusion.

7. All cells progress through basically the same cell cycle, including
   a. two phases.
   b. four active phases and a rest phase.
   c. three periods of rest and a splitting phase.
   d. four active phases.

Multiple Response

Select all that apply.

1. The amount of time that a cell takes to progress through the cell cycle is determined by which of the following?
   a. The acidity of the environment
   b. The genetic makeup of the cell
   c. The location of the cell in the body
   d. The number of ribosomes in the cell
   e. The cell response to contact inhibition
   f. The availability of nutrients and oxygen

2. Some substances will pass into the human cell by simple diffusion. Which of the following substances diffuse into the cell?
   a. Calcium
   b. Nitrogen
   c. Sodium
   d. Carbon dioxide
   e. Oxygen
   f. Potassium

3. Some substances require a channel or pore to enter a cell membrane. Which of the following substances use a channel to enter the cell?
   a. Calcium
   b. Urea
   c. Fat-soluble vitamins
   d. Sodium
   e. Oxygen
   f. Potassium

Matching

Match the phase of the cell cycle with the cell activity during that phase.

1. ____________ G_0 phase
2. ____________ G_1 phase
3. ____________ S phase
4. ____________ G_2 phase
5. ____________ M phase

A. Cell splits to form two identical daughter cells
B. Synthesis of DNA
C. Manufacture of substances needed to form mitotic spindles
D. Synthesis of substances needed for DNA production
E. Resting phase

Word Scramble

Unscramble the following letters to find basic cellular processes.

1. ifsnofidu ____________________
2. ctoyseondsi ____________________
3. ipysonictos ____________________
4. shipgoytacos ____________________
5. smooiss ____________________
6. tosimsi ____________________
7. vissape tatrrsopn ____________________
8. evicat protstran ____________________

Bibliography and References

Fox, S. (1991). *Perspectives on human biology.* Dubuque, IA: Wm. C. Brown.

Ganong, W. (2003). *Review of medical physiology* (21st ed.). Norwalk, CT: Appleton & Lange.

Gilman, A., Hardman, J. G., & Limbird, L. E. (Eds.). (2006). *Goodman and Gilman's the pharmacological basis of therapeutics* (11th ed.). New York: McGraw-Hill.

Guyton, A., & Hall, J. (2000). *Textbook of medical physiology* (10th ed.). Philadelphia: W. B. Saunders.

Porth, C. M. (2005). *Pathophysiology: Concepts of altered health states* (7th ed.). Philadelphia: Lippincott Williams & Wilkins.

CHAPTER 8

Anti-infective Agents

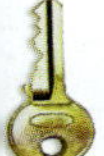

KEY TERMS

culture
prophylaxis
resistance
sensitivity testing
spectrum

LEARNING OBJECTIVES

Upon completion of this chapter, you will be able to:

1. Explain what is meant by selective toxicity.
2. Differentiate between broad-spectrum and narrow-spectrum drugs.
3. Define bacterial resistance to antibiotics.
4. Explain three ways to minimize bacterial resistance.
5. Describe three common adverse reactions associated with the use of antibiotics.

DRUG LIST

bacitracin
chloramphenicol
meropenem
polymyxin B
spectinomycin
vancomycin

Anti-infective agents are drugs that are designed to act selectively on foreign organisms that have invaded and infected the body of a human host. Ideally, these drugs would be toxic to the infecting organisms only and would have no effect on the host cells. In other words, they would possess selective toxicity—the ability to affect certain proteins or enzyme systems that are used by the infecting organism but not by human cells. Although human cells are different from the cells of invading organisms, they are somewhat similar, and no anti-infective drug has yet been developed that does not affect the host.

This chapter focuses on the principles involved in the use of anti-infective therapy. (The effects of anti-infectives on various age groups is discussed in Box 8.1.) The following chapters discuss specific agents that are used to treat particular infections: antibiotics, which are used to treat bacterial infections; antivirals; antifungals; antiprotozoals, which are used to treat infections caused by specific protozoa, including malaria; anthelmintics, which are used to treat infections caused by worms; and antineoplastics, which are used to treat cancers, diseases caused by abnormal cells.

Anti-infective Therapy

For centuries, people used various naturally occurring chemicals in an effort to treat disease. Often this was a random act that proved useful. For instance, the ancient Chinese found that applying moldy soybean curds to boils and infected wounds helped prevent infection or hastened cure. Their finding was, perhaps, a precursor to the penicillins used today.

The use of drugs to treat systemic infections is a relatively new concept. The first drugs used to treat systemic infections were developed in the 1920s. Paul Ehrlich was the first scientist to work on developing a synthetic chemical that would be effective only against infection-causing cells, not human cells. His research led the way for scientific investigation into anti-infective agents. In the late 1920s, scientists discovered penicillin in a mold sample; in 1935, the sulfonamides were introduced. Since then, the number of anti-infectives available for use has grown tremendously. However, many of the organisms that these drugs were designed to treat are rapidly learning to repel the effects of anti-infectives, so much work remains to deal with these emergent strains.

Mechanisms of Action

Anti-infective agents may act on the cells of the invading organisms in several different ways. The goal is interference with the normal function of the invading organism to prevent it from reproducing and to cause cell death without affecting host cells. Various mechanisms of action are briefly described here. The specific mechanism of action for each drug class is discussed in the chapters that follow.

- Some anti-infectives interfere with biosynthesis of the bacterial cell wall. Because bacterial cells have a slightly different composition than human cells, this is an effective way to destroy the bacteria without interfering with the host (Box 8.2). The penicillins work in this way.
- Some anti-infectives prevent the cells of the invading organism from using substances essential to their growth and development, leading to an inability to divide and eventually to cell death. The sulfonamides, the antimycobacterial drugs, and trimethoprim work in this way.

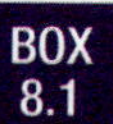

BOX 8.1 DRUG THERAPY ACROSS THE LIFESPAN

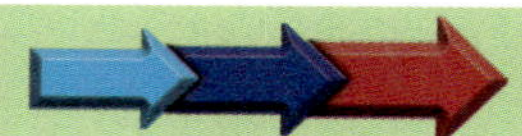

Anti-infective Agents

CHILDREN

Use anti-infectives with caution; early exposure can lead to early sensitivity.

Controversy is widespread regarding the use of antibiotics to treat ear infections, a common pediatric problem. Some believe that the habitual use of antibiotics for what might well be a viral infection has contributed greatly to the development of resistant strains.

Because children can have increased susceptibility to the gastrointestinal and nervous system effects of anti-infectives, monitor hydration and nutritional status carefully.

ADULTS

Adults often demand anti-infectives for a "quick cure" of various signs and symptoms. Drug allergies and the emergence of resistant strains can be a big problem with this group.

Pregnant and nursing women must use extreme caution in the use of anti-infectives. Many of them can affect the unborn baby and also cross into breast milk, leading to toxic effects in the neonate.

OLDER ADULTS

Older patients often do not present with the same signs and symptoms of infection that are seen in younger people.

Culture and sensitivity tests are important to determine the type and extent of many infections.

The older patient is susceptible to severe adverse gastrointestinal, renal, and neurological effects and must be monitored for nutritional status and hydration during drug therapy.

Anti-infectives that adversely affect the liver and kidneys must be used with caution in older patients, who may have decreased organ function.

BOX 8.2 Anti-infective Mechanism: Interference With Cell Wall Synthesis

Bacitracin (*Baci-IM, AK-Tracin, Baciguent*) is an antibiotic that interferes with the cell wall synthesis of susceptible staphylococcal bacteria. Adverse effects include nephrotoxicity and superinfection. Because of the development of resistant strains and more potent antibiotics, bacitracin is now indicated only for the treatment of respiratory infections in infants caused by susceptible staphylococci, treatment of eye infections, prevention of infections in minor skin wounds, and treatment of minor skin infections caused by susceptible strains of staphylococci. Bacitracin is available in intramuscular, ophthalmic, and topical preparations.

Usual Dosage

Infants <2.5 kg: 900 units/kg/day IM in three divided doses; >2.5 kg: 1000 units/kg/day IM in two to three divided doses

Ophthalmic use: ½-inch ribbon to affected eye, b.i.d. to q3–4h

Topical use: apply to affected area one to five times per day

- Many anti-infectives interfere with the steps involved in protein synthesis, a necessary function to maintain the cell and allow for cell division. The aminoglycosides, the macrolides, and chloramphenicol work in this way.
- Some anti-infectives interfere with DNA synthesis in the cell, leading to inability to divide and cell death. The fluoroquinolones work in this way.
- Other anti-infectives alter the permeability of the cell membrane to allow essential cellular components to leak out, causing cell death. Some antibiotics, antifungals, and antiprotozoal drugs work in this manner. These different methods appear in Figure 8.1.

Anti-infective Activity

The anti-infectives that are used today vary in their effectiveness against invading organisms; that is, the **spectrum** of activity varies. Some are so selective in their action that they are effective against only a few microorganisms with a very specific metabolic pathway or enzyme. These drugs are said to have a narrow spectrum of activity (Box 8.3). Other drugs interfere with biochemical reactions in many different kinds of microorganisms, making them useful in the treatment of a wide variety of infections. Such drugs are said to have a broad spectrum of activity.

Some anti-infectives are so active against the infective microorganisms that they actually cause the death of the cells they affect. These drugs are said to be bactericidal. Some anti-infectives are not as aggressive against invading organisms; they interfere with the ability of the cells to reproduce or divide. These drugs are said to be bacteriostatic. Several drugs are both bactericidal and bacteriostatic, often depending on the concentration of the drug that is present. Many of the adverse effects noted with the use of anti-infectives are associated with the aggressive properties of the drugs and their effect on the cells of the host as well as those of the pathogen.

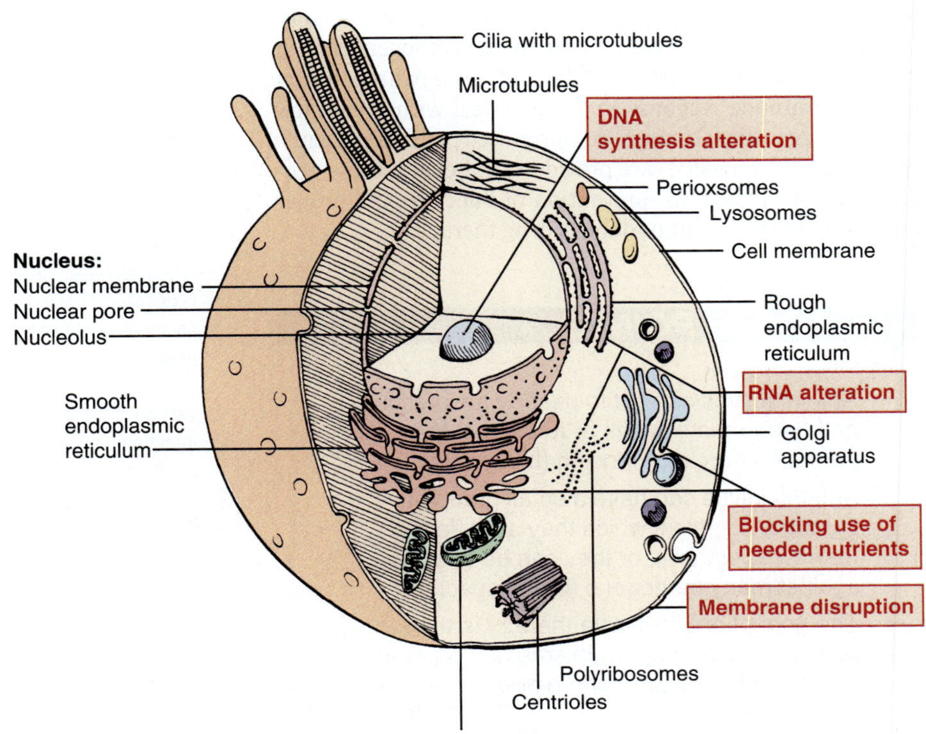

FIGURE 8.1 Anti-infectives can affect cells by disrupting the cell membrane, interfering with DNA synthesis, altering RNA, or blocking the use of essential nutrients.

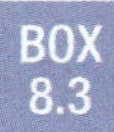

BOX 8.3 Narrow-Spectrum Antibiotic

Spectinomycin (*Trobicin*) is an example of an antibiotic with very specific effects. This drug interferes with protein synthesis, leading to cell death, only in susceptible strains of *Neisseria gonorrhoeae*. Spectinomycin is not known to be effective against any other bacterial species, and its use is limited to the treatment of specific gonococcal infections. The drug is given as one 2-g IM injection, which may be increased to a 4-g IM injection in areas where bacterial resistance is prevalent.

Human Immune Response

The goal of anti-infective therapy is reduction of the population of the invading organism to a point at which the human immune response can take care of the infection. If a drug were aggressive enough to eliminate all traces of any invading pathogen, it might be toxic to the host as well. The immune response (see Chapter 15) involves a complex interaction among chemical mediators, leukocytes, lymphocytes, antibodies, and locally released enzymes and chemicals. When this response is completely functional and all of the necessary proteins, cells, and chemicals are being produced by the body, it can isolate and eliminate foreign proteins, including bacteria, fungi, and viruses. However, if a person is immunocompromised for any reason (e.g., malnutrition, age, acquired immune deficiency syndrome [AIDS], use of immunosuppressant drugs), the immune system may be incapable of dealing effectively with the invading organisms. It is difficult to treat any infections in such patients for two reasons: (1) anti-infective drugs cannot totally eliminate the pathogen without causing severe toxicity in the host, and (2) these patients do not have the immune response in place to deal with even a few invading organisms. Immunocompromised patients present a real challenge to health care providers. In helping these people cope with infections, prevention of infection and proper nutrition are often as important as drug therapy.

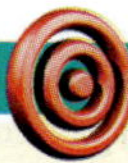

FOCUS POINTS

- Anti-infectives can act to destroy an infective pathogen (bactericidal) or to prevent the pathogen from reproducing (bacteriostatic).
- Anti-infectives can have a small group of pathogens against which they are effective (narrow spectrum), or they can be effective against many pathogens (broad spectrum).
- The goal of anti-infective therapy is the reduction of the invading organisms to a point at which the human immune response can take care of the infection.

Resistance

Because anti-infectives act on specific enzyme systems or biological processes, many microorganisms that do not use that system or process are not affected by a particular anti-infective drug. These organisms are said to have a natural or intrinsic **resistance** to that drug. When prescribing a drug for treatment of an infection, this innate resistance should be anticipated. The selected drug should be one that is known to affect the specific microorganism that is causing the infection.

Since the advent of anti-infective drugs, microorganisms that were once very sensitive to the effects of particular drugs have begun to develop acquired resistance to the agents (Box 8.4). This can result in a serious clinical problem. The emergence of resistant strains of bacteria and other organisms poses a threat: Anti-infective drugs may no longer control potentially life-threatening diseases, and uncontrollable epidemics may occur.

Acquiring Resistance

Microorganisms develop resistance in a number of ways, including the following:

- Producing an enzyme that deactivates the antimicrobial drug. For example, some strains of bacteria that were once controlled by penicillin now produce an enzyme called penicillinase, which inactivates penicillin before it can affect the bacteria. This occurrence led to the development of new drugs that are resistant to penicillinase.

BOX 8.4 Bacterial Resistance to an Anti-infective Drug

Vancomycin (*Vancocin, Vancoled*) is an antibiotic that interferes with cell wall synthesis in susceptible bacteria. It was developed as a result of a need for a drug that could be used both in patients who are intolerant to or allergic to penicillin and/or cephalosporins and in the treatment of patients with staphylococcal infections that no longer respond to penicillin or cephalosporins. This anti-infective drug can be used orally or intravenously to treat life-threatening infections when less toxic drugs cannot be used. It is used orally as prophylaxis against bacterial endocarditis in patients who cannot take penicillins or cephalosporins and to treat staphylococcal infections in people who cannot take these groups of drugs.

Because vancomycin may be highly toxic, its use is reserved for very special situations. It can cause renal failure, ototoxicity, superinfections, and a condition known as "red man syndrome," which is characterized by sudden and severe hypotension, fever, chills, paresthesias, and erythema or redness of the neck and back. When it is the only antibiotic that is effective against a specific bacteria, however, the benefits outweigh the risks.

Usual Dosage

Adult: 500 mg to 1 g PO or IV q6h for 7–10 days

Pediatric: 40 mg/kg/day PO or IV in four divided doses; do not exceed 2 g/day

- Changing cellular permeability to prevent the drug from entering the cell or altering transport systems to exclude the drug from active transport into the cell.
- Altering binding sites on the membranes or ribosomes, which then no longer accept the drug.
- Producing a chemical that acts as an antagonist to the drug.

Most commonly, the development of resistance depends on the degree to which the drug acts to eliminate the invading microorganisms that are most sensitive to its effects. The cells that remain may be somewhat resistant to the effects of the drug, and, with time, these cells form the majority in the population. These cells differ from the general population of the species because of slight variations in their biochemical processes or biochemicals. The drug does not cause a mutation of these cells; it simply allows the somewhat different cells to become the majority or dominant group after elimination of the sensitive cells. Other microbes may develop resistance through actual genetic mutation. A mutant cell survives the effects of an antibiotic and divides, forming a new colony of resistant microbes with a genetic composition that provides resistance to the anti-infective agent.

Preventing Resistance

Because the emergence of resistant strains of microbes is a serious public health problem that continues to grow, health care providers must work together to prevent the emergence of resistant pathogens. Exposure to an antimicrobial agent leads to the development of resistance, so it is important to limit the use of antimicrobial agents to the treatment of specific pathogens known to be sensitive to the drug being used.

Drug dosage is important in preventing the development of resistance. Doses should be high enough and the duration of drug therapy should be long enough to eradicate even slightly resistant microorganisms. The recommended dosage for a specific anti-infective agent takes this issue into account. Around-the-clock dosing eliminates the peaks and valleys in drug concentration and helps maintain a constant therapeutic level to prevent the emergence of resistant microbes during times of low concentration. The duration of drug use is critical to ensure that the microbes are completely, not partially, eliminated and are not given the chance to grow and develop resistant strains. It has proved to be difficult to convince people who are taking anti-infective drugs that the timing of doses and the length of time they continue to take the drug are important. Many people stop taking a drug once they start to feel better and then keep the remaining pills to treat themselves at some time in the future when they do not feel well. This practice favors the emergence of resistant strains. See Box 8.5 for tips on patient education.

Health care providers should also be cautious about the indiscriminate use of anti-infectives. Antibiotics are not effective in the treatment of viral infections or illnesses such as the common cold. However, many patients demand prescriptions for these drugs when they visit practitioners because they are convinced that they need to take something to feel better. Health care providers who prescribe anti-infectives without knowing the causative organism and which drugs might be appropriate are promoting the emergence of resistant strains of microbes. With many serious illnesses, including pneumonias for which the causative organism is suspected, antibiotic therapy may be started as soon as a culture is taken and before the results are known. Health care providers also tend to try newly introduced, more powerful drugs when a more established drug may be just as effective. Use of a powerful drug in this way leads to the rapid emergence of resistant strains to that drug, perhaps limiting its potential usefulness when it might be truly necessary.

BOX 8.5 FOCUS ON **CLINICAL SKILLS**

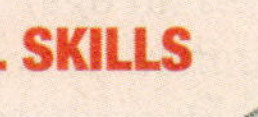

Teaching Patients

When teaching patients who are prescribed an anti-infective agent, it is important to always include some general points:

- This drug is prescribed for treating the particular infection that you have now. Do not use this drug to treat other infections.
- This drug needs to be taken as prescribed—for the correct number of times each day and for the full number of days. Do not stop taking the drug if you start feeling better. You need to take the drug for the full number of treatment days to assure that the infection has been destroyed.

Treatment of Systemic Infections

Many infections that once led to lengthy, organ-damaging, or even fatal illnesses are now managed quickly and efficiently with the use of systemic anti-infective agents. Before the introduction of penicillin to treat streptococcal infections, many people developed rheumatic fever with serious cardiac complications. Today, rheumatic fever and the resultant cardiac valve defects are seldom seen. Several factors should be considered before beginning one of these chemotherapeutic regimens to ensure that the patient obtains the greatest benefit possible with the fewest adverse effects. These factors include identification of the correct pathogen and selection of a drug that is most likely to (1) cause the least complications for that particular patient and (2) be most effective against the pathogen involved.

Identification of the Pathogen

Identification of the infecting pathogen is done by **culture** of a tissue sample from the infected area. Bacterial cultures are performed in a laboratory, where a swab of infected tissue is allowed to grow on an agar plate. Staining techniques and microscopic examination are used to identify the offending bacterium. When investigators search for parasitic sources of infection, stool can be examined for ova and parasites. Microscopic examination of other samples is also used to detect fungal and protozoal infections. The correct identification of the organism causing the infection is an important first step in determining which anti-infective drug should be used.

Sensitivity of the Pathogen

In many situations, health care providers use a broad-spectrum anti-infective agent that has been shown likely to be most effective in treating an infection with certain presenting signs and symptoms. In other cases of severe infection, a broad-spectrum antibiotic is started after a culture is taken but before the exact causative organism has been identified. Again, experience influences selection of the drug, based on the presenting signs and symptoms. In many cases, it is necessary to perform **sensitivity testing** on the cultured microbes. Sensitivity testing shows which drugs are capable of controlling the particular microorganism. This testing is especially important with microorganisms that have known resistant strains. In these cases, culture and sensitivity testing identify the causal pathogen and the most appropriate drug for treating the infection.

Combination Therapy

In some situations, a combination of two or more types of drugs effectively treats the infection. When the offending pathogen is known, combination drugs may be effective in interfering with its cellular structure in different areas or developmental phases.

Combination therapy may be used for several reasons:

- Combination therapy may allow the health care provider to use a smaller dosage of each drug, leading to fewer adverse effects but still having a therapeutic impact on the pathogen.
- Some drugs are synergistic, which means that they are more powerful when given in combination.
- Many microbial infections are caused by more than one organism, and each pathogen may react to a different anti-infective agent.
- Sometimes, the combined effects of the different drugs delay the emergence of resistant strains. This is important in the treatment of tuberculosis (a mycobacterial infection), malaria (a protozoal infection), and some bacterial infections. However, resistant strains seem more likely to emerge when fixed combinations are used over time, at least in some cases. Individualizing the combination seems to be more effective in destroying the pathogen without allowing time for the emergence of strains that are resistant to the drugs.

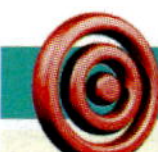

FOCUS POINTS

- Resistance of a pathogen to an anti-infective agent can be natural (the pathogen does not use the process the anti-infective works on) or acquired (the pathogen develops a process to oppose the anti-infective agent).
- The emergence of resistant strains is a serious public health problem.
- Health care providers need to be alert to preventing the emergence of resistant strains by not using antibiotics inappropriately, assuring that the anti-infective is taken at a high enough dose for a long enough period of time, and avoiding the use of newer, powerful anti-infectives if other drugs would be just as effective.
- Culture and sensitivity testing assures that the right drug is used for each infection.

Adverse Reactions to Anti-infective Therapy

Because anti-infective agents affect cells, it is always possible that the host cells will also be damaged (Box 8.6). No anti-infective agent has been developed that is completely free of adverse effects. The most commonly encountered adverse effects associated with the use of anti-infective

BOX 8.6 Serious Adverse Effects of Antibiotic Treatment

Chloramphenicol (*Chloromycetin*), an older antibiotic, prevents bacterial cell division in susceptible bacteria. Because of the potential toxic effects of this drug, its use is limited to serious infections for which no other antibiotic is effective. Chloramphenicol produces a "gray syndrome" in neonates and premature babies, which is characterized by abdominal distention, pallid cyanosis, vasomotor collapse, irregular respirations, and even death. In addition, the drug may cause bone marrow depression, including aplastic anemia that can result in death. These effects are seen even with the use of the ophthalmic and otic forms of the drug. Although the use of chloramphenicol is severely limited, it has stayed on the market because it is used to treat serious infections caused by bacteria that are not sensitive to any other antibiotic. It is available in oral, IV, ophthalmic, and otic forms.

Usual Dosage

Adult or pediatric: 50 mg/kg/day PO or IV in divided doses

Ophthalmic: instill ointment or solution as prescribed

Otic: 2–3 gtt into affected ear t.i.d.

agents are direct toxic effects on the kidney, gastrointestinal (GI) tract, and nervous system. Hypersensitivity reactions and superinfections also can occur.

Kidney Damage

Kidney damage occurs most frequently with drugs that are metabolized by the kidney and then eliminated in the urine. Such drugs, which have a direct toxic effect on the fragile cells in the kidney, can cause conditions ranging from renal dysfunction to full-blown renal failure. When patients are taking these drugs (e.g., aminoglycosides), they should be monitored closely for any sign of renal dysfunction. To prevent any accumulation of the drug in the kidney, patients should be well hydrated throughout the course of the drug therapy.

Gastrointestinal Toxicity

GI toxicity is very common with many of the anti-infectives. Many of these agents have direct toxic effects on the cells lining the GI tract, causing nausea, vomiting, stomach upset, or diarrhea, and such effects are sometimes severe (Box 8.7). There is also some evidence that the death of the microorganisms releases chemicals and toxins into the body, which can stimulate the chemoreceptor trigger zone (CTZ) in the medulla and induce nausea and vomiting.

In addition, some anti-infectives are toxic to the liver. These drugs can cause hepatitis and even liver failure. When patients are taking drugs known to be toxic to the liver (e.g., many of the cephalosporins), they should be monitored closely and the drug should be stopped at any sign of liver dysfunction.

Neurotoxicity

Some anti-infectives can damage or interfere with the function of nerve tissue, usually in areas where drugs tend to accumulate in high concentrations (Box 8.8). For example, the aminoglycoside antibiotics collect in the eighth cranial nerve and can cause dizziness, vertigo, and loss of hearing. Chloroquine, which is used to treat malaria and some other rheumatoid disorders, can accumulate in the retina and optic nerve and cause blindness. Other anti-infectives can cause dizziness, drowsiness, lethargy, changes in reflexes, and even hallucinations when they irritate specific nerve tissues.

Hypersensitivity Reactions

Allergic or hypersensitivity reactions reportedly occur with many antimicrobial agents. Most of these agents, which are protein bound for transfer through the cardiovascular system, are able to induce antibody formation in susceptible people. With the next exposure to the drug, immediate or delayed allergic responses may occur. Some of these drugs have demonstrated cross-sensitivity (e.g., penicillins, cephalosporins), and care must be taken to obtain a complete patient history before administering one of these drugs. It is important to determine what the allergic reaction was and when the patient experienced it (e.g., after first use of drug, after years of use). Some patients report having a drug allergy, but closer investigation indicates that their reaction actually constituted an anticipated effect or a known adverse effect to the drug. Proper interpretation

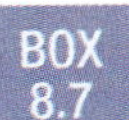

BOX 8.7 Severe Gastrointestinal Toxicity Resulting From Anti-Infective Treatment

Meropenem (*Merrem IV*), an IV antibiotic, inhibits the synthesis of bacterial cell walls in susceptible bacteria. It is used to treat intra-abdominal infections and some cases of meningitis caused by susceptible bacteria. Meropenem almost always causes very uncomfortable gastrointestinal effects; in fact, use of this drug has been associated with potentially fatal pseudomembranous colitis. It also results in headache, dizziness, rash, and superinfections. Because of its toxic effects on gastrointestinal cells, it is used only in those infections with proven sensitivity to meropenem and reduced sensitivity to less toxic antibiotics.

Usual Dosage

Adult: 1 g IV q8h

Pediatric: <3 mo: not recommended; >3 mo: 20–40 mg/kg IV q8h; if >50 kg, 1–2 g IV q8h

Geriatric: lower dose in accordance with creatinine clearance levels

BOX 8.8 Nerve Damage Caused by an Anti-infective Agent

Polymyxin B (generic), an older antibiotic, uses a surfactant-like reaction to enter the bacterial cell membrane and disrupt it, leading to cell death in susceptible gram-negative bacteria. This drug is available for IM, IV, or intrathecal use, as well as an ophthalmic agent for the treatment of infections caused by susceptible bacteria. Because of the actions of polymyxin B on cell membranes, however, it can be toxic to the human host, leading to nephrotoxicity, neurotoxicity (facial flushing, dizziness, ataxia, paresthesias, and drowsiness), and drug fever and rashes. Therefore, it is reserved for use in acute situations when the invading bacteria has been proven to be sensitive to polymyxin B and less sensitive to other, less toxic antibiotics.

Usual Dosage

Adult and pediatric: 15,000–25,000 units/kg/day IV may be divided into two doses *or*

25,000–30,000 units/kg/day IM divided into four to six doses *or*

50,000 units intrathecal daily for 3–4 days, then every other day for at least 2 wk *or*

1–2 gtt ophthalmic preparation in affected eye b.i.d. q4h

of this information is important to allow treatment of a patient with a drug to which the patient reported a supposed allergic reaction but which would be very effective against a known pathogen.

Superinfections

One offshoot of the use of anti-infectives, especially broad-spectrum anti-infectives, is destruction of the normal flora. When the normal flora is destroyed, opportunistic pathogens that were kept in check by the "normal" bacteria have the opportunity to invade tissues and cause infections. These opportunistic infections are called *superinfections*. Common superinfections include vaginal or GI yeast infections, which are associated with antibiotic therapy, and infections caused by *Proteus* and *Pseudomonas* throughout the body, which are a result of broad-spectrum antibiotic use. If patients receive drugs that are known to induce superinfections, they should be monitored closely and the appropriate treatment for any superinfection should be started as soon as possible.

Prophylaxis

Sometimes it is clinically useful to use anti-infectives as a means of **prophylaxis**, to prevent infections before they occur. For example, when patients anticipate traveling to an area where malaria is endemic, they may begin taking antimalarial drugs before the journey and periodically during the trip. Patients who are undergoing GI or genitourinary surgery, which might introduce bacteria from those areas into the system, often have antibiotics ordered immediately after the surgery and periodically thereafter, as appropriate, to prevent infection. Patients with known cardiac valve disease, valve replacements, and other conditions are especially prone to the development of subacute bacterial endocarditis because of the vulnerability of their heart valves. These patients use prophylactic antibiotic therapy as a precaution when undergoing invasive procedures, including dental work. Refer to the American Heart Association's recommended schedule for this prophylaxis.

Points to Remember

- Anti-infectives are drugs designed to act on foreign organisms that have invaded and infected the human host with selective toxicity, which means that they affect biological systems or structures that are found in the invading organisms but not in the host.
- The goal of anti-infective therapy is interference with the normal function of invading organisms to prevent them from reproducing and promotion of cell death without negative effects on the host cells. The infection should be eradicated with the least toxicity to the host and the least likelihood for development of resistance.
- Anti-infectives can work by altering the cell membrane of the pathogen, by interfering with protein synthesis, or by interfering with the ability of the pathogen to obtain needed nutrients.
- Anti-infectives also work to kill invading organisms or to prevent them from reproducing, thus depleting the size of the invasion to one that can be dealt with by the human immune system.
- Pathogens can develop resistance to the effects of anti-infectives over time when (1) mutant organisms that do not respond to the anti-infective become the majority of the pathogen population or (2) the pathogen develops enzymes to block the anti-infectives or alternative routes to obtain nutrients or maintain the cell membrane.
- An important aspect of clinical care involving anti-infective agents is preventing or delaying the development of resistance. This can be done by ensuring that the particular anti-infective agent is the drug of choice for the specific pathogen involved and that it is given in high enough doses for sufficiently long periods to rid the body of the pathogen.
- Culture and sensitivity testing of a suspected infection ensures that the correct drug is being used to treat the infection effectively. Culture and sensitivity testing should be performed before an anti-infective agent is prescribed.
- Anti-infectives can have several adverse effects on the human host, including renal toxicity, multiple GI effects, neurotoxicity, hypersensitivity reactions, and superinfections.
- Some anti-infectives are used as a means of prophylaxis when patients expect to be in situations that will expose them to a known pathogen, such as travel to an area where malaria is endemic, or oral or invasive GI surgery in a person who is susceptible to subacute bacterial endocarditis.

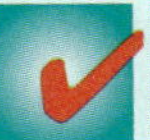

CHECK YOUR UNDERSTANDING

Answers to the questions in this chapter may be found in the Answer Key in the back of the book.

Multiple Choice

Select the best answer to the following.

1. Spectrum of activity of an anti-infective indicates
   a. the acidity of the environment in which they are most effective.
   b. the cell membrane type that the anti-infective affects.
   c. the anti-infective's effectiveness against different invading organisms.
   d. the resistance factor that bacteria have developed to this anti-infective.

2. The emergence of resistant strains of microbes is a serious public health problem. Health care providers can work to prevent the emergence of resistant strains by
   a. encouraging the patient to stop the antibiotic as soon as the symptoms are resolved, to prevent overexposure to the drug.
   b. encouraging the use of antibiotics when patients feel they will help.
   c. limiting the use of antimicrobial agents to the treatment of specific pathogens known to be sensitive to the drug being used.
   d. using the most powerful drug available to treat an infection, to ensure eradication of the microbe.

3. Sensitivity testing of a culture shows
   a. the drugs that are capable of controlling that particular microorganism.
   b. the patient's potential for allergic reactions to a drug.
   c. the offending microorganism.
   d. an immune reaction to the infecting organism.

4. GI toxicity is a very common adverse effect seen with anti-infective therapy. A patient experiencing GI toxicity might complain of
   a. elevated blood urea nitrogen (BUN).
   b. difficulty breathing.
   c. nausea, vomiting, or diarrhea.
   d. yellowish skin or sclera.

5. Superinfections can occur when anti-infective agents destroy the normal flora of the body. *Candida* infections are commonly associated with antibiotic use. A patient with this type of superinfection would exhibit
   a. difficulty breathing.
   b. vaginal discharge or white patches in the mouth.
   c. elevated BUN.
   d. dark lesions on the skin.

6. An example of an anti-infective used as a means of prophylaxis would be
   a. amoxicillin used to treat tonsillitis.
   b. penicillin used to treat an abscess.
   c. an antibiotic used before dental surgery.
   d. norfloxacin used to treat a bladder infection.

7. An important characteristic of any anti-infective drug is
   a. a broad spectrum of activity.
   b. a narrow spectrum of activity.
   c. resistance.
   d. selective toxicity.

Multiple Response

Select all that apply.

1. Bacterial resistance to an anti-infective could be the result of which of the following?
   a. Natural or intrinsic properties of the bacteria
   b. Changes in cellular permeability or cellular transport systems
   c. The production of chemicals that antagonize the drug
   d. Initial exposure to the anti-infective
   e. Combination of too many antibiotics for one infection
   f. Narrow spectrum of activity

2. Anti-infective drugs destroy cells that have invaded the body. They do not specifically destroy only the cell of the invader, and because of this, many adverse effects can be anticipated when an anti-infective is used. Which of the following adverse effects are often associated with anti-infective use?
   a. Superinfections
   b. Hypotension
   c. Renal toxicity
   d. Diarrhea
   e. Loss of hearing
   f. Constipation

Definitions

1. culture ____

____

2. prophylaxis ____

____

3. resistance ____

____

4. selective toxicity ______________________________

____

5. sensitivity testing ______________________________

____

6. spectrum ______________________________

____

Matching

Match the antibiotic with the appropriate description.

1. __________ polymyxin B
2. __________ meropenem
3. __________ chloramphenicol
4. __________ vancomycin
5. __________ spectinomycin
6. __________ bacitracin

A. Can cause potentially fatal pseudomembranous colitis
B. Associated with gray baby syndrome
C. Very toxic to human cells; nephrotoxicity, neurotoxicity common
D. Its use led to development of many resistant strains
E. Used for staphylococci infections in patients who cannot take penicillin or cephalosporins
F. Treatment of specific strains of *Neisseria gonorrhoeae*

Bibliography and References

Cohen, F. L., & Tartasky, D. (1997). Microbial resistance to drug therapy: A review. *American Journal of Infection Control, 25*(1), 51–64.

Degnan, R. (1997). Pharmacology in practice: Antibiotics. *RN, 60*(10), 49–55.

Drug facts and comparisons. (2006). St. Louis: Facts and Comparisons.

Gilman, A., Hardman, J. G., & Limbird, L. E. (Eds.). (2006). *Goodman and Gilman's the pharmacological basis of therapeutics* (11th ed.). New York: McGraw-Hill.

Karch, A. M. (2006). *2007 Lippincott's nursing drug guide.* Philadelphia: Lippincott Williams & Wilkins.

The medical letter on drugs and therapeutics. (2006). New Rochelle, NY: Medical Letter.

Porth, C. M. (2005). *Pathophysiology: Concepts of altered health states* (7th ed.). Philadelphia: Lippincott Williams & Wilkins.

CHAPTER 9

Antibiotics

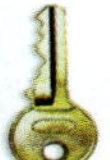

KEY TERMS

aerobic
anaerobic
antibiotic
bactericidal
bacteriostatic
gram negative
gram positive
synergy

LEARNING OBJECTIVES

Upon completion of this chapter, you will be able to:

1. Explain how an antibiotic is selected for use in a particular clinical situation.
2. Describe the therapeutic actions, indications, pharmacokinetics, contraindications, most common adverse reactions, and important drug–drug interactions associated with each of the classes of antibiotics: aminoglycosides, cephalosporins, fluoroquinolones, macrolides, lincosamides, monobactams, penicillins and penicillinase-resistant drugs, sulfonamides, tetracyclines, and antimycobacterials.
3. Discuss the use of antibiotics across the lifespan.
4. Compare and contrast the prototype drugs for each class of antibiotics with the other drugs in that class.
5. Outline the nursing considerations for patients receiving each class of antibiotic.

AMINOGLYCOSIDES

amikacin
P gentamicin
kanamycin
neomycin
streptomycin
tobramycin

CEPHALOSPORINS

P cefaclor
cefadroxil
cefazolin
cefdinir
cefditoren
cefepime
cefmetazole
cefoperazone
cefotaxime
cefotetan
cefoxitin
cefpodoxime
cefprozil
ceftazidime
ceftibuten
ceftizoxime
ceftriaxone
cefuroxime
cephalexin
cephradine
loracarbef

FLUOROQUINOLONES

P ciprofloxacin
gemifloxacin
levofloxacin
lomefloxacin
moxifloxacin
norfloxacin
ofloxacin
sparfloxacin

MACROLIDES

azithromycin
clarithromycin
dirithromycin
P erythromycin

LINCOSAMIDES

P clindamycin
lincomycin

MONOBACTAM ANTIBIOTICS

P aztreonam

PENICILLINS

P amoxicillin
ampicillin
carbenicillin
penicillin G benzathine
penicillin G potassium
penicillin G procaine
penicillin V
ticarcillin

PENICILLINASE-RESISTANT ANTIBIOTICS

nafcillin
oxacillin

SULFONAMIDES

cotrimoxazole
sulfadiazine
P sulfasalazine
sulfisoxazole

TETRACYCLINES

demeclocycline
doxycycline
minocycline
oxytetracycline
P tetracycline

ANTIMYCOBACTERIAL ANTIBIOTICS

Antituberculosis Drugs

capreomycin
cycloserine
ethambutol
ethionamide
P isoniazid
pyrazinamide
rifampin
rifapentine
streptomycin

Leprostatic Drugs

dapsone

OTHER ANTIBIOTICS

daptomycin
ertapenem
linezolid
quinupristin/dalfopristin
telithromycin
tigecycline

Antibiotics are chemicals that inhibit specific bacteria. Those substances that prevent the growth of bacteria are said to be **bacteriostatic**, and those that kill bacteria directly are said to be **bactericidal**. Several antibiotics are both bactericidal and bacteriostatic, depending on the concentration of the particular drug. Antibiotics are used to treat a wide variety of systemic and topical infections. Many new infections appear each year, and researchers are challenged to develop new antibiotics to deal with each new threat. Antibiotics are made in three ways: by living microorganisms, by synthetic manufacture, and in some cases, through genetic engineering. Discussed in this chapter are the major classes of antibiotics: aminoglycosides, cephalosporins, fluoroquinolones, lincosamides, macrolides, monobactams, penicillins and penicillinase-resistant drugs, sulfonamides, tetracyclines, and the disease-specific antimycobacterials, including the antitubercular and leprostatic drugs.

Bacteria and Antibiotics

Bacteria can invade the human body through many routes: for example, respiratory, gastrointestinal (GI), and skin. Once bacteria invade the body, the body becomes the host for the bacteria, supplying nutrients and enzymes that the bacteria need for reproduction. Unchallenged, the invading bacteria can multiply and send out other bacteria to further invade tissue.

The human immune response is activated when bacteria invade. Many of the signs and symptoms of an infection are related to the immune response as the body tries to rid itself of the foreign cells. Fever, lethargy, slow-wave sleep induction, and the classic signs of inflammation (i.e., redness, swelling, heat, and pain) all indicate that the body is responding to an invader.

The goal of antibiotic therapy is to decrease the population of the invading bacteria to a point at which the human immune system can effectively deal with the invader. To determine which antibiotic will effectively treat a specific infection, the causative organism must be identified. Culture and sensitivity testing is performed to identify the invading bacterial species by growing it in the laboratory and then determining the antibiotic to which that particular organism is most sensitive (i.e., which antibiotic best kills or controls the bacteria). Antibiotics have been developed to interfere with specific proteins or enzyme systems, so they are effective only against bacteria that use those proteins or enzymes.

Gram-positive bacteria are those whose cell wall retains a stain, known as Gram's stain, or resists decolorization with alcohol during culture and sensitivity testing. Gram-positive bacteria are commonly associated with infections of the respiratory tract and soft tissues. An example of a gram-positive bacterium is *Streptococcus pneumoniae,* a common cause of pneumonia. In contrast, **gram-negative** bacteria are those whose cell walls lose a stain or are decolorized by alcohol. These bacteria are frequently associated with infections of the genitourinary (GU) or GI tract. An example of a gram-negative bacterium is *Escherichia coli,* a common cause of cystitis. **Aerobic** bacteria depend on oxygen for survival, whereas **anaerobic** bacteria (e.g., those bacteria associated with gangrene) do not use oxygen.

If culture and sensitivity testing is not possible, either because the source of the infection is not identifiable or because the patient is too sick to wait for test results to determine the best treatment, clinicians attempt to administer a drug with a broad spectrum of activity against gram-positive or gram-negative bacteria or against anaerobic bacteria. Antibiotics that interfere with a biochemical reaction common to many organisms are known as broad-spectrum antibiotics. These drugs are often given at the beginning of treatment until the exact organism and sensitivity can be established. Because these antibiotics have such a wide range of effects, they are frequently associated with adverse effects. Human cells have many of the same properties as bacterial cells and can be affected in much the same way, so damage may occur to the human cells as well as the bacterial cells.

In choosing an antibiotic, clinicians also look for a drug with selective toxicity, or the ability to strike foreign cells with little or no effect on human cells. There is no perfect

BOX 9.1 **DRUG THERAPY ACROSS THE LIFESPAN**

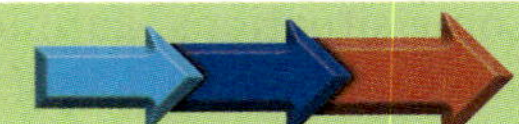

Antibiotics

CHILDREN

Children are very sensitive to the gastrointestinal and central nervous system (CNS) effects of most antibiotics, and more severe reactions can be expected when these drugs are used in children. It is important to monitor the hydration and nutritional status of children who are adversely affected by drug-induced diarrhea, anorexia, nausea, and vomiting. Superinfections can be a problem for small children as well. For example, thrush (oral candidiasis) is a common superinfection that makes eating and drinking difficult.

Many antibiotics do not have proven safety and efficacy in pediatric use, and extreme caution should be used when giving them to children. The fluoroquinolones, for instance, are associated with damage to developing cartilage and are not recommended for growing children.

Pediatric dosages of antibiotics should be double-checked to make sure that the child is receiving the correct dose, thereby improving the chance of eradicating the infection and decreasing the risk of adverse effects.

Antibiotic treatment of ear infections, a common pediatric problem, is controversial. Ongoing research suggests that judicious use of decongestants and anti-inflammatories may be just as successful as the use of antibiotics without the risk of development of resistant bacterial strains.

Parents, not wanting to see their child sick, may demand antibiotics as a cure-all whenever their child is fussy or feverish. Parent education is very important in helping to cut down the unnecessary use of antibiotics in children.

ADULTS

Many adults believe that antibiotics are a cure-all for any discomfort and fever. It is very important to explain that antibiotics are useful against only specific bacteria and actually can cause problems when used unnecessarily for viral infections, such as the common cold.

Adults need to be cautioned to take the entire course of the medication as prescribed and not to store unused pills for future infections or share antibiotics with symptomatic friends.

Pregnant and breast-feeding women should not take antibiotics unless the benefit clearly outweighs the potential risk to the fetus or neonate. Tetracyclines, for example, are associated with pitting of enamel in developing teeth and of calcium deposits in growing bones. These drugs can cause serious problems for neonates. Women of childbearing age should be advised to use barrier contraceptives if any of these drugs are used.

Many antibiotics interfere with the effectiveness of oral contraceptives, and unplanned pregnancies can occur.

OLDER ADULTS

In many instances, older adults do not present with the same signs and symptoms of infections as other patients. Therefore, assessing the problem and obtaining appropriate specimens for culture is especially important with this population.

Older patients may be more susceptible to the adverse effects associated with antibiotic therapy. Their hydration and nutritional status should be monitored closely, as should the need for safety precautions if CNS effects occur. If hepatic or renal dysfunction is expected (particularly in very old patients, those who may depend on alcohol, and those who are taking other hepatotoxic or nephrotoxic drugs), the dosage may need to be lowered and the patient should be monitored more frequently.

Elderly patients also need to be cautioned to complete the full course of drug therapy, even when they feel better, and not to save pills for self-medication at a future time.

antibiotic that is without effect on the human host, and this factor should be considered in antibiotic selection. Because various antibiotics have adverse effects that can be anticipated, they may be contraindicated in some patients, such as those who are immunocompromised, who have severe GI disease, or who are debilitated. (See Box 9.1 for antibiotics' effects across the lifespan.) The antibiotic of choice is one that affects the causative organism and leads to the fewest adverse effects for the patient involved.

In some cases, antibiotics are given in combination to promote **synergy**, so that their combined effect is greater than their effect if they are given individually. Use of synergistic antibiotics allows the patient to take a lower dose of each antibiotic to achieve the desired effect. Another possible benefit of combined therapy is that a lower dose of one of the antibiotics can be used, which helps reduce the adverse effects of that particular drug and makes it more useful in certain clinical situations. Or, one drug may "help" another become more effective (Box 9.2).

BOX 9.2 **Using Combination Drugs to Fight Resistant Bacteria**

Clavulanic acid protects certain beta-lactam antibiotics from breakdown in the presence of penicillinase enzymes.

A combination of amoxicillin and clavulanic acid (*Augmentin*) is commonly used to allow the amoxicillin to remain effective against certain strains of resistant bacteria (usual dosage, 250–500 mg PO q8h for adults or 20–40 mg/kg/day PO in divided doses for children). The theory behind the combination of ticarcillin and clavulanic acid (*Timentin*) is similar (usual dosage 3.1 g IM q4–6h for adults; safety not established for children).

Sulbactam is another drug that increases the effectiveness of antibiotics against certain resistant bacteria. When combined with ampicillin in the drug *Unasyn,* sulbactam inhibits many bacterial penicillinase enzymes, broadening the spectrum of the ampicillin. In this combination, sulbactam is also slightly antibacterial (usual adult dosage, 0.5–1 g sulbactam, with 1–2 g ampicillin IM or IV q6–8h).

In some situations, antibiotics are used as a means of prophylaxis, or prevention of potential infection. Patients who will soon be in a situation that commonly results in a specific infection (e.g., patients undergoing GI surgical procedures, which may introduce GI bacteria into the bloodstream or peritoneum) may be given antibiotics before they are exposed to the bacteria. Usually a large, one-time dose of an antibiotic is given to destroy any bacteria that enter the host immediately and thereby prevent a serious infection.

Bacteria and Resistance to Antibiotics

Bacteria have survived for hundreds of years because they can adapt to their environment. They do this by altering their cell wall or enzyme systems to become resistant to (i.e., protect themselves from) unfavorable conditions or situations. Many species of bacteria have developed resistance to certain antibiotics. For example, bacteria that were once very sensitive to penicillin have developed an enzyme called penicillinase, which effectively inactivates many of the penicillin-type drugs. New drugs had to be developed to effectively treat infections involving these once-controlled bacteria. Because these newer drugs are resistant to penicillinase, they can no longer be inactivated by the bacteria. Other drugs have been developed specifically to treat resistant infections. It is very important to use these drugs only when the identity and sensitivity of the offending bacterium have been established. Indiscriminate use of these new drugs can lead to the development of more resistant strains for which there is no effective antibiotic (Box 9.3).

The longer an antibiotic has been in use, the greater the chance that the bacteria will develop into a resistant strain. Efforts to control the emergence of resistant strains involve intensive education programs that advocate the use of antibiotics only when necessary and effective and not for treatment of viral infections such as the common cold (Box 9.4).

In addition, the use of antibiotics may result in the development of superinfections or overgrowth of resistant pathogens, such as bacteria, fungi, or yeasts, because antibiotics (particularly broad-spectrum agents) destroy bacteria in the flora that normally work to keep these opportunistic invaders in check. When "normal" bacteria are destroyed or greatly reduced in number, there is nothing to prevent the invaders from occupying the host. In most cases the superinfection is an irritating adverse effect (e.g., vaginal yeast infection, candidiasis, diarrhea), but in some cases, the superinfection can be more severe than the infection originally being treated. Treatment of the superinfection leads to new adverse effects and the potential for different superinfections. A vicious cycle of treatment and resistance is the result.

BOX 9.3 Antibiotics Developed Specifically for Treating Resistant Strains

Synercid

A new class of antibiotics, called streptogramins, became available in 1999. Two drugs in this new class, quinupristin and dalfopristin, are available only in a combination form called *Synercid.*

Together, they work synergistically and have been effective in treating vancomycin-resistant enterococci (VRE), resistant *Staphylococcus aureus,* and resistant *Staphylococcus epidermidis.* The drug is approved for VRE and methicillin-sensitive *S. aureus* (MSSA) infections.

The drug also seems to be active against penicillin-resistant pneumococcus. The usual dosage of this drug, for patients 16 years old and older, is 7.5 mg/kg IV q12h for 7 days. The drug should not be used unless the bacterium is clearly identified as being resistant to other antibiotics and sensitive to this one. Indiscriminate use of this new drug can lead to the development of even more invasive and resistant bacteria.

Linezolid

Linezolid (*Zyvox*) was introduced in 2000. This drug is indicated specifically for treatment of infections caused by vancomycin-resistant and methicillin-resistant strains of bacteria. It is available in intravenous and oral forms. The usual adult dosage is 600 mg PO, or it may be administered IV q12h for 10 to 14 days. This drug must also be used cautiously and only when a sensitive bacterial species has been clearly identified. It is the first oral drug approved for the treatment of diabetic foot ulcers. These drugs are part of a wide variety of compounds that are being investigated to deal with the increasing problem of resistant bacteria.

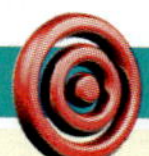

FOCUS POINTS

- The goal of antibiotic therapy is to reduce the population of the invading bacteria to a size that the human immune response can deal with.
- Bacteria can be classified as gram positive (frequently found in respiratory infections) or gram negative (frequently found in GI and GU infections). They can also be classified as anaerobic (not needing oxygen) or aerobic (dependent on oxygen).
- Culture and sensitivity testing assures that the correct antibiotic is chosen for each infection, a practice that may help decrease the number of emerging resistant strain bacteria.

Aminoglycosides

The aminoglycosides (see Table 9.1) are a group of powerful antibiotics used to treat serious infections caused by gram-negative aerobic bacilli. Because most of these drugs have potentially serious adverse effects, newer, less toxic drugs have

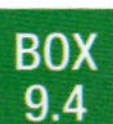

BOX 9.4 FOCUS ON THE **EVIDENCE**

Using Antibiotics Properly

In 2003, the Food and Drug Administration (FDA) and Centers for Disease Control (CDC) joined efforts to educate the public and health care providers about the dangers of inappropriate use of antibiotics. The evidence-based practice guidelines comprise data from many studies to outline the most efficacious use of antibiotics. To review some of the studies, review the references listed in the Bibliography and References section. Nurses should include some of the following points about the risks and dangers of antibiotic abuse in the patient education plan:

- Explain clearly that a particular antibiotic is effective against only certain bacteria and that a culture needs to be taken to identify the bacteria.
- Explain that bacteria can develop resistant strains that will not be affected by antibiotics in the future, so use of antibiotics now may make them less effective in situations in which they are really necessary.
- Ensure that patients understand the importance of taking the full course of medication as prescribed, even if they feel better. Stopping an antibiotic midway through a regimen often leads to the development of resistant bacteria. Using all of the medication will also prevent patients' saving unused medication to self-treat future infections or to share with other family members.
- Tell patients that allergies may develop with repeated exposures to certain antibiotics. In addition, explain to patients that saving antibiotics to take later, when they think they need them again, may lead to earlier development of an allergy, which will negate important tests that could identify the bacteria making them sick.
- Offer other medications, such as antihistamines, decongestants, or even chicken soup, to patients who request antibiotics; this may satisfy their need for something to take. Explaining that viral infections do not respond to antibiotics usually offers little consolation to patients who are suffering from a cold or the flu.

The publicity that many emergent, resistant strains of bacteria have received in recent years may help to get the message across to patients about the need to take the full course of an antibiotic and to use antibiotics only when they are the appropriate. To view the educational program developed by the FDA and the CDC for use with patients and the data behind these efforts, go to http://www.cdc.gov/drugresistance/community/.

replaced aminoglycosides in the treatment of less serious infections.

Amikacin (*Amikin*) is available for short-term intramuscular (IM) or intravenous (IV) use for serious gram-negative infections. The potential for nephrotoxicity and ototoxicity with amikacin is very high, so the drug is used only as long as absolutely necessary.

Gentamicin (*Garamycin*) is available in many forms: ophthalmic, topical, IV, intrathecal, impregnated beads on surgical wire, and liposomal injection. It covers a wide variety of infections, including pseudomonal diseases and once-rare infections seen in patients with acquired immune deficiency syndrome (AIDS).

Kanamycin (*Kantrex*), which is available in parenteral and oral forms, is used to treat hepatic coma when ammonia-producing bacteria in the GI tract cause serious illness. It is also used as an adjunctive therapy to decrease GI bacterial flora. Kanamycin should not be used for longer than 7 to 10 days because of its potential toxic effects, which include renal damage, bone marrow depression, and GI complications.

Neomycin (*Mycifradin*) is a slightly milder aminoglycoside that is used to suppress GI bacteria preoperatively and to treat hepatic coma. In topical form, neomycin is used to treat skin wounds and infections.

Streptomycin (generic), once a popular drug, is very toxic to the eighth cranial nerve and kidney. Today it is used as the fourth drug in combination therapy for tuberculosis. It can be used in severe infections if the organism has been shown to be sensitive to streptomycin and no less-toxic drugs can be used.

Tobramycin (*Nebcin, Tobrex*) is used for short-term IM or IV treatment of very serious infections. This drug is also available in an ophthalmic form for the treatment of ocular infections caused by susceptible bacteria.

Therapeutic Actions and Indications

The aminoglycosides are bactericidal. They inhibit protein synthesis in susceptible strains of gram-negative bacteria, which in turn leads to loss of functional integrity of the bacterial cell membrane, causing cell death (Figure 9.1). These drugs are used to treat serious infections caused by susceptible strains of gram-negative bacteria, including *Pseudomonas aeruginosa, E. coli, Proteus* species, the *Klebsiella–Enterobacter–Serratia* group, *Citrobacter* species, and *Staphylococcus* species such as *S. aureus*. Aminoglycosides are indicated for the treatment of serious infections that are susceptible to penicillin when penicillin is contraindicated, and they can be used in severe infections before culture and sensitivity tests have been completed.

Pharmacokinetics

The aminoglycosides are poorly absorbed from the GI tract but rapidly absorbed after IM injection, reaching peak levels within 1 hour. They are widely distributed throughout the body, crossing the placenta and entering breast milk. They should be used with great caution during pregnancy and lactation because of potential toxic effects on the fetus or neonate. Aminoglycosides are excreted unchanged in the urine and have an average half-life of 2 to 3 hours. Urine function should be tested daily when these drugs are used because they depend on the kidney for excretion and are toxic to the kidney; renal function can change daily while a patient is receiving the drug.

Table 9.1 DRUGS IN FOCUS

Aminoglycosides

Drug Name	Dosage/Route	Usual Indication
amikacin (*Amikin*)	15 mg/kg/day IM or IV divided into two or three equal doses; reduce dosage in renal failure	Treatment of serious gram-negative infections
P gentamicin (*Garamycin*)	Adult: 3 mg/kg/day IM or IV in three equal doses q8h; reduce dosage in renal failure Pediatric: 2–2.5 mg/kg/day q8h IV or IM	Treatment of Pseudomonas infections and a wide variety of gram-negative infections
kanamycin (*Kantrex*)	7.5 mg/kg q12h IM or 15 mg/kg/day IV divided into two to three equal doses given slowly	Treatment of hepatic coma and to decrease GI normal flora
neomycin (*Mycifradin*)	Adult: 15 mg/kg/day in divided doses q6h IM Pediatric: 50–100 mg/kg/day in divided doses PO for hepatic coma; do not use IM	Suppression of GI normal flora preoperatively; treatment of hepatic coma; topical treatment of skin wounds
streptomycin (*generic*)	Adult: 1–2 g/day IM in divided doses q6–12h Pediatric: 20–40 mg/kg/day IM in divided doses q6–12h	Fourth drug in combination therapy regimen for tuberculosis; treatment of severe infections with sensitive organisms
tobramycin (*Nebcin, Tobrex*)	Adult: 3 mg/kg/day in three equal doses IM or IV q8h; reduce dosage in renal failure Pediatric: 6–7.5 mg/kg/day in three to four equal doses q6–8h IV or IM	Short-term IV or IM treatment of serious infections; ocular infections caused by susceptible bacteria

Contraindications and Cautions

Aminoglycosides are contraindicated in the following conditions: known allergy to any of the aminoglycosides; renal or hepatic disease *that could be exacerbated by toxic aminoglycoside effects and that could interfere with drug metabolism and excretion, leading to higher toxicity;* pre-existing hearing loss, *which could be intensified by toxic drug effects on the auditory nerve;* active infection with herpes or mycobacterial infections *that could be worsened by the effects of an aminoglycoside on normal defense mechanisms;* myasthenia gravis or parkinsonism, *which often are*

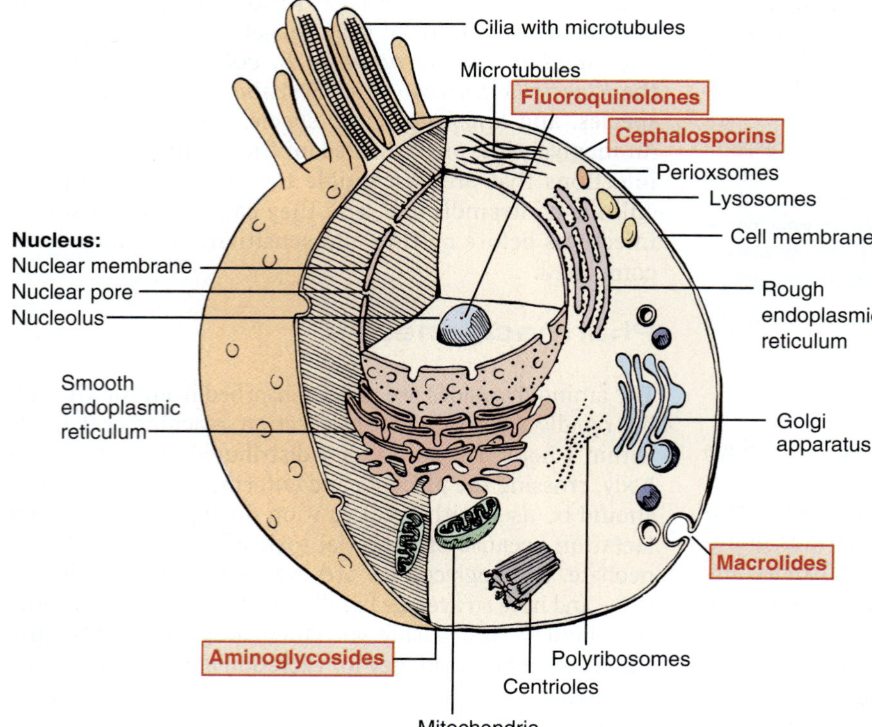

FIGURE 9.1 Sites of cellular action of aminoglycosides, cephalosporins, fluoroquinolones, and macrolides. Aminoglycosides disrupt the cell membrane. Cephalosporins cause bacteria to build weak cell walls when dividing. Fluoroquinolones interfere with the DNA enzymes needed for growth and reproduction. Macrolides change protein function by binding to the cell membrane to cause cell death or prevent cell division.

exacerbated by the effects of a particular aminoglycoside on the nervous system; lactation, *because aminoglycosides are excreted in breast milk and potentially could cause serious effects in the baby.* Caution should be used during pregnancy *because aminoglycosides are used to treat only severe infections, and the benefits of the drug should be carefully weighed against potential adverse effects on the fetus.*

Adverse Effects

The many serious adverse effects associated with aminoglycosides limit their usefulness. Central nervous system (CNS) effects include ototoxicity, possibly leading to irreversible deafness; vestibular paralysis resulting from drug effects on the auditory nerve; confusion; depression; disorientation; and numbness, tingling, and weakness related to drug effects on other nerves.

Renal toxicity, which may progress to renal failure, is caused by direct drug toxicity in the glomerulus, meaning that the drug molecules cause damage (e.g., obstruction) directly to the kidney. Bone marrow depression may result from direct drug effects on the rapidly dividing cells in the bone marrow, leading, for example, to immune suppression and resultant superinfections.

GI effects include nausea, vomiting, diarrhea, weight loss, stomatitis, and hepatic toxicity. These effects are a result of direct GI irritation, loss of bacteria of the normal flora with resultant superinfections, and toxic effects in the mucous membranes and liver as the drug is metabolized.

Cardiac effects can include palpitations, hypotension, and hypertension. Hypersensitivity reactions include purpura, rash, urticaria, and exfoliative dermatitis.

Clinically Important Drug–Drug Interactions

If aminoglycosides are taken in combination with potent diuretics, the incidence of ototoxicity, nephrotoxicity, and neurotoxicity increases. This combination should be avoided if at all possible.

If these antibiotics are given with anesthetics, nondepolarizing neuromuscular blockers, succinylcholine, or citrate anticoagulated blood, increased neuromuscular blockade with paralysis is possible. If a patient who has been receiving an aminoglycoside requires surgery, the fact that the aminoglycoside has been given should be indicated prominently on the chart. After surgery, the patient will require extended monitoring and support.

In addition, most aminoglycosides have a synergistic bactericidal effect when given with penicillins, cephalosporins, carbenicillin, or ticarcillin. In certain conditions, this synergism is used therapeutically to increase the effectiveness of treatment.

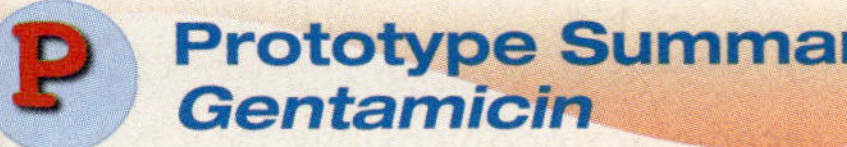

Indications: Treatment of serious infections caused by susceptible bacteria

Actions: Inhibits protein synthesis in susceptible strains of gram-negative bacteria, disrupting functional integrity of the cell membrane and causing cell death

Pharmacokinetics:

Route	Onset	Peak
IM, IV	Rapid	30–90 min

$T_{1/2}$: 2–3 hours; metabolized in the liver and excreted in the urine

Adverse effects: Sinusitis, dizziness, rash, fever, risk of nephrotoxicity

Nursing Considerations for Patients Receiving Aminoglycosides

Assessment: History and Examination

Screen for the following, *which are possible contraindications or cautions for use of the drug:* known allergy to any aminoglycoside (obtain specific information about the nature and occurrence of allergic reactions); history of renal or hepatic disease; preexisting hearing loss; active infection with herpes, vaccinia, varicella, or fungal or mycobacterial organisms; myasthenia gravis; parkinsonism; infant botulism; and current pregnancy or lactation status.

Physical assessment should be performed *to establish baseline data for assessing the effectiveness of the drug and the occurrence of any adverse effects associated with drug therapy.* Perform culture and sensitivity tests at the site of infection. Conduct orientation and reflex assessment as well as auditory testing *to evaluate any CNS effects of the drug.* Also assess vital signs: respiratory rate and adventitious sounds *to monitor for signs of infection or hypersensitivity reactions;* temperature *to assess for signs and symptoms of infection;* blood pressure *to monitor for cardiovascular effects of the drug.* Renal and hepatic function tests should be done *to determine baseline function of these organs and, possibly, the need to adjust dosage.*

Nursing Diagnoses

Patients who receive aminoglycosides may have the following nursing diagnoses related to drug therapy:

- Acute Pain related to GI, CNS effects of drug
- Disturbed Sensory Perception (Auditory) related to CNS effects of drug
- Risk for Infection related to bone marrow suppression
- Excess Fluid Volume related to nephrotoxicity
- Deficient Knowledge regarding drug therapy

Implementation With Rationale

- Check culture and sensitivity reports *to ensure that this is the drug of choice for this patient.*
- Ensure that the patient receives the full course of the aminoglycoside as prescribed, divided around the clock, *to increase effectiveness and decrease the risk for development of resistant strains of bacteria.*
- Monitor the site of infection and presenting signs and symptoms (e.g., fever, lethargy) throughout the course of drug therapy. *Failure of these signs and symptoms to resolve may indicate the need to reculture the site.* Arrange to continue drug therapy for at least 2 days after all signs and symptoms resolve.
- Monitor the patient regularly for signs of nephrotoxicity, neurotoxicity, and bone marrow suppression *to effectively arrange for discontinuation of drug or decreased dosage, as appropriate, if any of these toxicities occurs.*
- Provide safety measures *to protect the patient if CNS effects, such as confusion, disorientation, or numbness and tingling occur.*
- Provide small, frequent meals as tolerated; frequent mouth care; and ice chips or sugarless candy to suck if stomatitis and sore mouth are problems *to relieve discomfort. Also provide adequate fluids to replace fluid lost with diarrhea, if appropriate.*
- Ensure that the patient is hydrated at all times during drug therapy *to minimize renal toxicity from drug exposure.*
- Ensure that the patient is instructed about the appropriate dosage regimen and possible adverse effects *to enhance patient knowledge about drug therapy and to promote compliance.*

The patient should:

- Take safety precautions, such as changing position slowly and avoiding driving and hazardous tasks, if CNS effects occur.
- Try to drink a lot of fluids and to maintain nutrition (very important) even though nausea, vomiting, and diarrhea may occur.
- Avoid exposure to other infections (e.g., crowded areas, people with known infectious diseases).
- Report difficulty breathing, severe headache, loss of hearing or ringing in the ears, or changes in urine output to the health care provider.

Evaluation

- Monitor patient response to the drug (resolution of bacterial infection).
- Monitor for adverse effects (orientation and affect, hearing changes, bone marrow suppression, renal toxicity, hepatic dysfunction, GI effects).
- Evaluate the effectiveness of the teaching plan (patient can name drug, dosage, possible adverse effects to watch for, and specific measures to help avoid adverse effects).
- Monitor the effectiveness of comfort and safety measures and compliance with the therapeutic regimen.

Cephalosporins

The cephalosporins were first introduced in the 1960s. These drugs are similar to the penicillins in structure and in activity. Over time, four generations of cephalosporins have been introduced, each group with its own spectrum of activity, described in the following text and in Table 9.2).

First-generation cephalosporins are largely effective against the same gram-positive bacteria that are affected by penicillin G, as well as the gram-negative bacteria *Proteus mirabilis, E. coli,* and *Klebsiella pneumoniae* (*PEcK;* use these letters as a mnemonic device to remember which bacteria are susceptible to the first-generation cephalosporins).

Second-generation cephalosporins are effective against those strains, as well as *Haemophilus influenzae, Enterobacter aerogenes,* and *Neisseria* species. (Remember *HENPeCK.*) The second-generation drugs are less effective against gram-positive bacteria.

Third-generation cephalosporins are relatively weak against gram-positive bacteria but are more potent against the gram-negative bacilli as well, as *Serratia marcescens.* (Remember *HENPeCKS.*)

Fourth-generation cephalosporins are in development. The first drug of this group, cefepime (*Maxipime*), is active against gram-negative and gram-positive organisms, including cephalosporin-resistant staphylococci and *P. aeruginosa.*

Table 9.2 DRUGS IN FOCUS

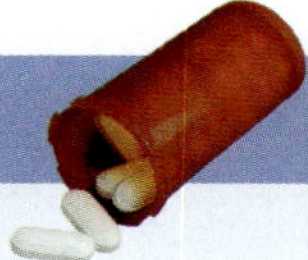

Cephalosporins

Drug Name	Dosage/Route	Usual Indications
First-Generation Cephalosporins		
cefadroxil (*Duricef*)	Adult: 1–2 g PO in a single or two divided doses; reduce dosage in renal impairment Pediatric: 30 mg/kg/day PO in divided doses q12h	Indicated for urinary tract infections (UTIs), pharyngitis, and tonsillitis caused by group A beta-hemolytic streptococci as well as skin infections
cefazolin (*Ancef, Zolicef*)	Adult: 250–500 mg IM or IV q4–8h; reduce dosage in renal impairment Pediatric: 25–50 mg/kg/day IM or IV in three or four divided doses	Respiratory tract, skin, GU, biliary tract, bone, joint, and myocardial infections as well as sepsis
cephalexin (*Keflex, Biocef*)	Adult: 250 mg PO q.i.d. Pediatric: 25–50 mg/kg/day PO in divided doses	Respiratory, skin, bone, and GU infections; used for otitis media in children
cephradine (*Velosef*)	Adult: 250–500 mg PO q6–12h; reduce dosage in renal impairment Pediatric: 25–100 mg/kg/day PO in divided doses q4–6h	Respiratory tract, skin, GU, biliary tract, bone, joint, and myocardial infections as well as sepsis and osteomyelitis; useful in situations in which a switch from parenteral to oral route is expected (e.g., preoperative prophylaxis followed by oral postoperative prophylaxis)
Second-Generation Cephalosporins		
P cefaclor (*Ceclor*)	Adult: 250 mg PO q8h—do not exceed 4 g/day; must be taken every 8–12 h around the clock Pediatric: 20 mg/kg/day PO in divided doses q8h; do not exceed 1 g/day	Respiratory tract infections, skin infections, UTIs, otitis media, typhoid fever, anthrax exposure
cefmetazole (*Zefazone*)	Adult: 2 g IV q6h for 5–14 days; reduce dosage in renal impairment Pediatric: safety not established	Used for severe infections; preoperative prophylaxis for cesarean section and abdominal, vaginal, biliary, or colorectal surgery
cefoxitin (*Mefoxin*)	Adult: 1–2 g IM or IV q6–8h; reduce dosage with renal impairment Pediatric: 80–160 mg/kg/day IM or IV in divided doses q4–6h	Used for severe infections; preoperative prophylaxis for cesarean section and abdominal, vaginal, biliary or colorectal surgery; more effective in gynecological and intra-abdominal infections than some other agents
cefprozil (*Cefzil*)	Adult: 250–500 mg PO q12h for 10 days—reduce dosage with renal impairment Pediatric: 7.5–20 mg/kg PO q12h for 10 days; for child 6 mo to 2 yr of age, 15 mg/kg PO q12h for 10 days	Pharyngitis, tonsillitis, otitis media, sinusitis, secondary bronchial infections, and skin infections
cefuroxime (*Ceftin, Zinacef*)	Adult: 250 mg PO b.i.d.; 750 mg to 1.5 g IM q8h; reduce dosage with renal impairment Pediatric: 125 mg PO b.i.d.; 50–100 mg/kg/day IM or IV in divided doses q6–8h	Wide range of infections, as listed for other second-generation drugs; also used to treat Lyme disease and preferred in situations involving an anticipated switch from parenteral to oral drug use
loracarbef (*Lorabid*)	Adult: 200–400 mg PO q12h; reduce dosage with renal impairment Pediatric: 15–30 mg/kg/day in divided doses q12h PO; should be taken every 12 hours for 7–14 days	Pharyngitis, tonsillitis, otitis media, sinusitis, UTIs, secondary bronchial infections, and skin infections
Third-Generation Cephalosporins		
cefdinir (*Omnicef*—a suspension form is available for children)	Adult: 300 mg PO q12h for 10 days; reduce dosage with renal impairment Pediatric: 7 mg/kg PO q12h	Respiratory infections, otitis media, sinusitis, laryngitis, bronchitis, skin infections
cefoperazone (*Cefobid*)	Adult: 2–4 g/day IM or IV in divided doses q12h; reduce dosage with hepatic impairment Pediatric: safety not established	Moderate to severe skin, urinary tract, and respiratory tract infections; pelvic inflammatory disease; intra-abdominal infections; peritonitis; septicemia
cefotaxime (*Claforan*)	Adult: 2–8 g/day IM or IV in divided doses q6–8h; reduce dosage with renal impairment Pediatric: 50–180 mg/kg/day IM or IV in divided doses q4–6h	Moderate to severe skin, urinary tract, and respiratory tract infections; pelvic inflammatory disease; intra-abdominal infections; peritonitis; septicemia; bone infections; CNS infections; preoperative prophylaxis
cefpodoxime (*Vantin*)	Adult: 100–400 mg PO q12h; reduce dosage with renal impairment Pediatric: 5 mg/kg PO q12h for 7–14 days	Respiratory infections, UTIs, gonorrhea, skin infections, and otitis media

(continued)

Table 9.2 DRUGS IN FOCUS *(Continued)*

Cephalosporins

Drug Name	Dosage/Route	Usual Indications
ceftazidime (*Ceptaz, Tazicef*)	Adult: 1 g q8–12h IM or IV; reduce dosage with renal impairment Pediatric: 30–50 mg/kg q8–12h IM or IV	Moderate to severe skin, urinary tract, and respiratory tract infections; intra-abdominal infections; septicemia; bone infections; CNS infections
ceftibuten (*Cedax*—available in a suspension form for children)	Adult: 400 mg PO every day for 10 days; reduce dosage with renal impairment Pediatric: 9 mg/kg/day PO for 10 days *Note*: once-a-day dosing increases compliance	Pharyngitis, tonsillitis, exacerbations of bronchitis, otitis media
ceftizoxime (*Cefizox*)	Adult: 1–2 g IM or IV q8–12h; reduce dosage with renal impairment Pediatric: 50 mg/kg IM or IV q6–8h	Respiratory, gynecological, pelvic inflammatory, intra-abdominal, skin, and bone and joint infections; also used for sepsis and meningitis
ceftriaxone (*Rocephin*)	Adult: 1–2 g/day IM or IV in divided doses b.i.d.–q.i.d. Pediatric: 50–75 mg/kg/day IV or IM in divided doses q12h	Moderate to severe skin, urinary tract, and respiratory tract infections; pelvic inflammatory disease; intra-abdominal infections; peritonitis; septicemia; bone infections; CNS infections; preoperative prophylaxis; unlabeled use for treatment of Lyme disease
Fourth-Generation Cephalosporins		
cefditoren (*Spectracef*)	Adult and Pediatric (>12 yr): 200–400 mg PO b.i.d.; reduce dosage with renal impairment	Acute exacerbations of chronic bronchitis; pharyngitis and tonsillitis; skin and skin structure infections
cefepime (*Maxipime*)	Adult: 0.5–2 g IM or IV q12h; must be injected for greatest effectiveness q12h for 7–10 days; reduce dosage with renal impairment Pediatric: 50 mg/kg per dose q12h IV or IM for 7–10 days	Moderate to severe skin, urinary tract, and respiratory tract infections

Therapeutic Actions and Indications

The cephalosporins are both bactericidal and bacteriostatic, depending on the dose used and the specific drug involved. In susceptible species, these agents basically interfere with the cell wall-building ability of bacteria when they divide; that is, they prevent the bacteria from biosynthesizing the framework of their cell walls. The bacteria with weakened cell walls swell and burst as a result of the osmotic pressure within the cell (see Figure 9.1).

Cephalosporins are indicated for the treatment of infections caused by susceptible bacteria. Selection of an antibiotic from this class depends on the sensitivity of the involved organism, the route of choice, and sometimes the cost involved. It is important to reserve cephalosporins for appropriate situations because cephalosporin-resistant bacteria are appearing in increasing numbers. Before therapy begins, a culture and sensitivity test should always be performed to evaluate the causative organism and appropriate sensitivity to the antibiotic being used.

Pharmacokinetics

The following cephalosporins are well absorbed from the GI tract: first-generation drugs cefadroxil, cephalexin, cephradine; second-generation drugs cefaclor, cefprozil, cefuroxime, and loracarbef; third-generation drugs cefdinir, cefpodoxime, and ceftibuten; and fourth-generation cefditoren and cefepime. The others are absorbed well after IM injection or IV administration. (Box 9.5 provides calculation practice using cefdinir.)

The cephalosporins are primarily metabolized in the liver and excreted in the urine. Caution must be used in patients with hepatic or renal impairment because either condition could alter drug metabolism and excretion. These drugs cross the placenta and enter breast milk. They should be used

BOX 9.5 FOCUS ON CALCULATIONS

Your patient is a 20-kg child with a severe case of tonsillitis. An order is written for cefdinir (*Omnicef*) 14 mg/kg/day PO for 10 days. The drug comes in an oral suspension 125 mg/mL. What should you administer at each dose?

The order is for 14 mg/kg, so 14 mg/kg × 20 kg = 280 mg. The available form is 125 mg/mL. Using the formula:

$$\frac{\text{amount of drug available}}{\text{volume available}} = \frac{\text{amount of drug prescribed}}{\text{volume to administer}}$$

$$\frac{125\ \text{mg}}{1\ \text{mL}} = \frac{280\ \text{mg}}{X}$$

$$125\ \text{mg}/X = 280\ \text{mg/mL}$$

$$X = \frac{280\ \text{mg/mL}}{125\ \text{mg}}$$

$$X = 2.24\ \text{mL}$$

during pregnancy and lactation only if the benefits clearly outweigh the potential risk of toxicity to the fetus or neonate.

Contraindications and Cautions

These drugs should not be used in patients with known allergies to cephalosporins or penicillins *because cross-sensitivity is common.* In addition, caution must be used in patients with renal failure because *the drugs are toxic to the kidneys,* and in pregnant or lactating patients because *potential effects on the baby are not known.*

Adverse Effects

The most common adverse effects of the cephalosporins involve the GI tract and include nausea, vomiting, diarrhea, anorexia, abdominal pain, and flatulence (common). Pseudomembranous colitis, a potentially dangerous disorder, has also been reported with some cephalosporins. A particular drug should be discontinued immediately at any sign of violent, bloody diarrhea or abdominal pain.

CNS symptoms include headache, dizziness, lethargy, and paresthesias. Nephrotoxicity is also associated with the use of cephalosporins, most particularly in patients who have a predisposing renal insufficiency. Other adverse effects include superinfections, which occur frequently because of the death of protective bacteria of the normal flora. Patients receiving parenteral cephalosporins should also be monitored for the possibility of phlebitis with IV administration or local abscess at the site of an IM injection.

Clinically Important Drug–Drug Interactions

The concurrent administration of cephalosporins with aminoglycosides increases the risk of nephrotoxicity. Patients who receive this combination should be monitored frequently, including evaluation of serum blood urea nitrogen (BUN) and creatinine levels.

Patients who receive oral anticoagulants in addition to cephalosporins may experience increased bleeding. They should be taught how to monitor for blood loss (e.g., bleeding gums, easy bruising) and should be aware that the dose of the oral anticoagulant may need to be reduced.

When a patient consumes alcohol while receiving cephalosporins or up to 72 hours after discontinuation of the drug, in many cases a disulfiram-like reaction occurs. A disulfiram-like reaction causes unpleasant symptoms such as flushing, throbbing headache, nausea and vomiting, chest pain, palpitations, dyspnea, syncope, vertigo, blurred vision, and, in extreme reactions, cardiovascular collapse, convulsions, or even death. Patients should be warned about this possible reaction and urged to refrain from drinking beverages or medications containing alcohol for 72 hours after the drug is stopped.

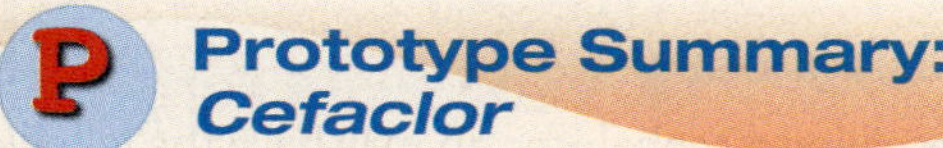

Prototype Summary: Cefaclor

Indications: Treatment of respiratory, dermatological, urinary tract, and middle ear infections caused by susceptible strains of bacteria

Actions: Inhibits the synthesis of bacterial cell walls, causing cell death in susceptible bacteria

Pharmacokinetics:

Route	Peak	Duration
Oral	30–60 min	8–10 h

$T_{1/2}$: 30–60 min; excreted unchanged in the urine

Adverse effects: Nausea, vomiting, diarrhea, rash, superinfection, bone marrow depression, risk for pseudomembranous colitis

Nursing Considerations for Patients Receiving Cephalosporins

Assessment: History and Examination

Screen for the following, *which are possible contraindications or cautions for use of the drug:* known allergy to any cephalosporin, penicillin, or any other allergens *because cross-sensitivity often occurs* (obtain specific information about the nature and occurrence of the allergic reactions); history of renal disease, *which could exacerbate nephrotoxicity related to the cephalosporin;* and current pregnancy or lactation status.

Physical assessment should be performed *to establish baseline data for assessing the effectiveness of the drug and the occurrence of any adverse effects associated with drug therapy.* Perform culture and sensitivity tests at the site of infection. Examine skin for any rash or lesions *to provide a baseline for possible adverse effects.* Note respiratory status—including rate, depth, and adventitious sounds—*to provide a baseline.* Check renal function test results, including BUN and creatinine clearance, *to assess the status of renal functioning and to detect the possible need to alter dosage.* Examine injection sites *to provide a baseline for determining adverse reactions or abscess formation.*

Nursing Diagnoses

Patients receiving a cephalosporin may have the following nursing diagnoses related to drug therapy:

- Acute Pain related to GI, CNS effects of drug
- Risk for Infection related to repeated injections
- Deficient Fluid Volume and Imbalanced Nutrition: Less Than Body Requirements, related to diarrhea
- Deficient Knowledge regarding drug therapy

Implementation With Rationale

- Check culture and sensitivity reports *to ensure that this is the drug of choice for this patient.*
- Monitor renal function test values before and periodically during therapy *to arrange for appropriate dosage reduction as needed.*
- Ensure that the patient receives the full course of the cephalosporin as prescribed, divided around the clock *to increase effectiveness and to decrease the risk of development of resistant strains.*
- Monitor the site of infection and presenting signs and symptoms (e.g., fever, lethargy) throughout the course of drug therapy. *Failure of these signs and symptoms to resolve may indicate the need to reculture the site.* Arrange to continue drug therapy for at least 2 days after the resolution of all signs and symptoms.
- Provide small, frequent meals as tolerated, frequent mouth care, and ice chips or sugarless candy to suck if stomatitis and sore mouth are problems *to relieve discomfort and provide nutrition, and adequate fluids to replace fluid lost with diarrhea.*
- Monitor patient for any signs of superinfection *to arrange for treatment if superinfection occurs.*
- Monitor injection sites regularly *to provide warm compresses and gentle massage to injection sites if painful or swollen.* If signs of phlebitis occur, remove IV line and reinsert in a different vein.
- Initiate safety measures, including adequate lighting, siderails on the bed, and assistance with ambulation *to protect the patient from injury if CNS effects occur.*
- Be sure to instruct the patient about the appropriate dosage schedule and about possible side effects *to enhance patient knowledge about drug therapy and to promote compliance.*

The patient should:

- Take safety precautions, including changing position slowly and avoiding driving and hazardous tasks, if CNS effects occur.
- Try to drink a lot of fluids and to maintain nutrition (very important) even though nausea, vomiting, and diarrhea may occur.
- Report difficulty breathing, severe headache, severe diarrhea, dizziness, or weakness to the health care provider.
- Avoid consuming alcoholic beverages while receiving cephalosporins and for at least 72 hours after completing the drug course because serious side effects could occur.

Evaluation

- Monitor patient response to the drug (resolution of bacterial infection).
- Monitor for adverse effects (orientation and affect; renal toxicity; hepatic dysfunction; GI effects; and local irritation, including phlebitis at injection and IV sites).
- Evaluate the effectiveness of the teaching plan (patient can name drug, dosage, possible adverse effects to expect, and specific measures to help avoid adverse effects).
- Monitor the effectiveness of comfort and safety measures and the patient's compliance with the regimen.

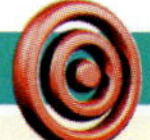

FOCUS POINTS

- Aminoglycosides inhibit protein synthesis in susceptible strains of gram-negative bacteria. They are reserved for use in serious infections because of potentially serious adverse effects.
- Monitor the patient on aminoglycosides for ototoxicity, renal toxicity, GI disturbances, bone marrow depression, and superinfections.
- Cephalosporins are a large group of antibiotics, similar to penicillin, that are effective against a wide range of bacteria.
- Monitor the patient on cephalosporins for GI upsets and diarrhea, pseudomembranous colitis, headache, dizziness, and superinfections.

Fluoroquinolones

The fluoroquinolones (Table 9.3) are a relatively new class of antibiotics with a broad spectrum of activity. These drugs, which are all made synthetically, are associated with relatively mild adverse reactions. The most widely

Table 9.3 DRUGS IN FOCUS

Fluoroquinolones

Drug Name	Dosage/Route	Usual Indication
P ciprofloxacin (*Cipro*)	Adult: 100–500 mg b.i.d. PO for up to 6 wk; reduce dosage in renal failure Pediatric: not recommended because of potential effects on developing cartilage	Treatment of infections caused by a wide spectrum of gram-negative bacteria
gemifloxacin (*Factive*)	Adult: 320 mg/day PO for 5–7 days	Treatment of acute exacerbations of chronic bronchitis, community-acquired pneumonia
levofloxacin (*Levaquin*)	Adult: 250–500 mg/day PO or IV; reduce dosage in renal impairment After exposure to anthrax: 500 mg/day PO or IV for 60 days	Treatment of respiratory, urinary tract, skin, and sinus infections caused by susceptible gram-negative bacteria in adults; treatment after exposure to anthrax
lomefloxacin (*Maxaquin*)	Adult: 400 mg/day PO for 10–14 days; reduce dosage with renal impairment	Treatment of lower respiratory tract and urinary tract infections in adults; preoperative and postoperative prophylaxis for transurethral prostate biopsies
moxifloxacin (*Avelox*)	Adult: 400 mg/day PO for 5–10 days; reduce dosage in renal impairment	Treatment of adults with sinusitis, bronchitis, or community-acquired pneumonia
norfloxacin (*Noroxin*)	Adult: 400 mg PO q12h for up to 28 days; reduce dosage in renal impairment	Treatment of various urinary tract infections
ofloxacin (*Floxin, Ocuflox*)	Adult: 200–400 mg q12h PO or IV for up to 10 days; reduce dosage in renal impairment	Treatment of respiratory, skin, and urinary tract infections; pelvic inflammatory disease; ocular infections; otic form available for otitis media
sparfloxacin (*Zagam*)	Adult: 400 mg PO on day 1, then 200 mg/day PO; reduce dosage in renal impairment	Treatment of community-acquired pneumonia and chronic bronchitis

used fluoroquinolone is ciprofloxacin (*Cipro*), which is effective against a wide spectrum of gram-negative bacteria. It is available in injectable, oral, and topical forms. In 2001 it was approved for prevention of anthrax infection in areas that might be exposed to germ warfare. It is also effective against typhoid fever.

Gemifloxacin (*Factive*) is an oral agent that is used for the treatment of acute exacerbations of chronic bronchitis and for treating community-acquired pneumonia.

Levofloxacin (*Levaquin*), which is available in oral and IV forms, may be used to treat respiratory, urinary tract, skin, and sinus infections caused by susceptible gram-negative bacteria. Because of its parenteral availability, it may be preferred for severe infections or for use when the patient cannot take oral drugs.

Lomefloxacin (*Maxaquin*) is an oral drug that can be used to treat lower respiratory tract infections, as well as many urinary tract infections. It is the drug of choice for preoperative and postoperative prophylaxis to prevent urinary tract infections after transurethral procedures or transrectal prostate biopsies.

Moxifloxacin (*Avelox*), an oral agent, is used to treat sinusitis, bronchitis, and pneumonia in adults.

Norfloxacin (*Noroxin*) is recommended only for treatment of various urinary tract infections caused by susceptible gram-negative bacteria.

Ofloxacin (*Floxin, Ocuflox*) can be given IV or orally to treat respiratory, skin, and urinary tract infections, as well as pelvic inflammatory disease. In addition, this drug is available as an ophthalmic agent for the treatment of ocular infections caused by susceptible bacteria.

Sparfloxacin (*Zagam*) is an oral agent used to treat community-acquired pneumonia and acute bronchitis caused by susceptible bacteria. Strains that have become resistant to the very frequently used ciprofloxacin may still be sensitive to these fluoroquinolones.

Therapeutic Actions and Indications

The fluoroquinolones enter the bacterial cell by passive diffusion through channels in the cell membrane. Once inside, they interfere with the action of DNA enzymes necessary for the growth and reproduction of the bacteria (see Figure 9.1). This leads to cell death because the bacterial DNA is damaged and the cell cannot be maintained. At the moment, the fluoroquinolones have the advantage of a unique way of disrupting bacterial activity. There is little cross-resistance with other forms of antibiotics. However, misuse of these drugs in the short time the class has been available has led to the existence of resistant strains of bacteria. Because so many resistant strains are emerging, infected tissue should always be cultured to determine the exact bacterial cause and sensitivity. These drugs have been associated with lesions in developing cartilage and therefore are not recommended for use in children younger than 18 years of age.

The fluoroquinolones are indicated for treating infections caused by susceptible strains of gram-negative bacteria, including *E. coli, P. mirabilis, K. pneumoniae, Enterobacter cloacae, Proteus vulgaris, Proteus rettgeri, Morganella morganii, Moraxella catarrhalis, H. influenzae, H. parainfluenzae, P. aeruginosa, Citrobacter freundii, S. aureus, Staphylococcus epidermidis,* some *Neisseria gonorrhoeae,* and group D streptococci. These infections frequently include urinary tract, respiratory tract, and skin infections.

Pharmacokinetics

The fluoroquinolones are absorbed from the GI tract, metabolized in the liver, and excreted in the urine and feces. Caution must be used in patients with renal or hepatic impairment, which could interfere with the metabolism and excretion of the drugs. They are widely distributed in the body. The fluoroquinolones cross the placenta and enter breast milk; they should be used during pregnancy and lactation only if the benefit outweighs the potential risk to the fetus or neonate.

Contraindications and Cautions

Fluoroquinolones are contraindicated in patients with known allergy to any fluoroquinolone and in pregnant or lactating women *because the drugs have unknown effects on fetuses and infants.* Caution should be used in the presence of renal dysfunction, *which could interfere with drug excretion,* and seizures, *which could be exacerbated by the drugs' effects on cell membrane channels.*

Adverse Effects

Several adverse effects are associated with fluoroquinolones. The most common are headache, dizziness, insomnia, and depression related to possible effects on the CNS membranes. GI effects include nausea, vomiting, diarrhea, and dry mouth, related to direct drug effect on the GI tract and possibly to stimulation of the chemoreceptor trigger zone (CTZ) in the CNS.

Immunological effects include bone marrow depression, which may be related to drug effects on the cells of the bone marrow that rapidly turn over. Other adverse effects include fever, rash, and photosensitivity, a potentially serious adverse effect that can cause severe skin reactions. Patients should be advised to avoid sun and ultraviolet light exposure and to use protective clothing and sunscreens.

Clinically Important Drug–Drug Interactions

When fluoroquinolones are taken concurrently with iron salts, sucralfate, mineral supplements, or antacids, the therapeutic effect of the fluoroquinolone is decreased. If this drug combination is necessary, administration of the two agents should be separated by at least 4 hours.

If fluoroquinolones are taken with drugs that increase the QTc interval or cause torsades de pointes (quinidine, procainamide, amiodarone, sotalol, erythromycin, terfenadine, pentamidine, tricyclics, phenothiazines), severe to fatal cardiac reactions are possible. These combinations should be avoided, but if they must be used, patients should be hospitalized with continual cardiac monitoring.

Combining fluoroquinolones with theophylline leads to increased theophylline levels because the two drugs use similar metabolic pathways. The theophylline dose should be decreased by one half, and serum theophylline levels should be monitored carefully. In addition, when fluoroquinolones are combined with nonsteroidal anti-inflammatory drugs (NSAIDs), an increased risk of CNS stimulation is possible. If this combination is used, patients should be monitored closely, especially those who have a history of seizures or CNS problems.

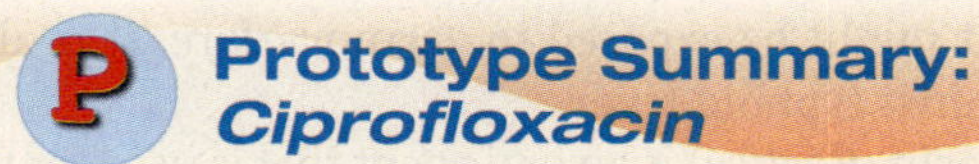

Indications: Treatment of respiratory, dermatological, urinary tract, ear, eye, bone, and joint infections; treatment after anthrax exposure, typhoid fever

Actions: Interferes with DNA replication in susceptible gram-negative bacteria, preventing cell reproduction

Pharmacokinetics:

Route	Onset	Peak	Duration
Oral	Varies	60–90 min	4–5 h
IV	10 min	30 min	4–5 h

$T_{1/2}$: 3.5–4 hours; metabolized in the liver, excreted in bile and urine

Adverse effects: Headache, dizziness, hypotension, nausea, vomiting, diarrhea, fever, rash

Nursing Considerations for Patients Receiving Fluoroquinolones

Assessment: History and Examination

Screen for the following, *which are possible contraindications or cautions for use of the drug:* known allergy to any fluoroquinolone (obtain specific information about the nature and occurrence of allergic reactions); history of renal disease, *which could interfere with excretion of the drug;* and current pregnancy or lactation status *because of potential adverse effects on the fetus or infant.*

Physical assessment should be performed *to establish baseline data for assessing the effectiveness of the drug and the occurrence of any adverse effects associated with drug therapy.* Perform culture and sensitivity tests at the site of infection. Examine the skin for any rash or lesions *to provide a baseline for possible adverse effects.* Conduct assessment of orientation, affect, and reflexes *to establish a baseline for any CNS effects of the drug.* Perform renal function tests, including BUN and creatinine clearance, *to evaluate the status of renal functioning and to assess necessary changes in dosage.*

Nursing Diagnoses

The patient receiving a fluoroquinolone may have the following nursing diagnoses related to drug therapy:

- Acute Pain related to GI, CNS, skin effects of drug
- Deficient Fluid Volume and Imbalanced Nutrition: Less Than Body Requirements, related to GI effects of drug
- Deficient Knowledge regarding drug therapy

Implementation With Rationale

- Check culture and sensitivity reports *to ensure that this is the drug of choice for this patient.*
- Monitor renal function tests before initiating therapy *to appropriately arrange for dosage reduction if necessary.*
- Ensure that the patient receives the full course of the fluoroquinolone as prescribed *to eradicate the infection and to help prevent the emergence of resistant strains.*
- Monitor the site of infection and presenting signs and symptoms (e.g., fever, lethargy, urinary tract signs and symptoms) throughout the course of drug therapy. *Failure of these signs and symptoms to resolve may indicate the need to reculture the site.* Arrange to continue drug therapy for at least 2 days after resolution of all signs and symptoms.
- Provide small, frequent meals as tolerated, frequent mouth care, and ice chips or sugarless candy to suck if dry mouth is a problem *to relieve discomfort and provide nutrition, and adequate fluids to replace those lost with diarrhea.*
- Implement safety measures, including adequate lighting, use of siderails, and assistance with ambulation *to protect patient from injury if CNS effects occur.*
- Ensure that the patient receives instructions about the appropriate dosage schedule and possible adverse effects *to enhance patient knowledge about drug therapy and to promote compliance.*

The patient should:

- Take safety precautions, including changing position slowly and avoiding driving and hazardous tasks, if CNS effects occur.
- Try to drink a lot of fluids and to maintain nutrition (very important), although nausea, vomiting, and diarrhea may occur.
- Avoid ultraviolet light and sun exposure, using protective clothing and sunscreens.
- Report difficulty breathing, severe headache, severe diarrhea, severe skin rash, fainting spells, and heart palpitations to the health care provider.

Evaluation

- Monitor patient response to the drug (resolution of bacterial infection).
- Monitor for adverse effects (orientation and affect, GI effects, photosensitivity).
- Evaluate the effectiveness of the teaching plan (patient can name drug, dosage, possible adverse effects to expect, and specific measures to help avoid adverse effects).
- Monitor the effectiveness of comfort and safety measures and compliance with the therapeutic regimen.

Macrolides

The macrolides are antibiotics that interfere with protein synthesis in susceptible bacteria. The macrolides include the following drugs (see also Table 9.4).

Erythromycin (*Ery-Tab, Eryc,* and others), the first macrolide to be developed, proved to be a good alternative for patients

Table 9.4 DRUGS IN FOCUS

Macrolides

Drug Name	Dosage/Route	Usual Indication
azithromycin (*Zithromax*)	Adult: 500 mg PO as a single dose on day 1, then 250 mg/day PO to a total dose of 1.5 g Pediatric: 10 mg/kg PO as a single dose on day 1, then 5 mg/kg PO on days 2–5	Treatment of mild to moderate respiratory infections and urethritis in adults and otitis media and pharyngitis/tonsillitis in children
clarithromycin (*Biaxin*)	Adult: 250–500 mg q12h PO for 7–14 days; reduce dosage with renal impairment Pediatric: 15 mg/kg/day PO given q12h for 10 days	Treatment of various respiratory, skin, sinus, and maxillary infections; effective against mycobacteria
dirithromycin (*Dynabac*)	Adults and Pediatric (>12 yr): 500 mg/day PO for 5–14 days Pediatric: (<12 yr): safety not established	Treatment of respiratory tract and skin infections
P erythromycin (*Ery-Tab, Eryc*)	Adult: 15–20 mg/kg/day IV or PO Pediatric: 30–50 mg/kg/day PO in divided doses	Treatment of infections in people allergic to penicillin, Legionnaire's disease, infections caused by *Corynebacterium diphtheriae*, ureaplasma species, syphilis, mycoplasma pneumonias, and chlamydial infections

who were allergic to penicillins. It is the drug of choice for the treatment of Legionnaire's disease, infections caused by *Corynebacterium diphtheriae,* ureaplasma, syphilis, mycoplasmal pneumonias, and chlamydial infections. It is readily absorbed from the GI tract and is metabolized in the liver with excretion mainly in the bile to feces. The half-life of erythromycin is 1.6 hours. It crosses the placenta and enters breast milk; it therefore should be used during pregnancy and lactation only if the benefit clearly outweighs the risk to the fetus or the neonate.

Azithromycin (*Zithromax*) is used for treating mild to moderate respiratory infections and urethritis in adults and is effective in treating otitis media, pharyngitis, and tonsillitis in children. It is absorbed from the GI tract and mainly excreted unchanged in the urine, making it necessary to monitor renal function when a patient is taking this drug. The half-life of azithromycin is 68 hours, making it useful for patients who have trouble remembering to take pills since it can be given once a day. It crosses the placenta and enters breast milk and therefore should be used during pregnancy and lactation only if the benefit clearly outweighs the risk to the fetus or neonate.

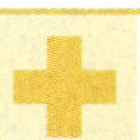

FOCUS ON PATIENT SAFETY

Many antibiotics used to treat childhood infections, such as otitis media and other upper respiratory infections (URIs), come in an oral suspension, suitable for children. The order for these solutions is usually written in teaspoons for the convenience of the parent who will be dispensing the medication. It is very important to make sure that the parent understands that the teaspoon in the prescription refers to a measuring teaspoon (5 mL). Inadvertent overdoses have been reported when parents used a flatware teaspoon to measure out the child's dose. Flatware teaspoons vary greatly in volume. If a parent calls to report that the medicine is all gone on day 4 and it was supposed to be given for 7 days, check to see how the medicine is being measured. Teaching the parent when the drug is first ordered can prevent problems during the course of treatment.

Clarithromycin (*Biaxin*) is an expensive oral agent that is effective in treating several respiratory, skin, sinus, and maxillary infections. In addition, it is effective against mycobacteria. It is readily absorbed from the GI tract and is metabolized in the liver for excretion in the urine. It is necessary to monitor renal function when a patient is taking this drug because it is excreted by the renal system. The half-life of clarithromycin is 3 to 7 hours. It crosses the placenta and enters breast milk and therefore should be used during pregnancy and lactation only if the benefit clearly outweighs the risk to the fetus or neonate.

Dirithromycin (*Dynabac*) is effective in treating susceptible upper and lower respiratory tract infections, skin infections, and pharyngitis/tonsillitis. It is absorbed from the GI tract, being converted from the prodrug dirithromycin to erythromycylamine in the intestinal wall. Most of the drug is excreted through the feces. It has a half-life of 2 to 36 hours. It also has the advantage of once-a-day dosing, which increases compliance in many cases. Dirithromycin crosses the placenta and enters breast milk; it should be used during pregnancy and lactation only if the benefit clearly outweighs the risk to the fetus or neonate.

Therapeutic Actions and Indications

The macrolides, which may be bactericidal or bacteriostatic, exert their effect by binding to the bacterial cell membrane and changing protein function (see Figure 9.1). This action can prevent the cell from dividing or cause cell death, depending on the sensitivity of the bacteria and the concentration of the drug.

Macrolides are indicated for treatment of the following conditions: acute infections caused by susceptible strains of *S. pneumoniae, Mycoplasma pneumoniae, Listeria monocytogenes,* and *Legionella pneumophila;* infections caused by group A beta-hemolytic streptococci; pelvic inflammatory disease caused by *N. gonorrhoeae;* upper respiratory tract infections caused by *H. influenzae* (with sulfonamides); infections caused by *C. diphtheriae* and *Corynebacterium minutissimum* (with antitoxin); intestinal amebiasis; and infections caused by *Chlamydia trachomatis.*

In addition, macrolides may be used as prophylaxis for endocarditis before dental procedures in patients with valvular heart disease who are allergic to penicillin. Topical macrolides are indicated for the treatment of ocular infections caused by susceptible organisms and for acne vulgaris, and they may also be used prophylactically against infection in minor skin abrasions and for the treatment of skin infections caused by sensitive organisms.

Contraindications and Cautions

Macrolides are contraindicated in patients with a known allergy to any macrolide *because cross-sensitivity occurs.* Ocular preparations are contraindicated for viral, fungal, or mycobacterial infections of the eye, *which could be exacerbated by loss of bacteria of the normal flora.* Caution should be used in patients with hepatic dysfunction *that could alter the metabolism of the drug;* in those with renal disease *that could interfere with the excretion of some of the drug;* in lactating women *because macrolides secreted in breast milk can cause diarrhea and superinfections in the infant;* and in pregnant women *because of potential adverse effects on the developing fetus.*

Adverse Effects

Relatively few adverse effects are associated with the macrolides. The most frequent ones, which involve the direct effects of the drug on the GI tract, are often uncomfortable enough to limit the use of the drug. These include abdominal cramping, anorexia, diarrhea, vomiting, and pseudomembranous colitis. Other effects include neurological symptoms such as confusion, abnormal thinking, and uncontrollable emotions, which could be related to drug effects on the CNS membranes; hypersensitivity reactions ranging from rash to anaphylaxis; and superinfections related to the loss of normal flora.

Clinically Important Drug–Drug Interactions

Increased serum levels of digoxin occur when digoxin is taken concurrently with macrolides. Patients who receive both drugs should have their digoxin levels monitored and dosage adjusted during and after treatment with the macrolide.

In addition, when oral anticoagulants, theophyllines, carbamazepine, or corticosteroids are administered concurrently with macrolides, the effects of these drugs reportedly increase as a result of metabolic changes in the liver. Patients who take any of these combinations may require reduced dosage of the particular drug and careful monitoring.

When cycloserine is taken with macrolides, increased serum levels of cycloserine have occurred, with a resultant risk of renal toxicity. This combination should be avoided if at all possible.

Clinically Important Drug–Food Interactions

Food in the stomach decreases the absorption of oral macrolides. Therefore, the antibiotic should be given on an empty stomach, 1 hour before or at least 2 to 3 hours after meals. A macrolide should be taken with a full, 8-oz glass of water.

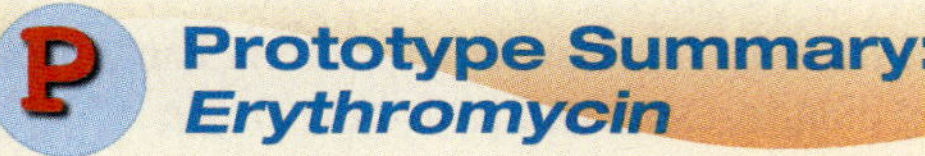

Prototype Summary: *Erythromycin*

Indications: Treatment of respiratory, dermatological, urinary tract, and GI infections caused by susceptible strains of bacteria

Actions: Binds to cell membranes causing a change in protein function and cell death; can be bacteriostatic or bactericidal

Pharmacokinetics:

Route	Onset	Peak
Oral	1–2 h	1–4 h
IV	Rapid	1 h

$T_{1/2}$: 3–5 hours; metabolized in the liver, excreted in bile and urine

Adverse effects: Abdominal cramping, vomiting, diarrhea, rash, superinfection, liver toxicity, risk for pseudomembranous colitis, potential for hearing loss

Nursing Considerations for Patients Receiving Macrolides

Assessment: History and Examination

Screen for the following, *which are possible contraindications or precautions for use of the drug:* known allergy to any macrolide (obtain specific information about the nature and occurrence of allergic reactions); history of liver disease *that could interfere with metabolism of the drug;* and current pregnancy or lactation status *because of potential adverse effects on the fetus or infant.*

Physical assessment should be performed *to establish baseline data for assessing the effectiveness of the drug and the occurrence of any adverse effects associated with drug therapy.* Obtain specimens for culture and sensitivity testing from the site of infection. Examine the skin for any rash or lesions *to provide a baseline for possible adverse effects.* Monitor temperature *to detect infection.* Conduct assessment of orientation, affect, and reflexes *to establish a baseline for any CNS effects of the drug.* Assess liver and renal function test values *to determine the status of renal and liver functioning and to determine any needed alteration in dosage.*

Nursing Diagnoses

The patient receiving a macrolide may have the following nursing diagnoses related to drug therapy:

- Acute Pain related to GI or CNS effects of the drug
- Risk for Infection related to potential for superinfections
- Deficient Knowledge regarding drug therapy

Implementation With Rationale

- Check culture and sensitivity reports *to ensure that this is the drug of choice for this patient.*
- Monitor hepatic and renal function test values before therapy begins *to arrange to reduce dosage as needed.*
- Ensure that the patient receives the full course of the macrolide as prescribed *to eradicate the infection and to help prevent the emergence of resistant strains.*
- Monitor the site of infection and presenting signs and symptoms (e.g., fever, lethargy, urinary tract signs and symptoms) throughout the course of drug therapy. *Failure of these signs and symptoms to resolve may indicate the need to reculture the site.* Arrange to continue drug therapy for at least 2 days after all signs and symptoms resolve.
- Provide small, frequent meals as tolerated *to ensure adequate nutrition with GI upset;* frequent mouth care and ice chips or sugarless candy to *suck to provide relief of discomfort if dry mouth is a problem;* and adequate fluids *to replace fluid lost with diarrhea.*
- Ensure ready access to bathroom facilities *to assist patients with problems associated with diarrhea.*
- Institute safety measures *to protect patient from injury if CNS effects occur.*
- Arrange for appropriate treatment of superinfections as needed *to decrease severity of infection and complications.*
- Ensure patient instruction about the appropriate dosage regimen and possible adverse effects *to enhance patient knowledge about drug therapy and to promote compliance.*

The patient should:

- Take safety precautions, including changing position slowly and avoiding driving and hazardous tasks, if CNS effects occur.
- Try to drink a lot of fluids and to maintain nutrition (very important) even though nausea, vomiting, and diarrhea may occur.
- Report difficulty breathing, severe headache, severe diarrhea, severe skin rash, and mouth or vaginal sores to a health care provider.

Evaluation

- Monitor patient response to the drug (resolution of bacterial infection).
- Monitor for adverse effects (orientation and affect, GI effects, superinfections).
- Evaluate the effectiveness of the teaching plan (patient can name the drug, dosage, possible adverse effects to expect, and specific measures to help avoid adverse effects).
- Monitor the effectiveness of comfort and safety measures and compliance with the regimen.

Lincosamides

The lincosamides (see Table 9.5) are similar to the macrolides but are more toxic. The lincosamides react at almost the same site in bacterial protein synthesis and are effective against the same strains of bacteria (Figure 9.2).

Clindamycin (*Cleocin*) is reserved for severe infections caused by the same strains of bacteria that are susceptible to macrolides. The drug is rapidly absorbed from the GI tract or from IM injections. Clindamycin has a half-life of 2 to 3 hours; it is metabolized in the liver and excreted in the urine and feces. Caution needs to be used in patients with hepatic or renal impairment, which could interfere with the metabolism and excretion of the drug. The drug crosses the placenta and enters breast milk; it should be used during pregnancy and lactation only if the benefit clearly outweighs the risk to the fetus or neonate. GI reactions, which are often severe, limit the usefulness of clindamycin. Severe pseudomembranous colitis has occurred as a result of treatment. However, for a serious infection caused by a susceptible bacterium, clindamycin may be the

Table 9.5 DRUGS IN FOCUS

Lincosamides

Drug Name	Dosage/Route	Usual Indications
clindamycin (*Cleocin*)	Adult: 150–300 mg PO q6h or 600–2700 mg/day in two to four equal doses; reduce dosage with renal impairment Pediatric: 8–25 mg/kg/day PO or 15–40 mg/kg/day IM or IV in three to four divided doses	Treatment of severe infections when penicillin or other less toxic antibiotics cannot be used
lincomycin (*Lincocin*)	Adult: 500 mg PO q6–8h, 600 mg IM q12–24h, or 600 mg to 1 g q8–12h; reduce dosage with renal impairment Pediatric: 30–60 mg/kg/day PO in three to four divided doses, 10 mg/kg IM q12–24h, or 10–20 mg/kg/day IV in divided doses	Treatment of severe infections when penicillin or other less toxic antibiotics cannot be used

drug of choice. It is available in parenteral and oral forms, as well as in topical and vaginal forms for the treatment of local infections.

Lincomycin (*Lincocin*) is indicated to treat severe infections when penicillin cannot be given and other, less toxic antibiotics, such as the macrolides, cannot be used. It is rapidly absorbed from the GI tract or from IM injections. Lincomycin is metabolized in the liver and excreted in the urine and feces. It has a half-life of 5 hours. Caution needs to be used in patients with hepatic or renal impairment, which could interfere with the metabolism and excretion of the drug. The drug crosses the placenta and enters breast milk; it should be used during pregnancy and lactation only if the benefit clearly outweighs the risk to the fetus or neonate. Severe GI reactions, including fatal pseudomembranous colitis, have occurred. Some other toxic effects that limit the usefulness of this drug are pain, skin infections, and bone marrow depression. Nursing care of patients taking these drugs is the same as for those taking macrolides, with additional precautions that include careful monitoring of GI activity and fluid balance and stopping the drug at the first sign of severe or bloody diarrhea.

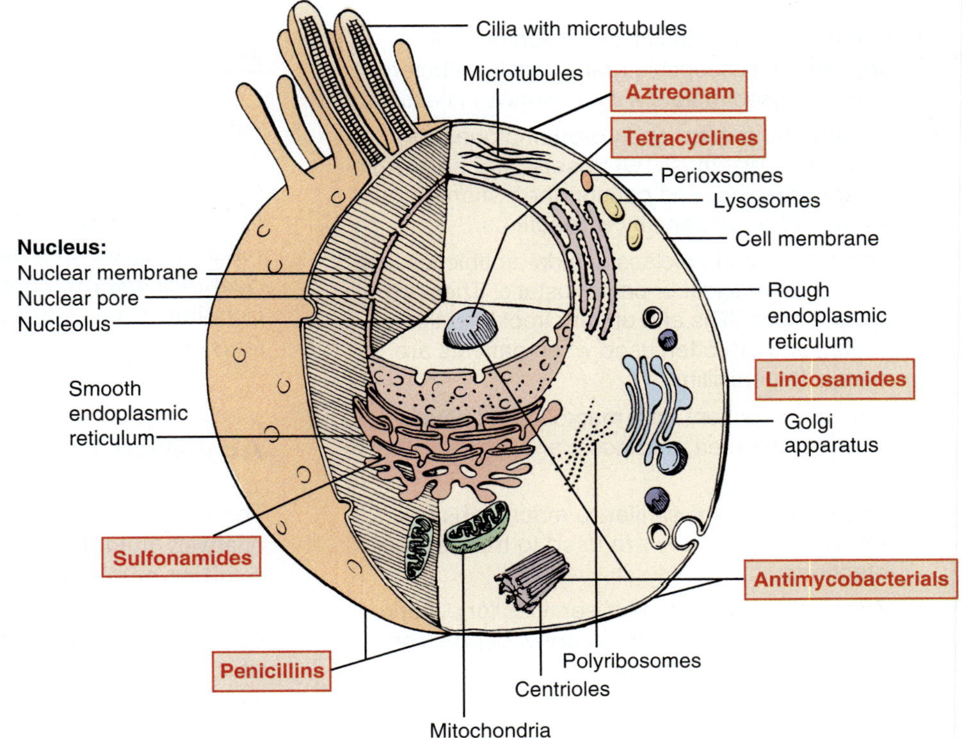

FIGURE 9.2 Sites of cellular action of lincosamides, aztreonam, penicillins, sulfonamides, tetracyclines, and antimycobacterial drugs. Lincosamides change protein function and prevent cell division or cause cell death. Aztreonam alters cell membranes to allow leakage of intracellular substances and causes cell death. Penicillins prevent bacteria from building their cells during division. Sulfonamides inhibit folic acid synthesis for RNA and DNA production. Tetracyclines inhibit protein synthesis, thereby preventing reproduction. Antimycobacterial drugs affect mycobacteria in three ways: They (1) affect the mycotic coat of the bacteria, (2) alter DNA and RNA, and (3) prevent cell division.

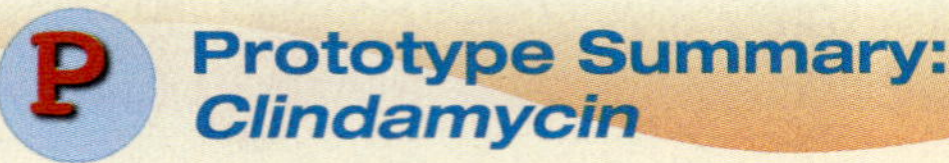

Prototype Summary: Clindamycin

Indications: Treatment of serious infections caused by susceptible strains of bacteria including some anaerobes; useful in septicemia and chronic bone and joint infections

Actions: Inhibits protein synthesis in susceptible bacteria, causing cell death

Pharmacokinetics:

Route	Onset	Peak	Duration
Oral	Varies	1–2 h	8–12 h
IM	20–30 min	1–3 h	8–12 h
IV	Immediate	Minutes	8–12 h
Topical	Minimal absorption occurs		

$T_{1/2}$: 2–3 hours; metabolized in the liver, excreted in the urine and feces

Adverse effects: Nausea, vomiting, diarrhea, pseudomembranous colitis, bone marrow suppression, hypotension, cardiac arrest with rapid IV infusion, rash, pain on injection, abscess at injection site

FOCUS POINTS

- Fluoroquinolones inhibit the action of DNA enzymes in susceptible gram-negative bacteria. They are used to treat a wide range of infections.
- Monitor the patient on fluoroquinolones for headache, dizziness, GI upsets, and bone marrow depression, and caution the patient about the risk of photosensitivity reactions.
- Macrolides are in a class of older antibiotics that can be bactericidal or bacteriostatic. They are used to treat URIs and urinary tract infections (UTIs), and are often used when patients are allergic to penicillin.
- Monitor the patient on a macrolide for nausea, vomiting, diarrhea, dizziness, and other CNS effects.
- Lincosamides are similar to macrolides but are more toxic. They are used to treat severe infections.
- Monitor the patient on lincosamides for pseudomembranous colitis, bone marrow depression, pain, and CNS effects.

Monobactam Antibiotics

The only monobactam antibiotic currently available for use is aztreonam (*Azactam*). Among the antibiotics, its structure is unique, and little cross-resistance occurs. Aztreonam is effective against gram-negative enterobacteria and has no effect on gram-positive or anaerobic bacteria (Table 9.6). The drug is a safe alternative for treating infections caused by susceptible bacteria in patients who may be allergic to penicillins or cephalosporins. Aztreonam is absorbed well after IM injection, reaching peak effect levels in 1 to 1.5 hours. Its half-life is 1.5 to 2 hours, and it is excreted unchanged in the urine. It crosses the placenta and enters breast milk; it therefore should be used during pregnancy and lactation only if the benefit clearly outweighs the potential risk to the fetus or neonate.

Therapeutic Actions and Indications

Aztreonam disrupts bacterial cell wall synthesis, which promotes leakage of cellular contents and cell death in susceptible bacteria (see Figure 9.2). The drug is indicated for the treatment of urinary tract, skin, intra-abdominal, and gynecological infections, as well as septicemia caused by susceptible bacteria, including *E. coli, Enterobacter, Serratia, Proteus, Salmonella, Providencia, Pseudomonas, Citrobacter, Haemophilus, Neisseria,* and *Klebsiella.* Aztreonam is available for IV and IM use only.

Contraindications and Cautions

Aztreonam is contraindicated with any known allergy to aztreonam. Caution should be used in patients with a history of acute allergic reaction to penicillins or cephalosporins *because of the possibility of cross-reactivity;* in those with renal or hepatic dysfunction *that could interfere with the clearance and excretion of the drug;* and in pregnant and lactating women *because of potential adverse effects on the fetus or neonate.*

Adverse Effects

The adverse effects associated with the use of aztreonam are relatively mild. Local GI effects include nausea, GI upset, vomiting, and diarrhea. Hepatic enzyme elevations related to direct drug effects on the liver may also occur. Other effects include inflammation, phlebitis, and discomfort at injection sites, as well as the potential for allergic response, including anaphylaxis.

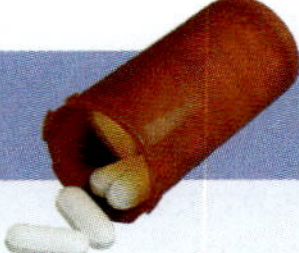

Table 9.6 DRUGS IN FOCUS

Monobactam Antibiotic

Drug Name	Dosage/Route	Usual Indications
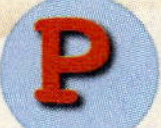 aztreonam (*Azactam*)	Adult: 500 mg to 1 g q8–12h IM or IV; reduce dosage in renal and hepatic impairment Pediatric: 30 mg/kg IM or IV q6–8h	Treatment of gram-negative enterobacterial infections, often as an alternative to penicillin

Prototype Summary: Aztreonam

Indications: Treatment of lower respiratory, dermatological, urinary tract, intra-abdominal, and gynecological infections caused by susceptible strains of gram-negative bacteria

Actions: Interferes with bacterial cell wall synthesis, causing cell death in susceptible gram-negative bacteria; is not effective against gram-positive or anaerobic bacteria

Pharmacokinetics:

Route	Onset	Peak	Duration
IM	Varies	60–90 min	6–8 h
IV	Immediate	30 min	6–8 h

$T_{1/2}$: 1.5–2 hours; excreted unchanged in the urine

Adverse effects: Nausea, vomiting, diarrhea, rash, superinfection, anaphylaxis, local discomfort at injection sites

Nursing Considerations for Patients Receiving Aztreonam

Assessment: History and Examination

Screen for the following, *which are possible contraindications or cautions for use of the drug:* known allergy to aztreonam (obtain specific information about the nature and occurrence of allergic reactions); history of acute allergic reactions to penicillins or cephalosporins; history of liver or kidney disease *that could interfere with clearance and excretion of the drug;* and current pregnancy or lactation status *because of potential adverse effects on the fetus or infant.*

Physical assessment should be performed *to establish baseline data for assessing the effectiveness of the drug and the occurrence of any adverse effects associated with drug therapy.* Obtain specimens for culture and sensitivity tests from the site of infection *to ensure that this is the most appropriate drug for this patient.* Monitor temperature *to detect infection.* Abdominal examination should be performed and liver and kidney function tests should be done *to determine any needed alteration in dosage.*

Nursing Diagnoses

The patient receiving aztreonam may have the following nursing diagnoses related to drug therapy:

- Acute Pain related to GI and local effects of drug
- Deficient Knowledge regarding drug therapy
- Deficient Fluid Volume (due to diarrhea)

Implementation With Rationale

- Check culture and sensitivity reports *to ensure that this is the drug of choice for this patient.*
- Monitor hepatic and renal function tests before therapy *to arrange to reduce dosage as needed.*
- Ensure that the patient receives the full course of aztreonam as prescribed *to eradicate the infection and to help prevent the emergence of resistant strains.*
- Monitor the site of infection and presenting signs and symptoms (e.g., fever, lethargy) throughout the course of drug therapy. *Failure of drug therapy to resolve these signs and symptoms may indicate the need to reculture the site.* Arrange to continue drug therapy for at least 2 days after the resolution of all signs and symptoms.
- Provide small, frequent meals as tolerated, frequent mouth care, and ice chips or sugarless candy to suck if dry mouth is a problem *to relieve discomfort and ensure nutrition.*

- Provide adequate fluids *to replace fluid lost with diarrhea.*
- Ensure ready access to bathroom facilities *to assist patients with problems associated with diarrhea.*
- Ensure that the patient is instructed about the route of administration and possible side effects *to enhance patient knowledge about drug therapy and to promote compliance.* The drug can be given only IV or IM, so the patient will not be responsible for administering the drug.

The patient should:

- Try to drink a lot of fluids and to maintain nutrition (very important), even though nausea, vomiting, and diarrhea may occur
- Report difficulty breathing, severe diarrhea, or mouth or vaginal sores to a health care provider.

Evaluation

- Monitor patient response to the drug (resolution of bacterial infection).
- Monitor for adverse effects (orientation and affect, GI effects, local inflammation).
- Evaluate the effectiveness of the teaching plan (patient can name the drug, dosage, possible adverse effects to expect, and specific measures to help avoid adverse effects).
- Monitor the effectiveness of comfort and safety measures and compliance with the regimen.

Penicillins and Penicillinase-Resistant Antibiotics

Penicillin was the first antibiotic introduced for clinical use. Sir Alexander Fleming used *Penicillium* molds to produce the original penicillin in the 1920s. Subsequent versions of penicillin were developed to decrease the adverse effects of the drug and to modify it to act on resistant bacteria.

With the prolonged use of penicillin, more and more bacterial species have synthesized the enzyme penicillinase to counteract the effects of penicillin. Researchers have developed a group of drugs with a resistance to penicillinase, which allows them to remain effective against bacteria that are now resistant to the penicillins (Table 9.7). The actual drug chosen depends on the sensitivity of the bacteria causing the infection, the desired and available routes, and the personal experience of the clinician with the particular agent. Culture and sensitivity tests should always be performed to ensure that the causative organism is sensitive to the penicillin selected for use. With the emergence of many resistant strains of bacteria, this has become increasingly important.

Therapeutic Actions and Indications

The penicillins and penicillinase-resistant antibiotics produce bactericidal effects by interfering with the ability of susceptible bacteria to build their cell walls when they are dividing (see Figure 9.2). These drugs prevent the bacteria from biosynthesizing the framework of the cell wall, and the bacteria with weakened cell walls swell and then burst from osmotic pressure within the cell. Because human cells do not use the biochemical process that the bacteria use to form the cell wall, this effect is a selective toxicity.

The penicillins are indicated for the treatment of streptococcal infections, including pharyngitis, tonsillitis, scarlet fever, and endocarditis; pneumococcal infections; staphylococcal infections; fusospirochetal infections; ratbite fever; diphtheria; anthrax; syphilis; and uncomplicated gonococcal infections. At high doses, these drugs are also used to treat meningococcal meningitis.

Pharmacokinetics

Most of the penicillins are rapidly absorbed from the GI tract, reaching peak levels in 1 hour. They are sensitive to the gastric acid levels in the stomach and should be taken on an empty stomach to ensure adequate absorption. Penicillins are excreted unchanged in the urine, making renal function an important factor in safe use of the drug. There are no adequate studies of use during pregnancy, so the drug should be used in pregnancy only if the benefit clearly outweighs the potential risk to the fetus. Penicillins enter breast milk and can cause diarrhea and adverse reactions in the baby. Use during lactation should be limited to situations in which the mother clearly would benefit from the drug.

Contraindications and Cautions

These drugs are contraindicated in patients with allergies to penicillin or cephalosporins or other allergens. Penicillin sensitivity tests are available if the patient's history of allergy is unclear and a penicillin is the drug of choice. Caution should be exercised in patients with renal disease (lowered doses are necessary *because excretion is reduced*), in those who are pregnant, and in lactating women (*diarrhea and superinfections may occur in the infant*).

Adverse Effects

The major adverse effects of penicillin therapy involve the GI tract. Common adverse effects include nausea, vomiting, diarrhea, abdominal pain, glossitis, stomatitis, gastritis, sore mouth, and furry tongue. These effects are primarily related to the loss of bacteria from the normal flora and the subsequent opportunistic infections that occur. Superinfections, including yeast infections, are also very common and are

Table 9.7 DRUGS IN FOCUS

Penicillins

Drug Name	Dosage/Route	Usual Indications
Penicillins		
penicillin G benzathine (*Bicillin, Permapen*)	Adult: 1.2–2.4 million units IM Pediatric: 900,000 to 1.2 million units IM as a single injection	Severe infections caused by sensitive organisms; treatment of syphilis and erysipeloid infections
penicillin G potassium (*Pfizerpen*)	Adult: 1–20 million units/day IM or IV, depending on condition Pediatric: 100,000 to 1 million units/day IM or IV	Treatment of severe infections; used for several days in some cases
penicillin G procaine (*Crysticillin-AS*)	Adult: 600,000 to 1.2 million units/day IM Pediatric: 50,000 units/kg/day IM	Treatment of moderately severe infections daily for 8–12 days
penicillin V (*Veetids*)	Adult: 250–500 mg q6–8h PO Pediatric: 15–62.5 mg/kg/day PO in divided doses q6–8h	Used for prophylaxis for bacterial endocarditis; Lyme disease, urinary tract infections
Extended-Spectrum Penicillins		
P amoxicillin (*Amoxil, Trimox*)	Adult: 250–500 mg PO q8h Pediatric: 20 mg/kg/day PO in divided doses q8h	Broad spectrum of uses for adults and children
ampicillin (*Principen*)	Adult: 250–500 mg IM or IV q6h, then 500 mg PO q6h when oral use is feasible Pediatric: 60 mg/kg/day IM or IV in four to six divided doses, then 250 mg PO q6h	Broad spectrum of activity; useful form if switch from parenteral to oral is anticipated; monitor for nephritis
carbenicillin (*Geocillin*)	Adult: 382–764 mg PO q.i.d Pediatric: safety not established	Treatment of UTIs in adults; not used in children
ticarcillin (*Ticar*)	Adult: 1g IM or direct IV q6h; reduce dosage with renal impairment Pediatric: 50–100 mg/kg/day IM or direct IV q6–8h	Severe infections caused by susceptible bacteria
Penicillin-Resistant Antibiotics		
nafcillin	Adult: 500–1000 mg IV q4h, 500 mg IM q6h, or 250–500 mg PO q4–6h Pediatric: 25 mg/kg IM b.i.d. or 25–50 mg/kg/day PO in four divided doses	Infections by penicillinase-producing staphylococci as well as group A hemolytic streptococci, plus *Streptococcus viridans*; drug of choice if switch to oral form is anticipated
oxacillin	Adult: 500 mg PO q4–6h or 250–500 mg IM or IV q4–6h Pediatric: 50 mg/kg/day IM, IV, or PO in equally divided doses q4–6h	Infections by penicillinase-producing staphylococci; streptococci; drug of choice if switch to oral form is anticipated

again associated with the loss of bacteria from the normal flora. Pain and inflammation at the injection site can occur with injectable forms of the drugs. Hypersensitivity reactions may include rash, fever, wheezing, and, with repeated exposure, anaphylaxis that can progress to anaphylactic shock and death.

Clinically Important Drug–Drug Interactions

If penicillins and penicillinase-resistant antibiotics are taken concurrently with tetracyclines, a decrease in the effectiveness of the penicillins results. This combination should be avoided if at all possible, or the penicillin dosages should be raised, which could increase the occurrence of adverse effects.

In addition, when the parenteral forms of penicillins and penicillinase-resistant drugs are administered in combination with any of the parenteral aminoglycosides, inactivation of the aminoglycosides occurs. These combinations should also be avoided.

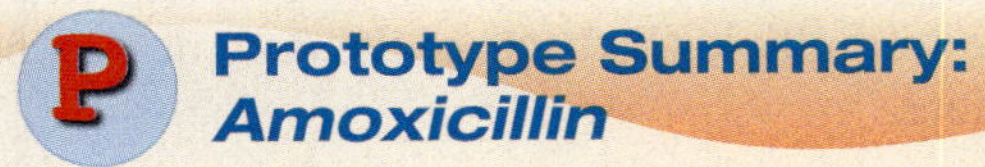

Prototype Summary: Amoxicillin

Indications: Treatment of infections caused by susceptible strains of bacteria, postexposure prophylaxis for anthrax, treatment of *Helicobacter* infections as part of combination therapy

Actions: Inhibits synthesis of the cell wall in susceptible bacteria, causing cell death

Pharmacokinetics:

Route	Onset	Peak	Duration
Oral	Varies	1 h	6–8 h

$T_{1/2}$: 1–1.4 hours; excreted unchanged in the urine

Adverse effects: Nausea, vomiting, diarrhea, glossitis, stomatitis, bone marrow suppression, rash, fever, superinfections, lethargy

Nursing Considerations for Patients Receiving Penicillins and Penicillinase-Resistant Antibiotics

Assessment: History and Examination

Screen for the following, *which are possible contraindications or cautions for use of the drug:* known allergy to any cephalosporins, penicillins, or other allergens *because cross-sensitivity often occurs* (obtain specific information about the nature and occurrence of allergic reactions); history of renal disease *that could interfere with excretion of the drug;* and current pregnancy or lactation status.

Physical assessment should be performed *to establish baseline data for evaluating the effectiveness of the drug and the occurrence of any adverse effects associated with drug therapy.* Perform culture and sensitivity tests at the site of infection *to ensure that this is the drug of choice for this patient.* Examine the skin and mucous membranes for any rashes or lesions *to provide a baseline for possible adverse effects.* Note respiratory status *to provide a baseline for the occurrence of hypersensitivity reactions.* Examine the abdomen *to monitor for adverse effects.* Evaluate renal function test findings, including BUN and creatinine clearance, *to assess the status of renal functioning and to determine any needed alteration in dosage.* Examine injection sites *to provide a baseline for determining adverse reactions or abscess formation.*

Nursing Diagnoses

The patient receiving a penicillin may have the following nursing diagnoses related to drug therapy:

- Acute Pain related to GI effects of drug
- Imbalanced Nutrition: Less Than Body Requirements related to multiple GI effects of the drug or to superinfections
- Deficient Knowledge regarding drug therapy

Implementation With Rationale

- Check culture and sensitivity reports *to ensure that this is the drug of choice for this patient.*
- Monitor renal function tests before and periodically during therapy *to arrange for dosage reduction as needed.*
- Ensure that the patient receives the full course of the penicillin as prescribed, in doses around the clock, *to increase effectiveness.*
- Explain storage requirements for suspensions and the importance of completing the prescribed therapeutic course even if signs and symptoms have disappeared, *to increase the effectiveness of the drug and decrease the risk of developing resistant strains.*
- Monitor the site of infection and presenting signs and symptoms (e.g., fever, lethargy) throughout the course of drug therapy. *Failure of these signs and symptoms to resolve may indicate the need to reculture the site.* Arrange to continue drug therapy for at least 2 days after the resolution of all signs and symptoms.
- Provide small, frequent meals as tolerated, ensure frequent mouth care, and offer ice chips or sugarless candy to suck if stomatitis and sore mouth are problems *to relieve discomfort and ensure nutrition.*
- Provide adequate fluids *to replace fluid lost with diarrhea.*
- Monitor the patient for any signs of superinfection *to arrange for treatment if superinfections occur.*
- Monitor injection sites regularly and *provide warm compresses and gentle massage to injection sites if painful or swollen.* If signs of phlebitis occur, remove the IV line and reinsert it in a different vein to continue the drug regimen.
- Be sure to instruct the patient regarding the appropriate dosage regimen and possible adverse effects *to enhance the patient's knowledge about drug therapy and promote compliance.*

The patient should:

- Try to drink a lot of fluids and to maintain nutrition (very important) even though nausea, vomiting, and diarrhea may occur.
- Report difficulty breathing, severe headache, severe diarrhea, dizziness, weakness, mouth sores, and vaginal itching or sores to a health care provider.

Box 9.6 contains a teaching checklist for penicillins.

Evaluation

- Monitor patient response to the drug (resolution of bacterial infection).
- Monitor for adverse effects (GI effects; local irritation, phlebitis at injection and IV sites; superinfections).
- Evaluate the effectiveness of the teaching plan (patient can name the drug, dosage, possible adverse effects to expect, and specific measures to help avoid adverse effects).
- Monitor the effectiveness of comfort and safety measures and compliance with the regimen (Critical Thinking Scenario 9-1).

BOX 9.6 **Patient Teaching Checklist: Penicillins**

- The penicillins are used to help destroy specific bacteria that are causing infections in the body. They are effective against only certain bacteria; they are not effective against viruses (such as cold germs) or other bacteria. To clear up a bacterial infection, the penicillins must act on the bacteria over a period of time, so it is very important to complete the full course of this penicillin to avoid recurrence of the infection.
- The drug should be taken on an empty stomach with a full 8-oz glass of water—1 hour before meals or 2 to 3 hours after meals is best. Do not use fruit juice, soft drinks, or milk to take your drug, because these foods may interfere with its effectiveness. (This does not apply to bacampicillin, amoxicillin, or penicillin V.)
- Common effects of these drugs include stomach upset, diarrhea, changes in taste, and change in the color of the tongue. Small, frequent meals may help. It is important to try to maintain good nutrition. These effects should go away when the drug is stopped.
- Report any of the following to your health care provider: hives, rash, fever, difficulty breathing, severe diarrhea.
- Tell any doctor, nurse, or other health care provider that you are taking this drug.
- Keep this drug and all medications out of the reach of children and pets.
- Do not share this drug with other people, and do not use this medication to self-treat other infections.
- It is very important that you complete the full course of your prescription, even if you feel better before you finish it.

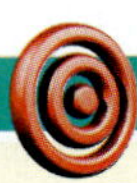

FOCUS POINTS

- The monobactam antibiotic aztreonam is effective against only gram-negative enterobacteria; it is safely used when patients are allergic to penicillin or cephalosporins.
- Monitor the patient on aztreonam for GI problems, liver toxicity, and pain at the injection site.
- The penicillins are one of the oldest classes of antibiotics, and many resistant strains have developed. The penicillinase-resistant antibiotics were created to combat bacteria that produce an enzyme to destroy the penicillin. Penicillins are used to treat a broad spectrum of infections, including respiratory and urinary tract infections.
- Monitor the patient on penicillin for nausea, vomiting, diarrhea, superinfections, and the possibility of hypersensitivity reactions.

Sulfonamides

The sulfonamides, or sulfa drugs (Table 9.8), are drugs that inhibit folic acid synthesis. Folic acid is necessary for the synthesis of purine and pyrimidines, which are precursors of RNA and DNA. For cells to grow and reproduce, they require folic acid. Humans cannot synthesize folic acid and depend on the folate found in their diet to obtain this essential substance. Bacteria are impermeable to folic acid and must synthesize it inside the cell.

Because of the emergence of resistant bacterial strains and the development of newer antibiotics, the sulfa drugs are not used much any more. However, they remain an inexpensive and effective treatment for urinary tract infections and trachoma, especially in developing countries and when cost is an issue.

Sulfadiazine (generic) is an oral agent with broad use in infections caused by susceptible bacteria. It is slowly absorbed from the GI tract, reaching peak levels in 3 to 6 hours.

Sulfisoxazole (*Gantrisin*) is used for a broad spectrum of infections caused by susceptible bacteria. This drug is also recommended by the Centers for Disease Control and Prevention (CDC) for the treatment of sexually transmitted diseases and has the unlabeled use of prophylaxis for recurrent otitis media. It is rapidly absorbed from the GI tract, reaching peak levels in 2 hours. After being metabolized in the liver, it is excreted in the urine with a half-life of 4.5 to 7.8 hours.

Sulfasalazine (*Azulfidine*) is a sulfapyridine that is carried by aminosalicylic acids (aspirin) that release the aminosalicylic acid in the colon. Sulfasalazine is used to treat ulcerative colitis and Crohn's disease because of the direct anti-inflammatory effect of the aspirin. In a delayed-release form, this sulfa drug is also used to treat rheumatoid arthritis that does not respond to other treatments. It is rapidly absorbed from the GI tract, reaching peak levels in 2 to 6 hours. After being metabolized in the liver, it is excreted in the urine with a half-life of 5 to 10 hours.

Cotrimoxazole (*Septra, Bactrim*) is a combination drug that contains sulfamethoxazole and trimethoprim, another antibacterial drug. This combination has proved to be very effective in the treatment of otitis media, bronchitis, urinary tract infections, and pneumonitis caused by *Pneumocystis carinii,* which is a serious problem in patients with compromised immune systems (e.g., those with AIDS). It is rapidly absorbed from the GI tract, reaching peak levels in 2 hours. After being metabolized in the liver, it is excreted in the urine with a half-life of 7 to 12 hours.

Therapeutic Actions and Indications

The sulfonamides competitively block para-aminobenzoic acid (PABA) to prevent the synthesis of folic acid in susceptible bacteria that synthesize their own folates for the production of RNA and DNA (see Figure 9.2). This includes gram-negative

CRITICAL THINKING SCENARIO 9-1

Antibiotics and Oral Contraceptives

THE SITUATION

G.S., a 27-year-old, married, female, graduate student is seen in the student health clinic a few weeks into the fall semester. She has developed a severe sinusitis and complains of head pressure, difficulty sleeping, fever, and muscle aches and pains. A culture is done, and the next day the culture and sensitivity report identifies the infecting organism as a strain of *Klebsiella* that is sensitive to tetracycline. G.S. returns to the clinic to get the prescription for tetracycline.

In talking with you, G.S. tells you that she began graduate school with plans to start a family in 2 years, after completing her program. She is a very organized person and has carefully planned her rigorous course work and her nonacademic activities so that almost every hour is scheduled. She states that she has successfully used low-dose oral contraceptives for 4 years and plans to continue this method of birth control.

CRITICAL THINKING

How do tetracyclines and some other antibiotics and oral contraceptives interact? What are the possible ramifications of continuing to take oral contraceptives during a pregnancy?

What nursing interventions are appropriate for G.S.?

What teaching points should be stressed with G.S.? Think about the nature of her personality and the problems that an unplanned pregnancy might cause. How can you help G.S. to cope with her infection, her drug regimen, and her rigorous schedule?

DISCUSSION

Several antibiotics, including tetracycline, are known to lead to the failure of oral contraceptives as evidenced by breakthrough bleeding and unplanned pregnancy. Although the exact way in which these drugs interact is incompletely understood, it is thought that the antibiotics destroy certain bacteria in the normal flora of the gastrointestinal (GI) tract. These bacteria are necessary for the breakdown and eventual absorption of the female hormones contained in the contraceptives. The 5 days of antibiotic treatment together with the time necessary for rebuilding the normal flora can be long enough for the hypothalamus to lose the negative feedback signal provided by the contraceptives that prevents ovulation and preparation of the uterus. Sensing the low hormone levels, the hypothalamus releases gonadotropin-releasing hormone, which leads to the release of follicle-stimulating hormone and luteinizing hormone, with subsequent ovulation.

G.S. will need a clear explanation and follow-up in written form about the risks of oral contraceptive failure while she is receiving tetracycline therapy. She should be encouraged to use an additional form of birth control during the course of her antibiotic use and to read all of the literature that comes with oral contraceptives as well as patient teaching information that should be provided with the antibiotic.

G.S. also may need a great deal of support and encouragement at this time. The sinus infection may increase her stress by interfering with her ability to stick to her rigid schedule. Discussing the possibility of an unplanned pregnancy may cause even more stress. The health clinic visit could be used as opportunity to allow G.S. to talk, to vent any frustrations and stress, and then to encourage her to make time for herself. The nurse should stress the importance of a good diet, which will assure that her body has the components she will need to fight this infection and to heal and to ward off other infections, as well as the importance of adequate rest and exercise. The nurse should also make sure that G.S. is receiving annual gynecologic exams and has been advised not to smoke.

All health care professionals who are involved with G.S. should consider the impact that an unplanned pregnancy could have on this very organized woman and use this as an example of the importance of clear, concise patient teaching in the administration of drug therapy.

NURSING CARE GUIDE FOR G.S.: TETRACYCLINE

Assessment: History and Examination

Allergy to any tetracycline

Hepatic or renal dysfunction

Pregnancy or lactation

Concurrent use of oral contraceptives, antacids, iron products, digoxin, or penicillins

General: site of infection, culture and sensitivity

Skin: color, lesions

Respiratory: respiration, adventitious sounds

GI: liver evaluation, bowel sounds, usual output

Laboratory data: liver and renal function tests, urinalysis

Antibiotics and Oral Contraceptives *(continued)*

Nursing Diagnoses

Acute Pain related to GI effects, superinfections

Imbalanced Nutrition, Less Than Body Requirements related to GI effects

Potential for Injury related to central nervous system (CNS) effects

Deficient Knowledge regarding drug therapy

Implementation

Perform culture and sensitivity tests before beginning therapy.

Administer drug on an empty stomach, 1 h before or 2 to 3 h after meals. Do not give with antacids, milk, or iron products.

Do not use outdated drug because of the risk of nephrotoxicity.

Monitor for and provide hygiene measures and treatment if superinfections occur.

Monitor nutritional status and fluid intake.

Provide ready access to bathroom facilities if diarrhea is a problem.

Provide support and reassurance for dealing with the drug effects and infection.

Provide patient teaching regarding drug name, dosage, adverse effects, precautions, warnings to report, and drugs that might cause a drug–drug interaction, including the need to use a second form of contraception if using oral contraceptives.

Evaluation

Evaluate drug effects: resolution of bacterial infections.

Monitor for adverse effects: GI effects, superinfections, CNS effects.

Monitor for drug–drug interactions: lack of effectiveness of oral contraceptives, lack of antibacterial effect with antacids or iron.

Evaluate effectiveness of patient teaching program.

Evaluate effectiveness of comfort and safety measures.

Patient Teaching for G.S.

- ☐ Tetracycline is an antibiotic that is specific for your infection. You should take it throughout the day for best results.
- ☐ Take this drug on an empty stomach, 1 hour before or 2 to 3 hours after meals, with a full glass of water.
- ☐ Do not take this drug with food, dairy products, iron preparations, or antacids.
- ☐ Take the full course of this antibiotic. Do not stop taking it if you feel better.
- ☐ Do not save tetracycline; outdated products can be very toxic to your kidneys.
- ☐ Oral contraceptives may become ineffective while you are taking this drug. If you rely on oral contraceptives for birth control, use a second form of contraceptive while on this drug.
- ☐ You may experience stomach upset or diarrhea.
- ☐ You may develop other infections in your mouth or vagina. (If this occurs, consult with your health care provider for appropriate treatment.)
- ☐ Tell any health care provider who is caring for you that you are taking this drug.
- ☐ Keep this, and all medications, out of the reach of children and pets.
- ☐ Report any of the following to your health care provider: changes in color of urine or stool, severe cramps, difficulty breathing, rash or itching, yellowing of the skin or eyes.

and gram-positive bacteria such as *C. trachomatis; Nocardia;* and some strains of *H. influenzae, E. coli,* and *P. mirabilis.* These drugs are used to treat trachoma (a leading cause of blindness), nocardiosis (which causes pneumonias, as well as brain abscesses and inflammation), urinary tract infections, and sexually transmitted diseases.

Pharmacokinetics

The sulfonamides are absorbed from the GI tract, metabolized in the liver, and excreted in the urine. The time to peak level and the half-life of the individual drug varies (described earlier). The sulfonamides are teratogenic; they are distributed into breast milk and should not be used during pregnancy or lactation.

Contraindications and Cautions

The sulfonamides are contraindicated with any known allergy to any sulfonamide, to sulfonylureas, or to thiazide diuretics *because cross-sensitivities occur;* during pregnancy *because the drugs can cause birth defects, as well as*

Table 9.8 DRUGS IN FOCUS

Sulfonamides

Drug Name	Dosage/Route	Usual Indications
sulfadiazine (*generic*)	Adult: 2–4 g PO loading dose, then 2–4 g/day PO in four to six divided doses Pediatric: 75 mg/kg PO, then 120–150 mg/kg/day PO in four to six divided doses	Treatment of a broad spectrum of infections
sulfisoxazole (*Gantrisin*)	Adult: 2–4 g PO loading dose, then 4–8 g/day PO in four to six divided doses Pediatric: 75 mg/kg PO, then 120–150 mg/kg/day PO in four to six divided doses	Treatment of a wide range of infections including various sexually transmitted diseases
P sulfasalazine (*Azulfidine*)	Adult: 3–4 g/day PO in evenly divided doses, then 500 mg PO q.i.d. Pediatric: 40–60 mg/kg/day PO in divided doses, then 20–30 mg/kg/day PO in four equally divided doses	Treatment of ulcerative colitis and Crohn's disease
cotrimoxazole (*Septra, Bactrim*)	Adult: 2 tablets PO q12h; reduce dosage with renal impairment Pediatric: 8 mg/kg/day trimethoprim plus 40 mg sulfamethoxazole PO q12h	Treatment of otitis media, bronchitis, urinary tract infections, and pneumonitis caused by *Pneumocystis carinii*

kernicterus; and during lactation *because of a risk of kernicterus, diarrhea, and rash in the infant.* Caution should be used in patients with renal disease or a history of kidney stones *because of the possibility of increased toxic effects of the drugs.*

Adverse Effects

Adverse effects associated with sulfonamides include GI effects such as nausea, vomiting, diarrhea, abdominal pain, anorexia, stomatitis, and hepatic injury, which are all related to direct irritation of the GI tract and the death of normal bacteria. Renal effects are related to the filtration of the drug in the glomerulus and include crystalluria, hematuria, and proteinuria, which can progress to a nephrotic syndrome and possible toxic nephrosis. CNS effects include headache, dizziness, vertigo, ataxia, convulsions, and depression (possibly related to drug effects on the nerves). Bone marrow depression may occur and is related to drug effects on the cells that turn over rapidly in the bone marrow.

Dermatological effects include photosensitivity and rash related to direct effects on the dermal cells. A wide range of hypersensitivity reactions may also occur.

Clinically Important Drug–Drug Interactions

If sulfonamides are taken with tolbutamide, tolazamide, glyburide, glipizide, acetohexamide, or chlorpropamide, the risk of hypoglycemia increases. If this combination is needed, the patient should be monitored and a dosage adjustment of the antidiabetic agent should be made. An increase in dosage will then be needed when sulfonamide therapy stops.

When sulfonamides are taken with cyclosporine, the risk of nephrotoxicity rises. If this combination is essential, the patient should be monitored closely and the sulfonamide stopped at any sign of renal dysfunction.

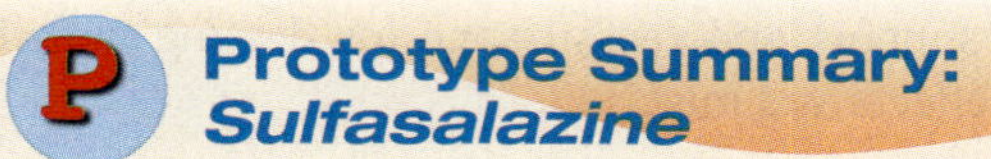

Prototype Summary: *Sulfasalazine*

Indications: Treatment of rheumatoid arthritis, arthritis, ulcerative colitis

Actions: Blocks PABA, an essential component of folic acid synthesis in susceptible gram-negative and gram-positive bacteria; two-thirds of the oral dose passes into the colon, where the sulfapyridine and aminosalicylic acid carrier split, giving a local anti-inflammatory agent to the colon

Pharmacokinetics:

Route	Onset	Peak
Oral	Varies	1.5–6 h; 6–24 h for the metabolite

$T_{1/2}$: 5–10 hours; metabolized in the liver, excreted in the urine

Adverse effects: Nausea, vomiting, diarrhea, hepatocellular necrosis, hematuria, bone marrow suppression, Stevens–Johnson syndrome, rash, photophobia, fever, chills

Nursing Considerations for Patients Receiving Sulfonamides

Assessment: History and Examination

Screen for the following, *which are possible contraindications or cautions for use of the drug:* known allergy to any sulfonamide, sulfonylureas, or thiazide diuretic *because cross-sensitivity often results* (obtain specific information about the nature and occurrence of allergic reactions); history of renal disease *that could interfere with excretion of the drug and lead to increased toxicity;* and current pregnancy or lactation status.

Physical assessment should be performed *to establish baseline data for assessing the effectiveness of the drug and the occurrence of any adverse effects associated with drug therapy.* Obtain specimens for culture and sensitivity tests at the site of infection *to ensure that this is the appropriate drug for this patient.* Examine skin and mucous membranes for any rash or lesions *to provide a baseline for possible adverse effects.* Note respiratory status *to provide a baseline for the occurrence of hypersensitivity reactions.* Conduct assessment of orientation, affect, and reflexes *to monitor for adverse drug effects* and examination of the abdomen *to monitor for adverse effects.* Monitor renal function test findings, including BUN and creatinine clearance, *to evaluate the status of renal functioning and to determine any needed alteration in dosage.* A complete blood count (CBC) also should be performed *to establish a baseline to monitor for adverse effects.*

Nursing Diagnoses

The patient receiving a sulfonamide may have the following nursing diagnoses related to drug therapy:

- Acute Pain related to GI, CNS, or skin effects of drug
- Disturbed Sensory Perception related to CNS effects
- Imbalanced Nutrition: Less Than Body Requirements related to multiple GI effects of the drug
- Deficient Knowledge regarding drug therapy

Implementation With Rationale

- Check culture and sensitivity reports *to ensure that this is the drug of choice for this patient and repeat cultures if response is not as anticipated.*
- Monitor renal function tests before and periodically during therapy *to arrange for a dosage reduction as necessary.*
- Ensure that the patient receives the full course of the sulfonamide as prescribed *to increase therapeutic effects and decrease the risk for development of resistant strains.*
- Administer the oral drug on an empty stomach 1 hour before or 2 hours after meals with a full glass of water *to promote adequate absorption of the drug.*
- Discontinue the drug immediately if hypersensitivity reactions occur *to prevent potentially fatal reactions.*
- Provide small, frequent meals and adequate fluids as tolerated; encourage frequent mouth care; and offer ice chips or sugarless candy to suck if stomatitis and sore mouth are problems *to relieve discomfort, ensure nutrition, and replace fluid lost with diarrhea.*
- Monitor CBC and urinalysis test results before and periodically during therapy *to check for adverse effects.*
- Be sure to instruct the patient about the appropriate dosage regimen, the proper way to take the drug (on an empty stomach with a full glass of water), and possible adverse effects, *to enhance patient knowledge about drug therapy and to promote compliance.*

The patient should:

- Avoid driving or operating dangerous machinery because dizziness, lethargy, and ataxia may occur.
- Try to drink a lot of fluids and maintain nutrition (very important), even though nausea, vomiting, and diarrhea may occur.
- Report to a health care provider any difficulty in breathing, rash, ringing in the ears, fever, sore throat, or blood in the urine.

Evaluation

- Monitor patient response to the drug (resolution of bacterial infection).
- Monitor for adverse effects (GI effects, CNS effects, rash, and crystalluria).
- Evaluate the effectiveness of the teaching plan (patient can name the drug, dosage, possible adverse effects to expect, and specific measures to help avoid adverse effects).
- Monitor the effectiveness of comfort and safety measures and compliance with the regimen.

Tetracyclines

The tetracyclines (Table 9.9) were developed as semisynthetic antibiotics based on the structure of a common soil mold. They work by inhibiting protein synthesis in susceptible bacteria. They are composed of four rings, which is how they got their name. Researchers have developed newer tetracyclines to increase absorption and tissue penetration. Widespread resistance to the tetracyclines has limited their use in recent years.

Tetracycline (*Sumycin* and others) is available in oral and topical forms for treatment of a wide variety of infections, including acne vulgaris and minor skin infections caused by susceptible organisms. When penicillin is contraindicated, tetracycline is often used. Tetracycline is also available as an ophthalmic agent to treat superficial ocular lesions caused by susceptible microorganisms and as a prophylactic agent for ophthalmia neonatorum caused by *N. gonorrhoeae* and *C. trachomatis.*

Demeclocycline (*Declomycin*) is available in oral form for treating a wide variety of infections. Like tetracycline, it is also often used when penicillin is contraindicated.

Doxycycline (*Doryx, Periostat,* and others) is available in oral and IV forms. Used for a wide variety of infections, this drug is recommended in the treatment of traveler's diarrhea, periodontal disease, acne, and some sexually transmitted diseases.

Minocycline (*Minocin*) is also available in IV and oral forms. It is used to treat severe infections caused by susceptible bacteria. In addition, minocycline is the drug of choice in treating meningococcal carriers (not the disease itself) and various uncomplicated GU and gynecological infections.

Oxytetracycline (*Terramycin*) is available for oral, IM, and IV use. It is used to treat a wide variety of infections caused by susceptible bacteria and when penicillin is contraindicated. Oxytetracycline is also used as an adjunctive therapy in the treatment of acute intestinal amebiasis.

Therapeutic Actions and Indications

The tetracyclines inhibit protein synthesis in susceptible bacteria, leading to the inability of the bacteria to multiply (see Figure 9.2). Because the affected protein is similar to a protein found in human cells, these drugs can be toxic to humans at high concentrations. Tetracyclines, which are effective against a wide range of bacteria, are indicated for treatment of infections caused by *rickettsiae, M. pneumoniae, Borrelia recurrentis, H. influenzae, Haemophilus ducreyi, Pasteurella pestis, Pasteurella tularensis, Bartonella bacilliformis, Bacteroides* species, *Vibrio* comma, *Vibrio* fetus, *Brucella* species, *E. coli, E. aerogenes, Shigella* species, *Acinetobacter calcoaceticus, Klebsiella* species, *Diplococcus pneumoniae,* and *S. aureus;* against agents that cause psittacosis, ornithosis, lymphogranuloma venereum, and granuloma inguinale; when penicillin is contraindicated in susceptible infections; and for treatment of acne and uncomplicated GU infections caused by *C. trachomatis.* Some of the tetracy-

Table 9.9 DRUGS IN FOCUS

Tetracyclines

Drug Name	Dosage/Route	Usual Indications
demeclocycline (*Declomycin*)	Adult: 150 mg PO q.i.d. or 300 mg PO b.i.d. Pediatric (>8 yr): 6–12 mg/kg/day PO in two to four divided doses	Treatment of a wide variety of infections when penicillin cannot be used
doxycycline (*Doryx, Periostat*)	Adult: 200 mg/day IV in two infusions of 1–4 h each *or* 100–300 mg/day PO Pediatric (>8 yr): 4.4 mg/kg/day PO	Treatment of a wide variety of infections, including traveler's diarrhea and sexually transmitted diseases; periodontal disease
minocycline (*Minocin*)	Adult: 200 mg IV, followed by 100 mg IV q12h, *or* 200 mg PO, then 100 mg PO q12h Pediatric (>8 yr): 4 mg/kg IV followed by 2 mg/kg IV or PO q12h	Treatment of meningococcal carriers and of various uncomplicated genitourinary and gynecological infections
oxytetracycline (*Terramycin*)	Adult: 250 mg/day IM, *or* 250–500 mg IV q12h, *or* 1–2 g/day PO in divided doses Pediatric (>8 yr): 15–25 mg/kg/day IM, *or* 12 mg/kg/day IV in divided doses, *or* 25–50 mg/kg/day PO in two to four divided doses	Treatment of a variety of infections caused by susceptible bacteria when penicillin is contraindicated; adjunct therapy in the treatment of acute intestinal amebiasis
P tetracycline (*Sumycin, Panmycin*)	Adult: 1–2 g/day PO in divided doses; topical applied generously to affected area Pediatric (>8 yr): 25–50 mg/kg/day PO in four divided doses	Treatment of a wide variety of infections, including acne vulgaris and minor skin infections caused by susceptible organisms; as an ophthalmic agent to treat superficial ocular lesions caused by susceptible microorganisms; as a prophylactic agent for ophthalmia neonatorum caused by *Neisseria gonorrhoeae* and *Chlamydia trachomatis*

clines are also used as adjuncts in the treatment of certain protozoal infections.

Pharmacokinetics

Tetracyclines are absorbed adequately, but not completely, from the GI tract. Their absorption is affected by food, iron, calcium, and other drugs in the stomach. Tetracyclines are concentrated in the liver and excreted unchanged in the urine, with half-lives ranging from 12 to 25 hours. These drugs cross the placenta and pass into breast milk. They should not be used in women who are pregnant or lactating or in children younger than 8 years of age because they can permanently discolor and damage enamel in developing teeth. They can also promote calcium complex formations in bone, which leads to decreased bone growth.

Contraindications and Cautions

Tetracyclines are contraindicated in patients with known allergy to tetracyclines or to tartrazine (i.e., in specific oral preparations that contain tartrazine) and during pregnancy and lactation *because of effects on the bones and teeth.*

Tetracyclines should be used with caution in children younger than 8 years of age *because they can potentially damage the bones and teeth.* They are also used with caution in patients with hepatic or renal dysfunction *because they are concentrated in the bile and excreted in the urine.* The ophthalmic preparation is contraindicated in patients who have fungal, mycobacterial, or viral ocular infections *because the drug kills not only the undesired bacteria, but also bacteria of the normal flora, which increases the risk for exacerbation of the ocular infection that is being treated.*

Adverse Effects

The major adverse effects of tetracycline therapy involve direct irritation of the GI tract and include nausea, vomiting, diarrhea, abdominal pain, glossitis, and dysphagia. Fatal hepatotoxicity related to the drug's irritating effect on the liver has also been reported. Skeletal effects involve damage to the teeth and bones. Because tetracyclines have an affinity for teeth and bones, they accumulate there, weakening the structure and causing staining and pitting of teeth and bones. Dermatological effects include photosensitivity and rash. Superinfections, including yeast infections, occur when bacteria of the normal flora are destroyed. Local effects, such as pain and stinging with topical or ocular application, are fairly common. Less frequent are hematological effects, such as hemolytic anemia and bone marrow depression secondary to the effects on bone marrow cells that turn over rapidly. Hypersensitivity reactions reportedly range from urticaria to anaphylaxis and also include intracranial hypertension.

Clinically Important Drug–Drug Interactions

When penicillin G and tetracyclines are taken concurrently, the effectiveness of penicillin G decreases. If this combination is used, the dose of the penicillin should be increased.

When oral contraceptives are taken with tetracyclines, the effectiveness of the contraceptives decreases. Therefore, patients who take oral contraceptives should be advised to use an additional form of birth control while receiving the tetracycline.

When methoxyflurane is combined with tetracycline, the risk of nephrotoxicity increases. If at all possible, this combination should be avoided. In addition, digoxin toxicity rises when tetracyclines are taken concurrently. Digoxin levels should be monitored and dosage adjusted appropriately during treatment and after tetracycline therapy is discontinued. Finally, decreased absorption of tetracyclines results from oral combinations with calcium salts, magnesium salts, zinc salts, aluminum salts, bismuth salts, iron, urinary alkalinizers, and charcoal.

Clinically Important Drug–Food Interactions

Because oral tetracyclines are not absorbed effectively if taken with food or dairy products, tetracyclines should be given on an empty stomach 1 hour before or 2 to 3 hours after any meal or other medication.

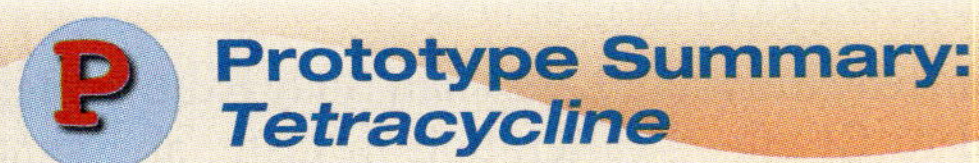

Prototype Summary: *Tetracycline*

Indications: Treatment of various infections caused by susceptible strains of bacteria; acne; when penicillin is contraindicated for eradication of susceptible organisms

Actions: Inhibits protein synthesis in susceptible bacteria, preventing cell replication

Pharmacokinetics:

Route	Onset	Peak
Oral	Varies	2–4 h
Topical	Minimal absorption occurs	

$T_{1/2}$: 6–12 hours; excreted unchanged in the urine

Adverse effects: Nausea, vomiting, diarrhea, glossitis, discoloring and inadequate calcification of primary teeth of fetus when used in pregnant women or of secondary teeth when used in children, bone marrow suppression, photosensitivity, superinfections, rash, local irritation with topical forms

Nursing Considerations for Patients Receiving Tetracyclines

Assessment: History and Examination

Screen for the following, *which are possible contraindications or cautions for use of the drug:* known allergy to any tetracycline or to tartrazine in certain oral preparations *because cross-sensitivity often occurs* (obtain specific information about the nature and occurrence of allergic reactions); any history of renal or hepatic disease *that could interfere with metabolism and excretion of the drug and lead to increased toxicity;* current pregnancy or lactation status; and age.

Physical examination should be performed *to establish baseline data for assessing the effectiveness of the drug and the occurrence of any adverse effects associated with drug therapy.* Perform culture and sensitivity tests at the site of infection *to ensure that this is the appropriate drug for this patient.* Conduct examination of the skin for any rash or lesions *to provide a baseline for possible adverse effects.* Note respiratory status *to provide a baseline for the occurrence of hypersensitivity reactions.* Evaluate renal and liver function test reports, including BUN and creatinine clearance, *to assess the status of renal and liver functioning, which helps to determine any needed changes in dosage.*

Nursing Diagnoses

The patient receiving a tetracycline may have the following nursing diagnoses related to drug therapy:

- Diarrhea related to drug effects
- Imbalanced Nutrition: Less Than Body Requirements related to GI effects, alteration in taste, and superinfections
- Impaired Skin Integrity related to rash and photosensitivity
- Deficient Knowledge regarding drug therapy

Implementation With Rationale

- Check culture and sensitivity reports *to ensure that this is the drug of choice for this patient.* Arrange for repeated cultures if response is not as anticipated.
- Monitor renal and liver function test results before and periodically during therapy *to arrange for a dosage reduction as needed.*
- Ensure that the patient receives the full course of the tetracycline as prescribed. The oral drug should be taken on an empty stomach 1 hour before or 2 hours after meals with a full 8-oz glass of water. Concomitant use of antacids or salts should be avoided because they interfere with drug absorption. *These precautions will increase drug effectiveness and decrease development of resistant strains of bacteria.*
- Discontinue the drug immediately if hypersensitivity reactions occur *to avoid the possibility of severe reactions.*
- Provide small, frequent meals as tolerated; frequent mouth care; and ice chips or sugarless candy to suck if stomatitis and sore mouth are problems *to relieve discomfort and ensure nutrition.* Also provide adequate fluids *to replace fluid lost with diarrhea.*
- Monitor for signs of superinfections *to arrange for treatment as appropriate.*
- Encourage the patient to apply sunscreen and wear clothing *to protect exposed skin from skin rashes and sunburn associated with photosensitivity reactions.*
- Be sure to instruct the patient about the appropriate dosage regimen, how to take the oral drug, and possible side effects *to enhance patient knowledge about drug therapy and to promote compliance.*

The patient should:

- Try to drink a lot of fluids and maintain nutrition (very important) even though nausea, vomiting, and diarrhea may occur.
- Use a barrier contraceptive method because oral contraceptives may not be effective while a tetracycline is being used.
- Know that superinfections may occur. Appropriate treatment can be arranged through the health care provider.
- Use sunscreens and protective clothing if sensitivity to the sun occurs.
- Know when to report dangerous adverse effects, such as difficulty breathing, rash, itching, watery diarrhea, cramps, or changes in color of urine or stool, to the health care provider.

Evaluation

- Monitor the patient's response to the drug (resolution of bacterial infection).
- Monitor for adverse effects (GI effects, rash, and superinfections).
- Evaluate the effectiveness of the teaching plan (patient can name the drug, dosage, possible adverse effects to expect, and specific measures to help avoid adverse effects).
- Monitor the effectiveness of comfort and safety measures and compliance with the regimen.

For related data, see Critical Thinking Scenario 9-1.

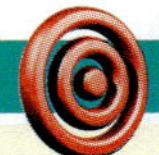

FOCUS POINTS

- Sulfonamides are older drugs; many strains have developed resistance to the sulfonamides, so they are not widely used any more.
- Monitor the patient on sulfonamides for CNS toxicity, nausea, vomiting, diarrhea, liver injury, renal toxicity, and bone marrow depression.
- Tetracyclines inhibit protein synthesis and prevent bacteria from multiplying. Tetracyclines can cause damage to developing teeth and bones and should not be used with pregnant women or children.
- Monitor the patient taking tetracyclines for GI effects, bone marrow depression, rash, and superinfections. Caution women that tetracyclines may make oral contraceptives ineffective.

Antimycobacterial Antibiotics

Mycobacteria, the group of bacteria that contain the pathogens that cause tuberculosis and leprosy, are classified on the basis of their ability to hold a stain even in the presence of a "destaining" agent such as acid. Because of this property, they are called "acid-fast" bacteria. The mycobacteria have an outer coat of mycolic acid that protects them from many disinfectants and allows them to survive for long periods in the environment. These slow-growing bacteria may need to be treated for several years before they can be eradicated.

Mycobacteria cause serious infectious diseases. The bacterium *Mycobacterium tuberculosis* causes tuberculosis, the leading cause of death from infectious disease in the world. For several years the disease was thought to be under control, but with the increasing number of people with compromised immune systems and the emergence of resistant bacterial strains, tuberculosis is once again on the rise.

Mycobacterium leprae causes leprosy, also known as Hansen's disease, which is characterized by disfiguring skin lesions and destructive effects on the respiratory tract. Leprosy is also a worldwide health problem; it is infectious when the mycobacteria invade the skin or respiratory tract of susceptible individuals. *Mycobacterium avium-intracellulare,* which causes mycobacterium avium complex (MAC), is seen in patients with AIDS or in other patients who are severely immunocompromised. Rifabutin (*Mycobutin*), which was developed as an antituberculosis drug, is most effective against *M. avium-intracellulare.*

Antituberculosis Drugs

Tuberculosis can lead to serious damage in the lungs, the GU tract, bones, and the meninges. Because *M. tuberculosis* is so slow growing, the treatment must be continued for 6 months to 2 years. The first-line drugs for treating tuberculosis are as follows:

- isoniazid [INH] (*Nydrazid*), which affects the mycolic acid coating of the bacterium
- rifampin (*Rifadin, Rimactane*), which alters DNA and RNA activity in the bacterium
- ethionamide (*Trecator SC*), which prevents cell division
- rifapentine (*Priftin*), which alters DNA and RNA activity, causing cell death

These drugs are used in combinations of two or more agents until bacterial conversion occurs or maximum improvement is seen. If the patient cannot take one or more of these drugs, or if the disease continues to progress because of the emergence of a resistant strain, the second-line drugs can be used:

- ethambutol (*Myambutol*), which inhibits cellular metabolism
- pyrazinamide (generic), which is both bactericidal and bacteriostatic

These drugs are used in combination with at least one other antituberculosis drug.

If therapeutic success is still not achieved, a third-line combination of two antituberculosis drugs can be tried:

- capreomycin (*Capastat*), whose mechanism of action is not known
- cycloserine (*Seromycin*), which inhibits cell wall synthesis and leads to cell death

Using the drugs in combination helps to decrease the emergence of resistant strains and to affect the bacteria at various phases during their long and slow life cycle. (See Table 9.10 for a listing of all the antituberculosis drugs.)

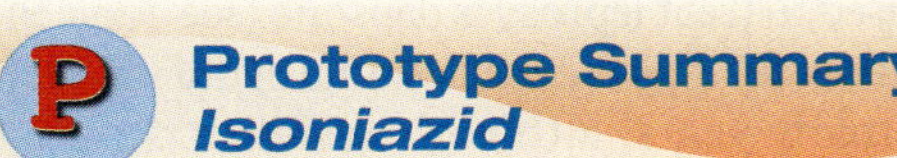

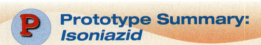

Prototype Summary: *Isoniazid*

Indications: Treatment of tuberculosis as part of combination therapy; prophylactic treatment of household members of recently diagnosed tuberculars

Actions: Interferes with lipid and nucleic acid synthesis in actively growing tubercle bacilli

Pharmacokinetics:

Route	Onset	Peak	Duration
Oral	Varies	1–2 h	24 h

$T_{1/2}$: 1–4 hours; metabolized in the liver, excreted in the urine

Adverse effects: Peripheral neuropathies, nausea, vomiting, hepatitis, bone marrow suppression, fever, local irritation at injection sites, gynecomastia, lupus syndrome

Table 9.10 DRUGS IN FOCUS

Antimycobacterial Drugs

Drug Name	Dosage/Route	Usual Indications
Antituberculosis Drugs		
capreomycin (*Capastat*)	Adult: 1 g/day IM for 60–120 days, followed by 1 g IM 2–3 times per wk for 18–24 mo; reduce dosage with renal impairment Pediatric: 15 mg/kg/day IM	Second-line drug for treatment of *Mycobacterium tuberculosis*
cycloserine (*Seromycin*)	Adult: 250 mg PO b.i.d. for 2 wk, then 500 mg to 1 g/day PO in divided doses Pediatric: safety not established	Second-line drug for treatment of *M. tuberculosis*
ethambutol (*Myambutol*)	Adult: 15 mg/kg/day PO as a single dose Pediatric: not recommended for children <13 yr	Second-line drug for treatment of *M. tuberculosis*
ethionamide (*Trecator S.C.*)	Adult: 15–20 mg/kg/day PO in divided doses with pyridoxine Pediatric: 10–20 mg/kg/day PO in divided doses with pyridoxine	First-line drug for treatment of *M. tuberculosis*
P isoniazid (INH) (*Nydrazid*)	Adult: 5 mg/kg/day PO Pediatric: 10–20 mg/kg/day PO	First-line drug for treatment of *M. tuberculosis*
pyrazinamide (*Generic*)	Adult and pediatric: 15–30 mg/kg/day PO	Second-line drug for treatment of *M. tuberculosis*
rifabutin (*Mycobutin*)	Adult: 300 mg PO daily Pediatric: safety not established	Treatment of *Mycobacterium avium-intracellulare* (MAC) in patients with advanced HIV infection
rifampin (*Rifadin, Rimactane*)	Adult: 600 mg PO or IV as a single daily dose Pediatric: 10–20 mg/kg/day PO or IV	First-line drug for treatment of *M. tuberculosis*
rifapentine (*Priftin*)	Adult: 600 mg PO 2 times per week for 2 mo Pediatric: safety not established	First-line drug for treatment of *M. tuberculosis*
Leprostatic Drugs		
dapsone (*Generic*)	Adult: 50–100 mg/day PO Pediatric: 1–2 mg/kg/day PO for 3 yr	Treatment of leprosy, *Pneumocystis carinii* pneumonia in AIDS patients, a variety of infections caused by susceptible bacteria and brown recluse spider bites

Leprostatic Drugs

The antibiotic used to treat leprosy is dapsone (see Table 9.10).

Dapsone (generic) has been the mainstay of leprosy treatment for many years, although resistant strains are emerging. Similar to the sulfonamides, dapsone inhibits folate synthesis in susceptible bacteria. In addition to its use in leprosy, dapsone is used to treat *P. carinii* pneumonia in AIDS patients and for a variety of infections caused by susceptible bacteria, as well as for brown recluse spider bites.

Recently, the hypnotic drug thalidomide (*Thalomid*) was approved for use in a condition that occurs after treatment for leprosy (Box 9.7).

Therapeutic Actions and Indications

Most of the antimycobacterial agents act on the DNA of the bacteria, leading to a lack of growth and eventually to bacterial death (see Figure 9.2). INH specifically affects the mycolic acid coat around the bacterium. Although many of the antimycobacterial agents are effective against other species of susceptible bacteria, their primary indications are in the treatment of tuberculosis or leprosy (as previ-

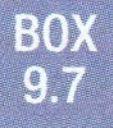

BOX 9.7 New Indication for Thalidomide

In the 1950s, the drug thalidomide became internationally known because it caused serious abnormalities (e.g., lack of limbs, defective limbs) in the fetuses of many women who received the drug during pregnancy to help them sleep and to decrease stress. This tragedy led to the recall of thalidomide in the United States and the establishment of more stringent standards for drug testing and labeling. In 1998, the Food and Drug Administration (FDA) approved the use of this controversial drug for the treatment of erythema nodosum leprosum, which is a painful inflammatory condition related to an immune reaction to dead bacteria that occurs after treatment for leprosy. It is also approved for use in the treatment of multiple myeloma, brain tumors, Crohn's disease, human immunodeficiency virus–wasting syndrome, and graft–host reaction in bone marrow transplant.

To take thalidomide, a woman must have a negative pregnancy test, receive instruction in using birth control, and sign a release stating that she understands the risks associated with the drug. These limits on the use of a drug were the first such restrictions ever ordered by the FDA.

Thalidomide (*Thalomid*) is given in doses of 100 to 300 mg/day PO at bedtime for at least 2 wk, followed by tapered dosage in 50-mg increments over the next 2 to 4 wk.

ously indicated). The antituberculosis drugs are always used in combination to affect the bacteria at various stages and to help to decrease the emergence of resistant strains.

Pharmacokinetics

The antimycobacterial agents are generally well absorbed from the GI tract, metabolized in the liver, and excreted in the urine. Caution should be used in patients with hepatic or renal dysfunction, which could interfere with the metabolism and excretion of the drugs. These drugs cross the placenta and enter breast milk; they should not be used during pregnancy and lactation unless the benefit to the mother clearly outweighs the potential risk to the fetus or neonate.

Contraindications and Cautions

Antimycobacterial drugs are contraindicated for patients with any known allergy to these agents; in those with severe renal or hepatic failure, *which could interfere with the metabolism or excretion of the drug;* in those with severe CNS dysfunction, *which could be exacerbated by the actions of the drug;* and in pregnancy *because of possible adverse effects on the fetus.* If an antituberculosis regimen is necessary during pregnancy, the combination of isoniazid, ethambutol, and rifampin is considered the safest.

Adverse Effects

CNS effects, such as neuritis, dizziness, headache, malaise, drowsiness, and hallucinations, are often reported and are related to direct effects of the drugs on neurons. These drugs also are irritating to the GI tract, causing nausea, vomiting, anorexia, stomach upset, and abdominal pain. Rifampin, rifabutin, and rifapentine cause discoloration of body fluids from urine to sweat and tears. Patients should be alerted that in many instances orange-tinged urine, sweat, and tears may stain clothing and permanently stain contact lenses. This can be frightening if the patient is not alerted to the possibility that it will happen. As with other antibiotics, there is always a possibility of hypersensitivity reactions, and the patient should be monitored on a regular basis.

Clinically Important Drug–Drug Interactions

When rifampin and INH are used in combination, the possibility of toxic liver reactions increases. Patients should be monitored closely.

Increased metabolism and decreased drug effectiveness occur as a result of administration of quinidine, metoprolol, propranolol, corticosteroids, oral contraceptives, oral anticoagulants, oral antidiabetic agents, digoxin, theophylline, methadone, phenytoin, verapamil, cyclosporine, or ketoconazole in combination with rifampin or rifabutin. Patients who are taking these drug combinations should be monitored closely and dosage adjustments made as needed.

Nursing Considerations for Patients Receiving Antimycobacterial Antibiotics

Assessment: History and Examination

Screen for the following, *which are possible contraindications or cautions for use of the drug:* known allergy to any antimycobacterial drug (obtain specific information about the nature and occurrence of allergic reactions); history of renal or hepatic disease, *which could interfere with metabolism and excretion of the drug and lead to toxicity;* history of CNS dysfunction, including seizure disorders and neuritis, *which could be exacerbated by adverse drug effects;* and current pregnancy status.

Physical examination should be performed *to establish baseline data for assessing the effectiveness of the drug and the occurrence of any adverse effects associated with drug therapy.* Obtain specimens for culture and sensitivity testing *to establish the sensitivity of the organism being treated.* Examine skin for any rash or lesions *to provide a baseline for possible adverse effects.* Evaluate CNS for orientation, affect, and reflexes *to establish a baseline and to monitor for adverse effects.* Note respiratory status *to provide a baseline for the occurrence of hypersensitivity reactions.* Evaluate renal and liver function tests, including BUN and creatinine clearance, *to assess the status of renal and liver functioning so as to determine any needed alteration in dosage.*

Nursing Diagnoses

The patient receiving an antimycobacterial drug may have the following nursing diagnoses related to drug therapy:

- Imbalanced Nutrition: Less Than Body Requirements, related to GI effects
- Disturbed Sensory Perception (Kinesthetic) related to CNS effects of the drug
- Acute Pain related to GI effects of drug
- Deficient Knowledge regarding drug therapy

Implementation With Rationale

- Check culture and sensitivity reports *to ensure that this is the drug of choice for this patient, and arrange repeated cultures if response is not as anticipated.*
- Monitor renal and liver function test results before and periodically during therapy *to arrange for dosage reduction as needed.*

- Ensure that the patient receives the full course of the drugs *to improve effectiveness and decrease the risk of development of resistant bacterial strains.* These drugs are taken for years and often in combination. Periodic medical evaluation and reteaching are often essential to ensure compliance.
- Discontinue the drug immediately if hypersensitivity reactions occur *to avert potentially serious reactions.*
- Encourage the patient to eat small, frequent meals as tolerated; perform frequent mouth care; and drink adequate fluids *to ensure adequate nutrition and hydration.* Monitor nutrition if GI effects become a problem.
- Ensure that the patient is instructed about the appropriate dosage regimen, use of drug combinations, and possible adverse effects *to enhance patient knowledge about drug therapy and to promote compliance.*

The patient should:

- Try to drink a lot of fluids to maintain nutrition (very important) even though nausea, vomiting, and diarrhea may occur.
- Use barrier contraceptives and understand that oral contraceptives may not be effective if antimycobacterial drugs are being used.
- Understand that normally some of these drugs impart an orange stain to body fluids. If this occurs, the fluids may stain clothing and tears may stain contact lenses.
- Report difficulty breathing, hallucinations, numbness and tingling, worsening of condition, fever and chills, or changes in color of urine or stool to a health care provider.

Evaluation

- Monitor patient response to the drug (resolution of mycobacterial infection).
- Monitor for adverse effects (GI effects, CNS changes, and hypersensitivity reactions).
- Evaluate the effectiveness of the teaching plan (patient can name the drug, dosage, possible adverse effects to expect, and specific measures to help avoid adverse effects).
- Monitor the effectiveness of comfort and safety measures and compliance with the regimen.

New Classes of Antibiotics

Four new classes of antibiotics are described in Boxes 9.8, 9.9, 9.10, and 9.11.

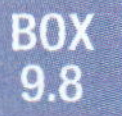

Telithromycin Approved for Respiratory Infections

Telithromycin (*Ketek*), the first drug in the new ketolide class of antibiotics, was approved for use in the United States in 2004. The drug has been in use in Europe since 2001. Telithromycin is effective against exacerbations of chronic bronchitis, acute bacterial sinusitis, and mild to moderate community acquired pneumonia. It is specifically effective against *Streptococcus pneumoniae* in patients older than 18 years. It is taken as an 800-mg oral dose once a day for 5 days, 7 to 10 days for community-acquired pneumonia. Patients should be monitored for pseudomembranous colitis, superinfections, and gastrointestinal discomfort.

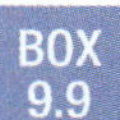

New Carbepenem Antibiotic Available for Parenteral Use

In late 2001, ertapenem (*Invanz*), a methyl-carbepenem antibiotic, was approved for use in treating community-acquired pneumonias, complicated skin and skin structure infections, and complicated intra-abdominal genitourinary, and pelvic infections. The carbepenem inhibits the synthesis of the bacterial cell wall, causing death of the bacteria. Its effectiveness against a wide range of bacteria may help to slow the emergence of resistant strains previously sensitive only to well-established antibiotics and may also provide successful treatment of some infections that are resistant to regularly used antibiotics. Ertapenem is given as 1 g IV or IM for 3 to 14 days, depending on the infection. It is not approved for use in children younger than 18 yr. It can cause allergic reactions in patients known to be allergic to penicillins or cephalosporins and is associated with gastrointestinal upset and possibly with pseudomembranous colitis. It is anticipated that other antibiotics in this class will be forthcoming if use of this drug proves successful.

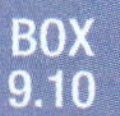

A Cyclic Lipopeptide Antibiotic: Daptomycin

The fall of 2003 saw the introduction of the first cyclic lipopeptide antibiotic, daptomycin (*Cubicin*). This class of drugs binds to bacterial cell membranes, causing a rapid depolarization of membrane potential. The loss of membrane potential leads to the inhibition of protein and DNA and RNA synthesis, which results in bacterial cell death. Daptomycin is approved for treating complicated skin and skin structure infections caused by susceptible gram-positive bacteria, including methicillin-resistant strains of *Staphylococcus aureus.* It must be given IV over 30 min, once each day for 7 to 14 days, which makes its use inconvenient. Patients should be monitored for pseudomembranous colitis and myopathies.

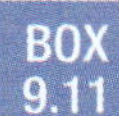

BOX 9.11 New Glycylcycline Antibiotic for IV Use

In 2005, the Food and Drug Administration approved tigecycline (*Tygacil*), the first drug of a new class of antibiotics called glycylcyclines. This antibiotic inhibits protein translation on ribosomes of certain bacteria, leading to their inability to maintain their integrity and culminating in the death of the bacterium. It is approved for use in the treatment of complicated skin and skin structure infections and intra-abdominal infections caused by susceptible bacteria. Caution should be used with a known allergy to tetracycline antibiotics, because a cross-sensitivity may occur. Women should be advised to use a barrier form of contraceptive when on this drug. Patients should be monitored for pseudomembranous colitis, rash, and superinfections. *Tygacil* is given as 100 mg IV followed by 50 mg IV q12h, infused over 30 to 60 min for 5 to 14 days.

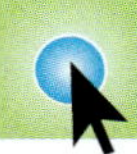

WEB LINKS

Health care providers, students, and patients may want to consult the following Internet resources:

http://www.chclibrary.org/micromed/00037050.html Information on aminoglycosides.

http://www.fhsu.edu/nursing/otitis Information on cephalosporins.

http://www.cellsalive.com/pen.htm Information on penicillins.

http://www.who.int/gtb/ Information on tuberculosis.

http://www.cpmc.columbia.edu/resources/tbcpp Information on resources for patients with tuberculosis.

http://www.leprosy.org Information on leprosy.

http://www.cdc.gov Information on infectious diseases, disease prevention, recommendations for treatment, and treatment schedules (CDC).

Points to Remember

- Antibiotics work by disrupting protein or enzyme systems within a bacterium, causing cell death (bactericidal) or preventing multiplication (bacteriostatic).
- The proteins or enzyme systems affected by antibiotics are more likely to be found or used in bacteria than in human cells.
- The goal of antibiotic therapy is to reduce the number of invading bacteria so that the normal immune system can deal with the infection.
- The primary therapeutic use of each antibiotic is determined by the bacterial species that are sensitive to that drug, the clinical condition of the patient receiving the drug, and the benefit-to-risk ratio for the patient.
- The longer an antibiotic has been available, the more likely it is that mutant bacterial strains resistant to the mechanisms of antibiotic activity will have developed.
- The most common adverse effects of antibiotic therapy involve the GI tract (nausea, vomiting, diarrhea, anorexia, abdominal pain) and superinfections (invasion of the body by normally occurring microorganisms that are usually kept in check by the normal flora).
- To prevent or contain the growing threat of drug-resistant strains of bacteria, it is very important to use antibiotics cautiously, to complete the full course of an antibiotic prescription, and to avoid saving antibiotics for self-medication in the future. A patient and family teaching program should address these issues, as well as the proper dosing procedure for the drug (even if the patient feels better) and the importance of keeping a record of any reactions to antibiotics.

CHECK YOUR UNDERSTANDING

Answers to the questions in this chapter may be found in the Answer Key in the back of the book.

Multiple Choice

Select the best answer to the following.

1. A bacteriostatic substance is one that
   a. directly kills any bacteria it comes in contact with.
   b. directly kills any bacteria that are sensitive to the substance.
   c. prevents the growth of any bacteria.
   d. prevents the growth of specific bacteria that are sensitive to the substance.

2. Gram-negative bacteria
   a. are mostly found in the respiratory tract.
   b. are mostly associated with soft tissue infections.
   c. are mostly found in the GI and GU tracts.
   d. accept a positive stain when tested.

3. Antibiotics that are used together to increase their effectiveness and limit the associated adverse effects are said to be
   a. broad spectrum.
   b. synergistic.
   c. bactericidal.
   d. anaerobic.

4. An aminoglycoside antibiotic might be the drug of choice in treating
   a. serious infections caused by susceptible strains of gram-negative bacteria.
   b. otitis media in an infant.
   c. cystitis in a woman who is 4 months pregnant.
   d. suspected pneumonia before the culture results are available.

5. Which of the following is not a caution for the use of cephalosporins?
   a. Allergy to penicillin
   b. Renal failure
   c. Allergy to aspirin
   d. Concurrent treatment with aminoglycosides

6. The fluoroquinolones
   a. are found freely in nature.
   b. are associated with severe adverse reactions.
   c. are widely used to treat gram-positive infections.
   d. are broad-spectrum antibiotics with few associated adverse effects.

7. Cipro, a widely used antibiotic, is an example of
   a. a penicillin.
   b. a fluoroquinolone.
   c. an aminoglycoside.
   d. a macrolide antibiotic.

8. A patient receiving a fluoroquinolone should be cautioned to anticipate
   a. increased salivation.
   b. constipation.
   c. photosensitivity.
   d. cough.

9. The goal of antibiotic therapy is
   a. to eradicate all bacteria from the system.
   b. to suppress resistant strains of bacteria.
   c. to reduce the number of invading bacteria so that the immune system can deal with the infection.
   d. to stop the drug as soon as the patient feels better.

10. The penicillins
   a. are bacteriostatic.
   b. are bactericidal, interfering with bacteria cell walls.
   c. are effective only if given intravenously.
   d. do not produce cross-sensitivity within their class.

Multiple Response

Select all that apply.

1. A young woman is found to have a soft tissue infection that is most responsive to tetracycline. Your teaching plan for this woman should include which of the following points?
   a. Tetracycline can cause gray baby syndrome.
   b. Do not use this drug if you are pregnant, because it can cause tooth and bone defects in the fetus.
   c. Tetracycline can cause severe acne.
   d. You should use a second form of contraception if you are using oral contraceptives because tetracycline can make them ineffective.
   e. This drug should be taken in the middle of a meal to decrease GI upset.
   f. You may experience a vaginal yeast infection as a result of this drug therapy.

2. In general, all patients receiving antibiotics should receive teaching that includes which of the following points?
   a. The need to complete the full course of drug therapy
   b. The possibility of oral contraceptive failure
   c. When to take the drug related to food and other drugs
   d. The need for screening blood tests
   e. Advisability of saving any leftover medication for future use
   f. How to detect superinfections and what to do if they occur

True or False

Indicate whether the following statements are true (T) or false (F).

_____ 1. Aerobic bacteria depend on oxygen for survival.

_____ 2. Bactericidal refers to a substance that prevents the replication of bacteria.

_____ 3. Bacteriostatic refers to a drug that causes the death of bacteria.

_____ 4. Anaerobic bacteria survive without oxygen.

_____ 5. Gram negative refers to bacteria that take a positive stain and are frequently associated with infections of the respiratory tract and soft tissues.

_____ 6. An antibiotic is a chemical that inhibits the growth of specific bacteria or causes the death of susceptible bacteria.

_____ 7. Antibiotics usually eradicate all of the bacteria that have entered the body.

_____ 8. Synergistic drugs are drugs that work together to increase a drug's effectiveness.

Web Exercise

Go to http://www.cdc.gov.

Select Health Topics A–Z, select the letter T, and then find tuberculosis. Develop an information sheet for a patient with tuberculosis, including teaching points, ways to remember to take the medication, family pointers, and drug effects.

Matching

Match the following antibiotics with the correct class.

1. ______________________ minocycline
2. ______________________ sulfasalazine
3. ______________________ capreomycin
4. ______________________ amikacin
5. ______________________ cefonicid
6. ______________________ erythromycin
7. ______________________ norfloxacin
8. ______________________ clindamycin
9. ______________________ ampicillin
10. ______________________ levofloxacin
11. ______________________ gentamicin
12. ______________________ dapsone

A. Aminoglycosides
B. Cephalosporins
C. Fluoroquinolones
D. Lincosamides
E. Penicillins
F. Sulfonamides
G. Tetracyclines
H. Leprostatic
I. Antimycobacterials
J. Macrolides

Bibliography and References

The choice of antibacterial drugs. (2001). *Medical Letter on Drugs and Therapeutics, 89,* 1111–1112.

Dowell, S. F., et al. (1998). Otitis media—Principles of judicious use of antimicrobial agents. *Pediatrics, 101,* 165–171.

Drug facts and comparisons. (2006). St. Louis: Facts and Comparisons.

Gilman, A., Hardman, J. G., & Limbird, L. E. (Eds.). (2006). *Goodman and Gilman's the pharmacological basis of therapeutics* (11th ed.). New York: McGraw-Hill.

Gonzales, R., Bartlett, J. G., Besser, R. E., Cooper, R. J., Hickner, J. M., Hoffman, J. R., Sande, M. A. (2001). Principles of appropriate antibiotic use for the treatment of acute respiratory tract infections in adults: Background, specific aims, and methods. *Annals of Internal Medicine, 134,* 479–486.

Karch, A. M. (2006). *2007 Lippincott's nursing drug guide.* Philadelphia: Lippincott Williams & Wilkins.

Porth, C. M. (2005). *Pathophysiology: Concepts of altered health states* (7th ed.). Philadelphia: Lippincott Williams & Wilkins.

Professional's guide to patient drug facts. (2006). St. Louis: Facts and Comparisons.

Rosenstan, et al. (1998). The common cold—Principles of judicious use of antimicrobial agents. *Pediatrics, 100,* 181–184.

CHAPTER 10

Antiviral Agents

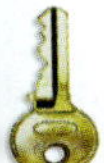

KEY TERMS

acquired immune deficiency syndrome (AIDS)

AIDS-related complex (ARC)

cytomegalovirus (CMV)

helper T cell

herpes

human immunodeficiency virus (HIV)

influenza A

interferons

nucleosides

protease inhibitors

reverse transcriptase inhibitors

virus

LEARNING OBJECTIVES

Upon completion of this chapter, you will be able to:

1. Discuss problems with treating viral infections in humans and the use of antivirals across the lifespan.
2. Describe characteristics of common viruses and the resultant clinical presentations of viral infections including a respiratory viral infection, a herpes infection, CMV, HIV/AIDS, hepatitis B.
3. Describe the therapeutic actions, indications, pharmacokinetics, contraindications, most common adverse reactions, and important drug–drug interactions associated with each of the classes of antivirals: agents for influenza A and respiratory viruses, agents for herpes and CMV, agents for HIV/AIDS, agents for hepatitis B, and topical agents.
4. Compare and contrast the prototype drugs for each class of antivirals with the other drugs within that class.
5. Outline the nursing considerations for patients receiving each class of antiviral agent.

AGENTS FOR INFLUENZA A AND RESPIRATORY VIRUSES

amantadine
oseltamivir
ribavirin
P rimantadine
zanamivir

AGENTS FOR HERPES AND CYTOMEGALOVIRUS

P acyclovir
cidofovir
famciclovir
foscarnet
ganciclovir
valacyclovir
valganciclovir

AGENTS FOR HIV AND AIDS

Reverse Transcriptase Inhibitors

delavirdine
efavirenz
emtricitabine
P nevirapine

Protease Inhibitors

amprenavir
atazanavir
fosamprenavir
indinavir
lopinavir
nelfinavir
ritonavir
saquinavir
tipranavir

Nucleosides

abacavir
didanosine
lamivudine

stavudine
tenofovir
zalcitabine
P zidovudine

Fusion Inhibitor
enfuvirtide

AGENTS FOR HEPATITIS B

P adefovir
entecavir

LOCALLY ACTIVE ANTIVIRAL AGENTS

docosanol
fomivirsen
ganciclovir
idoxuridine
imiquimod
penciclovir
trifluridine
vidarabine

Viruses cause a variety of conditions, ranging from warts, to the common cold and "flu," to diseases such as chickenpox and measles. A single virus particle is composed of a piece of DNA or RNA inside a protein coat. To carry on any metabolic processes, including replication, a virus must enter a cell. Once a virus has injected its DNA or RNA into its host cell, that cell is altered—that is, it is "programmed" to control the metabolic processes that the virus needs to survive. The virus, including the protein coat, replicates in the host cell (Figure 10.1). When the host cell can no longer carry out its own metabolic functions because of the viral invader, the host cell dies and releases the new viruses into the body to invade other cells.

Because viruses are contained inside human cells while they are in the body, it has proved difficult to develop effective drugs that destroy a virus without harming the human host. **Interferons** (see Chapter 15) are released by the host in response to viral invasion of a cell and prevent the replication of that particular virus. Some interferons that affect particular viruses are now available through genetic engineering programs. Other drugs that are used in treating viral infections have been effective against a limited number of viruses. Viruses that respond to some antiviral therapy include influenza A and some respiratory viruses, herpes viruses, cytomegalovirus (CMV), the human immunodeficiency virus (HIV) that causes acquired immune deficiency syndrome (AIDS), hepatitis B, and some viruses that cause warts and certain eye infections. Patients need to be cautioned against using certain alternative therapies while on antiviral medication (Box 10.1). (Box 10.2 discusses the use of antivirals across the lifespan.)

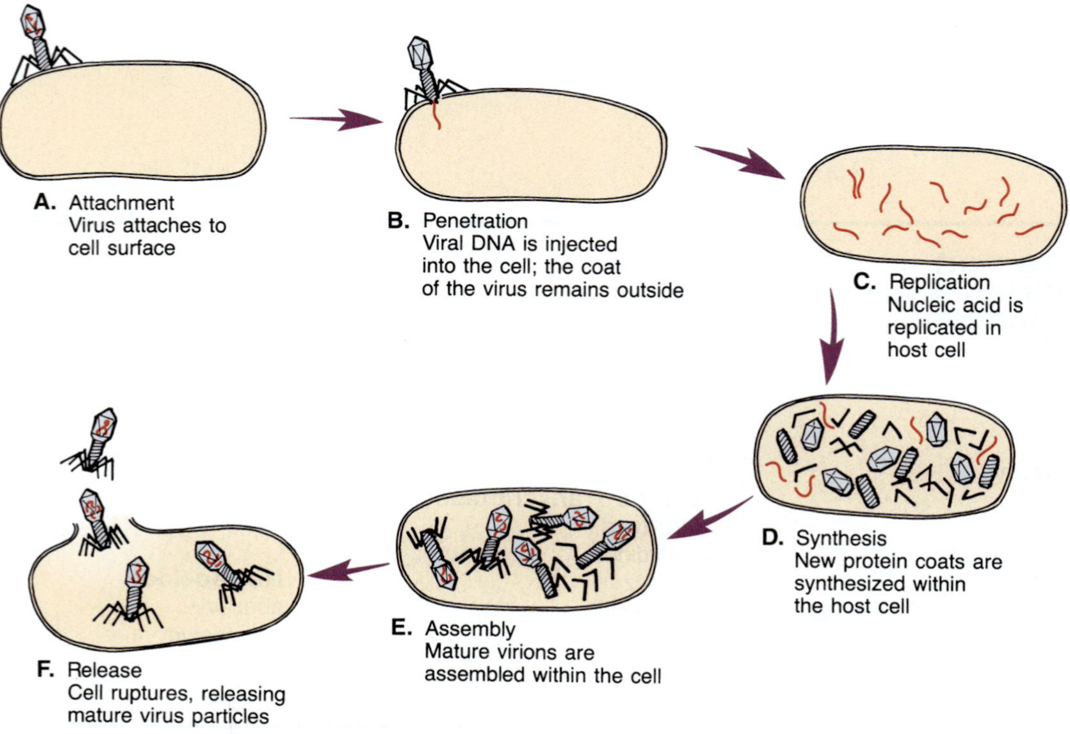
A. Attachment
Virus attaches to cell surface
B. Penetration
Viral DNA is injected into the cell; the coat of the virus remains outside
C. Replication
Nucleic acid is replicated in host cell
D. Synthesis
New protein coats are synthesized within the host cell
E. Assembly
Mature virions are assembled within the cell
F. Release
Cell ruptures, releasing mature virus particles

FIGURE 10.1 The stages in the replication cycle of a virus.

BOX 10.1 CULTURAL CONSIDERATIONS FOR DRUG THERAPY

Alternative Therapies and Antiviral Drugs

An increasing number of people in our culture are using alternative therapies as part of their daily regimen. St. John's wort is one of the more popular alternative therapies sold today. This herb has been used as an anti-inflammatory agent, as an antidepressant, as a diuretic, and as a treatment for gastritis and insomnia. Multimedia advertisements urge the use of St. John's wort to increase one's sense of well-being and to decrease depression "without the use of drugs." Many people with viral infections just do not feel well. They are tired, have muscle aches and pains, and feel feverish and low on energy. This herbal remedy seems to be aimed at these people. Unfortunately, St. John's wort has been shown to interact with many prescription drugs. When taken with St. John's wort, the protease inhibitors used in treating HIV were found to have decreased serum levels, leading to possible treatment failure. Because St. John's wort may induce the cytochrome P450 system in the liver, there is a possibility that it could increase the metabolism of many other antiviral drugs that are metabolized by that system and cause treatment failures with those drugs.

Patients may be reluctant to discuss their use of alternative therapies with the health care provider, because they want to maintain control over that aspect of their medical regimen or because they believe that the health care provider would not approve of the use of these therapies. It is important, when a patient is prescribed an antiviral agent, to ask specifically about the use of herbal or alternative medicines. Explain to the patient that antiviral drugs may interact with some herbal medicines and that it is important to try to avoid any adverse effects or drug failures.

Agents for Influenza A and Respiratory Viruses

Influenza A and other respiratory viruses, including influenza B and respiratory syncytial virus (RSV), invade the respiratory tract and cause the signs and symptoms of respiratory "flu."

Amantadine (*Symmetrel*) was first used to treat Parkinson's disease. However, patients who took amantadine did not get influenza during flu season. This drug is now used for both treatment and prevention of respiratory viral infections. It is slowly absorbed from the gastrointestinal (GI) tract, reaching peak levels in 4 hours. Excretion occurs unchanged through the urine, with a half-life of 15 hours. Because of its renal clearance, amantadine must be used at reduced doses and with caution in patients who have any renal impairment. Amantadine is embryotoxic in animals and crosses into breast milk; it should be used during pregnancy and lactation only if the benefits clearly outweigh the risks to the fetus or neonate.

Oseltamivir (*Tamiflu*) is effective in the treatment of uncomplicated influenza infections that have been symptomatic for less than 2 days. Oseltamivir is the only antiviral agent that has been shown to be effective in treating Avian flu. It is readily absorbed from the GI tract, extensively metabolized in the urine, and excreted in the urine with a half-life of 6 to 10 hours. The dosage should be reduced and the patient closely monitored if there is renal dysfunction. There are no adequate studies in pregnancy and lactation, so oseltamivir should be used during pregnancy and lactation only if the benefits clearly outweigh the risks to the fetus or neonate.

Ribavirin (*Virazole*) is effective against influenza A, RSV, and herpes viruses. This agent has been used in the treat-

BOX 10.2 DRUG THERAPY ACROSS THE LIFESPAN

Antivirals

CHILDREN

Children are very sensitive to the effects of most antiviral drugs, and more severe reactions can be expected when these drugs are used in children.

Many of these drugs do not have proven safety and efficacy in children, and extreme caution should be used.

Most of the drugs for prevention and treatment of influenza virus infections can be used, in smaller doses, for children.

Acyclovir is the drug of choice for children with herpes virus or cytomegalovirus infections.

The drugs used in the treatment of AIDS are frequently used in children, even when no scientific data are available, because of the seriousness of the disease. Dosage should be lowered according to body weight, and children must be monitored very closely for adverse effects on kidneys, bone marrow, and liver.

ADULTS

Adults need to know that these drugs are specific for the treatment of viral infections. The use of antibiotics to treat such infections can lead to the development of resistant strains and superinfections that can cause more problems.

Patients with HIV infection who are taking antiviral medications need to be taught that these drugs do not cure the disease, that opportunistic infections can still occur, and that precautions to prevent transmission of the disease need to be taken.

Pregnant women, for the most part, should not use these drugs unless the benefit clearly outweighs the potential risk to the fetus or neonate. Women of childbearing age should be advised to use barrier contraceptives if any of these drugs are used. Zidovudine has been safely used in pregnant women.

The Centers for Disease Control and Prevention advises that women with HIV infection should not breast-feed, to protect the neonate from the virus.

OLDER ADULTS

Older patients may be more susceptible to the adverse effects associated with these drugs; they should be monitored closely.

Patients with hepatic dysfunction are at increased risk for worsening hepatic problems and toxic effects of those drugs that are metabolized in the liver. Drugs that are excreted unchanged in the urine can be especially toxic to patients who have renal dysfunction. If hepatic or renal dysfunction is expected (extreme age, alcohol abuse, use of other hepatotoxic or nephrotoxic drugs), the dosage may need to be lowered and the patient should be monitored more frequently.

Table 10.1 DRUGS IN FOCUS

Influenza A and Respiratory Virus Drugs

Drug Name	Dosage/Route	Usual Indications
amantadine (*Symmetrel*)	Adult: 200 mg/day PO Pediatric (9–12 yr): 100 mg PO b.i.d. Pediatric (1–9 yr): 2–4 mg/lb PO daily	Treatment of Parkinson's disease; treatment and prevention of respiratory virus infections
oseltamivir (*Tamiflu*)	Adult: 75–150 mg PO b.i.d. for 5 days Pediatric (1–12 yr): 30–75 mg b.i.d. PO for 5 days	Treatment of uncomplicated influenza; treatment of Avian flu
ribavirin (*Rebetron*) (*Virazole*)	Adult: 400 mg/day PO in am with 600 mg/day PO in pm with 3 million International Units interferon alpha-2b Sub-Q 3 times per week Pediatric: 20 mg/mL in the reservoir for aerosol treatment over 12–18 h each day for 3–7 days	Treatment of chronic hepatitis C in patients who relapse after interferon-alpha therapy Treatment of influenza A, respiratory syncytial virus, and herpes virus infections
P rimantadine (*Flumadine*)	Adult: 100 mg PO b.i.d. Pediatric (≥10 yr): 5 mg/kg PO daily	Prevention and treatment of influenza A infections
zanamivir (*Relenza*)	Adult and children ≥7 yr: Two inhalations, b.i.d. (12 h apart) for 5 days	Treatment of uncomplicated influenza infections

ment of children with RSV and has been tested for use in several other viral conditions. It is available in a combination packet with interferon alfa-2b as an oral drug, *Rebetron,* for the treatment of chronic hepatitis C in children and adults. Ribavirin is absorbed well through the respiratory tract and has a half-life of 9.5 hours. It is teratogenic and is rated pregnancy category X. Women of childbearing age should be advised to use barrier contraceptives if they are taking this drug, although the drug is only used for adults with chronic hepatitis C.

Rimantadine (*Flumadine*), a synthetic agent, is used for the prevention and treatment of influenza A infections. It is absorbed from the GI tract with peak levels achieved in 6 hours. Rimantadine is extensively metabolized in the liver and excreted in the urine. Rimantadine is embryotoxic in animals and should be used during pregnancy only if the benefits clearly outweigh the risks. It should not be used by nursing mothers because it crosses into breast milk and can cause toxic reactions in the neonate. Use in children should be limited to prevention of influenza A infections.

Zanamivir (*Relenza*) was approved in 1999 to treat uncomplicated influenza infections in adults and in children older than 7 years of age who have had symptoms for less than 2 days. This drug must be delivered by a *Diskhaler* device, which comes with every prescription of zanamivir. It is absorbed through the respiratory tract and excreted unchanged in the urine with a half-life of 2.5 to 5.1 hours. Because of the renal excretion, the drug should be used cautiously in patients with any renal impairment. It should be used during pregnancy and lactation only if the benefits

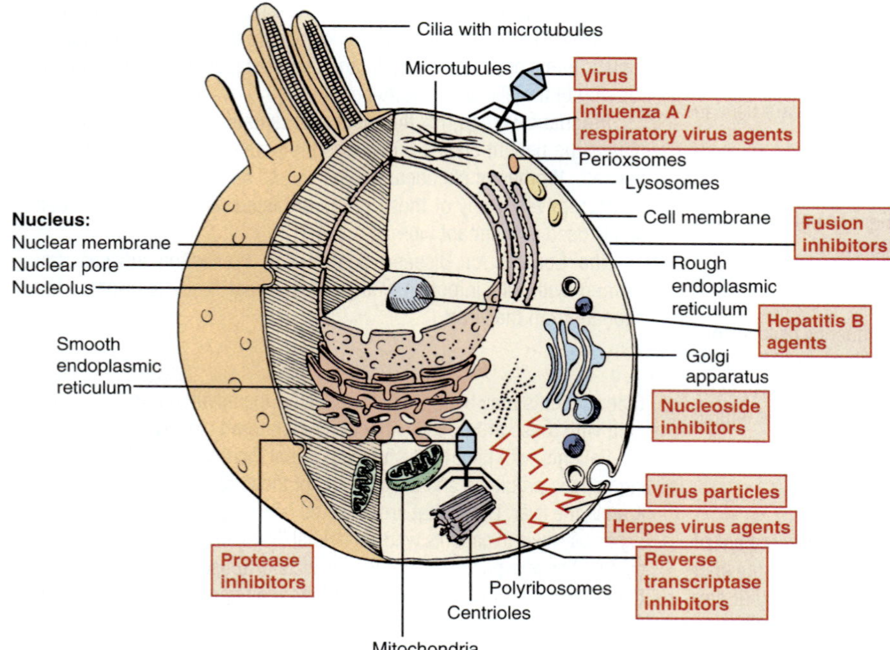

FIGURE 10.2 Agents for influenza A and respiratory viruses prevent shedding of the protein coat and entry of virus into the cell. Herpes virus agents alter viral DNA production. Agents that attempt to control HIV and AIDS work in the following ways: nucleosides interfere with HIV replication by blocking protein synthesis; reverse transcriptase inhibitors block the transfer of information that allows viral replication; protease inhibitors block protease within the virus, leading to immature, noninfective virus particles; fusion inhibitors prevent the virus from fusing with the cellular membrane, thereby preventing the HIV-1 virus from entering the cell. Antihepatitis B agents block DNA formation, preventing the formation of new viruses.

clearly outweigh the risks to the fetus or neonate. These drugs are described in detail in Table 10.1.

Therapeutic Actions and Indications

Although the exact mechanism of action of drugs that combat respiratory viruses is not known, it is believed that these agents prevent shedding of the viral protein coat and entry of the virus into the cell (Figure 10.2). This action prevents viral replication, causing viral death. These antiviral drugs are indicated for prevention of influenza A infection, which is especially important in health care workers and other high-risk individuals, and for reducing the severity of infection if it occurs.

Contraindications and Cautions

Caution should be used when giving these antiviral agents to patients with a known allergy; to pregnant or lactating women; or to patients with renal or liver disease, *which could alter metabolism and excretion of the drug.*

Adverse Effects

Use of these antiviral agents is frequently associated with various adverse effects that may be related to possible effects on dopamine levels in the brain. These adverse effects include light-headedness, dizziness, and insomnia; nausea; orthostatic hypotension; and urinary retention.

Clinically Important Drug–Drug Interactions

Patients who receive amantadine or rimantadine may experience increased atropine-like effects if either of these drugs is given with an anticholinergic drug.

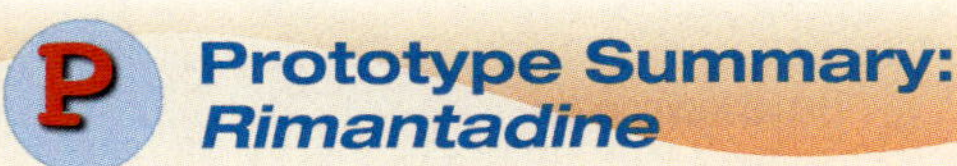

Prototype Summary: *Rimantadine*

Indications: Prophylaxis and treatment of illness caused by influenza A virus in adults; prophylaxis against influenza A virus in children

Actions: Inhibits viral replication, possibly by preventing the uncoating of the virus

Pharmacokinetics:

Route	Onset	Peak
Oral	Slow	6 h

$T_{1/2}$: 25.4 hours; excreted unchanged in the urine

Adverse effects: Light-headedness, dizziness, insomnia, nausea, dyspnea, orthostatic hypotension, depression

Nursing Considerations for Patients Receiving Influenza A and Respiratory Virus Drugs

Assessment: History and Examination

Patients who receive respiratory antiviral agents should be assessed for the following conditions, *which either are contraindications to the use of these drugs or necessitate precautionary measures:* known history of allergy to antivirals; history of liver or renal dysfunction *that might interfere with drug metabolism and excretion;* and current pregnancy or lactation status.

Physical assessment should be performed to *establish baseline data for evaluating the effectiveness of the drug and the occurrence of any adverse effects associated with drug therapy.* Include screening for orientation and reflexes *to evaluate any central nervous system (CNS) effects of the drug;* vital signs (respiratory rate, adventitious sounds, temperature) *to assess for signs and symptoms of the viral infection;* blood pressure *to monitor for orthostatic hypotension;* urinary output *to monitor genitourinary (GU) effects of the drug;* and renal and hepatic function tests *to determine baseline function of these organs.*

Nursing Diagnoses

The patient receiving a respiratory antiviral drug may have the following nursing diagnoses related to drug therapy:

- Acute Pain related to GI, CNS, or GU effects of drug
- Disturbed Sensory Perception (Kinesthetic) related to CNS effects of drug
- Deficient Knowledge regarding drug therapy

Implementation With Rationale

- Start drug regimen as soon after exposure to the virus as possible *to achieve best effectiveness and decrease the risk of complications of viral infection.*
- Administer influenza A vaccine before the flu season begins, if at all possible, *to prevent the disease and decrease the risk of complications.*
- Administer the full course of the drug *to obtain the full beneficial effects.*
- Provide safety provisions if CNS effects occur *to protect the patient from injury.*
- Instruct the patient about the appropriate dosage scheduling regimen; safety precautions, including changing position slowly and avoiding driving and hazardous tasks, to take if CNS effects occur; and the need to report any difficulty walking or talking *to enhance patient knowledge about drug therapy and to promote compliance.*

Evaluation

- Monitor patient response to the drug (prevention of respiratory flu-like symptoms; alleviation of flu-like symptoms).
- Monitor for adverse effects (orientation and affect, blood pressure, urinary output).
- Evaluate the effectiveness of the teaching plan (patient can name the drug, dosage, possible adverse effects to watch for, and specific measures to help avoid adverse effects).
- Monitor the effectiveness of comfort and safety measures and compliance with the regimen.

Agents for Herpes and Cytomegalovirus

Herpes viruses account for a broad range of conditions, including cold sores, encephalitis, shingles, and genital infections. **Cytomegalovirus (CMV)**, although slightly different from the herpes virus, can affect the eye, respiratory tract, and liver and reacts to many of the same drugs. A number of antiviral drugs are used to combat these infections (see Table 10.2).

Acyclovir (*Zovirax*) is specific for herpes virus infections. It is excreted unchanged in the urine and therefore must be used cautiously in the presence of renal impairment. Acyclovir crosses into breast milk and exposes the neonate to high levels of the drug, so extreme caution must be used during lactation.

Cidofovir (*Vistide*) is used to treat CMV retinitis in patients with AIDS only. It is associated with severe renal toxicity and granulocytopenia. Cidofovir is excreted unchanged in the urine and must be given with probenecid to increase renal clearance of the drug. The dosage must be decreased according to renal function and creatinine clearance. Use in children with AIDS should be very cautious because of potential carcinogenic effects and effects on fertility. If no other treatment option is available, monitor the child very closely.

Famciclovir (*Famvir*) is most effective in treating herpes infections. It is used to treat herpes zoster or shingles and for recurrent episodes of genital herpes. It is well absorbed from the GI tract, reaching peak levels in 2 to 3 hours. Famciclovir is metabolized in the liver and excreted in the urine and feces. Safety of use in children younger than 18 years of age has not been established.

Foscarnet (*Foscavir*) is available in intravenous (IV) form only. It can be highly toxic to the kidneys and is reserved for treatment of CMV retinitis in immunocompromised patients and for mucocutaneous acyclovir-resistant herpes simplex infections. About 90% of foscarnet is excreted unchanged in the urine, so it should be used cautiously and at reduced dosage in patients with renal impairment. Foscarnet has been shown to affect bone development and growth and should not be used in children unless the benefit clearly outweighs the risk and the child is monitored very closely.

Ganciclovir (*Cytovene*), which is available in IV and oral forms, is used for long-term treatment and prevention of CMV infections. Ganciclovir is primarily excreted unchanged in the feces with some urinary excretion. Ganciclovir is car-

Table 10.2 DRUGS IN FOCUS

Agents for Herpes Virus and Cytomegalovirus (CMV)

Drug Name	Dosage/Route	Usual Indications
P acyclovir (*Zovirax*)	Adult: 5–10 mg/kg q8h IV, IM, *or* Sub-Q, *or* 200 mg PO 5 times per day for 10 days and then 400 mg PO b.i.d. for 12 mo Pediatric: 250–500 mg/m^2 q8h IV, IM, *or* Sub-Q for 7–10 days, *or* 20 mg/kg q.i.d. PO for 5 days	Treatment of herpes virus infections
cidofovir (*Vistide*)	5 mg/kg IV (over 1 h) once weekly for 2 weeks, then every other week, with probenecid 2 g PO 3 h before and 1 g PO 2 h and 8 h after cidofovir infusion	Treatment of CMV retinitis in AIDS patients
famciclovir (*Famvir*)	Herpes zoster: 500 mg PO q8h for 7 days Genital herpes: 125 mg b.i.d. PO for 5 days	Treatment of herpes virus infections
foscarnet (*Foscavir*)	Adult: 40–60 mg/kg q8–12h IV given as a 2-h infusion Pediatric: safety and efficacy not established	Treatment of CMV and herpes simplex infections in immunocompromised patients
ganciclovir (*Cytovene*)	Adult: 5 m/kg q12h IV given over 1 h for 14–21 days then over 1 h daily 7 days/wk or 6 mg/kg/day for 5 days/wk for prophylaxis	Long-term treatment and prevention of CMV infection
valacyclovir (*Valtrex*)	Herpes zoster: 1 g PO t.i.d. for 7 days Genital herpes: 500 mg b.i.d. PO for 5 days	Treatment of herpes virus infections
valganciclovir (*Valcyfe*)	900 mg PO b.i.d. for 21 days, then 900 mg PO once a day for maintenance; reduce dosage with renal impairment	Treatment of CMV retinitis in AIDS patients

cinogenic and should be used only with extreme caution in children.

Valacyclovir (*Valtrex*) is an oral agent used for the treatment of herpes zoster and recurrent genital herpes; to decrease the risk of infection in healthy partners of herpes zoster patients; and for treatment of cold sores (herpes labialis) in adults. It is rapidly absorbed from the GI tract and metabolized in the liver to acyclovir. Excretion occurs through the urine, so caution should be used in patients with renal impairment. Safety for use in children has not been established.

Valganciclovir (*Valcyte*), which is the oral prodrug of ganciclovir, is used for the treatment of CMV retinitis in AIDS patients. It is primarily excreted unchanged in the feces with some urinary excretion. Valganciclovir is also carcinogenic and should be used only with extreme caution in children.

Therapeutic Actions and Indications

Drugs that combat herpes and CMV inhibit viral DNA replication by competing with viral substrates to form shorter, noneffective DNA chains (see Figure 10.2). This action prevents replication of the virus, but it has little effect on the host cells of humans because their DNA uses different substrates. These antiviral agents are indicated for treatment of the DNA viruses herpes simplex, herpes zoster, and CMV. Research has shown that they are very effective in immunocompromised individuals, such as patients with AIDS, those taking immunosuppressants, and those with multiple infections.

Pharmacokinetics

Of the agents used in the treatment of herpes and CMV, Cidofovir (*Vistide*) has proved embryotoxic in animals. For many of the other agents, no adequate studies have been completed during human pregnancy and lactation, but because of the toxicities of all of these drugs, they should be used during pregnancy and lactation only if the benefits clearly outweigh the potential risks to the fetus or neonate.

Contraindications and Cautions

Drugs indicated for the treatment of herpes and CMV should not be used during pregnancy or lactation or in patients with known allergies to antiviral agents; renal disease, *which could interfere with excretion of the drug;* or severe CNS disorders.

Adverse Effects

The adverse effects most commonly associated with these antivirals include nausea and vomiting, headache, depression, rash, and hair loss. Rash, inflammation, and burning often occur at sites of IV injection and topical application. Renal dysfunction and renal failure also have been reported.

Clinically Important Drug–Drug Interactions

The risk of nephrotoxicity increases when agents indicated for the treatment of herpes and CMV are used in combination with other nephrotoxic drugs.

The risk of drowsiness also rises when these antiviral agents are taken with zidovudine, an antiretroviral agent.

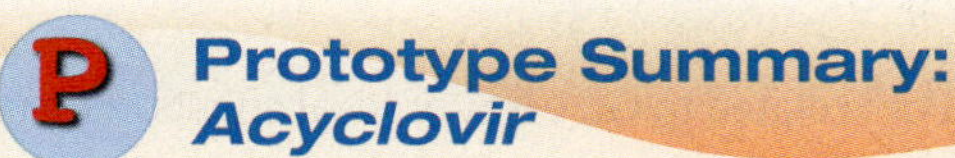

Prototype Summary: Acyclovir

Indications: Treatment of herpes simplex virus (HSV) 1 and 2 infections; treatment of severe genital HSV infections; treatment of HSV encephalitis; acute treatment of shingles and chickenpox; ointment for the treatment of genital herpes infections; cream for the treatment of cold sores (herpes labialis)

Actions: Inhibits viral DNA replication

Pharmacokinetics:

Route	Onset	Peak	Duration
Oral	Varies	1.5–2 h	Not known
IV	Immediate	1 h	8 h
Topical	Not generally absorbed systemically		

$T_{1/2}$: 2.5–5 hours; excreted unchanged in the urine

Adverse effects: Headache, vertigo, tremors, nausea, vomiting, rash

Nursing Considerations for Patients Receiving Agents for Herpes Virus and Cytomegalovirus

Assessment: History and Examination

Patients receiving DNA-active antiviral agents should be assessed for the following conditions, *which are cautions or contraindications to the use of these drugs:* any history of allergy to antivirals; renal dysfunction *that might interfere with the metabolism and excretion of the drug;* severe CNS disorders *that could be aggravated;* and pregnancy or lactation.

Physical assessment should be *performed to establish baseline data for assessing the effectiveness of the*

DNA-active antiviral drug and the occurrence of any adverse effects associated with drug therapy. Assess orientation and reflexes *to evaluate any CNS effects of the drug.* Examine skin (color, temperature, and lesions) *to monitor the effectiveness of the drug.* Evaluate renal function tests *to determine baseline function of the kidneys.*

Nursing Diagnoses

The patient receiving a DNA-active antiviral agent may have the following nursing diagnoses related to drug therapy:

- Acute Pain related to GI, CNS, or local effects of drug
- Disturbed Sensory Perception (Kinesthetic) related to CNS effects of drug
- Deficient Knowledge regarding drug therapy

Implementation With Rationale

- Ensure good hydration *to decrease the toxic effects on the kidneys.*
- Administer the drug as soon as possible after the diagnosis has been made *to improve effectiveness of the antiviral activity.*
- Ensure that the patient takes the complete course of the drug regimen *to improve effectiveness and decrease the risk of the emergence of resistant viruses.*
- Wear protective gloves when applying the drug topically *to decrease risk of exposure to the drug and inadvertent absorption.*
- Provide safety precautions if CNS effects occur (e.g., use of siderails, appropriate lighting, orientation, assistance) *to protect the patient from injury.*
- Warn the patient that GI upset, nausea, and vomiting can occur, *to prevent undue anxiety and increase awareness of the importance of nutrition.*
- Monitor renal function tests periodically during treatment *to detect and respond to renal toxicity as soon as possible.*
- Provide the patient with instructions about the drug *to enhance patient knowledge about drug therapy and to promote compliance.*

The patient should:

- Avoid sexual intercourse if genital herpes is being treated because these drugs do not cure the disease.
- Wear protective gloves when applying topical agents.
- Avoid driving and hazardous tasks if dizziness or drowsiness occurs.

Evaluation

- Monitor patient response to the drug (alleviation of signs and symptoms of herpes or CMV infection).
- Monitor for adverse effects (orientation and affect, GI upset, and renal function).
- Evaluate the effectiveness of the teaching plan (patient can name the drug, dosage, possible adverse effects to watch for, and specific measures to help avoid adverse effects).
- Monitor the effectiveness of comfort and safety measures and compliance with the regimen.

FOCUS POINTS

- Viruses are segments of RNA or DNA enclosed in a protein coat.
- A virus must enter a human cell to survive, making it difficult to treat without serious toxic effects for the host.
- Antiviral drugs that prevent the viral replication of respiratory viruses can be used to prevent or treat influenza A or other respiratory viruses.
- Drugs that interfere with viral DNA replication are used to treat herpes infections and CMV infections.
- These antiviral drugs are associated with GI upset and nausea, confusion, insomnia, and dizziness.

Agents for HIV and AIDS

The **human immunodeficiency virus (HIV)** attacks the **helper T cells** within the immune system. This virus enters the helper T cell and multiplies within the cell. When the cell ruptures, many new viruses are released to attack other helper T cells. The end result is that the immune system loses an important monitor that propels the immune reaction into full force when the body is invaded.

Loss of T-cell function causes **acquired immune deficiency syndrome (AIDS)** or **AIDS-related complex (ARC)**, diseases that are characterized by the emergence of a variety of opportunistic infections and cancers that occur when the immune system is depressed and unable to function properly. The HIV mutates over time, presenting a slightly different configuration with each new generation. Treatment of AIDS and ARC has been difficult for two reasons: (1) the length of time the virus can remain dormant within the T cells (i.e., months to years), and (2) the adverse effects of many potent drugs, which may include further depression of the immune system. At present, a combination of several different antiviral drugs is used to attack the virus at various points in its life cycle to achieve maximum effectiveness with the least amount of toxicity. The types of antiviral agents that are used to treat HIV infections are the reverse transcriptase inhibitors, the protease inhibitors, the nucleosides, and a new class of drugs called fusion inhibitors (Table 10.3). These drugs are known as antiretroviral agents. (See Box 10.3 for public education information regarding AIDS.)

Reverse Transcriptase Inhibitors

The **reverse transcriptase inhibitors** bind directly to HIV reverse transcriptase, blocking both RNA- and DNA-dependent DNA polymerase activities. They prevent the transfer of information that would allow the virus to replicate and survive.

Delavirdine (*Rescriptor*) must be used in combination therapy regimens because resistant strains develop rapidly when it is used alone. It is rapidly absorbed from the GI tract, with peak levels occurring within 1 hour. Delavirdine is extensively metabolized by the cytochrome P450 system in the liver and is excreted through the urine. Safety for use in children has not been established.

Efavirenz (*Sustiva*) is used in adults and children in combination with other antiretroviral agents. It is absorbed rapidly from the GI tract, reaching peak levels in 3 to 5 hours. Efavirenz is metabolized in the liver by the cytochrome P450 system and is excreted in the urine and feces with a half-life of 52 to 76 hours.

Emtricitabine (*Emtriva*) is used in patients older than 18 years in combination with other antiretroviral agents; it has the advantage of being a one-capsule-a-day therapy. Dosage needs to be reduced in renal impairment. It has been associated with severe and even fatal hepatomegaly with steatosis. Emtricitabine has a rapid onset and peaks in 1 to 2 hours. It has a half-life of 10 hours, and after being metabolized in the liver is excreted in the urine and feces.

Nevirapine (*Viramune*) is recommended for use in adults and children older than 2 months. After rapid GI absorption, nevirapine is metabolized by the cytochrome P450 system in the liver. Excretion is through the urine with a half-life of 45 hours. See Box 10.4 for information about the emergence of resistance to certain reverse transcriptase inhibitor combinations.

Pharmacokinetics

There are no adequate studies of reverse transcriptase inhibitors in pregnancy, so use should be limited to situations in which the benefits clearly outweigh any risks. It is suggested that women not breast-feed if they are infected with HIV.

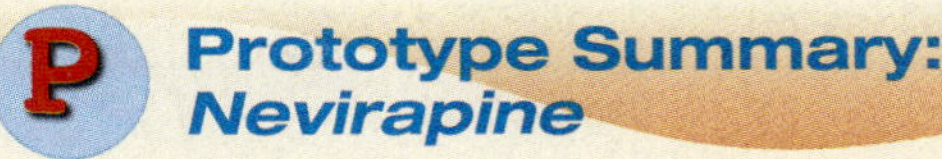

Prototype Summary: Nevirapine

Indications: Treatment of HIV-1 infected patients who have experienced clinical or immunologic deterioration, in combination with other antiretrovirals

Actions: Binds to HIV-1 reverse transcriptase and blocks replication of the HIV by changing the structure of the HIV enzyme

Pharmacokinetics:

Route	Onset	Peak
Oral	Rapid	4 h

$T_{1/2}$: 45 hours, then 25–30 hours; metabolized in the liver and excreted in the urine

Adverse effects: Headache, nausea, vomiting, diarrhea, rash, liver dysfunction, chills, fever

Protease Inhibitors

The **protease inhibitors** block protease activity within the HIV virus. Protease is essential for the maturation of an infectious virus; without it, an HIV particle is immature and noninfective. The protease inhibitors that are available for use include the following.

Amprenavir (*Agenerase*) was approved in 1999 for the treatment of adults and children with HIV in combination with other antiretroviral agents. It is rapidly absorbed from the GI tract, reaching peak levels within 1 hour. After undergoing metabolism in the liver, amprenavir is excreted in the urine and feces with a half-life of 7.1 to 10.6 hours. Because of the extensive hepatic metabolism, caution must be used in any patient with hepatic dysfunction. Box 10.5 provides calculation practice for using amprenavir.

Atazanivir (*Reyataz*) was approved in 2003 for treatment of adults with HIV infection, in combination with other antiretrovirals. It is not recommended for patients with severe hepatic impairment and should be used in reduced dosage with moderate hepatic impairment. It is rapidly absorbed from the GI tract and can be taken with food. After metabolism in the liver, it is excreted in the urine and feces with a half-life of 6.5 to 7.9 hours.

Fosamprenavir (*Lexiva*) was approved in 2004 for the treatment of HIV infection in adults, in combination with other antiretroviral agents. It is not recommended for use with ritonavir in protease-inhibitor experienced patients. It is rapidly absorbed after oral administration, reaching peak levels in 1.5 to 4 hours. It is metabolized in the liver

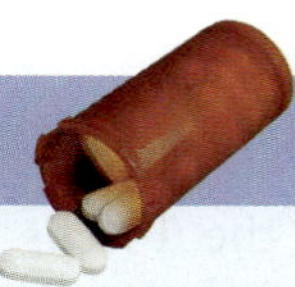

Table 10.3 DRUGS IN FOCUS

HIV and AIDS Drugs

Drug Name	Dosage/Route	Usual Indications
Reverse Transcriptase Inhibitors		
delavirdine (*Rescriptor*)	Adult: 400 mg PO t.i.d.	Part of combination therapy regimens for treatment of HIV in adults
efavirenz (*Sustiva*)	Adult: 600 mg/day PO Pediatric: dosage determined by age and weight	Treatment of adults and children with HIV in combination with other antiretroviral agents
emtricitabine (*Emtriva*)	Adult: 200 mg/day PO Renal impaired: reduce dosage based on function	Part of combination therapy for treatment of patients >8 years with HIV
P nevirapine (*Viramune*)	Adult: 200 mg/day PO for 14 days, then 200 mg PO b.i.d. Pediatric: 4 mg/kg PO for 14 days, then 4–7 mg/kg PO b.i.d.	Treatment of adults or children with HIV in combination with other antiretroviral agents
Protease Inhibitors		
amprenavir (*Agenerase*)	Adult: 1200 mg (8 tablets) PO b.i.d. Pediatric (13–16 yr): adult dose Pediatric (4–12 yr): 20 mg/kg PO b.i.d. (capsules) *or* 22.5 mg/kg PO b.i.d (solution)	Treatment of adults and children with HIV in combination with other antiretroviral agents
atazanavir (*Reyataz*)	Adult: 400 mg PO, q8h	Treatment of adults with HIV as part of combination therapy
fosamprenavir (*Lexiva*)	Adult: 1400 mg/day PO with 200 mg/day ritonavir PO *or* 700 mg PO b.i.d. with ritonavir 100 mg PO b.i.d.	Part of combination therapy for the treatment of HIV in adults
indinavir (*Crixivan*)	Adult: 800 mg PO q8h	Treatment of adults with HIV as part of combination therapy
lopinavir (*Kaletra*)	Adult: 3 capsules or 5 mL PO b.i.d. Pediatric (6 mo to 12 yr): 10–12 mg/kg PO b.i.d.	Treatment of adults and children with HIV in combination with other antiretroviral agents
nelfinavir (*Viracept*)	Adult: 750 mg PO t.i.d. Pediatric (2–13 yr): 20–30 mg/kg per dose PO t.i.d.	Combination therapy for the treatment of adults and children with HIV
ritonavir (*Norvir*)	Adult and Pediatric (>2 yr): 600 mg PO b.i.d.	Part of combination therapy for the treatment of adults and children with HIV
saquinavir (*Fortovase*) (*Invirase*)	*Fortovase*, Adult: Six 200-mg tablets PO t.i.d. *Invirase*, Adult: Three 200-mg tablets PO t.i.d.	Treatment of adults with HIV as part of combination therapy
tipranavir (*Aptivus*)	Adult: 300 mg/day PO with 200 mg ritonavir	Treatment of adults with HIV in combination with ritonavir
Nucleosides		
abacavir (*Ziagen*)	Adult: 300 mg PO b.i.d. Pediatric: 8 mg/kg PO b.i.d.	Combination therapy for the treatment of adults and children with HIV
didanosine (*Videx*)	Adult: 250–400 mg/day PO *or* 125–200 mg PO b.i.d. Pediatric: 120 mg/m^2 PO b.i.d.	Treatment of advanced infections in adults and children with HIV as part of combination therapy
lamivudine (*Epivir*)	Adult: 150 mg PO b.i.d.; for chronic hepatitis B, 100 mg PO q.d. Pediatric (3 mo–16 yr): 4 mg/kg PO b.i.d.	With other antiretroviral agents for the treatment of adults and children with HIV; as an oral solution for the treatment of chronic hepatitis B
stavudine (*Zerit, Zerit XR*)	Adult (≥60 kg): 40 mg PO b.i.d. Adult (30–60 kg): 30 mg PO b.i.d. Pediatric (≥30 kg): adult dosage Pediatric (<30 kg): 1 mg/kg per dose PO b.i.d.	Treatment of adults and children with HIV in combination with other antiretroviral agents
tenofovir (*Viread*)	Adult: 300 mg/day PO with food	Treatment of adults with HIV infection in combination with other antiretroviral drugs
zalcitabine (*Hivid*)	Adult: 0.75 mg PO q8h	Treatment of advanced infections in adults with HIV as part of combination therapy
P zidovudine [AZT] (*Retrovir, Aztec*)	Adult: 100 mg PO q4h Pediatric (3 mo to 12 yr): 180 mg/m^2 PO q6h Maternal: 100 mg PO 5 times per day until start of labor, then 2 mg/kg IV over 1 h, and then 1 mg/kg per hour IV until clamping of the cord	Treatment of symptomatic HIV in adults and children as part of combination therapy; prevention of maternal transmission of HIV
Fusion Inhibitor		
enfuvirtide (*Fuzeon*)	Adult: 90 mg PO b.i.d. by subcutaneous injection Pediatric 6–16 yr: 2 mg/kg b.i.d. by subcutaneous injection	Part of combination therapy in treatment of HIV patients with evidence of HIV replication despite antiretroviral therapy

BOX 10.3 FOCUS ON THE **EVIDENCE**

Public Education About AIDS

When AIDS was first diagnosed in the early 1980s, it was found in a certain population in New York City. The people in this group tended to be homosexuals, intravenous drug users, and debilitated persons with poor hygiene and nutrition habits. Originally, a number of health care practitioners thought that the disease was a syndrome of opportunistic infections that occurred in a population with repeated exposures to infections that naturally deplete the immune system. It was not until several years later that the human immunodeficiency virus (HIV) was identified. Since then, it has been discovered that HIV infection is rampant in many African countries. The infection also has spread throughout the United States in populations that are not homosexual or intravenous drug users and who have good nutrition and hygiene habits. As health care practitioners have learned, HIV is not particular about the body it invades. And once introduced into a body, it infects T cells and causes HIV infection.

The evidence shows that when a patient is diagnosed with HIV infection, the nurse faces a tremendous challenge for patient education and support. The patient and any significant others should be counseled about the risks of transmission and reassured about ways in which the virus is not transmitted. They will need to learn about drug protocols, T-cell levels, adverse drug effects, and anticipated progress of the disease. They also will need consistent support and a telephone number to call with questions at any time. Many communities have AIDS support groups and other resources that can be very helpful; the nurse can direct the patient to these resources as appropriate.

The combinations of drugs that are being used today and the constant development of more drugs make the disease less of a death sentence than it was in the past. The result, however, is that many people must take a large number of pills each day, at tremendous cost and inconvenience. Many people today do live for long periods with HIV infection. An AIDS vaccine is currently being studied and offers hope for preventing this disease in the future.

Public education is key for promoting the acceptance and support of patients with HIV infection or AIDS, who need a great deal of support and assistance. Nurses can be role models for dealing with HIV patients and can provide informal public education whenever the opportunity presents.

and excreted in urine and feces. Patients with mild to moderate hepatic dysfunction should receive a lower dose, and patients with severe hepatic dysfunction should not use this drug.

Indinavir (*Crixivan*) is available for treatment of adults and children older than 12 years with HIV. It is rapidly absorbed from the GI tract, reaching peak levels in 0.8 hours. Indinavir is metabolized in the liver by the cytochrome P450 system. It is excreted in the urine with a half-life of 1.8 hours. Patients with hepatic or renal impairment are at risk for increased toxic effects, and the dosage may need to be reduced. The safety of indinavir for use in children younger than 12 years has not been established.

BOX 10.4 FOCUS ON THE **EVIDENCE**

HIV Resistance

In late 2003, Gilead Sciences, Inc., notified health care professionals of a high rate of early virologic failure and the emergence of nucleoside reverse transcriptase inhibitor (NRTI) resistance-associated mutations. This was observed in a clinical study of HIV-infected, treatment-naive patients receiving a once-daily triple NRTI regimen containing didanosine enteric-coated beadlets (*Videx EC*), lamivudine (*Epivir*), and tenofovir disoproxil fumarate (*Viread*).

Based on these studies, tenofovir in combination with didanosine and lamivudine is not recommended when considering a new treatment regimen for therapy-naive or experienced patients with HIV infection. Patients currently on this regimen should be considered for treatment modification.

In a similar study, patients receiving unboosted *Reyataz* (atazanavir sulfate) and *Viread* (tenofovir) showed less decrease in viral concentrations and loss of virological response, which could show a possible resistance to *Reyataz.* For patients taking atazanavir and tenofovir, the Food and Drug Administration (FDA) advises that a boosted dose of atazanavir should be used to overcome a decrease in concentration of the drug that seems to occur when it is used with tenofovir.

Lopinavir (*Kaletra*) is used as a fixed combination drug that combines lopinavir and ritonavir. The ritonavir inhibits the metabolism of lopinavir, leading to increased lopinavir serum levels and effectiveness. This drug is approved for use in adults and children in combination with other antiretroviral agents for the treatment of HIV infection. It is readily absorbed from the GI tract and undergoes extensive hepatic metabolism by the cytochrome P450 system. Lopinavir is excreted in urine and feces.

BOX 10.5 FOCUS ON **CALCULATIONS**

The health care provider prescribes amprenavir (*Agenerase*) 20 mg/kg PO b.i.d. for a 14-year-old weighing 50 kg. The drug comes in 50- and 150-mg capsules. How many capsules should the child receive at each dose?

To figure out the ordered dose, perform the following calculation:

$$20 \text{ mg/kg} \times 50 \text{ kg} = 1000 \text{ mg/dose}$$

You want to give as few capsules as possible; therefore:

$$150 \text{ mg/capsule} = 1000 \text{ mg}/X$$

$$150 \text{ mg } X = 1000 \text{ mg capsules}$$

$$X = 6 \text{ capsules (150 mg)} + 100 \text{ mg}$$

You could give six 150-mg capsules and two 50-mg capsules, for a total of eight capsules.

Tipranavir (*Aptivus*) was approved in 2005 for the treatment of HIV infection in adults in combination with 200 mg ritonavir. It is taken orally with food, two 250-mg capsules each day with the ritonavir. It is slowly absorbed, reaching peak levels in 2.9 hours. It is metabolized in the liver with a half-life of 4.8 to 6 hours; excretion is through urine and feces. Tipranavir interacts with many other drugs, and its use must be carefully monitored based on other drugs in the overall drug regimen. Patients receiving tipranavir must have liver function monitored regularly because of the possibility of potentially fatal liver dysfunction.

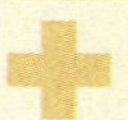

FOCUS ON PATIENT SAFETY

Name confusion has occurred between *Keppra* (levetiracetam), an antiepileptic drug, and *Kaletra* (lopinavir/ritonavir), the antiviral agent. When ordered in solution form, both are available in the same strength and appear the same. Serious effects occur when an epileptic patient receives the antiviral drug by mistake; seizures have developed. Problems would also occur if an HIV patient received the antiepileptic drug and did not have the antiviral protection. Use extreme caution when administering either of these drugs.

Nelfinavir (*Viracept*) must be given in combination with other drugs and can be used in the treatment of children with HIV. It is well absorbed from the GI tract, reaching peak levels in 2 to 4 hours. Nelfinavir is metabolized in the liver using the CY3A system, and caution must be used in patients with any hepatic dysfunction. It is primarily excreted in the feces, with a half-life of 3.5 to 5 hours. Because there is little renal excretion, this is considered a good drug for patients with renal impairment.

Ritonavir (*Norvir*) is used in combination with other antivirals and is available for use in adults and children. It is rapidly absorbed from the GI tract, reaching peak levels in 2 to 4 hours. Ritonavir undergoes extensive metabolism in the liver and is excreted in feces and urine. Many potentially serious toxic effects can occur when ritonavir is taken with nonsedating antihistamines, sedative/hypnotics, or antiarrhythmics because of the activity of ritonavir in the liver. Patients with hepatic dysfunction are at increased risk for serious effects when taking ritonavir and require a reduced dosage and close monitoring.

Saquinavir (*Fortovase, Invirase*) is used in combination regimens for adults. This drug is slowly absorbed from the GI tract and is metabolized in the liver by the cytochrome P450 mediator, so it must be used cautiously in the presence of hepatic dysfunction. It is primarily excreted in the feces with a short half-life. It has not been shown to be teratogenic, but use during pregnancy should be limited. Saquinavir crosses into breast milk, and women are advised not to breast-feed while taking this drug. The safety for use in children younger than 16 years of age has not been established.

Pharmacokinetics

Of the protease inhibitors listed, saquinavir (*Fortovase, Invirase*) is the only agent that has not been shown to be teratogenic; however, as mentioned, its use during pregnancy should be limited. Saquinavir crosses into breast milk, and women are advised not to breast-feed while taking this drug. For the other agents listed, there are no adequate studies in pregnancy, so use should be limited to situations in which the benefits clearly outweigh any risks. It is suggested that women not breast-feed if they are infected with HIV.

Nucleosides

Nucleosides interfere with HIV replication by inhibiting cell protein synthesis, leading to viral death. The nucleosides include the following agents.

Abacavir (*Ziagen*) is used in combination therapy in adults and children. Serious to fatal hypersensitivity reactions have occurred with this drug, and it must be stopped immediately at any sign of a hypersensitivity reaction (fever, chills, rash, fatigue, GI upset, flu-like symptoms). Patients exhibiting any signs of hypersensitivity should be listed with the Abacavir Hypersensitivity Registry, a drug follow-up registry that is maintained by the drug company and reported to the U.S. Food and Drug Administration. After rapid GI absorption, abacavir is metabolized in the liver and excreted in feces and urine.

Didanosine (*Videx*) is used to treat advanced infections in adults and children. It is rapidly destroyed in an acid environment and therefore must be taken in a buffered form. It reaches peak levels in 15 to 75 minutes. Didanosine undergoes intracellular metabolism with a half-life of 8 to 24 hours. Serious pancreatitis, hepatomegaly, and neurological problems have been reported with this drug, which is why its use should be limited to the treatment of advanced infections.

Lamivudine (*Epivir*) is recommended specifically for use with other antiretroviral agents; as an oral solution, *Epivir-HBV,* it is also recommended for the treatment of chronic hepatitis B. After rapid GI absorption, lamivudine is excreted primarily unchanged in the urine, with a half-life of 5 to 7 hours. Because excretion depends on renal function, dosage reduction is recommended in the presence of renal impairment.

Stavudine (*Zerit, Zerit XR*) is recommended specifically for use with other antiretroviral agents. It is rapidly absorbed from the GI tract, reaching peak levels in 1 hour. Most of the drug is excreted unchanged in the urine, making it important to reduce dosage and monitor patients carefully in the presence of renal dysfunction. It can be used for adults and children and is now available in an extended release form, allowing for once-a-day dosing.

Tenofovir (*Viread*) is a new drug that affects the virus at a slightly different point in replication—a nucleotide that becomes a nucleoside. It is used only in combination with other antiretroviral agents. It is rapidly absorbed from the GI tract, reaching peak levels in 45 to 75 minutes. Its metabolism is not known, but it is excreted in the urine. Severe hepatomegaly with steatosis has been reported with tenafovir, so it must be used with great caution in any patient with hepatic impairment or lactic acidosis. Patients also should be alerted that the drug may cause changes in body fat distribution, with loss of fat from arms, legs, and face and deposition of fat on the trunk, neck, and breasts.

Zalcitabine (*Hivid*) is used to treat advanced cases of HIV/AIDS in adults, as a monotherapy in adults who have become intolerant to zidovudine or who have progressive disease while taking zidovudine, and as combination therapy with zidovudine for the treatment of advanced HIV infection. After absorption from the GI tract, zalcitabine is excreted unchanged in the urine with a half-life of 2 hours. It is not advisable to use zalcitabine during pregnancy, and women of childbearing age should use barrier contraceptives while taking this drug. Safety for use in children younger than 13 years has not been established. Severe and even fatal adverse reactions, including neuropathies, lactic acidosis, pancreatitis, and hepatic toxicity, have occurred with this drug. Use should be limited to severe or recalcitrant cases.

Zidovudine [AZT] (*Aztec, Retrovir*) was one of the first drugs found to be effective in the treatment of AIDS. It is used to treat symptomatic disease in adults and children and to prevent maternal transmission of HIV. It is rapidly absorbed from the GI tract, with peak levels occurring within 30 to 75 minutes. Zidovudine is metabolized in the liver and excreted in the urine, with a half-life of 1 hour. Severe bone marrow suppression has occurred with this drug, which must be used very cautiously in patients with compromised bone marrow function. Patients with marked renal or hepatic impairment may require lower doses because of the role of these organs in metabolism and excretion. Zidovudine has been used safely during pregnancy.

Box 10.6 discusses combination drugs.

Pharmacokinetics

Of the nucleosides mentioned, zidovudine is the only agent that has been proven to be safe when used during pregnancy. Of the other agents, there have been no adequate studies in pregnancy, so use should be limited to situations in which the benefits clearly outweigh any risks. It is suggested that women not breast-feed if they are infected with HIV.

BOX 10.6 Fixed Combination Drugs for Treatment of HIV Infection

Patients who are taking combination drug therapy for HIV infection may have to take a very large number of pills each day. Keeping track of these pills and swallowing such a large number each day can be an overwhelming task. In an effort to improve patient compliance and make it easier for some of these patients, some anti-HIV agents are now available in combination products.

Combivir is a combination of 150 mg lamivudine and 300 mg zidovudine. The patient takes one tablet, twice a day. Because this is a fixed combination drug, it is not the drug of choice for patients who require a dosage reduction owing to renal impairment or adverse effects that limit dose tolerance.

Trizivir combines 300 mg abacavir, 150 mg lamivudine, and 300 mg zidovudine. The patient takes one tablet, twice a day. Because this is a fixed combination drug, it is not the drug of choice for patients who require a dosage reduction owing to renal impairment or adverse effects that limit dose tolerance. Patients taking *Trizivir* should be warned at the time the prescription is filled about the potentially serious hypersensitivity reactions associated with abacavir and should be given a written list of warning signs to watch for.

In 2004, two new combination products were approved to help make compliance with an HIV drug regimen easier. *Epzicom* (600 mg abacavir with 300 mg lamivudine) is taken as one tablet once a day. *Truvada* (200 mg emtricitabine with 300 mg tenofovir) is also a once-a-day tablet. Patient should be stabilized on each antiviral individually before being switched to the combination form.

2004 also saw the release of a combination package—ribavirin 200 mg with 3 million international units of interferon alfa-2b for the treatment of chronic hepatitis C. *Rebetron* combines the ribavirin capsules packaged with the subcutaneous preparation of interferon alfa-2b.

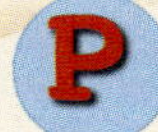

Prototype Summary: *Zidovudine*

Indications: Management of adults with symptomatic HIV infection in combination with other antiretrovirals; prevention of maternal–fetal HIV transmission

Actions: A thymidine analogue that is activated to a triphosphate form, which inhibits the replication of various retroviruses, including HIV

Pharmacokinetics:

Route	Onset	Peak
Oral	Varies	30–90 min
IV	Rapid	End of infusion

$T_{1/2}$: 30–60 min; metabolized in the liver and excreted in the urine

Adverse effects: Headache, insomnia, dizziness, nausea, diarrhea, fever, rash, bone marrow suppression

Fusion Inhibitors

A new class of drugs, called fusion inhibitors, was first introduced in 2003. The fusion inhibitor prevents the fusion of the virus with the human cellular membrane, which prevents the HIV-1 virus from entering the cell. This agent acts at a different site than do other HIV antivirals and is used in combination with drugs from the other classes to affect the virus at many points.

Enfuvirtide (*Fuzeon*) is used in combination with other antiretroviral agents to treat adults and children older than 6 years who have evidence of HIV-1 replication, despite ongoing antiretroviral therapy. It is given by subcutaneous injection and peaks in effect in 4 to 8 hours. After metabolism in the liver, it is recycled in the tissues and not excreted. The half-life of enfuvirtide is 3.2 to 4.4 hours. The drug has been associated with insomnia, depression, peripheral neuropathy, nausea, diarrhea, pneumonia, and injection site reactions.

Therapeutic Actions and Indications

The antiviral agents used to treat HIV and AIDS operate at various points in the life cycle of the virus and result in its death or inactivation (see Figure 10.2). Use of these drugs in combination can affect more viral particles and reduce the number of mutant viruses that are formed and spread to noninfected cells. These antiviral agents are indicated for the treatment of patients with documented AIDS or ARC who have decreased numbers of T cells and evidence of increased opportunistic infections.

Contraindications and Cautions

Because these drugs are used in the treatment of a potentially fatal disease with no known cure, there are no true contraindications to their use. Zidovudine is the drug of choice during pregnancy *to block maternal transmission of the virus.* Caution should be used with known allergies to any of these drugs; with hepatic or renal dysfunction, *which could lead to increased drug levels and toxicity;* and with pregnancy or lactation *because of potential adverse effects on the fetus or neonate.*

Adverse Effects

The adverse effects reported with the use of these drugs often are not distinguishable from the effects of the ongoing disease process. Adverse effects that are most often reported include the CNS effects of headache, dizziness, and myalgia; GI upset, including nausea, vomiting, and diarrhea; hepatic toxicity related to direct drug effects on the liver; fever and flu-like symptoms; rash (which is potentially fatal in some patients); and bone marrow depression, including agranulocytosis and anemia.

Clinically Important Drug–Drug Interactions

If nelfinavir is combined with pimozide, rifampin, triazolam, or midazolam, severe toxic effects and life-threatening arrhythmias may occur. Such combinations should be avoided.

Indinavir and nevirapine interact to cause severe toxicity. If these two drugs are given in combination, the dosages should be adjusted and the patient should be monitored closely.

Tenofovir can cause large increases in the serum level of didanosine. If both of these drugs are given, tenafovir should be given 2 hours before or 1 hour after didanosine.

Tipranavir has been shown to interact with many other drugs. Before administering tipranavir, it is important to check a drug guide to assess for potential interactions with other drugs being given.

When oral contraceptives are taken in combination with several of the antiviral agents, episodes of ineffective contraception may occur. Affected patients should be advised to use barrier contraceptives.

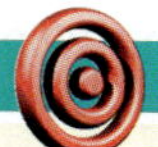

FOCUS POINTS

- The HIV virus infects helper T cells, leading to a loss of immune function and many opportunistic infections.
- Drugs used to treat HIV are given in combination to affect the virus at various points in the body: reverse transcriptase inhibitors block RNA and DNA activity in the cell; protease inhibitors prevent maturation of the virus; nucleosides prevent viral reproduction; and fusion inhibitors prevent the entry of the virus into the cell.
- Patients taking drugs to treat HIV need to take all of the medications continuously as prescribed and take precautions to prevent the spread of the disease to others.

Nursing Considerations for Patients Receiving Agents for HIV and AIDS

Assessment: History and Examination

Screen for the following conditions, *which are cautions or contraindications to the use of these drugs:* any history of allergy to antivirals; renal or hepatic dysfunction *that might interfere with the metabolism and excretion of the drug;* and pregnancy or lactation.

Physical assessment should be performed *to establish baseline data for assessing the effectiveness of the drug and the occurrence of any adverse effects associated with drug therapy.* Perform assessment of orientation and reflex *to evaluate any CNS effects of the drug.* Examine the skin (color, temperature, and lesions) *to monitor the effectiveness of the drug.* Check temperature *to monitor for infections.* Evaluate hepatic and renal function tests *to determine baseline function of the kidneys and liver.* Check results of a complete blood count (CBC) with differential *to monitor bone marrow activity* and T-cell number *to indicate effectiveness of the drugs.*

Nursing Diagnoses

The patient receiving drugs for HIV and AIDS may have the following nursing diagnoses related to drug therapy:

- Acute Pain related to GI, CNS, or dermatological effects of the drugs
- Disturbed Sensory Perception (Kinesthetic) related to CNS effects of the drugs
- Imbalanced Nutrition: Less Than Body Requirements, related to GI effects of the drugs
- Deficient Knowledge regarding drug therapy

Implementation With Rationale

- Monitor renal and hepatic function before and periodically during therapy *to detect renal or hepatic function changes and arrange to reduce dosage or provide treatment as needed.*
- Ensure that the patient takes the complete course of the drug regimen and takes all drugs included in a particular combination *to improve effectiveness of the drug and decrease the risk of emergence of resistant viral strains.*
- Administer drug around the clock, if indicated, *to provide the critical concentration needed for the drug to be effective.*
- Monitor nutritional status if GI effects are severe, and *take appropriate action to maintain nutrition.*
- Stop drug if severe rash occurs, especially if accompanied by blisters, fever, and so on, *to avert potentially serious reactions.*
- Provide safety precautions (e.g., the use of siderails, appropriate lighting, orientation, assistance) if CNS effects occur, *to protect patient from injury.*
- Teach the patient about the drugs prescribed *to enhance patient knowledge about drug therapy and to promote compliance.* Include as a teaching point the fact that these drugs do not cure the disease, so appropriate precautions should still be taken *to prevent transmission.*

The patient should:

- Have regular medical care.
- Have periodic blood tests, which are necessary to monitor the effectiveness and toxicity of the drug.
- Realize that GI upset, nausea, and vomiting may occur but that efforts must be taken to maintain adequate nutrition.
- Avoid driving and hazardous tasks if dizziness or drowsiness occurs.
- Report extreme fatigue, severe headache, difficulty breathing, or severe rash to a health care provider.

See Case Study and Focused Follow-up 10-1 for the antiviral agents used for HIV and AIDS.

Evaluation

- Monitor patient response to the drug (alleviation of signs and symptoms of AIDS or ARC and maintenance of T-cell levels).
- Monitor for adverse effects (orientation and affect, GI upset, renal and hepatic function, skin, levels of blood components).
- Evaluate the effectiveness of the teaching plan (patient can name the drug, dosage, possible adverse effects to watch for, and specific measures to help avoid adverse effects).
- Monitor the effectiveness of comfort and safety measures and compliance with the regimen (see Critical Thinking Scenario 10-1).

Drugs Used to Treat Hepatitis B

Hepatitis B is a serious to potentially fatal viral infection of the liver. The hepatitis B virus can be spread by blood or blood products, sexual contact, or contaminated needles or instruments. Health care workers are at especially high risk for encountering hepatitis B due to needle sticks. Hepatitis B has a higher mortality than other types of hepatitis and also brings with it the possibility of developing a chronic condition or becoming a carrier. In the past, hepatitis B was treated with interferons (see Chapter 17, Immune Modulators). In 2004 and 2005, two new drugs were approved specifically for treating chronic hepatitis B. Adefovir (*Hepsera*) and entecavir (*Baraclude*) are antiviral drugs that specifically inhibit reverse transcriptase in the hepatitis B virus and cause DNA chain termination, leading to blocked viral replication and decreased viral load (Table 10.4).

CRITICAL THINKING SCENARIO 10-1

Antiviral Agents for HIV and AIDS

The Situation

H.P. is a 34-year-old attorney who was diagnosed with AIDS, having had a positive HIV test 3 years ago. Although his T-cell count had been stabilized with treatment with zidovudine and efavirenz, it recently dropped remarkably. He presents with numerous opportunistic infections and Kaposi's sarcoma. H.P. admits that he has been under tremendous stress at work and at home in the past few weeks. He begins a combination regimen of lamivudine, zidovudine, ritonavir, and zalcitabine.

Critical Thinking

What are the important nursing implications in this case?

What role would stress play in the progress of this disease?

What specific issues should be discussed?

What other clinical implications should be considered?

Discussion

Combination therapy with antivirals has been found to be effective in decreasing some of the morbidity and mortality associated with HIV and AIDS. However, this treatment does not cure the disease. H.P. needs to understand that opportunistic infections can still occur and that regular medical help should be sought. He also needs to understand that these drugs do not decrease the risk of transmitting HIV by sexual contact or through blood contamination and he should be encouraged to take appropriate precautions.

It is important to make a dosing schedule for H.P., or even to prepare a weekly drug box, to ensure that all medications are taken as indicated. H.P. should also receive interventions to help him decrease his stress, because activation of the sympathetic nervous system during periods of stress depresses the immune system. Further depression of his immune system could accelerate the development of opportunistic infections and decrease the effectiveness of his antiviral drugs. Measures that could be used to decrease stress should be discussed and tried with H.P.

Discussing the adverse effects that H.P. may experience is important because gastrointestinal (GI) upset and discomfort may occur while he is taking all of these anti-HIV/AIDS medications. Small, frequent meals may help alleviate the discomfort. It is important that every effort be made to maintain H.P.'s nutritional state, and a nutritional consultation may be necessary if GI effects are severe. H.P. also may experience dizziness, fatigue, and confusion, which could cause more problems for him at work and may necessitate changes in his workload. Because some of the prescribed drugs must be taken around the clock, provisions may be needed to allow H.P. to take his drugs on time throughout the day. For example, he may need to wear an alarm wristwatch, establish planned breaks in his schedule at dosing times, or devise other ways to follow his drug regimen without interfering with his work schedule. The adverse effects and inconvenience of taking this many drugs may add to his stress. It is important that a health care provider work consistently with him to help him to manage his disease and treatment as effectively as possible.

Nursing Care Guide for H.P.: Antiviral Agents for HIV and AIDS

Assessment: History and Examination

Allergies to any of these drugs

Bone marrow depression

Renal or liver dysfunction

Skin: color, lesions, texture

CNS: affect, reflexes, orientation

GI: abdominal and liver evaluation

Hematological: CBC and differential; viral load; T-cell levels; renal and hepatic function tests

Nursing Diagnoses

Acute Pain related to GI, skin, CNS effects

Disturbed Sensory Perception (Kinesthetic) related to CNS effects

Imbalanced Nutrition: Less Than Body Requirements related to GI effects

Deficient Knowledge regarding drug therapy

Implementation

Monitor CBC and differential before and every 2 weeks during therapy.

Provide comfort and implement safety measures: assistance, temperature control, lighting control, mouth care, back rubs.

Antiviral Agents for HIV and AIDS *(continued)*

Provide small, frequent meals and monitor nutritional status.

Monitor for opportunistic infections and arrange treatment as indicated.

Provide support and reassurance for dealing with drug effects and discomfort.

Provide patient teaching regarding drug name, dosage, adverse effects, warnings, precautions, use of OTC or herbal remedies, and signs to report.

Evaluation

Evaluate drug effects: relief of signs and symptoms of AIDS and ARC; stabilization of T-cell levels.

Monitor for adverse effects: GI alterations, dizziness, confusion, headache, fever.

Monitor for drug–drug interactions as indicated for each drug.

Evaluate effectiveness of patient teaching plan.

Evaluate effectiveness of comfort and safety measures.

PATIENT TEACHING FOR H.P.

A combination of antiviral drugs has been prescribed to treat your HIV infection. These drugs work in combination to stop the replication of HIV, to control AIDS, and to maintain the functioning of your immune system. A schedule will be plotted out to show exactly when to take each of the drugs. It is very important that you take all of the drugs and that you stick to this schedule to ensure that the drugs can be effective and won't encourage the development of resistant strains of the virus.

These drugs are not a cure for HIV, AIDS, or AIDS-related complex (ARC). Opportunistic infections may occur, and regular medical follow-up should be sought to deal with the disease.

These drugs do not reduce the risk of transmission of HIV to others by sexual contact or by blood contamination; use appropriate precautions.

Common effects of these drugs include the following:

- ☐ *Dizziness, weakness, and loss of feeling:* Change positions slowly. If you feel drowsy, avoid driving and dangerous activities.
- ☐ *Headache, fever, muscle aches:* Analgesics may be ordered to alleviate this discomfort. Consult with your health care provider.
- ☐ *Nausea, loss of appetite, change in taste:* Small, frequent meals may help. It is important to try to maintain good nutrition. Consult your health care provider if this becomes a severe problem.
- ☐ Report any of the following to your health care provider: excessive fatigue, lethargy, severe headache, difficulty breathing, or skin rash.
- ☐ Avoid over-the-counter medications and herbal therapies; many of them interact with your drugs and may make them ineffective. If you feel that you need one of these, check with your health care provider first.
- ☐ Schedule regular medical evaluations, including blood tests, which are needed to monitor the effects of these drugs on your body and to adjust dosages as needed.
- ☐ Tell any doctor, nurse, or other health care provider that you are taking these drugs.
- ☐ Keep these drugs and all medications out of the reach of children. Do not share these drugs with other people.

Table 10.4 DRUGS IN FOCUS

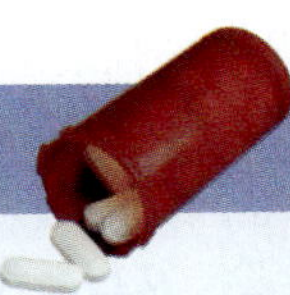

Hepatitis B drugs

Drug name	Dosage/Route	Usual Indications
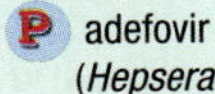 adefovir (*Hepsera*)	Adult: 10 mg/day PO Renal impairment: CrCl 20–40 mL/min—10 mg PO q48h CrCl 10–19 mL/min—10 mg PO q72h	Treatment of hepatitis B with evidence of active viral replication and persistent elevations in liver enzymes
entecavir (*Baraclude*)	Adults and children (≥16 yr): 0.5 mg/day; also receiving lamivudine: 1 mg/day Reduce dosage with renal impairment	Treatment of chronic hepatitis B in adults with evidence of active viral replication and persistent liver enzyme elevations

Therapeutic Actions and Indications

Adefovir and entecavir are indicated for the treatment of adults with chronic hepatitis B who have evidence of active viral replication and either evidence of persistent elevations in serum aminotransferases or histologically active disease. Both drugs decrease the viral load of hepatitis B by preventing viral replication through the blocking of reverse transcriptase.

Pharmacokinetics

These drugs are rapidly absorbed from the GI tract with peak effects occurring in 0.5 to 1.5 (entecavir) and 0.5 to 4 hours (adefovir). They are metabolized in the liver and excreted in the urine. The half-life of adefovir is 7.5 hours; entecavir has a half-life of 128 to 149 hours. It is not known if either of these drugs crosses the placenta or enters breast milk.

Contraindications and Cautions

These drugs are contraindicated with any known allergy to the drugs and with lactation, because of potential toxicity to the nursing baby. Caution should be used with renal impairment, pregnancy, and severe liver disease.

Adverse Effects

The adverse effects most frequently seen with these drugs are headache, dizziness, nausea, diarrhea, and elevated liver enzymes. Severe hepatomegaly with steatosis, sometimes fatal, has been reported with adefovir use. Lactic acidosis and renal impairment have been reported with both drugs. There is a risk that hepatitis B exacerbation could occur when the drugs are stopped.

Clinically Important Drug–Drug Interactions

There is an increased risk of renal toxicity if these drugs are taken with other nephrotoxic drugs. If such a combination is used, the patient should be closely monitored and the evaluation of risks versus benefits may need to be made if renal function begins to deteriorate.

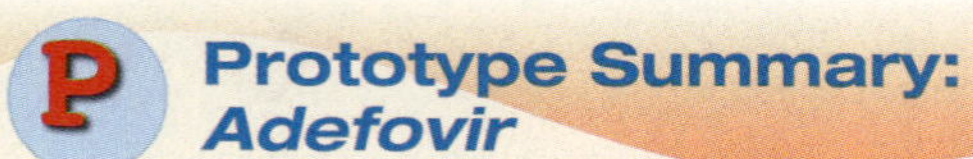

Prototype Summary: *Adefovir*

Indications: Treatment of chronic hepatitis B in adults with evidence of active viral replication and either evidence of persistent elevations in ALT or AST, or histologically active disease

Actions: Inhibits hepatitis B virus reverse transcriptase, causes DNA chain termination, and blocks viral replication

Pharmacokinetics:

Route	Onset	Peak	Duration
Oral	Rapid	0.6–4 h	Unknown

$T_{1/2}$: 7.5 hours; excreted in the urine

Adverse effects: Headache, asthenia, nausea, severe to fatal hepatomegaly with steatosis, nephrotoxicity, lactic acidosis, exacerbation of hepatitis B when discontinued

Nursing Considerations for Patients Receiving Agents for Hepatitis B

Assessment: History and Examination

Patients receiving agents to treat hepatitis B should be assessed for the following conditions, *which are cautions or contraindications to the use of these drugs:* any history of allergy to adefovir or entecavir; renal dysfunction, *which could be exacerbated by the nephrotoxic effects of these drugs;* severe liver impairment, *which could affect the metabolism and exacerbate the liver toxicity of these drugs;* and pregnancy and lactation, *because the potential effects of these drugs on the fetus or baby are not known.*

Physical assessment should be performed *to establish baseline data for assessing the effectiveness of these drugs and the occurrence of any adverse effects associated with drug toxicity.* Assess body temperature *to monitor underlying disease,* and orientation and reflexes *to assess for CNS changes.* Evaluate renal and liver function tests *to monitor for developing toxicity and for drug effectiveness.*

Nursing Diagnoses

The patient receiving an agent for chronic hepatitis B may have the following nursing diagnoses related to drug therapy:

- Acute Pain related to CNS and GI effects of the drug
- Imbalanced Nutrition: Less Than Body Requirements related to the GI effects of the drug
- Deficient Knowledge regarding drug therapy

Implementation With Rationale

- Monitor renal and hepatic function prior to and periodically during therapy *to detect renal or hepatic function changes and arrange to reduce dosage or provide treatment as needed.*
- Withdraw the drug and monitor the patient if patient develops signs of lactic acidosis or hepato-

toxicity, *because these adverse effects can be life threatening.*

- Caution patient to not run out of this drug, but to take it continually *because acute exacerbation of hepatitis B can occur when the drug is stopped.*
- Advise women of childbearing age to use barrier contraceptives *because the potential adverse effects of this drug on the fetus are not known.*
- Advise women who are breast-feeding to find another method of feeding the baby while using the drug, *because the potential toxic effects on the baby are not known.*
- Advise patients that these drugs do not cure the disease and there is still a risk of transferring the disease, *so the patient should continue to take appropriate steps to prevent transmission of hepatitis B.*
- Teach the patient about the drug prescribed, *to enhance patient knowledge about drug therapy and to promote compliance.*

The patient should:

- Have regular blood tests and medical follow-up.
- Take precautions to avoid running out of the drug, because the drug must be taken continually.
- Realize that GI upset, with nausea and diarrhea, is common with this drug.
- Report severe weakness, muscle pain, palpitations, yellowing of the eyes or skin, and trouble breathing.

Evaluation

- Monitor patient response to the drug (decreased viral load of hepatitis B).
- Monitor for adverse effects (liver or renal dysfunction, headache, nausea, diarrhea).
- Evaluate the effectiveness of the teaching plan (patient can name the drug, dosage, possible adverse effects to watch for, and specific measures to avoid adverse effects).
- Monitor the effectiveness of comfort and safety measures and compliance with the drug regimen.

Locally Active Antiviral Agents

Some antiviral agents are given locally to treat local viral infections. These agents include the following (see also Table 10.5):

- Idoxuridine (*Herplex*), which is applied directly to the eye and is used to treat herpes simplex keratitis
- Imiquimod (*Aldara*), which is applied locally for the treatment of genital and perianal warts
- Fomivirsen (*Vitravene*), which is injected into the eye to treat CMV retinitis in patients with AIDS
- Docosanol (*Abreva*), which is applied locally to treat oral and facial herpes simplex cold sores and fever blisters
- Ganciclovir (*Vitrasert*), which is implanted into the eye every 5 to 8 months for treatment of patients with CMV retinitis
- Penciclovir (*Denavir*), which is applied locally for the treatment of herpes labialis (cold sores) on the face and lips (not to be applied to mucous membranes)
- Trifluridine (*Viroptic*), which is applied locally to treat herpes simplex infections in the eye
- Vidarabine (*Vira-A*), which is used locally to treat herpes simplex infections of the eye that are not responsive to idoxuridine. Box 10.7 discusses how to apply these topical drugs.

Therapeutic Actions and Indications

These antiviral agents act on viruses by interfering with normal viral replication and metabolic processes. They are indicated for specific, local viral infections.

Contraindications and Cautions

Locally active antiviral drugs are not absorbed systemically, but caution should be used in patients with known allergic reactions to any topical drugs.

Adverse Effects

Because these drugs are not absorbed systemically, the adverse effects most commonly reported are local burning, stinging, and discomfort. These effects usually occur at the time of administration and pass with time.

Nursing Considerations for Patients Receiving Locally Active Antiviral Agents

Assessment: History and Examination

Patients receiving locally active antiviral agents should be assessed for any history of allergy to antivirals.

Physical assessment should be performed *to establish baseline data for evaluating the effectiveness of the drug and the occurrence of any adverse effects associated with drug therapy,* including inflammation at the site of infection.

Table 10.5 DRUGS IN FOCUS

Locally Active Antiviral Agents

Drug Name	Usual Indications
docosanol (*Abreva*)	Local treatment of oral and facial herpes simplex cold sores and fever blisters
fomivirsen (*Vitravene*)	Ophthalmic injection to treat cytomegalovirus (CMV) retinitis in patients with AIDS
ganciclovir (*Vitrasert*)	Implanted for treatment of CMV in patients with AIDS
idoxuridine (*Herplex*)	Ophthalmic agent used to treat herpes simplex keratitis (drug of choice)
imiquimod (*Aldara*)	Local treatment of genital and perianal warts
penciclovir (*Denavir*)	Local treatment of herpes labialis (cold sores) on the face and lips
trifluridine (*Viroptic*)	Ophthalmic ointment to treat herpes simplex infections in the eye
vidarabine (*Vira-A*)	Ophthalmic agent to treat herpes simplex infections of the eye that are not responsive to idoxuridine

Nursing Diagnoses

The patient receiving locally active antiviral drugs may have the following nursing diagnoses related to drug therapy:

- Acute Pain related to local effects of drug
- Deficient Knowledge regarding drug therapy

Implementation With Rationale

- Ensure proper administration of the drug *to improve effectiveness and decrease risk of adverse effects.*
- Stop the drug if severe local reaction occurs or if open lesions occur near the site of administration *to prevent systemic absorption.*
- Teach the patient about the drug being used *to enhance patient knowledge about drug therapy and to promote compliance.* Include as a teaching point the fact that these drugs do not cure the disease but should alleviate discomfort and prevent damage to healthy tissues. Encourage the patient to report severe local reaction or discomfort.

Evaluation

- Monitor patient response to the drug (alleviation of signs and symptoms of viral infection).
- Monitor for adverse effects (local irritation and discomfort).
- Evaluate the effectiveness of the teaching plan (patient can name the drug, the dosage, proper administration technique, and adverse effects to watch for and report to a health care provider).
- Monitor the effectiveness of comfort and safety measures and compliance with the regimen.

BOX 10.7 FOCUS ON CLINICAL SKILLS

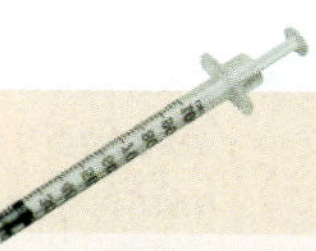

Before applying a topical drug, it is important to remember that these drugs are intended for topical, not systemic use.

1. Assess the affected area and make sure that there are no open lesions or abrasions that could allow for systemic absorption of the drug.
2. Clean the area to be treated and pat dry.
3. Apply the drug using gloves or an applicator to prevent exposure to the drug.
4. Always clean any old drug from the site before applying a new dose.
5. Make sure that the drug is applied only to affected areas and not spread to a wider area.

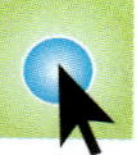

WEB LINKS

Health care providers and patients may want to consult the following Internet sources:

http://www.thebody.com Information on AIDS and HIV research, treatments, and resources.

http://www.cdc.gov Information on drug protocols and new HIV research.

http://www.critpath.org Information on AIDS.

http://www.aegis.com Health information for professionals and consumers.

Points to Remember

- Viruses are particles of DNA or RNA surrounded by a protein coat that survive by injecting their own DNA or RNA into a healthy cell and taking over its functioning.

- Because viruses are contained within human cells, it has been difficult to develop drugs that are effective antivirals and yet do not destroy human cells. Antiviral agents are available that are effective against only a few types of viruses.
- Influenza A and respiratory viruses cause the signs and symptoms of the common cold or "flu." The drugs that are available to prevent the replication of these viruses are used for prophylaxis against these diseases during peak seasons.
- Herpes viruses and CMV are DNA viruses that cause a multitude of problems, including cold sores, encephalitis, infections of the eye and liver, and genital herpes.
- Helper T cells are essential for maintaining a vigilant, effective immune system. When these cells are decreased in number or effectiveness, opportunistic infections occur. AIDS and ARC are syndromes of opportunistic infections that occur when the immune system is depressed.
- HIV, which specifically attacks helper T cells, may remain dormant in T cells for long periods and has been known to mutate easily.
- Antiviral agents that are effective against HIV and AIDS include reverse transcriptase inhibitors, protease inhibitors, nucleosides, and fusion inhibitors, all of which affect the way the virus communicates, replicates, or matures within the cell. These drugs are known as antiretroviral agents. They are given in combination to most effectively destroy the HIV virus and prevent mutation.
- Recently two drugs have been approved to treat hepatitis B infection.
- Some antivirals are available only for the local treatment of viral infections, including warts and eye infections. These drugs are not absorbed systemically.

CHECK YOUR UNDERSTANDING

Answers to the questions in this chapter may be found in the Answer Key in the back of the book.

Multiple Choice

Select the best answer to the following.

1. Viruses are known to cause
   a. tuberculosis.
   b. leprosy.
   c. the common cold.
   d. gonorrhea.
2. Virus infections have proved difficult to treat because
   a. viruses have a protein coat.
   b. viruses inject themselves into human cells to survive and to reproduce.
   c. viruses are bits of RNA or DNA.
   d. viruses easily resist drug therapy.
3. Naturally occurring substances that are released in the body in response to viral invasion are called
   a. antibodies.
   b. immunoglobulins.
   c. interferons.
   d. interleukins.
4. Herpes viruses cause a broad range of conditions but have not been identified as the causative agent in
   a. cold sores.
   b. shingles.
   c. genital infections.
   d. leprosy.
5. An important teaching point for the patient receiving an agent to treat herpes virus or CMV would be the following:
   a. stop taking the drug as soon as the lesions have disappeared.
   b. sexual intercourse is fine—as long as you are taking the drug, you are not contagious.
   c. drink plenty of fluids to decrease the drug's toxic effects on the kidneys.
   d. there are no associated GI adverse effects.
6. HIV (human immunodeficiency virus) attacks
   a. B clones.
   b. helper T cells.
   c. suppressor T cells.
   d. cytotoxic T cells.
7. Nursing interventions for the patient receiving antiviral drugs for the treatment of HIV probably would include
   a. monitoring renal and hepatic function periodically during therapy.
   b. administering the drugs just once a day to increase drug effectiveness.
   c. encouraging the patient to avoid eating if GI upset is severe.
   d. stopping the drugs and notifying the prescriber if severe rash occurs.
8. Locally active antiviral agents can be used to treat
   a. HIV infection.
   b. herpes simplex, keratitis, and warts.
   c. RSV.
   d. CMV systemic infections.

Multiple Response

Select all that apply.

1. When explaining to a client the reasoning behind using combination therapy in the treatment of HIV, the nurse would include which of the following points?
   a. The virus can remain dormant within the T cell for a very long time; they can mutate while in the T cell.
   b. Adverse effects of many of the drugs used to treat this virus include immune depression, so the disease could become worse.
   c. The drugs are cheaper if used in combination.
   d. The virus slowly mutates with each generation.
   e. Attacking the virus at many points in its life cycle has been shown to be most effective.
   f. Research has shown that using only one type of drug that targeted only one point in the virus life cycle led to more mutations and more difficulty in controlling the disease.

2. Appropriate nursing diagnoses related to the drug therapy for a patient receiving combination antiviral therapy for the treatment of HIV infection would include
   a. Disturbed Sensory Perception (Kinesthetic) related to the CNS effects of the drugs.
   b. Imbalanced Nutrition: More Than Body Requirements related to appetite stimulation.
   c. Congestive Heart Failure related to cardiac effects of the drugs.
   d. Adrenal Insufficiency related to endocrine effects of the drugs.
   e. Acute Pain related to GI, CNS, or dermatologic effects of the drugs.
   f. Deficient Knowledge regarding drug therapy.

Matching

Match the locally acting antiviral drug with the condition it is typically used to treat.

1. ____________________ imiquimod
2. ____________________ fomivirsen
3. ____________________ penciclovir
4. ____________________ trifluridine
5. ____________________ vidarabine

A. Herpes simplex eye infections
B. Cold sores on the face and lips
C. Genital and perianal warts
D. Cytomegalovirus (CMV) retinitis

Fill in the Blanks

1. A *Diskhaler* is used to deliver ______________ to treat uncomplicated influenza A infections in adults and children.

2. Children with respiratory syncytial virus (RSV) often respond very well to treatment with ____________.

3. Patients with Parkinson's disease who were treated with ____________ were found to have a decreased incidence of influenza. This drug is now used to treat and prevent influenza infections.

4. ____________ is available only in intravenous (IV) form and is very toxic to the renal system. It is effective in treating CMV retinitis in immune compromised patients and mucocutaneous acyclovir-resistant herpes simplex infections.

5. Herpes zoster and recurrent genital herpes are often treated with the oral agent ____________.

6. A very commonly used drug for the treatment of herpes infections is ____________ (*Zovirax*).

7. One of the first drugs approved for treating HIV infections that is still used frequently in combination therapy is ____________, known only as AZT in many communities.

8. A topical drug that is applied locally for the treatment of cold sores is ____________.

Bibliography and References

Centers for Disease Control and Prevention. (2001). USPHS/IDSA guidelines for the prevention of opportunistic infections in persons infected with HIV. U.S. Department of Health and Human Services. *MMWR Morbidity and Mortality Weekly Report, 46* (No. RR 12).

Drug facts and comparisons. (2006). St. Louis: Facts and Comparisons.

Gilman, A., Hardman, J. G., & Limbird, L. E. (Eds.). (2006). *Goodman and Gilman's the pharmacological basis of therapeutics* (11th ed.). New York: McGraw-Hill.

Guberski, R. D. (1997). Treatment of AIDS in adults: An update. *American Journal for Nurse Practitioners, 1*(1), 22–26.

Karch, A. M. (2006). *2007 Lippincott's nursing drug guide.* Philadelphia: Lippincott Williams & Wilkins.

Porth, C. M. (2005). *Pathophysiology: Concepts of altered health states* (7th ed.). Philadelphia: Lippincott Williams & Wilkins.

Professional's guide to patient drug facts. (2006). St. Louis: Facts and Comparisons.

CHAPTER 11

Antifungal Agents

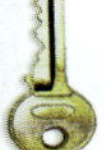

KEY TERMS

azoles

Candida

ergosterol

fungus

mycosis

tinea

LEARNING OBJECTIVES

Upon completion of this chapter, you will be able to:

1. Describe the characteristics of a fungus and a fungal infection.
2. Describe the therapeutic actions, indications, pharmacokinetics, contraindications, proper administration, most common adverse reactions, and important drug–drug interactions associated with systemic and topical antifungals.
3. Compare and contrast the prototype drugs for systemic and topical antifungals with the other drugs in each class.
4. Discuss the impact of using antifungals across the lifespan.
5. Outline the nursing considerations for patients receiving a systemic or topical antifungal.

SYSTEMIC ANTIFUNGALS

amphotericin B
caspofungin
P fluconazole
flucytosine
itraconazole
ketoconazole
micafungin
nystatin
terbinafine
voriconazole

TOPICAL ANTIFUNGALS

butenafine
butoconazole
ciclopirox
P clotrimazole
econazole
gentian violet
haloprogin
ketoconazole
miconazole
naftifine
oxiconazole
sertaconazole
terbinafine
tolnaftate
undecyclenic acid

Fungal infections in humans range from conditions such as the annoying "athlete's foot" to potentially fatal systemic infections. An infection caused by a **fungus** is called a **mycosis**. Fungi differ from bacteria in that the fungus has a rigid cell wall that is made up of chitin and various polysaccharides and a cell membrane that contains **ergosterol**. The composition of the protective layers of the fungal cell makes the organism resistant to antibiotics. Conversely, because of their cellular makeup, bacteria are resistant to antifungal drugs.

The incidence of fungal infections has increased with the rising number of immunocompromised individuals—patients with acquired immune deficiency syndrome (AIDS) and AIDS-related complex (ARC), those taking immunosuppressant drugs, those who have undergone transplantation surgery or cancer treatment, and members of the increasingly large elderly population, who are no longer able to protect themselves from the many fungi that are found throughout the environment (Box 11.1). For example, ***Candida***, a fungus that is normally found on mucous membranes, can cause yeast infections or "thrush" of the gastrointestinal (GI) tract and vagina in immunosuppressed patients.

Systemic Antifungals

The drugs used to treat systemic fungal infections (Table 11.1) can be toxic to the host and are not used indiscriminately. It is important to get a culture of the fungus causing the infection to ensure that the right drug is being used so that the patient is not put at additional risk from the toxic adverse effects associated with these drugs.

Amphotericin B (*Abelcet, AmBisome, Amphotec, Fungizone*), available in intravenous (IV) form, is a very potent drug with many unpleasant side effects that can cause renal failure. This drug is indicated for advanced and progressive systemic fungal infections, including aspergillosis, leishmaniasis, cryptococcosis, blastomycosis, moniliasis, coccidioidomycosis, histoplasmosis, and mucormycosis. Amphotericin B can also be used topically to treat resistant *Candida* infections. Because of the many adverse effects associated with this agent, its use is reserved for progressive, potentially fatal infections. Amphotericin B is excreted in the urine, with an initial half-life of 24 hours and then a 15-day half-life. Its metabolism is not fully understood. Amphotericin B has been used successfully during pregnancy, but it should be used cautiously. It crosses into breast milk and should not be used during lactation because of the potential risk to the neonate.

Caspofungin (*Cancidas*), available for IV use, is approved for the treatment of invasive aspergillosis in patients who are refractory to other treatments. This drug can be toxic to the liver; reduced doses must be used if a patient has known hepatic impairment. Caspofungin is slowly metabolized in the liver with half-lives of 9 to 11 hours, then 6 to 48 hours, and then 40 to 50 hours. It is bound to protein and widely distributed throughout the body. It is excreted through the urine. Concurrent use of cyclosporine is contraindicated unless the benefit clearly outweighs the risk of

BOX 11.1 DRUG THERAPY ACROSS THE LIFESPAN

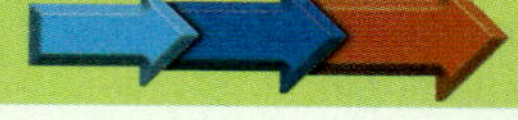

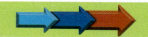

Antifungal Agents

CHILDREN

Children are very sensitive to the effects of most antifungal drugs, and more severe reactions can be expected when these drugs are used in children.

Many of these drugs do not have proven safety and efficacy in children, and extreme caution should be exercised when using them. Fluconazole, ketoconazole, and griseofulvin have established pediatric doses and would be drugs of choice if appropriate for a particular infection.

Topical agents should not be used over open or draining areas that would increase the risk of systemic absorption and toxicity. Occlusive dressings including tight diapers, should be avoided over the affected areas.

ADULTS

These drugs can be very toxic to the body, and their use should be reserved for situations in which the causative organism has been identified. Over-the-counter topical preparations are widely used, and patients should be cautioned to follow the instructions and to report continued problems to their health care provider.

Pregnant and nursing women should not use these drugs unless the benefit clearly outweighs the potential risk to the fetus or neonate. Women of childbearing age should be advised to use barrier contraceptives if any of these drugs are used. A severe fungal infection may threaten the life of the mother and/or fetus; in these situations, the potential risk of treatment should be carefully explained.

Topical agents should not be used over open or draining areas that would increase the risk of systemic absorption.

OLDER ADULTS

Older patients may be more susceptible to the adverse effects associated with these drugs and should be monitored closely.

Patients with hepatic dysfunction are at increased risk for worsening hepatic problems and toxic effects of many of these drugs (ketoconazole, itraconazole, griseofulvin). If hepatic dysfunction is expected (extreme age, alcohol abuse, use of other hepatotoxic drugs), the dosage may need to be lowered and the patient monitored more frequently.

Other agents are associated with renal toxicity (flucytosine, fluconazole, griseofulvin) and should be used cautiously in the presence of renal impairment. Patients at risk for renal toxicity should be monitored carefully.

Table 11.1 DRUGS IN FOCUS

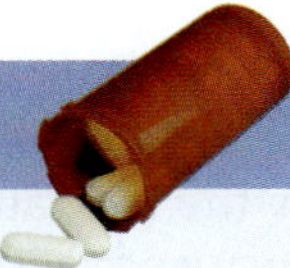

Systemic Antifungals

Drug Name	Dosage/Route	Usual Indications
amphotericin B (*Fungizone, Abelcet, Amphotec, AmBisome*)	0.25–1.5 mg/kg/day IV, based on the infection and its severity; also used topically	Treatment of aspergillosis, leishmaniasis, cryptococcosis, blastomycosis, moniliasis, coccidioidomycosis, histoplasmosis, and mucormycosis; topical treatment of resistant *Candida*
caspofungin acetate (*Cancidas*)	Adult: 70 mg/day IV loading dose then 50 mg/day IV infusion; dosage should be reduced to 35 mg/day IV infusion with hepatic impairment	Treatment of invasive aspergillosis in patients who are refractory or intolerant to other therapies
P fluconazole (*Diflucan*)	Adult: 200–400 mg PO on day 1, followed by 100 mg/day PO; IV route can be used, but do not exceed 200 mg/h Pediatric: 3–6 mg/kg PO; do not exceed 12 mg/kg	Treatment of candidiasis, cryptococcal meningitis, other systemic fungal infections; prophylaxis for reducing the incidence of candidiasis in bone marrow transplant recipients
flucytosine (*Ancobon*)	50–150 mg/kg/day PO in divided doses at 6-h intervals	Treatment of candidiasis, cryptococcosis
griseofulvin (*Fulvicin, Grifulvin V, Grisactin, Gris-PEG*)	*Tinea corporis, tinea cruris, and tinea capitis:* Adult: 500 mg (microsize) or 330–375 mg/day (ultramicrosize) PO *Tinea pedis and tinea unguium:* Adult: 0.75–1 g (microsize) or 660–750 mg (ultramicrosize) PO daily Pediatric (>2 yr): 11 mg/kg/day (microsize) or 7.3 mg (ultramicrosize) PO daily (not recommended for children ≤2 yr)	Treatment of tinea corporis, tinea pedis, tinea cruris, tinea barbae, tinea capitis, and tinea unguium
itraconazole (*Sporanox*)	Adult: 100–400 mg/day PO Pediatric: safety and efficacy not established	Treatment of blastomycosis, histoplasmosis, and aspergillosis
ketoconazole (*Nizoral*)	Adult: 200 mg/day PO, up to 400 mg/day PO in severe cases Pediatric (≥2 yr): 3.3–6.6 mg/kg/day PO Pediatric (<2 yr): safety not established Topical: as a shampoo	Treatment of aspergillosis, leishmaniasis, cryptococcosis, blastomycosis, moniliasis, coccidioidomycosis, histoplasmosis, and mucormycosis; topical treatment of mycoses, to reduce the scaling of dandruff
micafungin (*Mycamine*)	*Esophageal candidiasis:* Adult: 150 mg/day IV over 1 h for 6–30 days Prophylaxis: 50 mg/day IV over 1 h for about 19 days	Treatment of patients with esophageal candidiasis Prophylaxis of *Candida* infections in patients with hematopoietic stem cell transplant
nystatin (*Mycostatin, Nilstat, Nystex*)	500,000–1,000,000 units t.i.d. PO; continue for 48 h after resolution to prevent relapse; also used topically	Treatment of candidiasis
terbinafine (*Lamisil*)	250 mg/day PO for 6 wk (fingernail) or 12 wk (toenail)	Treatment of onychomycosis of the fingernail or toenail
voriconazole (*Vfend*)	Adult: 6 mg/kg IV q12h for two doses, then 4 mg/kg IV q12h; switch to oral dose as soon as possible >40 kg: 200 mg PO q12h <40 kg: 100 mg PO q12h	Treatment of invasive aspergillosis; treatment of serious fungal infections caused by *Scedosporium apiospermum, Fusarium* species

hepatic injury. Caspofungin is embryotoxic in animal studies and is known to enter breast milk; therefore, it should be used with great caution during pregnancy and lactation.

Flucytosine (*Ancobon*), available in an oral form, is a less toxic drug that is used for the treatment of systemic infections caused by *Candida* or *Cryptococcus*. It is well absorbed from the GI tract, with peak levels occurring in 2 hours. Most of the drug is excreted unchanged in the urine, and a small amount in the feces, with a half-life of 2.4 to 4.8 hours. Because the drug is excreted primarily in the urine, extreme caution is needed in the presence of renal impairment because drug accumulation and toxicity can occur. Because of the potential for adverse reactions in the fetus or neonate, flucytosine should be used during pregnancy and lactation only if the benefits clearly outweigh the risks. Safety for use in children has not been established.

Micafungin (*Mycamine*) is an intravenous drug used to treat esophageal candidiasis and to prevent *Candida* infections in patients undergoing hematopoietic stem cell transplants. It has a rapid onset, has a half-life of 14 to 17 hours, and is excreted in the urine. Potentially serious hypersensitivity reactions have occurred with this drug.

Patients should be monitored for bone marrow suppression. Because of the potential for adverse reactions in the fetus or the neonate, micafungin should be used during pregnancy and lactation only if the benefits clearly outweigh the risks.

Nystatin (*Mycostatin, Nilstat*) is used orally for the treatment of intestinal candidiasis. In addition, it is available in a number of topical preparations—oral suspension; troche; and vaginal suppository, cream, and ointment—for the treatment of local candidiasis, vaginal candidiasis, and cutaneous and mucocutaneous infections caused by *Candida* species. It is not absorbed from the GI tract and passes unchanged in the stool. It is not known whether nystatin crosses the placenta or enters breast milk, so it should not be used during pregnancy or lactation unless the benefits clearly outweigh the potential risks.

The "Azoles"

Another group of agents, called **azoles**, are newer drugs that are used to treat systemic fungal infections. Although they are less toxic than amphotericin B, they may also be less effective in very severe and progressive infections. The azoles include the following drugs.

Ketoconazole (*Nizoral*) is used orally to treat many of the same mycoses as amphotericin B. It works by blocking the activity of a steroid in the fungal wall and has the side effect of blocking the activity of human steroids, including testosterone and cortisol. Because of this action, ketoconazole is not the drug of choice for patients with endocrine or fertility problems. It has been associated with severe hepatic toxicity and should be avoided in patients with hepatic dysfunction. It is absorbed rapidly from the GI tract, with peak levels occurring within 1 to 3 hours. It is extensively metabolized in the liver and excreted through the feces. It strongly inhibits the cytochrome P450 (CYP450) enzyme system in the liver and is associated with many drug–drug interactions. This agent is also used topically as a shampoo to reduce the scaling associated with dandruff and as a cream to treat topical mycoses.

Fluconazole (*Diflucan*) is available in oral and IV preparations, so a patient who is seriously ill can be treated with the IV form and then switched to the oral form as his or her condition improves. Fluconazole, which is not associated with the endocrine problems seen with ketoconazole, is used to treat candidiasis, cryptococcal meningitis, and other systemic fungal infections. This drug has been used successfully as a prophylactic agent for reducing the incidence of candidiasis in bone marrow transplant recipients. Peak levels after administration occur within 1 to 2 hours. Most of the drug is excreted unchanged in the urine, making use with renal dysfunction difficult. Fluconazole also strongly inhibits the CYP450 liver enzyme system and may be associated with drug–drug interactions.

Itraconazole (*Sporanox*) is an oral agent used for the treatment of assorted systemic mycoses. This drug, which has been associated with hepatic failure, should not be used in patients with hepatic failure and should be used with caution in those with hepatic impairment. Itraconazole is slowly absorbed from the GI tract and is metabolized in the liver by the CYP450 system. It is excreted in the urine and feces.

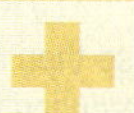

FOCUS ON PATIENT SAFETY

Ketoconazole (*Nizoral*), fluconazole (*Diflucan*), and itraconazole (*Sporanox*) have all been shown to be teratogenic in animals and should not be used in pregnancy or lactation unless the benefits clearly outweigh the potential risks.

Voriconazole (*Vfend*) is the newest of the systemic antifungals. It is available in oral and IV forms, making it useful for starting in a serious infection and switching to an oral form when the patient is able to take oral medications. It is used to treat invasive aspergillosis, as well as serious infections caused by *Scedosporium apiospermum* or *Fusarium* species, when the patient is intolerant or refractory to other therapy. Voriconazole should not be used with any other drugs that prolong the Qtc interval and can cause ergotism if taken with ergot alkaloids. (See Box 11.2 for information about hazardous interactions between voriconazole and herbal therapies.)

Terbinafine (*Lamisil*) is a similar drug that blocks the formation of ergosterol. It inhibits a CYP2D6 enzyme system, so it could be a better choice for patients who need to take drugs metabolized by the CYP450 system. Terbinafine is available as an oral drug for the treatment of onychomycosis of the toenail or fingernail. It is rapidly absorbed from the GI tract, extensively metabolized in the liver, and excreted in the urine.

Therapeutic Actions and Indications

All of the systemic antifungal drugs alter the cell permeability of the fungus, leading to cell death and prevention of replication (Figure 11.1). Some agents, including amphotericin B, nystatin, fluconazole, and itraconazole, bind to the ergosterol to open pores in the cell membrane. In contrast,

BOX 11.2 HERBAL AND ALTERNATIVE THERAPY

Patients being treated with voriconazole should be cautioned about the risk of ergotism if they combine this drug with ergot, an herb frequently used to treat migraine headache and menstrual problems. If the patient is using voriconazole, it should be suggested that ergot not be used until the antifungal therapy is finished.

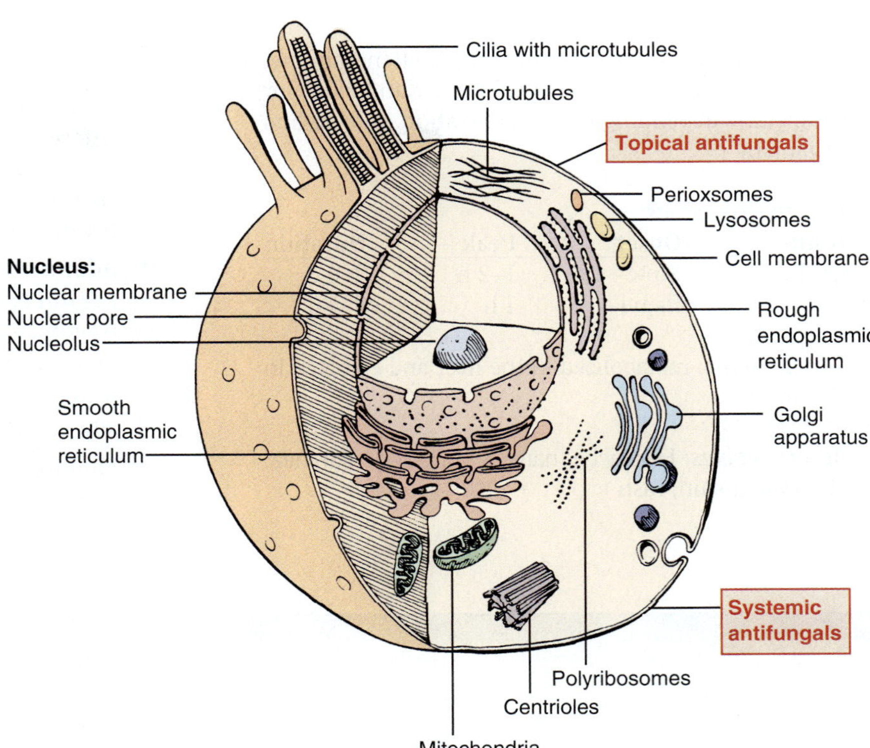

FIGURE 11.1 Sites of action of antifungal agents. Both systemic and topical antifungals alter fungal cell permeability, leading to prevention of replication and cell death.

ketoconazole and terbinafine impair the synthesis of ergosterol, allowing increased cell permeability and leakage of cellular components, leading to cell death. These agents are indicated for the treatment of systemic infections caused by susceptible fungi.

Contraindications and Cautions

Caution should be used when systemic antifungal agents are administered to anyone with a known allergy; during pregnancy and lactation (with the exception of terbinafine, use should be reserved for life-threatening infections); or to patients with renal or liver disease, *which could either alter drug metabolism and excretion or worsen as a result of the actions of the drug.*

Adverse Effects

Adverse effects frequently encountered with the use of systemic antifungal agents include central nervous system (CNS) effects, such as headache, dizziness, fever, shaking, chills, and malaise. GI effects include nausea, vomiting, dyspepsia, and anorexia. Hepatic dysfunction, which is seen more often with itraconazole, is associated with the toxic effects of the drug on the liver. Dermatological effects, such as rash and pruritus associated with local irritation, may occur. Renal dysfunction, which is more often seen with amphotericin B, is probably related to the drug effects on cell membranes.

Clinically Important Drug–Drug Interactions

Patients who receive amphotericin B should take neither other nephrotoxic drugs nor corticosteroids unless absolutely necessary *because of the increased risk of severe renal toxicity.*

The azole family of antifungal drugs can cause increased serum levels of the following agents: cyclosporine, digoxin, oral hypoglycemics, warfarin, oral anticoagulants, and phenytoin. Toxicity may occur *because the azoles inhibit the CYP450 liver enzyme system needed for metabolism of these drugs.* If these combinations cannot be avoided, patients should be closely monitored and dosage adjustments made.

Because the azoles have also been associated with potentially severe cardiovascular events when taken with lovastatin, simvastatin, triazolam, and midazolam, use of these drugs in combination with azoles should be avoided.

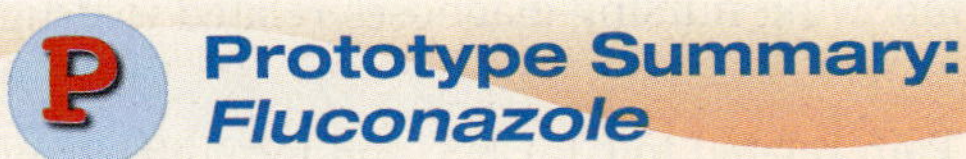

P Prototype Summary: *Fluconazole*

Indications: Treatment of oropharyngeal, esophageal, and vaginal candidiasis; cryptococcal meningitis; systemic fungal infections; prophylaxis to decrease incidence of candidiasis in bone marrow transplants

Actions: Binds to sterols in the fungal cell membrane, changing membrane permeability; fungicidal or fungistatic depending on concentration of drug and organism

Pharmacokinetics:

Route	Onset	Peak	Duration
Oral	Slow	1–2 h	2–4 d
IV	Rapid	1 h	2–4 d

$T_{1/2}$: 30 hours; metabolized in the liver and excreted in the urine

Adverse effects: Headache, nausea, vomiting, diarrhea, abdominal pain, rash

Nursing Considerations for Patients Receiving Systemic Antifungals

Assessment: History and Examination

Screen for the following, *which are cautions or contraindications for the use of these drugs:* history of allergy to antifungals; history of liver or renal dysfunction *that might interfere with metabolism and excretion of the drug;* and pregnancy or lactation.

Physical assessment should be performed *to establish baseline data for assessing the effectiveness of the drug and the occurrence of any adverse effects associated with drug therapy.* Perform a culture of the infected area *to make an accurate determination of the type and responsiveness of the fungus.* Assess orientation and reflexes *to evaluate any CNS effects of the drug.* Examine the skin for color and lesions *to check for dermatological effects of the drug.* Evaluate renal and hepatic function tests *to determine baseline function of these organs, to assess possible toxicity during drug therapy.*

Nursing Diagnoses

The patient receiving a systemic antifungal drug may have the following nursing diagnoses related to drug therapy:

- Acute Pain related to GI, CNS, and local effects of drug
- Disturbed Sensory Perception (Kinesthetic) related to CNS effects
- Deficient Knowledge regarding drug therapy

Implementation With Rationale

- Arrange for appropriate culture and sensitivity tests before beginning therapy *to ensure that the appropriate drug is being used.* However, in some cases, treatment can begin before test results are known because of the seriousness of the systemic infections.
- Administer the entire course of the drug *to get the full beneficial effects;* this may take as long as 6 months for some chronic infections.
- Monitor IV sites *to ensure that phlebitis does not occur.* Treat appropriately and restart IV at another site if phlebitis occurs.
- Monitor renal and hepatic function before and periodically during treatment *and arrange to stop drug if signs of organ failure occur.*
- Provide comfort and safety provisions if CNS effects occur (e.g., siderails and assistance with ambulation for dizziness and weakness, analgesics for headache, antipyretics for fever and chills, temperature regulation for fever) *to protect the patient from injury.*
- Provide small, frequent, nutritious meals if GI upset is severe. Monitor nutritional status and arrange a dietary consultation as needed *to ensure nutritional status.* GI upset may be decreased by taking an oral drug with food.
- Provide patient instruction *to enhance patient knowledge about drug therapy and to promote compliance.*

The patient should:

- Follow the appropriate dosage regimen.
- Take safety precautions, including changing position slowly and avoiding driving and hazardous tasks, if CNS effects occur.
- Take an oral drug with meals and try small, frequent meals if GI upset is a problem.
- Report to a health care provider any of the following: sore throat, unusual bruising and bleeding, or yellowing of the eyes or skin, all of which could indicate hepatic toxicity; severe nausea and vomiting, which could interfere with nutritional state and slow recovery; and severe local irritation with local application, which could indicate a sensitivity reaction and worsening of the infection.

Evaluation

- Monitor patient response to the drug (resolution of fungal infection).
- Monitor for adverse effects (orientation and affect, nutritional state, skin color and lesions, renal and hepatic function).

- Evaluate the effectiveness of the teaching plan (patient can name the drug, dosage, possible adverse effects to watch for, and specific measures to help avoid adverse effects).
- Monitor the effectiveness of comfort and safety measures and compliance with the regimen (see Critical Thinking Scenario 11-1).

FOCUS POINTS

- Fungi can cause many different infections in humans.
- Fungi differ from bacteria in that the fungus has a rigid cell wall that is made up of chitin and various polysaccharides and a cell membrane that contains ergosterol.
- Systemic antifungal drugs can be very toxic; extreme care should be taken to assure that the right drug is used to treat an infection and that the patient is monitored closely to prevent severe toxicity.
- Systemic antifungals are associated with many drug–drug interactions because of their effects on the liver. Monitor a patient closely when adding or removing a drug from a drug regimen if the patient is receiving a systemic antifungal.

Topical Antifungals

Some antifungal drugs are available only in topical forms for treating a variety of mycoses of the skin and mucous membranes. Fungi that cause these infections are called *dermatophytes*. These diseases include a variety of **tinea** infections, which are often referred to as ringworm, although the causal organism is a fungus, not a worm. Types of tinea include athlete's foot (tinea pedis), jock itch (tinea cruris), and yeast infections of the mouth and vagina often caused by *Candida*. Because the antifungal drugs reserved for use as topical agents (see Table 11.2) are often too toxic for systemic administration, care should always be taken when using them near open or draining wounds that might permit systemic absorption.

Gentian violet (generic), a very old agent, stains skin and clothing bright purple. In addition, it is very toxic when absorbed, so it cannot be used near active lesions.

Butenafine (*Mentax*) is applied only once a day for 4 weeks to treat tinea infections.

Butoconazole (*Gynazole I*), an over-the-counter (OTC) cream, is used to treat vaginal *Candida* infections.

Ciclopirox (*Loprox, Penlac Nail Lacquer*) is available as a cream or lotion for topical tinea infections and as a solution used specifically for fungal infections of the toenails and fingernails caused by *Trichophyton rubrum*.

Clotrimazole (*Lotrimin, Mycelex*), another OTC preparation, is used for treating oral and vaginal *Candida* infections and as a cream or lotion for treating tinea infections.

Econazole (*Spectazole*) is used to treat tinea infections. This drug can cause intense, local burning and irritation. It should be discontinued if these conditions become severe.

Haloprogin (*Halotex*) is a prescription cream or solution used to treat athlete's foot, jock itch, and ringworm infections.

Ketoconazole (*Nizoral*) in shampoo form is used to treat tinea corporis.

Miconazole (*Fungoid, Lotrimin AF, Monistat*) is available as an OTC product in several topical forms (vaginal suppository, cream, powder, and spray) for treatment of local, topical mycoses, including bladder and vaginal infections and athlete's foot.

Naftifine (*Naftin*) is a very powerful local antifungal agent that should not be used for longer than 4 weeks.

Oxiconazole (*Oxistat*) can be used for up to 1 month and is applied once daily or twice daily as needed.

Sertaconazole nitrate (*Ertaczo*) is applied between toes affected by tinea pedis and to the surrounding healthy tissue two times a day for 4 weeks.

Terbinafine (*Lamisil*) can be used for 1 to 4 weeks and is applied twice daily. This drug should be stopped when the fungal condition appears to be improved or if local irritation and pain become too great.

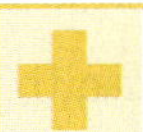

FOCUS ON **PATIENT SAFETY**

There have been several reports of name confusion between trade names, particularly *Lamisil* (terbinafine) the antifungal agent, and *Lamictal* (lamotrigine), an antiepileptic agent. Patients who needed Lamictal have been given the potentially toxic antifungal agent *Lamisil* with the result being seizures. Conversely, patients expecting to be treated for a serious systemic fungal infection received the antiepileptic preparation *Lamictal* and experienced CNS effects related to the drug. The Food and Drug Administration (FDA) has asked the manufacturers of these drugs to change the labels to bring attention to the differences. All health care providers should be especially cautious when using either one of the drugs and should alert the patient to the potential for errors and encourage the patient to be vigilant and to ask questions.

Tolnaftate (*Aftate, Tinactin*), an OTC drug, is very effective in the treatment of athlete's foot.

Undecyclenic acid (*Cruex, Desenex, Pedi-Dri*) is an OTC product that is recommended for athlete's foot, jock itch, diaper rash, and burning and chafing in the groin area.

CRITICAL THINKING SCENARIO 11-1

Poor Nutrition and Opportunistic Infections

The Situation

P.P., a 19-year-old woman and aspiring model, complains of abdominal pain, difficulty swallowing, and a very sore throat. The strict diets she has followed for long periods have sometimes amounted to a starvation regimen. In the past 18 months, she has received treatment for a variety of bacterial infections (e.g., pneumonia, cystitis) with a series of antibiotics.

P.P. appears to be a very thin, extremely pale young woman who looks older than her stated age. Her mouth is moist, and small, white colonies that extend down the pharynx cover the mucosa. A vaginal examination reveals similar colonies. Cultures are performed, and it is determined that she has mucocutaneous candidiasis. Ketoconazole (*Nizoral*) is prescribed, and P.P. is asked to return in 10 days for follow-up.

Critical Thinking

What are the effects of taking a variety of antibiotics on the normal flora? *Think about the possible cause of the mycosis.*

What happens to the immune system and to the skin and mucous membranes when a person's nutritional status becomes insufficient?

How is P.P.'s chosen profession affecting her health? What are the possible ramifications of suggesting that P.P. change her profession or her lifestyle?

What are the important nursing implications for P.P.? *Think about how the nurse can work with P.P. to ensure some compliance with therapy and a return to a healthy state.*

Discussion

Because of P.P.'s appearance, a complete physical examination should be performed before drug therapy is initiated. It is necessary to know baseline functioning to evaluate any underlying problems that may exist. Poor nutrition and total starvation result in characteristic deficiencies that predispose individuals to opportunistic infections and prevent their bodies from protecting themselves adequately through inflammatory and immune responses. In this case, the fact that liver changes often occur with poor nutrition is particularly important; such hepatic dysfunction may cause deficient drug metabolism and lead to toxicity.

An intensive program of teaching and support should be started for P.P., who should have an opportunity to vent her feelings and fears. She needs help accepting her diagnosis and adapting to the drug therapy and nutritional changes that are necessary for the effective treatment of this infection. She should understand the possible causes of her infection (poor nutrition and the loss of normal flora secondary to antibiotic therapy); the specifics of her drug therapy, including timing and administration; and adverse effects and warning signs that should be reported. P.P. should be monitored closely for adverse effects and should return for follow-up regularly while taking the ketoconazole. Nutritional counseling or referral to a dietitian for thorough nutritional teaching may prove beneficial.

The actual resolution of the fungal infection may occur only after a combination of prolonged drug and nutritional therapy. Because the required therapy will affect P.P.'s lifestyle tremendously, she will need a great deal of support and encouragement to make the necessary changes and to maintain compliance. A health care provider, such as a nurse whom P.P. trusts and with whom she can regularly discuss her concerns, may be an essential element in helping eradicate the fungal infection.

Nursing Care Guide for P.P.: Antifungal Agents

Assessment: History and Examination

Assess history of allergy to any antifungal drug. Also check history of renal or hepatic dysfunction and pregnancy or breast-feeding status.

Focus the physical examination on the following:

Local: culture of infected site

Skin: color, lesions, texture

GU: urinary output

GI: abdominal, liver evaluation

Hematological: renal and hepatic function tests

Nursing Diagnoses

Acute Pain related to GI, local, CNS effects

Disturbed Sensory Perception (Kinesthetic) related to CNS effects

Imbalanced Nutrition: Less Than Body Requirements related to GI effects

Deficient Knowledge regarding drug therapy

Poor Nutrition and Opportunistic Infections *(continued)*

Implementation

Culture infection before beginning therapy.

Provide comfort and implement safety measures (e.g., provide assistance and raise siderails). Ensure temperature control, lighting control, mouth care, and skin care.

Provide small, frequent meals and monitor nutritional status.

Provide support and reassurance for dealing with drug effects and discomfort.

Provide patient teaching regarding drug name, dosage, adverse effects, precautions, and warning signs to report.

Evaluation

Evaluate drug effects: relief of signs and symptoms of fungal infection.

Monitor for adverse effects: GI alterations, dizziness, confusion, headache, fever, renal or hepatic dysfunction, local pain, discomfort.

Monitor for drug–drug interactions as indicated for each drug.

Evaluate effectiveness of patient teaching program and of comfort and safety measures.

Patient Teaching for P.P.

- ☐ Ketoconazole is an antifungal drug that works to destroy the fungi that have invaded the body. Because of the way that antifungal drugs work, they may need to be taken over a long period of time.
- ☐ It is very important to take all of the prescribed medication.
- ☐ Common adverse effects of this drug include the following:
  - *Headache and weakness*—Change positions slowly. An analgesic may be ordered to help alleviate the headache. If you feel drowsy, avoid driving or dangerous activities.
  - *Stomach upset, nausea, and vomiting*—Small, frequent meals may help. Take the drug with food if appropriate, because this may decrease the gastrointestinal upset associated with these drugs. (Ketoconazole must be taken on an empty stomach at least 2 hours before taking a meal, antacids, milk products, or any other drugs.) Try to maintain adequate nutrition.
- ☐ Report any of the following to your health care provider: severe vomiting, abdominal pain, fever or chills, yellowing of the skin or eyes, dark urine or pale stools, or skin rash.
- ☐ Avoid over-the-counter medications. If you feel that you need one of these, check with your health care provider first.
- ☐ Take the full course of your prescription. Never use this drug to self-treat any other infection, and never give this drug to any other person.
- ☐ Tell any doctor, nurse, or other health care provider involved in your care that you are taking this drug.
- ☐ Keep this drug and all medications out of the reach of children.

Therapeutic Actions and Indications

The topical antifungal drugs work to alter the cell permeability of the fungus, causing prevention of replication and fungal death (see Figure 11.1). They are indicated only for local treatment of mycoses, including tinea infections. Because these agents are very toxic, they are not intended for systemic use, and they are not indicated for use near open lesions or wounds because of the increased risk of systemic absorption.

Contraindications and Cautions

Because these drugs are not absorbed systemically, contraindications are limited to known allergy to any of these drugs.

Adverse Effects

When these drugs are applied locally as a cream, lotion, or spray, local effects include irritation, burning, rash, and swelling. When they are taken as a suppository or troche, adverse effects include nausea, vomiting, and hepatic dysfunction (related to absorption of some of the drug by the GI tract) or urinary frequency, burning, and change in sexual activity (related to local absorption in the vagina).

Clinically Important Drug–Drug Interactions

Because these drugs are not generally absorbed systemically, there are no reported drug–drug interactions.

Table 11.2 DRUGS IN FOCUS

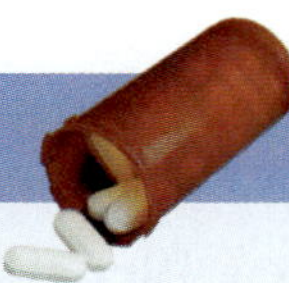

Topical Antifungals

Drug Name	Usual Indications
amphotericin B (*Fungizone*)	Treatment of cutaneous and mucocutaneous *Candida* infections
gentian violet (*generic*)	Treatment of topical mycosis
butenafine (*Mentax*)	Treatment of tinea infections
butoconazole (*Femstat 3*)	Available over the counter (OTC) for treatment of vaginal *Candida* infections
ciclopirox (*Loprox, Penlac, Nail Lacquer*)	Treatment of topical tinea infections; as solution for treatment of toenail and fingernail tinea infections
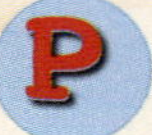 clotrimazole (*Lotrimin, Mycelex*)	Available OTC for treatment of oral and vaginal *Candida* infections; tinea infections
econazole (*Spectazole*)	Treatment of tinea infections
haloprogin (*Halotex*)	Treatment of athlete's foot, jock itch and ringworm infections
miconazole (*Monistat, Fungoid, Lotrimin*)	Treatment of local, topical mycoses, including bladder and vaginal infections and athlete's foot
naftifine (*Naftin*)	Short-term (up to 4 wk) treatment of severe topical mycosis
oxiconazole (*Oxistat*)	Short-term (up to 4 wk) treatment of topical mycosis
sertaconazole (*Ertaczo*)	Treatment of tinea pedis infections (up to 4 wk)
terbinafine (*Lamisil*)	Short-term (1–4 wk) treatment of topical mycosis
tolnaftate (*Tinactin, Aftate*)	Available OTC for treatment of athlete's foot
undecyclenic acid (*Cruex, Desenex, Pedi-Dri, Fungoid AF*)	Available OTC for treatment of athlete's foot, jock itch, diaper rash, burning and chafing in the groin area

Dosage/Route for all antifungals: Apply topically to affected area once or twice a day.

Prototype Summary: *Clotrimazole*

Indications: Treatment of oropharyngeal candidiasis (troche); prevention of oropharyngeal candidiasis in patients receiving radiation or chemotherapy; local treatment of vulvovaginal candidiasis (vaginal preparations); topical treatment of tinea pedia, tinea cruris, and tinea corporis

Actions: Binds to sterols in the fungal cell membrane, changing membrane permeability and allowing leakage of intracellular components, causing cell death

Pharmacokinetics: Not absorbed systemically; pharmacokinetics are unknown

Adverse effects: Troche: nausea, vomiting, abnormal liver function tests; topical: stinging, redness, urticaria, edema; vaginal: lower abdominal pain, urinary frequency, burning or irritation in the sexual partner

Nursing Considerations for Patients Receiving Topical Antifungals

Assessment: History and Examination

Patients who receive a topical antifungal agent should be assessed for any known allergy to any topical antifungal agent.

Physical assessment should be performed *to establish baseline data for assessment of the effectiveness of the drug and the occurrence of any adverse effects associated with drug therapy.* Perform culture and sensitivity testing of the affected area *to determine the causative fungus and appropriate medication.* Conduct local evaluation (e.g., color, temperature, lesions) *to monitor the effectiveness of the drug and to monitor for local adverse effects of the drug.*

Nursing Diagnoses

The patient receiving a topical antifungal drug may have the following nursing diagnoses related to drug therapy:

- Acute Pain related to local effects of drug
- Deficient Knowledge regarding drug therapy

Implementation With Rationale

- Culture the affected area before beginning therapy *to identify the causative fungus.*
- Ensure that the patient takes the complete course of the drug regimen *to achieve maximal results.*
- Ensure that the patient is using the correct method of administration depending on the route *to improve effectiveness and decrease risk of adverse effects:*
  - Troches should be dissolved slowly in the mouth.
  - Vaginal suppositories, creams, and tablets should be inserted high into the vagina with the patient remaining recumbent for at least 10 to 15 minutes after insertion.
  - Topical creams and lotions should be rubbed into the affected area after it has been cleansed with soap and water.
- Stop the drug if a severe rash occurs, especially if it is accompanied by blisters or if local irritation and pain are very severe. *This development may indicate a sensitivity to the drug or worsening of the condition being treated.*
- Provide patient instruction *to enhance patient knowledge about drug therapy and to promote compliance.*

The patient should:

- Know the correct method of drug administration.
- Know the length of time necessary to treat the infection adequately.
- Use clean, dry socks when treating athlete's foot, to help eradicate the infection.
- Avoid occlusive dressings because of the risk of increasing systemic absorption. Drugs should not be placed near open wounds or active lesions because these agents are not intended to be absorbed systemically.
- Report severe local irritation, burning, or worsening of the infection to a health care provider (refer to Case Study and Focused Follow-up 11-1).

Evaluation

- Monitor patient response to the drug (alleviation of signs and symptoms of the fungal infection).
- Monitor for adverse effects: rash, local irritation, and burning.
- Evaluate the effectiveness of the teaching plan (patient can name the drug, dosage, possible adverse effects to watch for, and specific measures to help avoid adverse effects).
- Monitor the effectiveness of comfort and safety measures and compliance with the regimen (see Case Study and Focused Follow-up 11-1).

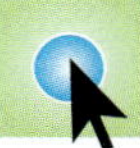

WEB LINKS

Health care providers and patients may want to consult the following Internet sources:

http://www.cdc.gov Information on drug protocols and fungal research.

http://www.athletesfoot.com Information about athlete's foot infections.

Points to Remember

- A fungus is a cellular organism with a hard cell wall that contains chitin and polysaccharides and a cell membrane that contains ergosterols.
- Any infection with a fungus is called a mycosis. Systemic fungal infections, which can be life-threatening, are increasing with the rise in the number of immunocompromised patients.
- Systemic antifungals alter the cell permeability, leading to leakage of cellular components. This causes prevention of cell replication and cell death.
- Because systemic antifungals can be very toxic, patients should be monitored closely while receiving them. Adverse effects may include hepatic and renal failure.
- Local fungal infections include vaginal and oral yeast infections (*Candida*) and a variety of tinea infections, including athlete's foot and jock itch.
- Topical antifungals are agents that are too toxic to be used systemically but are effective in the treatment of local fungal infections.
- Proper administration of topical antifungals improves their effectiveness. They should not be used near open wounds or lesions.
- Topical antifungals can cause serious local irritation, burning, and pain. The drug should be stopped if these conditions occur.

CHECK YOUR UNDERSTANDING

Answers to the questions in this chapter may be found in the Answer Key in the back of the book.

Multiple Choice

Select the best answer to the following.

1. A fungus is resistant to antibiotics because
   a. a fungus cell wall contains many protective layers, including folic acid and vitamin B.
   b. a fungus cell wall contains many protective layers, including chitin and ergosterol.
   c. a fungus does not reproduce by cell division.
   d. antibiotics affect only bacterial cell walls.

2. All systemic antifungal drugs function to
   a. break apart the fungus nucleus.
   b. interfere with fungus DNA production.
   c. alter cell permeability of the fungus, leading to cell death.
   d. prevent the fungus from absorbing needed nutrients.

3. Amphotericin B is associated with potentially serious nephrotoxicity and should not be given concurrently to a patient who is also taking
   a. digoxin.
   b. oral anticoagulants.
   c. phenytoin.
   d. corticosteroids.

4. Fungi that cause infections of the skin and mucous membranes are called
   a. mycoses.
   b. meningeal fungi.
   c. dermatophytes.
   d. worms.

5. Tinea infections include all of the following except
   a. athlete's foot.
   b. Rocky Mountain spotted fever.
   c. jock itch.
   d. vaginal yeast infections.

6. A woman with repeated vaginal yeast infections may be advised to have on hand
   a. tolnaftate.
   b. butenafine.
   c. clotrimazole.
   d. naftifine.

7. Care must be taken when using topical antifungal agents to prevent systemic absorption because
   a. the fungus is only on the surface.
   b. these drugs are too toxic to be given systemically.
   c. absorption would prevent drug effectiveness.
   d. these drugs can cause serious local burning and pain.

8. A patient with a severe case of athlete's foot is seen with lesions between the toes, which are oozing blood and serum. The patient would be noted to have a good understanding of teaching information if he reported:
   a. "I have to wear black socks and must be careful not to change them very often because it could pull more skin off of my feet."
   b. "I need to apply a thick layer of the antifungal cream between my toes, making sure that all of the lesions are full of cream."
   c. "I should wear white socks and keep my feet clean and dry. I should not use the antifungal cream in areas where I have open lesions."
   d. "After I apply the cream to my feet, I should cover my feet in plastic wrap for several hours to make sure the drug is absorbed."

Multiple Response

Select all that apply.

1. When administering an antifungal, the nurse would consider which of the following interventions to be appropriate?
   a. Ensuring that a culture of the affected area had been done
   b. Having the patient swallow the troche used for oral *Candida* infections
   c. Ensuring that the patient stays flat for at least 1 hour if receiving a vaginal suppository
   d. Monitoring the IV site to prevent phlebitis
   e. Keeping the patient NPO if GI upset occurs to prevent vomiting
   f. Providing antipyretics if fever occurs with IV antifungals

2. Teaching a client who is receiving an oral antifungal drug should include which of the following points?
   a. It is important that you complete the full course of your drug therapy.
   b. You can share this drug with other members of your family if they develop the same symptoms.
   c. If you feel drowsy or dizzy, you should avoid driving or operating dangerous machinery.
   d. If GI upset occurs, try to avoid eating and drinking as much as possible, to ensure that you do not vomit the drug and lose its effectiveness.

e. You should use over-the-counter drugs to counteract any adverse effects you experience—headache, fever, or rash.
f. Notify your health care provider if you experience yellowing of the skin or eyes, dark urine or light-colored stools, or fever and chills.

Web Exercise

The basketball coach at the local high school is concerned about an epidemic of athlete's foot that is affecting his entire team. Go on to the Internet to find information that will allow you to prepare a teaching protocol to help the coach with the treatment and prevention of this problem. Go to http://www.athletesfoot.com/ to get all types of information to help you prepare the teaching protocol; http://www.cdc.gov will give you information about available treatments and preventive measures that should be taken.

Fill in the Blanks

1. A fungus is a cellular organism with a ___________ cell wall that contains chitin and polysaccharides and a cell membrane that contains ___________.
2. Any infection with a fungus is called a(n) ___________.
3. Systemic antifungals can be very toxic; adverse effects may include ___________ and ___________ failure.
4. Vaginal and oral yeast infections are often caused by ___________.
5. Athlete's foot and jock itch are examples of ___________ infections.
6. Topical antifungals can be toxic and should not be absorbed ___________.
7. Topical antifungals should not be used near ___________ or lesions, which could increase absorption.
8. Topical antifungals can cause serious local ___________, ___________, and ___________.

Bibliography and References

Drug facts and comparisons. (2006). St. Louis: Facts and Comparisons.

Gilman, A., Hardman, J. G., & Limbird, L. E. (Eds.). (2006). *Goodman and Gilman's the pharmacological basis of therapeutics* (11th ed.). New York: McGraw-Hill.

Karch, A. M. (2006). *2007 Lippincott's nursing drug guide.* Philadelphia: Lippincott Williams & Wilkins.

Lewis, R. E., & Klepser, M. E. (1999). The changing face of nosocomial candidemia: Epidemiology, resistance and drug therapy. *American Journal of Health-System Pharmacy, 56,* 525–536.

Porth, C. M. (2005). *Pathophysiology: Concepts of altered health states* (7th ed.). Philadelphia: Lippincott Williams & Wilkins.

Professional's guide to patient drug facts. (2006). St. Louis: Facts and Comparisons.

CHAPTER 12

Antiprotozoal Agents

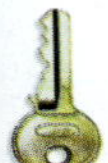

KEY TERMS

amebiasis

Anopheles mosquito

cinchonism

giardiasis

leishmaniasis

malaria

Plasmodium

Pneumocystis carinii pneumonia (PCP)

protozoa

trichomoniasis

trophozoite

trypanosomiasis

LEARNING OBJECTIVES

Upon completion of this chapter, you will be able to:

1. Outline the life cycle of the protozoan that causes malaria.
2. Describe the therapeutic actions, indications, pharmacokinetics, contraindications, proper administration, most common adverse reactions, and important drug–drug interactions associated with drugs used to treat malaria.
3. Describe other common protozoal infections, including cause and clinical presentation.
4. Compare and contrast the antimalarials with other drugs used to treat protozoal infections.
5. Outline the nursing considerations for patients receiving an antiprotozoal agent at all ages.

ANTIMALARIALS

P chloroquine
hydroxychloroquine
mefloquine
primaquine
pyrimethamine
quinine

OTHER ANTIPROTOZOALS

atovaquone
P metronidazole
nitazoxanide
pentamidine
tinidazole

Infections caused by **protozoa** are very common in several parts of the world. In tropical areas, where these types of illnesses are most prevalent, many people suffer multiple infestations at the same time. These infections are relatively rare in the United States, but with people traveling throughout the world in increasing numbers, it is not unusual to find an individual who returns home from a trip to Africa, Asia, or South America with fully developed protozoal infections. Protozoa thrive in tropical climates, but they may also survive and reproduce in any area where people live in very crowded and unsanitary conditions. This chapter focuses on protozoal infections that are caused by insect bites (malaria, trypanosomiasis, and leishmaniasis) and on those that result from ingestion or contact with the causal organism (amebiasis, giardiasis, and trichomoniasis). Box 12.1 discusses the use of antiprotozoals for various age groups affected by protozoal infections.

Malaria

Malaria is a parasitic disease that has killed hundreds of millions of people and even changed the course of history. The courses of several African battles and the building of the Panama Canal were altered by outbreaks of malaria. Even with the introduction of drugs for the treatment of this disease, it remains endemic in many parts of the world. Malaria is spread via the bite of an ***Anopheles* mosquito**, which harbors the protozoal parasite and carries it to humans. This is the only known method of disease transmission.

Four protozoal parasites, all in the genus ***Plasmodium***, have been identified as causes of malaria:

- *Plasmodium falciparum* is considered to be the most dangerous type of protozoan. Infection with this protozoan results in an acute, rapidly fulminating disease with high fever, severe hypotension, swelling and reddening of the limbs, loss of red blood cells, and even death.
- *Plasmodium vivax* causes a milder form of the disease, which seldom results in death.
- *Plasmodium malariae* is endemic in many tropical countries and causes very mild signs and symptoms in the population. It can cause more acute disease in travelers to endemic areas.
- *Plasmodium ovale,* which is rarely seen, seems to be in the process of being eradicated.

Part of the problem with malaria control is that the female mosquito, which is responsible for transmitting the disease, has developed a resistance to the insecticides designed to eradicate the mosquito. Widespread efforts at mosquito control were successful for a long period, with fewer cases of malaria seen each year. Because the insecticide-resistant mosquitoes continue to flourish, however, the incidence of malaria is again increasing. In addition, the protozoa that cause malaria have developed strains resistant to the usual antimalarial drugs. This combination of factors has led to a worldwide public health challenge.

Life Cycle of *Plasmodium*

The parasites that cause human malaria spend part of their life in the *Anopheles* mosquito and part in the human host

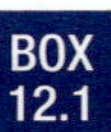

DRUG THERAPY ACROSS THE LIFESPAN

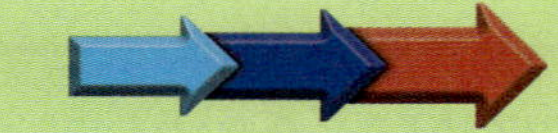

Antiprotozoal Agents

CHILDREN

Children are very sensitive to the effects of most antiprotozoal drugs, and more severe reactions can be expected when these drugs are used in children.

Many of these drugs do not have proven safety and efficacy in children, and extreme caution should be used. The dangers of infection resulting from travel to areas endemic with many of these diseases are often much more severe than the potential risks associated with cautious use of these drugs.

If a child needs to travel to an area with endemic protozoal infections, the CDC or local health department should be consulted about the safest possible preventative measures.

ADULTS

Adults should be well advised about the need for prophylaxis against various protozoal infections and the need for immediate treatment if the disease is contracted. It is very helpful to mark calendars as reminders of the days before, during, and after exposure on which the drugs should be taken.

Pregnant and nursing women should not use these drugs unless the benefit clearly outweighs the potential risk to the fetus or neonate. Women of childbearing age should be advised to use barrier contraceptives if any of these drugs are used. A pregnant woman traveling to an area endemic with protozoal infections should be advised of the serious risks to the fetus associated with both preventive therapy and treatment of acute attacks, as well as the risks associated with contracting the disease.

OLDER ADULTS

Older patients may be more susceptible to the adverse effects associated with these drugs. They should be monitored closely.

Patients with hepatic dysfunction are at increased risk for worsening hepatic problems and toxic effects of many of these drugs. If hepatic dysfunction is expected (extreme age, alcohol abuse, use of other hepatotoxic drugs), the dosage may need to be lowered and the patient monitored more frequently.

(Figure 12.1). When a mosquito bites a human who is infected with malaria, it sucks blood infested with gametocytes, which are male and female forms of the plasmodium. These gametocytes mate in the stomach of the mosquito and produce a zygote that goes through several phases before forming sporozoites (spore animals) that make their way to the mosquito's salivary glands. The next person who is bitten by that mosquito is injected with thousands of sporozoites. These animals travel through the bloodstream, where they quickly become lodged in the human liver and other tissues and invade the cells.

Inside human cells, the organisms undergo asexual cell division and reproduction. Over the next 7 to 10 days, these primary tissue schizonts grow and multiply within their invaded cells (as trophozoites). Merozoites are formed from the primary schizonts and then burst from invaded cells when they rupture because of overexpansion. These merozoites enter the circulation and invade red blood cells, in which they continue to divide until the blood cells also burst, sending more merozoites into the circulation to invade yet more red blood cells.

Eventually, there are a large number of merozoites in the body, as well as many ruptured and invaded red blood cells. At this point, the acute malarial attack occurs. The rupture of the red blood cells causes chills and fever related to the

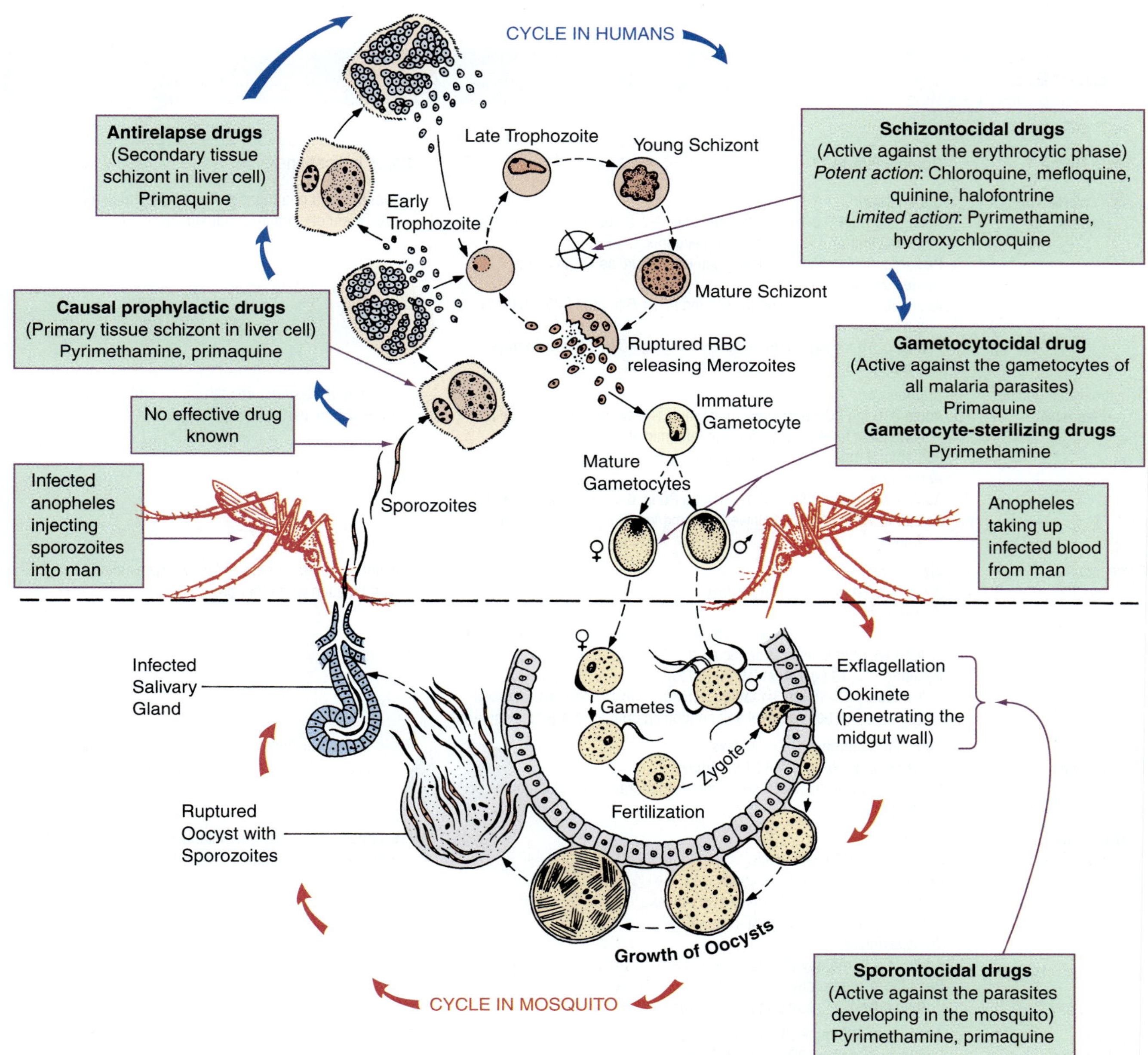

FIGURE 12.1 Types of antimalarial drugs in relation to the stages in the life cycle of *Plasmodium*.

pyrogenic effects of the protozoa and the toxic effects of the red blood cell components on the system. This cycle of chills and fever usually occurs about every 72 hours.

With *P. vivax* and *P. malariae* malaria, this cycle may continue for a long period. Many of the tissue schizonts lay dormant until they eventually find their way to the liver, where they multiply and then invade more red blood cells, again causing the acute cycle. This may occur for years in an untreated patient.

With *P. falciparum* malaria, there are no extrahepatic sites for the schizonts. If the patient survives an acute attack, no prolonged periods of relapse occur. The first attack of this type of malaria can destroy so many red blood cells that the patient's capillaries become clogged and the circulation to vital organs is interrupted, leading to death.

Antimalarials

Antimalarial drugs (Table 12.1) are usually given in combination form to attack the plasmodium at various stages of its life cycle. Using this approach, it is possible to prevent the acute malarial reaction in individuals who have been infected by the parasite.

Quinine (generic), the first drug found to be effective in the treatment of malaria, is now reserved for treatment of chloroquine-resistant infections in combination with other

Table 12.1 DRUGS IN FOCUS

Antimalarials

Drug Name	Dosage/Route	Usual Indications
P chloroquine (*Aralen*)	*Suppression:* Adult: 300 mg PO every week beginning 1–2 wk before exposure and continuing for 4 wk after leaving endemic area Pediatric: 5 mg/kg/wk PO, using same schedule as for an adult *Acute attacks:* Adult: 600 mg PO, followed by 300 mg PO in 6 h; then 300 mg PO on days 2 and 3 Pediatric: 10 mg/kg PO, followed by 5 mg/kg PO in 6 h and on days 2 and 3.	Prevention and treatment of *Plasmodium* malaria; treatment of extraintestinal amebiasis
hydroxychloroquine (*Plaquenil*)	*Suppression:* Adult: 310 mg PO every week, beginning 1–2 wk before exposure and continuing for 4 wk after leaving endemic area Pediatric: 5 mg/kg/wk, following adult schedule *Acute attack:* Adult: 620 mg PO, followed by 310 mg PO in 6 h and on days 2 and 3 Pediatric: 10 mg/kg PO, followed by 5 mg/kg PO in 6 h and on days 2 and 3	Treatment of *Plasmodium* malaria in combination with other drugs, particularly primaquine
mefloquine (*Lariam*)	*Treatment:* Adult: 1250 mg PO as a single dose *Prevention:* Adult: 250 mg PO once weekly, starting 1 wk before travel and continuing for 4 wk after leaving endemic area Pediatric: 15–19 kg,1/4 tablet; 20–30 kg, 1/2 tablet; 31–45 kg, 3/4 tablet; >45 kg, 1 tablet. Take once a week, starting 1 wk before travel and continuing until 4 wk after leaving area	Prevention and treatment of *Plasmodium* malaria in combination with other drugs
primaquine (*generic*)	Adult: 26.3 mg/day PO for 14 days Pediatric: 0.5 mg/kg/day PO for 14 days Begin therapy during last 2 wk of (or after) therapy with chloroquine or other drugs	Prevention of relapses of *P. vivax* and *P. malariae* infections; radical cure of *P. vivax* malaria
pyrimethamine (*Daraprim*)	*Prevention:* Adult: 25 mg PO every week Pediatric (>10 yr): same as adult Pediatric (4–10 yr): 12.5 mg PO every week Pediatric (<4 yr): 6.25 mg PO every week *Toxoplasmosis:* Adult: 50–75 mg/day PO with 1–4 g of a sulfonamide, for 4–5 wk Pediatric: 1 mg/kg/day PO, divided into two equal doses, for 2–4 days; then cut dose in half and continue for 1 mo	Prevention of *Plasmodium* malaria, in combination with other agents to suppress transmission; treatment of toxoplasmosis
quinine (*generic*)	Adult: 260–650 mg PO t.i.d. for 6–12 days Pediatric: 10 mg/kg PO q8h for 5–7 days	Treatment of chloroquine-resistant *Plasmodium* infections

agents. Quinine affects the DNA synthesis of the plasmodium, leading to an inability to reproduce effectively. The drug may lead to severe diarrhea and a condition called **cinchonism** (nausea, vomiting, tinnitus, and vertigo), which makes it less desirable than newer, less toxic drugs. Quinine is readily absorbed from the top of the small intestine, with peak serum levels occurring within 1 to 3 hours. It is metabolized in the liver, with a half-life of 4 to 5 hours, and is excreted in the urine. Quinine is toxic to the fetus and is classified as pregnancy category X. Barrier contraceptive use should be advised for women of childbearing age who need to take quinine.

Chloroquine (*Aralen*) is currently the mainstay of antimalarial therapy. This drug enters human red blood cells and changes the metabolic pathways necessary for the reproduction of the plasmodium. In addition, this agent is directly toxic to parasites that absorb it; it is acidic, and it decreases the ability of the parasite to synthesize DNA, leading to a blockage of reproduction. Chloroquine sometimes has serious adverse effects, such as hepatic toxicity, permanent eye damage, and blindness. Chloroquine is readily absorbed from the gastrointestinal (GI) tract, with peak serum levels occurring in 1 to 6 hours. It is concentrated in the liver, spleen, kidney, and brain and is excreted very slowly in the urine, primarily as unchanged drug. Use during pregnancy and lactation should be restricted to situations in which the benefit clearly outweighs the potential risk to the fetus or neonate.

Hydroxychloroquine (*Plaquenil*) inhibits parasite reproduction, and by blocking the synthesis of protein production, it can cause the death of the plasmodium. This drug is used in combination therapy, usually with primaquine, for greatest effectiveness. Hydroxychloroquine is readily absorbed from the GI tract, with peak serum levels occurring in 1 to 6 hours. It is excreted slowly in the urine, primarily as unchanged drug. Use during pregnancy and lactation should be restricted to situations where the benefit clearly outweighs the potential risk to the fetus or neonate.

Mefloquine (*Lariam*) increases the acidity of plasmodial food vacuoles, causing cell rupture and death. In combination therapy, mefloquine is used in malarial prevention, as well as treatment. Mefloquine is a mixture of molecules that are absorbed, metabolized, and excreted at different rates. The terminal half-life is 13 to 24 days. Metabolism occurs in the liver; caution should be used in patients with hepatic dysfunction. Pregnancy should be avoided during and for 2 months after completion of therapy. Mefloquine is teratogenic in preclinical studies. It also crosses into breast milk and can be very toxic to the baby. Breast-feeding should be discontinued if this drug is essential for therapy.

Primaquine (generic), another very old drug for treating malaria, similar to quinine, disrupts the mitochondria of the plasmodium. It also causes death of gametocytes and exoerythrocytic forms and prevents other forms from reproducing. Because of this action, it is especially useful in preventing relapses of *P. vivax* and *P. malariae* infections. Primaquine is readily absorbed and metabolized in the liver. Excretion occurs primarily in the urine. Safety for use during pregnancy has not been established.

Pyrimethamine (*Daraprim*) is used in combination with agents that act more rapidly to suppress malaria by blocking the use of folic acid in protein synthesis by the plasmodium, eventually leading to inability to reproduce and cell death. Pyrimethamine is readily absorbed from the GI tract, with peak levels occurring within 2 to 6 hours. It is metabolized in the liver and has a half-life of 4 days. It usually maintains suppressive concentrations in the body for about 2 weeks. As with other antiprotozoals, pyrimethamine should not be used during pregnancy or lactation unless the benefit clearly outweighs the potential risk to the fetus or neonate.

Fixed combination drugs for malaria prevention and treatment are discussed in Box 12.2. A cultural consideration related to some of these drugs is discussed in Box 12.3.

Therapeutic Actions and Indications

Research has demonstrated that the antimalarial agents are effective in interrupting plasmodial reproduction of protein synthesis in the red blood cell stage of the life cycle, as well as in the hepatic and gametocyte stages in some cases (Figure 12.2). Chemotherapeutic agents, which do not appear to affect the sporozoites, are used for prophylaxis and treatment of acute attacks of malaria caused by susceptible strains of *Plasmodium.*

Contraindications and Cautions

Contraindications to the use of antimalarials are the presence of known allergy to any of these drugs; liver disease or alcoholism, *both because of the parasitic invasion of the liver and because of the need for the hepatic metabolism to avoid reaching toxic levels;* and lactation *because the drugs can enter breast milk and could be toxic to the infant.* Caution should be used in patients with retinal disease or damage *because many of these drugs can affect vision and the retina, and the likelihood of problems increases if the retina is already damaged;* with psoriasis or porphyria *because of skin damage;* or with damage to mucous membranes, *which can occur as a result of the effects of the drug on proteins and protein synthesis.*

Adverse Effects

A number of adverse effects are encountered with the use of these antimalarial agents. Headache, dizziness, fever, shaking, chills, and malaise are associated with central nervous system (CNS) effects of the drugs and immune reaction to the release of the mitozoites. Nausea, vomiting, dyspepsia, and anorexia are associated with direct drug effects on the GI tract and effects on CNS control of vomiting related to cell death and protein changes. Hepatic dysfunction is associated with the toxic effects of the drug on the liver and the effects of the disease on the liver. Dermatological effects include rash, pruritus, and loss of hair associated with changes in protein synthesis. Visual changes, including possible blindness

BOX 12.2

Combination Drugs Used for Malaria Prevention and Treatment

Two fixed combination drugs are available for use in the prevention and treatment of malaria. Combining two different preparations in one drug may increase compliance by reducing the number of pills a patient has to take, and it conforms to the treatment protocol of taking drugs that effect the protozoa at different stages on their life cycle.

Fansidar is a combination of sulfadoxine and pyrimethamine. It is indicated for the treatment of *Plasmodium falciparum* malaria when chloroquine resistance is suspected. It is used for prophylaxis of malaria when travelers are going to areas in which chloroquine-resistant strains are known to be endemic. *Fansidar* is contraindicated in pregnancy, and women should be advised to use barrier contraceptives while taking it. Both of the constituent drugs cross into breast milk and can cause serious reactions in the neonate.

Usual dosage, acute attack

Adult: 2–3 tablets PO as a single dose

Pediatric (9–14 yr): 2 tablets PO as a single dose

Pediatric (4–8 yr): 1 tablet PO as a single dose

Pediatric (<4 yr): ½ tablet PO as a single dose

Usual dosage, prevention

Adult: 1 tablet PO every week or 2 tablets every other week

Pediatric (9–14 yr): ¾ tablet PO every week or 1½ tablets every other week

Pediatric (4–8 yr): ½ tablet PO every week or 1 tablet every other week

Pediatric (<4 yr): ¼ tablet PO every week or ½ tablet every other week

Preventive therapy should begin 1–2 days before exposure and should continue throughout and 4–6 wk after leaving the area.

Malarone and Malarone Pediatric combine atovaquone and proguanil. They are indicated for the prevention of *P. falciparum* malaria when chloroquine resistance has been reported. It is used for the treatment of uncomplicated *P. falciparum* malaria when chloroquine, halofantrine, and mefloquine have not proved successful, most likely because of resistance. This combination should be used in pregnancy and lactation only if the benefit clearly outweighs the potential risk to the fetus or neonate.

Usual dosage, acute attack:

Adult: 4 tablets PO as a single daily dose for 3 consecutive days

Pediatric (11–20 kg): 1 adult tablet PO daily for 3 consecutive days

Pediatric (21–30 kg): 2 adult tablets PO daily as a single daily dose for 3 consecutive days

Pediatric (31–40 kg): 3 adult tablets PO daily as a single daily dose for 3 consecutive days

Pediatric (>40 kg): 4 adult tablets PO daily as a single daily dose for 3 consecutive days

Prevention

Adult: 1 tablet PO daily

Pediatric (11–20 kg): 1 pediatric tablet PO daily

Pediatric (21–30 kg): 2 pediatric tablets PO daily

Pediatric (31–40 kg): 3 pediatric tablets PO daily

Pediatric (>40 kg): 1 adult tablet PO daily

Prevention should start 1–2 days before exposure and continue throughout and 7 days after leaving the area.

related to retinal damage from the drug and ototoxicity related to additional nerve damage, may occur. Cinchonism (nausea, vomiting, tinnitus, and vertigo) is more commonly seen with high levels of quinine and is related to drug effects in the CNS. This effect can be seen with any quinine-related drug if toxic levels occur.

BOX 12.3 CULTURAL CONSIDERATIONS FOR DRUG THERAPY

Potential for Hemolytic Crisis

Patients with glucose-6-phosphate dehydrogenase (G6PD) deficiency—which is more likely to occur in Greeks, Italians, and other people of Mediterranean descent—may experience a hemolytic crisis if taking the antimalarial agents chloroquine, primaquine, or quinine. Patients of Greek, Italian, or Mediterranean ancestry should be questioned about any history of potential G6PD deficiency. If no history is known, the patient should be tested before any of these drugs are prescribed. If testing is not possible and the drugs are needed, the patient should be monitored very closely and informed about the potential need for hospitalization and emergency services.

Clinically Important Drug–Drug Interactions

The patient who is receiving combinations of the quinine derivatives and quinine is at increased risk for cardiac toxicity and convulsions and should be checked very closely. Drug levels should be monitored and dosage adjustments made as needed.

Increased bone marrow suppression may occur if antifolate drugs (methotrexate, sulfonamides, etc.) are combined with pyrimethamine; pyrimethamine should be discontinued if signs of folate deficiency develop.

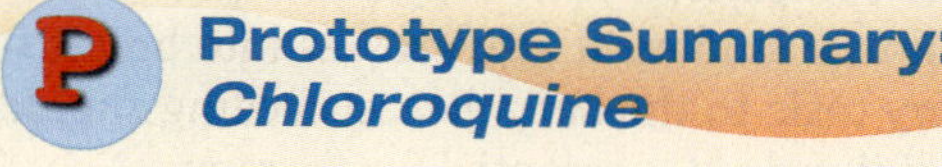

Prototype Summary: Chloroquine

Indications: Treatment and prophylaxis of acute attacks of malaria caused by susceptible strains of *Plasmodia;* treatment of extraintestinal amebiasis

Actions: Inhibits protozoal reproduction and protein synthesis

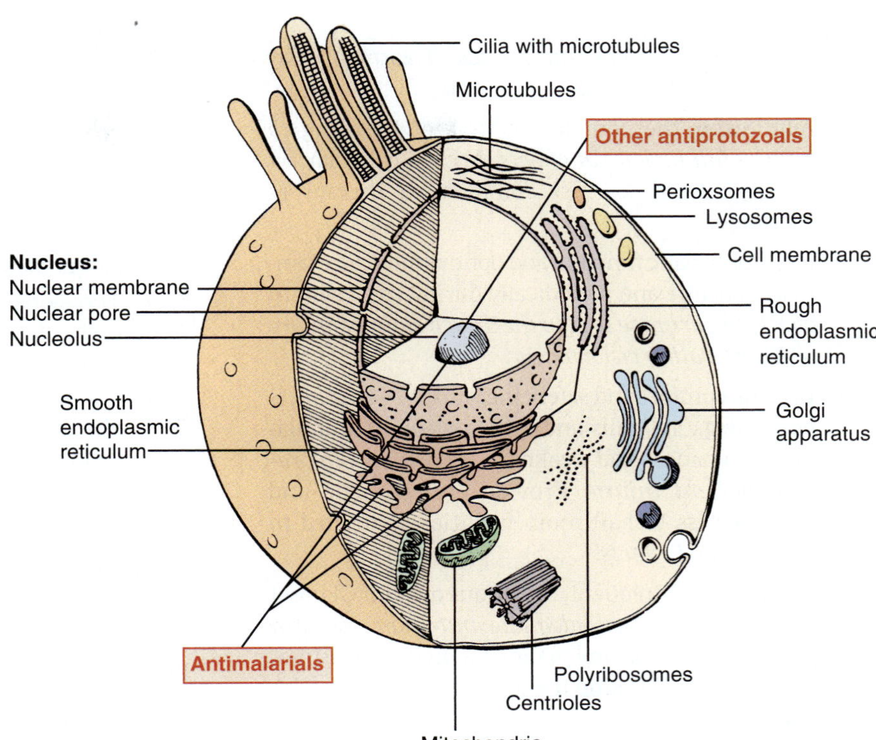

FIGURE 12.2 Sites of action of antimalarials and other antiprotozoals. Antimalarials block protein synthesis and cause cell death. Other antiprotozoals block DNA synthesis, prevent cell reproduction, and lead to cell death.

Pharmacokinetics:

Route	Onset	Peak	Duration
Oral	Varies	1–2 h	1 wk

$T_{1/2}$: 70–120 hours; metabolized in the liver and excreted in the urine

Adverse effects: Visual disturbances, retinal changes, hypotension, nausea, vomiting, diarrhea

Nursing Considerations for Patients Receiving Antimalarial Agents

Assessment: History and Examination

Screen for the following: history of allergy to any of the antimalarials; liver dysfunction or alcoholism *that might interfere with the metabolism and excretion of the drug;* porphyria or psoriasis, *which could be exacerbated by the drug effects;* retinal disease *that could increase the visual disturbances associated with these drugs;* pregnancy and lactation *because these drugs could affect the fetus and could enter the breast milk and be toxic to the infant.*

Physical assessment should be performed *to establish baseline data for assessment of the effectiveness of the drug and the occurrence of any adverse effects associated with drug therapy.* Assess CNS (reflexes and muscle strength). Perform retinal examination and auditory and ophthalmic screening *to detect cautions for drug use and to evaluate changes that occur as a result of drug therapy.* Perform liver evaluation and obtain liver function tests *to determine appropriateness of therapy and to monitor for toxicity.* Perform blood culture *to determine which Plasmodium species is causing the disease.* Conduct examination of the skin (lesions, color, temperature, and texture) *to monitor for adverse effects.*

Nursing Diagnoses

The patient receiving an antimalarial drug may have the following nursing diagnoses related to drug therapy:

- Acute Pain related to GI, CNS, and skin effects of drug
- Disturbed Sensory Perception (Kinesthetic, Visual) related to CNS effects
- Deficient Knowledge regarding drug therapy

Implementation With Rationale

- Arrange for appropriate culture and sensitivity tests before beginning therapy *to ensure proper drug for* susceptible *Plasmodium species.* Treatment may begin before test results are known.

- Administer the complete course of the drug *to get the full beneficial effects.* Mark a calendar for prophylactic doses. Use combination therapy as indicated.
- Monitor hepatic function and ophthalmologic examination before and periodically during treatment *to effectively arrange to stop the drug if signs of failure or deteriorating vision occur.*
- Provide comfort and safety measures if CNS effects occur (e.g., siderails and assistance with ambulation if dizziness and weakness are present) *to prevent patient injury.* Provide oral hygiene and ready access to bathroom facilities as needed *to cope with GI effects.*
- Provide small, frequent, nutritious meals if GI upset is severe *to ensure adequate nutrition.* Monitor nutritional status and arrange a dietary consultation as needed. Taking the drug with food may also decrease GI upset.
- Ensure that the patient is instructed concerning the appropriate dosage regimen *to enhance patient knowledge about drug therapy and to promote compliance.*

The patient should:

- Take safety precautions, including changing position slowly and avoiding driving and hazardous tasks, if CNS effects occur.
- Take the drug with meals and try small, frequent meals if GI upset is a problem.
- Report blurring of vision, which could indicate retinal damage; loss of hearing or ringing in the ears, which could indicate CNS toxicity; and fever or worsening of condition, which could indicate a resistant strain or noneffective therapy.

Evaluation

- Monitor patient response to the drug (resolution of malaria or prevention of malaria).
- Monitor for adverse effects (orientation and affect, nutritional state, skin color and lesions, hepatic function, and visual and auditory changes).
- Evaluate the effectiveness of the teaching plan (patient can name the drug, dosage, possible adverse effects to watch for, and specific measures to help avoid adverse effects).
- Monitor the effectiveness of comfort and safety measures and compliance with the regimen.

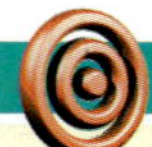

FOCUS POINTS

- A protozoan is a parasitic cellular organism. Its life cycle includes a parasitic phase inside human tissues or cells.
- Malaria is the most common protozoal infection. It is spread to humans by the bite of an *Anopheles* mosquito.
- The signs and symptoms of malaria are related to the destruction of red blood cells and toxicity to the liver.
- Treatment for malaria aims at attacking the parasite at the various stages of its development inside and outside the human body.

Other Protozoal Infections

Other protozoal infections that are encountered in clinical practice include amebiasis, leishmaniasis, trypanosomiasis, trichomoniasis, and giardiasis. These infections, which are caused by single-celled protozoa, are usually associated with unsanitary, crowded conditions and use of poor hygienic practices. Patients traveling to some other countries may encounter these infections, which also appear increasingly in the United States. (See Box 12.4 for a discussion of travel and tourism helping to spread pathogens.)

Amebiasis

Amebiasis, an intestinal infection caused by *Entamoeba histolytica,* is often known as amebic dysentery. *E. histolytica* has a two-stage life cycle (Figure 12.3). The organism exists in two stages: (1) a cystic, dormant stage, in which the protozoan can live for long periods outside the body or in the human intestine, and (2) a **trophozoite** stage in the ideal environment—the human large intestine.

The disease is transmitted while the protozoan is in the cystic stage in fecal matter, from which it can enter water and the ground. It can be passed to other humans who drink this water or eat food that has been grown in this ground. The cysts are swallowed and pass, unaffected by gastric acid, into the intestine. Some of these cysts are passed in fecal matter, and some of them become trophozoites that grow and reproduce. The trophozoites migrate into the mucosa of the colon, where they penetrate into the intestinal wall, forming erosions. These forms of *Entamoeba* release a chemical that dissolves mucosal cells, and eventually they eat away tissue until they reach the vascular system, which carries them throughout the body. The trophozoites lodge in the liver, lungs, heart, brain, and so on.

Early signs of amebiasis include mild to fulminate diarrhea. In the worst cases, if the protozoan is able to invade extra-intestinal tissue, it can dissolve the tissue and eventually cause

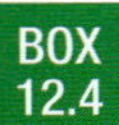

FOCUS ON THE **EVIDENCE**

World Travel and the Spread of Pathogens

Nowadays, people are traveling to more exotic areas of the world than ever before. Because of this, people are being exposed to more pathogens than ever before, and they also are potentially spreading pathogens to different areas of the world. Pathogens that are endemic in one area of the world, causing mild disease, can be quite devastating in a population that has not previously been exposed to that pathogen.

World health agencies and governments have established guidelines for prophylaxis and treatment of such diseases for travelers. People who are planning to travel out of the country should contact their local Health Department or the Centers for Disease Control and Prevention (CDC; website http://www.cdc/gov/travel) for the latest information on what prophylactic measures are required in the area they plan to visit and to learn about potential health hazards in that area. The information is updated frequently; treatment and prophylaxis suggestions are based on current clinical experience in the area and should be consulted regularly.

Patients who have been traveling to other areas of the world and who present with any illness should be questioned about where they traveled, what precautions (including prophylactic measures) were taken, and when they first experienced any signs or symptoms of illness. The CDC can be consulted about diagnosis and treatment guidelines for any tropical disease that is unfamiliar to a health care provider, as well as what precautions should be used in caring for such patients.

the death of the host. Some individuals can become carriers of the disease without having any overt signs or symptoms. These people seem to be resistant to the intestinal invasion but pass the cysts on in the stool.

Leishmaniasis

Leishmaniasis is a disease caused by a protozoan that is passed from sand flies to humans. The sand fly injects an asexual form of this flagellated protozoan, called a promastigote, into the body of a human, where it is rapidly attacked and digested by human macrophages. Inside the macrophages, the promastigote divides, developing many new forms called amastigotes, which keep dividing and eventually kill the macrophage, releasing the amastigotes into the system to be devoured by more macrophages. Thus, a cyclic pattern of infection is established. These amastigotes can cause serious lesions in the skin, the viscera, or the mucous membranes of the host.

Trypanosomiasis

Trypanosomiasis is caused by infection with *Trypanosoma.* Two parasitic protozoal species cause very serious and often fatal diseases in humans:

- African sleeping sickness, which is caused by *Trypanosoma brucei gambiense,* is transmitted by the tsetse fly. After the pathogenic organism has lived and grown in human blood, it eventually invades the CNS, leading to an acute inflammation that results in lethargy, prolonged sleep, and even death.
- Chagas' disease, which is caused by *Trypanosoma cruzi,* is almost endemic in many South American countries. This protozoan results in a severe cardiomyopathy that accounts for numerous deaths and disabilities in certain regions.

Trichomoniasis

Trichomoniasis, which is caused by another flagellated protozoan, *Trichomonas vaginalis,* is a common cause of vaginitis. This infection is usually spread during sexual intercourse by men who have no signs and symptoms of infection. In women, this protozoan causes reddened, inflamed vaginal mucosa, itching, burning, and a yellowish-green discharge.

Giardiasis

Giardiasis, which is caused by *Giardia lamblia,* is the most commonly diagnosed intestinal parasite in the United States. This protozoan forms cysts, which survive outside the body and allow transmission through contaminated water or food, and trophozoites, which break out of the cysts in the upper small intestine and eventually cause signs and symptoms of disease. Diarrhea, rotten egg-smelling stool, and pale and mucous-filled stool are commonly seen. Some patients experience epigastric distress, weight loss, and malnourishment as a result of the invasion of the mucosa.

Pneumocystis carinii Pneumonia

Pneumocystis carinii is an endemic protozoan that does not usually cause illness in humans. When an individual's immune system becomes suppressed, because of acquired immune deficiency syndrome (AIDS) or AIDS-related complex (ARC), the use of immunosuppressant drugs, or advanced age, this parasite is able to invade the lungs, leading to severe inflammation and the condition known as ***Pneumocystis carinii* pneumonia (PCP)**. This disease is the most common opportunistic infection in patients with AIDS.

Other Antiprotozoal Agents

Drugs that are available specifically for the treatment of these various protozoan infections include many of the malarial drugs; chloroquine is effective against extraintestinal amebiasis, and pyrimethamine is also effective in treating toxoplasmosis. Other drugs, including some tetracyclines and aminoglycosides, are used for treating these

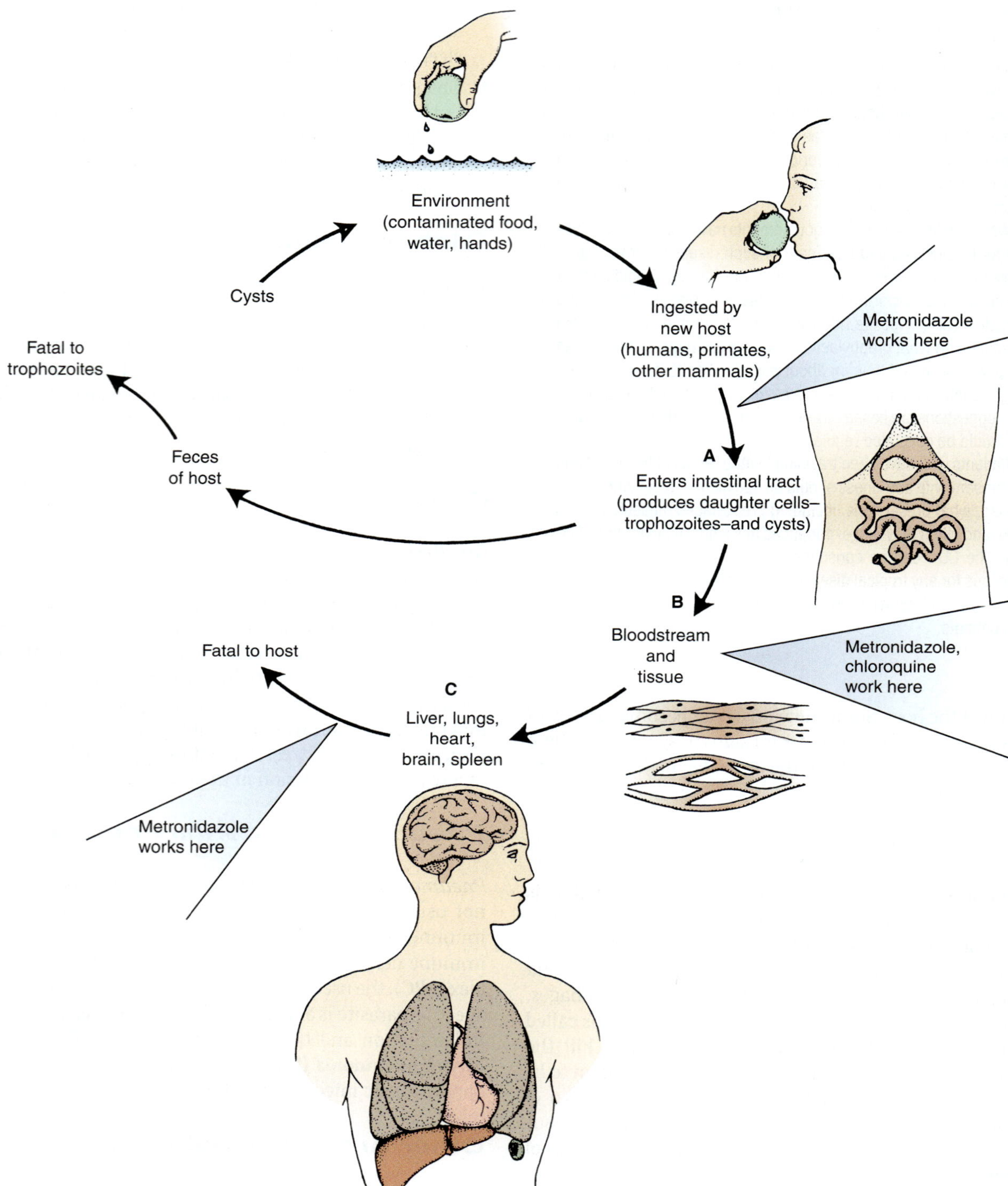

FIGURE 12.3 Life cycle of *Entamoeba histolytica* and the sites of action of metronidazole and chloroquine, which are used to treat amebiasis.

conditions at various stages of the disease (Table 12.2). Other antiprotozoals include the following agents.

- Atovaquone (*Mepron*), which is especially active against PCP, is slowly absorbed and is highly protein bound in circulation. It is excreted slowly through the feces, with a half-life of 67 to 76 hours. Use during pregnancy and lactation should be limited to those situations in which the benefit to the mother clearly outweighs the potential risks to the fetus or neonate. The safety and efficacy of atovaquone in children has not been established.
- Metronidazole (*Flagyl, MetroGel, Noritate*), which is used to treat amebiasis, trichomoniasis, and giardiasis, is well absorbed orally, reaching peak levels in 1 to 2 hours. It is metabolized in the liver with a half-life of 8 to 15 hours. Excretion occurs primarily through the urine. Metronidazole rapidly crosses the placenta and enters fetal circulation. It also passes into breast milk. Use during pregnancy and lactation should be restricted to those situations when the benefit clearly outweighs the risk to the fetus or neonate. Safety and efficacy in children has not been established.
- Nitazoxanide (*Alinia*) was approved in 2005 for the treatment of diarrhea caused by *Cryptosporidium parvum* (patients ≥1 year) or *Giardia lamblia* (patients 1 to 11 years). It is rapidly absorbed after oral administration, reaching peak levels in 1 to 4 hours. Nitazoxanide is metabolized in the liver and excreted in the urine and feces, and has a half-life of 8 to 12 hours. It is not known if nitazoxanide crosses the placenta or enters breast milk.
- Pentamidine (*NebuPent, Pentam 300*) is used as an inhalation agent and a systemic agent in the treatment of PCP and as a systemic drug in the treatment of trypanosomiasis and leishmaniasis. Pentamidine is readily absorbed through the lungs. Excretion occurs in the urine, with traces found in the urine for up to 6 weeks. The safety and efficacy of pentamidine during pregnancy and lactation, and for children, have not been established.
- Tinidazole (*Tindamax*) was approved in 2004 for the treatment of trichomoniasis, giardiasis, and amebiasis. It is rapidly absorbed after oral administration, reaching peak levels within 60 to 90 minutes. It is excreted in the urine with a half-life of 12 to 14 hours. Tinidazole crosses the placenta and enters breast milk. It should never be combined with alcohol and should be used cautiously with liver or renal dysfunction.

Table 12.2 DRUGS IN FOCUS

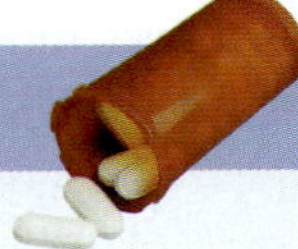

Antiprotozoal Agents

Drug Name	Dosage/Route	Usual Indications
atovaquone (*Mepron*)	*Prevention:* Adult and Pediatric (>13 yr): 1500 mg/day PO *Treatment:* Adult and Pediatric (>13 yr): 750 mg PO b.i.d. with meals for 12 days	Prevention and treatment of *Pneumocystis carinii* pneumonia
P metronidazole (*Flagyl, MetroGel, Noritate*)	*Amebiasis:* Adult: 750 mg PO t.i.d. for 5–10 days Pediatric: 35–50 mg/kg/day PO in three divided doses for 10 days *Trichomoniasis:* Adult: 2 g PO as one dose, or divided into two doses given on the same day or 250 mg PO t.i.d. for 7 days Pediatric: 5 mg/kg per dose PO t.i.d. for 7 days	Treatment of amebiasis, trichomoniasis, giardiasis
nitazoxanide (*Alinia*)	*Giardia:* Pediatric (12–47 mo): 100 mg PO q12h for 3 days Pediatric (4–11 yr): 200 mg PO q12h for 3 days *Cryptosporidium parvum:* Pediatric (1–11 yr): same as for *Giardia* Adults and Pediatric (≥12 yr): 500 mg PO q12h for 3 days	Treatment of diarrhea associated with *Cryptosporidium parvum* or *Giardia lamblia*
pentamidine (*Pentam 300, NebuPent*)	Inhalation: 300 mg once every 4 wk Injection: 4 mg/kg/day IM or IV for 14 days	As inhalation treatment of PCP; as a systemic agent in the treatment of trypanosomiasis and leishmaniasis
tinidazole (*Tindamax*)	*Trichomoniasis, giardiasis:* Adult: 2 g PO as a single dose with food Pediatric (≥3 yr): 50 mg/kg PO as a single dose with food *Amebiasis* Adult: 2 g/day PO with food for 3 days Pediatric (≥3 yr): 50 mg/kg/day PO with food, do not exceed 2 g/day	Treatment of trichomoniasis, giardiasis, amebiasis

Therapeutic Actions and Indications

These antiprotozoal agents act to inhibit DNA synthesis in susceptible protozoa, leading to the inability to reproduce and subsequent cell death (see Figure 12.2). These drugs are indicated for the treatment of infections caused by susceptible protozoa.

Contraindications and Cautions

Contraindications include the presence of any known allergy or hypersensitivity to any of these drugs and pregnancy *because drug effects on developing fetal DNA and proteins can cause fetal abnormalities and even death.* Caution should be used in the presence of CNS disease *because of possible exacerbation when the drug affects the CNS;* hepatic disease *because of possible exacerbation when hepatic drug effects occur;* candidiasis *because of the risk of superinfections;* and lactation, *because these drugs may pass into breast milk and could have severe adverse effects on the infant.*

Adverse Effects

Adverse effects that can be seen with these antiprotozoal agents include such CNS effects as headache, dizziness, ataxia, loss of coordination, and peripheral neuropathy related to drug effects on the neurons. GI effects include nausea, vomiting, diarrhea, unpleasant taste, cramps, and changes in liver function. Superinfections also can occur when the normal flora is disrupted.

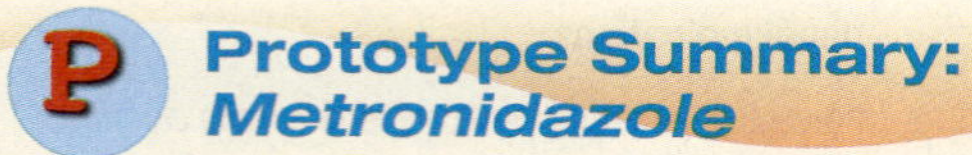

Prototype Summary: *Metronidazole*

Indications: Acute intestinal amebiasis, amebic liver abscess, trichomoniasis, acute infections caused by susceptible strains of anaerobic bacteria, and preoperative and postoperative prophylaxis for patients undergoing colorectal surgery

Actions: Inhibits DNA synthesis of specific anaerobes, causing cell death; mechanism of action as an antiprotozoal and amebicidal are not known

Pharmacokinetics:

Route	Onset	Peak
Oral	Varies	1–2 h
IV	Rapid	1–2 h

$T_{1/2}$: 6–8 hours; metabolized in the liver and excreted in the urine and feces

Adverse effects: Headache, dizziness, ataxia, nausea, vomiting, metallic taste, diarrhea, darkening of the urine

Nursing Considerations for Patients Receiving Antiprotozoal Agents

Assessment: History, Examination, and Physical Assessment

Screen for the following conditions: history of allergy to any of the antiprotozoals; liver dysfunction *that might interfere with metabolism and excretion of the drug or be exacerbated by the drug;* pregnancy, *which is a contraindication,* and lactation *because these drugs could enter the breast milk and be toxic to the infant;* CNS disease *that could be exacerbated by the drug;* and candidiasis *that could become severe as a result of the effects of these drugs on the normal flora.*

Physical assessment should be performed *to establish baseline data for determination of the effectiveness of the drug and the occurrence of any adverse effects associated with drug therapy.* Conduct an examination of the CNS *to check reflexes and of muscle strength to detect cautions for drug use and to evaluate changes that occur as a result of drug therapy.* Evaluate liver and liver function *tests to determine appropriateness of therapy and to monitor for toxicity.* Obtain cultures *to determine the exact protozoal species causing the disease.* Examine the skin and mucous membranes to check for lesions, color, temperature, and texture *to monitor for adverse effects and superinfections.*

Nursing Diagnoses

The patient receiving an antiprotozoal drug may have the following nursing diagnoses related to drug therapy:

- Acute Pain related to GI and CNS effects of drug
- Imbalanced Nutrition: Less Than Body Requirements related to severe GI effects of drug
- Disturbed Sensory Perception (Kinesthetic, Visual) related to CNS effects
- Deficient Knowledge regarding drug therapy

Implementation With Rationale

- Arrange for appropriate culture and sensitivity tests before beginning therapy *to ensure proper drug for susceptible organisms.* Treatment may begin before test results are known.
- Administer the complete course of the drug *to get the full beneficial effects.* Use combination therapy as indicated.
- Monitor hepatic function before and periodically during treatment *to arrange to effectively stop the drug if signs of failure or worsening liver function occur.*

- Provide comfort and safety measures if CNS effects occur, such as siderails and assistance with ambulation if dizziness and weakness are present, *to prevent injury to the patient.* Provide oral hygiene and ready access to bathroom facilities as needed *to cope with GI effects.*
- Arrange for treatment of superinfections as appropriate *to prevent severe infections.*
- Provide small, frequent, nutritious meals if GI upset is severe *to ensure proper nutrition.* Monitor nutritional status and arrange a dietary consultation as needed. Taking the drug with food may also decrease GI upset.
- Ensure that the patient is instructed about the appropriate dosage regimen *to enhance patient knowledge about drug therapy and to promote compliance.*

The patient should:

- Take safety precautions, including changing position slowly and avoiding driving and hazardous tasks, if CNS effects occur.
- Take the drug with meals and try small, frequent meals if GI upset is a problem.
- Report severe GI problems and interference with nutrition; fever and chills, which may indicate the presence of a superinfection; and dizziness, unusual fatigue, or weakness, which may indicate CNS effects (see Case Study and Focused Follow-up 12-1).

Evaluation

- Monitor patient response to the drug (resolution of infection and negative cultures for parasite).
- Monitor for adverse effects (orientation and affect, nutritional state, skin color and lesions, hepatic function, and occurrence of superinfections).
- Evaluate the effectiveness of the teaching plan (patient can name the drug, dosage, possible adverse effects to watch for, and specific measures to help avoid adverse effects).
- Monitor the effectiveness of comfort and safety measures and compliance with the regimen (see Critical Thinking Scenario 12-1).

CRITICAL THINKING SCENARIO 12-1

Coping With Amebiasis

The Situation

J.C., a 20-year-old male college student, reported to the university health center complaining of severe diarrhea, abdominal pain, and, most recently, blood in his stool. He had a mild fever and appeared to be dehydrated and very tired. The young man, who denied travel outside the country, reported eating most of his meals at the local beer joint, where he worked in the kitchen each night making pizza.

A stool sample for ova and parasites (O&P) was obtained, and a diagnosis of amebiasis was made. Metronidazole was prescribed. A public health referral was sent to find the source of the infection, which was the kitchen of the beer joint where J.C. worked. The kitchen was shut down until all the food, utensils, and environment passed state health inspection. Although a potential epidemic was averted (only three other cases of amebiasis were reported), the action of the public health officials added new stress to this student's life, because he was unemployed for several months.

Critical Thinking

What are the important nursing implications for J.C.? *Think about the usual nutritional state of a college student who eats most of his meals in a pizza place.*

What are the implications for recovery when a patient is malnourished and then has a disease that causes severe diarrhea, dehydration, and potential malnourishment? *Consider how difficult it will be for J.C. to be a full-time student while trying to cope with the signs and symptoms of his disease, as well as the adverse effects associated with his drug therapy and the need to maintain adequate nutrition to allow some healing and recovery.*

What potential problems could the added stress of being out of work have for J.C.? *Consider the physiological impact of stress, as well as the psychological problems of trying to cope with one more stressor.*

(continued)

Coping With Amebiasis *(continued)*

Discussion

J.C. needed a great deal of reassurance and an explanation of his disease. He learned that oral hygiene and small, frequent meals would help alleviate some of his discomfort until the metronidazole could control the amebiasis and that good hygiene and strict hand washing when the disease is active would help to prevent transmission. He was advised to watch for the occurrence of specific adverse drug effects, such as a possible severe reaction to alcohol (he was advised to avoid alcoholic beverages while taking this drug); gastrointestinal upset and a strange metallic taste (the importance of good nutrition to promote healing of the gastrointestinal tract was stressed); dizziness or light-headedness; and superinfections.

J.C. was scheduled for a follow-up examination for stool O&P and nutritional status. Metronidazole was continued until the stool sample came back negative. He needed and received a great deal of support and encouragement because he was far from home and the disease and the drug effects were sometimes difficult to cope with. The effects of stress—decreasing blood flow to the gastrointestinal tract, for example—can make it more difficult for patients such as J.C. to recover from this disease. Support and encouragement can be major factors in their eventual recovery. J.C. was given a telephone number to call if he needed information or support and a complete set of written instructions regarding the disease and the drug therapy.

Nursing Care Guide for J.C.: Metronidazole

Assessment: History and Examination

Allergies to metronidazole, renal or liver dysfunction

Concurrent use of barbiturates, oral anticoagulants, alcohol

Local: culture of stool for accurate diagnosis of infection

CNS: orientation, affect, vision, reflexes

Skin: color, lesions, texture

GI: abdominal, liver evaluation

Hematological: CBC, liver function tests

Nursing Diagnoses

Acute Pain related to GI, superinfection effects

Disturbed Sensory Perception (Kinesthetic, Visual) related to CNS effects

Imbalanced Nutrition: Less Than Body Requirements related to GI effects

Deficient Knowledge regarding drug therapy

Implementation

Culture infection before beginning therapy.

Provide comfort and safety measures: oral hygiene, safety precautions, treatment of superinfections, maintenance of nutrition.

Provide small, frequent meals and monitor nutritional status.

Provide support and reassurance for dealing with drug effects and discomfort.

Provide patient teaching regarding drug name, dosage, adverse effects, precautions, and warning signs to report and hygiene measures to observe.

Evaluation

Evaluate drug effects: resolution of protozoal infection.

Monitor for adverse effects: GI alterations, dizziness, confusion, CNS changes, vision loss, hepatic function, superinfections.

Monitor for drug–drug interactions with oral anticoagulants, alcohol, or barbiturates.

Evaluate effectiveness of patient teaching program.

Evaluate effectiveness of comfort and safety measures.

Patient Teaching for J.C.

You have been prescribed metronidazole to treat your amebic infection. This antiprotozoal drug acts to destroy certain protozoa that have invaded your body. Because it affects specific phases of the protozoal life cycle, it must be taken over a period of time to be effective. It is very important to take all the drug that has been ordered for you.

- ☐ This drug frequently causes stomach upset. If it causes you to have nausea, heartburn, or vomiting, take the drug with meals or a light snack.
- ☐ Common effects of this drug include the following:
  - *Nausea, vomiting, and loss of appetite:* Take the drug with food and have small, frequent meals.
  - *Superinfections of the mouth, skin:* These go away when the course of the drug has been completed. If they become uncomfortable, notify your health care provider for an appropriate solution.

Coping With Amebiasis *(continued)*

- *Dry mouth, strange metallic taste:* Frequent mouth care and sucking sugarless lozenges may help. This effect will also go away when the course of the drug is finished.
- *Intolerance to alcohol (nausea, vomiting, flushing, headache, and stomach pain):* Avoid alcoholic beverages or products containing alcohol while taking this drug.

☐ Report any of the following to your health care provider: sore throat, fever, or chills; skin rash or redness; severe gastrointestinal upset; and unusual fatigue, clumsiness, or weakness.

☐ Take the full course of your prescription. Never use this drug to self-treat any other infection or give it to any other person.

☐ Tell any doctor, nurse, or other health care provider that you are taking this drug.

☐ Keep this drug and all medications out of the reach of children.

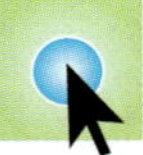

WEB LINKS

Health care providers and patients may want to consult the following Internet sources:

http://www.cdc.gov/travel/malinfo.htm Information on malaria, including information for travelers.

http://www.rph.wa.gov.au/labs/haem/malaria/ Information on malaria incidence, treatment, prevention, and support.

http://www.healthhubs.com/trypanosomiasis Information on trypanosomiasis.

http://www.vdh.state.va.us/epi/giarf.htm Information about giardiasis—support, treatment, prevention, and teaching.

http://www.cdc.gov/amebiasis/travel/diseases.htm Information about amebiasis prevention, incidence, and treatments.

Points to Remember

- A protozoan is a parasitic cellular organism. Its life cycle includes a parasitic phase inside human tissues or cells.
- Malaria, which occurs in many tropical parts of the world, has been spreading in recent years because of resistance to insecticides occurring in the *Anopheles* mosquito.
- Malaria is caused by *Plasmodium* protozoa, which must go through a cycle in the *Anopheles* mosquito before being passed to humans by the mosquito bite. Once inside a human, the protozoa invade red blood cells.
- The characteristic cyclic chills and fever of malaria occur when red blood cells burst, releasing more protozoa into the bloodstream.
- Malaria is treated with a combination of drugs that attack the protozoan at various stages in its life cycle.
- Amebiasis is caused by the protozoan *Entamoeba histolytica*, which invades human intestinal tissue after being passed to humans through unsanitary food or water.
- Leishmaniasis, a protozoan-caused disease, can result in serious lesions in the mucosa, viscera, and skin.
- Trypanosomiasis, which is caused by infection with a *Trypanosoma* parasite, may assume two forms. African sleeping sickness leads to inflammation of the CNS, and Chagas' disease results in serious cardiomyopathy.
- Trichomoniasis is caused by *Trichomonas vaginalis*. This common cause of vaginitis results in no signs or symptoms in men but serious vaginal inflammation in women.
- Giardiasis, which is caused by *Giardia lamblia*, is the most commonly diagnosed intestinal parasite in the United States. This disease may lead to serious malnutrition when the pathogen invades intestinal mucosa.
- *Pneumocystis carinii* is an endemic protozoan that does not usually cause illness in humans unless they become immunosuppressed. *P. carinii* pneumonia (PCP) is the most common opportunistic infection seen in AIDS patients.
- Patients receiving antiprotozoal agents should be monitored regularly to detect any serious adverse effects, including loss of vision, liver toxicity, and so on.

CHECK YOUR UNDERSTANDING

Answers to the questions in this chapter may be found in the Answer Key in the back of the book.

Multiple Choice

Select the best answer to the following.

1. Of the following protozoal infections, the one that is not caused by insect bites is
   a. malaria.
   b. trypanosomiasis.
   c. leishmaniasis.
   d. giardiasis.

2. Malaria is caused by the *Plasmodium* protozoan, which depends on
   a. a snail to act as intermediary in the life cycle of the protozoan.
   b. a mosquito and a red blood cell for maturation.
   c. a human liver cell for cell division and reproduction.
   d. stagnant water for maturation.

3. Drugs used to treat malaria are given in combination because
   a. they are less toxic that way.
   b. they are absorbed better if taken together.
   c. mosquitoes are less likely to bite a person who is taking combination drugs.
   d. the drugs can then affect the protozoan at various stages of the life cycle.

4. A patient traveling to an area of the world where malaria is known to be endemic should be taught to
   a. avoid drinking the water.
   b. begin prophylactic antimalarial therapy before traveling and continue it through the visit and for 2 to 3 weeks after the visit.
   c. take a supply of antimalarial drugs in case he or she gets a mosquito bite.
   d. begin prophylactic antimalarial therapy 2 weeks before traveling and stop the drugs on arrival at the destination.

5. Amebiasis or amebic dysentery
   a. is seen only in Third World countries.
   b. is caused by a protozoan that enters the body through an insect bite.
   c. is caused by a protozoan that can enter the body in the cyst stage in water or food, usually under unsanitary conditions.
   d. usually has no signs and symptoms.

6. Giardiasis is the most common intestinal parasite seen in the United States, and it
   a. does not respond to drug therapy.
   b. can invade the liver and cause death.
   c. is seen only in areas with no sanitation.
   d. is associated with rotten egg-smelling stool, diarrhea, and mucous-filled stool.

7. PCP (*Pneumocystis carinii* pneumonia) is not
   a. an endemic protozoan found in the human respiratory system.
   b. responsive to inhaled pentamidine.
   c. an opportunistic bacterial infection.
   d. frequently associated with immune suppression and AIDS.

8. Trypanosomiasis may assume two different forms:
   a. African sleeping sickness and Chagas' disease.
   b. elephantiasis and malaria.
   c. dysentery and African sleeping sickness.
   d. malaria and Chagas' disease.

9. A nurse would note that a patient had a good understanding of his antimalarial drug regimen if the patient reported
   a. "I keep these pills and take them only when I have been bitten by a mosquito."
   b. "I will need to take these pills daily for the rest of my life."
   c. "I will need to start taking these pills before my trip, the whole time I am on vacation, and for a period of time after I get back home."
   d. "I start taking these pills as soon as I arrive at my vacation destination."

Multiple Response

Select all that apply.

1. A mother calls in concerned that her son, a college freshman, has been diagnosed with giardiasis. The nurse would respond to the mother's concerns by telling her which of the following?
   a. You should have your son come home immediately so that he can be treated appropriately.
   b. This is a very rare disorder; it is not usually seen in this country.
   c. This is the most common protozoal infection seen in this country and is usually transmitted through food or water.
   d. This infection can be treated with oral drugs, and he should be able to get the drugs where his infection was diagnosed.

e. This is an infection that has to be treated quickly with IV medications.
f. Encourage your son to get the medicine and to try very hard to eat nutritious food.

Web Exercise

A friend of yours has won a trip around the world to many exotic places. You are asked if any immunizations are needed before the trip. Go to http://www.cdc.gov/travel and prepare a summary of suggested vaccinations or prophylactic measures that should be taken.

Matching

Match the following antiprotozoal drugs with the protozoal infection they are used to treat.

1. ____________________ primaquine
2. ____________________ atovaquone
3. ____________________ quinine
4. ____________________ pentamidine
5. ____________________ chloroquine
6. ____________________ metronidazole
7. ____________________ hydroxychloroquine
8. ____________________ tinidazole

A. Malaria
B. PCP infection
C. Trypanosomiasis and leishmaniasis
D. Trichomoniasis, giardiasis, amebiasis

Bibliography and References

Andrews, M., & Boyle, J. (2002). *Transcultural concepts in nursing care.* Philadelphia: Lippincott Williams & Wilkins.

Atkinson, W. L., Pickering, L. K., Schwartz, B., Weniger, B. G., Iskander, J. K., & Watson, J. C. (2002). General recommendations on immunization: Recommendations of the Advisory Committee on Immunization Practices and the American Academy of Family Physicians. *Morbidity and Mortality Weekly Report, 51*(RR02), 1–35.

Collins, W. E., & Jeffery, G. M. (2002). Extended clearance time after treatment of infections with *Plasmodium malariae* may not be indicative of resistance to chloroquine. *American Journal of Tropical Medicine & Hygiene, 67,* 406–410.

Drug facts and comparisons. (2006). St. Louis: Facts and Comparisons.

Gilman, A., Hardman, J. G., & Limbird, L. E. (Eds.). (2006). *Goodman and Gilman's the pharmacological basis of therapeutics* (11th ed.). New York: McGraw-Hill.

Karch, A. M. (2006). *2007 Lippincott's nursing drug guide.* Philadelphia: Lippincott Williams & Wilkins.

Porth, C. M. (2005). *Pathophysiology: Concepts of altered health states.* (7th ed.). Philadelphia: Lippincott Williams & Wilkins.

Professional's guide to patient drug facts. (2006). St. Louis: Facts and Comparisons.

CHAPTER 13

Anthelmintic Agents

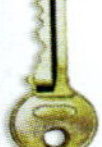

KEY TERMS

cestode
flatworm
helminth
nematode
pinworm
platyhelminth
roundworm
schistosomiasis
threadworm
trichinosis
whipworm

LEARNING OBJECTIVES

Upon completion of this chapter, you will be able to:

1. List the common worms that cause disease in humans.
2. Describe the therapeutic actions, indications, pharmacokinetics, contraindications, most common adverse reactions, and important drug-drug interactions associated with the anthelmintics.
3. Discuss the use of anthelmintics across the lifespan.
4. Compare and contrast the prototype drug mebendazole with other anthelmintics.
5. Outline the nursing considerations, including important teaching points to stress, for patients receiving an anthelmintic.

DRUG LIST

albendazole
ivermectin
P mebendazole
praziquantel
pyrantel
thiabendazole

About 1 billion people have worms in their gastrointestinal (GI) tract or other tissues, which makes helminthic infections among the most common of all diseases. These infestations are very common in tropical areas, but they are also often found in other regions, including countries such as the United States and Canada. With so many people traveling to many parts of the world, it is not uncommon for a traveler to pick up a helminthic infection in another country and inadvertently bring it home, where the worms are able to infect other individuals (Box 13.1). The **helminths** that most commonly infect humans are of two types: the **nematodes** or **roundworms**, and the **platyhelminthes** or **flatworms**.

Intestine-Invading Worms

Many of the worms that infect humans live only in the intestinal tract. Proper diagnosis of a helminthic infection requires a stool examination for ova (eggs) and parasites. Treatment of a helminthic infection entails the use of an anthelmintic drug. Another important part of therapy for helminthic infections involves the prevention of reinfection or spread of an existing infection. Measures such as thorough hand washing after use of the toilet; frequent laundering of bed linens and underwear in very hot, chlorine-treated water; disinfection of toilets and bathroom areas after each use; and good personal hygiene to wash away ova are important to the effectiveness of drug therapy and prevention of the spread of the disease.

Nematodes

Nematodes, or roundworms, include the commonly encountered **pinworms**, **whipworms**, **threadworms**, *Ascaris,* and hookworms. These worms cause diseases that range from mild to potentially deadly.

Pinworms

Pinworms, which stay in the intestine, cause little discomfort except for perianal itching or occasionally vaginal itching. Infection with pinworms is the most common helminthic infection among school-age children (Box 13.2).

Whipworms

Whipworms attach themselves to the wall of the colon; when large numbers of them are in the intestine, they cause colic and bloody diarrhea. In severe cases, whipworm infestation

BOX 13.1 CULTURAL CONSIDERATIONS FOR DRUG THERAPY

Travelers and Helminths

People who come from or travel to areas of the world where schistosomiasis is endemic should always be assessed for the possibility of infection with such a disease when seen for health care. Areas of the world in which this disease is endemic are mainly tropical settings, such as Puerto Rico, islands of the West Indies, Africa, parts of South America, the Philippines, China, Japan, and Southeast Asia. People traveling to these areas should be warned about wading, swimming, or bathing in freshwater streams, ponds, or lakes. For example, swimming in the Nile River is a popular attraction on Egyptian vacation tours; however, this activity may result in a lasting (unhappy) memory when the traveler returns home and is diagnosed with schistosomiasis. The nurse can suggest to patients who are planning a visit to one of these areas that they contact the Centers for Disease Control and Prevention (CDC) for health and safety guidelines, as well as signs and symptoms to watch for after returning home. The CDC can be reached on the World Wide Web at http://www.cdc.gov/travel.

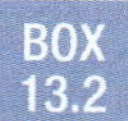

BOX 13.2 Managing Pinworm Infections

Infestation with worms can be a frightening and traumatic experience for most people. Seeing the worm can be an especially difficult experience. Some worm infestations are not that uncommon in this country, especially infestation with pinworms.

Pinworms can spread very rapidly among children in schools, summer camps, and other institutions. Once the infestation starts, careful hygiene measures and drug therapy are required to eradicate the disease. After the diagnosis has been made and appropriate drug therapy started, proper hygiene measures are essential. Some suggested hygiene measures that might help to control the infection include the following:

- Keep the child's nails cut short and hands well scrubbed, because reinfection results from the worm's eggs being carried back to the mouth after becoming lodged under the fingernails when the child scratches the pruritic perianal area.
- Give the child a shower in the morning to wash away any ova deposited in the anal area during the night.
- Change and launder undergarments, bed linens, and pajamas every day.
- Disinfect toilet seats daily and the floors of bathrooms and bedrooms periodically.
- Encourage the child to wash hands vigorously after using the toilet.

In some areas of the country, parents are asked to check for worm ova by pressing sticky tape against the anal area in the morning before bathing. The sticky tape is then pressed against a slide that can be taken or sent to a clinical laboratory for evaluation. It may take 5 to 6 weeks to get a clear reading with this method of testing. Some health care providers believe that the psychological trauma involved in doing this type of follow-up, especially with a school-age child, makes this task too onerous to ask parents to do. Instead, many believe that the ease of treating this relatively harmless disease makes it more prudent to continue to treat as prescribed and to forgo the follow-up testing.

It is important to reassure patients and families that these types of infections do not necessarily reflect negatively on their hygiene or lifestyle. It takes a coordinated effort among medical personnel, families, and patients to control a pinworm infestation.

may result in prolapse of the intestinal wall and anemia related to blood loss.

Threadworms

Threadworms are more pervasive than most of the other helminths. After burrowing into the wall of the small intestine, female worms lay eggs, which hatch into larvae that invade many body tissues, including the lungs, liver, and heart. In very severe cases, death may occur from pneumonia or from lung or liver abscesses that result from larval invasion.

Ascaris

Worldwide, *Ascaris* infection is the most prevalent helminthic infection. It may occur wherever sanitation is poor. Although many individuals have no idea that they have this infestation unless they see a worm in their stool, others become quite ill.

Initially, the individual ingests fertilized roundworm eggs, which hatch in the small intestine and then make their way to the lungs, where they may cause cough, fever, and other signs of a pulmonary infiltrate. The larvae then migrate back to the intestine, where they grow to adult size (i.e., about as long and as big around as an earthworm) and can cause abdominal distention and pain. In the most severe cases, intestinal obstruction by masses of worms can occur.

Hookworms

Hookworms attach themselves to the small intestine of infected individuals and suck blood from the walls of the intestine. This damages the intestinal wall and can cause severe anemia with lethargy, weakness, and fatigue. Malabsorption problems may occur as the small intestinal mucosa is altered. Treatment for anemia and fluid and electrolyte disturbances is an important part of the therapy for this infection.

Platyhelminths: Cestodes

The platyhelminths (flatworms) include the **cestodes** (tapeworms) that live in the human intestine and the flukes (schistosomes) that invade other tissues as part of their life cycle. Cestodes are segmented flatworms with a head, or scolex, and a variable number of segments that grow from the head; they sometimes form worms that are several yards long. Persons with a tapeworm may experience some abdominal discomfort and distention as well as weight loss because the worm eats ingested nutrients. Many infected patients require a great deal of psychological support when they excrete parts of the tapeworm or when the worm comes out the mouth or nose, which may occur occasionally.

Tissue-Invading Worm Infections

Some of the worms that invade the body exist outside the intestinal tract and can seriously damage the tissues they invade. Because of their location within healthy tissue, they can also be more difficult to treat.

Trichinosis

Trichinosis is the disease caused by ingestion of the encysted larvae of the roundworm, *Trichinella spiralis,* in undercooked pork. The larvae of this worm, which are deposited in the intestinal mucosa, pass into the bloodstream and are carried throughout the body. They can penetrate skeletal muscle and can cause an inflammatory reaction in cardiac muscle and in the brain. Fatal pneumonia, heart failure, and encephalitis may occur.

The best treatment for trichinosis is prevention. Because the larvae are ingested by humans in undercooked pork, freezing pork meat, monitoring the food eaten by pigs, and instructing people in the proper cooking of pork can be most beneficial.

Filariasis

Filariasis refers to infection of the blood and tissues of healthy individuals by worm embryos, which are injected by biting insects. These thread-like embryos, or filariae, can overwhelm the lymphatic system and cause massive inflammatory reactions. This may lead to severe swelling of the hands, feet, legs, arms, scrotum, or breast—a condition called elephantiasis.

Schistosomiasis

Schistosomiasis (Figure 13.1) is an infection by a fluke that is carried by a snail. This disease is a common problem in parts of Africa, Asia, and certain South American and Caribbean countries that have climates and snails conducive to the life cycle of schistosomes.

A description of the life cycle of schistosomes follows. The eggs, which are excreted in the urine and feces of infected individuals, hatch in fresh water into a form that infects a certain snail. Larvae, known as cercariae, develop in the snail, which sheds the cercariae back into the fresh-water pond or lake. People become infected when they come in contact with the infested water. The larvae attach to the skin and quickly burrow into the bloodstream and lymphatics. After they move into the lungs, and later the liver, they mature into adult worms that mate and migrate to the intestines and urinary bladder. The female worms then lay large numbers of eggs, which are expelled in the feces and urine, and the cycle begins again.

Signs and symptoms of infection with this helminth may include a pruritic rash where the larva attaches to the skin, which is often called swimmer's itch. About 1 or 2 months

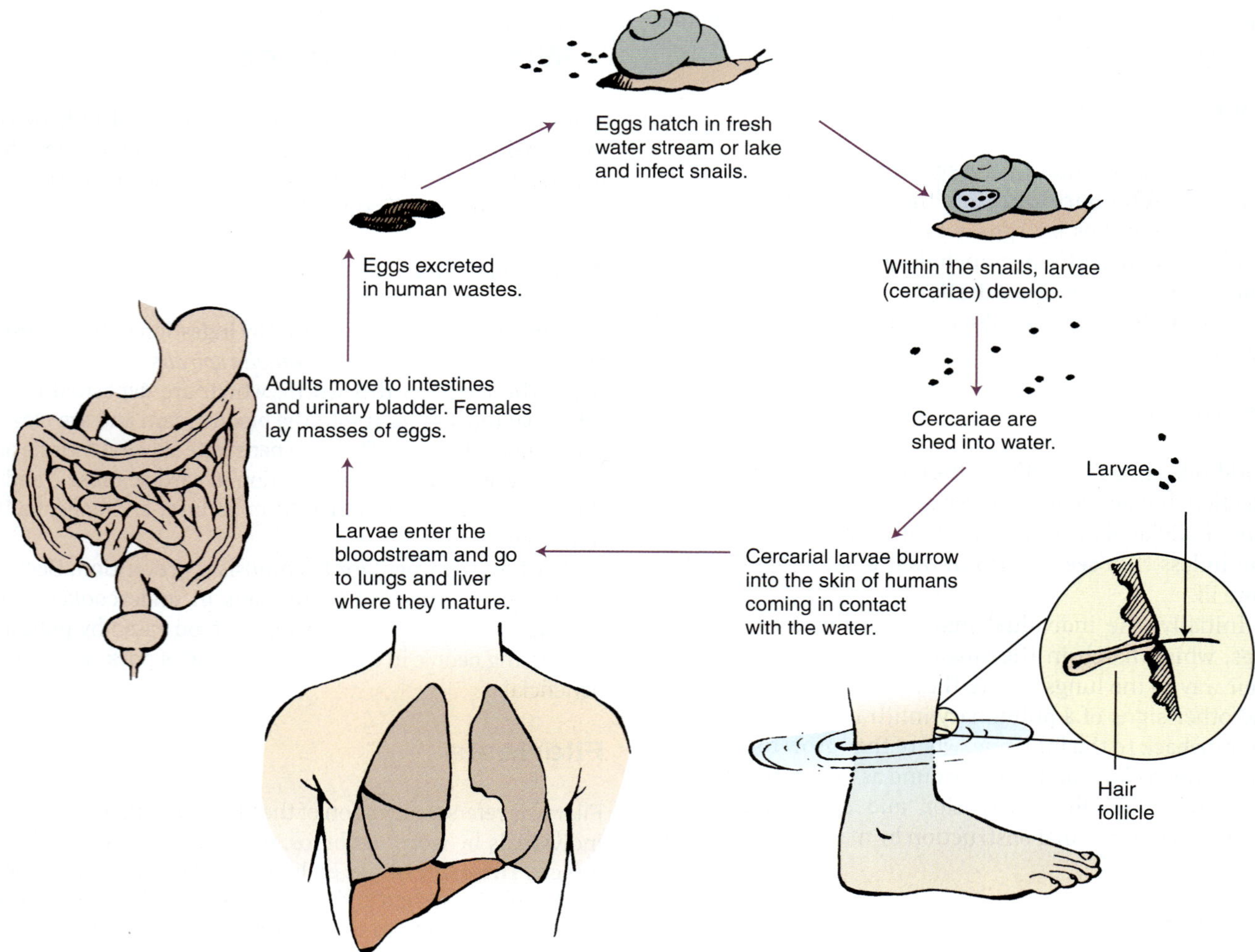

FIGURE 13.1 Life cycle of schistosomes.

later, affected individuals may experience several weeks of fever, chills, headache, and other symptoms. Chronic or severe infestation may lead to abdominal pain and diarrhea, as well as blockage of blood flow to areas of the liver, lungs, and central nervous system (CNS). These blockages can lead to liver and spleen enlargement, as well as signs of CNS and cardiac ischemia. (See Critical Thinking Scenario 13-1.)

FOCUS POINTS

- Helminths are worms that cause disease by invading the human body.
- Pinworms are the most frequent cause of helminth infection in the United States.
- Platyhelminths (flatworms) include tapeworms and flukes.
- Some helminths invade body tissues and can seriously damage lymphatic tissue, lungs, CNS, heart, or liver.

Anthelmintics

The anthelmintic drugs act on metabolic pathways that are present in the invading worm but absent or significantly different in the human host. (See Table 13.1 for a complete listing of anthelmintic drugs.) Mebendazole (*Vermox*), probably the most commonly used of all of the anthelmintics, is effective against pinworms, roundworms, whipworms, and hookworms. It is available in the form of a chewable tablet, and a typical 3-day course can be repeated in 3 weeks if needed. Because very little of the mebendazole is absorbed systemically, it has few adverse effects. The drug is not metabolized in the body, and most of it is excreted unchanged in the feces, although a small amount may be excreted in the urine. It should not be used during pregnancy because teratogenic effects do occur in rats, and there is a risk of possible fetal harm. Other anthelmintics cross into breast milk and can cause harm to the neonate, and it is not known whether mebendazole passes into breast milk; therefore, lactating women should be advised to select another way to feed the baby. (See Box 13.3 for

CRITICAL THINKING SCENARIO 13-1

Anthelmintics

The Situation

V.Y., a 33-year-old man from Vietnam, underwent a complete physical examination in preparation for a training job in custodial work at a local hospital. He was a refugee who had come to the United States 6 months ago as part of a church-sponsored resettlement program. In the course of the examination, it was found that he had a history of chronic diarrhea, hepatomegaly, pulmonary rales, and splenomegaly. Further tests indicated that he had chronic schistosomiasis. Because of V.Y.'s limited use of the English language, he was hospitalized so that his disease, which was unfamiliar to most of the associated health care providers, could be monitored. He was treated with praziquantel.

Critical Thinking

What are the important nursing implications for V.Y.? *Think about the serious limitations that are placed on medical care, particularly patient teaching, when the patient and the health care workers do not speak the same language.*

What innovative techniques could be used to teach this patient about the disease, the drugs, and the hygiene measures that are important for him to follow?

Are the other patients or workers in the hospital exposed to any health risks? What sort of educational program should be developed to teach them about this disease and to allay any fears or anxieties they may have?

What special interventions are needed to explain the drug therapy and any adverse effects or warning signs that V.Y. should be watching for?

Discussion

A language barrier can be a real handicap in the health care system. In many cases, pictures can assist communication. For example, the need for nutritious food is conveyed by using appropriate pictures of foods that should be eaten. Frequent reinforcement is necessary because the patient has no way of letting you know that he really understands the message that you are trying to convey. The patient is prepared for discharge through careful patient teaching that may involve pictures, calendars, and clocks so that he is given every opportunity to comply with his medical regimen.

In addition, the nursing staff should contact the local health department to determine whether the local sewer system can properly handle contaminated wastes. In this case, the staff learned from the Centers for Disease Control and Prevention that the snail's intermediate host does not live in this country, so the hazards posed by this waste are small, and normal disposal of the wastes should be appropriate.

V.Y. should also be observed for signs of adverse effects, although praziquantel is a relatively mild drug. Drug fever, abdominal pain, or dizziness may occur. If dizziness occurs, safety precautions, such as assistance with ambulation, use of siderails, and adequate lighting, need to be taken without alarming the patient.

Nursing Care Guide for V.Y.: Anthelmintic Agents

Assessment: History and Examination

Allergies to this drug, renal or liver dysfunction

Drug history: use of albendazole

Local: culture of infection

CNS: orientation, affect

Skin: color, lesions, texture

GI: abdominal and liver evaluation, including hepatic function tests

GU: renal function tests

Nursing Diagnoses

Acute Pain related to GI or CNS effects

Disturbed Personal Identity related to diagnosis and treatment

Fear related to communication problems, health issues

Deficient Knowledge regarding drug therapy

Implementation

Culture for ova and parasites before beginning therapy.

Provide comfort and safety measures: small, frequent meals; safety precautions; hygiene measures; maintenance of nutrition.

Monitor nutritional status as needed.

Provide support and reassurance to deal with drug effects, discomfort, and diagnosis.

(continued)

Anthelmintics *(continued)*

Provide patient teaching regarding drug name, dosage regimen, adverse effects and precautions to report, and hygiene measures to observe.

Evaluation

Evaluate drug effects: resolution of helminth infection.

Monitor for adverse effects: GI alterations, CNS changes, dizziness and confusion, renal and hepatic function.

Monitor for drug–drug interactions: concurrent use of albendazole.

Evaluate effectiveness of patient teaching program.

Evaluate effectiveness of comfort and safety measures.

Patient Teaching for V.Y.

- ☐ This drug is called an anthelmintic. It works to destroy certain helminths, or worms, that have invaded your body.
- ☐ It is important that you take the full course of the drug—three doses the first day, then retesting to repeat this course if needed to ensure that all of the worms, in all phases of their life cycle, have disappeared from your body.
- ☐ You may take this drug with meals or with a light snack to help decrease any stomach upset that you may experience. Swallow the tablets whole and avoid holding them in your mouth for any length of time because a very unpleasant taste may occur.
- ☐ Common effects of this drug include
  - *Nausea, vomiting, and loss of appetite:* Take the drug with food, and eat small, frequent meals.
  - *Dizziness and drowsiness:* If this occurs, avoid driving a car or operating dangerous machinery. Change positions slowly to avoid falling or injury.
- ☐ Report any of the following conditions to your health care provider: fever, chills, rash, headache, weakness, or tremors.
- ☐ Take all of the drug that has been prescribed. Never use this drug to self-treat any other infection or give it to any other person.
- ☐ Tell any doctor, nurse, or other health care provider that you are taking this drug.
- ☐ Keep this drug and all medications out of the reach of children.

Table 13.1 DRUGS IN FOCUS

Anthelmintics

Drug Name	Dosage/Route	Usual Indications
albendazole (*Albenza*)	*Hydatid disease:* ≥60 kg: 400 mg b.i.d. PO <60 kg: 15 mg/kg/day PO in divided doses, b.i.d., on a 28-day cycle followed by 14 days of rest, for a total of three cycles *Neurocysticercosis:* ≥60 kg: 400 mg b.i.d. PO <60 kg: 15/mg/kg/day PO in divided doses, b.i.d., for 8–30 days of treatment	Treatment of active lesions caused by pork tapeworm and cystic disease of the liver, lungs, and peritoneum caused by dog tapeworm
ivermectin (*Stromectol*)	150–200 mg/kg PO as a single dose	Treatment of threadworm disease or strongyloidiasis; onchocerciasis or river blindness
P mebendazole (*Vermox*)	100 mg PO morning and evening on 3 consecutive days *Enterobiasis:* 100 mg PO as a single dose	Treatment of diseases caused by pinworms, roundworms, whipworms, and hookworms
praziquantel (*Biltricide*)	3 doses of 20–25 mg/kg PO as a 1-day treatment	Treatment of a wide number of schistosomes or flukes
pyrantel (*Antiminth, Pin-Rid, Pin-X, Reese's Pinworm*)	11 mg/kg PO as a single dose; maximum dose, 1 g	Treatment of diseases caused by pinworms and roundworms
thiabendazole (*Mintezol*)	<150 lb: 10 mg/lb per dose PO, 2 doses per day ≥150 lb: 1.5 g/dose PO, 2 doses per day	Treatment of diseases caused by roundworms, hookworms, and whipworms

BOX 13.3

DRUG THERAPY ACROSS THE LIFESPAN

Anthelmintic Agents

CHILDREN

Culture of the suspected worm is important before beginning any drug therapy.

The more toxic drugs—albendazole, ivermectin, and praziquantel—should be avoided in children.

The most commonly used anthelmintic, mebendazole, comes in a chewable tablet that is convenient for use in children.

Nutritional status and hydration are major concerns with children taking these drugs who develop serious gastrointestinal effects.

ADULTS

Adults may be somewhat repulsed by the idea that they have a worm infestation, and they may be reluctant to discuss the needed lifestyle adjustments and treatment plans.

Pregnant and nursing women should not use these drugs unless the benefit clearly outweighs the potential risk to the fetus or neonate. If a severe helminth infestation threatens the mother, some of the drugs can be used as long as the mother is informed of the potential risk.

OLDER ADULTS

Older patients may be more susceptible to the central nervous system and gastrointestinal effects of some of these drugs. Dosage adjustment is needed for these agents.

Monitor hydration and nutritional status carefully.

more information about using anthelmintics with various age groups.)

Pyrantel (*Antiminth, Pin-Rid, Pin-X, Reese's Pinworm*) is an oral drug that is effective against pinworms and roundworms. Because this agent is given as a single dose, it may be preferred for patients who could have trouble remembering to take medications or following drug regimens. Pyrantel is poorly absorbed, and most of the drug is excreted unchanged in the feces, although a small amount may be found in the urine. It is not recommended for use during pregnancy or lactation, and safety has not been established for children younger than 2 years. Adverse effects associated with pyrantel include possible uncomfortable GI side effects and diarrhea.

Thiabendazole (*Mintezol*) may also be used in the treatment of roundworm, hookworm, and whipworm infections. However, it is not the drug of choice if one of the other drugs can be used because it is not as effective as other agents and can cause more uncomfortable adverse effects. Nevertheless, thiabendazole is the drug of choice for treatment of threadworm infections, and it can be used to alleviate the signs and symptoms of invasive trichinosis. It is readily absorbed from the GI tract, reaching peak levels in 1 to 2 hours. It is completely metabolized in the liver and primarily excreted in the urine. There are no established studies regarding use during pregnancy or lactation, so it is recommended that the drug not be used unless the benefit clearly outweighs the potential risk.

Albendazole (*Albenza*) is effective against active lesions caused by pork tapeworm and cystic disease of the liver, lungs, and peritoneum caused by dog tapeworm. A very powerful drug, albendazole has serious adverse effects, including renal failure and bone marrow depression. It should be used only after the causative worm has been identified. It is poorly absorbed from the GI tract, reaching peak plasma levels in about 5 hours. It is metabolized in the liver and primarily excreted in urine. Albendazole has been shown to be teratogenic in animal studies and should not be used during pregnancy or lactation. Women of childbearing age should be advised to use barrier contraceptives while taking this drug.

Ivermectin (*Stromectol*) is effective against the nematode that causes onchocerciasis, or river blindness, which is found in tropical areas of Africa, Mexico, and South America. The drug is also used to treat threadworm disease or strongyloidiasis. It is readily absorbed from the GI tract and reaches peak plasma levels in 4 hours. It is completely metabolized in the liver with a half-life of 16 hours; excretion is through the feces. Ivermectin should never be taken during pregnancy because it can cause serious fetal harm. Women of childbearing age should be advised to use barrier contraceptives while taking this drug. Ivermectin crosses into breast milk; the risk of toxic reactions in the neonate should be considered, and the drug should be used with caution during lactation.

Praziquantel (*Biltricide*) is very effective in the treatment of a wide number of schistosomes or flukes. This drug, which is taken in a series of three doses at 4- to 6-hour intervals, has relatively few adverse effects. The drug is rapidly absorbed from the GI tract and reaches peak plasma levels within 1 to 3 hours. It is metabolized in the liver with a half-life of 0.8 to 1.5 hours. Excretion of praziquantel occurs primarily through the urine. There are no adequate studies regarding the use of this drug during pregnancy, and it should be used cautiously. Praziquantel crosses into breast milk and should not be used during lactation; in addition, the baby should not be nursed for 72 hours after treatment is finished.

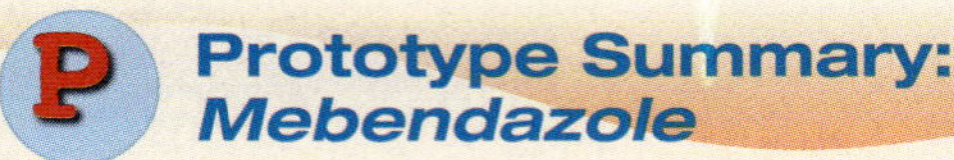

Prototype Summary: Mebendazole

Indications: Treatment of whipworm, pinworm, roundworm, and hookworm infections

Actions: Irreversibly blocks glucose uptake by susceptible helminths, depleting glycogen stores needed for survival and reproduction, causing the death of the helminth

Pharmacokinetics:

Route	Onset	Peak
Oral	Slow	2–4 h

$T_{1/2}$: 2.5–9 hours; metabolized in the liver and excreted in the feces

Adverse effects: Transient abdominal pain, diarrhea, fever

Therapeutic Actions and Indications

Anthelmintic agents are indicated for the treatment of infections by certain susceptible worms and are not interchangeable. Anthelmintics interfere with metabolic processes in particular worms, as noted previously (Figure 13.2).

Contraindications and Cautions

Contraindications to the use of anthelmintic drugs include the presence of known allergy to any of these drugs; lactation *because the drugs can enter breast milk and could be toxic to the infant;* and pregnancy (in most cases) *because of reported associated fetal abnormalities or death.* Caution should be used in the presence of renal or hepatic disease *that interferes with the metabolism or excretion of drugs that are absorbed systemically* and in cases of severe diarrhea and malnourishment, *which could alter the effects of the drug on the intestine and any pre-existing helminths.*

Adverse Effects

Adverse effects frequently encountered with the use of these anthelmintic agents are related to their absorption or direct action in the intestine. Mebendazole and pyrantel are not generally absorbed systemically and may cause abdominal discomfort, diarrhea, or pain. Anthelmintics that are absorbed systemically may cause the following effects: headache and dizziness; fever, shaking, chills, and malaise, associated with an immune reaction to the death of the worms; rash; pruritus; and loss of hair.

Changes in protein synthesis by the liver caused by Stevens–Johnson syndrome is associated with thiabendazole use and can be fatal. Also, renal failure and severe bone marrow depression are associated with albendazole, which is toxic to some human tissues. Patients taking this drug should be monitored carefully.

Clinically Important Drug-Drug Interactions

Combinations of theophylline and thiabendazole may lead to increased theophylline levels, and patients who take both of these drugs may require frequent monitoring and dosage reduction. The effects of albendazole, which are already severe, may increase if the drug is combined with dexamethasone, praziquantel, or cimetidine. These combinations should be avoided if at all possible; if they are necessary, patients should be monitored closely for occurrence of adverse effects.

Nursing Considerations for Patients Receiving Anthelmintics

Assessment: History and Examination

Screen for the following: history of allergy to any of the anthelmintics; hepatic or renal dysfunction *that might interfere with the metabolism and excretion of the drug;* pregnancy, *which is a contraindication to the use of some of these agents because of reported effects on the fetus;* and lactation *because these drugs could enter the breast milk and be toxic to the infant.*

Physical assessment should be performed to *establish baseline data for determining the effectiveness of the drug and the occurrence of any adverse effects associated with drug therapy.* Obtain a culture of stool for ova and parasites *to determine the infecting worm and establish appropriate treatment.* Examine reflexes and muscle strength *to evaluate changes that occur as a result of drug therapy.* Conduct hepatic evaluation, including liver function tests, and also renal function tests *to determine appropriateness of therapy and to monitor for toxicity.* Examine skin (lesions, color, temperature, and texture), *to monitor for adverse effects,* and abdomen, *to evaluate any changes from baseline related to the infection and to monitor for improvement and the possibility of adverse effects.*

Nursing Diagnoses

The patient receiving an anthelmintic drug may have the following nursing diagnoses related to drug therapy:

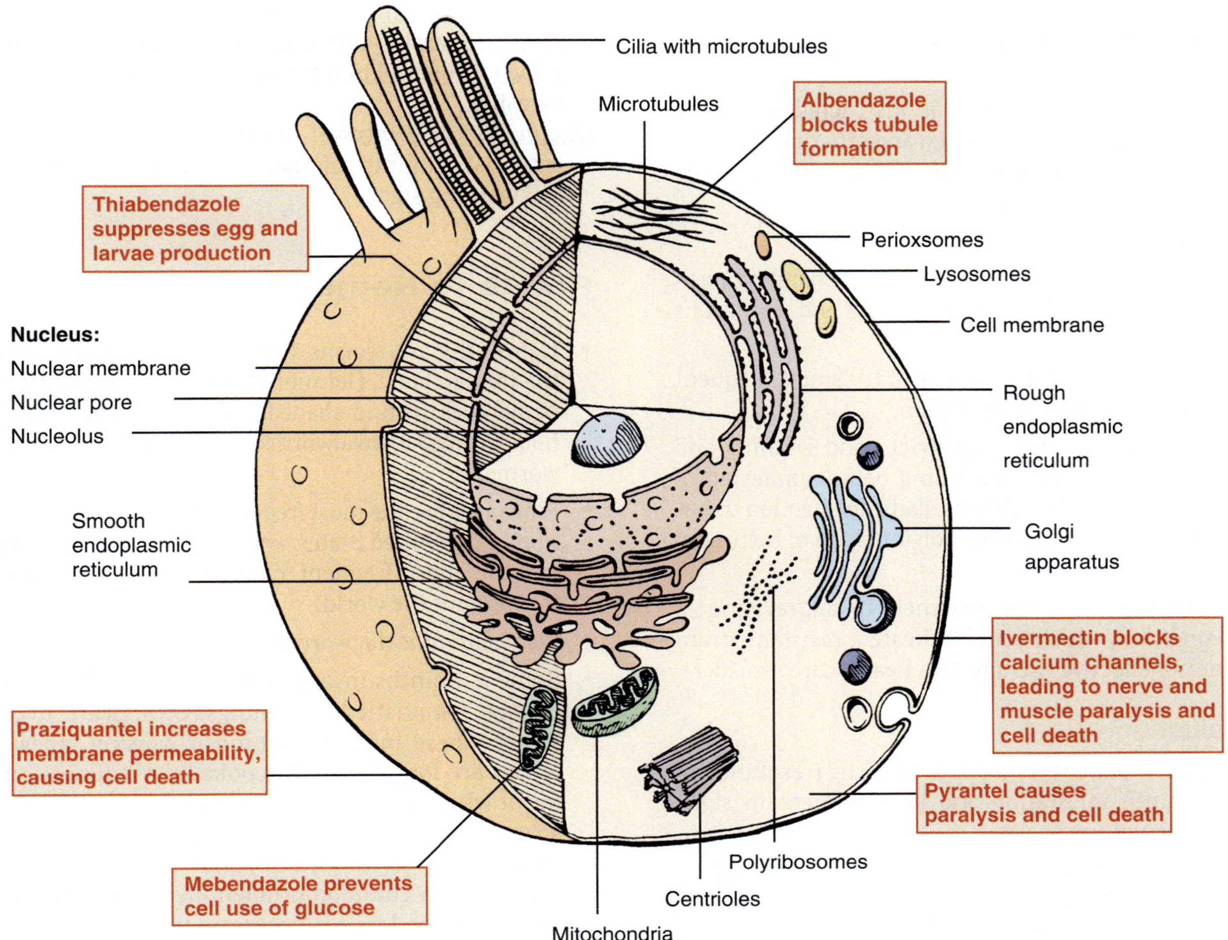

FIGURE 13.2 General structure of a cell, showing the sites of action of the anthelmintic agents. Mebendazole interferes with the ability to use glucose, leading to an inability to reproduce and cell death. Albendazole blocks tubule formation, resulting in cell death. Ivermectin blocks calcium channels, leading to nerve and muscle paralysis and cell death. Pyrantel is a neuromuscular polarizing agent that causes paralysis and cell death. Thiabendazole both suppresses egg and larva production and blocks a helminth-specific enzyme that promotes the development of eggs and larvae. Praziquantel increases membrane permeability, leading to a loss of intracellular calcium and muscular paralysis; it may also result in disintegration of the integument.

- Acute Pain related to GI, CNS, or skin effects of drug
- Disturbed Personal Identity related to diagnosis and treatment
- Deficient Knowledge regarding drug therapy

Implementation With Rationale

- Arrange for appropriate culture and sensitivity tests before beginning therapy *to ensure that the appropriate drug is being used.*
- Administer the complete course of the drug *to obtain the full beneficial effects.* Ensure that chewable tablets are chewed. The drug may be taken with food if necessary, but high-fat meals might interfere with drug effectiveness and should be avoided.
- Monitor hepatic and renal function before and periodically during treatment *to arrange to stop administration of albendazole if signs of failure occur.*
- Provide comfort and safety measures if CNS effects occur (e.g., siderails and assistance with ambulation in the presence of dizziness and weakness) *to protect patient from injury.* Provide oral hygiene and ready access to bathroom facilities as needed *to cope with GI effects.*
- Provide small, frequent, nutritious meals if GI upset is severe *to ensure adequate nutrition.* Monitor nutritional status and arrange a dietary consultation as

needed. Taking the drug with food may also decrease GI upset.

- Ensure that the patient is instructed about the appropriate dosage regimen and other measures *to enhance patient knowledge about drug therapy and to promote compliance.*

The patient should:

- Take safety precautions, including changing position slowly and avoiding driving and hazardous tasks, if CNS effects occur.
- Take the drug with meals and try small, frequent meals if GI upset is a problem.
- Note the importance of strict hand washing and hygiene measures, including daily laundering of underwear and bed linens, daily disinfection of toilet facilities, and periodic disinfection of bathroom floors.
- Report fever, severe diarrhea, or aggravation of condition, which could indicate a resistant strain or noneffective therapy, to a health care provider

Evaluation

- Monitor patient response to the drug (resolution of helminth infestation and improvement in signs and symptoms).
- Monitor for adverse effects (orientation and affect, nutritional state, skin color and lesions, hepatic and renal function, and abdominal discomfort and pain).
- Evaluate the effectiveness of the teaching plan (patient can name the drug, dosage, possible adverse effects to watch for, and specific measures to help avoid adverse effects).
- Monitor the effectiveness of comfort and safety measures and compliance with the regimen.

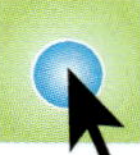

WEB LINKS

Health care providers and patients may want to consult the following Internet sources:

http://www.kidshealth.org/parent/infections/parasitic/pinworm.html Information on preventing and dealing with pinworm infections.

http://www.who.int/wormcontrol/en Information on schistosomiasis—incidence, precautions, treatments.

http://www.cdfound.to.it Information about other intestinal parasites.

http://www.cdc.gov/travel Information for travelers about potential helminth infestations, precautions, treatments, and warning signs.

Points to Remember

- Helminths are worms that cause disease by invading the human body. Helminths that affect humans include nematodes (round-shaped worms) such as pinworms, hookworms, threadworms, whipworms, and roundworms.
- Pinworms are the most frequent cause of helminth infection in the United States, and roundworms called *Ascaris* are the most frequent cause of helminth infections throughout the world.
- Platyhelminths (flatworms) include tapeworms and flukes.
- Some helminths invade body tissues and can seriously damage lymphatic tissue, lungs, CNS, heart, liver, and so on. These include trichinosis-causing tapeworms, which are found in undercooked pork; filariae, which occur when thread-like worm embryos clog up vascular spaces; and schistosomiasis-causing flukes, which can invade the liver, lungs, CNS, and other tissues. Schistosomiasis is a common problem in many tropical areas where the snail that is necessary in the life cycle of the fluke lives.
- Anthelmintic drugs affect metabolic processes that are either different in worms than in human hosts or are not found in humans. These agents all cause death of the worm by interfering with normal functioning.
- Prevention is a very important part of the treatment of helminths. Thorough hand washing; laundering of bed linens, pajamas, and underwear to destroy ova that are shed during the night; and disinfection of toilet facilities at least daily and of bathroom floors periodically help stop the spread of these diseases. In addition, proper sanitation and hygiene in food preparation and storage is essential for reducing the incidence of these infestations.
- Patient teaching is important for decreasing the stress and anxiety that may occur when individuals are diagnosed with a worm infestation.

CHECK YOUR UNDERSTANDING

Answers to the questions in this chapter may be found in the Answer Key in the back of the book.

Multiple Choice

Select the best answer to the following.

1. To ensure effective treatment of pinworm infections, the nurse should teach the patient and family to
   a. keep nails long so cutting will not introduce more infection.
   b. launder undergarments, bed linens, and pajamas every day.
   c. boil all drinking water.
   d. maintain a clear liquid diet for at least 7 to 10 days.

2. *Ascaris* infections are the most prevalent worldwide helminthic infections. If a patient is suspected of having an *Ascaris* infection, assessment of that patient would reveal
   a. cough, fever, and signs of pulmonary infestation.
   b. cardiac arrhythmias.
   c. seizures and disorientation.
   d. bloody diarrhea.

3. Schistosomiasis is an infection caused by
   a. a protozoan carried by a mosquito.
   b. improperly cooked pork.
   c. a fluke carried by a snail.
   d. eating food contaminated by fecal material.

4. A patient has traveled to Egypt and come home with schistosomiasis. The family is very concerned about spreading the disease. Important teaching information that could help the family would include which of the following:
   a. Strict hand washing will stop the spread of the disease.
   b. Isolating the patient will be necessary to stop the spread of the disease.
   c. Carefully cooking all of the patient's food will help to stop the spread of the disease.
   d. The snail that is needed for the life cycle of this worm does not live in this climate, and the disease cannot be spread without the snail.

5. Mebendazole is the most commonly used anthelmintic. It would be a drug of choice for treating
   a. pinworms, roundworms, whipworms, and hookworms.
   b. trichinosis and flukes.
   c. pork tapeworm and threadworms.
   d. all stages of schistosomal infections.

6. Patient teaching regarding the use of anthelmintics should include counseling about
   a. the use of oral contraceptives.
   b. the importance of maintaining nutrition during therapy.
   c. the use of oral anticoagulants.
   d. cardiac drug effects

7. Patients may experience anxiety about the diagnosis and treatment of helminthic infections. Teaching may help to alleviate this anxiety and should include
   a. what they may experience if the worms are passed from the body.
   b. focus on the cleanliness of the home
   c. measures to isolate the organism in the home
   d. criticism of their personal hygiene practices.

Multiple Response

Select all that apply.

1. An adult client is being treated with mebendazole for a pinworm infection. Appropriate nursing diagnoses that might apply to this patient would include
   a. Disturbed Personal Identity related to treatment.
   b. Abdominal distention related to worm infestation.
   c. Acute Pain related to GI effects.
   d. Risk for Social Isolation related to quarantine conditions.
   e. Impaired Physical Mobility related to muscle infestation.
   f. Deficient Knowledge related to drug therapy.

Definitions

Define the following terms.

1. cestode ______________________________

____

____

2. nematode ______________________________

____

____

3. pinworm ______________________________

____

____

4. roundworm ______________________________

____

____

5. schistosomiasis ______________________________

____

____

6. trichinosis ______________________________

____

____

7. threadworm ______________________________

____

____

8. whipworm ______________________________

____

____

Learning Activity

Prepare a patient teaching checklist for an individual who has been diagnosed with pinworms and has been prescribed mebendazole. The patient will be at home during treatment of this disease.

Bibliography and References

Andrews, M., & Boyle, J. (2002). *Transcultural concepts in nursing care.* Philadelphia: Lippincott Williams & Wilkins.

Drug facts and comparisons. (2006). St. Louis: Facts and Comparisons.

Gilman, A., Hardman, J. G., & Limbird, L. E. (Eds.). (2006). *Goodman and Gilman's the pharmacological basis of therapeutics* (11th ed.). New York: McGraw-Hill.

Karch, A. M. (2006). *2007 Lippincott's nursing drug guide.* Philadelphia: Lippincott Williams & Wilkins.

Professional's guide to patient drug facts. (2006). St. Louis: Facts and Comparisons.

CHAPTER 14

Antineoplastic Agents

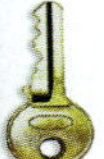

KEY TERMS

alopecia
anaplasia
angiogenesis
antineoplastic drug
autonomy
bone marrow suppression
carcinoma
metastasis
neoplasm
sarcoma

LEARNING OBJECTIVES

Upon completion of this chapter, you will be able to:

1. Describe the nature of cancer and the changes the body undergoes when cancer occurs.
2. Describe the therapeutic actions, indications, pharmacokinetics, contraindications, most common adverse reactions, and important drug–drug interactions associated with each class of antineoplastic agents: alkylating agents, antimetabolites, antineoplastic antibiotics, mitotic inhibitors, hormones and hormone modulators, cancer cell–specific agents, and miscellaneous agents.
3. Discuss the use of antineoplastic drugs across the lifespan.
4. Compare and contrast the prototype drugs for each class of antineoplastic agents with the other drugs in that class.
5. Outline the nursing considerations and teaching needs for patients receiving each class of antineoplastic agents.

ALKYLATING AGENTS

busulfan
carboplatin
carmustine
P chlorambucil
cisplatin
cyclophosphamide
ifosfamide
lomustine
mechlorethamine
melphalan
oxaliplatin
streptozocin
thiotepa

ANTIMETABOLITES

capecitabine
cladribine
clofarabine
cytarabine
floxuridine
fludarabine
fluorouracil
mercaptopurine
P methotrexate
pemetrexed
pentostatin
thioguanine

ANTINEOPLASTIC ANTIBIOTICS

bleomycin
dactinomycin
daunorubicin
P doxorubicin
epirubicin
idarubicin
mitomycin
mitoxantrone
valrubicin

MITOTIC INHIBITORS

docetaxel
etoposide
paclitaxel
teniposide
vinblastine
P vincristine
vinorelbine

HORMONES AND HORMONE MODULATORS

anastrazole
bicalutamide
estramustine
exemestane
flutamide
fulvestrant
goserelin
histrelin
letrozole

leuprolide
megestrol
nilutamide
P tamoxifen
testolactone
toremifene
triptorelin pamoate

CANCER CELL–SPECIFIC AGENTS

bortezomib
erlotinib
gefitinib
imatinib

MISCELLANEOUS ANTINEOPLASTIC AGENTS

altretamine
arsenic trioxide
asparaginase
bortezomib
dacarbazine
gemcitabine
hydroxyurea
irinotecan
mitotane
pegaspargase
porfimer
procarbazine
talc powder
temozolomide
topotecan
tretinoin

ANTINEOPLASTIC ADJUNCTIVE THERAPY

amifostine
dexrazoxane
leucovorin
mesna
rasburicase

One branch of chemotherapy involves drugs developed to act on and kill or alter human cells—the **antineoplastic drugs**, which are designed to fight **neoplasms**, or cancers. When chemotherapy is mentioned, most people think of cancer treatment. Antineoplastic drugs alter human cells in a variety of ways, and they are intended to have a greater impact on the abnormal cells that make up the neoplasm or cancer than on normal cells. This area of pharmacology, which has grown tremendously in recent years, now includes many drugs that act on or are part of the immune system; these substances fight the cancerous cells using components of the immune system instead of destroying cells directly (see Chapter 15). This chapter discusses the classic antineoplastic approach and those drugs that are used in cancer chemotherapy.

Neoplasms

Cancer is a disease that can strike a person at any age. It remains second only to coronary disease as the leading cause of death in the United States. Treatment of cancer can be a long and debilitating experience that leads to many disabilities in adults.

All cancers start with a single cell that is genetically different from the other cells in the surrounding tissue. This cell divides, passing along its abnormalities to daughter cells, eventually producing a tumor or neoplasm that has characteristics quite different from the original tissue (Figure 14.1). The cancerous cells exhibit **anaplasia**, a loss of cellular differentiation and organization, which leads to a loss of their ability to function normally. They also exhibit **autonomy**, growing without the usual homeostatic restrictions that regulate cell growth and control, which allows the cells to form a tumor.

Over time, these neoplastic cells grow uncontrollably, invading and damaging healthy tissue in the area and even undergoing **metastasis**, or traveling from the place of origin to develop new tumors in other areas of the body where conditions are favorable for cell growth (Figure 14.2). The abnormal cells release enzymes that generate blood vessels (**angiogenesis**) in the area to supply both oxygen and nutrients to the cells, thus contributing to their growth. Overall, the cancerous cells rob the host cells of energy and nutrients and block normal lymph and vascular vessels as the result of pressure and intrusion on normal cells, leading to a loss of normal cellular function.

The body's immune system can damage or destroy some neoplastic cells. T cells, which recognize the abnormal cells and destroy them; antibodies, which form in response to parts of the abnormal cell protein; interferons; and tissue necrosis factor (TNF) all play a role in the body's attempt to eliminate the abnormal cells before they become uncontrollable and threaten the life of the host. Once the neoplasm has grown and enlarged, it may overwhelm the immune system, which is no longer able to manage the problem.

Causes of Cancer

What causes the cells to mutate and become genetically different is not clearly understood. In some cases, a genetic predisposition to such a mutation can be found. Breast cancer, for example, seems to have a definite genetic link. In other cases, viral infection, constant irritation and cell turnover, and even stress have been blamed for the ensuing cancer. Stress reactions suppress the activities of the immune system (see Chapter 29), so if a cell is mutating while a person is under prolonged stress, research indicates that the cell has a better chance of growing into a neoplasm than when the person's immune system is fully active. Pipe smokers are at increased risk for development of tongue and mouth cancers because the heat and chemicals in the pipe are constantly destroying normal cells, which must be replaced rapidly, increasing the chances for development of a mutant cell. People living in areas with carcinogenic or cancer-causing

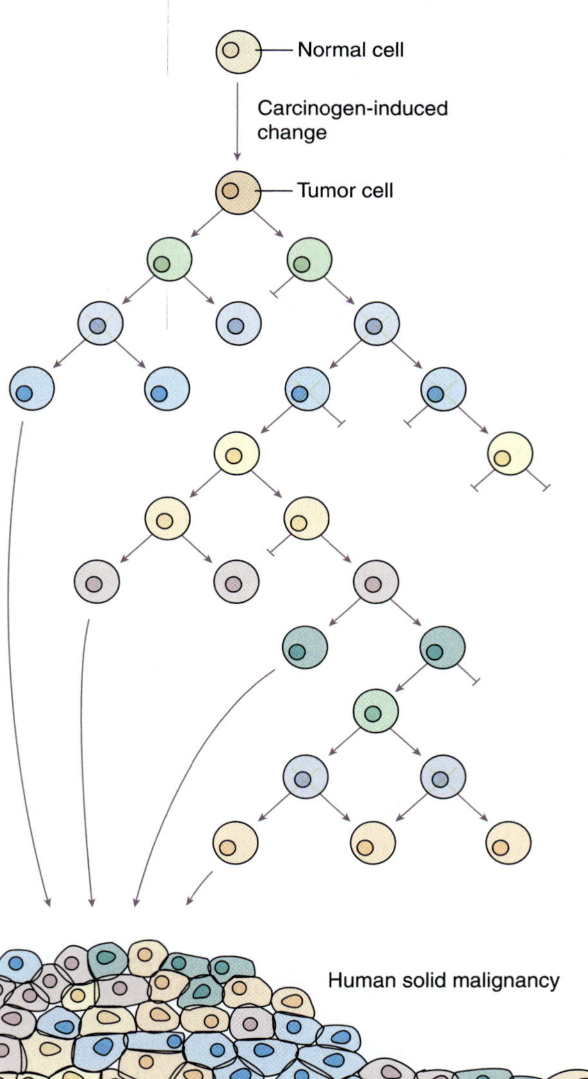

FIGURE 14.1 Tumor development from one cell, with somatic mutations occurring during cell division as the tumor grows.

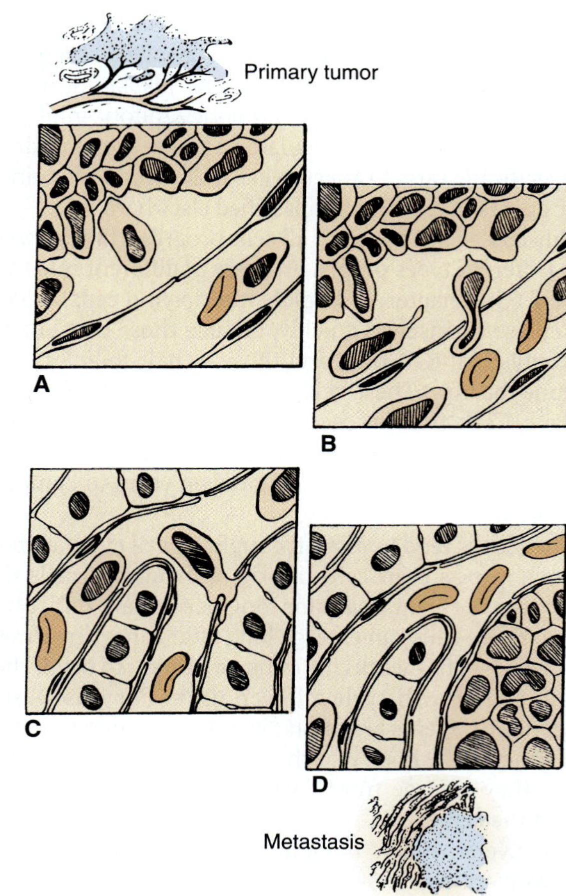

FIGURE 14.2 Metastasis of cancer cells. **(A)** Primary tumor grows and invades the surrounding tissues. **(B)** Tumor cells move into the endothelium and basement membrane of the surrounding capillary. **(C)** Shed tumor cells in lungs, brain, or liver become trapped and penetrate the capillary wall to establish themselves in this new environment. **(D)** Cancer cells proliferate at the new site, which requires a conducive environment with blood supply and nutrition.

chemicals in the air, water, or even the ground are at increased risk of developing mutant cells as a reaction to these toxic chemicals. Cancer clusters are often identified in such high-risk areas. Most likely, a mosaic of factors coming together in one person lead to development of the neoplasm.

Types of Cancer

Cancers can be divided into two groups: (1) solid tumors, and (2) hematological malignancies such as the leukemias and lymphomas, which occur in the blood-forming organs. Solid tumors may originate in any body organ and may be further divided into **carcinomas**, or tumors that originate in epithelial cells, and **sarcomas**, or tumors that originate in the mesenchyma and are made up of embryonic connective tissue cells. Examples of carcinomas include granular cell tumors of the breast, bronchogenic tumors arising in cells lining the bronchial tubes, and squamous and basal tumors of the skin. Sarcomas include osteogenic tumors, which form in the primitive cells of the bone, and rhabdomyosarcomas, which occur in striated muscles.

Antineoplastic Drugs

Antineoplastic drugs can work by affecting cell survival or by boosting the immune system in its efforts to combat the abnormal cells. Chapter 17 discusses the immune agents that are used to combat cancer. This chapter focuses on those drugs that affect cell survival. The antineoplastic drugs that are commonly used today include the alkylating agents, antimetabolites, antineoplastic antibiotics, mitotic inhibitors, hormones and hormone modulators, a new group of drugs that specifically target cancer cells, and a group of antineoplastic agents that cannot be classified elsewhere.

As discussed in Chapter 7, all cells progress through a cell cycle. Different types of cells progress at different rates (see Figure 7.6 in Chapter 7). Rapidly multiplying cells, or cells that replace themselves quickly, include those that line the gastrointestinal (GI) tract and those in hair follicles, skin, and bone marrow. These cells complete the cell cycle every few days. Cells that proceed very slowly through the cell cycle include those in the breasts, testicles, and ovaries. Some cells take weeks, months, or even years to complete the cycle.

Cancer cells tend to move through the cell cycle at about the same rate as their cells of origin; malignant cells that remain in a dormant phase for long periods are difficult to destroy. These cells can emerge long after cancer treatment has finished—after weeks, months, or years—to begin their division and growth cycle all over again. For this reason, antineoplastic agents are often given in sequence over periods of time, in the hope that the drugs will affect the cancer cells as they emerge from dormancy or move into a new phase of the cell cycle.

The adverse effects of cancer chemotherapy are often unpleasant and debilitating, and it is essential that patients understand the importance of returning every few weeks to go through the chemotherapy, with its adverse effects, over and over again.

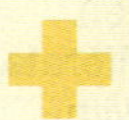

FOCUS ON PATIENT SAFETY

Because some adverse effects of therapy are so unpleasant, some patients try alternative and herbal therapies. For the patient's safety in such situations, the nurse should be prepared to alert the patient to advantages and disadvantages of these therapies (see Box 14.1)

Most cancer patients are not considered to be "cured" until they have been cancer-free for a period of 5 years because of the possibility of cancer cells emerging from dormancy and causing new tumors or problems. No cells have yet been identified that can remain dormant for longer than 5 years, so the chances of the emergence of one after that time are very slim. The goal of cancer therapy, much like that of anti-infective therapy, is to limit the offending cells enough so that the immune system can take care of them without causing too much toxicity to the host. However, this is a particularly difficult task when using antineoplastic drugs, because these agents are not specific to mutant cells; they also affect normal human cells. In most cases, antineoplastic drugs primarily affect rapidly multiplying human cells, which have many cells in many phases of the cell cycle (e.g., those in the hair follicles, GI tract, and bone marrow). Much research is being done to develop drugs that will affect the function of only the abnormal cells. Imatinib, released in 2001, is a drug that affects an enzyme used by very specific abnormal cells. Three other agents have been marketed that affect only mechanisms of cancer cells. It is anticipated that many more such drugs will be released in the near future.

BOX 14.1 CULTURAL CONSIDERATIONS FOR DRUG THERAPY

Alternative Therapies and Cancer

The diagnosis of cancer and the sometimes devastating effects of cancer treatment often drive patients to seek out alternative therapies, either as adjuncts to traditional cancer therapy or sometimes instead of traditional therapy. Because Asian-Americans and Pacific Islanders often see drug therapy and other cancer therapies as part of the yin/yang belief system, they may turn to a variety of herbal therapies to balance their systems.

The nurse should be aware of some potential interactions that may occur when alternative therapies are used:

- *Echinacea*—may be hepatotoxic; increases the risk of hepatotoxicity when taken with antineoplastics that are hepatotoxic
- *Ginkgo*—inhibits blood clotting, which can cause problems after surgery or with bleeding neoplasms
- *Saw palmetto*—may increase the effects of various estrogen hormones and hormone modulators; advise patients taking such drugs to avoid this herb
- *St. John's wort*—can greatly increase photosensitivity, which can cause problems with patients who have received radiation therapy or are taking drugs that cause other dermatological effects; has been shown to interfere with the effectiveness of some antineoplastic agents

If a patient has an unexpected reaction to a drug being used, ask about whether they are using alternative therapies. Many of these agents are untested, and interactions and adverse effects are not well documented.

Some antineoplastic drugs influence fertility as a result of toxic effects on ova and sperm production. In addition, these agents are usually selective for rapidly growing cells, so they are dangerous during pregnancy. Because of the possible occurrence of serious fetal effects, pregnancy is a contraindication to the use of antineoplastic drugs.

Cancer treatment is aimed at destroying cancer cells through several methods, including surgery to remove them, stimulation of the immune system to destroy them, radiation therapy to destroy them, and drug therapy to kill them during various phases of the cell cycle. To do this effectively, and without too much damage to the host, combination therapy is often most successful. Surgery followed by radiation, chemotherapy, or both is very effective with some cancers. A collection of chemotherapeutic agents that work at different phases of the cell cycle is frequently most effective in treating many cancers.

Many antineoplastic drugs often cause another adverse effect, cancer itself, because they cause cell death, leading to the need for cell growth and the increased risk of mutant cell development. In addition, they jeopardize the immune system by causing **bone marrow suppression**, inhibiting the blood-forming components of the bone marrow and interfering with the body's normal protective actions against abnormal cells. Other specific adverse effects may occur with particular drugs. The patient's hematological profile must always be assessed for toxic effects.

A cancerous mass may be so large that no therapy can arrest its growth without killing the host. In such cases, cancer chemotherapeutic agents are used as palliative therapy to shrink the size of the tumor and alleviate some of the signs and symptoms of the cancer, decreasing pain and increasing function. Here the goal of drug therapy is not to cure the disease but to try to improve the patient's quality of life in a situation in which there is no cure. The effect of the antineoplastic agents on people of different ages is discussed in Box 14.2. Some emerging antineoplastic agents are discussed in Box 14.3.

BOX 14.3 FOCUS ON THE **EVIDENCE**

New Drugs for the Battle Against Cancer

Arsenic trioxide *(Trisenox),* known as a poison in forensic medicine, has been approved for the induction and remission of promyelocytic leukemia (PML) in patients whose disease is refractory to conventional therapy and whose leukemia is characterized by t(15:17) translocation of PML/RAR-alpha gene expression. It is given intravenously at a rate of 0.15 mg/kg/day until bone marrow remission occurs and then 0.15 mg/kg/day starting 3 to 6 wk after induction. The patient needs to be screened carefully for toxic reactions.

Other drugs are under development that target specific areas of the human genome. In the future, antineoplastic drugs may be able to target abnormal cells and not affect the healthy cells. This could relieve the suffering of many patients undergoing cancer chemotherapy.

Several familiar drugs are being studied for their ability to block angiogenesis. By blocking the development of new blood vessels to feed the tumor, the growing cells in the tumor will lack nutrition and oxygen and will not be able to survive. Celecoxib (*Celebrex*), an anti-inflammatory drug, is being studied in various cancer combination drug trials for this effect. Some low-molecular-weight heparins, such as dalteparin (*Fragmin*), are also being studied for this effect.

BOX 14.2 **DRUG THERAPY ACROSS THE LIFESPAN**

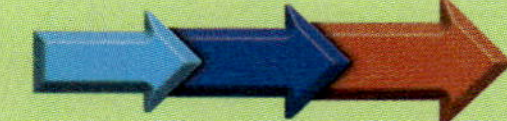

Antineoplastic Agents

CHILDREN

Antineoplastic protocols have been developed for the treatment of most pediatric cancers. Combination therapy is stressed to eliminate as many of the mutant cells as possible. Dosage and timing of these combinations is crucial.

Double checking of dosage, including recalculating desired dose and verifying the drug amount with another nurse, is good practice when giving these toxic drugs to children.

Children need to be monitored closely for hydration and nutritional status. The nutritional needs of a child are greater than those of an adult, and this needs to be considered when formulating a care plan.

Children need support and comfort and also need to be allowed to explore and learn like any other children. Body image problems, lack of energy and the need to protect the child from exposure to infection can isolate a child receiving antineoplastic agents. The total care plan of the child needs to include social, emotional, and intellectual stimulation.

Monitor bone marrow activity very carefully, and adjust the dosage accordingly.

ADULTS

The adult receiving antineoplastic drugs is confronted with many dilemmas that the nurse needs to address. Changes in body image are common with loss of hair, skin changes, gastrointestinal complaints, and weight loss. Fear of the diagnosis and the treatment is also common with these patients. Networking support systems and providing teaching, reassurance, and comfort can have a tremendous impact on the success of the drug therapy.

Pregnant and nursing women should not receive these drugs, which are toxic to the developing cells of the fetus. Pregnant women who are diagnosed with cancer are in a difficult situation: the drug therapy can have serious adverse effects on the fetus, and not using the drug therapy can be detrimental to the mother. Education, support, and referrals to appropriate specialists are important. Nursing women should find another method of feeding the baby, to prevent the adverse effects to the fetus that occur when these drugs cross into breast milk. Use of barrier contraceptives is urged when these drugs are being used by women of childbearing age.

OLDER ADULTS

Older adults may be more susceptible to the CNS and gastrointestinal effects of some of these drugs. Older patients should be monitored for hydration and nutritional status regularly. Safety precautions should be instituted if CNS effects occur, including increased lighting, assistance with ambulation, and use of supports.

Many older patients have decreased renal and/or hepatic function. Many of these drugs depend on the liver and kidney for metabolism and excretion. Renal and liver function tests should be done before (baseline) and periodically during the use of these drugs, and dosage should be adjusted accordingly.

Protecting these patients from exposure to infection and injury is a very important aspect of their nursing care. Older patients are naturally somewhat immunosuppressed because of age, and giving drugs that further depress the immune system can lead to infections that are serious and difficult to treat. Monitor blood counts carefully, and arrange for rest or reduced dosage as indicated.

Alkylating Agents

Alkylating agents produce their cytotoxic effects by reacting chemically with portions of the RNA, DNA, or other cellular proteins, and they are most potent when they bind with cellular DNA. The oldest drugs in this class are the nitrogen mustards, and modifications of the structure of these drugs have led to the development of the nitrosoureas. Because alkylating agents can affect cells even in the resting phase, these drugs are said to be non–cell cycle-specific (Figure 14.3). They are most useful in the treatment of slow-growing cancers, which have many cells in the resting phase.

Therapeutic Actions and Indications

The alkylating agents work by disrupting cellular mechanisms that affect DNA, causing cell death. They are effective against various lymphomas; leukemias; myelomas; some ovarian, testicular, and breast cancers; and some pancreatic cancers. Table 14.1 lists the various alkylating agents, their indications and dosages, and specific information about each drug. These agents are not used interchangeably.

Pharmacokinetics

The alkylating agents vary in their degree of absorption, and little is known about their distribution in the tissues. They are metabolized and sometimes activated in the liver, with many of these agents using the cytochrome P450 systems, and they are excreted in the urine, so caution must be used in patients with hepatic or renal dysfunction. Their use during pregnancy and lactation is contraindicated because of the potential harm to the neonate.

Contraindications and Cautions

Caution should be used when giving alkylating agents to any individual with a known allergy to any of the alkylating agents; during pregnancy or lactation, *when these drugs are contraindicated because of potential severe effects on the neonate;* with bone marrow suppression, *which is often the index for redosing and dosing levels;* or with suppressed renal or hepatic function, *which may interfere with metabolism or excretion of these drugs and often indicates a need to change the dosage.*

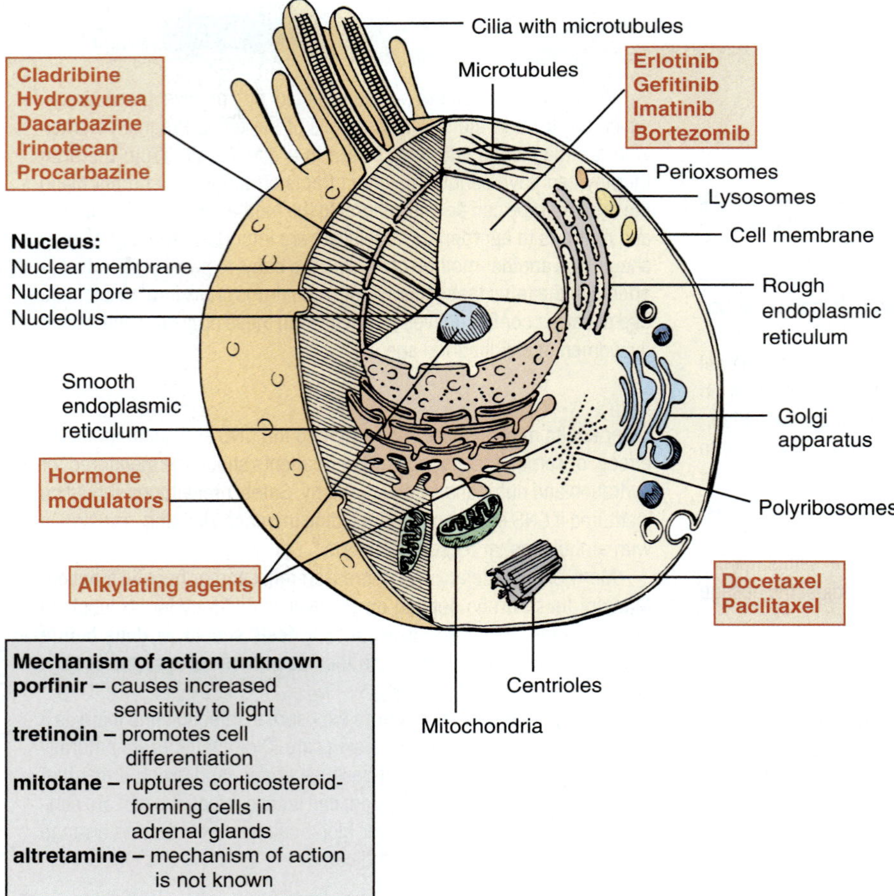

FIGURE 14.3 Sites of action of non–cell cycle-specific antineoplastic agents. Hormone modulators react with specific receptor sites to block cell growth and activity. Docetaxel and paclitaxel inhibit microtubular reorganization. Cladribine and hydroxyurea block DNA synthesis; dacarbazine blocks DNA and RNA synthesis; irinotecan disrupts DNA strands; procarbazine inhibits DNA, RNA, and protein synthesis; gefitinib, erlotinib, and imatinib inhibit protein tyrosine kinase; bortezomib is an aromase inhibitor.

Table 14.1 DRUGS IN FOCUS

Alkylating Agents

Drug Name	Dosage/Route	Usual Indications
busulfan (*Busulfex, Myleran*)	Induction: 4–8 mg/day PO Maintenance: 1–3 mg/day PO Injection: 0.8 mg/kg as a 2-h IV infusion q6h for 4 d via a central venous catheter	Treatment of chronic myelogenous leukemia; not effective in blastic phase or without the Philadelphia chromosome **Special considerations:** Dosing monitored by effects on bone marrow; always push fluids to decrease toxic renal effects; alopecia is common
carboplatin (*Paraplatin*)	360 mg/m² IV on day 1 every 4 wk; reduce dosage as needed based on blood counts and with renal impairment	Palliative treatment of returning ovarian cancer after prior chemotherapy; initial treatment of ovarian cancer with other chemotherapy; may be useful in several other cancers **Special considerations:** Dosage and timing determined by bone marrow response; alopecia is common
carmustine (*BiCNU, Gliadel*)	150–200 mg/m² IV every 6 wk as a single dose or divided daily injections; wafers implanted into brain at time of surgery	Treatment of brain tumors, Hodgkin's disease, and multiple myelomas; available in implantable wafer form for treatment of glioblastoma **Special considerations:** Dosage determined by bone marrow toxicity; usually not repeated for 6 wk; often used in combination therapy
P chlorambucil (*Leukeran*)	0.1–0.2 mg/kg/day PO for 3–6 wk; or 0.4 mg/kg PO every 2 wk with maintenance dose of 0.03–0.1 mg/kg/day PO	Treatment of lymphomas and leukemias including Hodgkin's disease; being considered for the treatment of rheumatoid arthritis and other conditions **Special considerations:** Toxic to liver and bone marrow; dosing based on bone marrow response
cisplatin (*Platinol-AQ*)	20–50 mg/m²/day IV, once every 3 wk used in combination with other antineoplastic agents	Combination therapy for metastatic testicular or ovarian tumors, advanced bladder cancers **Special considerations:** Neurotoxic, nephrotoxic, and can cause serious hypersensitivity reactions
cyclophosphamide (*Cytoxan, Neosar*)	Induction: 40–50 mg/kg/day IV over 2–5 days, or 1–5 mg/kg/day PO Maintenance: 1–5 mg/kg/day PO, or 10–15 mg/kg IV q7–10 days	Treatment of lymphoma, myelomas, leukemias, and other cancers in combination with other drugs **Special considerations:** Hemorrhagic cystitis is a potentially fatal side effect; alopecia is common
ifosfamide (*Ifex*)	1.2 g/m²/day IV for 5 consecutive days; repeat every 3 wk	Combination therapy as a third-line agent in treating germ cell testicular cancers; being tested for treatment of other cancers **Special considerations:** Alopecia is common
lomustine (*CeeNU*)	130 mg/m² PO as a single dose every 6 wk; adjust dosage based on blood counts	Palliative combination therapy for Hodgkin's disease and primary and metastatic brain tumors **Special considerations:** Immune suppression and gastrointestinal effects are common
mechlorethamine (*Mustargen*)	0.4 mg/kg IV for each course; usually repeated every 3–6 wk	Nitrogen mustard; palliative treatment in Hodgkin's disease, leukemia, bronchial carcinoma, other cancers; injected for treatment of effusions secondary to cancer metastases **Special considerations:** Gastrointestinal toxicity, bone marrow suppression, and impaired fertility are common
melphalan (*Alkeran*)	*Multiple myeloma:* 6 mg/day PO for 2–3 wk, then a rest period, *or* 16 mg/m² IV at 2-wk intervals for four doses, then at 4-wk intervals *Ovarian cancer:* 0.2 mg/kg/day PO for 5 days; repeat course every 4–5 wk	Nitrogen mustard; palliative treatment for multiple myeloma, ovarian cancers **Special considerations:** Oral route is preferred; pulmonary fibrosis, bone marrow suppression, and alopecia are common
oxaliplatin (*Eloxatin*)	85 mg/m² IV with leucovorin, followed by 5-FU, at 2-wk cycles, *or* 1000 mg/m² IV at weekly intervals	Treatment of metastatic carcinoma of the colon or rectum when disease progresses after standard therapy **Special considerations:** Premedicate with antiemetics and dexamethasone; monitor for potentially dangerous anaphylactic reactions
streptozocin (*Zanosar*)	500 mg/m² IV for 5 consecutive days, usually given every week, *or* 1000 mg/m³ IV at weekly intervals	Treatment of metastatic islet cell carcinoma of the pancreas **Special considerations:** Gastrointestinal and renal toxicity are common; causes infertility; wear rubber gloves to avoid drug contact with the skin—if contact occurs, wash with soap and water
thiotepa (*Thioplex*)	0.3–0.4 mg/kg IV at 1–4-wk intervals	Treatment of adenocarcinoma of the breast and uterus and papillary carcinoma of the bladder; available intrathecally to treat effusion **Special considerations:** Infertility, rash, gastrointestinal toxicity, dizziness, headache, and bone marrow suppression are common

Adverse Effects

Adverse effects frequently encountered with the use of these alkylating agents are listed here; see Table 14.1 for a list of the most common adverse effects specific to each agent. Amifostine (*Ethyol*) and mesna (*Mesnex*) are cytoprotective (cell-protecting) drugs that may be given to limit certain effects of cisplatin and ifosfamide, respectively (Box 14.4).

Hematological effects include bone marrow suppression, with leukopenia, thrombocytopenia, anemia, and pancytopenia, secondary to the effects of the drugs on the rapidly multiplying cells of the bone marrow. GI effects include nausea, vomiting, anorexia, diarrhea, and mucous membrane deterioration, all of which are related to the drugs' effects on the rapidly multiplying cells of the GI tract. Hepatic toxicity and renal toxicity may occur, depending on the exact mechanism of action. **Alopecia**, or hair loss, related to effects on the hair follicles, may also occur. All drugs that cause cell death can cause a potentially toxic increase in uric acid levels. In 2004, a new drug was introduced to manage uric acid levels in pediatric patients (Box 14.5).

Clinically Important Drug–Drug Interactions

Alkylating agents that are known to cause hepatic or renal toxicity should be used cautiously with any other drugs that have similar effects. In addition, drugs that are toxic to the liver may adversely affect drugs that are metabolized in the liver or that act in the liver (e.g., oral anticoagulants). Specific drug–drug interactions for each agent should be checked in your nursing drug guide.

BOX 14.4 Drugs That Protect Cells from Alkylating Agents

Amifostine *(Ethyol)* is a cytoprotective (cell-protecting) drug that preserves healthy cells from the toxic effects of cisplatin. It is thought to react to the specific acidity and vascularity of nontumor cells to protect them, and it may also act as a scavenger of free radicals released by cells that have been exposed to cisplatin. Amifostine is given at a dose of 910 mg/m^2 q.i.d. as a 15-min IV infusion starting within 30 min after starting cisplatin therapy; timing is very important to its effectiveness. Now approved for use to prevent the renal toxicity associated with the use of cisplatin in patients with advanced ovarian cancer, amifostine is under investigation as an agent to protect lung fibroblasts from the effects of paclitaxel. Because amifostine is associated with severe nausea and vomiting, concurrent administration of an antiemetic is recommended. It also can cause hypotension, and patients should be monitored closely for this condition.

Mesna *(Mesnex)* is a cytoprotective agent that is used to reduce the incidence of hemorrhagic cystitis caused by ifosfamide or cyclophosphamide. Mesna, which is known to react chemically with urotoxic metabolites of ifosfamide, is given intravenously at the time of the ifosfamide injection at a dose that is 20% of the ifosfamide dose, and is repeated 4 h and 8 h afterward. Because mesna has been associated with nausea and vomiting, an antiemetic may be useful.

BOX 14.5 Drug to Manage Rising Uric Acid Levels Associated With Tumor Lysis

Rasburicase (*Elitek*) was approved in 2004 for the management of plasma uric acid levels in pediatric patients with leukemia, lymphoma, and solid tumor malignancies who are receiving antineoplastic therapy associated with tumor lysis and subsequent elevated serum uric acid levels. It is administered as a single daily IV infusion of 0.15–0.2 mg/kg over 30 min for 5 days. Chemotherapy should be started 4–24 h after the first dose of rasburicase. Uric acid levels should be monitored frequently, using prechilled, heparinized vials that are kept in an ice-water bath. This analysis should be done within 4 h of each rasburicase dose.

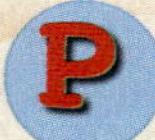

Prototype Summary: Chlorambucil

Indications: Palliative treatment of chronic lymphocytic leukemia, malignant lymphomas, and Hodgkin's disease

Actions: Alkylates cellular DNA, interfering with the replication of susceptible cells

Pharmacokinetics:

Route	Onset	Peak	Duration
Oral	Varies	1 h	15–20 h

$T_{1/2}$: 60–90 min, metabolized in the liver and excreted in the urine

Adverse effects: Tremors, muscle twitching, confusion, nausea, hepatotoxicity, bone marrow suppression, sterility, cancer

Nursing Considerations for Patients Receiving Alkylating Agents

Assessment: History and Examination

Screen for the following, *which will alert you to specific cautions or contraindications to the use of the drug:*

- History of allergy to any of the alkylating agents
- Bone marrow suppression
- Renal or hepatic dysfunction
- Pregnancy or lactation

Physical assessment should be performed *to establish baseline data for determining the effective-*

ness of the drug and the occurrence of any adverse effects associated with drug therapy. Include screening for orientation and reflexes *to evaluate any central nervous system (CNS) effects;* respiratory rate and adventitious sounds *to monitor the disease* and *to evaluate for respiratory or hypersensitivity effects;* pulse, rhythm, and auscultation *to monitor for systemic or cardiovascular effects;* and bowel sounds and mucous membrane status *to monitor for GI effects.* Evaluate the complete blood count (CBC) with differential and renal and liver function tests *to monitor for dosage adjustment as needed* and *to evaluate toxic drug effects.*

See Critical Thinking Scenario 14-1 for a full discussion of assessing and evaluating antineoplastic therapy with breast cancer.

Nursing Diagnoses

The patient receiving an alkylating agent may have the following nursing diagnoses related to drug therapy:

- Acute Pain related to GI, CNS, skin effects of drug
- Disturbed Body Image related to alopecia, skin effects, impaired fertility
- Fear, Anxiety related to diagnosis and treatment
- Deficient Knowledge regarding drug therapy

Implementation With Rationale

- Arrange for blood tests before, periodically during, and for at least 3 weeks after therapy *to monitor bone marrow function.* Discontinue the drug or reduce the dose as needed.
- Administer medication according to scheduled protocol and in combination with other drugs as indicated *to improve effectiveness.*
- Ensure that the patient is well hydrated *to decrease risk of renal toxicity.*
- Protect the patient from exposure to infection; limit invasive procedures *when bone marrow suppression limits the patient's immune/inflammatory responses.*
- Provide small, frequent meals, frequent mouth care, and dietary consultation as appropriate *to maintain nutrition when GI effects are severe.* Antiemetics may be helpful in some cases. (See Box 14.6.)
- Arrange for proper head covering at extremes of temperature if alopecia occurs; a wig, scarf, or hat *is important for maintaining body temperature.* If alopecia is an anticipated effect of drug therapy, advise the patient to obtain a wig or head covering before the condition occurs *to promote self-esteem and a positive body image.*
- Provide patient teaching *to enhance patient knowledge about drug therapy and to promote compliance regarding:*
  - The appropriate dosage regimen, including dates to return for further doses.
  - The importance of covering the head at extremes of temperature.
  - The need to try to maintain nutrition if GI effects are severe.
  - The need to avoid exposure to infection.
  - The need to plan appropriate rest periods, because fatigue and weakness are common effects of the drugs.
  - The possibility of impaired fertility; the patient may wish to consult a health care provider.
  - The importance of not taking the drugs during pregnancy and of using barrier contraceptives.

Evaluation

- Monitor patient response to the drug (alleviation of cancer being treated, palliation of signs and symptoms of cancer).
- Monitor for adverse effects (bone marrow suppression, GI toxicity, neurotoxicity, alopecia, renal or hepatic dysfunction).
- Evaluate the effectiveness of the teaching plan (patient can name the drug, dosage, possible adverse effects to watch for, and specific measures to help avoid adverse effects).

FOCUS POINTS

- Cancers arise from a single abnormal cell that multiplies and grows.
- Cancer cells lose their normal function (anaplasia), develop characteristics that allow them to grow in an uninhibited way (autonomy), and have the ability to travel to other sites in the body that are conducive to their growth (metastasis). They also have the ability to grow new blood vessels to feed the tumor (angiogenesis).
- The goal of cancer chemotherapy is to decrease the size of the neoplasm so that the human immune system can deal with it.
- Alkylating agents affect cellular RNA or DNA, are cell cycle nonspecific, and are most effective against slow-growing tumors.

CRITICAL THINKING SCENARIO 14-1

Antineoplastic Therapy and Breast Cancer

THE SITUATION

A 34-year-old white woman, B.P., is a school teacher with two young daughters. She noticed a slightly painful lump under her arm when showering. About 2 weeks later, she found a mass in her right breast. Initial patient assessment found that she had no other underlying medical problems, had no allergies, and took no medications. Her family history was most indicative: Many of the women in her family—her mother, two grandmothers, three aunts, two older sisters, and one younger sister—died of breast cancer when they were in their early 30s. All data from the initial examination, including an evaluation of the lump in the upper outer quadrant of her breast and the presence of a fixed axillary node, were recorded as baseline data for further drug therapy and treatment. B.P. underwent a radical mastectomy with biopsy report for grade IV infiltrating ductal carcinoma (28 of 35 lymph nodes were positive for tumor) and then radiation therapy. Then she began a 1-year course of doxorubicin, cyclophosphamide, and paclitaxel (AC/Paclitaxel/sequential)

CRITICAL THINKING

What are the important nursing implications for B.P.? *Think about the outlook for B.P., based on her biopsy results and her family history.*

What are the effects of high levels of stress on the immune system and the body's ability to fight cancer?

What impact will this disease have on B.P.'s job and her family? *Think about the adverse drug effects that can be anticipated.* How can good patient teaching help B.P. to anticipate and cope with these many changes and unpleasant effects?

What future concerns should be addressed or at least approached at this point in the treatment of B.P's disease? What are the implications for her two daughters? How may a coordinated health team work to help the daughters cope with their mother's disease, as well as the prospects for their future?

DISCUSSION

The extent of B.P.'s disease, as evidenced by the biopsy results, does not signify a very hopeful prognosis. In this case, the overall nursing care plan should take into account not only the acute needs related to surgery and drug therapy, but also future needs related to potential debilitation and even the prospect of death. Immediate needs include comfort and teaching measures to help B.P. deal with the mastectomy and recovery from the surgery. She should be given an opportunity to vent her feelings and thoughts in a protected environment. Efforts should be made to help her to organize her life and plans around her radiation therapy and chemotherapy.

The adverse effects associated with the antineoplastic agents she will be given should be explained and possible ways to cope should be discussed. These effects include the following:

Alopecia—B.P. should be reassured that her hair will grow back, but she will need to cover her head in extremes of temperature. Purchasing a wig before the hair loss begins may be a good alternative to trying to remember later what her hair was like.

Nausea and vomiting—These effects will most often occur immediately after the drugs are given. Antiemetics may be ordered, but they are frequently not very effective.

Bone marrow suppression—This will make B.P. more susceptible to disease, which could be a problem for a teacher and a mother with young children. Ways to avoid contact and infection, as well as warning signs to report immediately, should be discussed.

Mouth sores—Stomatitis and mucositis are common problems. Frequent mouth care is important. The patient should be encouraged to maintain fluid intake and nutrition.

Because the antineoplastic therapy will be a long-term regimen, it might help to prepare a calendar of drug dates for use in planning other activities and events. All of B.P.'s treatment should be incorporated into a team approach that helps B.P. and her family deal with the impact of this disease and its therapy, as well as with the potential risk to her daughters. B.P.'s daughters are in a very high-risk group for this disease, so the importance of frequent examinations as they grow up needs to be stressed. In some areas of the country, health care providers are encouraging prophylactic mastectomies for women in this very high-risk group.

NURSING CARE GUIDE FOR B.P.: ANTINEOPLASTIC AGENTS

Assessment: History and Examination

Allergies to any of these drugs, renal or hepatic dysfunction, pregnancy or lactation, bone marrow suppression, or GI ulceration

Antineoplastic Therapy and Breast Cancer *(continued)*

Concurrent use of: ketoconazole, diazepam, verapamil, quinidine, dexamethasone, cisplatin, cyclosporine, teniposide, etoposide, vincristine, testosterone, or digoxin, which could interact with these drugs

Local: evaluation of injection site

CNS: orientation, affect, reflexes

Skin: color, lesions, texture

GI: abdominal, liver evaluation

Laboratory tests: CBC with differential; renal and hepatic function tests

Nursing Diagnoses

Acute Pain related to GI, CNS, skin effects

Imbalanced Nutrition: Less Than Body Requirements related to GI effects

Disturbed Body Image related to diagnosis, therapy, adverse effects

Deficient Knowledge regarding drug therapy

Implementation

Ensure safe administration of the drug.

Provide comfort and safety measures: mouth and skin care, rest periods, safety precautions, antiemetics as needed, maintenance of nutrition, and head covering.

Provide support and reassurance to deal with drug effects, discomfort, and diagnosis.

Provide patient teaching regarding drug name, dosage, adverse effects, precautions to take, signs and symptoms to report, and comfort measures to observe.

Evaluation

Evaluate drug effects: resolution of cancer.

Monitor for adverse effects: GI toxicity, bone marrow suppression, CNS changes, renal and hepatic damage, alopecia, extravasation of drug.

Monitor for drug–drug interactions as listed.

Evaluate effectiveness of patient teaching program.

Evaluate effectiveness of comfort and safety measures.

Patient Teaching for B.P.:

Antineoplastic agents work to destroy cells at various phases of their life cycle. The drugs are given in combination to affect the cells at these various stages. These drugs are prescribed to kill cancer cells that are growing in the body. Because these drugs also affect normal cells, they sometimes cause many adverse effects. Your drug combination includes doxorubicin, cyclophosphamide, and paclitaxel.

- ☐ These drugs are given in a 21-day cycle, followed by a rest period. You will need to mark your calendar with the treatment days and rest days. You will need to have regular blood tests to follow the effects of these drugs on your blood cells.
- ☐ Common adverse effects of these drugs include:
  - *Nausea and vomiting*—Antiemetic drugs and sedatives may help. Your health care provider will be with you to help if these effects occur.
  - *Loss of appetite*—It is very important to keep up your strength. Tell people if there is something that you would be interested in eating—anything that appeals to you. Alert someone if you feel hungry, regardless of the time of day.
  - *Loss of hair*—Your hair will grow back, although its color or consistency may be different from what it was originally. It may help to purchase a wig before you lose your hair so that you can match appearance if you would like to. Hats and scarves may also be worn. It is very important to keep your head covered in extremes of temperature and to protect yourself from sun, heat, and cold. Because much of the body's heat can be lost through the head, not protecting yourself could cause serious problems.
  - *Mouth sores*—Frequent mouth care is very helpful. Try to avoid very hot or spicy foods.
  - *Fatigue, malaise*—Frequent rest periods and careful planning of your day's activities can be very helpful.
  - *Bleeding*—You may bruise more easily than you normally do, and your gums may bleed while you are brushing your teeth. Special care should be taken when shaving or brushing your teeth. Avoid activities that might cause an injury, and avoid medications that contain aspirin.
  - *Susceptibility to infection*—Avoid people with infections or colds, and avoid crowded, public places. In some cases, the people who are caring for you may wear gowns and masks to protect you from their germs. Avoid working in your garden, because soil can be full of bacteria.

(continued)

Antineoplastic Therapy and Breast Cancer *(continued)*

- ☐ Report any of the following to your health care provider: bruising and bleeding, fever, chills, sore throat, difficulty breathing, flank pain, and swelling in your ankles or fingers.
- ☐ Take the full course of your prescription. It is very important to take the complete regimen that has been ordered for you. Cancer cells grow at different rates, and they go through rest periods during which they are not susceptible to the drugs. The disease must be attacked over time to eradicate the problem.
- ☐ Tell any doctor, nurse, or other health care provider that you are taking this drug.
- ☐ Try to maintain a balanced diet while you are taking this drug. Drink 10 to 12 glasses of water each day during the drug therapy.
- ☐ Use a barrier contraceptive while you are taking this drug. These drugs can cause serious effects to a developing fetus, and precautions must be taken to avoid pregnancy. If you think that you are pregnant, consult your health care provider immediately.
- ☐ You need to have periodic blood tests and examinations while you are taking this drug. These tests help guard against serious adverse effects and may be needed to determine the next dose of your drug.

BOX 14.6 Antiemetics and Cancer Chemotherapy

Antineoplastic drugs can directly stimulate the chemoreceptor trigger zone (CTZ) in the medulla to induce nausea and vomiting. These drugs also cause cell death, which releases many toxins into the system—and which in turn stimulate the CTZ. Because patients expect nausea and vomiting with the administration of antineoplastic agents, the higher cortical centers of the brain can stimulate the CTZ to induce vomiting just at the thought of the chemotherapy.

A variety of antiemetic agents have been used in the course of antineoplastic therapy. Sometimes a combination of drugs is most helpful. It should also be remembered that an accepting environment, plenty of comfort measures (e.g., environmental control, mouth care, ice chips), and support for the patient can help decrease the discomfort associated with the emetic effects of these drugs. Antihistamines to decrease secretions and corticosteroids to relieve inflammation are useful as adjunctive therapies.

Drugs that are known to help in treating antineoplastic chemotherapy-induced nausea and vomiting include the following:

- Dronabinol (*Marinol*) is a synthetic derivative of delta-9-tetrahydrocannabinol, the active ingredient in marijuana; this is not usually a first-line drug because of associated CNS effects. The usual dosage is 5 mg/m^2 PO 1–3 h before chemotherapy and repeated q2–4h after chemotherapy.
- Ondansetron (*Zofran*), granisetron (*Kytril*), and palonosetron (*Aloxi*) block serotonin receptors in the CTZ and are among the most effective antiemetics, especially if combined with a corticosteroid such as dexamethasone. The usual dosage is three 0.15-mg/kg doses IV or 8 mg PO t.i.d. starting 30 min before chemotherapy (ondansetron) or 10 mg/kg IV or 1 mg PO b.i.d. (granisetron), or 0.25 mg IV over 30 seconds, starting 30 min before chemotherapy (palonosetron).
- Aprepitant (*Emend*) blocks human substance P/neurokinin 1 receptors in the CNS, blocking the nausea and vomiting caused by severely emetogenic antineoplastic drugs without effects on dopamine, serotonin, or norepinephrine. The usual dosage is 125 mg PO 1 h before chemotherapy (day 1) and 80 mg PO once daily in the morning on days 2 and 3; given in combination with 12 mg dexamethasone PO on day 1 and 8 mg dexamethasone PO on days 2 to 4 and 32 mg ondansetron IV on day 1 only.
- Two benzodiazepines, alprazolam (*Xanax*), 0.5 mg PO t.i.d., and lorazepam (*Ativan*), 2–6 mg/day PO, seem to be effective in directly blocking the CTZ to relieve nausea and vomiting caused by cancer chemotherapy; they are especially effective when combined with a corticosteroid.
- Haloperidol (*Haldol*), 0.5–2.0 mg PO t.i.d. or 2–25 mg IM or IV, is a dopaminergic blocker that also is believed to have direct CTZ effects.
- Metoclopramide (*Reglan*), 2 mg/kg IV over at least 30 min, calms the activity of the GI tract; it is especially effective if combined with a corticosteroid, an antihistamine, and a centrally acting blocker such as haloperidol or lorazepam.
- Prochlorperazine (*Compazine*), 5–10 mg PO t.i.d. to q.i.d. or 5–10 mg IM, is a phenothiazine that has been found to have strong antiemetic action in the CNS; it can be given by a variety of routes.

Nausea and vomiting are unavoidable aspects of many chemotherapeutic regimens. However, treating the patient as the chemotherapy begins, using combination regimens, and providing plenty of supportive and comforting nursing care can help to alleviate some of the distress associated with these adverse effects.

Antimetabolites

Antimetabolites are drugs that have chemical structures similar to those of various natural metabolites that are necessary for the growth and division of rapidly growing neoplastic cells and normal cells. Antimetabolites replace those needed metabolites and thereby prevent normal cellular function. The use of these drugs has been somewhat limited because of the ability of neoplastic cells to develop resistance to these agents rather rapidly. For this reason, these drugs are usually administered as part of a combination therapy.

Therapeutic Actions and Indications

The antimetabolites inhibit DNA production in cells that depend on certain natural metabolites to produce their DNA. Many of these agents inhibit thymidylate synthetase, DNA polymerase, or folic acid reductase, all of which are needed for DNA synthesis. They are considered to be S phase-specific in the cell cycle. They are most effective in rapidly dividing cells, in which they prevent cell replication, leading to cell death (Figure 14.4). The antimetabolites are indicated for the treatment of various leukemias, including some GI and basal cell cancers. Table 14.2 lists the antimetabolites, their indications, and specific information about each drug. Methotrexate is also indicated for the treatment of rheumatoid arthritis and psoriasis.

Pharmacokinetics

Methotrexate is absorbed well from the GI tract and is excreted unchanged in the urine. Patients with renal impairment may require reduced dosage and increased monitoring when taking methotrexate. Methotrexate readily crosses the blood–brain barrier. Cytarabine, clofarabine, floxuridine, fluorouracil, and pemetrexed are not absorbed well from the GI tract and need to be administered by a different route. They are metabolized in the liver and excreted in the urine, making it important to monitor patients with hepatic or renal impairment who are receiving these drugs. Mercaptopurine and thioguanine are absorbed slowly from the GI tract and are metabolized in the liver and excreted in the urine. All of these agents are contraindicated during pregnancy and lactation because of the potential risk to the neonate.

Contraindications and Cautions

Caution should be used when administering antimetabolites to any individual with a known allergy to any of the antimetabolites; during pregnancy and lactation, *when these drugs are contraindicated because of potential severe effects on the neonate;* with bone marrow suppression, *which is often the index for redosing and dosing levels;* with renal or hepatic dysfunction, *which might interfere with the metabolism or excretion of these drugs and often indicates a need to change the dosage;* and with known GI ulcerations or ulcerative diseases *that might be exacerbated by the effects of these drugs.*

Adverse Effects

Adverse effects frequently encountered with the use of the antimetabolites are listed here. To counteract the effects of treatment with one antimetabolite, methotrexate, the drug leucovorin is sometimes given (Box 14.7).

Hematological effects include bone marrow suppression, with leukopenia, thrombocytopenia, anemia, and pancytopenia, secondary to the effects of the drugs on the rapidly multiplying cells of the bone marrow. Toxic GI effects include nausea, vomiting, anorexia, diarrhea, and mucous membrane deterioration, all of which are related to drug effects on the rapidly multiplying cells of the GI tract. CNS effects include headache, drowsiness, aphasia, fatigue, malaise, and dizziness. Patients should be advised to take precautions if these conditions occur. As with alkylating agents, effects of the antimetabolites may include possible hepatic toxicity or renal toxicity depending on the exact mechanism of action. Alopecia may also occur.

Clinically Important Drug-Drug Interactions

Antimetabolites that are known to cause hepatic or renal toxicity should be used with care with any other drugs known to have the same effect. In addition, drugs that are toxic to the liver may adversely affect drugs that are metabolized in the liver or that act in the liver (e.g., oral anticoagulants). Specific drug–drug interactions for each agent should be checked in your nursing drug guide.

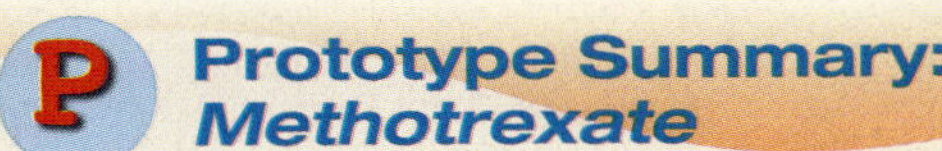

Prototype Summary: Methotrexate

Indications: Treatment of gestational choriocarcinoma, chorioadenoma destruens, hydatidiform, meningeal leukemia; symptomatic control of severe psoriasis; rheumatoid arthritis; juvenile rheumatoid arthritis.

Actions: Inhibits folic acid reductase, leading to inhibition of DNA synthesis and inhibition of cellular replication; affects the most rapidly dividing cells.

Pharmacokinetics:

Route	Onset	Peak
Oral	Varies	1–4 h
IV	Rapid	0.5–2 h

$T_{1/2}$: 2–4 hours, excreted unchanged in the urine

Adverse effects: Fatigue, malaise, rashes, alopecia, ulcerative stomatitis, hepatic toxicity, severe bone marrow suppression, interstitial pneumonitis, chills, fever, anaphylaxis

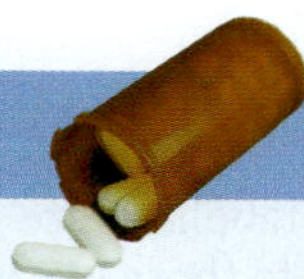

Table 14.2 DRUGS IN FOCUS

Antimetabolites

Drug Name	Dosage/Route	Usual Indications
capecitabine (*Xeloda*)	2500 mg/m²/day PO in two divided doses for 2 wk, then 1 wk rest, for three cycles	Treatment of metastatic breast cancer with resistance to paclitaxel or anthracyclines; treatment of metastatic colorectal cancer as first-line therapy treatment of breast cancer with docetaxel in patients with metastatic disease **Special considerations:** Severe diarrhea can occur—monitor hydration and nutrition; monitor for bone marrow suppression
cladribine (*Leustatin*)	0.09 mg/kg/day IV for 7 consecutive days	Treatment of active hairy cell leukemia **Special considerations:** Severe bone marrow depression can occur—monitor patient closely and reduce dosage as needed; fever is common, especially early in treatment
clofarabine (*Clolar*)	52 mg/m² by IV infusion over 2 h daily for 5 days; repeat every 2–6 wk, based on baseline function	Treatment of patients 1–21 yr of age with acute lymphocytic leukemia (ALL) after at least two relapses on other regimens **Special considerations:** GI toxicity, bone marrow suppression, and infection are common
cytarabine (*Ara-C, Cytosar-U*)	200 mg/m²/day by continuous IV infusion for 5 days, repeat every 2 wk	Treatment of meningeal and myelocytic leukemias; used in combination with other agents; lymphomatous meningitis; non-Hodgkin's lymphoma in children **Special considerations:** GI toxicity and cytarabine syndrome (fever, myalgia, bone pain, chest pain, rash, conjunctivitis, and malaise) are common—this syndrome sometimes responds to corticosteroids; alopecia may occur
floxuridine (*FUDR*)	0.1–0.6 mg/kg/day via intra-arterial line	Palliative management of GI adenocarcinoma metastatic to the liver in patients who are not candidates for surgery **Special considerations:** Administer by intra-arterial line only; bone marrow suppression, GI toxicity, neurotoxicity, and alopecia are common
fludarabine (*Fludara*)	25 mg/m²/day IV for 5 days; repeat every 28 days	Treatment of chronic lymphocytic leukemia (CLL); unresponsive B cell CLL with no progress with at least one other treatment **Special considerations:** CNS toxicity can be severe; GI toxicity, respiratory complications, renal failure, and a tumor lysis syndrome are common
fluorouracil (*Adrucil, Efudex, Fluoroplex*)	12 mg/kg/day IV on days 1–4, then 6 mg/kg IV on days 6, 8, 10, and 12	Palliative treatment of various GI cancers; topical treatment of basal cell carcinoma and actinic and solar keratoses **Special considerations:** GI toxicity, bone marrow suppression, alopecia, and skin rash are common; avoid occlusive dressings with topical forms; wash hands thoroughly after coming in contact with drug
mercaptopurine (*Purinethol*)	2.5 mg/kg/day PO for 4 wk; then re-evaluate	Remission induction and maintenance therapy in acute leukemias **Special considerations:** Bone marrow toxicity and GI toxicity are common; hyperuricemia is a true concern—ensure that the patient is well hydrated during therapy
P methotrexate (*Folex, Rheumatrex*)	Dosage varies with route and disease being treated; 15–30 mg PO or IM is common	Treatment of leukemias, psoriasis, rheumatoid arthritis, and choriocarcinomas **Special considerations:** Hypersensitivity reactions can be severe; liver toxicity and GI complications are common; monitor for bone marrow suppression and increased susceptibility to infections; dose pack available for the oral treatment of psoriasis and rheumatoid arthritis
pemetrexed (*Alimta*)	500 mg/m² IV over 10 min on day 1 with 75 mg/m² cisplatin IV over 2 h; repeat cycle every 21 days	Treatment of malignant mesothelioma in patients whose disease is unresectable or who are not candidates for surgery; locally advanced or metastatic non–small cell lung cancer as a single agent after other chemotherapy **Special considerations:** Pretreat with corticosteroids, folic acid, and vitamin B_{12}; monitor for bone marrow suppression and GI effects.
pentostatin (*Nipent*)	4 mg/m² IV every other week	Hairy cell leukemia in adults if refractory to interferon-alpha therapy **Special considerations:** Associated with severe renal, hepatic, CNS, and pulmonary toxicities—monitor patient closely and reduce dosage accordingly; 3–6 mo of interferon-alpha therapy should be tried before using pentostatin
thioguanine (*generic*)	2 mg/kg/day PO for 4 wk; then dosage may be increased if tolerated well	Remission induction and maintenance of acute leukemias alone or as part of combination therapy **Special considerations:** Bone marrow suppression, GI toxicity, miscarriage, and birth defects have been reported; monitor bone marrow status to determine dosage and redosing; ensure that the patient is well hydrated during therapy to minimize hyperuricemia—patient may respond to allopurinol and urine alkalinization

BOX 14.7 A Drug That Protects Against an Antimetabolite

Leucovorin (*Wellcovorin*) is an active form of folic acid that is used to "rescue" normal cells from the adverse effects of methotrexate therapy in the treatment of osteosarcoma. This drug is also used to treat folic acid deficiency conditions such as sprue, nutritional deficiency, pregnancy, and lactation. Leucovorin is given orally or intravenously at the time of methotrexate therapy and for the next 72 h at a dose of 12–15 g/m² PO or IV followed by 10 mg/m² PO q6h for 72 h. Use of this drug has been associated with pain at the injection site.

Nursing Considerations for Patients Receiving Antimetabolites

Assessment: History and Examination

Screen for the following, *which will alert you to cautions and contraindications for the use of the drug:* history of allergy to the specific antimetabolite; bone marrow suppression; renal or hepatic dysfunction; pregnancy or lactation; and GI ulcerative disease.

Physical assessment should be performed *to establish baseline data for determining the effectiveness of the drug and the occurrence of any adverse effects associated with drug therapy.* Include screening for orientation and reflexes *to evaluate any CNS effects;* respiratory rate and adventitious sounds *to monitor the disease and to evaluate for respiratory or hypersensitivity effects;* pulse, rhythm, and cardiac auscultation *to monitor for systemic or cardiovascular effects;* and bowel sounds and mucous membrane status *to monitor for GI effects.* Evaluate the CBC with differential and renal and liver function tests *to monitor for dosage adjustment as needed and to evaluate toxic drug effects.*

Nursing Diagnoses

The patient receiving an antimetabolite may have the following nursing diagnoses related to drug therapy:

- Acute Pain related to GI, CNS, skin effects of drug
- Disturbed Body Image related to alopecia, skin effects, impaired fertility
- Fear, Anxiety related to diagnosis and treatment
- Deficient Knowledge regarding drug therapy

Implementation with Rationale

- Arrange for blood tests to monitor bone marrow function before, periodically during, and for at least 3 weeks after therapy *to arrange to discontinue the drug or reduce the dose as needed.*
- Administer medication according to scheduled protocol and in combination with other drugs as indicated *to improve effectiveness of drug therapy.*
- Ensure that the patient is well hydrated *to decrease risk of renal toxicity.*
- Provide small, frequent meals; frequent mouth care; and dietary consultation as appropriate *to maintain nutrition when GI effects are severe.* Antiemetics may be helpful in some cases. (See Box 14.5.)
- Arrange for proper head covering at extremes of temperature if alopecia occurs; a wig, scarf, or hat *is important for maintaining body temperature.* If alopecia is an anticipated effect of drug therapy, advise the patient to obtain a wig or head covering before the condition occurs *to promote self-esteem and a positive body image.*
- Protect the patient from exposure to infections, *because bone marrow suppression will limit immune/inflammatory responses.*
- Provide patient teaching *to enhance patient knowledge about drug therapy and to promote compliance regarding:*
  - The appropriate dosage regimen, including dates to return for further doses.
  - The need to try to maintain nutrition if GI effects are severe.
  - The importance of covering the head at extremes of temperature if alopecia is anticipated.
  - The need to plan appropriate rest periods because fatigue and weakness are common effects of the drugs.
  - The importance of avoiding crowded places, sick people, and working in soil, to avoid infection.
  - Possible dizziness, headache, and drowsiness; if these occur, the patient should avoid driving or using dangerous equipment.
  - The possibility of impaired fertility; the patient may wish to consult a health care provider.
  - The importance of not taking the drugs during pregnancy and of using barrier contraceptives.

Evaluation

- Monitor patient response to the drug (alleviation of cancer being treated, palliation of signs and symptoms of cancer, palliation of rheumatoid arthritis or psoriasis).

- Monitor for adverse effects (bone marrow suppression, GI toxicity, neurotoxicity, alopecia, renal or hepatic dysfunction).
- Evaluate the effectiveness of the teaching plan (patient can name the drug, dosage, possible adverse effects to watch for, and specific measures to help avoid adverse effects).
- Monitor the effectiveness of comfort and safety measures and compliance with the regimen

Antineoplastic Antibiotics

Antineoplastic antibiotics are not selective only for bacterial cells; they are also toxic to human cells. Because these drugs tend to be more toxic to cells that are multiplying rapidly, they are useful in the treatment of certain cancers. These cell cycle–specific drugs interfere with cellular DNA, disrupting it and causing cell death (see Figure 14.4). Some antineoplastic antibiotics break up DNA links, and others prevent DNA synthesis. Like other antineoplastics, the main adverse effects of these drugs are seen in cells that multiply rapidly: cells in the bone marrow, GI tract, and skin.

Therapeutic Actions and Indications

The antineoplastic antibiotics are cytotoxic and interfere with DNA synthesis by inserting themselves between base pairs in the DNA chain and causing a mutant DNA molecule, leading to cell death. Table 14.3 lists the various antineoplastic antibiotics, their indications, and specific information about each drug. Their potentially serious adverse effects may limit their usefulness in patients with pre-existing diseases and in those who are debilitated and therefore more susceptible to these effects.

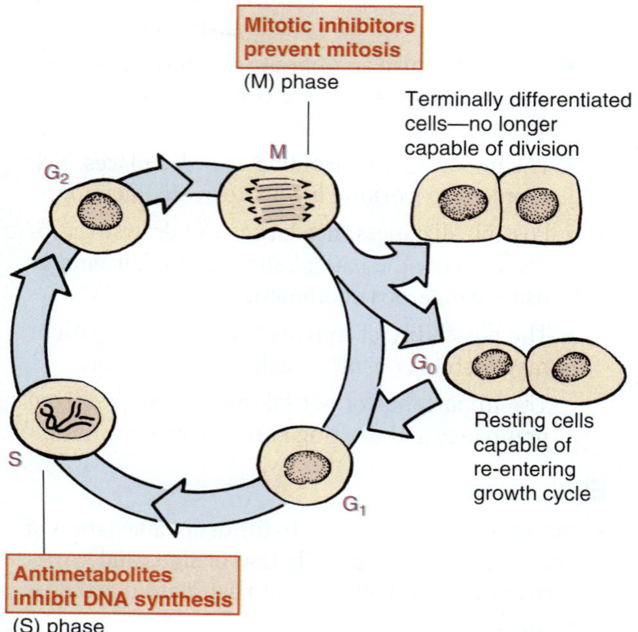

FIGURE 14.4 Sites of action of cell cycle–specific antineoplastic agents.

Pharmacokinetics

The antineoplastic antibiotics are not absorbed well from the GI tract and are given IV or injected into specific sites. They are metabolized in the liver and excreted in the urine at various rates. Many of them have very long half-lives (45 hours for idarubicin, more than 5 days for mitoxantrone). Daunorubicin and doxorubicin do not cross the blood–brain barrier, but they are widely distributed in the body and are taken up by the heart, lungs, kidneys, and spleen. All of these agents are contraindicated for use during pregnancy and lactation because of the potential risk to the neonate.

Contraindications and Cautions

Caution should be used when giving antineoplastic antibiotics to an individual with a known allergy to the antibiotic or related antibiotics and during pregnancy and lactation. Care should also be taken in patients with the following conditions: bone marrow suppression, *which is often the index for redosing and dosing levels;* suppressed renal or hepatic function, *which might interfere with the metabolism or excretion of these drugs and often indicates a need to change the dosage;* known GI ulcerations or ulcerative diseases, *which may be exacerbated by the effects of these drugs;* pulmonary problems with bleomycin or mitomycin, or cardiac problems with idarubicin or mitoxantrone, *which are specifically toxic to these systems.*

Adverse Effects

Adverse effects frequently encountered with the use of these antibiotics include bone marrow suppression, with leukopenia, thrombocytopenia, anemia, and pancytopenia, secondary to the effects of the drugs on the rapidly multiplying cells of the bone marrow. Toxic GI effects include nausea, vomiting, anorexia, diarrhea, and mucous membrane deterioration, all of which are related to drug effects on the rapidly multiplying cells of the GI tract. As with the alkylating agents and antimetabolites, effects of antineoplastic antibiotics may include renal or hepatic toxicity, depending on the exact mechanism of action. Alopecia may also occur. Specific drugs are toxic to the heart and lungs; Box 14.8 discusses a cardioprotective drug that interferes with the effects of doxorubicin.

Table 14.3 DRUGS IN FOCUS

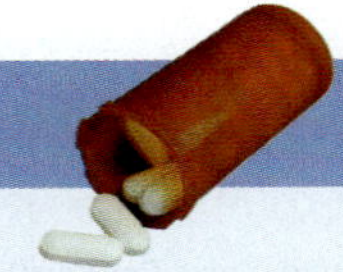

Antineoplastic Antibiotics

Drug Name	Dosage/Route	Usual Indications
bleomycin (*Blenoxane*)	0.25–0.5 units/kg IM, IV, or Sub-Q once or twice weekly	Palliative treatment of squamous cell carcinomas, testicular cancers, and lymphomas; used to treat malignant pleural effusion **Special considerations:** GI toxicity, severe skin reactions, and hypersensitivity reactions may occur; pulmonary fibrosis can be a serious problem—baseline and periodic chest radiographs and pulmonary function tests are necessary.
dactinomycin (*Cosmegen*)	Adult: 0.5 mg/day IV for up to 5 days Pediatric: 0.015 mg/kg/day IV for up to 5 days or a total dose of 2.5 mg/m²/wk	Part of combination drug regimen in the treatment of a variety of sarcomas and carcinomas; potentiates the effects of radiation therapy **Special considerations:** Bone marrow suppression and GI toxicity, which may be severe, limit the dose; effects may not appear for 1 to 2 wk; local extravasation can cause necrosis and should be treated with injectable corticosteroids, ice to the area, and restarting of the IV line in a different vein
daunorubicin (*DaunoXome*)	40 mg/m² IV, infused over 1 h; repeat every 2 wk	First-line treatment of advanced HIV infection and associated Kaposi's sarcoma **Special considerations:** Complete alopecia is common, and GI toxicity and bone marrow suppression may also occur; severe necrosis may occur at sites of local extravasation—immediate treatment with corticosteroids, normal saline, and ice may help; if ulcerations occur, a plastic surgeon should be called
P doxorubicin (*Adriamycin*)	60–75 mg/m² as a single IV dose; repeat every 21 days	Treatment of a number of leukemias and cancers; used to induce regression; available in a liposomal form for treatment of AIDS-associated Kaposi's sarcoma **Special considerations:** Complete alopecia is common; GI toxicity and bone marrow suppression may occur; severe necrosis may occur at sites of local extravasation—immediate treatment with corticosteroids, normal saline and ice may help; if ulcerations occur, a plastic surgeon should be called; toxicity is dose related—an accurate record of each dose received is important in determining dosage. Severe pulmonary toxicity, alopecia, and injection site and GI toxicity occur.
epirubicin (*Ellence*)	100–120 mg/m² IV given in repeated 3–4-wk cycles all on day 1 or divided on days 1 and 8	Adjunctive therapy in patients with evidence of axillary node tumor involvement after resection of primary breast cancer. **Special considerations:** May cause cardiotoxicity and delayed cardiomyopathy; monitor for myelosuppression and hyperuricemia; severe local cellulitis and tissue necrosis can occur with extravasation.
idarubicin (*Idamycin*)	12 mg/m²/day IV for 3 days with cytarabine	Combination therapy for treatment of acute myeloid leukemia in adults **Special considerations:** May cause severe bone marrow suppression, which regulates dosage; associated with cardiac toxicity, which can be severe; GI toxicity and local necrosis with extravasation are also common; severe necrosis may occur at sites of local extravasation—immediate treatment with corticosteroids, normal saline, and ice may help; if ulcerations occur, a plastic surgeon should be called; it is essential to monitor heart and bone marrow function to protect the patient from potentially fatal adverse effects
mitomycin (*Mutamycin, Mutozytrex*)	*Mutamycin* 20 mg/m² IV as a single dose at 6–8-wk intervals *Mutozytrex:* 15 mg/m² as a single IV dose every 6–8 wks based on bone marrow status	Treatment of disseminated adenocarcinoma of the stomach and pancreas **Special considerations:** Severe pulmonary toxicity, alopecia, and injection site and GI toxicity occur
mitoxantrone (*Novantrone*)	12 mg/m²/day IV for 1–3 days *Multiple sclerosis:* 12 mg/m² IV as a short infusion every 3 mo	Part of combination therapy in the treatment of adult leukemias; treatment of bone pain in advanced prostatic cancer; reduction of neurological disability and frequency of relapses in chronic, progressive, relapsing multiple sclerosis **Special considerations:** Severe bone marrow suppression may occur and limits dosage; alopecia, GI toxicity, and congestive heart failure often occur; avoid direct skin contact with the drug—use gloves and goggles; monitor bone marrow activity and cardiac activity to adjust dosage or discontinue drug as needed
valrubicin (*Valstar*)	800 mg intravesically once a week for 6 wk	Intravesical therapy for carcinoma in situ of the bladder if refractory to bacille Calmette-Guérin (BCG) therapy (orphan drug) **Special considerations:** Use goggles and gloves when handling, avoid contact with eyes; severe bladder spasms have occurred, use caution with history of irritable bowel syndrome, do not clamp bladder catheter in place

BOX 14.8 A Cardioprotective Antineoplastic Drug

Dexrazoxane (*Zinecard*), a powerful intracellular chelating agent, is a cardioprotective drug that interferes with the cardiotoxic effects of doxorubicin. The associated adverse effects are difficult to differentiate from those attributable to doxorubicin. This agent is approved for use to prevent the cardiomyopathy associated with doxorubicin in doses greater than 300 mg/m^2 in women with metastatic breast cancer. Dexrazoxane is given intravenously in a dosage proportional to (10 times greater than) the doxorubicin dose 30 min before the doxorubicin is administered.

Clinically Important Drug–Drug Interactions

Antimetabolites that are known to cause hepatic or renal toxicity should be used with care with any other drugs known to have the same effect. Drugs that result in toxicity to the heart or lungs should be used with caution with any other drugs that produce that particular toxicity. Specific drug–drug interactions for each agent are listed in your nursing drug guide.

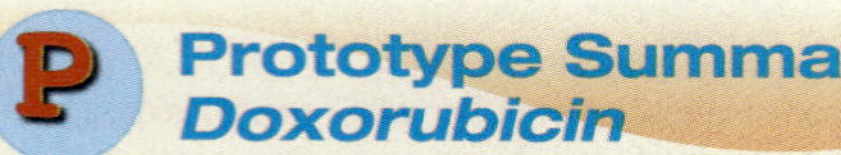

Prototype Summary: Doxorubicin

Indications: To produce regression in acute lymphoblastic lymphoma, acute myeloblastic leukemia, Wilm's tumor, neuroblastoma, soft tissue and bone sarcoma, breast carcinoma, ovarian carcinoma, thyroid carcinoma, Hodgkin's and non-Hodgkin's lymphomas, bronchogenic carcinoma; also to treat AIDS-related Kaposi's sarcoma

Actions: Binds to DNA and inhibits DNA synthesis in susceptible cells, causing cell death

Pharmacokinetics:

Route	Onset	Peak	Duration
IV	Rapid	2 h	24–36 h

$T_{1/2}$: 12 min, then 3.3 hours, then 29.6 hours; metabolized in the liver and excreted in the bile, feces, and urine

Adverse effects: Cardiac toxicity, complete but reversible alopecia, nausea, vomiting, mucositis, red urine, myelosuppression, fever, chills, rash

Nursing Considerations for Patients Receiving Antineoplastic Antibiotic Agents

Assessment: History and Examination

Screen for the following, *which could be cautions or contraindications to the use of the drug:* history of allergy to the antibiotic in use, bone marrow suppression, renal or hepatic dysfunction, respiratory or cardiac disease, pregnancy or lactation, and GI ulcerative disease.

Physical assessment should be performed *to establish baseline data for determining the effectiveness of the drug and the occurrence of any adverse effects associated with drug therapy.* Include screening for orientation and reflexes *to evaluate any CNS effects;* respiratory rate and adventitious sounds *to monitor the disease and evaluate for respiratory or hypersensitivity effects;* pulse, rhythm, cardiac auscultation, and baseline electrocardiogram *to monitor for systemic or cardiovascular effects;* and bowel sounds and mucous membrane status *to monitor for GI effects.* Evaluate the CBC with differential and renal and liver function tests *to monitor for dosage adjustment as needed and to evaluate toxic drug effects.*

Nursing Diagnoses

The patient receiving an antineoplastic antibiotic may have the following nursing diagnoses related to drug therapy:

- Acute Pain related to GI, CNS, local effects of drug
- Disturbed Body Image related to alopecia, skin effects
- Fear, Anxiety related to diagnosis and treatment
- Deficient Knowledge regarding drug therapy

Implementation with Rationale

- Arrange for blood tests to monitor bone marrow function before, periodically during, and for at least 3 weeks after therapy *to arrange to discontinue the drug or reduce the dose as needed.* Monitor cardiac and respiratory function as well as clotting times as appropriate for the drug being used *to arrange to discontinue the drug or reduce the dose as needed.*
- Protect the patient from exposure to infection *because bone marrow suppression will decrease immune/inflammatory reactions.*

- Administer medication according to scheduled protocol and in combination with other drugs as indicated *to improve effectiveness of drug therapy.*
- Ensure that the patient is well hydrated *to decrease risk of renal toxicity.*
- Provide small, frequent meals; frequent mouth care; and dietary consultation as appropriate *to maintain nutrition when GI effects are severe.* Antiemetics may be helpful in some cases. (See Box 14.5.)
- Arrange for proper head covering at extremes of temperature if alopecia occurs; a wig, scarf, or hat *is important for maintaining body temperature.* If alopecia is an anticipated effect of drug therapy, advise the patient to obtain a wig or head covering before the condition occurs *to promote self-esteem and a positive body image.*
- Provide patient teaching *to enhance patient knowledge about drug therapy and to promote compliance regarding:*
  - The appropriate dosage regimen, including dates to return for further doses.
  - The need to try to maintain nutrition if GI effects are severe.
  - The importance of covering the head at extremes of temperature if alopecia is anticipated.
  - The need to plan appropriate rest periods because fatigue and weakness are common effects of the drugs.
  - The need to avoid crowded places, sick people, and working in soil, to prevent infection.
  - Possible dizziness, headache, and drowsiness; if these occur, the patient should avoid driving or using dangerous equipment.
  - The possibility of impaired fertility; the patient may wish to consult a health care provider.
  - The importance of not taking the drugs during pregnancy and of using barrier contraceptives.

Evaluation

- Monitor patient response to the drug (alleviation of cancer being treated and palliation of signs and symptoms of cancer).
- Monitor for adverse effects (bone marrow suppression, GI toxicity, neurotoxicity, alopecia, renal or hepatic dysfunction, and cardiac or respiratory dysfunction).
- Evaluate the effectiveness of the teaching plan (patient can name the drug, dosage, possible adverse effects to watch for, and specific measures to help avoid adverse effects).

Mitotic Inhibitors

Mitotic inhibitors are drugs that kill cells as the process of mitosis begins (see Figure 14.4). These cell-cycle–specific agents inhibit DNA synthesis. Like other antineoplastics, the main adverse effects of the mitotic inhibitors occur with cells that rapidly multiply: those in the bone marrow, GI tract, and skin.

Therapeutic Actions and Indications

The mitotic inhibitors interfere with the ability of a cell to divide; they block or alter DNA synthesis, thus causing cell death. They work in the M phase of the cell cycle. These drugs are used for the treatment of a variety of tumors and leukemias. Table 14.4 lists the mitotic inhibitors, their indications, and specific information about each drug. These drugs are not interchangeable, and each has a specific use.

Pharmacokinetics

Generally, these drugs are not well absorbed from the GI tract and are given intravenously. They are metabolized in the liver and excreted primarily in the feces, making them safer for use in patients with renal impairment than the antineoplastics that are cleared through the kidney. They should not be used during pregnancy or lactation because of the potential risk to the neonate.

Contraindications and Cautions

Caution should be used when giving these drugs to anyone with a known allergy to the drug or related drugs and during pregnancy and lactation. Care should also be taken in patients with the following conditions: bone marrow suppression, *which is often the index for redosing and dosing levels;* renal or hepatic dysfunction, *which could interfere with the metabolism or excretion of these drugs and often indicates a need to change the dosage;* and known GI ulcerations or ulcerative diseases, *which may be exacerbated by the effects of these drugs.*

Adverse Effects

Adverse effects frequently encountered with the use of mitotic inhibitors include bone marrow suppression, with leukopenia, thrombocytopenia, anemia, and pancytopenia, secondary to the effects of the drugs on the rapidly multiplying cells of the bone marrow. GI effects include nausea, vomiting, anorexia, diarrhea, and mucous membrane deterioration. As with the other antineoplastic agents, effects of the mitotic inhibitors may include possible hepatic or renal toxicity, depending on the exact mechanism of action. Alopecia may also occur. These drugs also cause necrosis and cellulitis if extravasation occurs, so injection sites should be regularly monitored and appropriate action taken as needed (Box 14.9).

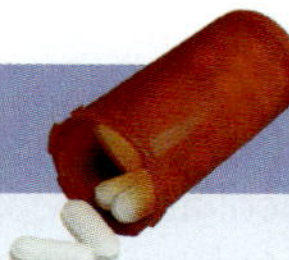

Table 14.4 DRUGS IN FOCUS

Mitotic Inhibitors

Drug Name	Dosage/Route	Usual Indications
docetaxel (*Taxotere*)	60–100 mg/m² IV over 1 h every 3 wk	Treatment of breast cancer and non–small cell lung cancer **Special considerations:** Monitor patient closely—deaths have occurred during use; severe fluid retention can occur—premedicate with corticosteroids and monitor for weight gain; skin rash and nail disorders are usually reversible; monitor patients closely during use
etoposide (*Toposar, VePesid*)	35–100 mg/m²/day IV for 4–5 days	Treatment of testicular cancers refractory to other agents; non-small cell long carcinomas **Special considerations:** Fatigue, GI toxicity, bone marrow depression and alopecia are common side effects; avoid direct skin contact with the drug, use protective clothing and goggles; monitor bone marrow function to adjust dosage; rapid fall in blood pressure can occur during IV infusion—monitor patient carefully
paclitaxel (*Taxol, Onxol*)	135–175 mg/m²/day IV over 3 h every 3 wk	Treatment of advanced ovarian cancer, breast cancer, non–small cell lung cancer, and AIDS-related Kaposi's sarcoma **Special considerations:** Anaphylaxis and severe hypersensitivity reactions have occurred—monitor very closely during administration; also monitor for bone marrow suppression; cardiovascular toxicity and neuropathies have occurred
teniposide (*Vumon*)	165–250 mg/m² IV weekly in combination with other drugs	In combination with other drugs for induction therapy in childhood acute lymphoblastic leukemia **Special considerations:** GI toxicity, CNS effects, bone marrow suppression, and alopecia are common effects; avoid direct skin contact with the drug—use protective clothing and goggles; monitor bone marrow function to adjust dosage; rapid fall in blood pressure can occur during IV infusion—monitor patient carefully
vinblastine (*Velban*)	Adult: 3.7 mg/m² IV once weekly Pediatric: 2 mg/m² IV once weekly Dosage may then be increased based on leukocyte count and patient response	Palliative treatment of various lymphomas and sarcomas; advanced Hodgkin's disease; alone or as part of combination therapy for the treatment of advanced testicular germ cell cancers **Special considerations:** GI toxicity, CNS effects, and total loss of hair are common; antiemetics may help; avoid contact with drug, and monitor injection sites for reactions
P vincristine (*Oncovin, Vincasar*)	Adult: 1.4 mg/m² IV at weekly intervals Pediatric: 2 mg/m² IV once weekly	Treatment of acute leukemia, various lymphomas, and sarcomas **Special considerations:** Extensive CNS effects are common, GI toxicity, local irritation at injection IV site, and hair loss commonly occur; syndrome of inappropriate secretion of antidiuretic hormone (SIADH) has been reported—monitor urine output and arrange for fluid restriction and diuretics as needed.
vinorelbine (*Navelbine*)	30 mg/m² IV once weekly, based on granulocyte count	First-line treatment of unresectable advanced non–small cell lung cancer; stage IV non–small cell lung cancer and stage III non–small cell lung cancer with cisplatin **Special considerations:** GI and CNS toxicity are common; total loss of hair, local reaction at injection site, and bone marrow depression also occur; prepare a calendar with return dates for the series of injections; avoid extravasation but arrange for hyaluronidase infusion if it occurs; antiemetics may be helpful if reaction is severe

Clinically Important Drug–Drug Interactions

Mitotic inhibitors that are known to be toxic to the liver or the CNS should be used with care with any other drugs known to have the same adverse effect. Specific drug–drug interactions for each agent are listed in your nursing drug guide.

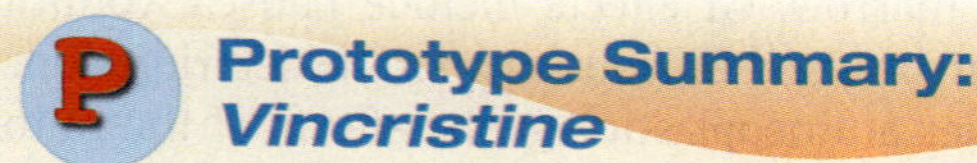

Prototype Summary: Vincristine

Indications: Acute leukemia, Hodgkin's disease, non-Hodgkin's lymphoma, rhabdomyosarcoma, neuroblastoma, Wilm's tumor

Actions: Arrests mitotic division at the stage of metaphase; exact mechanism of action is not understood

Pharmacokinetics:

Route	Onset	Peak
IV	Varies	15–30 min

$T_{1/2}$: 5 min, then 2.3 hours, then 85 hours; metabolized in the liver and excreted in the feces and urine

Adverse effects: Ataxia, cranial nerve manifestations, neuritic pain, muscle wasting, constipation, leukopenia, weight loss, loss of hair, death

BOX 14.9 FOCUS ON **CLINICAL SKILLS**

Preventing and Treating Extravasation

When an IV antineoplastic drug extravasates, or infiltrates into the surrounding tissue, serious tissue damage can occur. These drugs are toxic to cells, and the resulting tissue injury can result in severe pain, scarring, nerve and muscle damage, infection, and in very severe cases even amputation of the limb.

Prevention is the best way to deal with extravasation. Interventions that can help to prevent extravasation include the following: use a distal vein, avoid small veins on the wrist or digits; never use an existing line unless it is clearly open and running well; start the infusion with plain 5% dextrose in water (D5W) and monitor for any sign of extravasation; check the site frequently and ask the patient to report any discomfort in the area; if at all possible, do not use an infusion pump to administer one of these drugs because it will continue to deliver the drug under pressure and can cause a severe extravasation.

If extravasation occurs, there are specific antidotes to use with some antineoplastic drugs. The antidote is usually administered through the IV line to allow it to infiltrate the same tissue, but if the line has been pulled, a tuberculin syringe can be used to inject the antidote subcutaneously into the tissue surrounding the infiltrated area.

Drug	Antidote and Suggested Dosage
etoposide teniposide vinblastine vincristine	hyaluronidase (*Wydase*), 0.2 mL Sub-Q; then apply heat to disperse drug and alleviate pain
daunorubicin doxorubicin vinblastine vincristine	8.4% sodium bicarbonate, 5 mL; flush area with normal saline, apply cold compress; local infiltration with corticosteroids may also be ordered at 25 to 50 mg/mL of extravasate; if ulceration occurs, a plastic surgery consultation should be obtained
mechlorethamine	isotonic sodium thiosulfate (1/6 M), 10 mL infused immediately, then apply an ice compress for 6–12 h
dactinomycin	50 mg ascorbic acid injection; flush area with normal saline and apply cold compresses; consider use of an injectable corticosteroid if reaction is severe

Nursing Considerations for Patients Receiving Mitotic Inhibitors

Assessment: History and Examination

Screen for the following, *which could be cautions or contraindications to the use of the drug:* history of allergy to the drug used (or related drugs), bone marrow suppression, renal or hepatic dysfunction, pregnancy or lactation, and GI ulcerative disease.

Physical assessment should be performed *to establish baseline data for determining the effectiveness of the drug and the occurrence of any adverse effects associated with drug therapy.* Include screening for orientation and reflexes *to evaluate any CNS effects;* skin, *to evaluate for lesions,* hair and hair distribution, *to monitor for adverse effects;* respiratory rate and adventitious sounds *to monitor the disease and to evaluate for respiratory or hypersensitivity effects;* and bowel sounds and mucous membrane status *to monitor for GI effects.* Evaluate the CBC with differential and renal and liver function tests *to monitor for dosage adjustment as needed and to evaluate toxic drug effects.* Regular evaluation of injection sites should be performed *to check for signs of extravasation or inflammation.*

Nursing Diagnoses

The patient receiving a mitotic inhibitor may have the following nursing diagnoses related to drug therapy:

- Acute Pain related to GI, CNS, local effects of drug
- Disturbed Body Image related to alopecia, skin effects
- Fear, Anxiety related to diagnosis and treatment
- Deficient Knowledge regarding drug therapy

Implementation With Rationale

- Arrange for blood tests to monitor bone marrow function before, periodically during, and for at least 3 weeks after therapy *to arrange to discontinue the drug or reduce the dose as needed.*
- Avoid direct skin or eye contact with the drug. Wear protective clothing and goggles while preparing and administering the drug *to prevent toxic reaction to the drug.*
- Administer medication according to scheduled protocol and in combination with other drugs as indicated *to improve effectiveness of drug therapy.*
- Ensure that the patient is well hydrated *to decrease risk of renal toxicity.*
- Monitor injection sites *to arrange appropriate treatment for extravasation, local inflammation, or cellulitis.*
- Protect the patient from exposure to infection *because bone marrow suppression will decrease immune/inflammatory responses.*
- Provide small, frequent meals; frequent mouth care; and dietary consultation as appropriate *to maintain nutrition if GI effects are severe.* Antiemetics may be helpful in some cases. (See Box 14.5.)

- Arrange for proper head covering at extremes of temperature if alopecia or epilation occurs; a wig, scarf, or hat *is important for maintaining body temperature.* If alopecia is an anticipated effect of drug therapy, advise the patient to obtain a wig or head covering before the condition occurs *to promote self-esteem and a positive body image.*
- Provide patient teaching to enhance patient knowledge about drug therapy and *to promote compliance regarding:*
  - The appropriate dosage regimen, including dates to return for further doses.
  - The need to try to maintain nutrition if GI effects are severe.
  - The importance of covering the head at extremes of temperature if alopecia is anticipated.
  - The need to plan appropriate rest periods because fatigue and weakness are common effects of the drugs.
  - The need to avoid crowded areas, sick people, and working in the soil, to prevent infections.
  - Possible dizziness, headache, and drowsiness; if these occur, the patient should avoid driving or using dangerous equipment.
  - The possibility of impaired fertility; the patient may wish to consult a health care provider.
  - The importance of not taking the drugs during pregnancy and of using barrier contraceptive.

Evaluation

- Monitor patient response to the drug (alleviation of cancer being treated and palliation of signs and symptoms of cancer).
- Monitor for adverse effects (bone marrow suppression, GI toxicity, neurotoxicity, alopecia, renal or hepatic dysfunction, and local reactions at the injection site).
- Evaluate the effectiveness of the teaching plan (patient can name the drug, dosage, possible adverse effects to watch for, and specific measures to help avoid adverse effects).

FOCUS POINTS

- Antimetabolites inhibit DNA production by inhibiting metabolites needed for synthesis of DNA in susceptible cells.
- Antimetabolites are S-phase–specific and are used for some leukemias, as well as some GI and basal cell cancers.
- Antineoplastic antibiotics are toxic to rapidly dividing cells. These drugs are cell-cycle–specific, affecting the S phase.
- Mitotic inhibitors kill cells during the M phase and are used to treat a variety of cancers.
- Bone marrow suppression, alopecia, and toxic GI effects are common with all three of these types of drugs.

Hormones and Hormone Modulators

Some cancers, particularly those involving the breast tissue, ovaries, uterus, prostate, and testes, are sensitive to estrogen stimulation. Estrogen receptor sites on the tumor react with circulating estrogen, and this reaction stimulates the tumor cells to grow and divide. Several antineoplastic agents are used to block or interfere with these receptor sites so as to prevent growth of the cancer and in some situations to actually cause cell death. Some hormones are used to block the release of gonadotropic hormones in breast or prostate cancer if the tumors are responsive to gonadotropic hormones. Others may block androgen receptor sites directly and are useful in the treatment of advanced prostate cancers.

Therapeutic Actions and Indications

The hormones and hormone modulators used as antineoplastics are receptor site–specific or hormone-specific to block the stimulation of growing cancer cells that are sensitive to the presence of that hormone (see Figure 14.3). These drugs are indicated for the treatment of breast cancer in postmenopausal women or in other women without ovarian function, and some are indicated for the treatment of prostatic cancers that are sensitive to hormone manipulation. Table 14.5 lists the hormones and hormone modulators, their uses, and specific information about each drug.

Pharmacokinetics

These drugs are readily absorbed from the GI tract, metabolized in the liver, and excreted in the urine. Caution must be used with any patient who has hepatic or renal impairment. These drugs cross the placenta and enter into breast milk and are contraindicated during pregnancy and lactation because of toxic effects on the neonate.

Contraindications and Cautions

Caution should be used when giving hormones and hormone modulators to anyone with a known allergy to any of these

Table 14.5 DRUGS IN FOCUS

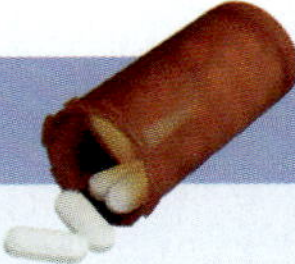

Hormones and Hormone Modulators

Drug Name	Dosage/Route	Usual Indications
anastrazole (*Arimidex*)	1 mg/day PO	Treatment of advanced breast cancer in post-menopausal women after tamoxifen therapy; first-line treatment of postmenopausal women with locally advanced breast cancer **Actions:** Antiestrogen drug; blocks estradiol production without effects on adrenal hormones **Special considerations:** GI effects, signs and symptoms of menopause—hot flashes, mood swings, edema, vaginal dryness and itching—as well as bone pain and back pain, treatable with analgesics, may occur; monitor lipid concentrations in patients at risk for high cholesterol level
bicalutamide (*Casodex*)	50 mg/day PO	In combination with a luteinizing hormone for the treatment of advanced prostate cancer **Actions:** Antiandrogen drug that competitively binds androgen receptor sites **Special considerations:** Gynecomastia and breast tenderness occur in 33% of patients; GI complaints are common. Pregnancy category X.
estramustine (*Emcyt*)	10–16 mg/kg/day PO in three to four divided doses for 30–90 days, then re-evaluate	Palliative for treatment of metastatic and progressive prostate cancer **Actions:** Binds to estrogen steroid receptors, causing cell death **Special considerations:** GI toxicity, rash, bone marrow depression, breast tenderness, and cardiovascular toxicity are common adverse effects; 30–90 days of therapy may be required before effects are seen; monitor cardiovascular, liver, and bone marrow function throughout therapy
exemestane (*Aromasin*)	25 mg/day PO with meals	Treatment of advanced, metastatic breast cancer in postmenopausal women whose disease has progressed after tamoxifen therapy. **Actions:** Inactivates steroid aromatase, lowering circulating estrogen levels and preventing the conversion of androgens to estrogen. **Special considerations:** Avoid use in premenopause, or with liver or renal dysfunction; hot flashes, headache, GI upset, anxiety, and depression are common.
flutamide (*Eulexin*)	250 mg PO t.i.d. given 8 h apart	With a luteinizing hormone for treatment of locally confined and metastatic prostate cancer **Actions:** Antiestrogenic drug, inhibits androgen uptake and binding on target cells **Special considerations:** May cause liver toxicity, so liver function should be monitored regularly; associated with impaired fertility and cancer development; urine may become greenish; protect patient from exposure to the sun—photosensitivity is common
fulvestrant (*Faslodex*)	250 mg IM at 1-mo intervals	Treatment of hormone receptor-positive metastatic breast cancer in postmenopausal women with disease progression after antiestrogen therapy. **Actions:** Competitively binds to estrogen receptors, downregulating the estrogen receptor protein in breast cancer cells. **Special considerations:** Pregnancy category X; hot flashes, depression, headache, and GI upset are common; mark calendar with monthly injection dates; injection site reactions may occur.
goserelin (*Zoladex*)	3.6–10.8 mg implant, Sub-Q, every 28 days to 12 wk	Treatment of advanced prostatic and breast cancers; management of endometriosis **Actions:** Synthetic luteinizing hormone that inhibits pituitary release of gonadotropic hormones **Special considerations:** 3.6-mg dose is effective in decreasing the signs and symptoms of endometriosis; associated with hypercalcemia and bone density loss—monitor serum calcium levels regularly; impairs fertility and is carcinogenic; monitor male patients for possible ureteral obstruction, especially during the first month
histrelin (*Vantas*)	50-mg implant every 12 mo	Palliative treatment of advanced prostate cancer **Actions:** Inhibits gonadotropic secretion; decreases follicle-stimulating hormone and luteinizing hormone levels and testosterone levels **Special considerations:** Must be surgically implanted and removed; hot flashes very common; monitor implantation site
letrozole (*Femara*)	2.5 mg/day PO	Treatment of advanced breast cancer in postmenopausal women with disease after antiestrogen therapy **Actions:** Prevents the conversion of precursors to estrogens in all tissues **Special considerations:** GI toxicity, bone marrow depression, alopecia, hot flashes, and CNS depression are common effects; discontinue drug at any sign that the cancer is progressing

(continued)

Table 14.5 DRUGS IN FOCUS *(Continued)*

Hormones and Hormone Modulators

Drug Name	Dosage/Route	Usual Indications
leuprolide (*Lupron*)	3.7–30 mg by injection, implant, or depot every 1–4 mos, depending on preparation used	Treatment of advanced prostate cancer; also used to treat precocious puberty and endometriosis **Actions:** A natural luteinizing hormone that blocks the release of gonadotropic hormones **Special considerations:** Monitor cancer patient's prostate-specific antigen levels periodically; monitor bone density and serum calcium levels; warn patient that he may have difficulty voiding the first few weeks and may experience bone pain, hot flashes, and pain at injection site
megestrol (*Megace*)	*Breast cancer:* 160 mg/day PO *Endometrial cancer:* 40–320 mg/day PO	Palliative treatment of advanced breast or endometrial cancer **Actions:** Blocks luteinizing hormone release; efficacy not understood **Special Considerations:** Monitor for thromboembolic events and weight gain; not for use during pregnancy
nilutamide (*Nilandron*)	300 mg/day PO for 30 days, then 150 mg/day PO	With surgical castration for treatment of metastatic prostate cancer **Actions:** Antiestrogenic drug, inhibits androgen uptake and binding on target cells **Special considerations:** May cause liver toxicity, and liver function test results should be monitored regularly; associated with interstitial pneumonitis—baseline and periodic chest radiographs should be obtained, and discontinue drug at first sign of dyspnea
P tamoxifen (*Nolvadex*)	20–40 mg/day PO	In combination therapy with surgery to treat breast cancer; treatment of advanced breast cancer in men and women; first drug approved for the prevention of breast cancer in women at high risk for breast cancer **Actions:** Antiestrogen, competes with estrogen for receptor sites in target tissues **Special considerations:** Signs and symptoms of menopause are common effects; CNS depression, bone marrow depression, and GI toxicity are also common; can change visual acuity and cause corneal opacities and retinopathy—pretherapy and periodic ophthalmic examinations are indicated
testolactone (*Teslac*)	250 mg PO q.i.d.	Treatment of breast cancer in postmenopausal women and in premenopausal women in whom ovarian function has been terminated **Actions:** Synthetic androgen; antineoplastic effects in postmenopausal women with breast cancer are not clearly understood—thought to act via competitive reaction for estrogen receptor sites **Special considerations:** GI effects and hypercalcemia are common reactions; virilization—hirsutism, deepening of voice, clitoral enlargement, facial hair growth, altered libido—is often an unacceptable reaction that limits drug use in some women; monitoring of serum calcium is important during the course of the therapy; a class III controlled substance
toremifene (*Fareston*)	60 mg/day PO	Treatment of advanced breast cancer in women with estrogen receptor–positive disease **Actions:** Binds to estrogen receptors and prevents growth of breast cancer cells **Special considerations:** Signs and symptoms of menopause are common effects; CNS depression and GI toxicity are also common
triptorelin pamoate (*Trelstar Depot*)	3.75-mg IM depot monthly or 11.25-mg IM depot every 3 mo	Treatment of advanced prostatic cancer. **Actions:** Analog of LHRH, causes a decrease in FHS and LH levels, leading to a suppression of testosterone production. **Special considerations:** Monitor PSA and testosterone levels regularly; sexual dysfunction, urinary tract symptoms, bone pain, and hot flashes are common; schedule depot injections and mark calendars for patient.

drugs; during pregnancy, *when blocking of estrogen effects or any gonadotropic effects can lead to fetal death and serious problems for the mother;* and during lactation. Care should also be taken in patients with bone marrow suppression, *which is often the index for redosing and dosing levels,* and in those with renal or hepatic dysfunction, *which could interfere with the metabolism or excretion of these drugs and often indicates a need to change the dosage.* Hypercalcemia is a contraindication to the use of toremifene, *which is known to increase calcium levels.*

Adverse Effects

Adverse effects frequently encountered with the use of these drugs involve the effects that are seen when estrogen is blocked or inhibited. Menopause-associated effects include hot flashes, vaginal spotting, vaginal dryness, moodiness, and depression. Other effects include bone marrow suppression and GI toxicity, including hepatic dysfunction. Hypercalcemia is also encountered as the calcium is pulled out of the bones without estrogen activity to promote calcium deposition.

Clinically Important Drug–Drug Interactions

If hormones and hormone modulators are taken with oral anticoagulants, there is often an increased risk of bleeding. Care should also be taken with any drugs that might increase serum lipid levels.

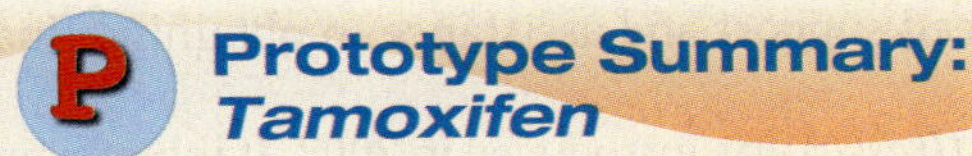

Prototype Summary: Tamoxifen

Indications: Treatment of metastatic breast cancer, reduction of risk of invasive breast cancer in women with ductal carcinoma in situ, reduction in occurrence of contralateral breast cancer in patients receiving adjuvant tamoxifen therapy, reduction in incidence of breast cancer in women at high risk for breast cancer, treatment of McCune-Albright syndrome, and treatment of precocious puberty in female patients 2–10 years of age

Actions: Competes with estrogen for binding sites in target tissues, such as the breast; a potent antiestrogenic agent

Pharmacokinetics:

Route	Onset	Peak
Oral	Varies	4–7 h

$T_{1/2}$: 7–14 days; metabolized in the liver and excreted in the feces

Adverse effects: Hot flashes, rash, nausea, vomiting, vaginal bleeding, menstrual irregularities, edema, pain, cerebrovascular accident, pulmonary emboli

Nursing Considerations for Patients Receiving Hormones and Hormone Modulators

Assessment: History and Examination

Screen for the following, *which could be cautions or contraindications to the use of the drug:* history of allergy to the drug in use or any related drugs, bone marrow suppression, renal or hepatic dysfunction, pregnancy or lactation, hypercalcemia, and hypercholesterolemia.

Physical assessment should be performed *to establish baseline data for determining the effectiveness of the drug and the occurrence of any adverse effects associated with drug therapy.* Include screening for orientation and reflexes *to evaluate any CNS effects;* skin, *to evaluate for lesions;* hair and hair distribution *to monitor for adverse drug effects;* blood pressure, pulse, and perfusion *to evaluate the status of the cardiovascular system and monitor for adverse drug effects;* and bowel sounds and mucous membrane status *to monitor for GI effects.* Evaluate the CBC with differential, serum calcium levels, and renal and liver function tests *to monitor for dosage adjustment as needed and to evaluate toxic drug effects.*

Nursing Diagnoses

The patient receiving a hormone or hormone modulator may have the following nursing diagnoses related to drug therapy:

- Acute Pain related to GI, CNS, menopausal effects of drug
- Disturbed Body Image related to antiestrogen effects, virilization
- Fear, Anxiety related to diagnosis and treatment
- Deficient Knowledge regarding drug therapy

Implementation With Rationale

- Arrange for blood tests to monitor bone marrow function before and periodically during therapy *to discontinue the drug or reduce the dose as needed.*
- Provide small, frequent meals; frequent mouth care; and dietary consultation as appropriate *to maintain nutrition when GI effects are severe.*
- Provide comfort measures *to help the patient cope with menopausal signs and symptoms* such as hygiene measures, temperature control, and stress reduction. Reduce the dosage if these effects become severe or intolerable.
- Advise the patient of the need to use barrier contraceptive measures while taking these drugs *to avert serious fetal harm.*
- Provide patient teaching *to enhance patient knowledge about drug therapy and to promote compliance regarding:*
  - The appropriate dosage regimen, including dates to return for further doses.
  - Maintenance of nutrition even if GI effects are severe.
  - Not taking these drugs during pregnancy and using barrier contraceptives.
  - Staying in a cool environment.
  - Practicing good hygiene and skin care and using stress reduction to cope with menopausal effects.

Evaluation

- Monitor patient response to the drug (alleviation of cancer being treated and palliation of signs and symptoms of cancer being treated).
- Monitor for adverse effects (bone marrow suppression, GI toxicity, menopausal signs and symptoms, hypercalcemia, and cardiovascular effects).
- Evaluate the effectiveness of the teaching plan (patient can name the drug, dosage, possible adverse effects to watch for, and specific measures to help avoid adverse effects).

Cancer Cell-Specific Agents

Imatinib mesylate (*Gleevec*) was approved in 2001 for the treatment of adults with chronic myeloid leukemia (CML) who are in blast crisis, accelerated phase, or chronic phase after failure with interferon-alpha therapy; it has since also been approved for use in the treatment of patients with CD117 positive unresectable or metastatic malignant GI stromal tumors (GIST). This oral antineoplastic drug is a protein tyrosine kinase inhibitor that selectively inhibits the Bcr-Abl tyrosine kinase created by the Philadelphia chromosome abnormality in CML; this inhibits proliferation and induces apoptosis in the Bcr-Abl–positive cell lines as well as fresh leukemic cells, thereby inhibiting tumor growth in CML patients in blast crisis. It also inhibits the CD117 site in GIST patients. Because of its specific effects on these tumor cells, it is not associated with adverse effects on normal human cells. The adverse effects associated with this drug include GI upset, muscle cramps, fluid retention, and skin rash. The bone marrow suppression, alopecia, and severe GI effects associated with more traditional antineoplastic therapy do not occur.

Imatinib is slowly absorbed from the GI tract, reaching peak levels in 2 to 4 hours. It is extensively metabolized in the liver, with a half-life of 18 and then 40 hours. Caution should be used with known hepatic dysfunction and when using drugs affected by the cytochrome P450 enzyme system. St. John's wort decreases the effectiveness of this drug and should be avoided. This drug crosses the placenta and is in pregnancy category D. Women of child-bearing age should be advised to use barrier contraceptives while taking this drug. It can enter breast milk, and it should be used during lactation only if the benefits to the mother clearly outweigh the risks to the baby.

Patients who have CML and who have been switched to this drug after traditional chemotherapy have been amazed at how good they feel and how much they have recovered. Long-term effects are not yet known because the drug is relatively new. It is being researched for possible use in other cancers. The down side to this drug is the cost. It is estimated that 1 year of treatment with the drug (which needs to be taken continually) costs the patient between $30,000 and $35,000. Novartis, the drug company that manufactures *Gleevec,* has set up a patient assistance program with a sliding-scale price reduction based on income. They do not want patients to have to pay more than 20% of their annual income for the drug. Patients prescribed this drug may need support and assistance in obtaining financial help.

Gefitinib (*Iressa*) was introduced in 2003. It inhibits tyrosine kinases, including ones associated with epidermal growth factor receptors. It is indicated as monotherapy for the treatment of patients with locally advanced or metastatic non–small cell lung cancer after failure with platinum-based or docetaxel chemotherapies. This drug has been associated with potentially severe interstitial lung disease and various eye symptoms. Table 14.6 discusses these two drugs. In 2005, the U.S. Food and Drug Administration (FDA) announced that postmarketing studies did not support the use of gefitinib. Patients taking the drug did not live longer than patients using less toxic therapy. The Iressa Access Program was put into place in mid-2005 to ensure the proper use of the drug, limiting its availability to only those patients who had done well on gefitinib therapy. Initiation of *Iressa* therapy is no longer supported.

In 2003, the FDA approved bortezomib (*Velcade*) for the treatment of multiple myeloma in patients whose disease had progressed after two other standard therapies. This drug inhibits proteasome in human cells, a large protein complex that works to maintain cell homeostasis and protein production. Without it, the cell loses homeostasis and dies. This drug was shown to delay tumor growth in selected tumors. It is given intravenously, is metabolized in the liver by the cytochrome P450 system, and is excreted in feces and urine. The half-life varies with the disease being treated, ranging from 9 to 15 hours. It should not be used during pregnancy, following fetal abnormalities in animal studies. It may cross into breast milk, so nursing mothers should find another method of feeding the baby. This drug can cause peripheral neuropathies, hypotension, and bone marrow suppression. Renal and liver function should be monitored closely. Since it is metabolized by the cytochrome P450 system, there is potential for numerous drug interactions. Check your drug guide before administering this drug with any other drugs.

In late 2004, the FDA approved erlotinib (*Tarceva*), a drug that inhibits cell epidermal growth factor receptors. This growth factor is found on normal and cancerous cells. Erlotinib is approved for the treatment of non–small cell lung cancer that is locally advanced after failure of at least one other standard drug regimen. This drug is rapidly absorbed orally, reaching peak levels in 4 hours. It is metabolized in the liver, requiring caution in patients with hepatic

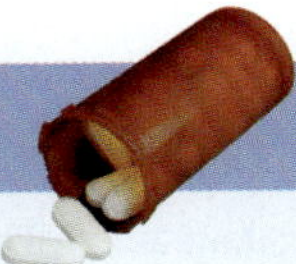

Table 14.6 DRUGS IN FOCUS

Cancer Cell–Specific Agents

Drug Name	Dosage/Route	Usual Indications
bortezomib (*Velcade*)	1.3 mg/m² by bolus IV injection on days 1, 4, 8, and 11, followed by 10 days of rest	Treatment of multiple myeloma in patients with disease progression after two other therapies **Actions:** Blocks cellular homeostasis by inhibiting proteasome, causing cell death and delaying tumor growth **Special considerations:** May cause peripheral neuropathies, hypotension, and bone marrow suppression; do not use during pregnancy
erlotinib (*Tarceva*)	150 mg/day PO 1 h before or 2 h after meal	Treatment of locally advanced or metastatic non–small cell lung cancer after failure of at least one other drug regimen **Actions:** Inhibits tyrosine kinase associated with epidermal growth factor, expressed on surface of normal and cancer cells **Special considerations:** Serious to fatal interstitial lung disease—monitor with hepatic impairment; do not use during pregnancy
gefitinib (*Iressa*)	250 mg/day PO	Monotherapy for non–small cell lung cancer in patients with locally advanced disease and no response to platinum-based or docetaxel therapy; use limited to patients doing well on therapy—not for new use. **Actions:** Inhibits various tyrosine kinases, including ones associated with epidermal growth factor. **Special considerations:** Interstitial lung disease may occur; monitor pulmonary function closely; eye changes may require stopping the drug for a while; do not use during pregnancy; numerous drug–drug interactions are possible.
imatinib (*Gleevec*)	*Chronic phase CML:* 400 mg/day PO, may be increased to 600 mg/day if needed *Blast crisis CML:* 600 mg/day PO, may increase to 400 mg PO b.i.d. *First-line CML treatment:* 400 mg/day PO *GIST:* 400–600 mg/day PO	Treatment of CML patients in blast crisis or in chronic phase after interferon alpha therapy; treatment of patients with Kit-positive malignant GI stromal tumors (GIST); first-line treatment of CML. **Actions:** Inhibits the Bcr-Abl tyrosine kinase, inhibiting cell proliferation and blocking tumor growth. **Special considerations:** Administer with a meal and a full glass of water; arrange for small, frequent meals if GI upset is a problem; provide analgesics for headache and muscle pain; monitor CBC and for edema to arrange for dosage reduction if needed; patient should receive consultation to deal with high cost of drug.

impairment; is excreted in the feces and urine; and has a half-life of 36 hours. Erlotinib has been associated with maternal toxicity and fetal death in animals and should not be used during pregnancy. It is not known whether it crosses into breast milk, but because of the potential for severe toxicity in the baby, another method of feeding the baby should be used during drug therapy. This drug is associated with severe to fatal interstitial lung disease, severe diarrhea, and severe skin reactions. It is metabolized by the cytochrome P450 system and could interact with any other drugs that use that system.

Miscellaneous Antineoplastic Agents

Many other agents that do not fit into one of the previously discussed groups are used as antineoplastics to cause cell death. These drugs are used for treating a wide variety of cancers. Table 14.7 lists the unclassified antineoplastic drugs, their indications, and anticipated adverse effects. Specific information about each drug may be obtained in your nursing drug guide. (See Figure 14.3 for sites of action of the miscellaneous antineoplastic agents.)

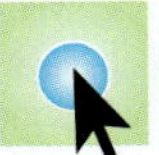

WEB LINKS

Health care providers and patients may want to consult the following Internet sources:

http://cancer.gov/cancer_information Information on cancer, including research, protocols, and new information, maintained by the National Cancer Institute of the National Institutes of Health.

http://cancerguide.org Information on cancer care and general patient education.

www.angio.org Information on angiogenesis research and clinical studies.

http://www.cancer.org Information on numerous cancer connections, support groups, treatment, and resources.

http://www.acor.org Information about online resources related to all types of cancer.

http://www.ons.org Information about the Oncology Nursing Society.

Table 14.7 DRUGS IN FOCUS

Miscellaneous Antineoplastics

Drug Name	Dosage/Route	Usual Indications
altretamine (*Hexalen*)	260 mg/m²/day PO for 14–21 days in a 28-day cycle	Single agent used in the palliative treatment of persistent or recurrent ovarian cancer **Actions:** Cytotoxic; mechanism of action unknown **Special considerations:** Severe bone marrow depression and peripheral sensory neuropathy as well as severe GI toxicity can limit the use of this drug; a 14-day rest may alleviate the side effects sufficiently to allow redosing
arsenic trioxide (*Trisenox*)	Induction: 0.15 mg/kg/day IV until remission Consolidation: continue 3–6 wk after inducting for up to 25 doses	Induction and consolidation in patients with acute promyelocytic leukemia (APL) who are refractory to or relapsed from standard therapy **Actions:** Causes damage to fusion proteins and DNA failure leading to cell death **Special considerations:** Monitor for cardiac toxicity; do not use during pregnancy
asparaginase (*Elspar*)	1000–6000 units/m² IM or IV and specific days as part of a specific combination regimen	As part of combination therapy to induce remission in children with acute lymphocytic leukemia **Actions:** An enzyme that hydrolyzes the amino acid asparagine, which is needed by malignant cells for protein synthesis; inhibits cell proliferation; most effective in G_1 phase of the cell cycle **Special considerations:** Can cause severe bone marrow depression, renal toxicity, and fatal hyperthermia; hypersensitivity reactions to this drug are common, and patients should be tested and desensitized, if necessary, before using the drug
bortezomib (*Velcade*)	1.3 mg/m²/dose by bolus IV injection twice weekly for 2 wk, followed by 10 days of rest; repeat cycle	Treatment of multiple myeloma in patients who have received at least two prior therapies and have progression of disease **Actions:** Inhibits proteasome in mammalian cells, disrupting normal homeostasis within the cell and causing cell death **Special considerations:** Sensory peripheral neuropathy occurs; provide for patient protection; monitor CBC and adjust for bone marrow suppression; nausea, vomiting, and diarrhea are common; antidiarrheals and antiemetics should be considered
dacarbazine (*DTIC-Dome*)	2–4.5 mg/kg/day IV for 10 days, repeat at 4-wk intervals; or 150–250 mg/m²/day IV for 5 days in combination with other drugs	Treatment of metastatic malignant melanoma and as second-line therapy in combination with other drugs for the treatment of Hodgkin's disease **Actions:** Inhibits DNA and RNA synthesis, causing cell death; cell-cycle nonspecific **Special considerations:** Bone marrow depression, GI toxicity and severe photosensitivity are common effects; extravasation can cause tissue necrosis or cellulitis—use extreme care and monitor injection sites regularly
gemcitabine (*Gemzar*)	1000 mg/m² IV over 30 min, once a week for 7 wk, then 3 wk of treatment followed by 1 wk of rest	First-line treatment of locally advanced or metastatic adenocarcinoma of the pancreas in patients who have received fluorouracil (5-FU); with cisplatin for advanced non–small cell lung cancer **Actions:** S-phase cell-cycle specific; causes cell death by disrupting DNA and RNA synthesis **Special considerations:** Can cause severe bone marrow depression, GI toxicity, pain, and alopecia; interstitial pneumonitis
hydroxyurea (*Hydrea*)	20–30 mg/kg PO daily	Inhibits enzymes essential for the synthesis of DNA, causing cell death **Actions:** Treatment of melanoma, ovarian cancer, chronic myelocytic leukemia; in combination therapy for primary squamous cell cancers of the head and neck; also used in the treatment of sickle cell anemia **Special considerations:** Can cause bone marrow depression, headache, rash, GI toxicity, and renal dysfunction; encourage patient to drink 10–12 glasses of water each day while taking this drug
irinotecan (*Camptosar*)	125 mg/m² IV over 90 min, once a week for 4 wk, followed by 2 wk of rest; repeat every 6 wk	Treatment of metastatic colon or rectal cancer after treatment with 5-FU **Actions:** Disrupts DNA strands during DNA synthesis, causing cell death **Special considerations:** Can cause severe bone marrow depression, which regulates dose of the drug; causes GI toxicity, dyspnea, and alopecia
mitotane (*Lysodren*)	2–6 mg PO in divided doses t.i.d. to q.i.d. to a maximum of 9–10 g/day	Treatment of inoperable adrenocortical carcinoma **Actions:** Cytotoxic to corticosteroid-forming cells of the adrenal gland **Special considerations:** Can cause GI toxicity, CNS toxicity with vision and behavioral changes, adrenal insufficiency; monitor for adrenal insufficiency and arrange for replacement therapy as indicated
pegasparagase (*Oncaspar*)	2500 International units/m² IM or IV q14d	Treatment of acute lymphocytic leukemia in patients who are hypersensitive to asparaginase **Actions:** An enzyme that hydrolyzes the amino acid asparaginase, which is needed by malignant cells for protein synthesis; inhibits cell proliferation; most effective in G_1 phase of the cell cycle

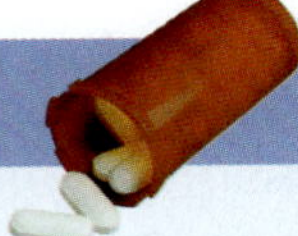

Table 14.7 DRUGS IN FOCUS (Continued)

Miscellaneous Antineoplastics

Drug Name	Dosage/Route	Usual Indications
		Special considerations: Can cause potentially fatal hyperthermia, bone marrow depression, renal toxicity, and pancreatitis, monitor patient regularly, and arrange decreased dosage as appropriate if toxic effects occur
porfimer (*Photofrin*)	2 mg/kg IV over 3–5 min; may repeat in 40–50 h and again in 96–120 h	Photosensitizing agent that is used with laser light to decrease tumor size in patients with obstructive esophageal cancers not responsive to laser treatment alone **Actions:** Taken up by cells, causing radical reactions when cells are exposed to laser light, causing cell death. **Special considerations:** Has been associated with pleural effusion and fistula; associated with GI and cardiac toxicity; must be given in conjunction with scheduled laser treatment, with at least 30 days between treatments; protect patient from exposure to light with protective clothing for 30 days after treatment (sunscreens are not effective); avoid direct contact with the drug—protective clothing and goggles are suggested
procarbazine (*Matulane*)	Adult: 2–6 mg/kg/day PO; base the dose on bone marrow response Pediatric: 50 mg/m²/day, adjust based on bone marrow response	Used in combination therapy for treatment of stage III and IV Hodgkin's disease **Actions:** Inhibits DNA, RNA, and protein synthesis, leading to cell death **Special considerations:** Bone marrow toxicity; GI toxicity and skin lesions also limit use in some patients; severity of adverse effects regulates the dose of the drug
talc powder (*Sclerosol*)	4–8-g spray through open thoracotomy or during thoracoscopy	Prevention of recurrence of malignant pleural effusion **Actions:** Induces the inflammatory response, promoting adhesion of the pleura and preventing accumulation of fluid **Special considerations:** Monitor for cardiac and respiratory effects; no actual antineoplastic actions
temozolomide (*Temodar*)	75 mg/m²/day PO with radiation	Treatment of refractory astrocytoma or glioblastoma in patients refractory to other treatments **Actions:** Prevents proliferation of tumor cells by affecting DNA and guanine-rich links **Special considerations:** Monitor bone marrow closely; especially toxic in women and elderly
topotecan (*Hycamtin*)	1.5 mg/m²/day IV for 5 days; as part of a 2-day course; minimum of four courses	Treatment of patients with metastatic ovarian cancer after failure of other agents **Actions:** Damages DNA strand, causing cell death during cell division **Special considerations:** Can cause severe bone marrow depression, which regulates the dose of the drug; total alopecia, GI toxicity, and CNS effects may also limit the use of the drug; analgesics may be helpful
tretinoin (*Vesanoid*)	45 mg/m²/day PO for 30 days	Used to induce remission in APL; can cause severe respiratory and cardiac toxicity, including myocardial infarction and cardiac arrest **Actions:** Promotes cell differentiation and the repopulation of the bone marrow with normal cells in patients with APL **Special considerations:** GI toxicity, pseudotumor cerebri (papilledema, headache, nausea, vomiting, visual changes), skin rash, and fragility may limit use in some patients; discontinue drug at first sign of toxic effects; use for induction of remission only—then other chemotherapeutic agents should be used

Points to Remember

- Cancers arise from a single abnormal cell that multiplies and grows.
- Cancers can manifest as diseases of the blood and lymph tissue or as growth of tumors arising from epithelial cells (carcinomas) or from mesenchymal cells and connective tissue (sarcomas).
- Cancer cells lose their normal function (anaplasia), develop characteristics that allow them to grow in an uninhibited way (autonomy), have the ability to travel to other sites in the body that are conducive to their growth (metastasis), and can stimulate the production of blood vessels to bring nutrients to the growing tumor (angiogenesis).
- Antineoplastic drugs affect both normal cells and cancer cells by disrupting cell function and division at various points in the cell cycle; new drugs are being developed, such as kinase inhibitors, to target cancer cell–specific functions.
- Cancer drugs are usually most effective against cells that multiply rapidly (i.e., proceed through the cell cycle quickly). These cells include most neoplasms, bone marrow cells, cells in the GI tract, and cells in the skin or hair follicles.
- The goal of cancer chemotherapy is to decrease the size of the neoplasm so that the human immune system can deal with it.
- Antineoplastic drugs are often given in combination so that they can affect cells in various stages of the cell

cycle, including cells that are emerging from rest or moving to a phase of the cycle that is disrupted by these drugs.

- Adverse effects associated with antineoplastic therapy include effects caused by damage to the rapidly multiplying cells, such as bone marrow suppression, which may limit the drug use; GI toxicity, with nausea, vomiting, mouth sores, and diarrhea; and alopecia (hair loss).
- Chemotherapeutic agents should not be used during pregnancy or lactation because they may result in potentially serious adverse effects on the rapidly multiplying cells of the neonate.

CHECK YOUR UNDERSTANDING

Answer to the questions in this chapter may be found in the Answer Key in the back of the book.

Multiple Choice

Select the best answer to the following.

1. Many properties of neoplastic cells are different from those of normal cells, with the exception of
   a. anaplasia.
   b. metastasis.
   c. mitosis.
   d. autonomy.

2. Carcinomas are tumors that
   a. originate in the mesenchyma and are made up of embryonic connective tissue cells.
   b. originate in the bone marrow and affect the blood.
   c. originate in the striated muscle.
   d. originate in epithelial cells.

3. The goal of traditional antineoplastic drug therapy is to
   a. reduce the size of the mass of abnormal cells so that the immune system can take care of destroying them.
   b. eradicate all of the abnormal cells that have developed.
   c. destroy all cells of the originating type.
   d. stimulate the immune system to destroy the neoplastic cells.

4. Cancer can be a difficult disease to treat because
   a. cells no longer progress through the normal cell cycle.
   b. cells can develop resistance to drug therapy.
   c. cells can remain in the dormant state for long periods and emerge months to years later.
   d. the exact cause of cancer is not known.

5. Antineoplastic drugs destroy human cells. They are most likely to cause cell death among healthy cells that
   a. have poor cell membranes.
   b. are rapidly turning over and progress through their cell cycle rapidly.
   c. are in dormant tissues.
   d. are across the blood–brain barrier.

6. Cancer treatment usually occurs in several different treatment phases. In assessing appropriateness of another round of chemotherapy for a particular patient, the nurse would evaluate
   a. hair loss.
   b. bone marrow function.
   c. anorexia.
   d. heart rate.

7. It is important to explain to women that chemotherapeutic agents should not be used during pregnancy because
   a. the tendency to cause nausea and vomiting will be increased.
   b. of potentially serious adverse effects on the rapidly multiplying cells of the fetus.
   c. bone marrow toxicity could alter hormone levels.
   d. patients may be weakened by the drug regimen.

8. Most cancer drugs are most effective against
   a. slowly growing cells.
   b. cells in the dormant phase of the cell cycle.
   c. cells that multiply rapidly and go through the cell cycle quickly.
   d. cells that have moved from their normal site in the body.

Multiple Response

Select all that apply.

1. Patient teaching can be very important in helping the client receiving cancer chemotherapy. It is important for the nurse to stress which of the following points?
   a. The importance of keeping the head covered at extremes of temperature
   b. The need to use barrier contraceptives because of the risk of serious fetal effects
   c. The importance of avoiding exposure to infection because the ability to heal or to fight infection is impaired

d. The importance of avoiding food if nausea or vomiting is a problem
e. The importance of avoiding digging in the dirt without protective coverings because of the many pathogens that live in the dirt that could cause infection
f. The importance of taking periodic rest periods during the day because you will feel tired when your red blood cell count falls

2. Hair loss, or alopecia, is an adverse effect of many antineoplastic agents. If a client is receiving a drug that usually causes alopecia, it is important that the nurse do which of the following?
   a. Warn the patient that alopecia will occur.
   b. Encourage the patient to arrange for an appropriate head covering at extremes of temperature.
   c. Advise the patient to lie with the legs elevated and head low to promote circulation and prevent hair loss.
   d. Encourage the patient to arrange for a wig or other head covering before the hair loss occurs.
   e. Advise the patient that people will stare and can be rude when hair loss occurs.
   f. Make arrangements for the patient to attend a support group before hair loss happens.

Matching

Match the word with the appropriate definition.

1. ______________________ anaplasia
2. ______________________ alopecia
3. ______________________ carcinoma
4. ______________________ metastasize
5. ______________________ neoplasm
6. ______________________ sarcoma
7. ______________________ autonomy
8. ______________________ antineoplastic

A. Tumors in the mesenchyma, composed of embryonic connective tissue cells
B. Drugs used to combat cancer
C. Tumors starting in epithelial cells
D. Loss of organization and structure
E. To travel throughout the body via lymph and circulation
F. New growth or cancer
G. Loss of hair
H. Loss of normal controls and reactions that limit cell growth and spreading

Word Scramble

Unscramble the following words to form the names of commonly used antineoplastic agents.

1. tlvniinsaeb ______________________
2. mcenualtirs ______________________
3. cnbporatali ______________________
4. psnitilac ______________________
5. fnxiometa ______________________
6. embyloeni ______________________
7. nezabacadri ______________________
8. pdeteosoi ______________________

Bibliography and References

Baquiran, D. C. (2001). *Lippincott's cancer chemotherapy handbook* (2nd ed.). Philadelphia: Lippincott Williams & Wilkins.

DeVita, V. T., Hellman, S., & Rosenberg, S. A. (2005). *Cancer: Principles and practice of oncology* (7th ed.). Philadelphia: Lippincott Williams & Wilkins.

Drug facts and comparisons. (2006). St. Louis: Facts and Comparisons.

Gilman, A., Hardman, J. G., & Limbird, L. E. (Eds.). (2006). *Goodman and Gilman's the pharmacological basis of therapeutics* (11th ed.). New York: McGraw-Hill.

Grochow, L. B., & Ames, M. M. (1998). *A clinician's guide to chemotherapy pharmacokinetics and pharmacodynamics.* Baltimore: Williams & Wilkins.

Karch, A. M. (2006). *2007 Lippincott's nursing drug guide.* Philadelphia: Lippincott Williams & Wilkins.

Navarro, T. M. (1998). Chemotherapy extravasation. *American Journal of Nursing, 98*(11), 38.

Porth, C. M. (2005). *Pathophysiology: Concepts of altered health states* (7th ed.). Philadelphia: Lippincott Williams and Wilkins.

Professional's guide to patient drug facts. (2006). St. Louis: Facts and Comparisons.

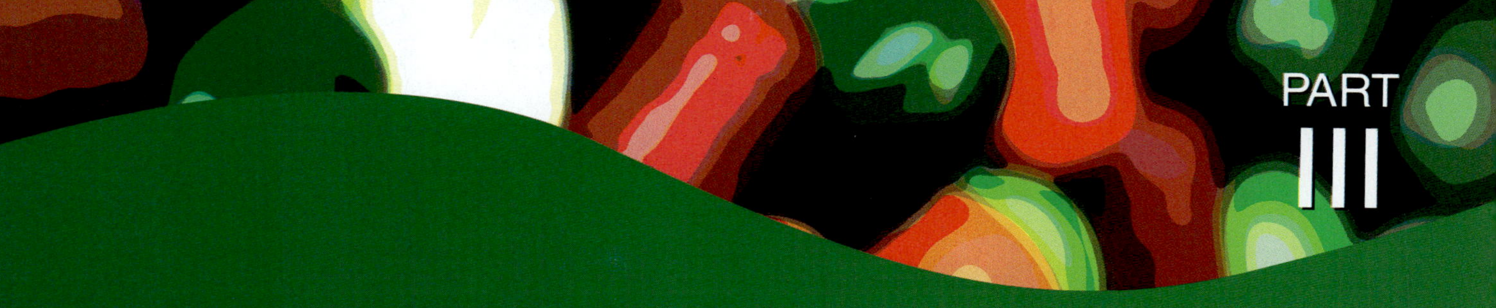

PART III

Drugs Acting on the Immune System

CHAPTER 15

Introduction to the Immune Response and Inflammation

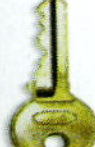

KEY TERMS

antibodies
antigen
arachidonic acid
autoimmune disease
B cells
calor
chemotaxis
complement
dolor
Hageman factor
interferons
interleukins
kinin system
leukocytes
lymphocytes
macrophages
myelocytes
phagocytes
phagocytosis
pyrogen
rubor
T cells
tumor

LEARNING OBJECTIVES

Upon completion of this chapter, you will be able to:

1. List four natural body defenses against infection.
2. Outline the sequence of events in the inflammatory response.
3. Correlate the events in the inflammatory response with the clinical picture of inflammation.
4. Describe the cells associated with the body's fight against infection and their basic functions.
5. Outline the sequence of events in an antibody-related immune reaction and correlate these events with the clinical presentation of such a reaction.

The body has many defense systems in place to keep it intact and to protect it from external stressors. These stressors can include bacteria, viruses, other foreign pathogens or nonself-cells, trauma, and exposure to extremes of environmental conditions. The same defense systems that protect the body also help to repair it after cellular trauma or damage. Understanding the basic mechanisms involved in these defense systems helps to explain the actions of the drugs that affect the immune system and inflammation.

Body Defenses

The body's defenses include barrier defenses, cellular defenses, the inflammatory response, and the immune response.

Barrier Defenses

Certain anatomical barriers exist to prevent the entry of foreign pathogens and to serve as important lines of defense in protecting the body.

Skin

The skin is the first line of defense. The skin acts as a physical barrier to protect the internal tissues and organs of the body. Glands in the skin secrete chemicals that destroy or repel many pathogens. The skin sloughs off daily, making it difficult for any pathogen to colonize on the skin. Finally, an array of normal flora bacteria live on the skin and destroy many disease-causing pathogens.

Mucous Membranes

Mucous membranes line the areas of the body that are exposed to external influences but do not have the benefit of skin protection. These body areas include the respiratory tract, which is exposed to air; the gastrointestinal (GI) tract, which is exposed to anything ingested by mouth; and the genitourinary (GU) tract, which is exposed to many pathogens from the rectal area. Like the skin, the mucous membrane is a physical barrier to invasion. It also secretes a sticky mucus, which traps invaders and inactivates them for later destruction and removal by the body. The mucus works much like flypaper trapping flies.

In the respiratory tract, the mucous membrane is lined with tiny, hair-like processes called *cilia*. The cilia sweep any captured pathogens or foreign materials upward toward the mouth, either to be swallowed or to cause irritation to the area and be removed by a cough or a sneeze.

In the GI tract, the mucous membrane serves as a protective coating, preventing erosion of GI cells by the acidic environment of the stomach, the digestive enzymes of the small intestine, and the waste products that accumulate in the large intestine. The mucous membrane also secretes mucus that serves as a lubricant throughout the GI tract to facilitate movement of the food bolus and of waste products.

In the GU tract, the mucous membrane provides direct protection against injury and trauma and traps any pathogens in the area for destruction by the body.

Gastric Acid

The stomach secretes acid in response to many stimuli. The acidity of the stomach not only aids digestion, but also destroys many would-be pathogens that are either ingested or swallowed after removal from the respiratory tract.

Major Histocompatibility Complex

The body's last barrier of defense is the ability to distinguish between self-cells and foreign cells. All of the cells and tissues of each person are marked for identification as part of that individual's genetic code. No two people have exactly the same code. In humans, the genetic identification code is carried on a chromosome and is called the major histocompatibility complex (MHC). The MHC produces several proteins called histocompatibility antigens, or human leukocyte antigens (HLAs), that are found on the cell membrane and allow the body to recognize cells as being self-cells. Cells that do not have these proteins are identified as foreign and are destroyed by the body.

Cellular Defenses

Any foreign pathogen that manages to get past the barrier defenses will encounter the human immune system, or mononuclear phagocyte system (MPS). Previously called the reticuloendothelial system, the MPS is composed of the thymus gland, the lymphatic tissue, leukocytes, lymphocytes, and numerous chemical mediators.

Leukocytes

Stem cells in the bone marrow produce two types of white blood cells or **leukocytes**: lymphocytes and myelocytes. The **lymphocytes** are the key components of the immune system and consist of T cells, B cells, and natural killer cells (see later discussion of the immune response). The **myelocytes** can develop into a number of different cell types that are important in both the basic inflammatory response and the immune response. Myelocytes include neutrophils, basophils, eosinophils, and monocytes, or macrophages (Figure 15.1).

Neutrophils

Neutrophils are polymorphonuclear leukocytes that are capable of diapedesis (moving outside of the bloodstream) and **phagocytosis** (engulfing and digesting foreign material). When the body is injured or invaded by a pathogen, neutrophils are rapidly produced and move to the site of the insult to attack the foreign substance. Because neutrophils are able to engulf and digest foreign material, they are called **phagocytes**. Phagocytes are able to identify nonself-cells by

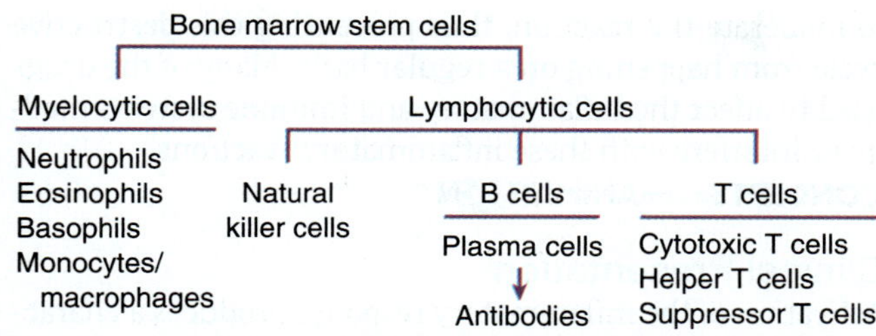

FIGURE 15.1 Types of white blood cells, or leukocytes, produced by the body.

use of the MHC, and they can engulf these cells or mark them for destruction by cytotoxic T cells.

Basophils

Basophils are myelocytic leukocytes that are not capable of phagocytosis. They are full of chemical substances that are important for initiating and maintaining an immune or inflammatory response. These substances include histamine, heparin, and other chemicals used in the inflammatory response.

Eosinophils

Eosinophils are circulating myelocytic leukocytes whose exact function is not understood. They are often found at the site of allergic reactions and may be responsible for removing the proteins and active components of the immune reaction from the site of an allergic response.

Monocytes/Macrophages

Monocytes or mononuclear phagocytes are also called **macrophages**. They are mature leukocytes that are capable of phagocytizing an **antigen** (foreign protein). They also can process antigens and present them to active lymphocytes for destruction. Macrophages can be circulating phagocytes, or they can be fixed in specific tissues, such as the Kupffer cells in the liver, the cells in the alveoli of the respiratory tract, and the microglia in the central nervous system (CNS), GI, circulatory, and lymph tissues. These cells are active phagocytes and can release chemicals that are necessary to elicit a strong inflammatory reaction. Macrophages help remove foreign material from the body, including pathogens, debris from dead cells, and necrotic tissue from injury sites, so that the body can heal. These cells respond to chemical mediators (released by other cells that are active in the inflammatory and immune responses) to increase the intensity of a response and to facilitate the body's reaction. Figure 15.2 shows what these five different types of cells look like.

Mast Cells

Mast cells are fixed basophils that do not circulate; they are found in the respiratory and GI tracts and in the skin. They release many of the chemical mediators of the inflammatory and immune responses when they are stimulated by local irritation.

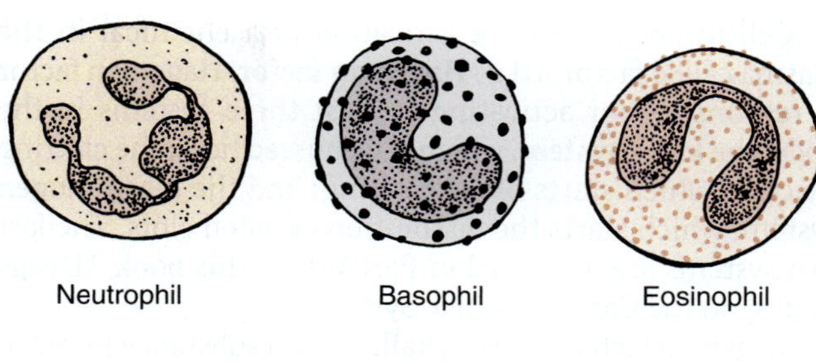

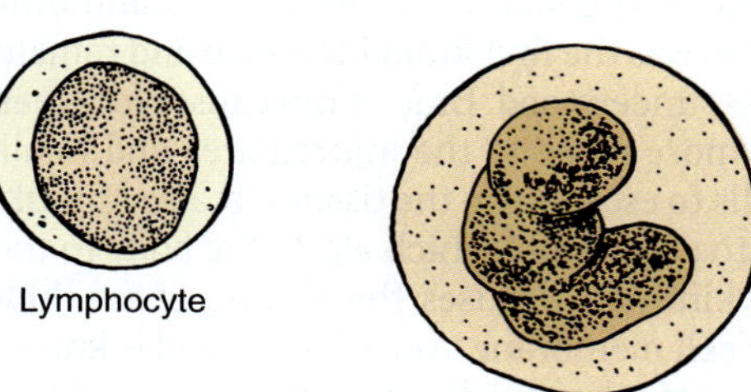

FIGURE 15.2 Appearance of various types of leukocytes.

Tissue and Gland Connections

Lymphoid tissues that play an important part in the cellular defense system include the lymph nodes, spleen, thymus gland (a bipolar gland located in the middle of the chest, which becomes smaller with age), bone marrow, and lymphoid tissue throughout the respiratory and GI tracts. The bone marrow and the thymus gland are important for creation of the cellular components of the MPS and also have a role in their differentiation and regulation. The lymph nodes and lymphoid tissue store concentrated populations of leukocytes and lymphocytes in positions that facilitate their surveillance for and destruction of foreign proteins. Other cells travel through the cardiovascular and lymph systems to search for foreign proteins or to reach the sites of injury or pathogen invasion.

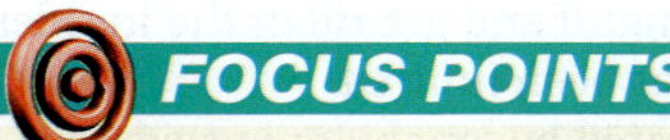

FOCUS POINTS

- The body has several defense mechanisms in place to protect it from injury or foreign invasion. Among them are barrier protectors, such as the skin, mucous membranes, normal flora, and gastric acid, and cellular protectors, such as the lymphocytes (T and B cells), the myelocytes (neutrophils, eosinophils, basophils, and macrophages), and mast cells.

The Inflammatory Response

The inflammatory response is the local reaction of the body to invasion or injury. Any insult to the body that injures cells or tissues sets into action a series of events and chemical reactions.

Cell injury causes the activation of a chemical in the plasma called factor XII or **Hageman factor**. Hageman factor is responsible for activating at least three systems in the body: the **kinin system**, which is discussed here; the clotting cascade, which starts blood clotting; and the plasminogen system, which starts the dissolution of blood clots. The last two systems are discussed in Part VIII of this book, "Drugs Acting on the Cardiovascular System."

Hageman factor activates kallikrein, a substance found in the local tissues, which causes the precursor substance kininogen to be converted to bradykinin and other kinins. Bradykinin was the first kinin identified and remains the one that is best understood. Bradykinin causes local vasodilation to bring more blood to the injured area and to allow white blood cells to escape into the tissues. It also stimulates nerve endings to cause pain, which alerts the body to the injury.

Bradykinin also causes the release of **arachidonic acid** from the cell membrane. Arachidonic acid is known to cause the release of other substances called autacoids. These substances act like local hormones—they are released from cells, cause an effect in the immediate area, and then are broken down. These autacoids include the following:

- Prostaglandins, some of which augment the inflammatory reaction and some of which block it
- Leukotrienes, some of which can cause vasodilation and increased capillary permeability and some of which can block the reactions
- Thromboxanes, which cause local vasoconstriction and facilitate platelet aggregation and blood coagulation

While this series of Hageman factor-initiated events is proceeding, another locally mediated response is occurring. Injury to a cell membrane causes the local release of histamine. Histamine causes vasodilation, which brings more blood and blood components to the area; changes capillary permeability, making it easier for neutrophils and blood chemicals to leave the bloodstream and enter the injured area; and stimulates pain perception. These activities bring neutrophils to the area to engulf and get rid of the invader, or to remove the cell that has been injured.

Some leukotrienes activated by arachidonic acid have a property called **chemotaxis**, which is the ability to attract neutrophils and to stimulate them and other macrophages in the area to be very aggressive. As the neutrophils become active and other chemicals are released into the area, they can injure or destroy local cells. The destruction of a cell results in the release of various lysosomal enzymes from the cell. These enzymes lyse or destroy cell membranes and cellular proteins. They are an important part of biological recycling and the breakdown of once-living tissues after death. In the case of an inflammatory reaction, they can cause local cellular breakdown and further inflammation, which can develop into a vicious cycle leading to cell death.

Many inflammatory diseases, such as rheumatoid arthritis and systemic lupus erythematosus, are examples of these uncontrolled cycles. The prostaglandins and leukotrienes are important to the inflammatory response because they act to moderate the reaction, thus preventing this destructive cycle from happening on a regular basis. Many of the drugs used to affect the inflammatory and immune systems modify or interfere with these inflammatory reactions.

CONCEPTS in action ANIMATION

Clinical Presentation

Activation of the inflammatory response produces a characteristic clinical picture. The Latin words **calor** (heat), **tumor** (swelling), **rubor** (redness), and **dolor** (pain) describe a typical inflammatory reaction. Calor, or heat, occurs because of the increased blood flow to the area. Tumor, or swelling, occurs because of the fluid that leaks into the tissues as a result of the change in capillary permeability. Rubor, or redness, is related again to the increase in blood flow caused by the vasodilation. Dolor, or pain, comes from the activation of pain fibers by histamine and the kinin system. These signs and symptoms occur anytime a cell is injured (Figure 15.3).

For example, if you scratch the top of your hand and wait for about a minute, the direct line of the scratch will be red (rubor) and raised (tumor). If you feel it gently, it will be warmer than the surrounding area (calor). You should also experience a burning sensation or discomfort at the site of the scratch (dolor). Invasion of the lungs by bacteria can produce pneumonia. If the lungs could be examined closely, they would also show the signs and symptoms of inflammation. They would be very red from increased blood flow; fluid would start to leak out of the capillaries (often this can be heard as rales); the patient would complain of chest discomfort; and the increased blood flow to the area of infection would make it appear hot or very active on a scan. No matter what the cause of the insult, the body's local response is the same.

Once the inflammatory response is under way and neutrophils become active, engulfing and digesting injured cells or the invader, they release a chemical that is a natural **pyrogen**, or fever-causing substance. This pyrogen resets specific neurons in the hypothalamus to maintain a higher body temperature, seen clinically as a fever. The higher temperature acts as a catalyst to many of the body's chemical reactions, making the inflammatory and immune responses more effective. Treating fevers remains a controversial subject because lowering a fever decreases the efficiency of the immune and inflammatory responses.

The leukotrienes (activated through the kinin system) affect the brain to induce slow-wave sleep, which is thought to be important for saving energy to fight the invader. They also cause myalgia and arthralgia (muscle and joint pain)—common signs and symptoms of various inflammatory diseases—which also cause reduced activity and save energy. All of these chemical responses make up the total clinical picture of an inflammatory reaction.

The Immune Response

More specific invasion can stimulate a more specific response through the immune system. The lymphocytes produced in the bone marrow by the stem cells can develop into T lym-

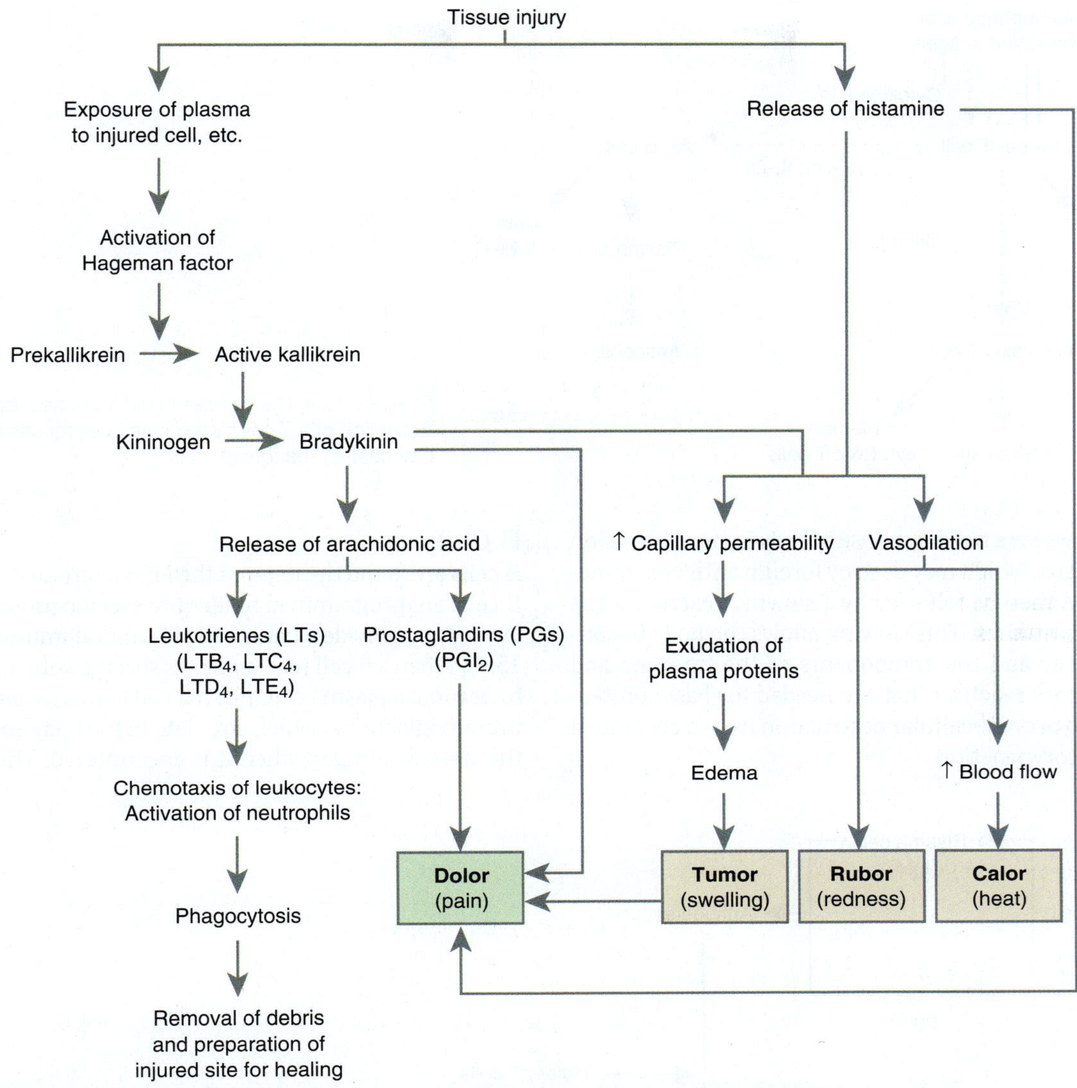

FIGURE 15.3 The inflammatory response in relation to the four cardinal signs of inflammation.

phocytes (so named because they migrate from the bone marrow to the thymus gland for activation and maturation) or B lymphocytes (so named because they are activated in the bursa of Fabricius in the chicken, although the specific point of activation in humans has not been identified). Other identified lymphocytes include natural killer cells and lymphokine-activated killer cells. These cells are aggressive against neoplastic or cancer cells and promote rapid cellular death. They do not seem to be programmed for specific identification of cells. Research in the area of lymphocyte identification is relatively new and continues to grow. There may be other lymphocytes with particular roles in the immune response that have not yet been identified.

T Cells

T cells are programmed in the thymus gland and provide what is called cell-mediated immunity (Figure 15.4). T cells develop into at least three different cell types.

1. *Effector or cytotoxic T cells* are found throughout the body. These T cells are aggressive against nonself-cells, releasing cytokines, or chemicals, that can either directly destroy a foreign cell or mark it for aggressive destruction by phagocytes in the area by eliciting an inflammatory response. These nonself-cells have membrane-identifying antigens that are different from those established by the person's MHC. They may be the body's own cells that have been invaded by a virus, which changes the cell membrane; neoplastic cancer cells; or transplanted foreign cells.
2. *Helper T cells* respond to the chemical indicators of immune activity and stimulate other lymphocytes, including B cells, to be more aggressive and responsive.
3. *Suppressor T cells* respond to rising levels of chemicals associated with an immune response to suppress or slow the reaction. The balance of the helper and suppressor

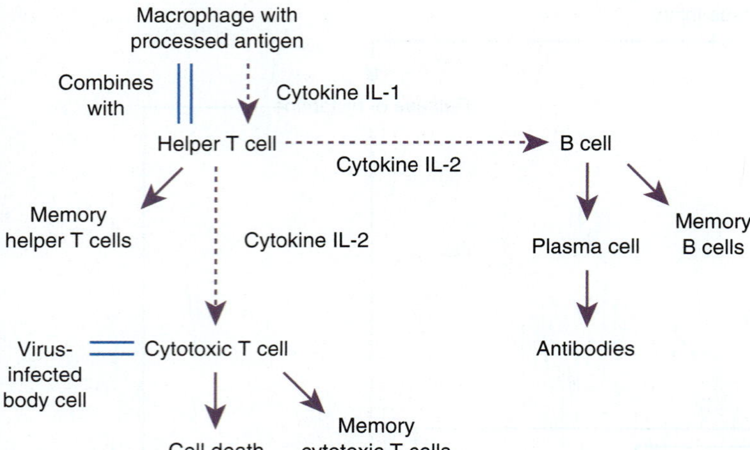

FIGURE 15.4 The cell-mediated immune response. Activation of a T cell by a nonself-cell results in responses that destroy the foreign cell.

T cells allows for a rapid response to body injury or invasion by pathogens, which may destroy foreign antigens immediately and then be followed by a slowing reaction if the invasion continues. This slowing allows the body to conserve energy and the components of the immune and inflammatory reaction that are needed for basic protection and to prevent cellular destruction from a continued inflammatory reaction.

B Cells

B cells are found throughout the MPS in groups called clones. B cells are programmed to identify specific proteins, or antigens. They provide what is called humoral immunity (Figure 15.5). When a B cell reacts with its specific antigen, it changes to become a plasma cell. Plasma cells produce **antibodies**, or immunoglobulins, which circulate in the body and react with this specific antigen when it is encountered. This is a direct

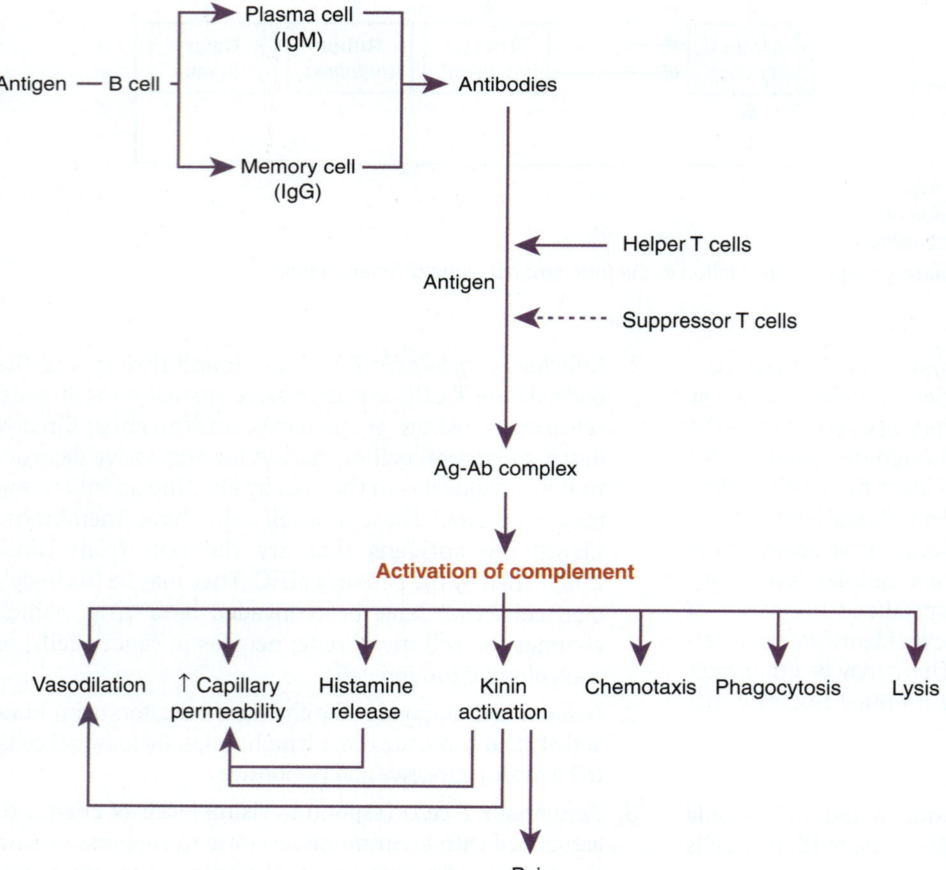

FIGURE 15.5 The humoral immune response.

chemical reaction. When the antigen and antibody react, they form an antigen–antibody complex. This new structure reveals a new receptor site on the antibody that activates a series of plasma proteins in the body called **complement**.

Complement proteins react in a cascade fashion to form a ring around the antigen–antibody complex. The complement can destroy the antigen by altering the membrane to allow an osmotic inflow of fluid that bursts the cell. They also induce chemotaxis (attraction of phagocytic cells to the area), increase the activity of phagocytes, and release histamine. Histamine release causes vasodilation, which increases blood flow to the area and brings in all of the components of the inflammatory reaction to destroy the antigen. The antigen–antibody–complement complex precipitates out of the circulatory system and deposits in various sites, including end arteries in joints, the eye, the kidney, and the skin. The signs and symptoms of the inflammatory response can be seen where the antigen–antibody complexes are deposited. Chickenpox eruptions are an example of an antigen–antibody–complement complex that deposits in the skin and causes a local inflammatory reaction.

The initial formation of antibodies, or primary response, takes several days. Once activated, the B cells form memory cells that will produce antibodies for immediate release in the future if the antigen is encountered. The antibodies are released in the form of immunoglobulins. Five different types of immunoglobulins have been identified. The first one that is released is called immunoglobulin M (IgM), and it contains the antibodies produced at the first exposure to the antigen. IgG, another form of immunoglobulin, contains antibodies made by the memory cells that circulate and enter the tissue; most of the immunoglobulin found in the serum is IgG. IgA is found in tears, saliva, sweat, mucus, and bile. It is secreted by plasma cells in the GI and respiratory tracts and in epithelial cells. These antibodies react with specific pathogens that are encountered in exposed areas of the body. IgE is present in small amounts and seems to be related to allergic responses and to the activation of mast cells. IgD is another identified immunoglobulin whose role has not been determined.

This process of antibody formation, called acquired or active immunity, is a lifelong reaction. For example, a person exposed to chickenpox will have a mild respiratory reaction when the virus (varicella) first enters the respiratory tract. There will then be a 2- to 3-week incubation period as the body is forming IgM antibodies and preparing to attack any chickenpox virus that appears. The chickenpox virus enters a cell and multiplies. The cell eventually ruptures and ejects more viruses into the system. When this happens, the body is ready to respond with the immediate release of antibodies, and a full-scale antigen–antibody response is seen throughout the body. Fever, myalgia, arthralgia, and skin lesions are all part of the immune response to the virus. Once all of the invading chickenpox viruses have been destroyed, or have entered the CNS to safely hibernate away from the antibodies, the clinical signs and symptoms resolve. (Varicella can enter the CNS and stay dormant for many years. The antibodies are not able to cross into the CNS, and the virus remains unaffected while it stays there.)

The B memory cells will continue to make a supply of immunoglobulin, IgG, for use with any future exposure to the chickenpox virus. That exposure usually does not evolve into a clinical case because the viruses are destroyed immediately on entering the body and do not have a chance to multiply. Older patients with weakened immune systems, people who are immunosuppressed, and individuals who have depleted their immune system fighting an infection are at risk for development of shingles if they had chickenpox earlier in their lives. The dormant virus, which has aged and changed somewhat, is able to leave the CNS along a nerve root because the immunosuppressed body is slow to respond. The antibodies do eventually respond to the varicella, and the signs and symptoms of shingles occur as the virus is attacked along the nerve root. Figure 15.6 outlines this entire process.

B clones cluster in areas where they are most likely to encounter the specific antigen that they have been programmed to recognize. For example, pathogens or antigens that are introduced into the body via the respiratory tract will meet up with the B cells in the tonsils and upper respiratory tract; antigens that enter the body through the GI tract will meet their B cells situated in the esophagus and GI tract. Theorists believe that the B cells are programmed genetically and are formed by the time of birth. Clones of B cells contain similar cells. The introduction of an antigen to which there are no preprogrammed B cells could result in widespread disease because the body would have no way of responding. A big concern of space travel has always been the introduction of a completely new antigen to the earth; for this reason, long periods of decontamination have been used after rocks or debris are brought back to earth. Germ warfare research is ongoing in some countries to develop an antigen that has not been seen before and to which people would have no response.

Other Mediators

Several other factors also play an important role in the immune reaction. **Interferons** are chemicals that are secreted by cells that have been invaded by viruses and possibly by other stimuli. The interferons prevent viral replication and also suppress malignant cell replication and tumor growth.

Interleukins are chemicals secreted by active leukocytes to influence other leukocytes. Interleukin 1 (IL-1) stimulates T and B cells to initiate an immune response. IL-2 is released from active T cells to stimulate production of more T cells and to increase the activity of B cells, cytotoxic cells, and natural killer cells. Interleukins also cause fever, arthralgia, myalgia, and slow-wave sleep induction—all things that help the body to conserve energy for use in fighting off the invader. Several other factors released by lymphocytes and basophils have been identified. These include interleukins such as B-cell growth factor, macrophage-activating factor, macrophage-inhibiting factor, platelet-activating factor, eosinophil chemotactic factor, and neutrophil chemotactic factor. The thymus gland also releases a number of hormones that aid in the maturation of

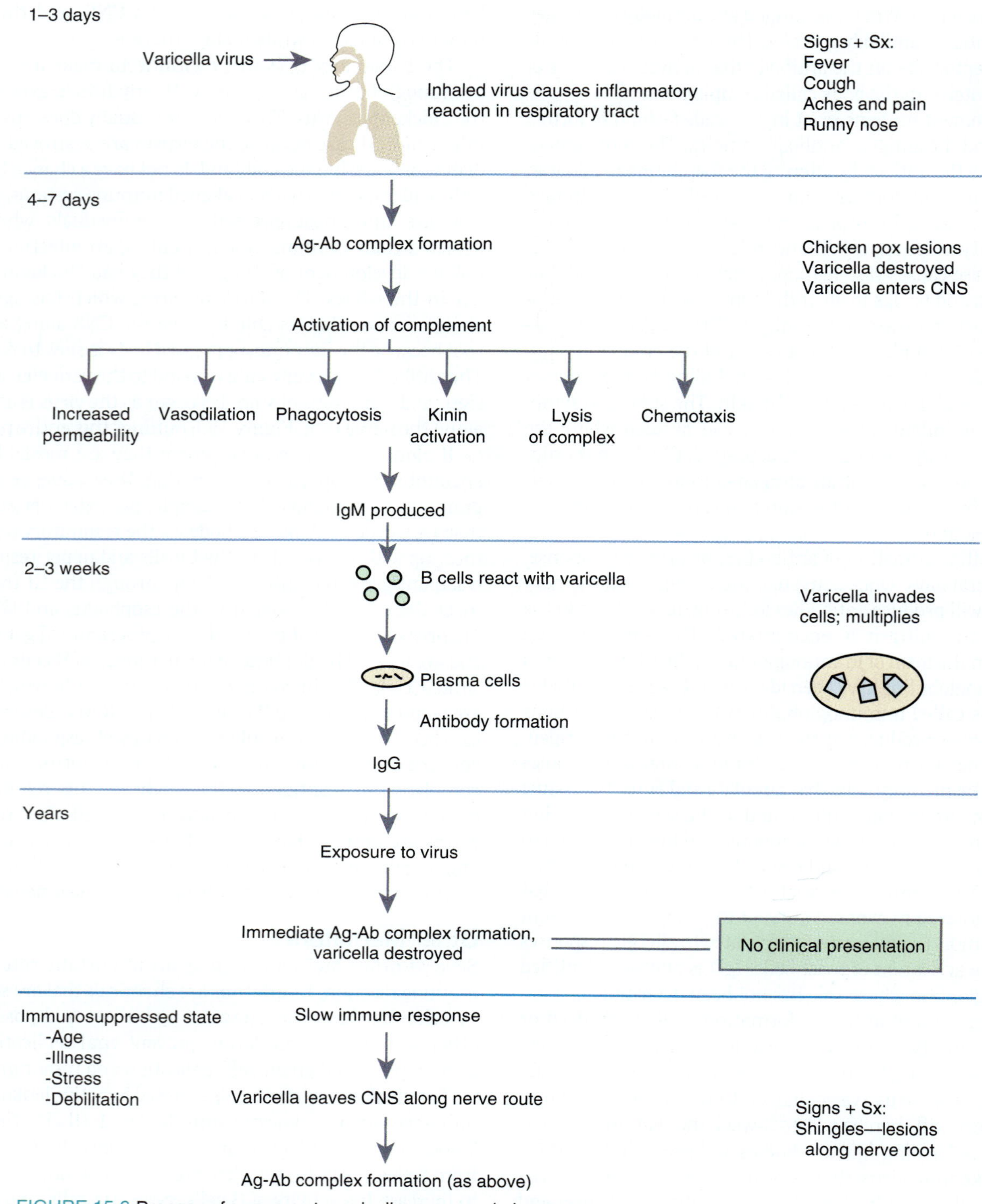

FIGURE 15.6 Process of response to varicella exposure in humans.

T cells and that circulate in the body to stimulate and communicate with T cells. Thymosin, a thymus hormone that has been replicated, is important in the maturation of T cells and cell-mediated immunity. Research is ongoing on the use of thymosin in certain leukemias and melanomas to stimulate the immune response.

Tumor necrosis factor (TNF), a cytokine, is a chemical released by macrophages that inhibits tumor growth and can actually cause tumor regression. It also works with other chemicals to make the inflammatory and immune responses more aggressive and efficient. Research is ongoing to determine the therapeutic effectiveness of TNF. TNF receptor sites are now available for injection into patients with acute rheumatoid arthritis. These receptor sites react with TNF released by the macrophages in this inflammatory disease. All of these chemicals act as communication factors within the immune system, allowing the coordination of the immune response.

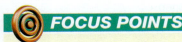

CONCEPTS in action ANIMATION

Interrelationship of the Immune and Inflammatory Responses

The immune and inflammatory responses work together to protect the body and to maintain a level of homeostasis within the body. Helper T cells stimulate the activity of B cells and effector T cells. Suppressor T cells monitor the chemical activity in the body and act to suppress B-cell and T-cell activity when the foreign antigen is under control. Both B cells and T cells ultimately depend on an effective inflammatory reaction to achieve the end goal of destruction of the foreign protein or cell (Figure 15.7).

FOCUS POINTS

- The response to the inflammatory stimuli involves local vasodilation, increased capillary permeability, and the stimulation of pain fibers. These reactions alert the person to the injury and bring an increased blood flow to the area.
- The clinical presentation of an inflammatory reaction is heat, redness, swelling, and pain (e.g., calor, rubor, tumor, and dolor).
- The immune response provides a specific reaction to foreign cells or proteins.
- T cells can be cytotoxic, destroying nonself-cells; helper, augmenting an immune reaction; or suppressor, dampening the immune response to save energy and prevent cell damage.

Pathophysiology Involving the Immune System

Several conditions can arise that cause problems involving the immune system. These conditions, many of which are treated by drugs that stimulate or suppress the immune system, include neoplasm, viral invasion, autoimmune disease, and transplant rejection.

Neoplasms

Neoplasms occur when mutant cells escape the normal surveillance of the immune system and begin to grow and

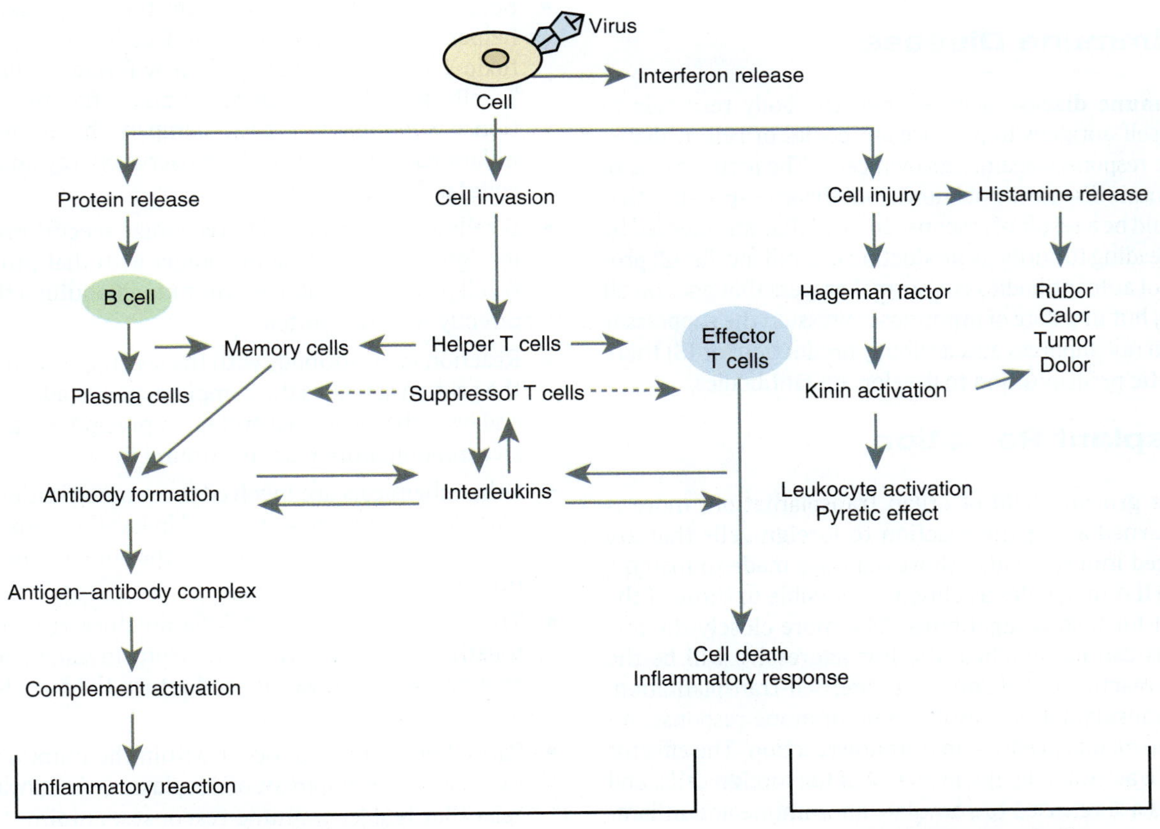

FIGURE 15.7 Interrelationship of immune and inflammatory reactions.

multiply. This can happen in many ways. For example, aging causes a decreased efficiency of the immune system, allowing some cells to escape. Location of the mutant cells can present a problem for getting lymphocytes to an area to respond. Mutant cells in breast tissue, for example, are not well perfused with blood and may escape detection until they are quite abundant. "Sneaking through" of a cell can occur. Sometimes cells are able to avoid detection by the T cells until the growing mass of cells is so large that the immune system cannot deal with it. Tumors can produce blocking antibodies that cover the antigen receptor sites on the tumor and prevent recognition by cytotoxic T cells. A weakly antigenic tumor may develop; such a tumor elicits a mild response from the immune system and somehow tricks the T cells into allowing it to survive.

Viral Invasion of Cells

Viruses are parasites that can survive only by invading a host cell that provides the nourishment necessary for viral replication. Invasion of a cell alters the cell membrane and the antigenic presentation of the cell (the MHC). This change can activate cellular immunity, or it can be so subtle that the immune system's response to the cell is mild or absent. In some cases the response activates a cellular immune reaction to normal cells similar to the one that was invaded. This is one theory for the development of autoimmune disease.

Autoimmune Disease

Autoimmune disease occurs when the body responds to specific self-antigens to produce antibodies or cell-mediated immune responses against its own cells. The actual cause of autoimmune disease is not known, but theories speculate that (1) it could be a result of response to a cell that was invaded by a virus, leading to antibody production to similar cells; (2) production of autoantibodies is a normal process that goes on all the time, but in a state of immunosuppression the suppressor T cells do not suppress autoantibody production; or (3) there is a genetic predisposition to develop autoantibodies.

Transplant Rejection

With the growing field of organ transplantation, more is being learned about the reaction to foreign cells that are introduced into the body. Effort is always made to match a donor's HLA molecules as closely as possible to those of the recipient for histocompatibility. The more closely the foreign cells can be matched, the less aggressive will be the immune reaction to the donated tissue. Self-transplantation, or autotransplantation, results in no immune response. All other transplants produce an immune reaction. The effector T cells are activated by the presence of the foreign cells, and cytokines are released to stimulate an immune and inflammatory reaction and to destroy the foreign cells.

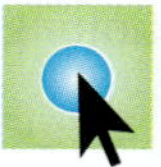

WEB LINKS

Health care providers and patients may want to consult the following Internet sources:

http://www.keratin.com/am/amindex.shtml Detailed review of the immune system.

http://www.thebody.com/step/immune.html Travel through the virtual immune system.

Points to Remember

- The body has several defense mechanisms in place to protect it from injury or foreign invasion: the skin, mucous membranes, normal flora, gastric acid, and the inflammatory and immune responses.
- The inflammatory response is a general response to any cell injury.
- The inflammatory response involves activation of Hageman factor to stimulate the kinin system and release of histamine from injured cells to generate local inflammatory responses.
- The clinical presentation of an inflammatory reaction is heat, redness, swelling, and pain (i.e., calor, rubor, tumor, and dolor).
- Several types of T cells exist: effector or cytotoxic T cells, helper T cells, and suppressor T cells. Effector or cytotoxic T cells immediately destroy foreign cells. Helper T cells stimulate the immune and inflammatory reactions. Suppressor T cells dampen the immune and inflammatory responses to conserve energy and prevent cellular damage.
- B cells are programmed to recognize specific proteins or foreign antigens. Once in contact with that protein, the B cell produces antibodies (immunoglobulins) that react directly with the protein.
- Reaction of an antibody with the specific receptor site on the protein activates the complement cascade of proteins and lyses the associated protein or precipitates an aggressive inflammatory reaction around it.
- Other chemicals are involved in communication among parts of the immune system and in local response to invasion. Any of these chemicals has the potential to alter the immune response.
- The T cells, B cells, and inflammatory reaction work together to protect the body from invasion, limit the response to that invasion, and return the body to a state of homeostasis.
- Patient problems that occur within the immune system include the development of neoplasms, viral invasions of cells that trigger immune responses, autoimmune diseases, and rejections of transplanted organs.

CHECK YOUR UNDERSTANDING

Answers to the questions in this chapter may be found in the Answer Key in the back of the book.

Multiple Choice

Select the best answer to the following.

1. Antibodies
   a. are carbohydrates.
   b. are secreted by activated T cells.
   c. are not found in circulating gamma globulins.
   d. are effective only against specific antigens.

2. B and T cells are similar in that they both
   a. secrete antibodies.
   b. play important roles in the immune response.
   c. are activated in the thymus gland.
   d. release cytotoxins to destroy cells.

3. Which of the following is not a cytokine?
   a. Interleukin 2
   b. Antibody
   c. Tumor necrosis factor
   d. Interferon

4. As part of the nonspecific defense against infection
   a. blood flow and vascular permeability to proteins increase throughout the circulatory system.
   b. particles in the respiratory tract are engulfed by phagocytes.
   c. B cells are released from the bone marrow.
   d. neutrophils release lysosomes, heparin, and kininogen into the extracellular fluid.

5. B cells respond to an initial antigen challenge by
   a. reducing in size.
   b. immediately producing antigen-specific antibodies.
   c. producing a large number of cells that are unlike the original B cell.
   d. producing new cells that become plasma cells and memory cells.

6. Treating fevers remains a controversial subject because
   a. fevers make people feel ill.
   b. higher temperatures act as catalysts to many of the body's chemical reactions, so the inflammatory and immune responses are more effective.
   c. higher temperatures can suppress the body's normal metabolism.
   d. higher temperatures can alter the body's hormone levels, particularly progesterone.

7. T cells are programmed in the thymus gland and can become any of the following *except*
   a. cytotoxic T cells.
   b. helper T cells.
   c. suppressor T cells.
   d. antibody-secreting T cells.

8. Interleukins are
   a. chemicals released when a virus enters a cell.
   b. chemicals secreted by activated leukocytes to influence other leukocytes.
   c. part of the kinin system.
   d. activated by arachidonic acid.

Multiple Response

Select all that apply.

1. Which of the following statements could be used to describe a neutrophil?
   a. They possess the property of phagocytosis.
   b. When activated, they release a pyrogen that causes fever.
   c. When the body is injured, they are produced rapidly and in large numbers.
   d. They are not capable of movement outside the circulatory system.
   e. They are most often seen in response to an allergic reaction.
   f. They float around in the blood and release chemicals in response to injury.

2. The inflammatory response is activated whenever cell injury occurs. An inflammatory response would involve which of the following activities?
   a. Activation of Hageman factor
   b. Vasodilation in the area of the injury
   c. Generalized edema and tumor development
   d. Changes in capillary permeability to allow proteins to leak out of the capillaries
   e. Activation of complement
   f. Production of interferon

True or False

Indicate whether the following statements are true (T) or false (F).

_____ 1. You are walking in a daisy field and get stung by what looks like a wasp. You should apply ice to the area to contain the venom.

_____ 2. You have a hard, reddened, warm area on your arm. You should apply ice to the affected area to keep the hardness, redness, and warmth from spreading.

_____ 3. You have a hard, reddened, warm area on your arm. You should apply heat to the area to increase the blood flow to provide inflammatory and immune factors to the site.

_____ 4. Having your tonsils removed will prevent further upper respiratory infections.

_____ 5. Basophils are the first white blood cells at the site of an injury.

_____ 6. All white blood cells possess the property of phagocytosis.

_____ 7. Chemotaxis is the ability to move within the tissues.

_____ 8. Plasma cells are large and active B cells.

_____ 9. The thymus gland is responsible for the activation and programming of the B cells.

_____ 10. Applying ice to an injection site will decrease the pain of the injection but will also decrease the absorption of the injected substance.

Definitions

Define the following terms.

1. interleukin ______________________________
____

2. rubor ______________________________
____

3. pyrogen ______________________________
____

4. antibody ______________________________
____

5. chemotaxis ______________________________
____

6. dolor ______________________________
____

7. neutrophil ______________________________
____

8. antigen ______________________________
____

Bibliography and References

Ganong, W. (2003). *Review of medical physiology* (21st ed.). Norwalk, CT: Appleton & Lange.

Gilman, A., Hardman, J. G., & Limbird, L. E. (Eds.). (2006). *Goodman and Gilman's the pharmacological basis of therapeutics* (11th ed.). New York: McGraw-Hill.

Guyton, A., & Hall, J. (2000). *Textbook of medical physiology* (10th ed.). Philadelphia: W. B. Saunders.

Karch, A. M. (2006). *2007 Lippincott's nursing drug guide.* Philadelphia: Lippincott Williams & Wilkins.

Peakman, M., & Vergani, D. (1997). *Basic and clinical immunology.* New York: Churchill-Livingstone.

Porth, C. M. (2005). *Pathophysiology: Concepts of altered health states* (7th ed.). Philadelphia: Lippincott Williams & Wilkins.

Stites, D. P., Terr, A. I., & Parslow, T. G. (Eds.). (1997). *Medical immunology* (9th ed.). Stamford, CT: Appleton & Lange.

CHAPTER 16

Anti-inflammatory Agents

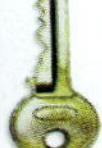

KEY TERMS

analgesic

anti-inflammatory

antipyretic

chrysotherapy

nonsteroidal anti-inflammatory drugs (NSAIDs)

salicylates

LEARNING OBJECTIVES

Upon completion of this chapter, you will be able to:

1. Describe the sites of action of the various anti-inflammatory agents.
2. Describe the therapeutic actions, indications, pharmacokinetics, contraindications, most common adverse reactions, and important drug–drug interactions associated with each class of anti-inflammatory agents: salicylates, nonsteroidal anti-inflammatory drugs, and miscellaneous agents.
3. Discuss the use of anti-inflammatory drugs across the lifespan.
4. Compare and contrast the prototype drugs for each class of anti-inflammatory drugs with the other drugs in that class.
5. Outline the nursing considerations and teaching needs for patients receiving each class of anti-inflammatory agents.

SALICYLATES

P aspirin
balsalazide
choline magnesium trisalicylate
choline salicylate
mesalamine
olsalazine
salsalate
sodium thiosalicylate

NONSTEROIDAL ANTI-INFLAMMATORY DRUGS

celecoxib
diclofenac
diflunisal
etodolac
fenoprofen
flurbiprofen
P ibuprofen
indomethacin
ketoprofen
ketorolac
mefenamic acid
meloxicam
nabumetone
naproxen
oxaprozin
piroxicam
sulindac
tolmetin

RELATED DRUGS

P acetaminophen
anakinra
auranofin
P aurothioglucose
etanercept
gold sodium thiomalate
hyaluronidase derivatives
leflunomide
penicillamine
sodium hyaluronate

The inflammatory response is designed to protect the body from injury and pathogens. It employs a variety of potent chemical mediators to produce the reaction that helps to destroy pathogens and promote healing. As the body reacts to these chemicals, it produces some signs and symptoms of disease, such as swelling, pain, fever, aches, and pains. Occasionally, the inflammatory response becomes a chronic condition and can actually result in body damage, leading to increased inflammatory reactions. **Anti-inflammatory** agents generally block or alter the chemical reactions associated with the inflammatory response to stop one or more of the signs and symptoms of inflammation.

Anti-inflammatory Agents

Several different types of drugs are used as anti-inflammatory agents. Corticosteroids (discussed in Chapter 36) are used systemically to block the inflammatory and immune systems. Blocking these important protective processes may produce many adverse effects, including decreased resistance to infection and neoplasms. Corticosteroids also are used topically to produce a local anti-inflammatory effect without as many adverse effects. Antihistamines (discussed in Chapter 54) are used to block the release of histamine in the initiation of the inflammatory response. In this chapter, discussion of anti-inflammatory agents focuses on salicylates, nonsteroidal anti-inflammatory drugs, and other related drugs. (See Box 16.1 for information on using these drugs with various age groups, and Box 16.2 for problems that some African Americans have with anti-inflammatory drugs.)

Salicylates are popular anti-inflammatory agents, not only because of their ability to block the inflammatory response, but also because of their **antipyretic** (fever-blocking) and **analgesic** (pain-blocking) properties. They are generally available without prescription and are relatively nontoxic when used as directed.

Nonsteroidal anti-inflammatory drugs (NSAIDs) are some of the most widely used drugs in the United States. They provide strong anti-inflammatory and analgesic effects yet do not have the adverse effects that are associated with the corticosteroids.

Acetaminophen also is a widely used agent. It has antipyretic and analgesic properties but does not have the anti-inflammatory effects of the salicylates or the NSAIDs.

Because many anti-inflammatory drugs are available over the counter (OTC), there is a potential for abuse and overdosing. In addition, patients may take these drugs and block the signs and symptoms of a present illness, thus potentially causing the misdiagnosis of a problem. Patients also may combine these drugs and unknowingly induce toxicity. All of these drugs have adverse effects that can be dangerous if toxic levels of drug circulate in the body.

BOX 16.1 DRUG THERAPY ACROSS THE LIFESPAN

Anti-inflammatory Agents

CHILDREN

Children are more susceptible to the GI and CNS effects of these drugs. Care must be taken to make sure that the child receives the correct dose of any anti-inflammatory agent. This can be a problem because many of these drugs are available in OTC pain, cold, flu, and combination products. Parents need to be taught to read the label to find out the ingredients and the dosage they are giving the child.

Acetaminophen is probably the most used anti-inflammatory drug for children. Care must be taken to avoid overdosage, which can cause severe hepatotoxicity.

Aspirin and choline magnesium trisalicylate are the only salicylates recommended for children. They should not be used when any risk of Reye's syndrome exists.

Ibuprofen, naproxen, tolmetin, meloxicam, and, in some cases, indomethacin are the NSAIDs approved for use in children.

Children with arthritis may receive treatment with gold salts or etanercept; they must be monitored very closely for toxic effects.

ADULTS

Adults need to be cautioned about the presence of these drugs in many OTC products and taught to be aware of exactly what they are taking to avoid serious toxic effects. They should also be cautioned to report OTC drug use to their health care provider when they are receiving any other prescription drug, to avoid possible drug–drug interactions and the masking of signs and symptoms of disease.

Pregnant and nursing women should not use these drugs unless the benefit clearly outweighs the potential risk to the fetus or neonate. The salicylates, NSAIDs, and gold products have potentially severe adverse effects on the neonate and possibly the mother. Acetaminophen can be used cautiously if a pain preparation or antipyretic are needed. Nondrug measures should be taken when at all possible to decrease the potential risk. These women also need to be urged to avoid OTC drugs unless they are suggested by their health care providers.

OLDER ADULTS

Older patients may be more susceptible to the CNS and GI effects of some of these drugs. Dosage adjustment is not needed for many of these agents.

Geriatric warnings have been associated with naproxen, ketorolac, and ketoprofen because of reports of increased toxicity when they are used by older patients. These NSAIDs should be avoided if possible.

Gold salts, used to treat arthritis, which is more common in older patients, are particularly toxic for geriatric patients. Accumulations in tissues can lead to increased renal, GI, and even liver problems. If gold is used in this group, the dosage should be reduced and the patient monitored very closely for toxic effects.

BOX 16.2 CULTURAL CONSIDERATIONS FOR DRUG THERAPY

Sensitivity to Anti-inflammatory Drugs

African Americans have a documented decreased sensitivity to the pain-relieving effects of many of the anti-inflammatory drugs. They do, however, have an increased risk of developing gastrointestinal adverse effects to these drugs, including acetaminophen. This should be taken into consideration when using these drugs as analgesics. Increased dosages may be needed to achieve a pain-blocking effect, but the increased dosage will put these patients at an even greater risk for development of the adverse GI effects associated with these drugs. These patients should be monitored closely, and efforts should be made to decrease pain using nondrug measures such as positioning, environmental control, physical therapy, warm soaks, and so on. If African American patients are prescribed anti-inflammatory drugs, they should be educated about the signs and symptoms of gastrointestinal bleeding and what to report. They also should be monitored regularly for any adverse reactions to these drugs.

Salicylates

Salicylates are some of the oldest anti-inflammatory drugs used. They were extracted from willow bark, poplar trees, and other plants by ancient peoples to treat fever, pain, and what we now call inflammation. The synthetic salicylates include the following drugs (see also Table 16.1):

Aspirin (*Bayer, Empirin,* and others) is one of the most widely used drugs for treating inflammatory conditions; it is available OTC.

Balsalazide (*Tricosal*) is a new drug that is delivered intact to the colon, where it delivers a local anti-inflammatory effect for patients with ulcerative colitis.

Choline magnesium trisalicylate (*Tricosal*) is used for mild pain and fevers and to treat arthritis.

Choline salicylate (*Arthropan*) is used to treat mild pain and fevers, as well as arthritis; it is available only as an OTC drug.

Mesalamine (*Pentasa* and others) is a unique compound that releases aspirin in the large intestine for a direct anti-inflammatory effect in ulcerative colitis or other conditions involving inflammation of the large intestine.

Olsalazine (*Dipentum*) is a drug that is converted to mesalamine in the colon and has the same direct anti-inflammatory effects.

Salsalate (*Argesic* and others) is used to treat pain, fever, and inflammation.

Sodium thiosalicylate (*Rexolate*) is used mainly for episodes of acute gout and muscular pain, and to treat rheumatic fever.

A person who does not respond to one salicylate may respond to a different one.

Table 16.1 DRUGS IN FOCUS

Salicylates

Drug Name	Dosage/Route	Usual Indications
P aspirin (*Bayer, Empirin,* others)	Adult: 325–650 mg PO or PR q4h *Myocardial infarction (MI):* 300–325 mg PO Pediatric: 65–100 mg/kg/day PO or PR in four to six divided doses; if <2 yr of age, consult with prescriber	Treatment of fever, pain, inflammatory conditions; at low dose to prevent the risk of death and MI in patients with history of MI, prevention of transient ischemic attacks
balsalazide (*Colazal*)	Three 750-mg capsules PO t.i.d. for 8 wk	Treatment of mildly to moderately acute ulcerative colitis in adults
choline magnesium trisalicylate (*Tricosal*)	Adult: 1.5–3 g/day PO in two to three divided doses Pediatric: 50 mg/kg/day PO in two divided doses	Relief of mild pain, fevers; treatment of arthritis
choline salicylate (*Arthropan*)	Adult and children (>12 yr): 870 mg PO q3–4h	Relief of mild pain, fevers; treatment of arthritis
mesalamine (*Pentasa,* others)	800 mg PO t.i.d. for 6 wk; or 4 g/60 mL rectal suspension daily at bedtime or 500 mg suppository PR, retained for 1–3 h b.i.d.	Treatment of ulcerative colitis and other inflammatory bowel disease in adults
olsalazine (*Dipentum*)	1 g/day PO in two divided doses	Treatment of ulcerative colitis and other inflammatory bowel disease in adults
salsalate (*Argesic,* others)	3000 mg/day PO in divided doses	Treatment of pain, fever, inflammation in adults
sodium thiosalicylate (*Rexolate*)	50–150 mg IM q3–6h	Relief of gout, muscular pain; treatment of rheumatic fever in adults

Therapeutic Actions and Indications

Salicylates inhibit the synthesis of prostaglandin, an important mediator of the inflammatory reaction (Figure 16.1). The antipyretic effect of salicylates may be related to blocking of a prostaglandin mediator of pyrogens (chemicals that cause an increase in body temperature and that are released by active white blood cells) at the thermoregulatory center of the hypothalamus. At low levels, aspirin also affects platelet aggregation by inhibiting the synthesis of thromboxane A_2, a potent vasoconstrictor that normally increases platelet aggregation and blood clot formation. At higher levels, aspirin inhibits the synthesis of prostacyclin, a vasodilator that inhibits platelet aggregation.

Salicylates are indicated for the treatment of mild to moderate pain, fever, and numerous inflammatory conditions, including rheumatoid arthritis and osteoarthritis. (See Box 16.3 and Critical Thinking Scenario 16-1 for more on rheumatoid arthritis.) Aspirin at low doses is indicated for the prevention of transient ischemic attack (TIA) and stroke in adults with a history of emboli. It also is indicated to reduce the risk of death and myocardial infarction (MI) in patients with a history of MI or unstable angina.

Pharmacokinetics

Salicylates are readily absorbed directly from the stomach, reaching peak levels within 5 to 30 minutes. They are metabolized in the liver and excreted in the urine, with a half-life of 15 minutes to 12 hours, depending on the salicylate involved. Salicylates cross the placenta and enter breast milk; they are not indicated for use during pregnancy or lactation because of the potential adverse effects on the neonate and associated bleeding risks for the mother.

Contraindications and Cautions

Salicylates are contraindicated in the presence of known allergy to salicylates, other NSAIDs (more common with a history of nasal polyps, asthma, or chronic urticaria), or tartrazine (a dye that has a cross-sensitivity with aspirin); bleeding abnormalities, *because of the changes in platelet aggregation associated with these drugs;* impaired renal function, *because the drug is excreted in the urine;* chickenpox or influenza, *because of the risk of Reye's syndrome in children and teenagers;* surgery or other invasive procedures scheduled within 1 week, *because of the risk of increased bleeding;* and pregnancy or lactation, *because of the potential adverse effects on the neonate or mother.*

Adverse Effects

The adverse effects associated with salicylates may be the result of direct drug effects on the stomach (nausea, dyspepsia, heartburn, epigastric discomfort) and on clotting

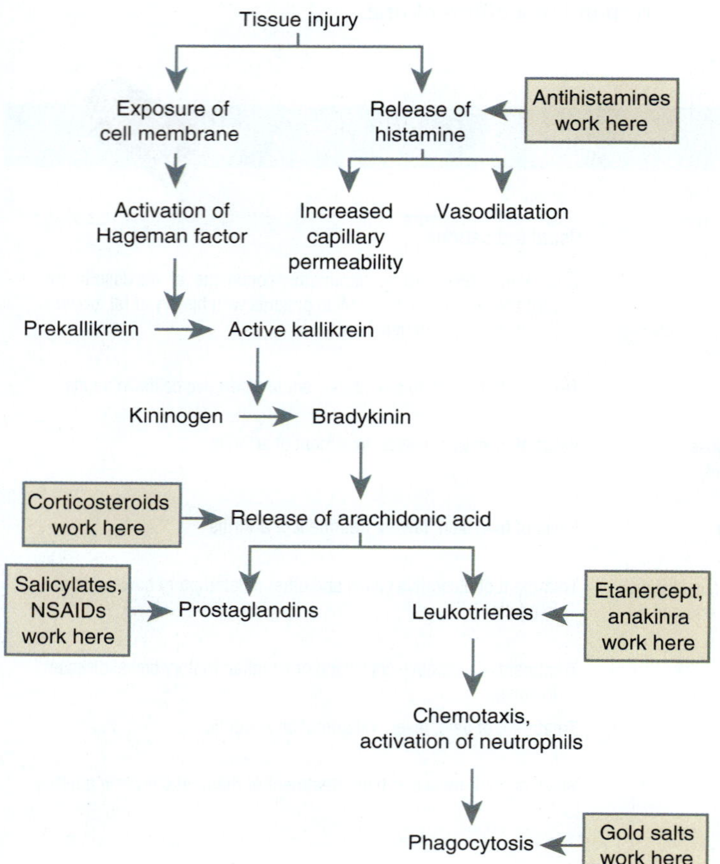

FIGURE 16.1 Sites of action of anti-inflammatory agents.

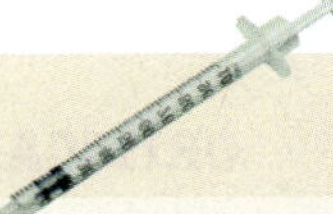

BOX 16.3 FOCUS ON **CLINICAL SKILLS**

Rheumatoid Arthritis

Pathophysiology

Rheumatoid arthritis is a chronic, systemic disease that affects people of all ages. It is considered to be an autoimmune disease. Patients with rheumatoid arthritis have high levels of rheumatoid factor (RF), an antibody to immunoglobulin G (IgG). RF interacts with circulating IgG to form immune complexes, which tend to deposit in the synovial fluid of joints as well as in the eye and other small vessels. The formation of the immune complex activates complement and precipitates an inflammatory reaction. During the immune reaction, lysosomal enzymes are released that destroy the tissues surrounding the joint. This destruction of normal tissue causes a further inflammatory reaction, and a cycle of destruction and inflammation ensues. Over time, the joint becomes severely damaged and the synovial space fills with scar tissue.

Effects of Disease

The patient with rheumatoid arthritis is in chronic pain, related to the release of the chemicals involved in the inflammatory process and the pressure of the swelling tissues in the joint capsule. At this time there is no cure for rheumatoid arthritis. Treatment is aimed at relieving the signs and symptoms of inflammation and delaying the progressive damage to the joints. The patient with this disease will progressively lose the use of the joint, which affects mobility as well as the ability to carry on the activities of daily living. Depression is not an uncommon side effect to this disease.

Clinical Skills

Specific nursing interventions can help to alleviate some of the signs and symptoms of rheumatoid arthritis and help the patient to cope with the disease. These interventions include physical therapy; range-of-motion exercises; application of hot and cold packs to the joints; weight-bearing exercises; spacing activities throughout the day to make the most of energy and movement reserves; and assistance devices for normal daily activities (e.g., big handles on utensils and pens to help patients do things for themselves when they cannot grasp small handles). Thorough teaching about drug regimens can also help prevent adverse effects and increase compliance.

Patients may have to progress through a series of drugs as various agents lose their effectiveness. Aspirin, NSAIDs, gold therapy, and more potent antiarthritis drugs may all be used at one time or another. The patient with rheumatoid arthritis will profit from a relationship with a consistent, reliable health care provider who listens, offers support, and has knowledge of new drugs and treatments to improve the quality of life. Many community support and information groups are available as resources to patients—and to health care providers who work with these patients. For a listing of available resources in your area, contact the Arthritis Foundation: http://www.arthritis.org.

systems (blood loss, bleeding abnormalities). Salicylism can occur with high levels of aspirin; dizziness, ringing in the ears, difficulty hearing, nausea, vomiting, diarrhea, mental confusion, and lassitude can occur. Acute salicylate toxicity may occur at doses of 20 to 25 g in adults or 4 g in children. Signs of salicylate toxicity include hyperpnea; tachypnea; hemorrhage; excitement; confusion; pulmonary edema; convulsions; tetany; metabolic acidosis; fever; coma; and cardiovascular, renal, and respiratory collapse.

Clinically Important Drug–Drug Interactions

The salicylates interact with many other drugs, primarily because of alterations in absorption, effects on the liver, or extension of the therapeutic effects of the salicylate or the interacting drug (or both). The list of interacting drugs in each drug monograph in a nursing drug guide should be consulted and the prescriber consulted before adding or removing a salicylate from any drug regimen.

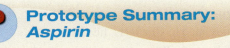

P Prototype Summary: *Aspirin*

Indications: Treatment of mild to moderate pain, fever, inflammatory conditions; reduction of risk of TIA or stroke; reduction of risk of MI

Actions: Inhibits the synthesis of prostaglandins; blocks the effects of pyrogens at the hypothalamus; inhibits platelet aggregation by blocking thromboxane A_2

Pharmacokinetics:

Route	Onset	Peak	Duration
Oral	5–30 min	0.25–2 h	3–6 h
Rectal	1–2 h	4–5 h	6–8 h

$T_{1/2}$: 15 minutes to 12 hours; metabolized in the liver and excreted in the urine

Adverse effects: Nausea, vomiting, heartburn, epigastric discomfort, occult blood loss, dizziness, tinnitus, acidosis

Nursing Considerations for Patients Receiving Salicylates

Assessment: History and Examination

Screen for any of the following, *which could be contraindications or cautions for the use of the drug:* known allergies to any salicylates, NSAIDs, or tartrazine; renal

CRITICAL THINKING SCENARIO 16-1

Aspirin and Rheumatoid Arthritis

THE SITUATION

G.T. is an 82-year-old man on a fixed income with a 14-year history of rheumatoid arthritis. He is seen in the clinic for evaluation of his arthritis and to address his complaint that his medicines are not helping him. On examination, it is found that G.T.'s range of motion, physical examination of joints, and overall presentation have not changed since his last visit. G.T. states that he had been taking aspirin, as prescribed, for his arthritis. But he read that aspirin can cause severe stomach problems, so he had switched to *Ecotrin* (an aspirin and antacid combination). This drug was much more expensive than he could handle on his fixed income, so he had started taking the drug only once every 3 days.

CRITICAL THINKING

Think about the pathophysiology of rheumatoid arthritis and how the drugs ordered act on the inflammatory process. How can the nurse best explain the disease and the drug regimen to this patient?

What could be contributing to G.T.'s perception that his condition has worsened?

What nursing interventions would be appropriate to help G.T. cope with his disease and his need for medication?

DISCUSSION

G.T. should be offered encouragement and support to deal with his progressive disease and the drug regimen required. The fact that his physical status has not changed but he perceives that the disease is worse may reflect other underlying problems that are making it more difficult for him to cope with chronic pain and limitations. The nurse should explore his social situation, any changes in his living situation, and support services. An examination should be done to determine whether other physical problems have emerged that could be adding to his sense that things are getting worse. The actions of aspirin on the arthritic process should be reviewed in basic terms, with emphasis on the importance of preventing further damage and maintaining high enough levels of aspirin to control the arthritis signs and symptoms. Pictures of the process involved in rheumatoid arthritis may help—the simpler the better in most cases.

G.T. also should be taught that all aspirin is the same, so it is acceptable to buy the cheapest generic aspirin. He can check the expiration date to make sure that the drug is fresh and still therapeutic and check that it does not smell like vinegar. Tell G.T. that the expensive combination product that G.T. has been using has not been proven to be any more effective at helping arthritis or at decreasing adverse effects than generic aspirin.

If G.T. has been having gastrointestinal complaints with the aspirin, he can be encouraged to take the drug with food and to have small, frequent meals to keep stomach acid levels at a more steady state. If G.T. has not been having any gastrointestinal complaints, he should be asked to report any immediately. The importance of the placebo effect cannot be overlooked with this patient. Many patients actually state that they feel better when they are using well-recognized, brand-name products. With support and encouragement, G.T. can be helped to follow his prescribed drug regimen and delay further damage from his arthritis.

NURSING CARE GUIDE FOR G.T.: ASPIRIN AND RHEUMATOID ARTHRITIS

Assessment

History and Examination

Allergies to aspirin; renal or hepatic impairment; ulcerative GI disease, peptic ulcer, hearing impairment, blood dyscrasias

Concurrent use of anticoagulants, steroids, ascorbic acid, phenylbutazone, alcohol, furosemide, acetazolamide, methazolamide, antacids, methotrexate, valproic acid, sulfonylureas, insulin, captopril, beta-adrenergic blockers, probenecid, sulfinpyrazone, spironolactone, nitroglycerin

Neurologic: orientation, reflexes, affect

Musculoskeletal system: ROM, joint assessment

Skin: color, lesions

CV: pulse, cardiac auscultation, blood pressure, perfusion

GI: liver evaluation, bowel sounds

Lab tests: CBC, liver and renal function tests

Nursing Diagnoses

Acute Pain related to GI effects, headache

Disturbed Sensory Perception (Auditory, Kinesthetic) related to CNS effects

Deficient Knowledge regarding drug therapy

Aspirin and Rheumatoid Arthritis *(continued)*

Implementation

Ensure proper administration of the drug.

Administer with food if GI upset occurs.

Provide support and comfort measures to deal with adverse effects: small, frequent meals; safety measures if CNS effects occur; measures for headache; bowel training as needed.

Provide patient teaching regarding drug name, dosage, side effects, precautions, and warnings to report; supplementary measures to help decrease arthritis pain.

Evaluation

Evaluate drug effects: decrease in signs and symptoms of inflammation.

Monitor for adverse effects: CNS changes, rash, GI upset, GI bleeding

Monitor for drug–drug interactions as listed.

Evaluate effectiveness of patient teaching program.

Evaluate effectiveness of comfort/safety measures.

Patient Teaching for G.T.

- ☐ Your doctor has prescribed aspirin to help relieve the signs and symptoms of your rheumatoid arthritis. Aspirin works as an anti-inflammatory drug. It works in the body to decrease inflammation and to relieve the signs and symptoms of inflammation, such as pain, swelling, heat, tenderness, and redness. It does not cure your arthritis, but will help you to live with it more comfortably.
- ☐ Take your aspirin exactly as prescribed, every day. It is important to take the drug every day so that the blood levels of the aspirin are high enough to be effective. Do not use any aspirin that has a vinegar odor.
- ☐ Some of the following adverse effects may occur:
  - *Nausea, vomiting, abdominal discomfort:* Taking the drug with food or eating small, frequent meals may help. If these effects persist, consult with your health care provider.
  - *Diarrhea, constipation:* These effects may decrease over time; ensure ready access to bathroom facilities and consult with your health care provider for possible treatment.
  - *Drowsiness, dizziness, blurred vision:* Avoid driving or performing tasks that require alertness if you experience any of these problems.
  - *Headache:* If this becomes a problem, consult with your health care provider. Do not self-treat with more aspirin or other analgesics.
- ☐ Tell any health care provider who is taking care of you that you are taking this drug.
- ☐ Avoid using other over-the-counter preparations while you are taking this drug. If you feel that you need one of these drugs, consult with your health care provider for the most appropriate choice. Many of these drugs may also contain aspirin and could cause an overdose.
- ☐ Report any of the following to your health care provider: fever, rash, GI pain, nausea, itching, or black or tarry stools.
- ☐ Keep this drug and all medications out of the reach of children.

disease; bleeding disorders; chicken pox; influenza; and pregnancy or lactation.

Include screening *for baseline status before beginning therapy and for any potential adverse effects:* the presence of any skin lesions; temperature; orientation, reflexes, eighth cranial nerve function, and affect; pulse, blood pressure, perfusion; respirations and adventitious sounds; liver evaluation; bowel sounds; and complete blood count (CBC), liver and renal function tests, urinalysis, stool guaiac, and clotting times.

Nursing Diagnoses

The patient receiving salicylates may have the following nursing diagnoses related to drug therapy:

- Acute Pain related to central nervous system (CNS) and gastrointestinal (GI) effects
- Ineffective Breathing Pattern if toxic effects occur
- Disturbed Sensory Perception (Auditory, Kinesthetic) if toxic effects occur
- Deficient Knowledge regarding drug therapy

Implementation With Rationale

- Administer with food if GI upset is severe; provide small, frequent meals *to alleviate GI effects.*
- Administer drug as indicated; monitor dosage *to avoid toxic levels.*

- Monitor for severe reactions *to avoid problems and provide emergency procedures* (gastric lavage, induction of vomiting, charcoal) if they occur.
- Arrange for supportive care and comfort measures (rest, environmental control) *to decrease body temperature or to alleviate inflammation.*
- Ensure that the patient is well hydrated during therapy *to decrease the risk of toxicity.*
- Provide thorough patient teaching, including measures to avoid adverse effects and warning signs of problems, as well as proper administration, *to increase knowledge about drug therapy and to increase compliance with drug regimen.*
- Offer support and encouragement *to deal with the drug regimen.*

Evaluation

- Monitor patient response to the drug (improvement in condition being treated, relief of signs and symptoms of inflammation).
- Monitor for adverse effects (GI upset, CNS changes, bleeding).
- Evaluate effectiveness of teaching plan (patient can name drug, dosage, adverse effects to watch for, specific measures to avoid adverse effects).
- Monitor effectiveness of comfort measures and compliance with the drug regimen.

FOCUS POINTS

- Salicylates block prostaglandin activity, which decreases the inflammatory response and relieves the signs and symptoms of inflammation.
- Salicylates can cause GI irritation, eighth cranial nerve stimulation, and salicylism—ringing in the ears, acidosis, nausea, vomiting, diarrhea, mental confusion, and lassitude.

Nonsteroidal Anti-inflammatory Drugs

The NSAIDs are a drug class that has become one of the most commonly used types in the United States. This group of drugs includes the following agents (see also Table 16.2).

Propionic Acids

- Fenoprofen (*Nalfon*) is used to treat pain and manage arthritis.
- Flurbiprofen (*Ansaid*) is used for the long-term management of arthritis and as a topical preparation for managing pain after eye surgery.
- Ibuprofen (*Motrin, Advil,* and others) is used as an OTC pain medication and for long-term management of arthritis pain and dysmenorrhea; it is the most widely used of the NSAIDs.
- Ketoprofen (*Orudis*) is available for short-term management of pain and as a topical agent to relieve ocular itching caused by seasonal rhinitis.
- Naproxen (*Naprosyn*) is available for OTC pain relief and to treat arthritis and dysmenorrhea.
- Oxaprozin (*Daypro*) is very successfully used to manage arthritis.

Acetic Acids

- Diclofenac (*Voltaren, Cataflam*) is used to treat acute and long-term pain associated with inflammatory conditions.
- Etodolac (*Lodine*) is widely used for arthritis pain.
- Indomethacin (*Indocin*) is available in oral, topical, and rectal preparations for the relief of moderate to severe pain associated with inflammatory conditions and in intravenous form to promote closure of the patent ductus arteriosus in premature infants.
- Ketorolac (*Toradol*) is used for short-term management of pain and topically to relieve ocular itching.
- Nabumetone (*Relafen*) is used to treat acute and chronic arthritis pain.
- Sulindac (*Clinoril*) is used for long- and short-term treatment of the signs and symptoms of various inflammatory conditions.
- Tolmetin (*Tolectin*) is used to treat acute attacks of rheumatoid arthritis and juvenile arthritis (Box 16.4).

Fenamates

- Mefenamic acid (*Ponstel*) is used only for short-term treatment of pain.
- Piroxicam (*Feldene*) is used to treat acute and chronic arthritis.
- Diflunisal (*Dolobid*) is used for moderate pain and for the treatment of arthritis.

Oxicam Derivative

Meloxicam (*Mobic*) is used for the relief of the signs and symptoms of juvenile arthritis, osteoarthritis, and rheumatoid arthritis.

Cyclooxygenase-2 Inhibitor

Celecoxib (*Celebrex*) is used for the acute and long-term treatment of arthritis, particularly in patients who cannot tolerate the GI effects of other NSAIDs; for acute pain in adults; for ankylosing spondylitis; and for primary

Table 16.2 DRUGS IN FOCUS

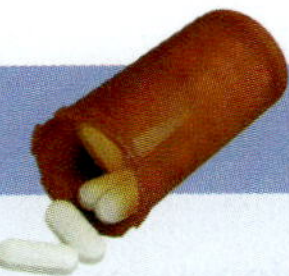

Nonsteroidal Anti-inflammatory Drugs

Drug Name	Dosage/Route	Usual Indications
celecoxib (*Celebrex*)	Initially: 100–200 mg PO b.i.d. 400 mg, then 200 mg PO b.i.d. for acute pain; 400 mg PO b.i.d. for FAP	Treatment of acute and chronic arthritis in adults; acute pain; primary dysmenorrhea; reduction of the number of colorectal polyps in familial adenomatous polyposis (FAP); ankylosing spondylitis
diclofenac (*Voltaren, Cataflam*)	100–200 mg/day PO 25–50 mg b.i.d. to q.i.d. PO	Treatment of acute and chronic pain associated with inflammatory conditions in adults
diflunisal (*Dolobid*)	500–1000 mg/day PO in two divided doses	Treatment of moderate pain, arthritis in adults
etodolac (*Lodine*)	800–1200 mg/day PO in divided doses; 200–400 mg q6–8h PO for pain management	Treatment of arthritis pain in adults; management of chronic pain (ER formulation)
fenoprofen (*Nalfon*)	200–600 mg PO t.i.d. or q.i.d.	Treatment of pain, arthritis in adults
flurbiprofen (*Ansaid*)	200–300 mg PO in divided doses; ophthalmic solution: 1 gtt q30min beginning 2 h after surgery	Long-term management of arthritis; topically to manage pain after eye surgery in adults
P ibuprofen (*Motrin, Advil, others*)	Adult: 400–800 mg PO t.i.d. to q.i.d. Pediatric: 30–40 mg/kg/day PO in three to four divided doses for arthritis; 5–10 mg/kg PO q6–8h for fever	Treatment of pain, arthritis, dysmenorrhea, juvenile arthritis
indomethacin (*Indocin*)	Adult: 75–150 mg/day PO in three to four divided doses Pediatric (>2 yr): in special circumstances, 2 mg/kg/day PO in divided doses	Relief of moderate to severe pain in PO, topical, and PR forms; closure of patent ductus arteriosus in premature infants (given IV)
ketoprofen (*Orudis*)	25–75 mg PO t.i.d. to q.i.d.; reduce dosage with hepatic or renal impairment; SR form: 200 mg/day PO	Short-term management of pain; long-term management of arthritis (SR form); ophthalmic form to relieve ocular itching
ketorolac (*Toradol*)	10 mg PO q4–6h, or 30–60 mg IM, switching to oral form as soon as possible, or 30 mg IV as a single dose Ophthalmic: 1 gtt to affected eye q.i.d. Reduce dosage with renal impairment and in patients >65 yr	Short-term management of pain in adults; topically to relieve ocular itching
mefenamic acid (*Ponstel*)	500 mg PO, then 250 mg PO q6h as needed	Short-term treatment of pain in adults and children >14 yr; primary dysmenorrhea
meloxicam (*Mobic*)	Adult: 7.5 mg/day PO to a maximum of 15 mg/day Pediatric: 0.125 mg/kg/day PO to a maximum of 7.5 mg/day	Treatment of osteoarthritis, rheumatoid arthritis, and juvenile arthritis
nabumetone (*Relafen*)	1000 mg/day PO as a single dose	Treatment of acute and chronic arthritis pain in adults
naproxen (*Naprosyn*)	Adult: 250–500 mg PO b.i.d.; do not give >200 mg q12h for geriatric patients Pediatric: 10 mg/kg/day PO in two divided doses for juvenile arthritis; do not give OTC versions to children <12 yr without consulting health care provider	Treatment of pain, arthritis, dysmenorrhea, juvenile arthritis
oxaprozin (*Daypro*)	1200 mg PO daily	Treatment of arthritis in adults
piroxicam (*Feldene*)	20 mg/day PO as a single dose	Treatment of acute and chronic arthritis in adults
sulindac (*Clinoril*)	150–200 mg PO b.i.d.	Treatment of various inflammatory conditions in adults
tolmetin (*Tolectin*)	Adult: 400 mg PO t.i.d.; 600–800 mg/day in three to four doses for maintenance Pediatric: 20 mg/kg/day PO in three to four divided doses	Treatment of acute flares of rheumatoid and juvenile arthritis

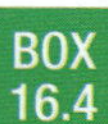

FOCUS ON THE EVIDENCE

Cyclooxygenase-2 Inhibitors

In late 2004, Merck voluntarily withdrew their cyclooxygenase-2 (COX-2) inhibitor, rofecoxib (*Vioxx*), from the market following release of a mid-study finding that the use of the drug over an 18-month period led to a significant increase in cardiovascular (CV) mortality in the those taking the drug compared with a placebo group. The study, called the APPROVe study (Adenomatous Polyp Prevention on Vioxx), was targeted at testing whether the blocking of such growth factors as angiogenesis could decrease cancer risk in a specific population. The study participants took 25 mg of *Vioxx* each day for 18 months (the halfway point in the study) when the finding of increased CV events was announced and the study was stopped. The CV outcomes were not noted earlier than 18 months. Interestingly, other studies, including a 4-year study of the effects on Alzheimer's disease, did not show a significant difference in CV events between the placebo and drug groups. Yet, in the VIGOR (*Vioxx* Gastrointestinal Outcomes Research) study, in which rofecoxib was compared with naproxen (another NSAID) for 12 months, increased CV events were noted in the rofecoxib group after only 2 months.

The U.S. Food and Drug Administration (FDA) formed a committee to study the COX-2 inhibitors and then all of the NSAIDs on the market to see if there were any problems in oversight of drug safety and to make recommendations about the future use of these drugs.

Valdecoxib (*Bextra*) was withdrawn from the market at FDA request after the committee reviewed data. A small study did show an increase in CV events, including death, when *Bextra* was used immediately in postoperative patients recovering from coronary artery bypass graft (CABG) surgery. The drug was not proven to be especially more effective than other NSAIDs for relieving pain, and already had a black-box warning about the increased possibility of severe skin reactions, including Stevens–Johnson syndrome. With those facts in mind and the possibility of a COX-2 link to increased CV events, the FDA believed that the benefits of marketing the drug did not outweigh the potential risks for using the drug.

Celecoxib (*Celebrex*) remains on the market. The APC study (Adenoma Prevention with Celecoxib) did show a two- to threefold increase in CV events among patients using the drug compared with placebo over 33 months. There did seem to be a dose correlation, with more events in the group using a higher dose. A nearly identical study, the PreSAP trial (Prevention of Spontaneous Adenomatous Polyps), showed no increase in CV events in the group using celecoxib. A small study, the ADAPT (Alzheimer's Disease Anti-inflammatory Prevention Trial), did not appear to show an increase in CV events in the patients in that study.

The media helped to fuel a real concern about the safety of any anti-inflammatory medication. The questions remain: Were the CV events related to dosage, length of drug use, or the underlying conditions of the patients being studied? Were the CV events a direct effect of the COX-2 inhibitor? Would these same events have occurred if the drug were used at the dosages approved and for the approved length of time? More long-term, controlled studies are needed to answer these questions. In the meantime, the FDA has recommended that valdecoxib and rofecoxib stay off the market until appropriate guidelines and controls are in place for their return; that all NSAIDs' packaging information include warnings that there is potential risk for increased CV events as well as the risk of gastrointestinal bleeding, and that health care providers use caution in recommending these drugs to anyone with an established CV risk; that all prescription NSAIDs be contraindicated in patients immediately after CABG surgery; and that the prescribing information for celecoxib include a black-box warning referencing the available data about increased CV risk. Two new COX-2 inhibitors being studied, lumiracoxib and etoricoxib, will be carefully reviewed for data on the incidence of increased CV events before they will be considered for approval.

Specialists treating patients with chronic pain have petitioned to have the FDA return rofecoxib and valdecoxib to the market, citing patients who could only obtain relief using those drugs. Some patients only respond to these particular NSAIDs, and these specialists feel that the patients should have a choice, being informed of the risks, to continue their use to relieve pain. Clearly, more long-term studies are needed. The nurse may be asked about this controversy and what recommendations are in place by patients who want relief from pain but really want to understand the risks to their health. To get a complete summary of the research, the report to the FDA, and current recommendations and research, go to www.fda.gov and click on NSAIDs under Hot Topics on the right side of the page. This site is updated regularly and offers information geared to patients and to health care professionals.

dysmenorrhea. Celecoxib is also being studied for its potential ability to block angiogenesis in various cancers.

The choice of NSAID depends on personal experience and the patient's response to the drug. A patient may have little response to one NSAID and a huge response to another. It may take several trials to determine the drug of choice for any particular patient (Box 16.4).

Therapeutic Actions and Indications

The anti-inflammatory, analgesic, and antipyretic effects of the NSAIDs are largely related to inhibition of prostaglandin synthesis (see Figure 16.1). The NSAIDs block two enzymes, known as cyclooxygenase-1 (COX-1) and cyclooxygenase-2 (COX-2). COX-1 is present in all tissues and seems to be involved in many body functions, including blood clotting, protecting the stomach lining, and maintaining sodium and water balance in the kidney. COX-1 turns arachidonic acid into prostaglandins as needed in a variety of tissues. COX-2 is active at sites of trauma or injury when more prostaglandins are needed, but it does not seem to be involved in the other tissue functions. By interfering with this part of the inflammatory reaction, NSAIDs block inflammation before all of the signs and symptoms can develop. Most NSAIDs also block various other functions of the prostaglandins, including protection of the stomach lining, regulation of blood clotting, and water and salt balance in the kidney. The COX-2 inhibitors are thought to act only at sites of trauma and injury to more specifically block the inflammatory reaction.

The adverse effects associated with most NSAIDs are related to blocking of both of these enzymes and changes in the functions that they influence—GI integrity, blood clotting, and sodium and water balance. The COX-2 inhibitors are designed to affect only the activity of COX-2, the enzyme that becomes active in response to trauma and injury. They do not interfere with COX-1, which is needed for normal functioning of these systems. Consequently, these drugs should not have the associated adverse effects seen when both COX-1 and COX-2 are inhibited. Experience has shown that the COX-2 inhibitors still have some effect on these other functions, and patients should still be evaluated for GI effects, changes in bleeding time, and water retention. Recent studies suggest that they may block some protective responses in the body, such as vasodilation and inhibited platelet clumping, which could lead to cardiovascular problems.

The NSAIDs are indicated for relief of the signs and symptoms of rheumatoid arthritis and osteoarthritis, for relief of mild to moderate pain, for treatment of primary dysmenorrhea, and for fever reduction.

Pharmacokinetics

The NSAIDs are rapidly absorbed from the GI tract, reaching peak levels in 1 to 3 hours. They are metabolized in the liver and excreted in the urine. NSAIDs cross the placenta and cross into breast milk. Therefore, they are not recommended during pregnancy and lactation because of the potential adverse effects on the fetus or neonate.

Contraindications and Cautions

The NSAIDs are contraindicated in the presence of allergy to any NSAID or salicylate, and celecoxib is also contraindicated in the presence of allergy to sulfonamides. Additional contraindications are cardiovascular dysfunction or hypertension, *because of the varying effects of the prostaglandins;* peptic ulcer or known GI bleeding, *because of the potential to exacerbate the GI bleeding;* and pregnancy or lactation, *because of potential adverse effects on the neonate or mother*. Caution should be used with renal or hepatic dysfunction, *which could alter the metabolism and excretion of these drugs,* and with any other known allergies, *which indicate increased sensitivity*.

Adverse Effects

Patients receiving NSAIDs often experience nausea, dyspepsia, GI pain, constipation, diarrhea, or flatulence caused by direct GI effects of the drug. The potential for GI bleeding often is a cause of discontinuation of the drug. Headache, dizziness, somnolence, and fatigue also occur frequently and could be related to prostaglandin activity in the CNS. Bleeding, platelet inhibition, and even bone marrow depression have been reported with chronic use and probably are related to the blocking of prostaglandin activity. Rash and mouth sores may occur, and anaphylactoid reactions leading to fatal anaphylactic shock have been reported in cases of severe hypersensitivity.

Clinically Important Drug–Drug Interactions

There often is a decreased diuretic effect when these drugs are taken with loop diuretics; there is a potential for decreased antihypertensive effect of beta-blockers if these drugs are combined; and there have been reports of lithium toxicity, especially when combined with ibuprofen. Patients who receive these combinations should be monitored closely, and appropriate dosage adjustments should be made by the prescriber.

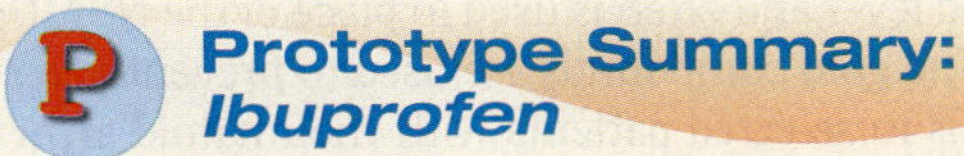

Prototype Summary: Ibuprofen

Indications: Relief of the signs and symptoms of rheumatoid arthritis and osteoarthritis; relief of mild to moderate pain; treatment of primary dysmenorrhea; fever reduction

Actions: Inhibits prostaglandin synthesis by blocking cyclooxygenase-1 and -2 receptor sites, leading to an anti-inflammatory effect, analgesia, and antipyretic effects

Pharmacokinetics:

Route	Onset	Peak	Duration
Oral	30 min	1–2 h	4–6 h

$T_{1/2}$: 1.8 to 2.5 hours; metabolized in the liver and excreted in the urine

Adverse effects: Headache, dizziness, somnolence, fatigue, rash, nausea, dyspepsia, bleeding, constipation

Nursing Considerations for Patients Receiving NSAIDs

Assessment: History and Examination

Screen for any of the following, *which could be contraindications or cautions for the use of the drug:* known allergies to any salicylates, NSAIDs, or tartrazine; pregnancy or lactation; hepatic or renal disease; cardiovascular dysfunction; hypertension; and GI bleeding or peptic ulcer.

Include *screening for baseline status before beginning therapy and for any potential adverse effects:* presence of any skin lesions; temperature; orientation, reflexes, and affect; pulse, blood pressure, and perfusion; respirations and adventitious sounds; liver evaluation; bowel sounds; and CBC, liver and renal function tests, urinalysis, stool guaiac, and serum electrolytes.

Nursing Diagnoses, Implementation, and Evaluation

Refer to the Nursing Considerations section for the salicylates.

Related Drugs

Other drugs used to treat inflammatory conditions include acetaminophen (*Tylenol*), gold compounds, and other antiarthritic drugs. Acetaminophen is used to treat moderate to mild pain and fever and often is used in place of the NSAIDs or salicylates. The gold compounds are used to prevent and suppress arthritis in selected patients with rheumatoid arthritis. The other antiarthritic drugs (Table 16-3) are specifically used to block the inflammation and tissue damage of rheumatoid arthritis.

Acetaminophen

Therapeutic Actions and Indications

Acetaminophen acts directly on the thermoregulatory cells in the hypothalamus to cause sweating and vasodilation; this in turn causes the release of heat and lowers fever. The mechanism of action related to the analgesic effects of acetaminophen has not been identified.

Acetaminophen is indicated for the treatment of pain and fever associated with a variety of conditions, including influenza; for the prophylaxis of children receiving diphtheria–pertussis–tetanus (DPT) immunizations (aspirin may mask Reye's syndrome in children); and for the relief of musculoskeletal pain associated with arthritis.

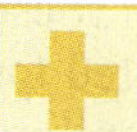

FOCUS ON PATIENT SAFETY

Acetaminophen Toxicity: With thousands of acetaminophen toxicities reported every year, the Federal Drug Administration and the Institute for Safe Medication Practices have launched a campaign to educate health care providers, patients, and parents about the risk associated with acetaminophen use. Acetaminophen is found in numerous OTC products for treating pain, colds, flu, and allergies. These products are available without a prescription. Many people are unaware of their potential hazards, and they do not report the use of these products to their health care provider, even when specifically asked about drug use.

Table 16.3 DRUGS IN FOCUS

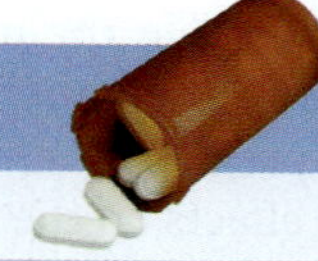

Anti-inflammatory and Antiarthritis Agents

Drug Name	Dosage/Route	Usual Indications
P acetaminophen (*Tylenol*)	Adult: 1000 mg PO t.i.d. to q.i.d. *or* 325–650 mg PR q4–6h Pediatric: adjust dosage based on age	Relief of pain and fever in a variety of situations
anakinra (*Kineret*)	Adult: 100 mg/day Sub-Q	Reduction of signs and symptoms of rheumatoid arthritis in patients ≥18 yr if one or more other arthritis agents have failed
auranofin (*Ridaura*)	Adult: 6 mg/day PO; monitor geriatric patients carefully Pediatric: 0.1–0.15 mg/kg/day PO	Long-term therapy for rheumatic disorders
P aurothioglucose (*Solganal*)	Adult: 10 mg IM, then two doses of 25 mg IM, then two doses of 50 mg IM; then 50 mg IM every 3–4 wk; monitor geriatric patients carefully Pediatric: one-quarter the adult dose	Injected drug for early treatment of rheumatic disorders
etanercept (*Enbrel*)	Adult: 25 mg Sub-Q two times per week or 50 mg Sub-Q once a week Pediatric (4–17 yr): 0.4 mg/kg Sub-Q two times per week with 72–96 h between doses; not recommended for patients <4 yr	Reduction of signs and symptoms of severe rheumatoid arthritis in patients whose disease is unresponsive to other therapy; prevention of damage early in the disease; ankylosing spondylosis; psoriatic arthritis
gold sodium thiomalate (*Aurolate*)	Adult: 10 mg IM, then 25 mg IM every other week; use caution in geriatric patients Pediatric: 10 mg IM, then 1 mg/kg IM every other week	Injected drug for early treatment of rheumatic disorders
hylan G-F 20 (*Synvisc*)	2 mL once a week for 3 wk injected into the affected knee	Relief of pain in the knees of arthritis patients whose disease is unresponsive to conventional treatment
leflunomide (*Arava*)	100 mg PO daily for 3 days, then 20 mg PO daily	Treatment of active rheumatoid arthritis, to relieve signs and symptoms and to slow progression of disease in adults
penicillamine (*Depen*)	125–250 mg PO daily	Treatment of severe, active rheumatoid arthritis in adults whose disease is unresponsive to conventional therapy
sodium hyaluronate (*Hyalgan*)	2 mg once a week for 5 wk injected into the affected knee	Relief of pain in the knees of arthritis patients whose disease is unresponsive to conventional treatment

Patients, or parents, seeking relief from the signs and symptoms associated with the common cold or flu infection may take more than one of these products, hoping to relieve a stuffy nose, headache, or cough by combining products containing acetaminophen. Many people do not read the product labels, relying instead on the advertised use. The consequence is thousands of reports of people overdosing on acetaminophen while following the dosage guidelines. In addition, patients who take liquid forms of these products may use an inaccurate measuring device (like a flatware teaspoon) and inadvertently overdose. Health care providers need to be alert for signs and symptoms of acetaminophen toxicity—initially nausea, vomiting, and GI upset. They need to ask patients specifically about whether they are using OTC products to reduce pain, control coughs, or help them sleep through the night.

The education of parents and patients about this potential hazard should not wait until a disaster occurs but should be incorporated into regular well visits. Patients should be taught how to read labels, monitor dosage, and measure liquid medications, what signs and symptoms of overdose to watch for, and what to do if any occur.

Pharmacokinetics

Acetaminophen is rapidly absorbed from the GI tract, reaching peak levels in 0.5 to 2 hours. It is extensively metabolized in the liver and excreted in the urine, with a half-life of about 2 hours. Caution should be used in patients with hepatic or renal impairment, which could interfere with metabolism and excretion of the drug, leading to toxic levels. Acetaminophen crosses the placenta and enters breast milk; it should be used cautiously during pregnancy or lactation because of the potential adverse effects on the fetus or neonate.

Contraindications and Cautions

Acetaminophen is contraindicated in the presence of allergy to acetaminophen. It should be used cautiously in pregnancy or lactation and in hepatic dysfunction or chronic alcoholism *because of associated toxic effects on the liver.*

Adverse Effects

Adverse effects associated with acetaminophen use include headache, hemolytic anemia, renal dysfunction, skin rash, and fever. Hepatotoxicity is a potentially fatal adverse effect that is usually associated with chronic use and overdose and is related to direct toxic effects on the liver.

Clinically Important Drug–Drug Interactions

There is an increased risk of bleeding with oral anticoagulants because of effects on the liver; of toxicity with chronic ethanol ingestion because of toxic effects on the liver; and of hepatotoxicity with barbiturates, carbamazepine, hydantoins, rifampin, or sulfinpyrazone. These combinations should be avoided, but if they must be used, appropriate dosage adjustment should be made and the patient should be monitored closely.

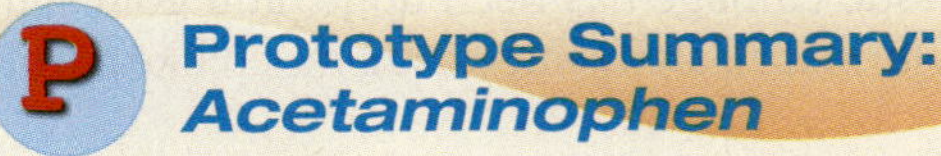

Prototype Summary: Acetaminophen

Indications: Treatment of mild to moderate pain, fever, or signs and symptoms of the common cold or flu; musculoskeletal pain associated with arthritis and rheumatic disorders

Actions: Acts directly on the hypothalamus to cause vasodilation and sweating, which will reduce fever; mechanism of action as an analgesic is not understood

Pharmacokinetics:

Route	Onset	Peak	Duration
Oral	Varies	0.5–2 h	3–6 h

$T_{1/2}$: 1 to 3 hours; metabolized in the liver and excreted in the urine

Adverse effects: Rash, fever, chest pain, liver toxicity and failure, bone marrow suppression

FOCUS POINTS

- NSAIDs block prostaglandin synthesis at cyclo-oxygenase-1 and -2 sites. This blocks inflammation but also blocks protection of the stomach lining, as well as the kidneys' regulation of water.
- There are many different NSAIDs. If one does not work for a particular patient, another one might.
- Acetaminophen causes vasodilation and heat release, lowering fever and working to relieve pain.
- Acetaminophen can cause liver failure. It is found in many OTC products. Patients need to be taught to avoid toxic doses of acetaminophen.

Gold Compounds

Some patients with rheumatic inflammatory conditions do not respond to the usual anti-inflammatory therapies, and their conditions worsen despite weeks or months of standard pharmacologic treatment. Some of these patients respond to treatment with gold salts, also known as **chrysotherapy**. The gold salts that are currently available for use include auranofin (*Ridaura*), an oral agent used for long-term therapy; aurothioglucose (*Solganal*), an injected drug that is recommended for treatment early in the disease, before too much tissue damage has been done; and gold sodium thiomalate (*Aurolate*), an injected drug much like aurothioglucose.

Therapeutic Actions and Indications

Gold salts are absorbed by macrophages, which results in inhibition of phagocytosis (see Figure 16.1). Because phagocytosis is blocked, the release of lysosomal enzymes is inhibited and tissue destruction is decreased. This action allows gold salts to suppress and prevent some arthritis and synovitis. Gold salts are indicated to treat selected cases of rheumatoid and juvenile rheumatoid arthritis in patients whose disease has been unresponsive to standard therapy. These drugs do not repair damage; they prevent further damage and so are most effective if used early in the disease.

Pharmacokinetics

The gold salts are absorbed at varying rates, depending on their route of administration. They are widely distributed throughout the body but seem to concentrate in the hypothalamic-pituitary-adrenocortical (HPA) system and in the adrenal and renal cortices. The gold salts are excreted in urine and feces. These drugs cross the placenta and cross into breast milk. They have been shown to be teratogenic in animal studies and should not be used during pregnancy or lactation. Barrier contraceptives should be recommended to women of childbearing age, and another method of feeding the baby should be used if gold therapy is needed in a lactating woman.

Contraindications and Cautions

Gold salts can be quite toxic and are contraindicated in the presence of any known allergy to gold, severe diabetes, congestive heart failure, severe debilitation, renal or hepatic impairment, hypertension, blood dyscrasias, recent radiation treatment, history of toxic levels of heavy metals, and pregnancy or lactation.

Adverse Effects

A variety of adverse effects are common with the use of gold salts and are probably related to their deposition in the tissues and effects at that local level: stomatitis, glossitis, gingivitis, pharyngitis, laryngitis, colitis, diarrhea, and other GI inflammation; gold bronchitis and interstitial pneumonitis; bone marrow depression; vaginitis and nephrotic syndrome; dermatitis, pruritus, and exfoliative dermatitis; and allergic reactions ranging from flushing, fainting, and dizziness to anaphylactic shock.

Clinically Important Drug–Drug Interactions

These drugs should not be combined with penicillamine, antimalarials, cytotoxic drugs, or immunosuppressive agents other than low-dose corticosteroids because of the potential for severe toxicity.

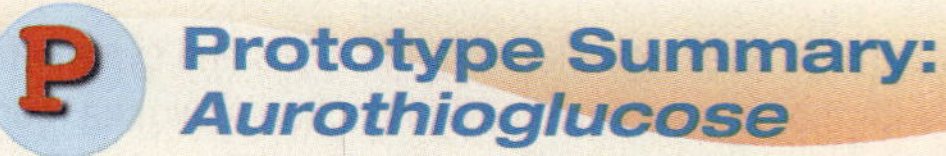

Indications: Treatment of selected cases of adult and juvenile rheumatoid arthritis, most effective early in disease

Actions: Taken up by macrophages, which inhibits phagocytosis and release of lysosomal enzymes that cause damage associated with inflammation

Pharmacokinetics:

Route	Onset	Peak
IM	Slow	4–6 h

$T_{1/2}$: 3 to 7 days; excreted in the urine and feces

Adverse effects: Dermatitis, nausea, vomiting, stomatitis, anemia, interstitial pneumonitis, acute tubular necrosis

Other Antiarthritis Drugs

Six other drugs have become available to relieve the pain and suffering of patients with acute rheumatoid arthritis that is no longer responsive to conventional therapy: etanercept (*Enbrel*), leflunomide (*Arava*), penicillamine (*Depen*), hyaluronidase derivative (*Synvisc*), sodium hyaluronate (*Hyalgan*), and anakinra (*Kineret*). Methotrexate (see Chapter 14) has also been used to treat rheumatoid arthritis when patients do not respond to standard therapy.

Therapeutic Actions and Indications

Etanercept (*Enbrel*) contains genetically engineered tumor necrosis factor (TNF) receptors derived from Chinese hamster ovary cells. These receptors react with free-floating TNF released by active leukocytes in autoimmune inflammatory disease to prevent the damage caused by TNF. Etanercept is indicated for subcutaneous use to reduce the signs and symptoms of active rheumatoid arthritis and prevent damage in the early stages of the disease; for treating juvenile rheumatoid arthritis; for treating ankylating spondylosis; and for treating psoriatic arthritis. A warning has been issued stating that the drug has been associated with the development of serious CNS problems, including multiple sclerosis. It can also cause severe myelosuppression and increased risk of infections and cancer development. Patients who use this drug need to be monitored very closely.

Leflunomide (*Arava*) directly inhibits an enzyme, dihydroorotate dehydrogenase (DHODH), that is active in the autoimmune process that leads to rheumatoid arthritis, preventing the signs and symptoms of inflammation and blocking the structural damage this inflammation can cause. Leflunomide is indicated for the treatment of active rheumatoid arthritis to relieve symptoms and to slow the progression of the disease. It has been associated with severe hepatic toxicity, and the patient's liver function needs to be monitored closely.

Penicillamine (*Depen*) lowers the immunoglobulin M (IgM) rheumatoid factor levels in patients with acute rheumatoid arthritis, relieving the signs and symptoms of inflammation. It may take 2 to 3 months of therapy before a response is noted.

Hyaluronidase derivatives, such as hylan G-F 20 (*Synvisc*) and sodium hyaluronate (*Hyalgan*) have elastic and viscous properties. These drugs are injected directly into the joints of patients with severe rheumatoid arthritis of the knee. They seem to cushion and lubricate the joint and relieve the pain associated with degenerative arthritis. They are given weekly for 3 to 5 weeks.

Anakinra (*Kineret*) is the newest of the antiarthritis drugs. This drug is an interleukin-1 receptor antagonist. It blocks the increased interleukin-1, which is responsible for the degradation of cartilage in rheumatoid arthritis. This drug must be given each day by subcutaneous injection and is often used in combination with other antiarthritis drugs.

Contraindications and Cautions

These drugs are contraindicated in the presence of allergy to the drugs or to the animal products from which they were derived (Chinese hamster products in etanercept; chicken products in hylan G-F 20 and sodium hyaluronate); pregnancy or lactation, *because of the potential for adverse effects on the fetus or neonate;* acute infection, *because of the blocking of normal inflammatory pathways;* and liver or renal impairment, *which could be exacerbated by these drugs.*

Adverse Effects

A variety of adverse effects are common with the use of these drugs, including local irritation at injection sites (anakinra, etanercept, hyaluronidase derivatives, and sodium hyaluronate), pain with injection, and increased risk of infection. Leflunomide is associated with potentially fatal hepatic toxicity and rashes. Penicillamine is associated with a potentially fatal myasthenic syndrome, bone marrow depression, and assorted hypersensitivity reactions. Etanercept is associated with severe bone marrow suppression, as well as serious CNS disorders, including multiple sclerosis.

Clinically Important Drug-Drug Interactions

Hyaluronidase derivatives, such as sodium hyaluronate should not be injected at the same time as local anesthetics.

Because leflunomide can cause severe liver dysfunction if combined with other hepatotoxic drugs, this combination should be avoided.

The absorption of penicillamine is decreased if taken with iron salts or antacids; if these are given together, they should be separated by at least 2 hours.

Anakinra and etanercept should not be used together because of an increased risk of serious infections.

Nursing Considerations for Patients Receiving Other Related Drugs

Nursing considerations for patients receiving the drugs listed in this section are similar to those for patients receiving other anti-inflammatory drugs. Details related to each individual drug can be found in the specific drug monograph in your nursing drug guide.

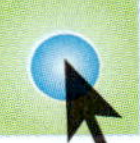

WEB LINKS

Health care providers and patients may want to consult the following Internet sources:

http://www.arthritis.org Information on arthritis—disease, treatments, research.

http://www.fda.gov Information on drug research and development and warnings.

http://www.nlm.nih.gov/medlineplus/arthritis.htm Information on research, advances, advice, and patient teaching protocols.

Points to Remember

- The inflammatory response, which is important for protecting the body from injury and invasion, produces many of the signs and symptoms associated with disease, including fever, aches and pains, and lethargy.
- Chronic or excessive activity by the inflammatory response can lead to the release of lysosomal enzymes and tissue destruction.
- Anti-inflammatory drugs block various chemicals associated with the inflammatory reaction. Anti-inflammatory drugs also may have antipyretic (fever-blocking) and analgesic (pain-blocking) activities.
- Salicylates block prostaglandin activity. NSAIDs block prostaglandin synthesis. Acetaminophen causes vasodilation and heat release, lowering fever and working to relieve pain. Gold salts prevent macrophage phagocytosis, lysosomal release, and tissue damage. Etanercept contains TNF receptors to deactivate TNF and slow progression of

autoimmune diseases. Leflunomide deactivates an enzyme active in autoimmune disease. Penicillamine is a chelating agent that lowers levels of IgM rheumatoid factor in acute rheumatoid arthritis. Hyaluronidase derivatives and sodium hyaluronate are viscous and elastic hyaluronic acid derivatives that lubricate arthritic knees and stop some of the pain of inflammation. Anakinra is an interleukin-1 receptor antagonist that blocks the degradation of cartilage in rheumatoid arthritis.

- Salicylates can cause acidosis and eighth cranial nerve damage. NSAIDs are most associated with GI irritation and bleeding. Acetaminophen can cause serious liver toxicity. The gold salts cause many systemic inflammatory reactions. Other antiarthritis drugs are associated with local injection site irritation and increased susceptibility to infection. Leflunomide is associated with severe hepatic toxicity.
- Many anti-inflammatory drugs are available OTC, and care must be taken to prevent abuse or overuse of these drugs.

CHECK YOUR UNDERSTANDING

Answers to the questions in this chapter may be found in the Answer Key in the back of the book.

Multiple Choice

Select the best answer to the following.

1. An analgesic is a drug that
   a. reduces fever.
   b. reduces swelling.
   c. reduces redness.
   d. reduces pain.

2. An antipyretic is a drug that can
   a. block pain.
   b. block swelling.
   c. block fever.
   d. block inflammation.

3. Salicylates are very popular anti-inflammatory agents for all of the following reasons, *except*
   a. they have antipyretic properties.
   b. they have analgesic properties.
   c. they are available without a prescription.
   d. they must be given parenterally.

4. The NSAIDs affect the COX-1 and COX-2 enzymes. By blocking COX-2 enzymes, the NSAIDs block inflammation and the signs and symptoms of inflammation at the site of injury or trauma. By blocking COX-1 enzymes, these drugs block
   a. fever regulation.
   b. prostaglandins that protect the stomach lining.
   c. swelling in the periphery.
   d. liver function.

5. Your patient has been receiving ibuprofen for many years to relieve the pain of osteoarthritis. Assessment of the patient should include
   a. an electrocardiogram.
   b. CBC with differential.
   c. respiratory auscultation.
   d. renal evaluation.

6. Patients taking NSAIDs should be taught to avoid the use of OTC medications without checking with their prescriber because
   a. many of the OTC preparations contain NSAIDs and inadvertent toxicity could occur.
   b. no one should take more than one type of pain reliever at a time.
   c. increased GI upset could occur.
   d. there is a risk of Reye's syndrome.

7. Chronic or excessive activity by the inflammatory response can lead to
   a. loss of white blood cells.
   b. coagulation problems.
   c. release of lysosomal enzymes and tissue destruction.
   d. adrenal suppression.

8. A patient with rheumatoid arthritis who is on a fixed income and who is being treated with aspirin should be advised
   a. to use only brand-name aspirin.
   b. to use only enteric-coated aspirin.
   c. to use generic aspirin, checking the expiration date before use.
   d. to switch to one of the NSAIDs.

Multiple Response

Select all that apply.

1. A client is being treated for severe rheumatoid arthritis. The nurse could anticipate treatment with which of the following.
   a. Etanercept—tumor necrosis factor
   b. Gold therapy
   c. Hylan G-F 20—hylans with elastic properties
   d. Ketoprofen
   e. Interferon beta-2a
   f. Methotrexate

2. The nurse notes an order for oxaprozin (*Daypro)* for the treatment of arthritis. Before administering the drug, the nurse would assess the patient for which problems that could be cautions or contraindications?
   a. Headaches
   b. Dysmenorrhea
   c. Active peptic ulcer disease
   d. Chronic obstructive pulmonary disease
   e. Renal impairment
   f. Bleeding disorders

Web Exercise

You are caring for a patient who has newly diagnosed rheumatoid arthritis. The family is involved and supportive and would like information on the disease and treatment options and any new information. Go to http://www.arthritis.org and prepare an information sheet for this patient and family using data from that site.

Matching

Match the word with the appropriate definition.

1. ______________________ anti-inflammatory
2. ______________________ antipyretic
3. ______________________ analgesic
4. ______________________ salicylates
5. ______________________ NSAIDs
6. ______________________ pyrogens
7. ______________________ chrysotherapy

A. Treatment with gold salts
B. Nonsteroidal anti-inflammatory drugs
C. Block the prostaglandin system to prevent inflammation
D. Blocking the effects of the inflammatory response
E. Blocking pain sensation
F. Substances that elevate the body's temperature
G. Blocking fever

Bibliography and References

Acetaminophen toxicity. ISMP Safety Alert (Aug. 7, 2002); p. 1.

Agrawal, N. M., & Aziz, K. (1998). Prevention of gastrointestinal complications with nonsteroidal antiinflammatory drugs. *Journal of Rheumatology, 51*(Suppl.), 17–20.

Cash, J. M., & Wilder, R. L. (1995). Refractory rheumatoid arthritis: Therapeutic options. *Rheumatic Diseases Clinics North America, 21*(1), 1–18.

Drug facts and comparisons. (2006). St. Louis: Facts & Comparisons.

Gilman, A., Hardman, J. G., & Limbird, L. E. (Eds.). (2006). *Goodman and Gilman's the pharmacological basis of therapeutics* (11th ed.). New York: McGraw-Hill.

Hill, J., Thorpe, R., & Bird, H. (2003). Outcomes for patients with RA—a rheumatology nurse practitioner clinic compared to standard outpatient care. *J Musculoskeletal Care, 1*(1), 5–20.

Karch, A. M. (2006). *2007 Lippincott's nursing drug guide.* Philadelphia: Lippincott Williams & Wilkins.

Lancaster, C. (1995). Effective nonsteroidal antiinflammatory drugs devoid of gastrointestinal side effects: Do they really exist? *Digestive Diseases and Sciences, 13*(Suppl. 1), 40–47.

Porth, C. M. (2005). *Pathophysiology: Concepts of altered health states* (7th ed.). Philadelphia: Lippincott Williams & Wilkins.

The medical letter on drugs and therapeutics. (2006). New Rochelle, NY: Medical Letter.

CHAPTER 17

Immune Modulators

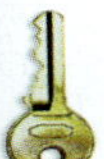

KEY TERMS

immune stimulant

immune suppressant

monoclonal antibodies

recombinant DNA technology

LEARNING OBJECTIVES

Upon completion of this chapter, you will be able to:

1. Describe the sites of actions of the various immune modulators.
2. Describe the therapeutic actions, indications, pharmacokinetics, contraindications, most common adverse reactions, and important drug–drug interactions associated with each class of immune modulator: interferons, interleukins, T- and B-cell modulators, immune suppressants, interleukin receptor antagonists, and monoclonal antibodies.
3. Discuss the use of immune modulators across the lifespan.
4. Compare and contrast the prototype drugs for each class of immune modulators with the other drugs in that class and with drugs in other classes.
5. Outline the nursing considerations and teaching needs for patients receiving each class of immune modulator.

IMMUNE STIMULANTS

Interferons

interferon alfa-2a

P interferon alfa-2b

interferon alfacon-1

interferon alfa-n3

interferon beta-1a

interferon beta-1b

interferon gamma-1b

peginterferon alfa-2a

peginterferon alfa-2b

Interleukins

P aldesleukin

oprelvekin

T- and B-cell Modulators

levamisole

IMMUNE SUPPRESSANTS

T- and B-cell Suppressors

alefacept

azathioprine

P cyclosporine

glatiramer acetate

mycophenolate

pimecrolimus

sirolimus

tacrolimus

Interleukin Receptor Antagonist

anakinra

Monoclonal Antibodies

adalimumab

alemtuzumab

basiliximab

bevacizumab

cetuximab

daclizumab

efalizumab

erlotinib

gemtuzumab

ibritumomab

infliximab

P muromonab-CD3

natalizumab

omalizumab

palivizumab

pegaptanib

rituximab

tositumomab

trastuzumab

As the name implies, immune modulators are used to modify the actions of the immune system. **Immune stimulants** are used to energize the immune system when it is exhausted from fighting prolonged invasion or needs help fighting a specific pathogen or cancer cell. **Immune suppressants** are used to block the normal effects of the immune system in cases of organ transplantation (in which nonself-cells are transplanted into the body and destroyed by the immune reaction) and in autoimmune disorders (in which the body's defenses recognize self-cells as foreign and work to destroy them).

The knowledge base about the actions and components of the immune system is growing and changing daily. As new discoveries are made and interactions understood, new applications will be found for modulating the immune system in a variety of disorders. (See Box 17.1 for their use in a variety of age groups. Box 17.2 discusses the use of immune modulators during pregnancy.)

BOX 17.2 Focus on Gender Considerations: Immune Modulators and Pregnancy

Generally, immune modulators are contraindicated for use during pregnancy and lactation, largely because these drugs have been associated with fetal abnormalities, increased maternal and fetal infections, and suppressed immune responses in nursing babies. Female patients should be informed of the risk of using these drugs during pregnancy and receive counseling in the use of barrier contraceptives. (The use of barrier contraceptives is advised because the effects of oral contraceptives may be altered by liver changes or by changes in the body's immune response, potentially resulting in unexpected pregnancy.)

If a patient taking immune modulators becomes pregnant or decides that she wants to become pregnant, she should discuss this with her health care provider and review the risks associated with use of the drug or drugs being taken. The monoclonal antibodies should be used with caution during pregnancy and lactation. Because long-term studies of most of these drugs are not yet available, it may be prudent to advise patients taking these drugs to avoid pregnancy if possible.

Immune Stimulants

Immune stimulants include the interferons, which are naturally released from human cells in response to viral invasion; the interleukins, synthetic compounds much like the interleukins that communicate between lymphocytes, which stimulate cellular immunity and inhibit tumor growth; and a T- and B-cell modulator called levamisole (*Ergamisol*), which restores immune function and also stimulates immune system activity (Figure 17.1).

Interferons

Interferons are naturally produced and released by human cells that have been invaded by viruses. They may also be released from cells in response to other stimuli. A number of interferons are available for use today. Several are produced by **recombinant DNA technology**, including interferon alfa-2a (*Roferon-A*), interferon alfa-2b (*Intron-A*), inter-

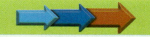

BOX 17.1 DRUG THERAPY ACROSS THE LIFESPAN

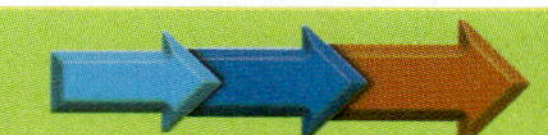

Immune Modulators

CHILDREN

Most of the drugs that affect the immune system are not recommended for use in children or have not been tested in children. The exceptions—interferon alfa-2b, azathioprine, cyclosporine, tacrolimus, and palivizumab—should be used cautiously, monitoring the child frequently for infection, GI, renal, hematological, or CNS effects.

The immune suppressants (azathioprine, cyclosporine, and tacrolimus) are usually needed in higher doses for children than for adults to achieve the same therapeutic effect.

Protecting the child from infection and injury is a very important part of the care of a child taking an immune modulator. This can be a great challenge with an active child.

ADULTS

Both the adult patient who is receiving a parenteral immune modulator and a significant other should learn the proper technique for injection, disposal of needles, and special storage precautions for the drug. It is important to stress ways to avoid exposure to infection and injury to prevent further complications. The patient should be encouraged to seek regular follow-up and medical care.

Immune modulators are contraindicated during pregnancy and lactation because of the potential for adverse effects on the fetus or neonate and complications for the mother. Women of childbearing age should be advised to use barrier contraceptives while taking these drugs and, if breast-feeding, should be counseled to find another method of feeding the baby. Some of these drugs impair fertility, and the patient should be advised of this fact before taking the drug.

OLDER ADULTS

Older patients may be more susceptible to the effects of the immune modulators, partly because the aging immune system is less efficient and less responsive.

These patients need to be monitored closely for infection, GI, renal, hepatic, and CNS effects. Baseline renal and liver function tests can help to determine whether a decreased dosage will be needed before beginning therapy.

Because these patients are more susceptible to infection, they need to receive extensive teaching about ways to avoid infection and injury.

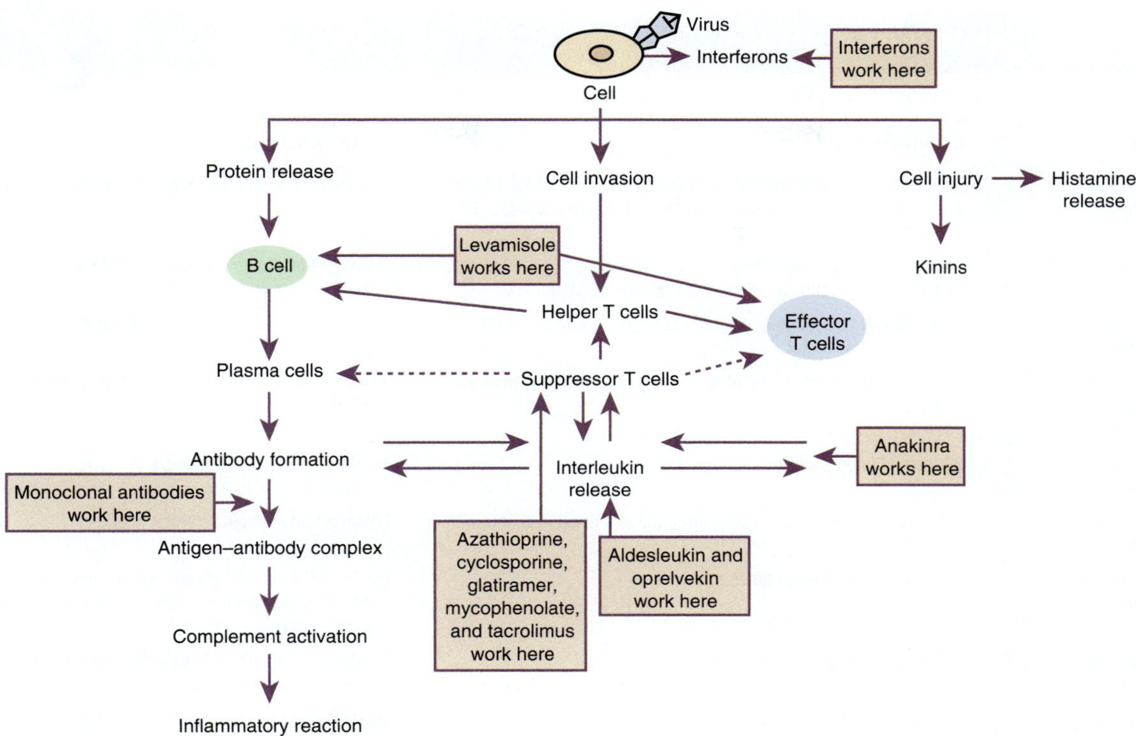

FIGURE 17.1 Sites of action of the immune modulators.

feron alfacon-1 (*Infergen*), peginterferon alfa-2a (*Pegasys*), peginterferon alfa-2b (*Peg-Intron*), and interferon beta-1b (*Betaseron*). Interferon alfa-n3 (*Alferon N*) is produced by harvesting human leukocytes and is injected directly into warts, a viral infection. Interferon beta-1a (*Avonex*) is produced from Chinese hamster ovary cells. Interferon gamma-1b (*Actimmune*) is produced by *Escherichia coli* bacteria. The interferon of choice depends on the condition being treated (Table 17.1).

Therapeutic Actions and Indications

Interferons act to prevent virus particles from replicating inside other cells. They also stimulate interferon receptor sites on noninvaded cells to produce antiviral proteins, which prevent viruses from entering the cell. In addition, interferons have been found to inhibit tumor growth and replication. Interestingly, interferon gamma-1b also acts like an interleukin, stimulating phagocytes to be more aggressive.

Interferons are indicated for treating selected leukemias (alfa-2a, alfa-2b); multiple sclerosis (beta-1a, beta-1b); intralesional treatment of warts (alfa-n3, alfa-2b); chronic hepatitis B or chronic hepatitis C (alfa-2b); chronic hepatitis C (alfacon-1, peginterferons); acquired immune deficiency syndrome (AIDS)-related Kaposi's sarcoma (alfa-2a, alfa-2b, and unlabeled uses for several other interferons); and severe infections caused by chronic granulomatous disease (gamma-1b). Most of the interferons are being tested for the treatment of various cancers and AIDS-related problems.

Pharmacokinetics

The interferons are generally well absorbed after subcutaneous or intramuscular injection. They are broken down in the tissues and seem to be excreted primarily through the kidneys. Many of them are teratogenic in animals and therefore should not be used during pregnancy. Use of barrier contraceptives is advised for women of childbearing age. It is not known whether these drugs cross into breast milk, but because of the potential adverse effects on the baby, it is advised that the drugs not be used during lactation unless the benefits to the mother clearly outweigh any risks to the baby.

Contraindications and Cautions

The use of interferons is contraindicated in the presence of known allergy to any interferon or product components and during pregnancy and lactation *because of the potential risk to the fetus or neonate.* Caution should be used in the presence of known cardiac disease *because hypertension and arrhythmias have been reported with the use of these drugs;* with myelosuppression *because these drugs may further suppress the bone marrow;* and with central nervous system (CNS) dysfunction of any kind *because of the potential for CNS depression and personality changes that have been reported.*

Adverse Effects

The adverse effects associated with the use of interferons are related to the immune or inflammatory reaction that is being

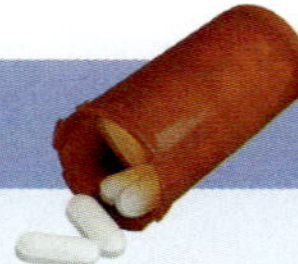

Table 17.1 DRUGS IN FOCUS

Interferons

Drug Name	Dosage/Route	Usual Indications
interferon alfa-2a (*Roferon-A*)	*Leukemia:* 3 million international Units/day Sub-Q or IM for 16–24 wk *Kaposi's sarcoma:* 36 million International Units/day Sub-Q or IM for 10–12 wk	Treatment of leukemias, Kaposi's sarcoma in adults
P interferon alfa-2b (*Intron-A*)	Adult: dosage varies widely based on indication Pediatric: for hepatitis B, adjust adult dosage to weight	Treatment of leukemias, Kaposi's sarcoma, warts, hepatitis B, malignant melanoma
interferon alfacon-1 (*Infergen*)	9 mcg Sub-Q as a single dose three times per week for 24 wk	Treatment of chronic hepatitis C in adults
interferon alfa-n1 interferon alfa-n3 (*Alferon N*)	250,000 International Units intralesionally two times per week for 8 wk	Intralesional treatment of warts; AIDS-related complex, AIDS orphan drug indication
interferon beta-1a (*Avonex*)	30 mcg IM once a week	Treatment of multiple sclerosis in adults
interferon beta-1b (*Betaseron*)	0.25 mg Sub-Q every other day; discontinue if disease is unremitting >6 mo	Treatment of multiple sclerosis in adults
interferon gamma-1b (*Actimmune*)	50 mcg/m^2 Sub-Q three times per week	Treatment of serious, chronic granulomatous disease in adults; delaying time to disease progression in severe, malignant osteopetrosis
peginterferon alfa-2a (*Pegasys*)	180 mcg Sub-Q once a week for 48 wk	Treatment of adults with hepatitis C who have compensated liver disease
peginterferon alfa-2b (*Peg-Intron*)	1 mcg/kg Sub-Q once a week for 1 yr	Treatment of chronic hepatitis C in adults

stimulated (e.g., lethargy, myalgia, arthralgia, anorexia, nausea). Other commonly seen adverse effects include headache, dizziness, bone marrow depression, depression and suicidal ideation, photosensitivity, and liver impairment.

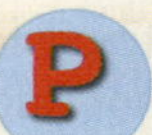

Prototype Summary: Interferon Alfa-2b

Indications: Hairy cell leukemia, malignant melanoma, AIDS-related Kaposi's sarcoma, chronic hepatitis B and C, intralesional treatment of condylomata acuminata in patients 18 years of age or older

Actions: Inhibits the growth of tumor cells and enhances the immune response

Pharmacokinetics:

Route	Onset	Peak
IM, Sub-Q	Rapid	3–12 h
IV	Rapid	End of infusion

$T_{1/2}$: 2 to 3 hours; metabolized in the kidney, excretion is unknown

Adverse effects: Dizziness, confusion, rash, dry skin, anorexia, nausea, bone marrow suppression, flu-like syndrome

Interleukins

Interleukins (Table 17.2) are chemicals produced by T cells to communicate between leukocytes. Interleukin-2 stimulates cellular immunity by increasing the activity of natural killer cells, platelets, and cytokines. Two interleukin-2 preparations are available for use. Aldesleukin (*Proleukin*) is a human interleukin produced by recombinant DNA technology using *E. coli* bacteria. Oprelvekin (*Neumega*) is a newer agent, released in 1998, that is also produced by DNA technology.

Therapeutic Actions and Indications

Natural interleukin-2 is produced by helper T cells to activate cellular immunity and inhibit tumor growth by increasing lymphocyte numbers and their activity. When interleukins are administered, there are increases in the number of natural killer cells and lymphocytes, in cytokine activity, and in the number of circulating platelets. Aldesleukin is indicated for the treatment of specific renal carcinomas and is also being investigated for use in the treatment of AIDS and AIDS-related disorders. Oprelvekin is indicated for the prevention of severe thrombocytopenia (an abnormal decrease in the number of platelets) after myelosuppressive chemotherapy in select patients.

Pharmacokinetics

The interleukins are rapidly distributed after injection and are primarily cleared from the body by the kidneys. They were shown to be embryocidal and teratogenic in animal studies

Table 17.2 DRUGS IN FOCUS

Interleukins

Drug Name	Dosage/Route	Usual Indications
P aldesleukin (*Proleukin*)	Two 5-day cycles of 600,000 International Units/kg IV q8h given over 15 min	Treatment of specific renal carcinomas in adults
oprelvekin (*Neumega*)	50 mcg/kg/day Sub-Q starting 1 day after chemotherapy and continuing for 14–21days	Prevention of severe thrombocytopenia after myelosuppressive chemotherapy

and should not be used during pregnancy. Use of barrier contraceptives is recommended for women of childbearing age who require one of these drugs. It is not clear whether the drugs cross into breast milk, but it is recommended that they not be used during lactation; if they must be used, another method of feeding the baby must be chosen because of the potential for adverse effects in the baby.

Contraindications and Cautions

Interleukins are contraindicated in the presence of any allergy to an interleukin or *E. coli*-produced product and during pregnancy and lactation. Caution should be used with renal, liver, or cardiovascular impairment *because of the adverse effects of the drugs.*

Adverse Effects

The adverse effects associated with the interleukins can be attributed to their effect on the body during inflammation (e.g., lethargy, myalgia, arthralgia, fatigue, fever). Respiratory difficulties, CNS changes, and cardiac arrhythmias also have been reported, and the patient should be monitored for these effects and the drug stopped if they do occur.

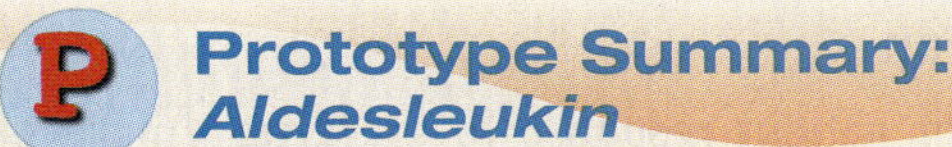

Prototype Summary: Aldesleukin

Indications: Metastatic renal cell carcinoma in adults; orphan drug use: treatment of metastatic melanomas

Actions: Activates human cellular immunity and inhibits tumor growth through increases in lymphocytes, platelets, and cytokines

Pharmacokinetics:

Route	Onset	Peak	Duration
IV	5 min	13 min	3–4 h

$T_{1/2}$: 85 min; metabolized in the kidney and excreted in the urine

Adverse effects: Mental status changes, dizziness, hypotension, sinus tachycardia, arrhythmias, pruritus, nausea, vomiting, diarrhea, anorexia, gastrointestinal (GI) bleed, bone marrow suppression, respiratory difficulties, fever, chills, pain

T- and B-Cell Modulator

The drug levamisole (*Ergamisol*) is an immune stimulant that restores suppressed immune function in certain situations (Table 17.3).

Therapeutic Actions and Indications

Levamisole stimulates B cells, which in turn stimulate antibody formation, enhance T-cell activity, and increase the activity of both monocytes and macrophages. Levamisole is indicated for the treatment of Dukes' stage C colon cancer after surgical resection and in conjunction with fluorouracil therapy. With further research, the indications may be expanded to include other carcinomas.

Pharmacokinetics

Levamisole is readily absorbed from the GI tract, reaching peak levels in 1.5 to 2 hours. It is extensively metabolized in

Table 17.3 DRUGS IN FOCUS

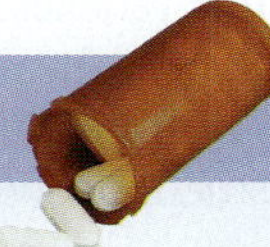

T- and B-Cell Modulator

Drug Name	Dosage/Route	Usual Indications
levamisole (*Ergamisol*)	50 mg PO q8h given with fluorouracil	Treatment of Dukes' stage C colon cancer after resection in adults

the liver and excreted in the urine, with a half-life of 16 hours. Levamisole was embryotoxic in animal studies and should not be used during pregnancy. Women of childbearing age should be advised to use barrier contraceptives. It is not known whether levamisole crosses into breast milk, but because of the potentially severe adverse effects it could have on a neonate, it is recommended that the drug not be used during lactation.

Contraindications and Cautions

Levamisole is contraindicated in the presence of any known allergy to levamisole or its components and in pregnancy and lactation *because of possible adverse effects to the fetus or neonate.*

Adverse Effects

The most common adverse effects seen with levamisole are related to immune stimulation (so-called flu-like effects: fatigue, lethargy, myalgia, arthralgia, fever). Other adverse effects that have been reported include GI upset, nausea, taste perversions, and diarrhea; dizziness, headache, and depression; bone marrow depression; dermatitis; and hair loss.

Clinically Important Drug–Drug Interactions

There is a possibility of a disulfiram-type reaction if this drug is combined with alcohol. Patients should be cautioned to avoid this combination. There also is a possibility of increased phenytoin levels and toxicity if levamisole is combined with phenytoin. If such a combination cannot be avoided, phenytoin levels should be monitored and appropriate dosage reductions made.

Nursing Considerations for Patients Receiving Immune Stimulants

Assessment: History and Examination

Screen for any of the following conditions, *which would contraindicate or require cautious use of the drug:* known allergies to any of these drugs or their components; pregnancy or lactation; hepatic, renal, or cardiac disease; bone marrow depression; and CNS disorders, including seizures.

Include screening *for baseline status before beginning therapy and for any potential adverse effects:* presence of any skin lesions; weight; temperature; orientation, reflexes; pulse, blood pressure, electrocardiogram (ECG), heart rhythm; liver evaluation; complete blood count (CBC), liver and renal function tests; and assessment of condition being treated.

Nursing Diagnoses

The patient receiving immune stimulants may have the following nursing diagnoses related to drug therapy:

- Acute Pain related to CNS, GI, and flu-like effects
- Imbalanced Nutrition: Less Than Body Requirements related to flu-like effects
- Anxiety related to diagnosis and drug therapy
- Deficient Knowledge regarding drug therapy

Implementation With Rationale

- Arrange for laboratory tests before and periodically during therapy, including CBC and differential, *to monitor for drug effects and adverse effects.*
- Administer drug as indicated; instruct the patient and a significant other if injections are required *to ensure that the drug will be given even if the patient is not able to administer it.*
- Monitor for severe reactions and *arrange to discontinue drug immediately if they occur.*
- Arrange for supportive care and comfort measures for flu-like symptoms (e.g., rest, environmental control, acetaminophen) *to help the patient cope with the drug effects.* Ensure that the patient is well hydrated during therapy *to prevent severe adverse effects.*
- Instruct female patients in the use of barrier contraceptives *to avoid pregnancy during therapy because of the potential for adverse effects on the fetus.*
- Provide thorough patient teaching, including measures to avoid adverse effects, warning signs of problems, and proper administration, *to increase knowledge about drug therapy and to increase compliance with the drug regimen.*
- Offer support and encouragement *to deal with the diagnosis and the drug regimen.*

Evaluation

- Monitor patient response to the drug (improvement in condition being treated).
- Monitor for adverse effects (flu-like symptoms, GI upset, CNS changes, bone marrow depression).
- Evaluate the effectiveness of the teaching plan (patient can name drug, dosage, adverse effects to watch for, specific measures to avoid adverse effects).
- Monitor the effectiveness of comfort measures and compliance with the regimen.

FOCUS POINTS

- Immune stimulants assist the immune system to fight specific pathogens or cancer cells; in doing so they cause flu-like symptoms.

- Interferons are used to treat various cancers and warts.
- Interleukins stimulate cellular immunity and inhibit tumor growth.

Immune Suppressants

Immune suppressants often are used in conjunction with corticosteroids, which block the inflammatory reaction and decrease initial damage to cells. They are especially beneficial in cases of organ transplantation and in the treatment of autoimmune diseases. The immune suppressants include T- and B-cell suppressors, an interleukin receptor antagonist, and **monoclonal antibodies**—antibodies produced by a single clone of B cells that react with specific antigens.

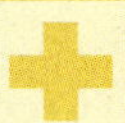

FOCUS ON **PATIENT SAFETY**

Because patients receiving immune suppressants are at high risk for infection and cancers, they need to be forewarned to avoid situations in which exposure to infection may be high (e.g., crowds, working in the soil, visiting hospitals or sick friends, consorting with children during flu and cold season). They should also avoid activities that may cause injury, which leads to infection. Protective strategies include wearing masks and heavy gloves, delaying vaccinations, knowing the signs and symptoms of infection that warrant medical care, and obtaining regular physical examinations and screenings for diseases of developing neoplasms.

T- and B-Cell Suppressors

Several T- and B-cell immune suppressors are available for use (Table 17.4). Only one, cyclosporine (*Sandimmune, Neoral*), is used to suppress rejection in a variety of transplantation scenarios. It also is the most commonly used immune suppressant. *Neoral* is also used to treat rheumatoid arthritis and psoriasis. It is well absorbed from the GI tract, reaching peak levels in 1 to 2 hours. Cyclosporine is extensively metabolized in the liver by the cytochrome P450 system and is primarily excreted in the bile. The half-life of the drug is about 19 hours for *Sandimmune* and 8.4 hours for *Neoral*. Cyclosporine was embryotoxic in animal studies and crosses into breast milk. The drug should not be used during pregnancy or lactation, and women of childbearing age should be advised to use barrier contraceptives.

Alefacept (*Amevive*) is used to treat adult patients with severe, chronic psoriasis who are candidates for systemic therapy or phototherapy. It is rapidly absorbed and can be given IM or IV. It reaches peak levels in 4 to 6 hours and has a half-life of 270 hours. This drug binds to leukocytes and lymphocyte antigens. Alefacept is teratogenic in animal studies and should be used during pregnancy only if the benefit clearly outweighs the risk to the fetus. The drug enters breast milk and should not be used during lactation.

Azathioprine (*Imuran*) is used specifically to prevent rejection in renal homotransplants and to treat rheumatoid arthritis (an autoimmune disorder) in selected patients. It is rapidly absorbed from the GI tract, reaching peak levels in 1 to 2 hours. This drug is catabolized in the liver and red blood cells. It was highly teratogenic in animal studies and crosses into breast milk. Because of the potential effects on the fetus or neonate, the drug should not be used during pregnancy or lactation, and women of childbearing age should be advised to use barrier contraceptives.

Glatiramer acetate (*Copaxone*) is used specifically to reduce the number of relapses in multiple sclerosis, which is thought to be related to an autoimmune reaction. Little is known about the pharmacokinetics of this drug. Some of it is immediately hydrolyzed on injection, some enters the lymph system, and some may actually reach the systemic circulation. Because it is not known whether this drug crosses the placenta or crosses into breast milk, use during pregnancy and lactation should be reserved for those situations in which the benefit to the mother clearly outweighs the potential risk to the fetus or neonate.

Mycophenolate (*CellCept*) is an oral drug that is used with cyclosporine and corticosteroids to prevent organ rejection after renal, hepatic, or heart transplantation. It is readily absorbed and immediately metabolized to its active metabolite. Most of the metabolized drug is then excreted in the urine. Caution should be used if serious renal impairment exists, and the dosage should be lowered. Mycophenolate was teratogenic in animal studies, and women of childbearing age should be advised to use barrier contraceptives whenever this drug is used. It is not known whether mycophenolate crosses into human breast milk, but because of the potential for adverse effects in the baby, it should not be used during lactation.

Sirolimus (*Rapamune*) is used to prevent organ rejection in patients receiving renal transplants and should be used with cyclosporine and corticosteroids. It is being studied for use in the treatment of psoriasis. Sirolimus is rapidly absorbed from the GI tract, reaching peak levels in 1 hour. It is extensively metabolized in the liver, partly by the cytochrome P450 system. Reduced dosage may be needed if hepatic impairment is present. The drug is then excreted primarily in the feces. Sirolimus was embryotoxic in animal studies and should not be used during pregnancy unless the benefit to the mother clearly outweighs the potential risks to the fetus. It is not known whether sirolimus crosses into breast milk, but because of the potential for serious adverse effects in the baby, the drug should not be used during lactation.

Tacrolimus (*Prograf*) is used to prevent liver or renal transplant rejection and is being studied for use in multiple other transplant scenarios. This drug is rapidly absorbed from the GI tract, reaching peak levels in 1.5 to 3.5 hours. It

Table 17.4 DRUGS IN FOCUS

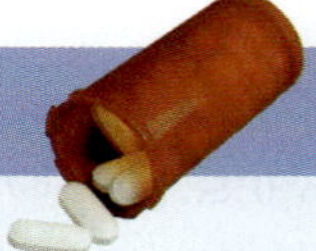

T- and B-Cell Suppressors

Drug Name	Dosage/Route	Usual Indications
alefacept (*Amevive*)	7.5 mg IV bolus once a week or 15 mg IM once a week, in 12-wk cycles	Treatment of adults with moderate to severe chronic plaque psoriasis who are candidates for systemic therapy or phototherapy
azathioprine (*Imuran*)	Adult: 3–5 mg/kg/day PO for prevention of rejection; maintenance: 1–3 mg/kg/day PO *Rheumatoid arthritis:* 1–2.5 mg/kg/day PO Reduce dosage with renal impairment Pediatric: 3–5 mg/kg/day IV or PO to prevent rejection; maintenance: 1–3 mg/kg/day PO	Prevention of rejection in renal homotransplants; treatment of rheumatoid arthritis
P cyclosporine (*Sandimmune*)	15 mg/kg PO as a single oral dose 4–12 h before transplantation, then 5–10 mg/kg/day PO Pediatric: larger doses may be needed to achieve therapeutic levels	Suppression of rejection in a variety of transplant situations; rheumatoid arthritis, psoriasis (*Neoral*)
(*Neoral*)	9–15 mg/kg PO as a single oral dose 4–12 h before transplantation, then 5–10 mg/kg/day PO—titrate down *Rheumatoid arthritis:* 2.5 mg/kg/day PO in two divided doses *Psoriasis:* 2.5 mg/kg PO b.i.d.	
glatiramer acetate (*Copaxone*)	20 mg/day Sub-Q	Reduction of the number of relapses in multiple sclerosis in adults
mycophenolate (*CellCept*)	1–1.5 mg PO b.i.d.; may be started IV during transplantation, with switch to oral route as soon as possible	Prevention of rejection after renal, hepatic, or heart transplantation in adults
pimecrolimus (*Elidel*)	Apply thin layer to affected area b.i.d.	Treatment of mild to moderate atopic dermatitis in patients >2 yr; limit use
sirolimus (*Rapamune*)	6 mg PO as soon after transplant as possible; then 2 mg/day PO Children (<13 yr): 3 mg/m^2 PO loading dose, then 1 mg/m^2/day PO	Prevention of rejection after renal transplantation
tacrolimus (*Prograf*)	0.1–0.2 mg/kg/day PO in two divided doses; may begin as continuous IV infusion of 0.03–0.05 mg/kg/day, with switch to oral form as soon as possible Pediatric: may require higher doses to achieve therapeutic levels	Prevention of rejection after renal or liver transplantation
tacrolimus (*Protopic*)	Apply thin layer to affected area b.i.d.	Treatment of moderate to severe atopic dermatitis; continue for 1 wk after resolution

is extensively metabolized in the liver by the cytochrome P450 system and is excreted in the urine. Lower doses of the drug may be needed in the presence of hepatic or renal impairment, which would interfere with the metabolism and excretion of the drug. Tacrolimus crosses the placenta and has been associated with hyperkalemia and renal dysfunction in the fetus. Avoid use in pregnancy unless the benefit to the mother clearly outweighs the risk to the fetus. It crosses into breast milk and is contraindicated during lactation because of the potential for serious adverse effects on the baby. Ongoing drug studies continue to explore unlabeled uses of many of these agents to prevent other transplant rejections.

Therapeutic Actions and Indications

The exact mechanism of action of the T- and B-cell suppressors is not clearly understood. It has been shown that they do block antibody production by B cells, inhibit suppressor and helper T cells, and modify the release of interleukins and of T-cell growth factor (see Figure 17.1).

The T- and B-cell suppressors are indicated for the prevention and treatment of specific transplant rejections. Azathioprine and cyclosporine have also been approved for the treatment of rheumatoid arthritis. Many of the T- and B-cell suppressors are used to treat a variety of autoimmune disorders and other transplant rejections as unlabeled uses for the drugs.

Contraindications and Cautions

The use of T- and B-cell suppressors is contraindicated in the presence of any known allergy to the drug or its components, and during pregnancy and lactation *because of the potential adverse effects on the fetus or neonate.* Caution should be used with renal or hepatic impairment, *which could interfere with the metabolism or excretion of the drug,* and in the presence of known neoplasms, *which potentially could spread with immune system suppression.*

Adverse Effects

Patients receiving these drugs are at increased risk for infection and for the development of neoplasms because of their blocking effect on the immune system. Other potentially dangerous adverse effects include hepatotoxicity, renal toxicity, renal dysfunction, and pulmonary edema. Patients may experience headache, tremors, secondary infections such as acne, GI upset, diarrhea, and hypertension.

Clinically Important Drug–Drug Interactions

There is an increased risk of toxicity if these drugs are combined with other drugs that are hepatotoxic or nephrotoxic. Extreme care should be used if such combinations are necessary. Other reported drug–drug interactions are drug specific (consult a drug guide or drug handbook).

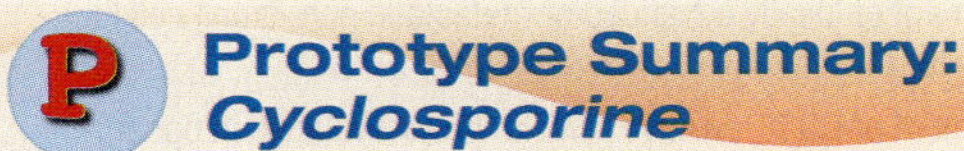

Prototype Summary: Cyclosporine

Indications: Prophylaxis for organ rejection in kidney, liver, and heart transplants (used with corticosteroids); treatment of chronic rejection in patients previously treated with other immunosuppressants; treatment of rheumatoid arthritis and recalcitrant psoriasis

Actions: Reversibly inhibits immunocompetent lymphocytes; inhibits T-helper cells and T-suppressor cells, lymphokine production, and release of interleukin-2 and T-cell growth factor

Pharmacokinetics:

Route	Onset	Peak
Oral	Varies	3.5 h
IV	Rapid	1–2 h

$T_{1/2}$: 19 to 27 hours; metabolized in the liver and excreted in the bile and urine

Adverse effects: Tremor, hypertension, gum hyperplasia, renal dysfunction, diarrhea, hirsutism, acne, bone marrow suppression

Interleukin Receptor Antagonist

Anakinra (*Kineret*) specifically antagonizes human interleukin-1 receptors, blocking the activity of interleukin-1. Interleukin-1 levels are elevated in response to inflammation or immune reactions and are thought to be responsible for the degradation of cartilage that occurs in rheumatoid arthritis.

Therapeutic Actions and Indications

Anakinra is used to reduce the signs and symptoms of moderately to severely active rheumatoid arthritis in patients 18 years of age and older who have not responded to the traditional antirheumatic drugs.

Pharmacokinetics

The recommended dosage is 100 mg/d by subcutaneous injection. Anakinra is absorbed slowly, reaching peak effects in 3 to 7 hours. It is metabolized in the tissues with a 4- to 6-hour half-life. The drug may cross the placenta and may enter breast milk. It is excreted in the urine.

Contraindications and Cautions

Anakinra is contraindicated with any known allergy to *E. coli*-produced products or to anakinra itself. It should be used with caution during pregnancy and lactation and in patients with renal impairment, immunosuppression, or any active infection. There is an increased risk of infection whenever this drug is used, and the patient needs to be protected from exposure to infections and monitored closely after any invasive procedures. Immunizations cannot be given while the patient is on this drug.

Patients need to be instructed in proper subcutaneous injection technique and cautioned to store the drug in the refrigerator. They also need to be aware of the drug's expiration date.

Adverse Effects

Headache, sinusitis, nausea, diarrhea, upper respiratory and other infections, and injection site reactions are among the most common adverse effects.

Clinically Important Drug–Drug Interactions

Patients who are also receiving etanercept (*Enbrel*) must be monitored very closely because severe and even life-threatening infections have occurred.

Monoclonal Antibodies

Antibodies that attach to specific receptor sites are being developed to respond to very specific situations. Every year, several new monoclonal antibodies are marketed, exemplifying the rapid pace with which these agents are being developed and approved for clinical use. (See Table 17.5 for a list of these antibodies.)

Therapeutic Actions and Indications

Muromonab-CD3 (*Orthoclone OKT3*), the first monoclonal antibody approved for use, is a T-cell–specific antibody that is available as an intravenous (IV) agent. It reacts as an antibody to human T cells, disabling the T cells and acting as an immune suppressor (see Figure 17.1). Muromonab is indicated for the treatment of acute allograft rejection in patients undergoing renal transplantation. It also is indicated for the

Table 17.5 DRUGS IN FOCUS

Monoclonal Antibodies

Drug Name	Dosage/Route	Usual Indications
adalimumab (*Humira*)	40 mg Sub-Q every other week; if also taking methotrexate, may require 40 mg Sub-Q once a week	Reduction of signs and symptoms and inhibition of structural damage in adults who have moderate to severe rheumatoid arthritis and who have not responded to other drugs
alemtuzumab (*Campath*)	3 mg/day IV as a 2-h infusion; increase slowly to maintenance dose of 30 mg/day IV three times per week for up to 12 wk	Treatment of B-cell chronic lymphocytic leukemia in patients who have been treated with alkylating agents and have failed fludarabine therapy
basiliximab (*Simulect*)	20 mg IV twice—first dose within 24 h of transplantation then at 4 days	Prevention of renal transplant rejection
bevacizumab (*Avastin*)	5 mg/kg IV every 14 days	With 5-FU, first-line treatment of patients with metastatic colon or rectal cancer
cetuximab (*Erbitux*)	400 mg/m^2 IV over 2 h, weekly maintenance of 250 mg/m^2 IV over 1 h	Treatment of advanced epidermal growth factor expressing colorectal cancer
daclizumab (*Zenapax*)	1 mg/kg IV for five doses, the first within 24 h of transplantation, and the last within 14 days after transplantation	Prevention of renal transplant rejection
efalizumab (*Raptiva*)	0.7 mg/kg Sub-Q conditioning dose, then 1 mg/kg Sub-Q once a week	Treatment of adult patients with chronic moderate to severe plaque psoriasis who are candidates for systemic therapy
erlotinib (*Tarceva*)	150 mg/day PO	Treatment of locally advanced or metastatic non–small cell lung cancer after failure of other therapies
gemtuzumab (*Mylotarg*)	9 mg/m^2 IV over 2 h, two doses given 14 days apart	Treatment of CD33-positive AML in the first relapse in patients >60 yr who are not candidates for cytotoxic chemotherapy
ibritumomab (*Zevalin*)	2 mg antibody labeled with 0.3 or 0.4 mCi/kg yttrium-90 IV	Treatment of B-cell non-Hodgkin's lymphoma in conjunction with rituximab
infliximab (*Remicade*)	5 mg/kg IV over 2 h; may be repeated at 2 wk and 6 wk	To decrease the signs and symptoms of Crohn's disease in patients who do not respond to other therapy; treatment of rheumatoid arthritis and psoriatic arthritis
P muromonab-CD3 (*Orthoklone OKT3*)	5 mg/day IV for 10–14 days infused as an IV bolus over <1 min	Prevention of renal transplant rejection; treatment of steroid-resistant rejection of heart and liver transplants in adults
natalizumab (*Tysabri*)	300 mg IV over 1 h, every 4 weeks	Monotherapy for the treatment of patients with relapsing forms of multiple sclerosis to delay the accumulation of physical disability and reduce the frequency of clinical exacerbations
omalizumab (*Xolair*)	0.15 mg/kg/day Sub-Q	Treatment of asthma with a very strong allergic component and seasonal allergic rhinitis not well controlled with traditional medications
palivizumab (*Synagis*)	15 mg/kg IM as a single dose at the start of RSV season	Prevention of serious respiratory syncytial virus (RSV) infection in high-risk children
pegaptanib (*Macugen*)	0.3 mg once every 6 wk by intravitreous injection	Treatment of neovascular (wet) age-related macular degeneration
rituximab (*Rituxan*)	375 mg/m^2 IV once weekly for four doses	Treatment of relapsed follicular B-cell non-Hodgkin's lymphoma; CD20–positive follicular non-Hodgkin's lymphoma
tositumomab with iodine 131 tositumomab (*Bexxar*)	450 mg IV in 50 mL 0.9% sodium chloride over 60 min, then 35 mg iodine 131 tositumomab over 30 min; repeat based on response	CD20–positive follicular non-Hodgkin's lymphoma when disease is refractory to rituximab and relapsed following chemotherapy
trastuzumab (*Herceptin*)	4 mg/kg IV over 90 min, then 2 mg/kg IV once a week over at least 30 min	Treatment of metastatic breast cancer with tumors that over-express human epidermal growth factor receptor 2 (HER2)

treatment of steroid-resistant acute allograft rejection in those receiving heart or liver transplants.

Adalimumab (*Humira*) is a monoclonal antibody specific for human tumor necrosis factor. It keeps the inflammatory reaction in check by reacting with and deactivating the free-floating tumor necrosis factor released by active leukocytes. It is used for reducing the signs and symptoms and preventing the structural damage associated with rheumatoid arthritis.

Alemtuzumab (*Campath*) is a monoclonal antibody that is specific for lymphocyte receptor sites; it is used for the treatment of B-cell chronic lymphocytic leukemia in patients who have been treated with alkylating agents and have failed fludarabine therapy.

Basiliximab (*Simulect*) and daclizumab (*Zenapax*) are monoclonal antibodies to interleukin-2 receptor sites on activated T lymphocytes; they react with those sites and block cellular response to allograft transplants. They are approved for use in preventing renal transplant rejection and are used in conjunction with cyclosporine and corticosteroids.

Bevacizumab (*Avastin*) is a monoclonal antibody used with fluorourocil (5-FU) as an antineoplastic agent for the first-line treatment of patients with metastatic colon or rectal cancer.

Cetuximab (*Erbitux*) is a monoclonal antibody specific to epidermal growth factor receptor sites. It is used for the treatment of advanced epidermal growth factor–expressing colorectal cancer.

Efalizumab (*Raptiva*) is a monoclonal antibody specific for an antigen on human leukocytes. It prevents the adhesion of leukocytes to certain other cells. It is used for the treatment of adult patients with moderate to severe plaque psoriasis who are candidates for systemic therapy. This drug is associated with increased susceptibility to infections and reduced platelet counts and bleeding.

Erlotinib (*Tarceva*) is an oral agent for the treatment of locally advanced or metastatic non–small cell lung cancer. Its use is reserved for patients whose disease has progressed after other therapies.

Gemtuzumab (*Mylotarg*) is an antibody to CD33 sites found in acute myelocytic leukemia. It is given IV to treat the first relapse in patients 60 years of age or older who are not candidates for cytotoxic chemotherapy. Fever is common after infusion of the drug, and it is important to make sure that the patient is well hydrated.

Ibritumomab (*Zevalin*) is an antibody to specific sites on activated B lymphocytes. It is used for the treatment of follicular B-cell non-Hodgkin's lymphoma in patients no longer responding to rituximab. Ibritumomab is used in combination with radiation therapy.

Infliximab (*Remicade*) is a monoclonal antibody to tumor necrosis factor. It is used to decrease the signs and symptoms of Crohn's disease in patients who do not respond to conventional therapy and for the treatment of fistulating Crohn's disease. It also is approved for use with methotrexate in the treatment of progressing moderate to severe rheumatoid arthritis.

Natalizumab (*Tysabri*) is a monoclonal antibody that was approved for decreasing the frequency of clinical exacerbations of multiple sclerosis. The manufacturer stopped marketing the drug weeks after its release because of reports of CNS complications. It was returned to the market in June, 2006.

Omalizumab (*Xolair*) is a monoclonal antibody used for the treatment of asthma with a strong allergic component, and for patients with seasonal rhinitis that is not well controlled with traditional medications. It is an antibody to immunoglobulin E, an important factor in allergic reactions.

Palivizumab (*Synagis*) is a monoclonal antibody to the antigenic site on respiratory syncytial virus (RSV); it inactivates that virus. It is used to prevent RSV disease in high-risk children.

Pegaptanib (*Macugen*) is a monoclonal antibody that is injected into the intravitreous fluid of the eye, once every 6 weeks. It is specific for the treatment of neovascular (wet) age-related macular degeneration.

Rituximab (*Rituxan*) is a monoclonal antibody to specific sites on activated B lymphocytes; it is used in the treatment of CD 20-positive, follicular B-cell non-Hodgkin's lymphoma.

Tositumomab combined with iodine 131 tositumomab (*Bexxar*) is given to treat CD20-positive, follicular B-cell non-Hodgkin's lymphoma patients whose disease is refractory to rituximab and who have relapsed on therapy. There is a high risk of cytopenia with this drug, and it is pregnancy category X.

Trastuzumab (*Herceptin*) is a monoclonal antibody that reacts with human epidermal growth factor receptor 2 (HER2), a genetic defect that is seen in certain metastatic breast cancers. It is used in the treatment of metastatic breast cancer in tumors that overexpress HER2.

Pharmacokinetics

Monoclonal antibodies must be injected. They are processed by the body like other antibodies. It is not known whether they cross the placenta or enter breast milk, but because of the potential for adverse effects, they should not be used during pregnancy or lactation unless the benefit clearly outweighs the potential risk to the fetus or neonate.

Contraindications and Cautions

Monoclonal antibodies are contraindicated in the presence of any known allergy to the drug or to murine products, and in the presence of fluid overload. They should be used cautiously with fever (treat the fever before beginning therapy), previous administration of the monoclonal antibody (*serious hypersensitivity reactions can occur with repeat administration*), and pregnancy or lactation.

Adverse Effects

The most serious adverse effects associated with the use of monoclonal antibodies are acute pulmonary edema (dyspnea, chest pain, wheezing), which is associated with severe fluid retention, and cytokine release syndrome (flu-like symptoms that can progress to third-spacing of fluids and shock). Other adverse effects that can be anticipated include fever, chills, malaise, myalgia, nausea, diarrhea, vomiting, and increased susceptibility to infection.

Clinically Important Drug–Drug Interactions

Use caution and arrange to reduce the dosage if a monoclonal antibody is combined with any other immunosuppressant drug because severe immune suppression with increased infections and neoplasms can occur.

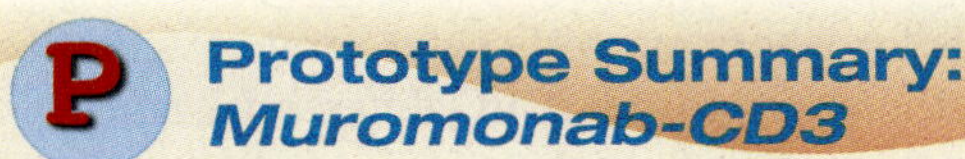

Indications: Treatment of acute allograft rejection in renal transplant patients; treatment of steroid-resistant acute allograph rejection in cardiac and hepatic transplant patients

Actions: Monoclonal antibody to the antigen of human T cells; functions as an immunosuppressant by enabling T cells

Pharmacokinetics:

Route	Onset	Peak	Duration
IV	Minutes	2–7 days	7 days

$T_{1/2}$: 47 to 100 hours; metabolized in the tissues

Adverse effects: Malaise, tremors, vomiting, nausea, diarrhea, acute pulmonary edema, dyspnea, fever, chills, increased susceptibility to infection

Nursing Considerations for Patients Receiving Immune Suppressants

Assessment: History and Examination

Screen for the following, *which could be contraindications or cautions to use of the drug:* any known allergies to any of these drugs or their components; pregnancy or lactation; renal or hepatic impairment; and history of neoplasm.

Include screening *for baseline status before beginning therapy and for any potential adverse effects:* presence of any skin lesions; weight; temperature; orientation, reflexes; pulse, blood pressure, ECG; liver evaluation; CBC, liver, and renal function tests; and assessment of condition being treated.

Nursing Diagnoses

The patient receiving immune suppressants may have the following nursing diagnoses related to drug therapy:

- Acute Pain related to CNS, GI, and flu-like effects
- Risk for Infection related to immune suppression
- Imbalanced Nutrition: Less Than Body Requirements, related to nausea and vomiting
- Deficient Knowledge regarding drug therapy

Implementation With Rationale

- Arrange for laboratory tests before and periodically during therapy, including CBC, differential, and liver and renal function tests, *to monitor for drug effects and adverse effects.*
- Administer the drug as indicated; instruct the patient and a significant other if injections are required *to ensure proper administration of the drug.*
- Protect the patient from exposure to infections and maintain strict aseptic technique for any invasive procedures *to prevent infections during immunosuppression.*
- Arrange for supportive care and comfort measures for flu-like symptoms (rest, environmental control, acetaminophen) *to decrease patient discomfort and increase therapeutic compliance.*
- Monitor nutritional status during therapy; provide small, frequent meals, mouth care, and nutritional consultation as necessary *to ensure adequate nutrition.*
- Instruct female patients in the use of barrier contraceptives *to avoid pregnancy during therapy because of the risk of adverse effects to the fetus.*
- Provide thorough patient teaching, including measures to avoid adverse effects, warning signs of problems, and proper administration, *to increase knowledge about drug therapy and to increase compliance with the drug regimen.*
- Offer support and encouragement *to help the patient deal with the diagnosis and the drug regimen.*

Evaluation

- Monitor patient response to the drug (prevention of transplant rejection; improvement in autoimmune disease or cancer; prevention of RSV disease; improvement in signs and symptoms of Crohn's disease or rheumatoid arthritis).
- Monitor for adverse effects (flu-like symptoms, GI upset, increased infections, neoplasms, fluid overload).
- Evaluate the effectiveness of the teaching plan (patient can name drug, dosage, adverse effects to watch for, specific measures to avoid adverse effects).
- Monitor the effectiveness of comfort measures and compliance to the regimen (Critical Thinking Scenario 17-1).

WEB LINKS

Health care providers and patients may want to consult the following Internet sources:

http://www.oncolink.upenn.edu Information on cancers (including leukemias and Kaposi's sarcoma) and treatments.

http://www.nmss.org Information on multiple sclerosis (updates, treatments, contact groups).

http://www.fda.gov/cber Information on drug research and development, new approvals, alerts, and warnings.

CRITICAL THINKING SCENARIO 17-1

Holistic Care for a Transplantation Patient

The Situation

After waiting on a transplant list for 4 years, T.B. received a human heart transplant to replace his heart, which had been severely damaged by cardiomyopathy. Before getting the transplant, T.B. was bedridden, on oxygen, and near death. The transplant has given T.B. a "new lease on life," and he is determined to do everything possible to stay healthy and improve his activity and lifestyle. Currently, he is being maintained on cyclosporine, mycophenolate, and corticosteroids.

Critical Thinking

What important teaching facts would help T.B. to achieve his goal? *Think about the psychological impact of the heart transplant and the "new lease on life."*

What activity, dietary, and supportive guidelines should be outlined for T.B.?

What impact will T.B.'s drug regimen have on his plans?

How can all of the aspects of his condition and medical care be coordinated to give T.B. the best possible advantages for the future?

Discussion

T.B.'s medical regimen will include a very complicated combination of rehabilitation, nutrition, drug therapy, and prevention. T.B. should know the risks of transplant rejection and the measures that will be used to prevent it. He also should know the names of his medications and when to take them, the signs and symptoms of rejection to watch for, and what to do if they occur. T.B. must understand the need to prevent exposure to infections and the precautions required, such as avoiding crowded areas and people with known diseases, avoiding injury, and taking steps to maintain cleanliness and avoid infection if an injury occurs.

The medications that T.B. is taking may cause him to experience flu-like symptoms, which can be quite unpleasant. A restful, quiet environment may help to decrease his stress. Acetaminophen may be ordered to help alleviate the fever, aches, and pains.

T.B. also may experience gastrointestinal upset, nausea, and vomiting related to drug effects. A nutritional consultation may be requested to help T.B. maintain a good nutritional state. Frequent mouth care and small, frequent meals may help. Proper nutrition will help T.B. to recover, heal, and maintain his health.

T.B.'s primary health care provider will need to work with the transplantation surgeon, rehabilitation team, nutritionist, and cardiologist to coordinate a total program that will help T.B. to avoid problems and make the most of his transplanted heart.

Nursing Care Guide for T.B.: Cyclosporine, Mycophenolate, and Corticosteroids

Assessment: History and Examination

- Assess for history of allergies to any immune suppressant, renal or hepatic impairment, history of neoplasm, concurrent use of cholestyramine, theophylline, phenytoin, other nephrotoxic drugs, digoxin, lovastatin, diltiazem, metoclopramide, nicardipine, amiodarone, androgens, azole antifungals, macrolides; grapefruit juice.
- Review physical examination findings, including orientation, reflexes, affect (neurological); temperature and weight (general); pulse, cardiac auscultation, blood pressure, edema, electrocardiogram (cardiovascular); liver evaluation (GI); and laboratory test results (complete blood count, liver and renal function tests, condition being treated)

Nursing Diagnoses

Acute Pain related to CNS, GI, flu-like symptoms

Risk for Infection related to immune suppression

Imbalanced Nutrition: Less Than Body Requirements related to GI effects

Deficient Knowledge regarding drug therapy

Implementation

Arrange for laboratory tests before and periodically during therapy.

Administer drug as indicated.

Protect patient from exposure to infection.

Provide supportive and comfort measures to deal with adverse effects.

(continued)

Holistic Care for a Transplantation Patient *(continued)*

Monitor nutritional status and intervene as needed.

Provide patient teaching regarding the drugs and their dosage, adverse effects, precautions, and warning signs to report to care provider.

Evaluation

Evaluate drug effects: prevention of transplant rejection, improvement of autoimmune disease.

Monitor for adverse effects: infection, flu-like symptoms, GI upset, fluid overload, neoplasm.

Monitor for drug–drug interactions and drug–food interactions.

Evaluate effectiveness of patient teaching program and of comfort and safety measures.

Patient Teaching for T.B.: Cyclosporine, Mycophenolate, and Corticosteroids

- ☐ You will need to take a combination of drugs to prevent your body from rejecting your new organ. These drugs include cyclosporine, mycophenolate, and corticosteroids. They suppress the activity of your immune system and prevent your body from rejecting any transplanted tissue.
- ☐ You should never stop taking your drugs without consulting your health care provider. If your prescription is low or you are unable to take the medication for *any* reason, notify your health care provider.
- ☐ You should not take your cyclosporine with grapefruit juice.
- ☐ Some of the following adverse effects may occur:
  - *Nausea, vomiting:* Taking the drug with food and eating small frequent meals may help. It is very important that you maintain good nutrition. A consult with a nutritionist may be needed to help you if these GI problems are severe.
  - *Diarrhea:* This may not decrease; ensure ready access to bathroom facilities.
  - *Flu-like symptoms:* Rest and a cool, peaceful environment may help; acetaminophen may be ordered to help relieve discomfort.
  - *Rash, mouth sores:* Frequent skin and mouth care may ease these effects.
- ☐ You will be more susceptible to infection because your body's normal defenses will be decreased. You should avoid crowded places, people with known infections, and working in soil. If you notice any signs of illness or infection, notify your health care provider immediately.
- ☐ Tell any doctor, nurse, or other health care provider involved in your care that you are taking these drugs.
- ☐ You will need to schedule periodic blood tests and perhaps biopsies while you are being treated with these drugs.
- ☐ Report any of the following to your health care provider: unusual bleeding or bruising, fever, sore throat, mouth sores, fatigue, and any other signs of infection or injury.
- ☐ Keep your medications safely out of the reach of children and pets and do not share medications with anyone else.

Points to Remember

- Immune stimulants boost the immune system when it is exhausted from fighting off prolonged invasion or needs help fighting a specific pathogen or cancer cell.
- Immune suppressants are used to depress the immune system when needed to prevent transplant rejection or severe tissue damage associated with autoimmune disease.
- Interferons are naturally released from cells in response to viral invasion; they are used to treat various cancers and warts.
- Interleukins stimulate cellular immunity and inhibit tumor growth; they are used to treat very specific cancers.
- Adverse effects seen with immune stimulants are related to the immune response (flu-like symptoms, including fever, myalgia, lethargy, arthralgia, and fatigue).
- Immune suppressants are used in a variety of specific transplantation situations. Research is ongoing to extend the use of various immune suppressants to other situations, including various autoimmune disorders.
- Increased susceptibility to infection and increased risk of neoplasm are potentially dangerous effects associated with the use of immune suppressants. Patients need to be protected from infection, injury, and invasive procedures.

CHECK YOUR UNDERSTANDING

Answers to the questions in this chapter may be found in the Answer Key in the back of the book.

Multiple Choice

Select the best answer to the following.

1. You would *not* expect to use an immune suppressant when working with
   a. treatment of transplant rejection.
   b. treatment of autoimmune disease.
   c. reduction of the number of relapses in multiple sclerosis.
   d. treatment of aggressive cancers.

2. Interferon alfa-n3 (*Alferon N*) would be the drug of choice for
   a. treatment of leukemias.
   b. treatment of multiple sclerosis.
   c. intralesional treatment of warts.
   d. treatment of Kaposi's sarcoma.

3. Patient teaching for a patient receiving an interferon would include
   a. proper use of oral contraceptives.
   b. use of aspirin to control adverse effects.
   c. importance of exercise and cardiovascular workouts.
   d. proper methods for drawing up and injecting the drug.

4. Patients who are receiving an immune stimulant may experience any of the clinical signs of immune response activity, including
   a. flu-like symptoms (arthralgia, myalgia, fatigue, anorexia).
   b. diarrhea.
   c. constipation.
   d. headache.

5. Organ transplants are often rejected by the body because the T cells recognize the transplanted cells as foreign and try to destroy them. Treatment with an immune suppressant would
   a. activate antibody production.
   b. stimulate interleukin release.
   c. stimulate thymus secretions.
   d. block the inflammatory reaction and initial damage to the transplanted cells.

6. You might use a monoclonal antibody in treating
   a. warts.
   b. herpes zoster.
   c. metastatic breast cancers with tumors that overexpress HER2.
   d. Kaposi's sarcoma.

Multiple Response

Select all that apply.

1. The nurse is assigned to care for a client who is receiving immune suppressants. The nurse would continually assess the client for which of the following anticipated adverse effects?
   a. Development of cancers
   b. Increased risk of infection
   c. Cardiac standstill
   d. Development of secondary infections
   e. Increased bleeding tendencies
   f. Hepatomegaly

2. Teaching points that the nurse would incorporate into the care of a client receiving cylosporine would include which of the following?
   a. Use barrier contraceptives to avoid pregnancy.
   b. If mouth sores occur, try to restrict eating as much as possible.
   c. Dilute the solution with milk, chocolate milk, or orange juice and drink immediately.
   d. Avoid drinking grapefruit juice when on this drug.
   e. Stop taking the drug if GI upset or fever occurs.
   f. Refrigerate the oral solution.

Definitions

Define the following terms.

1. autoimmune ______________________________
   ____
   ____

2. interferon ______________________________
   ____
   ____

3. interleukin ______________________________
   ____
   ____

4. monoclonal antibodies ______________________________
____
____

5. immune suppressant ______________________________
____
____

Fill in the Blanks

1. ______________ ______________ are specific antibodies produced by a single clone of B cells to react with a specific antigen.

2. The following monoclonal antibodies are used in the prevention of renal transplant rejection: ______________, ______________, and ______________.

3. Infliximab is used to treat ______________ disease in patients who do not respond to other therapy.

4. Palivizumab was developed for the prevention of ______________ ______________ ______________ in children who are at high-risk.

5. Treatment of metastatic breast cancer with tumors that overexpress human epidermal growth factor receptor 2 (HER2) is specifically the indication for ______________.

6. ______________ is used for the treatment of relapsed follicular B-cell non-Hodgkin's lymphoma B lymphocytes.

7. The treatment of asthma with a strong allergic component is the main indication for ______________.

8. ______________ is specifically used to treat B-cell chronic lymphocytic leukemia.

Bibliography and References

Drug facts and comparisons. (2006). St. Louis: Facts & Comparisons.

Gilman, A., Hardman, J. G., & Limbird, L. E. (Eds.). (2006). *Goodman and Gilman's the pharmacological basis of therapeutics* (11th ed.). New York: McGraw-Hill.

Karch, A. M. (2006). *2007 Lippincott's nursing drug guide.* Philadelphia: Lippincott Williams & Wilkins.

Porth, C. M. (2005). *Pathophysiology: Concepts of altered health states* (7th ed.). Philadelphia: Lippincott Williams & Wilkins.

The medical letter on drugs and therapeutics. (2006). New Rochelle, NY: Medical Letter.

CHAPTER 18

Vaccines and Sera

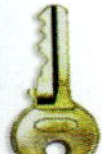

KEY TERMS

active immunity

antitoxins

immune sera

immunization

passive immunity

serum sickness

vaccine

LEARNING OBJECTIVES

Upon completion of this chapter, you will be able to:

1. Define the terms active immunity and passive immunity.
2. Describe the therapeutic actions, indications, pharmacokinetics, contraindications, most common adverse reactions, and important drug–drug interactions associated with each vaccine, immune serum, antitoxin, and antivenin.
3. Discuss the use of vaccines and sera across the lifespan, including recommended immunization schedules.
4. Compare and contrast the prototype drugs for each class of vaccine and immune serum with others in that class.
5. Outline the nursing considerations and teaching needs for patients receiving a vaccine or immune serum.

VACCINES

Bacterial Vaccines

BCG
haemophilus influenza b conjugate vaccine
haemophilus influenza b conjugate vaccine and hepatitis B surface antigen
meningococcal polysaccharide vaccine
meningococcal polysaccharide diphtheria toxoid conjugate vaccine
pneumococcal vaccine, polyvalent
pneumococcal 7-valent conjugate vaccine
typhoid vaccine

Toxoids

diphtheria and tetanus oxoids, combined, absorbed
diphtheria and tetanus toxoids and acellular pertussis vaccine, absorbed
diphtheria and tetanus toxoids and acellular pertussis and *Haemophilus influenza* B conjugate vaccines
diphtheria and tetanus toxoids and acellular pertussis, absorbed, and hepatitis B (recombinant) and inactivated poliovirus vaccines, combined

Viral Vaccines

hepatitis A vaccine, inactivated
hepatitis A vaccine, inactivated, with hepatitis B recombinant vaccine
hepatitis B vaccine
influenza virus vaccine
influenza virus vaccine, intranasal
Japanese encephalitis vaccine
measles virus vaccine, live attenuated
P measles, mumps, rubella vaccine
mumps virus vaccine, live
poliovirus vaccine, inactivated
rabies vaccine
rubella virus vaccine
rubella and mumps virus vaccine, live
smallpox vaccine
varicella virus vaccine
yellow fever vaccine

IMMUNE SERA

anti-thymocyte immune globulin
cytomegalovirus immune globulin
hepatitis B immune globulin
P immune globulin, intramuscular
immune globulin, intravenous
lymphocyte immune globulin
rabies immune globulin
respiratory syncytial virus immune globulin
RHO immune globulin
RHO immune globulin, microdose
tetanus immune globulin
vaccinia immune globulin
varicella zoster immune globulin

ANTITOXINS AND ANTIVENINS

antivenin (crotalidae) polyvalent
antivenin (micrurus fulvius)
black widow spider antivenin
crotalidae polyvalent immune fab

Vaccines, immune sera, and antitoxins are usually referred to as *biologicals.* They are used to stimulate the production of antibodies, to provide preformed antibodies to facilitate an immune reaction, or to react specifically with the toxins produced by an invading pathogen. Prudent, prophylactic medical care requires the routine administration of certain vaccines to prevent diseases before they occur. Box 18.1 discusses the use of biologicals among various age groups.

Immunity

Immunity is a state of relative resistance to a disease that develops after exposure to the specific disease-causing agent. People are not born with immunity to diseases, so they must acquire immunity by stimulating B-cell clones to form plasma cells, and then antibodies.

Active immunity occurs when the body recognizes a foreign protein and begins producing antibodies to react with that specific protein or antigen. After plasma cells are formed to produce antibodies, specific memory cells that produce the same antibodies are created. If the specific foreign protein is introduced into the body again, these memory cells react immediately to release antibodies. This type of immunity is thought to be lifelong.

Passive immunity occurs when preformed antibodies are injected into the system and react with a specific antigen. These antibodies come from animals that have been infected with the disease or from humans who have had the disease and have developed antibodies. The circulating antibodies act the same as those produced from plasma cells, recognizing the foreign protein and attaching to it, rendering it harmless. Unlike active immunity, passive immunity is limited. It lasts only as long as the circulating antibodies last because the body does not produce its own antibodies. In some cases, the host human produces antibodies to the circulating injected antibodies. This results in **serum sickness**, a massive immune reaction. Signs and symptoms of serum sickness include fever, arthritis, flank pain, myalgia, and arthralgia.

Immunization

Immunization is the process of artificially stimulating active immunity by exposing the body to weakened or less toxic proteins associated with specific disease-causing organisms. The goal is to cause an immune response without having the patient suffer the full course of a disease. Children routinely are immunized against many infections that were once quite devastating (Figure 18.1 and Box 18.2). For example, smallpox was one of the first diseases against which children were immunized. Today, smallpox is considered to be eradicated worldwide. Concerns over biological terrorism have renewed interest in this disease, and smallpox vaccine is available for

BOX 18.1 DRUG THERAPY ACROSS THE LIFESPAN

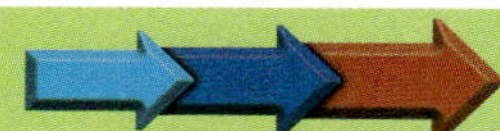

Biologicals

CHILDREN

Routine immunizations for children has become a standard of care in this country. Parents should receive written records of immunizations given to their children to assure continuity of care. The parent should be asked to report adverse reactions to any immunization. Sensitive children may receive divided doses of their immunizations to help prevent adverse reactions.

Simple comfort measures—warm soaks at the injection site, acetaminophen to reduce fever or aches and pains, comfort from parents or caregivers—will help the child deal with the immunization experience.

Parent education is a very important aspect of the immunization procedure. Parents may need reassurance and educational materials when concerns about the safety of immunizations arise.

ADULTS

There are a number of reasons why adults should receive certain immunizations. For example, adults who are traveling to areas with high risk for particular diseases—and who may not have previously been exposed to those diseases—are advised to be immunized.

In addition, adults with chronic diseases are advised to be immunized yearly with an influenza vaccine, and once with a pneumococcal pneumonia vaccine. These vaccines provide some protection against diseases that can prove dangerous for people with chronic lung, cardiovascular, or endocrine disorders. The influenza vaccine changes yearly, depending on predictions of which flu strain might be emergent in that year. The pneumonia vaccine contains 23 strains and is believed to offer lifetime protection.

Tetanus shots also are recommended for adults every 10 years, or with any injury that potentially could precipitate a tetanus infection.

OLDER ADULTS

Older patients are at greater risk for severe illness from influenza and pneumococcal infections. The yearly flu shot and the pneumococcal vaccine should be stressed for this group.

A tetanus booster every 10 years will also help to protect older adults from exposure to that illness. Ask the patient about any adverse reaction to previous tetanus boosters, and weigh the risk against the possible exposure to tetanus.

If an older patient is traveling to an area where a particular disease is endemic and the risk of exposure is great, the Centers for Disease Control and Prevention should be contacted to determine whether the appropriate vaccine is acceptable for use in the older patient.

Recommended Childhood and Adolescent Immunization Schedule UNITED STATES • 2006

Vaccine ▼ / Age ►	Birth	1 mo	2 mos	4 mos	6 mos	12 mos	15 mos	18 mos	24 mos	4-6 yrs	11-12 yrs	13-14 yrs	15 yrs	16-18 yrs
Hepatitis B[1]	HepB	HepB		*HepB[1]*		HepB					HepB series			
Diphtheria, Tetanus, Pertussis[2]			DTaP	DTaP	DTaP		DTaP			DTaP	Tdap		Tdap	
Haemophilus influenzae type b[3]			Hib	Hib	*Hib[3]*	Hib								
Inactivated Poliovirus			IPV	IPV		IPV				IPV				
Measles, Mumps, Rubella[4]						MMR				MMR		MMR		
Varicella[5]							Varicella				Varicella			
Meningococcal[6]						Vaccines within broken line are for selected populations				MPSV4	MCV4		MCV4 / MCV4	
Pneumococcal[7]			PCV	PCV	PCV	PCV			PCV		PPV			
Influenza[8]						Influenza (Yearly)					Influenza (Yearly)			
Hepatitis A[9]										HepA series				

This schedule indicates the recommended ages for routine administration of currently licensed childhood vaccines, as of December 1, 2005, for children through age 18 years. Any dose not given at the recommended age should be given at any subsequent visit when indicated and feasible.

Indicates age groups that warrant special effort to administer those vaccines not previously administered. Additional vaccines may be licensed and recommended during the year. Licensed combination vaccines may be used whenever any components of the combination are indicated and other components of the vaccine are not contraindicated and if approved by the Food and Drug Administration for that dose of the series. Providers should consult the respective ACIP statement for detailed recommendations. Clinically significant adverse events that follow immunization should be reported to the Vaccine Adverse Event Reporting System (VAERS). Guidance about how to obtain and complete a VAERS form is available at www.vaers.hhs.gov or by telephone, 800-822-7967.

- Range of recommended ages
- Catch-up immunization
- 11–12-year-old assessment

FIGURE 18.1 Recommended immunization schedule for children and adults. (Source: Centers for Disease Control (CDC) and Prevention and the American Academy of Pediatrics, 2006).

people who might be at high risk for exposure to a potential attack by terrorists using smallpox.

Diphtheria, pertussis, tetanus, haemophilus B influenza, hepatitis B, hepatitis A, chickenpox, polio, meningitis, measles, mumps, and rubella are all standard childhood immunizations today. The use of vaccines is not without controversy. Severe reactions, although rare, have occurred. The central reporting of adverse effects or suspected adverse effects may help to clarify concerns about reactions to immunizations. Adults may also require immunizations in certain situations: exposure, travel to an area endemic in a disease they have not had and have not been immunized against, and occupations that are considered high risk (see Figure 18.1). People who receive allergy shots to help them cope with the signs and symptoms of allergic reactions are receiving antigenic proteins that stimulate antibody production to prevent the allergic response (Box 18.3).

Vaccines

The word **vaccine** comes from the Latin word for smallpox, *vaccinia*. Vaccines are immunizations containing weakened or altered protein antigens that stimulate formation of antibodies against a specific disease (Figure 18.2). They are used to promote active immunity. Box 18.4 discusses vaccines and the use of biological weapons.

Vaccines can be made from chemically inactivated microorganisms or from live, weakened viruses or bacteria. Toxoids are vaccines that are made from the toxins produced by the microorganism. The toxins are altered so that they are no longer poisonous but still have the recognizable protein antigen that will stimulate antibody production.

The particular vaccine that is used depends on the possible exposure a person will have to a particular disease and

UNITED STATES • OCTOBER 2005–SEPTEMBER 2006

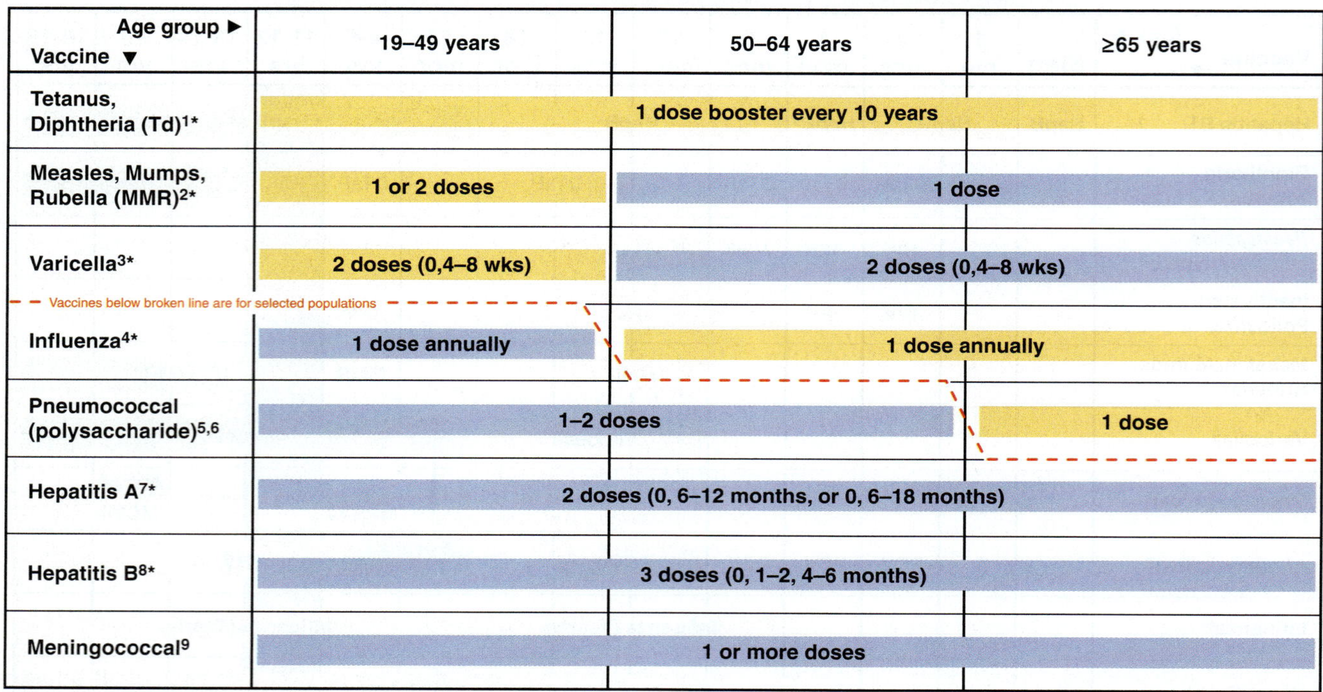

Vaccine ▼ / Age group ►	19–49 years	50–64 years	≥65 years
Tetanus, Diphtheria (Td)[1]*	1 dose booster every 10 years		
Measles, Mumps, Rubella (MMR)[2]*	1 or 2 doses	1 dose	
Varicella[3]*	2 doses (0,4–8 wks)	2 doses (0,4–8 wks)	
Influenza[4]*	1 dose annually	1 dose annually	
Pneumococcal (polysaccharide)[5,6]	1–2 doses		1 dose
Hepatitis A[7]*	2 doses (0, 6–12 months, or 0, 6–18 months)		
Hepatitis B[8]*	3 doses (0, 1–2, 4–6 months)		
Meningococcal[9]	1 or more doses		

Vaccines below broken line are for selected populations

NOTE: These recommendations must be read along with the footnotes.

* Covered by the Vaccine Injury Compensation Program.

For all persons in this category who meet the age requirements and who lack evidence of immunity (e.g., lack documentation of vaccination or have no evidence of prior infection)

Recommended if some other risk factor is present (e.g., based on medical, occupational, lifestyle, or other indications)

This schedule indicates the recommended age groups and medical indications for routine administration of currently licensed vaccines for persons aged ≥19 years. Licensed combination vaccines may be used whenever any components of the combination are indicated and when the vaccine's other components are not contraindicated. For detailed recommendations, consult the manufacturers' package inserts and the complete statements from the ACIP (www.cdc.gov/nip/publications/acip-list.htm).

Report all clinically significant postvaccination reactions to the Vaccine Adverse Event Reporting System (VAERS). Reporting forms and instructions on filing a VAERS report are available by telephone, 800-822-7967, or from the VAERS web site at www.vaers.hhs.gov.

Information on how to file a Vaccine Injury Compensation Program claim is available at www.hrsa.gov/osp/vicp or by telephone, 800-338-2382. To file a claim for vaccine injury, contact the U.S. Court of Federal Claims, 717 Madison Place, N.W., Washington, DC 20005, telephone 202-357-6400.

Additional information about the vaccines listed above and contraindications for vaccination is also available at www.cdc.gov/nip or from the CDC–INFO Contact Center at 800-CDC-INFO (232-4636) in English and Spanish, 24 hours a day, 7 days a week.

FIGURE 18.1 *(continued)*

the age of the person. Some vaccines are used only in children, and some cannot be used in infants. (Box 18.5 contains a discussion of childhood vaccinations and autism.) Some vaccines require booster doses—doses that are given a few months after the initial dose to further stimulate antibody production. In many cases, antibody titers (levels of the antibody in the serum) can be used to evaluate a person's response to an immunization and determine the need for a booster dose. Table 18.1 lists the various vaccines, and Critical Thinking Scenario 18-1 discusses how to educate a parent about vaccines.

Therapeutic Actions and Indications

Vaccines stimulate active immunity in people who are at high risk for development of a particular disease. The vaccine needed for a patient depends on the exposure that person will have to the pathogen. Exposure is usually determined by where the person lives, travel plans, and work or family environment exposures. Vaccines are thought to provide lifelong immunity to the disease against which the patient is being immunized.

BOX 18.2 CULTURAL CONSIDERATIONS FOR DRUG THERAPY

Pediatric Immunization

It is well-documented that by preventing potentially devastating diseases, society prevents unneeded suffering and death, and saves valuable citizens for the future. Pediatric immunization has helped to greatly decrease the incidence of most childhood diseases and has prevented associated complications. In the United States, routine immunization is considered standard medical practice.

Ensuring that every child has the opportunity to receive the recommended immunizations has become a political as well as a social issue. The cost of preventing a disease that most people have never even seen may be difficult to justify to families who have trouble putting food on the table. Widespread campaigns to provide free immunizations and health screening to all children have addressed this problem but have not been totally successful.

In addition, periodic reports of severe or even fatal reactions to standard immunizations alarm many parents about the risks of immunizations. These parents need facts as well as reassurance about modern efforts to prevent and screen for these reactions.

Public education efforts should be directed at providing parents with information about pediatric immunization and encouraging them to act on that information. Nurses are often in the ideal position to provide this information, during prenatal visits, while screening for other problems, or even standing in line at a grocery store. It is important for nurses to be well versed on the need for standard immunizations and screening to prevent severe reactions. The Centers for Disease Control and Prevention (http://www.cdc.gov) offers current information and updates for health care providers, as well as patient teaching materials that can be printed for easy reference.

BOX 18.3 FOCUS ON CLINICAL SKILLS

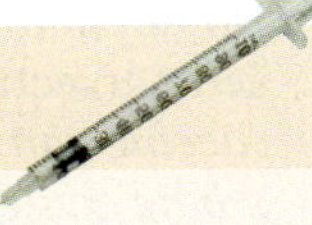

Use of Allergenic Extracts

Many people receive "allergy shots" or injections of allergenic extracts. These extracts contain various antigens based on specific standardizations. The exact action of these extracts is not completely understood, but it has been shown that after injection, specific immunoglobulin G (IgG) antibodies appear in the serum. These antibodies compete with IgE for the receptor site on a specific antigen that is the cause of the allergy. (IgE is the immune globulin that is associated with allergic reactions; these antibodies react with mast cells, causing the release of histamine and other inflammatory chemicals when they have combined with the antigen). After repeated exposure to the antigens, the levels of IgG antibodies increase and the circulating levels of IgE seem to decrease, leading to less allergic response. It may take 4 to 6 months of subcutaneous injections of the allergenic extract every 3 to 14 days to achieve relief from the symptoms of the allergic reaction. The IgG levels remain high for weeks or sometimes months, but the individual response varies widely. Many people are maintained with a weekly injection once the desired response has been achieved.

Contraindications and Cautions

The use of vaccines is contraindicated in the presence of immune deficiency *because the vaccine could cause disease and the body would not be able to respond as anticipated if in an immunodeficient state;* during pregnancy *because of potential effects on the fetus and on the success of the pregnancy;* with known allergies to any of the components of the vaccine (refer to each individual vaccine for specifics, sometimes including eggs, where some pathogens are cultured); or in patients who are receiving immune globulin or who have received blood or blood products within the last 3 months *because a serious immune reaction could occur.*

Caution should be used any time a vaccine is given to a child with a history of febrile convulsions or cerebral injury, or in any condition in which a potential fever would be dangerous. Caution also should be used in the presence of any acute infection.

Adverse Effects

Adverse effects of vaccines are associated with the immune or inflammatory reaction that is being stimulated: moderate fever, rash, malaise, chills, fretfulness, drowsiness, anorexia, vomiting, and irritability. Pain, redness, swelling, and even nodule formation at the injection site are also common. In rare instances, severe hypersensitivity reactions have been reported.

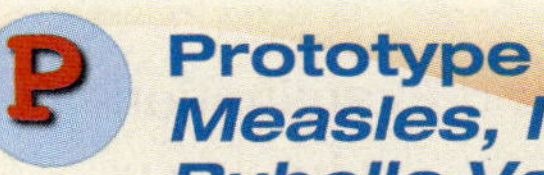

Prototype Summary: *Measles, Mumps, and Rubella Vaccine*

Indications: Active immunization against measles, mumps, and rubella in children older than 15 months and adults

Actions: Attenuated measles, mumps, and rubella viruses produce a modified infection and stimulate active immune reaction with the production of antibodies to these viruses

Pharmacokinetics:

Route	Onset	Peak
IM	Rapid	3–12 h

$T_{1/2}$: Unknown; metabolized in the tissues, excretion is unknown

Adverse effects: Moderate fever, rash, burning or stinging wheal or flare at site of injection, febrile convulsions and high fever are rare, Guillain-Barré syndrome, ocular palsies

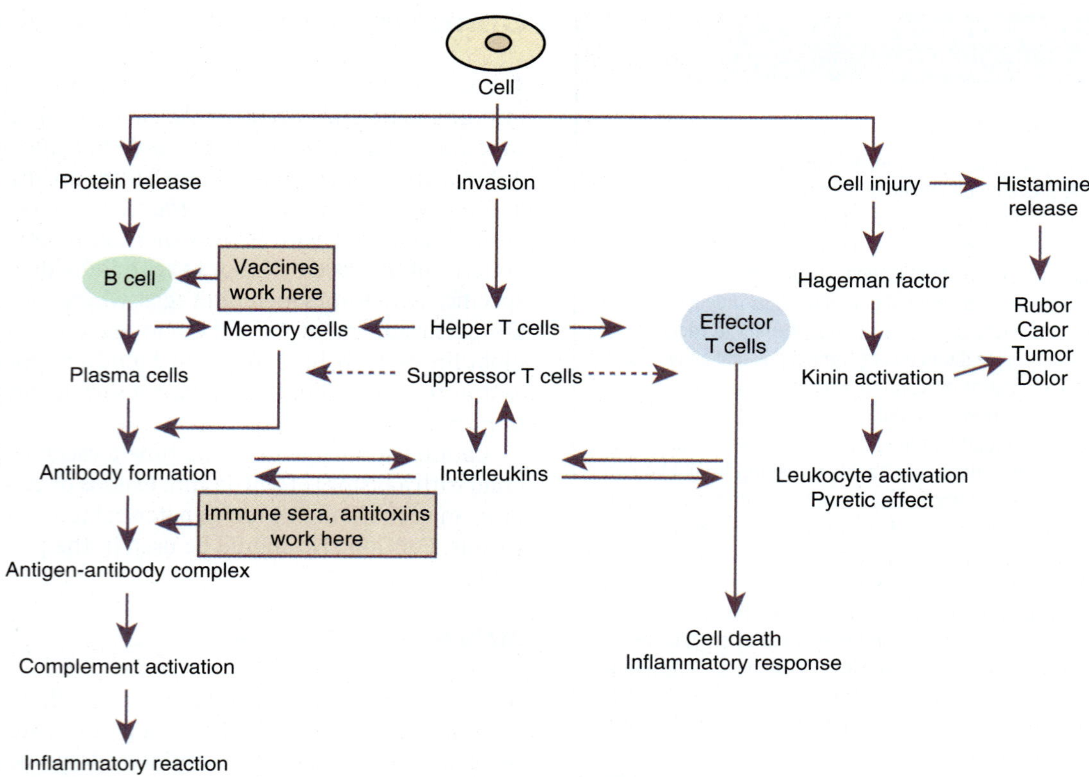

FIGURE 18.2 Sites of action of vaccines, immune sera, and antitoxins.

Nursing Considerations for Patients Receiving Vaccines

Assessment: History and Examination

Screen for any of the following, *which could be contraindications or cautions for use of the drug:* known allergies to any vaccines or to the components of the one being used; pregnancy; recent administration of immune globulin or blood products; immune deficiency; and acute infection.

Include screening *for baseline status before beginning therapy and for any potential adverse effects:* presence of any skin lesions; temperature; affect; range of motion; pulse, blood pressure, perfusion; respirations and adventitious sounds.

Nursing Diagnoses

The patient receiving a vaccine may have the following nursing diagnoses related to drug therapy:

- Acute Pain related to injection, gastrointestinal (GI), and flu-like effects
- Ineffective Tissue Perfusion if severe reaction occurs
- Deficient Knowledge regarding drug therapy

Implementation With Rationale

- Do not use to treat acute infection; *a vaccine is only used to prevent infection with future exposures.*
- Do not administer if the patient exhibits signs of acute infection or immune deficiency *because the vaccine can cause a mild infection and can exacerbate acute infections.*
- Do not administer if the patient has received blood, blood products, or immune globulin within the past 3 months *because a severe immune reaction could occur.*
- Arrange for proper preparation and administration of the vaccine; check on the timing and dosage of each injection *because dosage, preparation, and timing vary with individual vaccines.*
- Maintain emergency equipment on standby, including epinephrine, *in case of severe hypersensitivity reaction.*
- Arrange for supportive care and comfort measures for flu-like symptoms (rest, environmental control, acetaminophen) and for injection discomfort (local heat application, anti-inflammatories, resting arm) *to promote patient comfort.*
- Be aware that children should not receive aspirin to treat the discomforts associated with the immu-

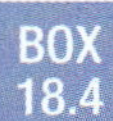

BOX 18.4 Vaccines and Biological Weapons

The events of September 11, 2001, and the subsequent war on terrorism have heightened awareness of several diseases that might be in development as biological weapons. Anthrax, plague, tularemia, smallpox, botulism, and a variety of viral hemorrhagic fevers are all considered to be likely biological warfare weapons.

Anthrax

A vaccine is available in the United States made from inactivated cell-free filtrate of an avirulent strain of the anthrax bacillus. It is available only for military use. Active production stopped in 1998, but production and supply issues were made high priorities. Ciprofloxacin and, in sensitive cases, doxycycline and penicillins are effective in treating postexposure cases. The vaccine is given and repeated in 2 and 4 weeks, along with the appropriate antibiotic, to patients who have been exposed.

Plague

Plague is easily spread from person to person, and without treatment can progress rapidly to respiratory failure and death. There is currently no vaccine for plague; a whole-cell vaccine that was used for many years is no longer available. Research is ongoing using a pneumonic plague vaccine that has successfully protected animals. Several drugs have been found to be life-saving with plague—streptomycin, doxycycline, ciprofloxacin, and chloramphenicol.

Smallpox

Smallpox was considered eradicated since no new cases had been seen in 20 years. Smallpox is highly transmissible and has a 30% mortality rate in unvaccinated people. Immunization against smallpox ended in the 1970s. There is now a commercially available vaccine, but use is somewhat limited because of questions raised during studies of the vaccine. It is given to military personnel and people thought to be at high risk. It is currently thought that the vaccine is no longer effective after 20 years, although there is no definite evidence that previously vaccinated people have no protection. The smallpox vaccine uses live virus, placed in punctures made in the skin. After exposure, vaccination given within the first 3 to 4 days can prevent the disease. If it has been 7 days or longer since exposure, the vaccine and a vaccinia immune globulin should be used, if any are available. So far no drugs are thought to be effective in treating smallpox. Early studies have, however, shown cidofovir to be effective in vitro.

Tularemia

Tularemia in an aerosolized form can cause systemic and respiratory illness with a 35% mortality rate. It is not passed from person to person. There is no vaccine available, but doxycycline and ciprofloxacin can be used after exposure, and gentamicin has been effective after symptoms appear.

Botulism

Botulism, produced by *Clostridium botulinum,* can be aerosolized or used to contaminate food. The toxin it produces causes cranial nerve palsies that can result in muscle paralysis and respiratory failure. A botulinum toxoid is available through the Centers for Disease Control and Prevention for the military and high-risk workers. Antitoxin is also available for patients with specific exposures, and research is ongoing with an equine antitoxin effective against all seven serotypes of botulism that is thought to cause fewer hypersensitivity reactions than what is currently available.

Viral Hemorrhagic Fever

Lassa, Marburg, Junin, and Ebola viruses cause hemorrhagic fevers with mortality rates as high as 90%. No vaccines are currently available for these agents, although the United States Army has had success with a vaccine for Junin. Ribavirin has been effective in some cases of Lassa fever and has been effective orally for postexposure prophylaxis. It is being studied for effectiveness with these other viruses. Currently there is no established treatment, and this area is one of the highest priorities for combating possible biological warfare.

nization. *Aspirin can mask warning signs of Reye's syndrome, a potentially serious disease.*

- Provide thorough patient teaching, including measures to avoid adverse effects, warning signs of problems, and the need to keep a written record of immunizations, *to increase knowledge about drug therapy and to increase compliance with the drug regimen.*
- Provide a written record of the immunization, including the need to return for booster immunizations and timing of the boosters, if necessary, *to increase patient compliance with medical regimens.*

Evaluation

- Monitor patient response to the drug (prevention of disease, appropriate antibody titer levels).
- Monitor for adverse effects (flu-like symptoms; GI upset; local pain, swelling, nodule formation at injection site).
- Evaluate the effectiveness of the teaching plan (patient can name drug, dosage, adverse effects to watch for, has written record of immunizations).
- Monitor the effectiveness of comfort measures and adherence to the regimen.

BOX 18.5 FOCUS ON THE **EVIDENCE**

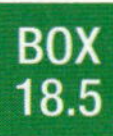

Studies Find No Link Between MMR Vaccine and Autism

The Immunization Safety Review Committee Board of Health Promotion and Disease Prevention of the Institute of Medicine under the auspices of the Centers for Disease Control and Prevention and the National Institutes of Health has concluded that there is no evidence to support a linkage between the use of measles–mumps–rubella (MMR) vaccine and the development of autism (a psychiatric neurological impairment affecting children and marked by deficits in communication and social attachment). The media, however, continue to pursue this possible connection, raising concerns for parents about the use of vaccines in children.

Among materials studied by the Institute of Medicine were questionnaires about reported symptoms and the timing of the vaccination and Vaccine Adverse Event Reporting System (VAERS) reports. The information obtained will help determine a need for other research, and it will also be used to educate parents. Parents can be referred to www.cdc.gov; click on vaccine safety to get current information and to review the research that has been done.

Source: Immunization Safety Review Committee. (2004). *Immunization safety review: Vaccines and autism.* Washington, DC: National Academies Press.

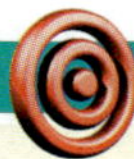

FOCUS POINTS

- Immunity is a state of relative resistance to a disease that develops only after exposure to the specific disease-causing agent.
- Active immunity occurs when a person's body is stimulated to make antibodies against specific proteins.
- Vaccines provide active immunity by stimulating production of antibodies to a specific protein, which may produce the signs and symptoms of a mild immune reaction, but protects the person from the more devastating effects of disease.

Immune Sera and Antitoxins

As explained earlier, passive immunity can be achieved by providing preformed antibodies to a specific antigen. These antibodies are found in immune sera, which may contain antibodies to toxins, venins, bacteria, viruses, or even red blood cell antigenic factors. The term **immune sera** is usually used to refer to sera that contain antibodies to specific bacteria or viruses. The terms **antitoxin** and antivenin are used to refer to immune sera that have antibodies to very specific toxins that might be released by invading pathogens or to venom that might be injected through spider or snake bites. Table 18.2 lists the various available immune sera and antitoxins.

Therapeutic Actions and Indications

Immune sera are used to provide passive immunity to a specific antigen or disease. They also may be used as prophylaxis against specific diseases after exposure in patients who are immunosuppressed. In addition, immune sera may be used to lessen the severity of a disease after known or suspected exposure (see Figure 18.2 for sites of action of immune sera and antitoxins).

Contraindications and Cautions

Immune sera are contraindicated in the presence of a history of severe reaction to any immune sera or to products similar to the components of the sera. They should be used with caution during pregnancy *because of potential risk to the fetus;* with coagulation defects or thrombocytopenia; or with a known history of previous exposure to the immune sera *because increased risk of hypersensitivity reaction occurs with each use.*

Adverse Effects

Adverse effects can be attributed either to the effect of immune sera on the immune system (rash, nausea, vomiting, chills, fever) or to allergic reactions (chest tightness, falling blood pressure, difficulty breathing). Local reactions are very common (swelling, tenderness, pain, muscle stiffness at the injection site).

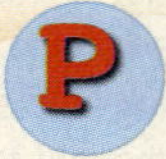

Prototype Summary: *Immune Globulin, Intramuscular*

Indications: Prophylaxis against hepatitis A, measles, varicella, rubella; prophylaxis for patients with immunoglobulin deficiency

Actions: Provides preformed antibodies to hepatitis A, measles, varicella, rubella, and perhaps other antigens, providing a passive, short-term immunity

Pharmacokinetics:

Route	Onset	Peak
IM	Slow	2–5 days

$T_{1/2}$: Unknown; metabolized in the tissues, excretion is unknown

Adverse effects: Tenderness, muscle stiffness at site of injection; urticaria, angioedema, nausea, vomiting, chills, fever, chest tightness

(text continues on page 294)

Table 18.1 DRUGS IN FOCUS

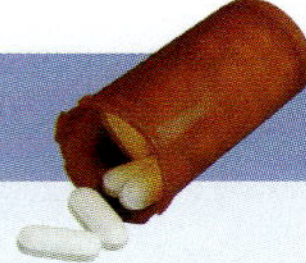

Vaccines

Drug Name	Dosage/Route	Usual Indications
Bacterial Vaccines		
BCG (*TICE BCG*)	0.2–0.3 mL percutaneously	Prevention of tuberculosis with high risk of exposure
haemophilus influenza b conjugate vaccine (*HibTITER, Liquid PedvaxHIB, ActHIB*)	0.5 mL IM; ages vary with preparation	Active immunization against *Haemophilus influenza* type B infection in infants and children
haemophilus influenza b conjugate vaccine and hepatitis B surface antigen (*Comvax*)	Three 0.5-mL IM injections at 2, 4, and 6 mo with 0.5 mL booster at 15–18 mo	Immunization of children against haemophilus B and hepatitis B infections
meningococcal polysaccharide vaccine (*Menomune-A/C/Y/W-135*)	0.5 mL Sub-Q	Immunization against meningococcal infections in endemic areas
meningococcal polysaccharide diphtheria toxoid conjugate vaccine (*Menactra*)	0.5 mL IM	Active immunization of people aged 11–55 yr to prevent invasive meningococcal disease
pneumococcal vaccine, polyvalent (*Pneumovax 23*)	0.5 mL Sub-Q or IM, not recommended for children <2 yr of age	Immunization against pneumococcal infections
pneumococcal 7-valent conjugate vaccine (*Prevnar*)	7–11 mo: three 0.5-mg IM doses at least 4 wk apart and the last one at >1 yr 12–23 mo: two 0.5-mg IM doses 2 mo apart 24 mo–9 yr: one 0.5-mg IM dose	Prevention of invasive pneumococcal disease in infants and children
typhoid vaccine (*Vivotif Berna Typhim VI*)	Two doses of 0.5 mL Sub-Q at intervals ≥4 wk with booster given every 3 yr, *or* one capsule PO on days 1, 3, 5, and 7	Immunization against typhoid fever
Toxoids		
diphtheria and tetanus toxoids, combined, adsorbed (*DT, Td*)	Two IM injections of 0.5 mL at intervals of 4–8 wk, with booster of 0.5 mL in 6–12 mo	Immunization of adults and children >7 yr of age against diphtheria and tetanus
diphtheria and tetanus toxoids and acellular pertussis vaccine, adsorbed (*DTaP, Tripedia, Infanix, Adacel, Boostrix*)	0.5 mL IM at 18 mo, at least 6 mo after DTwP as the fourth dose, then 0.5 mL IM at 4–6 yr *Booster:* 10–18 yr (*Boostrix*)*:* 0.5 mL IM 11–64 yr (*Adacel*)*:* 0.5 mL IM	Immunization of children against diphtheria, tetanus, and pertussis as the fourth and fifth doses of the immunization series Booster for adolescents and adults
diphtheria and tetanus toxoids and acellular pertussis and *Haemophilus influenza* type B conjugate vaccines (*DTaP-HIB*) (*TriHIBit*)	0.5 mL IM at 15–18 mo	Active immunization of children aged 15–18 mo as the fourth dose when being immunized with *ActHIB* or DTP
diphtheria and tetanus toxoids and acellular pertussis, adsorbed, and hepatitis B (*recombinant*) and inactivated poliovirus vaccine, combined (*Pediatrix*)	0.5 mL IM, three doses at 8-wk intervals or completion of series in combined form	Active immunization against diphtheria, tetanus, pertussis, hepatitis B, and poliovirus in infants with HBsAg-negative mothers
Viral Vaccines		
hepatitis A vaccine, inactivated (*Havrix, Vaqta*)	Adult: 1 mL IM with a booster dose in 6–12 mo Pediatric: 0.5 mL IM with a repeat dose in 6–12 mo	Immunization of adults and children against hepatitis A infection
hepatitis A vaccine, inactivated, with hepatitis B recombinant vaccine (*Twinrix*)	1 mL IM followed by booster doses at 1 mo and 6 mo	Immunization against hepatitis A and hepatitis B infections in people ≥18 yr of age

(continued)

Table 18.1 DRUGS IN FOCUS *(Continued)*

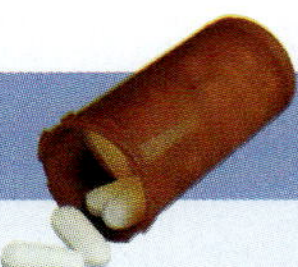

Vaccines

Drug Name	Dosage/Route	Usual Indications
Viral Vaccines		
hepatitis B vaccine (*Energix-B, Recombivax-HB*)	0.5–1 mL IM followed by 0.5–1 mL IM at 1 mo and 6 mo	Immunization against hepatitis B infections in susceptible people and in infants born to mothers with hepatitis B
influenza virus vaccine (*Fluzone, Fluvirin*)	Adult: 0.5 mL IM Pediatric: 0.25–0.5 mL IM repeated in 4 wk	Prophylaxis in adults and children at high risk for complications of influenza infections
influenza virus vaccine, intranasal (*FluMist*)	9–49 yr: 0.5 mL intranasal once each flu season 5–8 yr not previously vaccinated with *FluMist:* two doses of 0.5 mL each intranasally given 60 days apart 5–8 yr previously vaccinated with *FluMist:* 0.5 mL intranasally once per flu season	Active immunization to prevent disease caused by influenza A and B viruses
Japanese encephalitis vaccine (*JE-VAX*)	1 mL Sub-Q on days 0, 7, and 30 1–3 yr: 0.5 mL Sub-Q on days 0, 7 and 30	Immunization of persons >1 yr of age who reside in or will travel to endemic areas
measles virus vaccine (*Attenuvax*)	0.5 mL Sub-Q	Immunization against measles
P measles, mumps, rubella vaccine (*MMR-II*)	0.5 mL Sub-Q	Immunization against measles, mumps, and rubella in adults and children >15 mo of age
measles, mumps, rubella, varicella virus vaccine (*ProQuad*)	0.5 mL Sub-Q	Simultaneous immunization against measles, mumps, rubella, and varicella in children aged 12 mo to 12 yr
measles and rubella virus vaccine, live (*M-R-Vax II*)	0.5 mg Sub-Q	Immunization against measles and rubella in children ≥15 mo of age
mumps virus vaccine (*Mumpsvax*)	0.5 mL Sub-Q	Immunization against mumps in persons >12 mo of age
poliovirus vaccine, inactivated (*IPOL*)	0.5 mL Sub-Q at 2, 4, and 12–15 mo; booster when starting school Adult: 0.5 mL Sub-Q, two doses at intervals of 1–2 mo, with a third dose 6–12 mo later	Immunization against polio infections in adults and children
rabies vaccine (*Imovax Rabies, RabAvert*)	*Pre-exposure:* 1 mL IM on days 0, 7, 21, and 28 *Postexposure:* 1 mL IM on days 0, 3, 7, 21, and 28	Pre-exposure immunization against rabies for high-risk people; postexposure antirabies regimen with rabies immune globulin
rubella virus vaccine (*Meruvax II*)	One dose Sub-Q (>1000 times the median tissue culture infective dose [$TCID_{50}$])	Immunization against rubella in adults and children >12 mo of age
rubella and mumps vaccine, live (*Biavax II*)	0.5 mg Sub-Q	Immunization against rubella and mumps in children >12 mo, preferably at 15 mo
smallpox vaccine (*Dryvax*)	One drop of live virus in two to three prepared punctures on the upper arm; inspect after 6–8 days; a scab should form, leaving a scar; if only a mild reaction occurs, repeat vaccination using 15 punctures in the area where a drop of vaccine is placed	Active immunization against smallpox disease
varicella virus vaccine (*Varivax*)	0.5 mL Sub-Q, followed by 0.5 mL Sub-Q 4–8 wk later	Immunization against chickenpox infections in adults and children ≥12 mo of age
yellow fever vaccine (*YF-Vax*)	Children 1–12 yr: 0.5 mL Sub-Q 0.5 mL Sub-Q booster every 10 yr	Immunization of travelers to areas where yellow fever is endemic

CRITICAL THINKING SCENARIO 18-1

Educating a Parent About Vaccines

The Situation

S.D. is a 25-year-old, first-time mother who has brought her 2-month-old daughter to the well-baby clinic for a routine evaluation. The baby is found to be healthy, growing well, and within normal parameters for her age. At the end of the visit, the nurse prepares to give the baby the first of her routine immunizations. S.D. becomes concerned and expresses fears about paralysis and infant deaths associated with immunizations.

Critical Thinking

What information should S.D. be given about immunizations?

What nursing interventions would be appropriate at this time? *Think of ways to explain the importance of immunizations to S.D. while supporting her concerns for the welfare of her baby.*

How can this experience be incorporated into a teaching plan for S.D. and her baby?

Discussion

S.D. should be reassured before the baby is immunized. The nurse can tell her that in the past, paralysis and infant deaths were reported, but that efforts continue to make the vaccines pure. Careful monitoring of the child and the child's response to each immunization can help avoid such problems. Reassure S.D. that the immunizations will prevent her daughter from contracting many, sometimes deadly, diseases. Praise S.D.'s efforts for researching information that might affect her baby and for asking questions that could have an impact on her child and her understanding of her care.

The recommended schedule of immunizations should be given to S.D. so that she is aware of what is planned and how the various vaccines are spaced and combined. She should be encouraged to monitor the baby after each injection for fever, chills, and flu-like reactions. When she gets home, she can medicate the baby with acetaminophen to avert many of these symptoms before they happen. (S.D. should be advised not to give the baby aspirin, which could cover up Reye's syndrome, a potentially serious disorder.) S.D. also should be told that the injection site might be sore, swollen, and red, but that this will pass in a couple of days. S.D. can ease the baby's discomfort by applying warm soaks to the area for about 10 to 15 minutes every 2 hours.

S.D. should be encouraged to write down all of the immunizations that the baby has had and to keep this information handy for easy reference. She should also be encouraged to record any adverse effects that occur after each immunization. If reactions are uncomfortable, it is possible to split doses of future immunizations.

The nurse should give S.D. a chance to vent her concerns and fears. First-time parents may be more anxious than experienced ones when dealing with issues involving a new baby. To alleviate S.D.'s anxiety, the nurse should provide a telephone number that S.D. can call if the baby seems to be having a severe reaction or if S.D. wants to discuss any questions or concerns. She should feel that support is available for any concern that she may have. Because this interaction is likely to form the basis for future interactions with S.D., it is important to establish a sense of respect and trust.

Nursing Care Guide for S.D.'s Baby: Vaccines

Assessment: History and Examination

Allergies to the serum base, acute infection, immunosuppression

General: temperature

CV: pulse, cardiac auscultation, blood pressure, edema, perfusion

Respiratory: respirations, adventitious sounds

Skin: lesions

Joints: range of motion

Nursing Diagnoses

Acute Pain related to infection and flu-like symptoms

Ineffective Tissue Perfusion if severe reaction occurs

Deficient Knowledge regarding drug therapy

Implementation

Ensure proper preparation and administration of vaccine within appropriate time frame.

(continued)

Educating a Parent About Vaccines *(continued)*

Provide supportive and comfort measures to deal with adverse effects: anti-inflammatory/antipyretic, local heat application, small meals, rest, and a quiet environment.

Provide parent teaching regarding drug name, adverse effects and precautions, and warning signs to report.

Provide emergency life support if needed for acute reaction.

Evaluation

Evaluate drug effects: serum titers reflecting immunization (if appropriate).

Monitor for adverse effects: pain, flu-like symptoms, local discomfort.

Evaluate effectiveness of parent teaching program.

Evaluate effectiveness of comfort and safety measures.

Evaluate effectiveness of emergency measures if needed.

Patient Teaching for S.D.

- ☐ This immunization will help your baby to develop antibodies to protect her against diphtheria, tetanus, and pertussis. The baby will develop antibodies to these diseases, and this will prevent the baby from contracting one of these potentially deadly diseases in the future.
- ☐ The injection site might be sore and painful. Heat applied to the area may help this discomfort and speed the baby's recovery.
- ☐ Adverse effects that the baby might experience include fever, muscle aches, joint aches, fatigue, malaise, crying, and fretfulness. Acetaminophen may help these discomforts; check with your health care provider for the correct dose to use for the baby. Rest, small meals, and a quiet environment may also help the baby to feel better.
- ☐ The adverse effects should pass within 2 to 3 days. If they seem to be causing undue discomfort or persist longer than a few days, notify your health care provider.
- ☐ Booster immunizations are required for this immunization. Your baby should receive a booster immunization at your next well-baby checkup. Keep a written record of this immunization.
- ☐ Please contact your health care provider if you have any questions or concerns.

Nursing Considerations for Patients Receiving Immune Sera or Antitoxins

Assessment: History and Examination

Screen for the following, *which could be contraindications or cautions to the use of the drug:* any known allergies to any of these drugs or their components; pregnancy; previous exposure to the serum being used; thrombocytopenia; coagulation disorders; and immunization history.

Include screening *for baseline status before beginning therapy and for any potential adverse effects:* presence of any skin lesions; temperature; orientation, reflexes; pulse, blood pressure, respirations, and adventitious sounds.

Nursing Diagnoses

The patient receiving immune sera may have the following nursing diagnoses related to drug therapy:

- Acute Pain related to local, GI, and flu-like effects
- Ineffective Tissue Perfusion related to possible severe reactions
- Deficient Knowledge regarding drug therapy

Implementation With Rationale

- Do not administer to any patient with a history of severe reaction to immune globulins or to the components of the drug being used *because severe immune reactions can occur.*
- Administer the drug as indicated. *Preparation varies with each product; always check manufacturer's guidelines.*
- Monitor for severe reactions and *have emergency equipment ready.*
- Arrange for supportive care and comfort measures for flu-like symptoms (rest, environmental control, acetaminophen) and for the local reaction (heat to injection site, anti-inflammatories) *to promote patient comfort.*
- Provide thorough patient teaching, including measures to avoid adverse effects and warning signs of problems, *to improve patient compliance.*

Table 18.2 DRUGS IN FOCUS

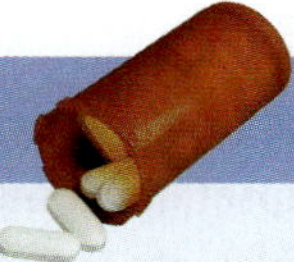

Immune Sera

Drug Name	Dosage/Route	Usual Indications
anti-thymocyte immune globulin (*Thymoglobulin*)	1.5 mg/kg/day for 7–14 days as 6-h infusion for the first dose and ≥4 h for each subsequent dose	Treatment of renal transplant acute rejection in conjunction with immunosuppression
cytomegalovirus immune globulin (*CytoGam*)	15 mg/kg IV over 30 min increased to 30 mg/kg IV over 30 min, then 60 mg/kg IV to a max of 150 mg/kg; infuse at 72 h, at 2 wk, and then at 4, 6, 8, 12, and 16 wk after transplantation	Attenuation of primary cytomegalovirus disease after renal transplantation
hepatitis B immune globulin (*BayHep B Nabi-HB*)	0.06 mL/kg IM, repeated at 3 mo and 6 mo	Postexposure prophylaxis against hepatitis B
P immune globulin, intramuscular (*BayGam*, others)	Dosage varies with exposure; check manufacturer's instructions	Prophylaxis after exposure to hepatitis A, measles, varicella, or rubella
immune globulin, intravenous (*Gamimune N, Gammagard,* and others)	Dosage varies with indication and preparation; always check manufacturer's instructions	Prophylaxis after exposure to hepatitis A, measles, varicella, or rubella; bone marrow and other transplants; Kawasaki's disease; chronic lymphocytic leukemia; treatment of patients with immunoglobulin deficiency
lymphocyte immune globulin (*Atgam*)	Adult: 10–30 mg/kg/day IV Pediatric: 5–25 mg/kg/day IV for aplastic anemia	Management of allograft rejection in renal transplantation; treatment of aplastic anemia
rabies immune globulin (*BayRab, Imogam Rabies*)	20 International Units/kg IM	Protection against rabies in nonimmunized patients exposed to rabies
respiratory syncytial virus immune globulin (*RespiGAM*)	1.5 mL/kg/h for 15 min, then 3 mL/kg/h for 15 min, then 6 mL/kg/h to a total monthly infusion of 750 mg/kg	Prevention of respiratory syncytial virus infection in children <24 mo of age with bronchopulmonary dysplasia or premature birth
RHO immune globulin (*BayRho-D Full Dose, RhoGAM*)	One vial IM within 72 h after delivery	Prevention of sensitization to the Rh factor
RHO immune globulin, microdose (*BayRho-D Mini-Dose, MICRhoGAM*)	One vial IV within 72 h after delivery	Prevention of sensitization to the Rh factor
tetanus immune globulin (*Bay Tet*)	250 units IM	Passive immunization against tetanus at time of injury
vaccinia immune globulin IV (*VIGIV*)	2 mL/kg (100 mg/kg) IV	Treatment and management of vaccinia infections
varicella zoster immune globulin (*Varicella Zoster Immune Globulin*)	125 units/10 kg IM, to a maximum of 625 units	Passive immunization against varicella zoster in immunosuppressed patients exposed to disease
Antitoxins and Antivenins		
antivenin (crotalidae polyvalent) (*generic*)	20–40 mL IV, up to 100–150 mL in severe cases	Neutralizes the venom of pit vipers, rattlesnakes, and copperheads
antivenin (micrurus fulvius) (*generic*)	30–50 mL IV, flush with fluids after antivenin has infused	Neutralizes the venom of coral snakes
Black widow spider antivenin (*Antivenin*)	25 mL IM or IV in 10–50 mL saline over 15 min	Treatment of symptoms of black widow spider bites
crotalidae polyvalent immune fab (*CroFab*)	Four to six vials IV given diluted over 60 min	Treatment of rattlesnake bites

- Provide a written record of immune sera use and encourage the patient or family to keep that information *to ensure proper medical treatment and to avert future reactions.*

Evaluation

- Monitor the patient's response to the drug (improvement in disease signs and symptoms, prevention of severe disease).

- Monitor for adverse effects (flu-like symptoms, GI upset, local inflammation and pain).
- Evaluate the effectiveness of the teaching plan (patient can name drug, dosage, adverse effects to watch for, specific measures to avoid adverse effects, need to retain written record of injection).
- Monitor the effectiveness of comfort measures and compliance with the regimen.

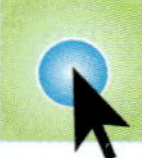

WEB LINKS

Health care providers and patients may want to consult the following Internet sources:

http://www.travelhealth.com Patients traveling to various parts of the world can obtain information on vaccines that are needed and food and travel precautions.

http://www.cdc.gov Annual updates on immunization guidelines.

Points to Remember

- Immunity (relative resistance to a disease) may be active or passive. Active immunity results from the body making antibodies against specific proteins for immediate release if that protein re-enters the body. Passive immunity results from preformed antibodies to a specific protein, which offers protection against the protein only for the life of the circulating antibodies.
- Immunizations are given to stimulate active immunity in a person who is at high risk for exposure to specific diseases. Immunizations are a standard part of preventive medicine.
- Vaccines contain weakened or partial proteins from specific antigens that stimulate the production of antibodies to that protein, thus providing active immunity.
- Immune sera provide preformed antibodies to specific proteins for people who have been exposed to them or are at high risk for exposure.
- Serum sickness, a massive immune reaction, occurs more frequently with immune sera than with vaccines. Patients need to be monitored for any history of hypersensitivity reactions, and emergency equipment should be available.
- Patients should be advised to keep a written record of all immunizations or immune sera used. Booster doses may be needed to further stimulate antibody production.

CHECK YOUR UNDERSTANDING

Answers to the questions in this chapter may be found in the Answer Key in the back of the book.

Multiple Choice

Select the best answer to the following.

1. Vaccines are used to stimulate
   a. passive immunity to a foreign protein.
   b. active immunity to a foreign protein.
   c. serum sickness.
   d. a mild disease in healthy people.

2. Common adverse effects associated with routine immunizations would *not* include
   a. difficulty breathing.
   b. fever and rash.
   c. drowsiness and fretfulness.
   d. pain, redness, swelling, and nodule formation at the site of injection.

3. A 6-month-old child would *not* be a candidate for
   a. diphtheria, tetanus, pertussis (DTaP) vaccine.
   b. *H. influenza* B vaccine.
   c. poliovirus vaccine.
   d. chickenpox vaccine.

4. Every fall, older adults and people who are at high risk for complications of influenza should receive a flu vaccine. This is repeated every year because
   a. the immunity wears off after a year.
   b. the strains of virus predicted to cause the flu change every year.
   c. a booster shot will activate the immune system.
   d. older people do not produce good antibodies.

5. You should check a patient's record to make sure that tetanus booster shots have been given
   a. only with exposure to anaerobic bacteria.
   b. every 2 years.
   c. every 5 years.
   d. every 10 years.

6. A nurse suffers a needle stick after injecting a patient with suspected hepatitis B. The nurse should
   a. have repeated titers to determine whether she was exposed to hepatitis B and, if she was, have hepatitis immune globulin.

b. immediately receive hepatitis immune globulin and begin hepatitis B vaccines if she has not already received them.
c. start antibiotic therapy immediately.
d. go on sick leave until all screening tests are negative.

7. A patient is to receive immune globulin after exposure to hepatitis A. The patient has a previous history of allergies to various drugs. Before giving the immune globulin, the nurse should
   a. make sure that emergency equipment is readily available in case of a massive immune reaction.
   b. premedicate the patient with aspirin.
   c. make sure all of the patient's vaccinations are up to date.
   d. make sure the patient has a ride home.

Multiple Response

Select all that apply.

1. A public education campaign to stress the importance of childhood immunizations should include which of the following points?
   a. Prevention of potentially devastating diseases outweighs the discomfort and risks of immunization.
   b. Routine immunization is standard practice in the United States.
   c. The practice of routine immunizations has virtually wiped out many previously deadly or debilitating diseases.
   d. The risk of severe adverse reactions is on the rise and is not being addressed.
   e. If you have a family history of autism, you should not have your child immunized.
   f. The discomfort associated with the immunization can be treated with OTC drugs and passes quickly.

2. A mother brings her child to his 18-month well-baby visit. The nurse would not give the child his routine immunizations in which of the following situations?
   a. He cried at his last immunization.
   b. He developed a fever or rash after his last immunization.
   c. He currently has a fever and symptoms of a cold.
   d. He is allergic to aspirin.
   e. He is currently taking oral corticosteroids.
   f. His siblings are all currently being treated for a viral infection.

3. When assessing the medical record of an older adult to evaluate the status of his immunizations, the nurse would be looking for evidence of which of the following?
   a. Yearly pneumococcal vaccination
   b. Yearly flu vaccination
   c. Tetanus booster every 10 years
   d. Tetanus booster every 5 years
   e. MMR vaccine if born after 1957
   f. Varicella vaccine, only if evidence of having had chickenpox as a child

Web Exercise

Your patient, a new mother, has arrived at the clinic with her 2-week-old baby for routine postpartum health care. She has been watching a television talk show about the hazards of vaccinations and asks some good questions about vaccinating her baby. Go to the Internet and find some useful information that can be printed out to help your patient understand vaccinations and to make good decisions about her child's health care. www.cdc.gov might be a good place to start.

True or False

Indicate whether the following statements are true (T) or false (F).

_____ 1. Tetanus vaccines will provide active immunity against tetanus toxins.

_____ 2. Active immunity occurs when the host is stimulated to make antibodies to a specific antigen.

_____ 3. Gamma globulin provides a good form of passive immunity to patients exposed to a specific antigen.

_____ 4. Vaccines are used to promote active immunity.

_____ 5. Vaccines are only used to prevent infection with future exposures.

_____ 6. Serious reactions have occurred to routine immunizations in the past.

_____ 7. Patients will not experience any discomfort after an immunization injection.

_____ 8. Serum sickness—a massive immune reaction—occurs more frequently with vaccines than with immune sera.

Bibliography and References

AMA drug evaluations. (2006). Chicago: American Medical Association.
Drug facts and comparisons. (2006). St. Louis: Facts & Comparisons.
Gilman, A., Hardman, J. G., & Limbird, L. E. (Eds.). (2006). *Goodman and Gilman's the pharmacological basis of therapeutics* (11th ed.). New York: McGraw-Hill.
Halsey, R. A., et al. (2001). A review: MMR vaccine and autism spectrum disorders: Report of the AAP technical review panel. *Pediatrics, 107(5),* 1–23.
Karch, A. M. (2006). *2007 Lippincott's nursing drug guide.* Philadelphia: Lippincott Williams & Wilkins.
Porth, C. M. (2005). *Pathophysiology: Concepts of altered health states* (7th ed.). Philadelphia: Lippincott Williams & Wilkins.
The medical letter on drugs and therapeutics. (2006). New Rochelle, NY: Medical Letter.

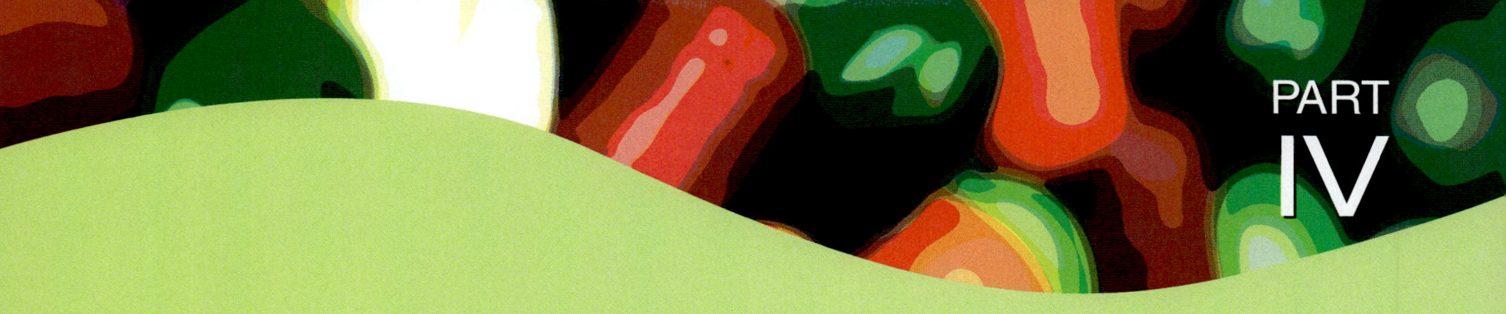

PART IV

Drugs Acting on the Central and Peripheral Nervous Systems

CHAPTER 19

Introduction to Nerves and the Nervous System

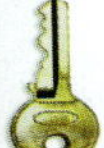

KEY TERMS

action potential
afferent
axon
dendrite
depolarization
effector
efferent
engram
forebrain
hindbrain
limbic system
midbrain
neuron
neurotransmitter
repolarization
Schwann cell
soma
synapse

LEARNING OBJECTIVES

Upon completion of this chapter, you will be able to:

1. Label the parts of a neuron and describe the functions of each part.
2. Describe an action potential, including the roles of the various electrolytes involved.
3. Explain what a neurotransmitter is, including its origins and functions at the synapse.
4. Describe the function of the cerebral cortex, cerebellum, hypothalamus, thalamus, midbrain, pituitary gland, medulla, spinal cord, and reticular activating system.
5. Discuss what is known about learning and the impact of emotion on that process.

The nervous system is responsible for controlling the functions of the human body, analyzing incoming stimuli, and integrating internal and external responses. The nervous system is composed of the central nervous system (the brain and spinal cord) and the peripheral nervous system (PNS). The PNS is composed of sensory receptors that bring information into the central nervous system (CNS) and motor nerves that carry information away from the CNS to facilitate response to stimuli. The autonomic nervous system, which is discussed in Chapter 29, uses components of the CNS and PNS to regulate automatic or unconscious responses to stimuli.

The structural unit of the nervous system is the nerve cell, or **neuron**. The billions of nerve cells that make up the nervous system are organized to allow movement; realization of various sensations; response to internal and external stimuli; and learning, thinking, and emotion. The mechanisms that are involved in all of these processes are not clearly understood. The actions of drugs that are used to affect the functioning of the nerves and the responses that these drugs cause throughout the nervous system provide some of the current theories about the workings of the nervous system.

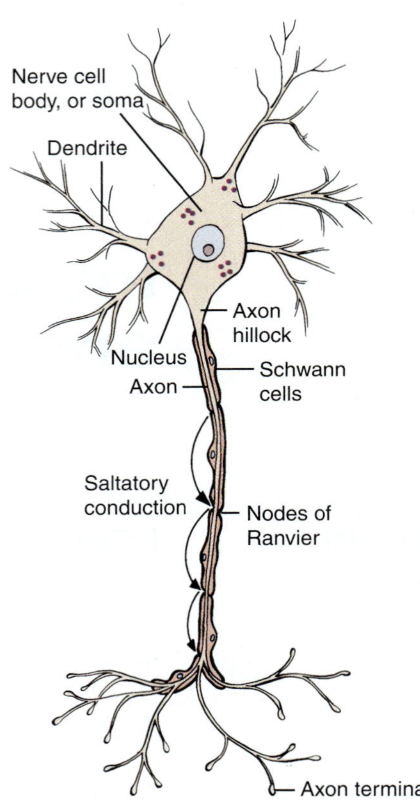

FIGURE 19.1 The neuron, functional unit of the nervous system.

Physiology of the Nervous System

The nervous system operates through the use of electrical impulses and chemical messengers to transmit information throughout the body and to respond to internal and external stimuli. The properties and function of the neuron provide the basis for all nervous system function.

Neurons

As noted previously, the neuron is the structural unit of the nervous system. The human body contains about 14 billion neurons. About 10 billion of these are located in the brain, and the remainder make up the spinal cord and PNS.

Neurons have several distinctive cellular features. Each neuron is made up of a cell body, or **soma**, which contains the cell nucleus, cytoplasm, and various granules and other particles (Figure 19.1). Short, branch-like projections that cover most of the surface of a neuron are known as **dendrites**. These structures, which provide increased surface area for the neuron, bring information into the neuron from other neurons.

One end of the nerve body extends into a long process that does not branch out until the very end of the process. This elongated process is called the nerve **axon**, and it emerges from the soma at the axon hillock (see Figure 19.1). The axon of a nerve can be extremely tiny, or it can extend for several feet. The axon carries information from a nerve to be transmitted to **effector** cells—cells in a muscle, a gland, or another nerve. This transmission occurs at the end of the axon, where the axon branches out in what is called the axon terminal.

The axons of many nerves are packed closely together in the nervous system and look like cable or fiber tracts. **Afferent** fibers are nerve axons that run from peripheral receptors into the CNS. In contrast, **efferent** fibers are nerve axons that carry nerve impulses from the CNS to the periphery to stimulate muscles or glands. (An easy way to remember the difference between afferent and efferent is to recall that efferent fibers exit from the CNS.)

It is currently thought that neurons are unable to reproduce; so, if nerves are destroyed, they are lost. If dendrites and axons are lost, nerves regenerate those structures; however, for this regeneration to occur, the soma and the axon hillock must remain intact. For a clinical example, consider a person who has closed a car door on his or her finger. Sensation and movement may be lost or limited for a certain period, but because the nerve bodies for most of the nerves in the hand are located in ganglia (groups of nerve bodies) in the wrist, they are able to regenerate the damaged axon or dendrites. Over time, sensation and full movement should return.

Research on possible ways to stimulate the reproduction of nerves is under way. Although scientists have used nerve growth factor with fetal cell implants to stimulate some nerve growth, it is currently assumed that nerves are unable to reproduce.

Action Potential

Nerves send messages by conducting electrical impulses called **action potentials**. Nerve membranes, which are capable of conducting action potentials along the entire membrane, send messages to nearby neurons or to effector cells that may be located inches to feet away via this electrical communication system. Like all cell membranes, nerve membranes have various channels or pores that control the movement of substances into and out of the cell. Some of these channels allow the movement of sodium, potassium, and calcium. When cells are at rest, their membranes are impermeable to sodium. However, the membranes are permeable to potassium ions.

The sodium–potassium pump that is active in the membranes of neurons is responsible for this property of the membrane. This system pumps sodium ions out of the cell and potassium ions into the cell. At rest, more sodium ions are outside the cell membrane and more potassium ions are inside. Electrically, the inside of the cell is relatively negative compared with the outside of the membrane, which establishes an electrical potential along the nerve membrane. When nerves are at rest, this is referred to as the resting membrane potential of the nerve.

Stimulation of a neuron causes **depolarization** of the nerve, which means that the sodium channels open in response to the stimulus, and sodium ions rush into the cell, following the established concentration gradient. If an electrical monitoring device is attached to the nerve at this point, a positive rush of ions is recorded. The electrical charge on the inside of the membrane changes from relatively negative to relatively positive. This sudden reversal of membrane potential, called the action potential (Figure 19.2), lasts less than a microsecond. Using the sodium–potassium pump, the cell then returns that section of membrane to the resting membrane potential, a process called **repolarization**. The action potential generated at one point along a nerve membrane stimulates the generation of an action potential in adjacent portions of the cell membrane, and the stimulus travels the length of the cell membrane.

CONCEPTS in action ANIMATION

Nerves can respond to stimuli several hundred times per second, but for a given stimulus to cause an action potential, it must have sufficient strength and must occur when the nerve membrane is able to respond—that is, when it has repolarized. A nerve cannot be stimulated again while it is depolarized. The balance of sodium and potassium across the cell membrane must be re-established.

Nerves require energy (i.e., oxygen and glucose) and the correct balance of the electrolytes sodium and potassium to maintain normal action potentials and transmit information into and out of the nervous system. If an individual has anoxia or hypoglycemia, the nerves might not be able to maintain the sodium–potassium pump, and that individual may become severely irritable or too stable (not responsive to stimuli).

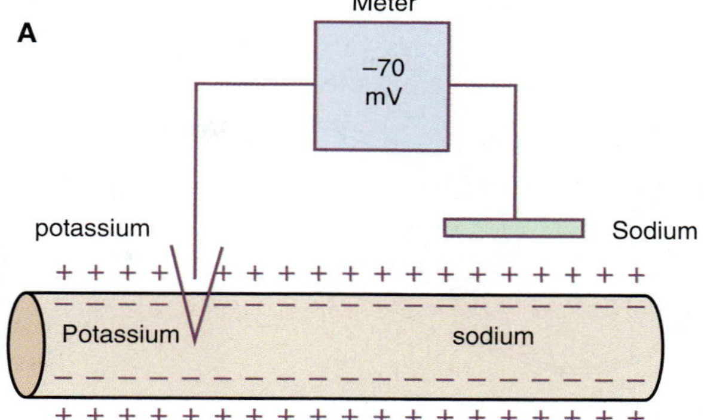

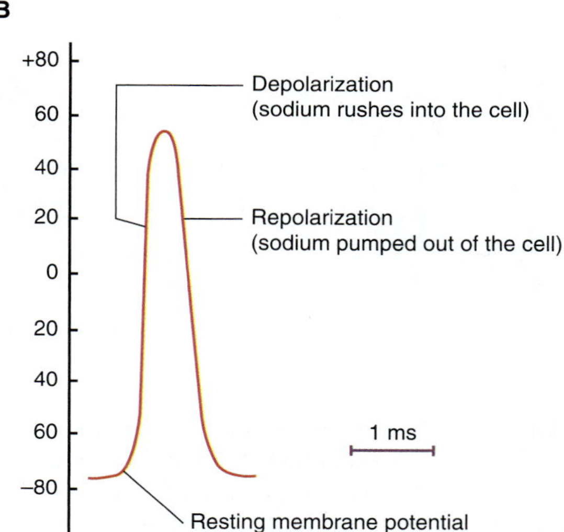

FIGURE 19.2 The action potential. **(A)** A segment of an axon showing that, at rest, the inside of the membrane is relatively negatively charged and the outside is positively charged. A pair of electrodes placed as shown would record a potential difference of about –70 mV; this is the resting membrane potential. **(B)** An action potential of about 1 msec that would be recorded if the axon shown in **A** were brought to threshold. At the peak of the action potential, the charge on the membrane reverses polarity.

Long nerves are myelinated: they have a myelin sheath that speeds electrical conduction and protects the nerves from the fatigue that results from frequent formation of action potentials. Even though many of the tightly packed nerves in the brain do not need to travel far to stimulate another nerve, they are myelinated. The effect of this myelination is not understood.

Myelinated nerves have **Schwann cells**, which are very resistant to electrical stimulation (Figure 19.3), located at specific intervals along the axons. The Schwann cells wrap themselves around the axon in jelly-roll fashion. Between the Schwann cells are areas of uncovered nerve membrane called the nodes of Ranvier. So-called "leaping" nerve conduction occurs along these exposed nerve fibers. An action potential excites one section of nerve membrane, and the electrical impulse then "skips" from one node to the next,

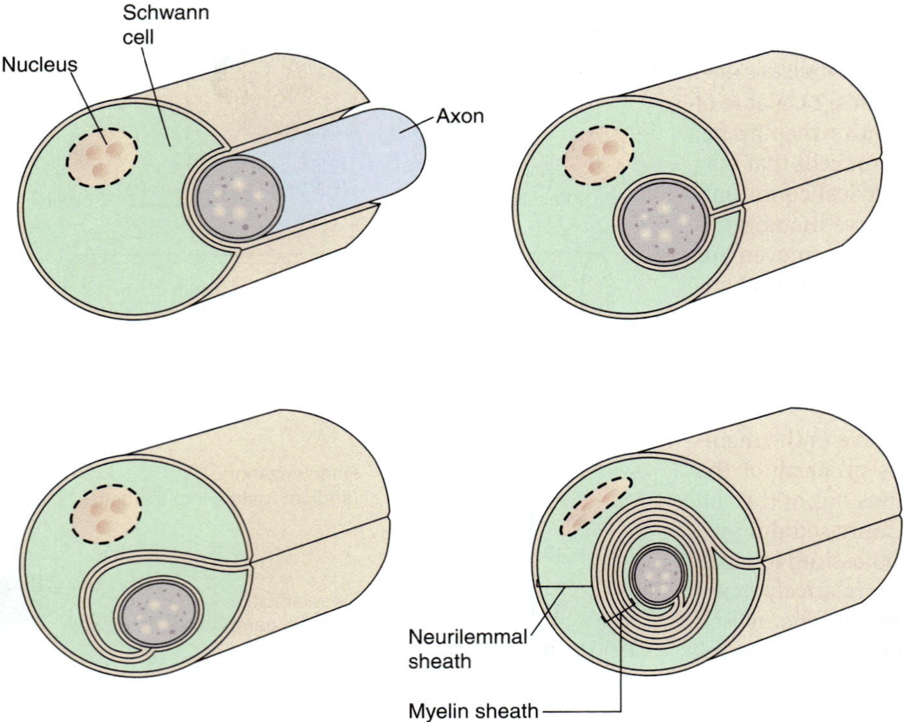

FIGURE 19.3 Formation of a myelin sheath in a peripheral axon. Successive wrappings of the Schwann cell membranes form the sheath, with most of the Schwann cell cytoplasm left outside the myelin. Therefore, the neurilemmal death of Schwann cells is outside the myelin sheath.

generating an action potential. Because the membrane is forming fewer action potentials, the speed of conduction is much faster and the nerve is protected from exhaustion or using up energy to form multiple action potentials. This node-to-node mode of conduction is termed *saltatory* or *leaping transmission.*

If the Schwann cells become enlarged or swollen and block the nodes of Ranvier, conduction does not occur because the electrical impulse has a limited firing range. A stimulus may simply be "lost" along the nerve, as in the neuromuscular disease multiple sclerosis. Believed to be an autoimmune disorder that attacks Schwann cells and leads to swelling and scarring of these cells, this disease is characterized by a progressive loss of nerve response and muscle function.

Nerve Synapse

When the electrical action potential reaches the end of an axon, the electrical impulse comes to a halt. At this point the stimulus no longer travels at the speed of electricity. The transmission of information between two nerves or between a nerve and a gland or muscle is chemical. Nerves communicate with other nerves or effectors at the nerve **synapse** (Figure 19.4). The synapse is made up of a presynaptic nerve, the synaptic cleft, and the postsynaptic effector cell. The nerve axon, called the presynaptic nerve, releases a chemical called a **neurotransmitter** into the synaptic cleft, and the neurotransmitter reacts with a very specific receptor site on the postsynaptic cell to cause a reaction.

Neurotransmitters

Neurotransmitters stimulate postsynaptic cells either by exciting or by inhibiting them. The reaction that occurs when a neurotransmitter stimulates a receptor site depends on the specific neurotransmitter that it releases and the receptor site it activates. A nerve may produce only one type of neurotransmitter, using building blocks such as tyrosine or choline from the extracellular fluid, often absorbed from dietary sources. The neurotransmitter, packaged into vesicles, moves to the terminal membrane of the axon, and when the nerve is stimulated the vesicles contract and push the neurotransmitter into the synaptic cleft. The calcium channels in the nerve membrane are open during the action potential, and the presence of calcium causes the contraction. When the cell repolarizes, calcium leaves the cell, and the contraction stops. Once released into the synaptic cleft, the neurotransmitter reacts with very specific receptor sites to cause a reaction.

To return the effector cell to a resting state so that it can be stimulated again, if needed, neurotransmitters must be inactivated. Neurotransmitters may be either reabsorbed by the presynaptic nerve in a process called reuptake (a recycling effort by the nerve to reuse the materials and save resources) or broken down by enzymes in the area (e.g., monoamine oxidase breaks down the neurotransmitter norepinephrine; the enzyme acetylcholinesterase breaks down the neurotransmitter acetylcholine). Several neurotransmitters have been identified. As research continues, other neurotransmitters may be discovered, and the actions of known neurotransmitters will be better understood.

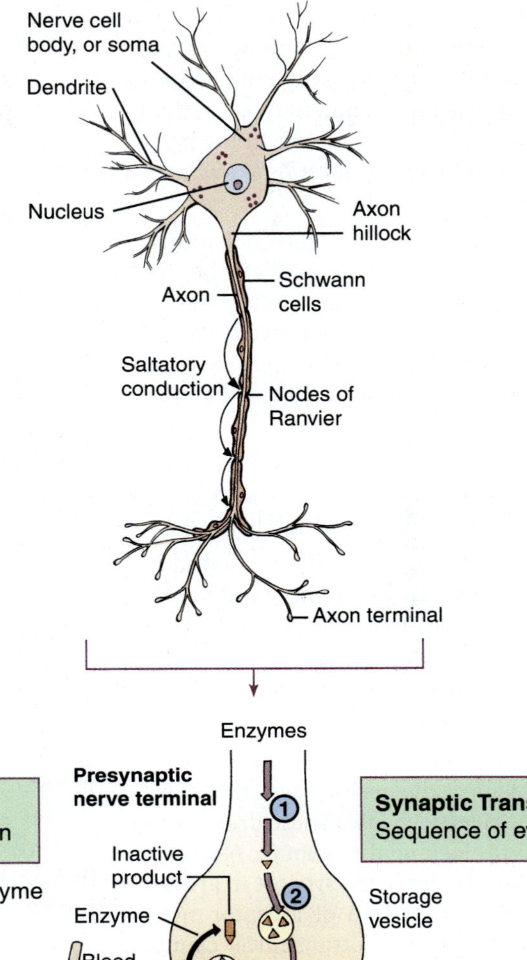

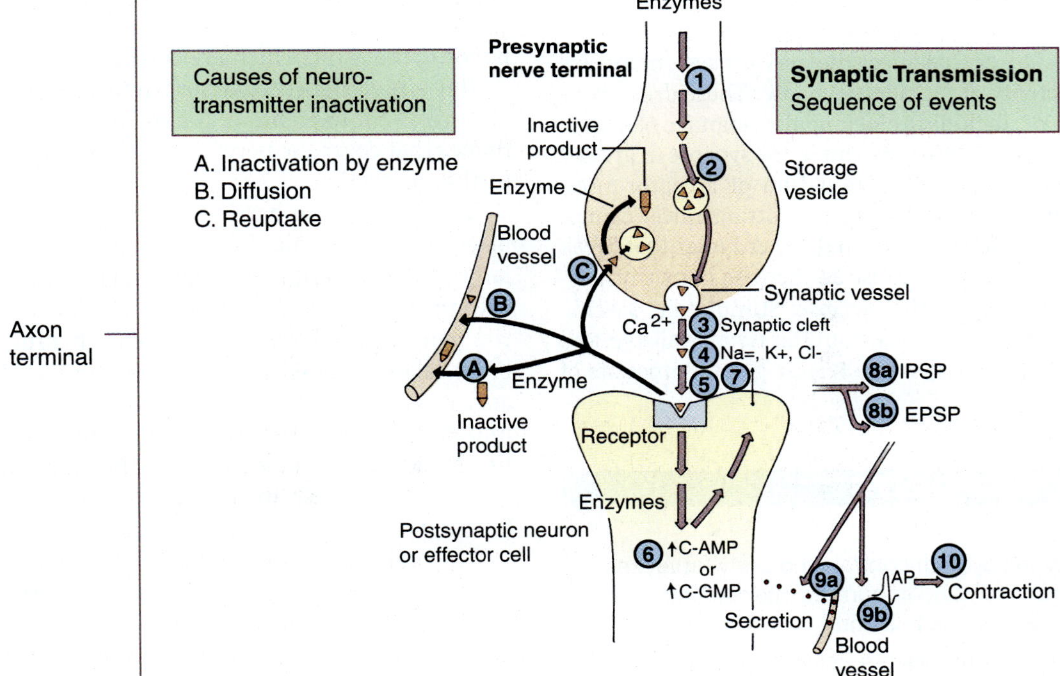

FIGURE 19.4 The sequence of events in synaptic transmission: **(1)** synthesis of the neurotransmitter; **(2)** uptake of the neurotransmitter into storage vesicles; **(3)** release of the neurotransmitter by an action potential in the presynaptic nerve; **(4)** diffusion of the neurotransmitter across the synaptic cleft; **(5)** combination of the neurotransmitter with a receptor; **(6)** a sequence of events leading to activation of second messengers within the postsynaptic nerve; **(7)** change in permeability of the postsynaptic membrane to one or more ions, causing **(8a)** an inhibitory postsynaptic potential or **(8b)** an excitatory postsynaptic potential. Characteristic responses of the postsynaptic cell are as follows: **(9a)** the gland secretes hormones; **(9b)** the muscle cells have an action potential; and **(10)** the muscle contracts. The action of the neurotransmitter is terminated by one or more of the following processes: **(A)** inactivation by an enzyme; **(B)** diffusion out of the synaptic cleft and removal by the vascular system; and **(C)** reuptake into the presynaptic nerve followed by storage in a synaptic vesicle or deactivation by an enzyme.

The following are selected neurotransmitters:

- *Acetylcholine,* which communicates between nerves and muscles, is also important as the preganglionic neurotransmitter throughout the autonomic nervous system and as the postganglionic neurotransmitter in the parasympathetic nervous system and in several pathways in the brain.
- *Norepinephrine* and *epinephrine* are catecholamines, which are released by nerves in the sympathetic branch of the autonomic nervous system and are classified as hormones when they are released from cells in the adrenal medulla. These neurotransmitters also occur in high levels in particular areas of the brain, such as the limbic system.
- *Dopamine,* which is found in high concentrations in certain areas of the brain, is involved in the coordination of impulses and responses, both motor and intellectual.
- *Gamma-aminobutyric acid (GABA),* which is found in the brain, inhibits nerve activity and is important in preventing overexcitability or stimulation such as seizure activity.
- *Serotonin,* which is also found in the limbic system, is important in arousal and sleep, as well as in preventing depression and promoting motivation.

Many of the drugs that affect the nervous system involve altering the activity of the nerve synapse. These drugs have several functions, including blocking the reuptake of neurotransmitters so that they are present in the synapse in greater quantities and cause more stimulation of receptor sites; blocking receptor sites so that the neurotransmitter cannot stimulate the receptor site; blocking the enzymes that break down neurotransmitters to cause an increase in neurotransmitter concentration in the synapse; stimulating specific receptor sites when the neurotransmitter is not available; and causing the presynaptic nerve to release greater amounts of the neurotransmitter.

FOCUS POINTS

- The nervous system controls the body, analyzes external stimuli, and integrates internal and external responses to stimuli.
- The neuron, comprising a cell body, dendrites and an axon, is the functional unit of the nervous system. Dendrites route information to the nerve, and axons take the information away.
- Nerves transmit information by way of action potentials. An action potential is a sudden change in membrane charge from negative to positive that is triggered when stimulation of a nerve opens sodium channels and allows positive sodium ions to flow into the cell.
- When sodium ions flow into a nerve, the nerve membrane depolarizes. Mechanically, this is recorded as a flow of positive electrical charges. Repolarization immediately follows, with the sodium–potassium pump in the cell membrane pumping sodium and potassium ions out of the cell, leaving the inside of the membrane relatively negative to the outside.
- At the end of the axon, neurons communicate with chemicals called neurotransmitters, which are produced by the nerve. Neurotransmitters are released into the synapse when the nerve is stimulated; they react with a very specific receptor site to cause a reaction and are immediately broken down or removed from the synapse.

Central Nervous System

The CNS consists of the brain and the spinal cord, the two parts of the body that contain the vast majority of nerves. The bones of the vertebrae protect the spinal cord, and the bones of the skull, which are corrugated much like an egg carton and designed to absorb impact, protect the brain (Figure 19.5). In addition, the meninges, which are membranes that cover the nerves in the brain and spine, furnish further protection.

The blood–brain barrier, a functioning boundary, also plays a defensive role. It keeps toxins, proteins, and other large structures out of the brain and prevents their contact with the sensitive and fragile neurons. The blood–brain barrier represents a therapeutic challenge to drug treatment of brain-related disorders because a large percentage of drugs are carried bound to plasma proteins and are unable to cross into the brain. When a patient is suffering from a brain infection, antibiotics cannot cross into the brain until the infection is so severe that the blood–brain barrier can no longer function.

The brain has a unique blood supply to protect the neurons from lack of oxygen and glucose. Two arteries, the carotids, branch off the aortic arch and go up into each side of the brain at the front of the head, and two other arteries, the vertebrals, enter the back of the brain to become the basilar arteries. These arteries all deliver blood to a common vessel at the bottom of the brain called the circle of Willis, which distributes the blood to the brain as it is needed (Figure 19.6). The role of the circle of Willis becomes apparent when an individual has an occluded carotid artery. Although the passage of blood through one of the carotid arteries may be negligible, the areas of the brain on that side will still have a full blood supply because of the blood sent to those areas via the circle of Willis.

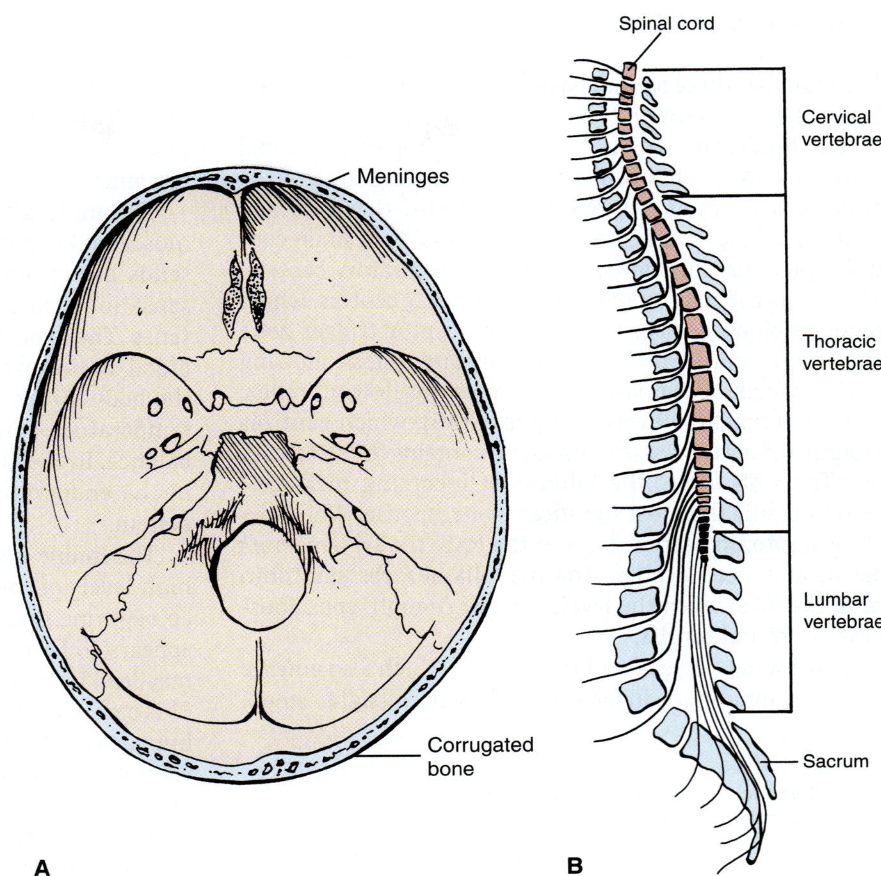

FIGURE 19.5 Bony and membranous protection of the brain **(A)** and the spine **(B)**.

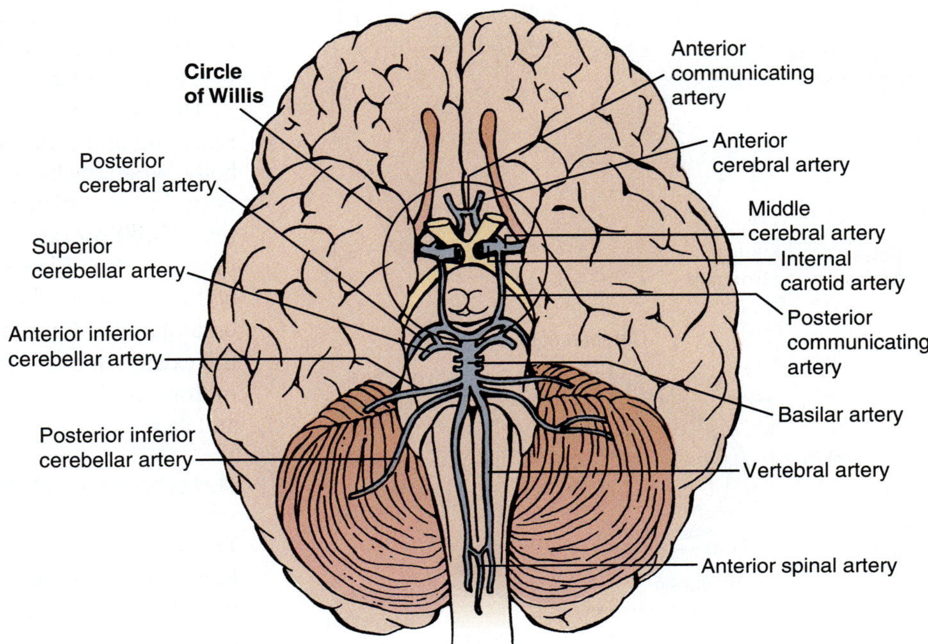

FIGURE 19.6 The protective blood supply of the brain: the carotid, vertebral, and basilar arteries join to form the circle of Willis.

Anatomy of the Brain

The brain has three major divisions: the hindbrain, the midbrain, and the forebrain (Figure 19.7).

The **hindbrain**, which runs from the top of the spinal cord into the midbrain, is the most primitive area of the brain and contains the brainstem, where the pons and medulla oblongata are located. These areas of the brain control basic, vital functions, such as the respiratory centers, which control breathing; the cardiovascular centers, which regulate blood pressure; the chemoreceptor trigger zone and emetic zone, which control vomiting; the swallowing center, which coordinates the complex swallowing reflex; and the reticular activating system (RAS), which controls arousal and awareness of stimuli and contains the sleep center. The RAS filters the billions of incoming messages, selecting only the most significant for response. When levels of serotonin become high in the RAS, the system shuts down, and sleep occurs. The medulla absorbs serotonin from the RAS; when the levels are low enough, consciousness or arousal results.

The cranial nerves (see Figure 19.7), which also emerge from the hindbrain, involve *specific* senses (sight, smell, hearing, balance, taste) and some muscle activity of the head and neck (e.g., chewing, eye movement). The cerebellum, a part of the brain that looks like a skein of yarn and lies behind the other parts of the hindbrain, coordinates the motor function that regulates posture, balance, and voluntary muscle activity.

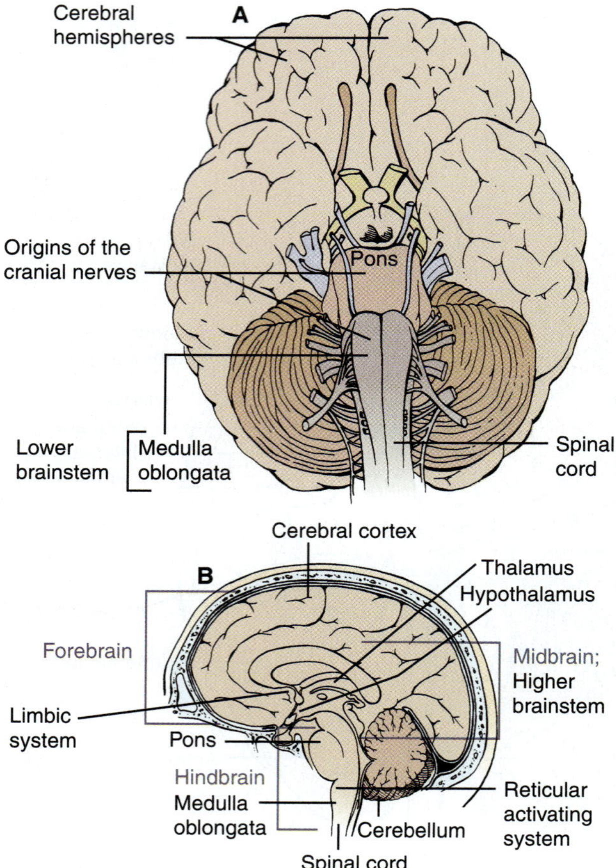

FIGURE 19.7 Anatomy of the brain. **(A)** A view of the underside of the brain. **(B)** The medial or midsagittal view of the brain.

The **midbrain** contains the thalamus, the hypothalamus, and the limbic system (see Figure 19.7). The thalamus sends direct information into the cerebrum to transfer sensations, such as cold, heat, pain, touch, and muscle sense. The hypothalamus, which is poorly protected by the blood–brain barrier, acts as a major sensor for activities in the body. Areas of the hypothalamus are responsible for temperature control, water balance, appetite, and fluid balance. In addition, the hypothalamus plays a central role in the endocrine system and in the autonomic nervous system.

The **limbic system** is an area of the brain that contains high levels of three neurotransmitters: epinephrine, norepinephrine, and serotonin. Stimulation of this area, which appears to be responsible for the expression of emotions, may lead to anger, pleasure, motivation, stress, and so on. This part of the brain seems to be largely responsible for the human aspect of brain function. Drug therapy aimed at alleviating emotional disorders such as depression and anxiety often involves attempting to alter the levels of epinephrine, norepinephrine, and serotonin.

The **forebrain** is made up of two cerebral hemispheres joined together by an area called the corpus callosum. These two hemispheres contain the sensory neurons, which receive nerve impulses, and the motor neurons, which send them. They also contain areas that coordinate speech and communication and seem to be the area where learning takes place (see Figures 19.7 and 19.8).

Different areas of the brain appear to be responsible for receiving and sending information to specific areas of the body. When the brain is viewed at autopsy, it looks homogenous, but scientists have mapped the general areas that are responsible for sensory response, motor function, and other functions (see Figure 19.8). In conjunction with the cerebellum, groups of ganglia or nerve cell bodies called the basal ganglia, located at the bottom of the brain, make up the extrapyramidal motor system. This system coordinates motor activity for unconscious activities such as posture and gait.

Anatomy of the Spinal Cord

The spinal cord is made up of 31 pairs of spinal nerves. Each spinal nerve has two components or roots. These mixed nerve parts include a sensory fiber (called the dorsal root) and a motor fiber (called the ventral root). The spinal sensory fibers bring information into the CNS from the periphery. The motor fibers cause movement or reaction.

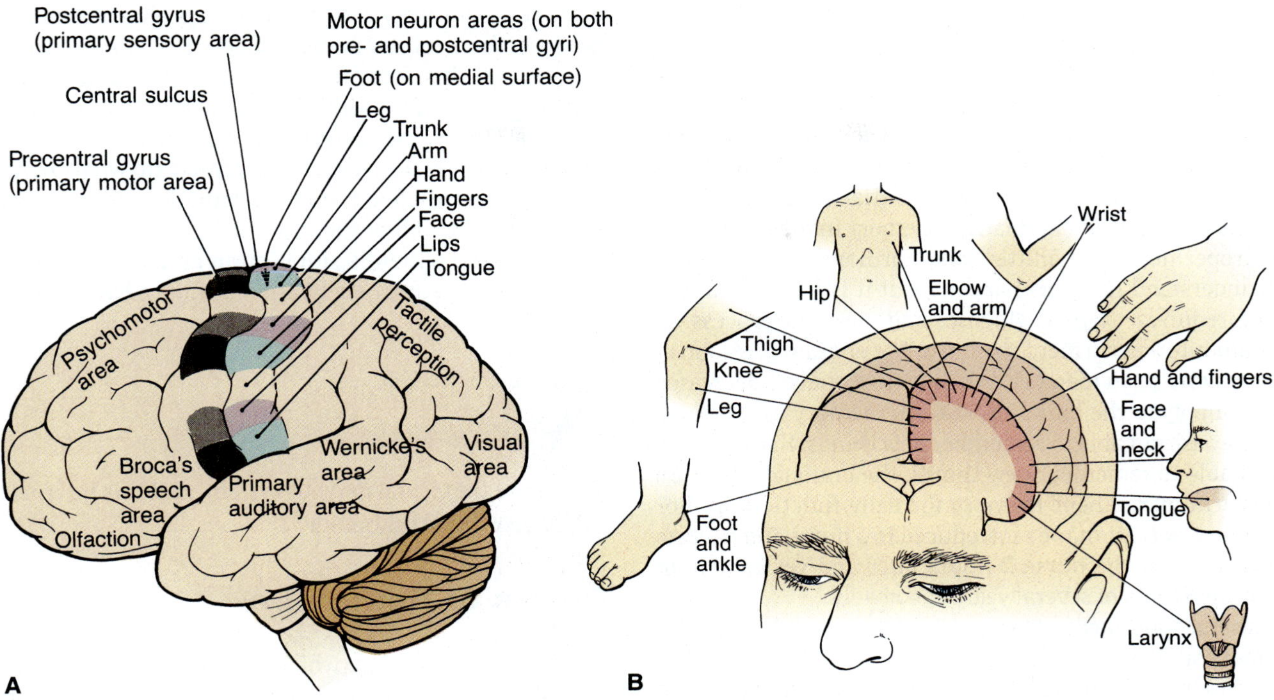

FIGURE 19.8 Functional areas of the brain. **(A)** Topographical organization of functions of control and interpretation in the cerebral cortex. **(B)** Areas of the brain that control specific areas of the body. Size indicates relative distribution of control.

Functions of the Central Nervous System

The brain is responsible for coordinating reactions to the constantly changing external and internal environment. In all animals, the function of this organ is essentially the same. The human component involving emotions, learning, and conscious response takes the human nervous system beyond a simple reflex system and complicates the responses seen to any stimulus.

Sensory Functions

Millions of sensory impulses are constantly streaming into the CNS from peripheral receptors. Many of these impulses go directly to specific areas of the brain designated to deal with input from particular areas of the body or from the senses. The responses that occur as a result of these stimuli can be altered by efferent neurons that respond to emotions through the limbic system, to learned responses stored in the cerebral cortex, or to autonomic input mediated through the hypothalamus.

The intricacies of the human brain can change the response to a sensation depending on the situation. People may react differently to the same stimulus. For example, if an individual drops a can on his or her foot, the physiological response is one of pain and a stimulation of the sympathetic branch of the autonomic nervous system. If the person is alone or in a very comfortable environment (e.g., fixing dinner at home), he or she may scream, swear, or jump around. But if that person is in the company of other people (e.g., a cooking teacher working with a class), he or she may be much more dignified and quiet.

Motor Functions

The sensory nerves that enter the brain react with related motor nerves to cause a reaction mediated by muscles or glands. The motor impulses that leave the cortex are further regulated or coordinated by the pyramidal system, which coordinates voluntary movement, and the extrapyramidal system, which coordinates unconscious motor activity that regulates control of position and posture. For example, some drugs may interfere with the extrapyramidal system and cause tremors, shuffling gait, and lack of posture and position stability. Motor fibers from the cortex cross to the other side of the spinal cord before emerging to interact with peripheral effectors. In this way, motor stimuli coming from the right side of the brain affect motor activity on the left side of the body. For example, an area of the left cortex may send an impulse down to the spinal cord that reacts with an interneuron, crosses to the other side of the spinal cord, and causes a finger on the right hand to twitch.

Intellectual and Emotional Functions

The way that the cerebral cortex uses sensory information is not clearly understood, but research has demonstrated that the two hemispheres of the brain process information in different ways. The right side of the brain is the more artistic side, concerned with forms and shapes, and the left side is more analytical, concerned with names, numbers, and processes. Why the two hemispheres are different and how they develop differently is not known.

When learning takes place, distinct layers of the cerebral cortex are affected, and an actual membrane change occurs in a neuron to store information in the brain permanently. Learning begins as an electrical circuit called an **engram**, a reverberating circuit of action potentials that eventually becomes a long-term, permanent memory in the presence of the proper neurotransmitters and hormones. Scientists do not understand how this happens, but it is known that the nerve requires oxygen, glucose, and sleep to process an engram into a permanent memory. The engram is responsible for short-term memory. When patients have a decreased blood supply to the brain, short-term memory may be lost, and they are not able to remember new things. Because they are unable to remember new things, the brain falls back on long-term, permanent memory for daily functioning. For example, a patient may be introduced to a nurse and have no recollection of the nurse 2 hours later and yet be able to recall the events of several years ago vividly.

Several substances appear to affect learning. Antidiuretic hormone (ADH), which is released during reactions to stress, increases learning. In situations in which a person is trying to learn, it may help to feel slightly stressed. Too much stress prevents learning, however. A patient who is a little nervous about upcoming surgery seems to display a better mastery of facts about the surgery and postoperative procedures than either one who is very stressed and scared or one who appears to show no interest or concern. Oxytocin also seems to increase actual learning. Because childbirth is the only known time that oxytocin levels increase, the significance of this is not understood. Nurses who work with maternity patients should know that women in labor will very likely remember the smallest details about the whole experience and should use whatever opportunity is made available to do teaching.

In addition, the limbic system appears to play an important role in how a person learns and reacts to stimuli. The emotions associated with a memory as well as with the present have an impact on stimulus response. The placebo effect is a documented effect of the mind on drug therapy: If a person perceives that a drug will be effective, it is much more likely to actually be effective. This effect, which uses the actions of the cerebrum and the limbic system, can have a tremendous impact on drug response. Events that are perceived as stressful by some patients may be seen as positive by other patients.

Clinical Significance of Drugs That Act on the Nervous System

The features of the human nervous system, including the complexities of the human brain, sometimes make it difficult to predict the exact reaction of a particular patient to a given drug. When a drug is used to affect the nervous system, the occurrence of many systemic effects is always a possibility because the nervous system affects the entire body. The chapters in this section address the individual classes of drugs used to treat disorders of the nervous system, including their adverse effects. An understanding of the actions of specific drugs makes it easier to anticipate what therapeutic and adverse effects might occur. In addition, nurses should consider all of the learned, cultural, and emotional aspects of the patient's situation in an attempt to provide optimal therapeutic benefit and minimal adverse effects.

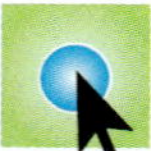

WEB LINK

To explore the virtual nervous system, visit this Internet site: http://www.InnerBody.com

Points to Remember

- The nervous system, which consists of the CNS and the PNS, is responsible for control of the human body, analysis of stimuli coming into the system, and integration of internal and external responses to stimuli.
- Although nerves do not reproduce, they can regenerate injured parts if the soma and axon hillock remain intact.
- Efferent nerves take information out of the CNS to effector sites; afferent nerves are sensory nerves that take information into the CNS.
- Nerves transmit information by way of electrical charges called action potentials. An action potential is a sudden change in membrane charge from negative to positive. It is caused when stimulation of a nerve opens sodium channels and allows positive sodium ions to flow into the cell.
- When the transmission of action potentials reaches the axon terminal, it causes the release of chemicals called neurotransmitters, which cross the synaptic cleft to stimulate an effector cell, which can be another nerve, a muscle, or a gland.
- A neurotransmitter must be produced by a nerve (each nerve can produce only one kind); it must be released into the synapse when the nerve is stimulated; it must react with a very specific receptor site to cause a reaction; and it must be immediately broken down or removed from the synapse so that the cell can be ready to be stimulated again.
- Much of the drug therapy in the nervous system involves receptor sites and the release or reuptake and breakdown of neurotransmitters.
- The CNS consists of the brain and spinal cord, which are protected by bone and meninges. To ensure blood flow to the brain if a vessel should become damaged, the brain

also has a protective blood supply moderated by the circle of Willis.

- The hindbrain, the most primitive area of the brain, contains the centers that control basic, vital functions. The pons, the medulla, and the reticular activating system (RAS), which regulates arousal and awareness, are all located in the hindbrain. The cerebellum, which helps coordinate motor activity, is found at the back of the hindbrain.
- The midbrain consists of the hypothalamus, the thalamus, and the limbic system. The limbic system is responsible for the expression of emotion, and the thalamus and hypothalamus coordinate internal and external responses and direct information into the cerebral cortex.
- The cerebral cortex consists of two hemispheres, which regulate the communication between sensory and motor neurons and are the sites of thinking and learning.
- The mechanisms of learning and processing learned information are not understood. Emotion-related factors influence the human brain, which handles stimuli and responses in complex ways.
- Much remains to be learned about the human brain and how drugs influence it. The actions of many drugs that have known effects on human behavior are not understood.

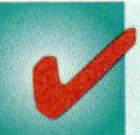

CHECK YOUR UNDERSTANDING

Answers to the questions in this chapter may be found in the Answer Key in the back of the book.

Multiple Choice

Select the best answer to the following.

1. The cerebellum
   a. initiates voluntary muscle movement.
   b. helps regulate the tone of skeletal muscles.
   c. if destroyed, would result in the loss of all voluntary skeletal activity.
   d. contains the centers responsible for the regulation of body temperature.

2. At those regions of the nerve membrane where myelin is present, there is
   a. low resistance to electrical current.
   b. high resistance to electrical current.
   c. high conductance of electrical current.
   d. energy loss for the cell.

3. The nerve synapse
   a. is not resistant to electrical current.
   b. cannot become exhausted.
   c. has a synaptic cleft.
   d. transfers information at the speed of electricity.

4. Which of the following could result in the initiation of an action potential?
   a. Depolarizing the membrane
   b. Decreasing the extracellular potassium concentration
   c. Increasing the activity of the sodium–potassium active transport system
   d. Stimulating the nerve with a threshold electrical stimulus during the absolute refractory period of the membrane

5. Neurotransmitters are
   a. produced in the muscle to communicate with nerves.
   b. the chemicals used to stimulate or suppress effectors at the nerve synapse.
   c. usually found in the diet.
   d. nonspecific in their action on various nerves.

6. The limbic system is an area of the brain that
   a. is responsible for coordination of movement.
   b. is responsible for the special senses.
   c. is responsible for the expression of emotions.
   d. controls sleep.

7. The most primitive area of the brain, the brainstem, contains areas responsible for
   a. vomiting, swallowing, respiration, arousal, and sleep.
   b. learning.
   c. motivation and memory.
   d. taste, sight, hearing, and balance.

8. A clinical indication of poor blood supply to the brain, particularly to the higher levels where learning takes place, would be
   a. loss of long-term memory.
   b. loss of short-term memory.
   c. living in the past.
   d. insomnia.

Multiple Response

Select all that apply.

1. In explaining the importance of a constant blood supply to the brain, the nurse would tell the student which of the following?
   a. Energy is needed to maintain nerve membranes and cannot be produced without oxygen.

b. Carbon dioxide must constantly be removed to maintain the proper pH.
c. Little glucose is stored in nerve cells, so a constant supply is needed.
d. The brain needs a constant supply of insulin and thyroid hormone.
e. The brain swells easily and needs the blood supply to reduce swelling.
f. Circulating aldosterone levels maintain the fluid balance in the brain.

2. The blood–brain barrier could be described by which of the following?
   a. It is produced by the cells that make up the meninges.
   b. It is regulated by the microglia in the CNS.
   c. It is weaker in certain parts of the brain.
   d. It is uniform in its permeability throughout the CNS.
   e. It is an anatomical structure that can be punctured.
   f. It is more likely to block the entry of proteins into the CNS.

Matching

Match the word with the appropriate definition.

1. ____________ action potential
2. ____________ afferent
3. ____________ axon
4. ____________ dendrite
5. ____________ depolarization
6. ____________ effector
7. ____________ efferent
8. ____________ engram
9. ____________ forebrain
10. ____________ hindbrain

A. Motor neurons
B. Long projection from a neuron that carries information from one nerve to another nerve or effector
C. Neurons or groups of neurons that bring information to the CNS
D. The brainstem
E. Upper level of the brain
F. Short-term memory
G. The electrical signal by which neurons send information
H. Muscle, a gland, or another nerve stimulated by a nerve
I. Reversing the membrane charge from negative to positive
J. Short projection on a neuron that transmits information

Definitions

Define the following terms

1. neuron ____
2. neurotransmitter ____
3. limbic system ____
4. Schwann cell ____
5. myelination ____
6. soma ____
7. synapse ____
8. repolarization ____

Bibliography and References

Fox, S. (1991). *Perspectives on human biology.* Dubuque, IA: Wm. C. Brown.

Ganong, W. (2003). *Review of medical physiology* (21st ed.). Norwalk, CT: Appleton & Lange.

Gilman, A., Hardman, J. G., & Limbird, L. E. (Eds.). (2006). *Goodman and Gilman's the pharmacological basis of therapeutics* (11th ed.). New York: McGraw-Hill.

Guyton, A., & Hall, J. (2000). *Textbook of medical physiology* (10th ed.). Philadelphia: W. B. Saunders.

Karch, A. M. (2006). *2007 Lippincott's nursing drug guide.* Philadelphia: Lippincott Williams & Wilkins.

Porth, C. M. (2005). *Pathophysiology: Concepts of altered health states* (7th ed.). Philadelphia: Lippincott Williams & Wilkins.

CHAPTER 20

Anxiolytic and Hypnotic Agents

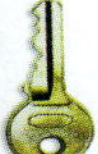

KEY TERMS

anxiety
anxiolytic
barbiturate
benzodiazepine
hypnosis
hypnotic
sedation
sedative

LEARNING OBJECTIVES

Upon completion of this chapter, you will be able to:

1. Define the states that are affected by anxiolytic or hypnotic agents.
2. Describe the therapeutic actions, indications, pharmacokinetics, contraindications, most common adverse reactions, and important drug–drug interactions associated with each class of anxiolytic or hypnotic agent: benzodiazepines, barbiturates, and miscellaneous agents.
3. Discuss the use of anxiolytic or hypnotic agents across the lifespan.
4. Compare and contrast the prototype drugs for each class of anxiolytic or hypnotic drug with the other drugs in that class.
5. Outline the nursing considerations and teaching needs for patients receiving each class of anxiolytic or hypnotic agent.

BENZODIAZEPINES

alprazolam
chlordiazepoxide
clonazepam
clorazepate
(P) diazepam
estazolam
flurazepam
lorazepam
oxazepam
quazepam
temazepam
triazolam

BARBITURATES

amobarbital
butabarbital
mephobarbital
pentobarbital
(P) phenobarbital
secobarbital

OTHER ANXIOLYTIC AND HYPNOTIC DRUGS

buspirone
chloral hydrate
dexmedetomidine
diphenhydramine
eszopiclone
meprobamate
paraldehyde
promethazine
ramelteon
zaleplon
zolpidem

The drugs discussed in this chapter are used to alter an individual's responses to the environment. They have been called **anxiolytics**, because they can prevent feelings of tension or fear; **sedatives**, because they can calm patients and make them unaware of their environment; **hypnotics**, because they can cause sleep; and minor tranquilizers, because they can produce a state of tranquility in anxious patients. In the past, a given drug would simply be used at different dosages to yield each of these effects. Further research into how the brain reacts to outside stimuli has resulted in the increased availability of specific agents that produce particular goals and avoid unwanted adverse effects. Use of these drugs also varies across the lifespan (Box 20.1).

States Affected by Anxiolytic and Hypnotic Drugs

Anxiety

Anxiety is a feeling of tension, nervousness, apprehension, or fear that usually involves unpleasant reactions to a stimulus, whether actual or unknown. Anxiety is often accompanied by signs and symptoms of the sympathetic stress reaction (see Chapter 29), which may include sweating, fast heart rate, rapid breathing, and elevated blood pressure. Mild anxiety, a not uncommon reaction, may serve as a stimulus or motivator in some situations. A person who feels anxious about being alone in a poorly lit parking lot at night may be motivated to take extra safety precautions. When anxiety becomes overwhelming or severe, it can interfere with the activities of daily living and lead to medical problems related to chronic stimulation of the sympathetic nervous system. A severely anxious person may, for example, be afraid to leave the house or to interact with other people. In these cases, treatment is warranted. Anxiolytic drugs are drugs that are used to lyse or break the feeling of anxiety (Table 20.1).

Sedation

The loss of awareness and reaction to environmental stimuli is termed **sedation.** This condition may be desirable in patients who are restless, nervous, irritable, or overreacting to stimuli. Although sedation is anxiolytic, it may frequently lead to drowsiness. For example, sedative-induced drowsiness is a concern for outpatients who need to be alert and responsive in their normal lives. On the other hand, this tiredness may be desirable for patients who are about to undergo surgery or other procedures and who are receiving medical

BOX 20.1 DRUG THERAPY ACROSS THE LIFESPAN

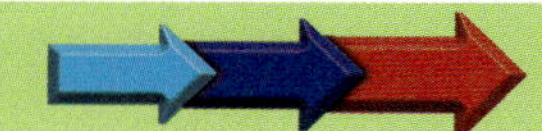

Anxiolytic and Hypnotic Agents

CHILDREN

Use of anxiolytic and hypnotic drugs with children is challenging. The response of the child to the drug may be unpredictable; inappropriate aggressiveness, crying, irritability, and tearfulness are common.

Of the benzodiazepines, only chlordiazepoxide, clonazepam, clorazepate, and diazepam have established pediatric dosages. Some of the others are used in pediatric settings, and dosage may be calculated using age and weight.

The barbiturates, being older drugs, have established pediatric dosages. These drugs must be used with caution because of the often unexpected responses. Children must be monitored very closely for CNS depression and excitability.

Chloral hydrate and paraldehyde are approved for use in children. The potential for adverse effects and the unpleasant taste and odor of paraldehyde make them less desirable as sleep agents. The antihistamines diphenhydramine and promethazine are more popular for use in helping to calm children and to induce rest and sleep. Care must be taken to assess for possible dried secretions and effects on breathing. Dosage must be calculated carefully.

ADULTS

Adults using these drugs for the treatment of insomnia need to be cautioned that they are for short-term use only. The reason for the insomnia should be sought (e.g., medical, hormonal, or anxiety problems). Other methods for helping to induce sleep—established routines, quiet activities before bed, a back-rub or warm bath—should be encouraged before drugs are prescribed. Adults receiving anxiolytics also may need referrals for counseling and diagnosis of possible causes. Adults should be advised to avoid driving and making legal decisions when taking these drugs.

Liver function should be evaluated before and periodically during therapy.

These drugs are contraindicated during pregnancy and lactation because of the potential for adverse effects on the fetus and possible sedation of the baby. The antihistamines, which have not been associated with congenital malformations, may be the safest to use, with caution, if an anxiolytic or hypnotic drug must be used.

OLDER ADULTS

Older patients may be more susceptible to the adverse effects of these drugs, from unanticipated CNS effects to increased sedation, dizziness, and even hallucinations. Dosages of all of these drugs should be reduced and the patient should be monitored very closely for toxic effects and to provide safety measures if CNS effects do occur.

Baseline liver and renal function tests should be performed, and these values should be monitored periodically for any changes that would indicate a need to decrease dosage further or to stop the drug.

Nondrug measures to reduce anxiety and to help induce sleep are important with older patients. The patient should be screened for physical problems, neurological deterioration, or depression, which could contribute to the insomnia or anxiety.

Table 20.1 DRUGS IN FOCUS

Benzodiazepines*

Drug Name	Dosage/Route	Usual Indications
alprazolam (*Xanax*)	0.25–0.5 mg PO t.i.d. up to 1–10 mg/day PO have been used; reduced dosage in elderly	Anxiety; panic attacks **Onset:** 30 min **Duration:** 4–6 h **Special considerations:** Taper after long-term therapy
chlordiazepoxide (*Librium*)	Adult: 5–25 mg PO t.i.d. to q.i.d.; or 50–100 mg IV or IM; may be repeated; reduce dosage with older patients Pediatric (>6 yr): 5 mg PO b.i.d. to q.i.d.; 25–50 mg IV or IM	Anxiety; alcohol withdrawal; preoperative anxiolytic **Onset:** 10–15 min **Duration:** 2–3 days **Special considerations:** Monitor injection sites
clonazepam (*Klonopin*)	Adult: 1.5 mg/day PO in divided doses; up to 20 mg/day Pediatric: 0.01–0.03 mg/kg/day PO in two to three divided doses, up to 0.1–0.3 mg/kg/day	Seizures; panic attacks; restless leg syndrome; neuralgias; acute manic episodes **Onset:** varies **Duration:** weeks
clorazepate (*Tranxene*)	Adult: 15–60 mg/day in divided doses; 7.5–15 mg/day PO for elderly patients Pediatric: (9–12 yr): 7.5 mg PO b.i.d. as adjunct therapy for epilepsy	Anxiety; alcohol withdrawal; partial seizures **Onset:** rapid **Duration:** days **Special considerations:** Taper dosage
P diazepam (*Valium*)	Adult: 2–10 mg PO b.i.d. to q.i.d.; or 0.2 mg/kg PR; or 2–30 mg IM b.i.d. or IV; 2–2.5 mg PO b.i.d. for elderly patients Pediatric: 1–2.5 mg PO t.i.d. to q.i.d.; 0.3–0.5 mg/kg PR; or 1–3 mg IM or IV	Anxiety; alcohol withdrawal; muscle relaxant; antiepileptic; antitetanus; preoperative anxiolytic **Onset:** 5–60 min **Duration:** 3 h **Special considerations:** Monitor injection sites; drug of choice if route change is anticipated; taper after long-term therapy
estazolam (*ProSom*)	1 mg PO at bedtime; start with 0.5 mg for elderly or debilitated patient	Hypnotic; treatment of insomnia **Onset:** 45–60 min **Duration:** 2 h **Special considerations:** Monitor liver and renal function, CBC if used long-term
flurazepam (*Dalmane*)	30 mg PO at bedtime; 15 mg PO at bedtime for elderly or debilitated patients	Hypnotic; treatment of insomnia **Onset:** varies **Duration:** 30–60 min **Special considerations:** Monitor liver and renal function, CBC in long-term use
lorazepam (*Ativan*)	2–6 mg/day PO in divided doses; or 0.05 mg/kg IM; or 0.044 mg/kg IV	Anxiety; preanesthesia anxiolytic **Onset:** 1–30 min **Duration:** 12–24 h **Special considerations:** Monitor injection sites; reduce dosage of narcotics given with this drug
oxazepam (*Serax*)	10–15 mg PO t.i.d. to q.i.d	Anxiety; alcohol withdrawal **Onset:** slow **Duration:** 2–4 h **Special considerations:** Preferred for elderly
quazepam (*Doral*)	15 mg PO at bedtime	Hypnotic; treatment of insomnia **Onset:** varies **Duration:** 4–6 h **Special considerations:** Monitor liver and renal function, CBC if used for long-term therapy; taper after long-term therapy
temazepam (*Restoril*)	15–30 mg PO at bedtime	Hypnotic; treatment of insomnia **Onset:** varies **Duration:** 4–6 h **Special considerations:** Taper after long-term therapy
triazolam (*Halcion*)	0.125–0.5 mg PO at bedtime	Hypnotic; treatment of insomnia **Onset:** varies **Duration:** 2–4 h **Special considerations:** Monitor liver and renal function, CBC; taper after long-term therapy

*Onset of action and duration are important in selecting the correct drug for a particular use.

support. The choice of an anxiolytic drug depends on the situation in which it will be used, keeping the related adverse effects in mind.

Hypnosis

Extreme sedation results in further central nervous system (CNS) depression and sleep, or **hypnosis**. Hypnotics are used to help people fall asleep by causing sedation. Drugs that are effective hypnotics act on the reticular activating system (RAS) and block the brain's response to incoming stimuli. Hypnosis, therefore, is the extreme state of sedation, in which the person no longer senses or reacts to incoming stimuli.

Benzodiazepines

Benzodiazepines, the most frequently used anxiolytic drugs, prevent anxiety without causing much associated sedation. In addition, they are less likely to cause physical dependence than many of the older sedatives/hypnotics that are used to relieve anxiety. Table 20.1 lists the currently available benzodiazepines, including common indications and specific information about each drug. Box 20.2 provides an exercise in calculating dosage for a pediatric patient.

Therapeutic Actions and Indications

The benzodiazepines act in the limbic system and the RAS to make gamma-aminobutyric acid (GABA) more effective, causing interference with neuron firing (Figure 20.1). GABA stabilizes the postsynaptic cell. This leads to an anxiolytic effect at doses lower than those required to induce sedation and hypnosis. The exact mechanism of action is not clearly understood.

The benzodiazepines are indicated for the treatment of the following conditions: anxiety disorders, alcohol withdrawal, hyperexcitability and agitation, and preoperative relief of anxiety and tension to aid in balanced anesthesia.

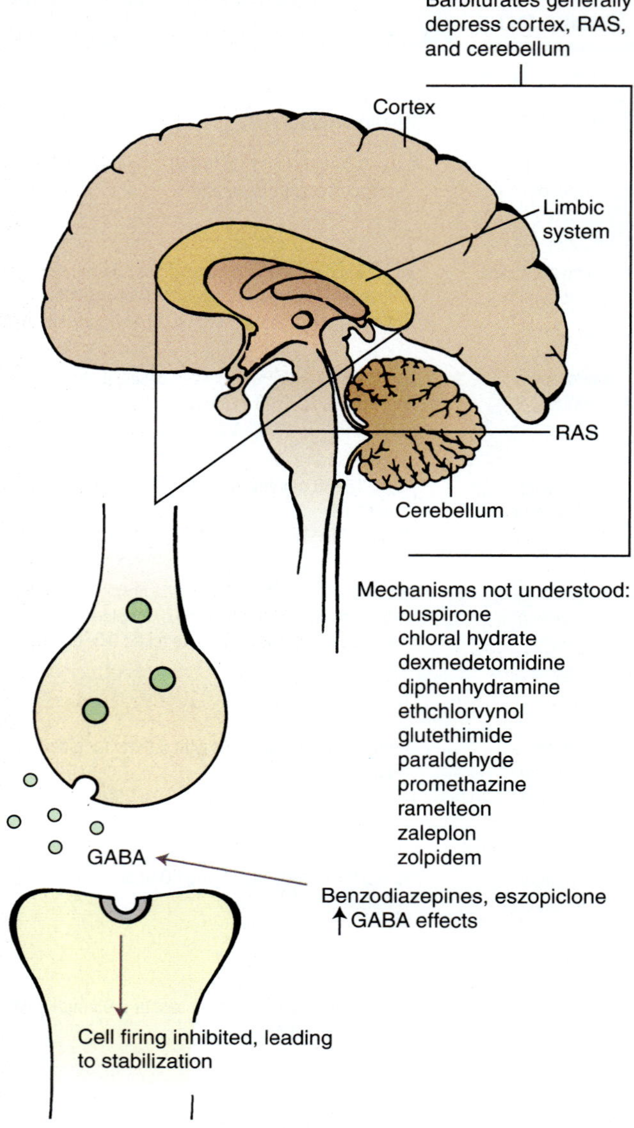

FIGURE 20.1 Sites of action of the benzodiazepines and barbiturates.

BOX 20.2 FOCUS ON CALCULATIONS

Your 3-year-old patient, weighing 25 kg, is prescribed chloral hydrate as a hypnotic at bedtime. The order reads: 50 mg/kg/day PO at bedtime. The drug comes in a syrup form as 500 mg/5 mL. How much syrup would you give as the bedtime dose?

First, figure out what the correct dose would be:

$$50 \text{ mg/kg} \times 25 \text{ kg} = 1250 \text{ mg}$$

Set up the equation using available form = prescribed dose:

$$500 \text{ mg/5 mL} = 1250 \text{ mg/dose}$$

Then, cross-multiply:

$$500 \text{ mg (dose)} = 6250 \text{ mg (mL)}$$
$$\text{dose} = 6250 \text{ mg (mL)}/500 \text{ mg}$$
$$\text{dose} = 12.5 \text{ mL}$$

Because this is a child, it is good practice to ask another nurse to calculate the correct dosage and then compare your work, so you can double-check the accuracy of your calculations.

Pharmacokinetics

The benzodiazepines are well absorbed from the gastrointestinal (GI) tract, with peak levels achieved in 30 minutes to 2 hours. They are lipid soluble and well distributed throughout the body, crossing the placenta and entering breast milk. The benzodiazepines are metabolized extensively in the liver. Patients with liver disease must receive a smaller dose and be monitored closely. Excretion is primarily through the urine.

Contraindications and Cautions

Contraindications to benzodiazepines include allergy to any benzodiazepine; psychosis, *which could be exacerbated by sedation;* and acute narrow-angle glaucoma, shock, coma, or acute alcoholic intoxication, *all of which could be exacerbated by the depressant effects of these drugs.*

In addition, these sedative/hypnotics are contraindicated in pregnancy *because a predictable syndrome of cleft lip or palate, inguinal hernia, cardiac defects, microcephaly, or pyloric stenosis occurs when they are taken in the first trimester.* Neonatal withdrawal syndrome may also result. Breast-feeding is also a contraindication *because of potential adverse effects on the neonate (e.g., sedation).*

Caution should be used in elderly or debilitated patients *because of the possibility of unpredictable reactions* and in cases of renal or hepatic dysfunction, *which may alter the metabolism and excretion of these drugs, resulting in direct toxicity.* Dosage adjustments usually are needed for such patients. Box 20.3 provides information about the effect of benzodiazepines in African American patients.

Adverse Effects

The adverse effects of benzodiazepines are associated with the impact of these drugs on the central and peripheral nervous systems. Nervous system effects include sedation, drowsiness, depression, lethargy, blurred vision, headaches, apathy, light-headedness, and confusion. In addition, mild paradoxical excitatory reactions may occur during the first 2 weeks of therapy.

Several other kinds of adverse effects may occur. GI conditions such as dry mouth, constipation, nausea, vomiting, and elevated liver enzymes may result. Cardiovascular problems may include hypotension, hypertension, arrhythmias, palpitations, and respiratory difficulties. Hematological conditions such as blood dyscrasias and anemia are possible. Genitourinary (GU) effects include urinary retention and hesitancy, loss of libido, and changes in sexual functioning. Because phlebitis, local reactions, and thrombosis may occur at local injection sites, such sites should be monitored. Abrupt cessation of these drugs may lead to a withdrawal syndrome characterized by nausea, headache, vertigo, malaise, and nightmares.

Clinically Important Drug–Drug Interactions

The risk of CNS depression increases if benzodiazepines are taken with alcohol or other CNS depressants, so such combinations should be avoided. In addition, the effects of benzodiazepines increase if they are taken with cimetidine, oral contraceptives, or disulfiram. If any of these drugs are used with benzodiazepines, patients should be monitored and the appropriate dosage adjustments made.

Finally, the impact of benzodiazepines may be decreased if they are given with theophyllines or ranitidine. If either of these drugs is used, dosage adjustment may be necessary.

BOX 20.3 CULTURAL CONSIDERATIONS FOR DRUG THERAPY

Benzodiazepine Levels

Special care should be taken when anxiolytic or hypnotic drugs are given to African Americans. About 15% to 20% of African Americans are genetically predisposed to delayed metabolism of benzodiazepines. As a result, they may develop high serum levels of these drugs, with increased sedation and an increased incidence of adverse effects.

If an anxiolytic or hypnotic agent is the drug of choice for an African American individual, the smallest possible dose should be used, and the patient should be monitored very closely during the first week of treatment. Dosage adjustments are necessary to achieve the most effective dose with the fewest adverse effects.

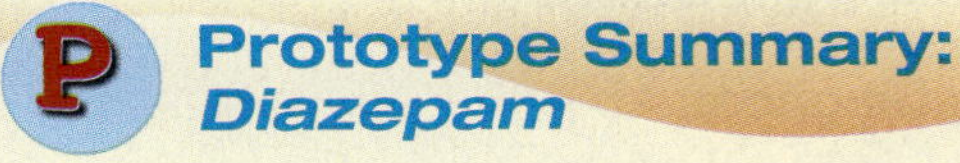

Prototype Summary: Diazepam

Indications: Management of anxiety disorders, acute alcohol withdrawal, muscle relaxation, treatment of tetanus, antiepileptic adjunct in status epilepticus, preoperative relief of anxiety and tension

Actions: Acts in the limbic system and reticular formation to potentiate the effects of GABA, an inhibitory neurotransmitter; may act in spinal cord and supraspinal sites to produce muscle relaxation

Pharmacokinetics:

Route	Onset	Peak	Duration
Oral	30–60 min	1–2 h	3 h
IM	15–30 min	30–45 min	3 h
IV	1–5 min	30 min	15–60 min
Rectal	Rapid	1.5 h	3 h

$T_{1/2}$: 20–80 hours, metabolized in the liver, excreted in urine

Adverse effects: Mild drowsiness, depression, lethargy, apathy, fatigue, restlessness, bradycardia, tachycardia, constipation, diarrhea, incontinence, urinary retention, changes in libido, drug dependence with withdrawal syndrome

Nursing Considerations for Patients Receiving Benzodiazepines

Assessment: History and Examination

Screen for the following conditions, *which could be contraindications or cautions to the use of the drug:* any known allergies to benzodiazepines; impaired liver or kidney function, *which could alter the metabolism and excretion of a particular drug;* any condition *that might be exacerbated by the depressant effects of the drugs* (e.g., glaucoma, coma, psychoses, shock, acute alcohol intoxication); and pregnancy and lactation.

Include screening for baseline status before beginning therapy *to check for occurrence of any potential adverse effects.* Assess for the following: temperature and weight; skin color and lesions; affect, orientation, reflexes, and vision; pulse, blood pressure, and perfusion; respiratory rate, adventitious sounds, and presence of chronic pulmonary disease; and bowel sounds on abdominal examination. Laboratory tests should include renal and liver function tests and complete blood count (CBC). Refer to Critical Thinking Scenario 20-1 for a full discussion of nursing care for a patient dealing with anxiety.

Nursing Diagnoses

The patient receiving a benzodiazepine may have the following nursing diagnoses related to drug therapy:

- Disturbed Thought Processes and Disturbed Sensory Perception (Visual, Kinesthetic) related to CNS effects
- Risk for Injury related to CNS effects
- Disturbed Sleep Pattern related to CNS effects
- Deficient Knowledge regarding drug therapy

Implementation With Rationale

- Do not administer intra-arterially *because serious arteriospasm and gangrene could occur.* Monitor injection sites carefully for local reactions to institute treatment as soon as possible.
- Do not mix intravenous (IV) drugs in solution with any other drugs *to avoid potential drug–drug interactions.*
- Give parenteral forms only if oral forms are not feasible or available, and switch to oral forms, *which are safer and less likely to cause adverse effects,* as soon as possible.
- Give IV drugs slowly *because these agents have been associated with hypotension, bradycardia, and cardiac arrest.*
- Arrange to reduce the dosage of narcotic analgesics in patients receiving a benzodiazepine *to decrease potentiated effects and sedation.*
- Maintain patients who receive parenteral benzodiazepines in bed for a period of at least 3 hours. Do not permit ambulatory patients to operate a motor vehicle after an injection *to ensure patient safety.*
- Monitor hepatic and renal function as well as CBC during long-term therapy *to detect dysfunction and to arrange to taper and discontinue drug if dysfunction occurs.*
- Taper dosage gradually after long-term therapy, especially in epileptic patients. *Acute withdrawal could precipitate seizures in these patients. It may also cause withdrawal syndrome.*
- Provide comfort measures *to help patients tolerate drug effects,* such as having them void before dosing, instituting a bowel program as needed, giving food with the drug if GI upset is severe, environmental control (lighting, temperature, stimulation), safety precautions (use of siderails, assistance with ambulation), and orientation.
- Provide thorough patient teaching, including drug name, prescribed dosage, measures for avoidance of adverse effects, and warning signs that may indicate possible problems. Instruct patients about the need for periodic monitoring and evaluation *to enhance patient knowledge about drug therapy and to promote compliance.*
- Offer support and encouragement *to help the patient cope with the diagnosis and the drug regimen.*
- If necessary, use flumazenil (Box 20.4), the benzodiazepine antidote, *for treatment of overdose.*

Evaluation

- Monitor patient response to the drug (alleviation of signs and symptoms of anxiety; sleep; sedation).
- Monitor for adverse effects (sedation, hypotension, cardiac arrhythmias, hepatic or renal dysfunction, blood dyscrasias).
- Evaluate effectiveness of teaching plan (patient can give the drug name, dosage, possible adverse effects to watch for, specific measures to help avoid adverse effects, and the importance of continued follow-up).
- Monitor effectiveness of comfort measures and compliance with regimen (Critical Thinking Scenario 20-1).

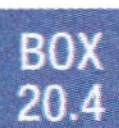

BOX 20.4 **A Benzodiazepine Antidote**

Flumazenil (*Romazicon*), a benzodiazepine antidote, acts by inhibiting the effects of the benzodiazepines at the gamma-aminobutyric acid (GABA) receptors. It is used for three purposes: to treat benzodiazepine overdose, to reverse the sedation caused by benzodiazepines that are used as adjuncts for general anesthesia, and to reverse sedation produced for diagnostic tests or other medical procedures.

Flumazenil, which is available for IV use only, is injected into the tubing of a running IV. The drug has a rapid onset of action that peaks 5 to 10 minutes after administration. It is metabolized in the liver. Because this drug has a half-life of about 1 hour, it may be necessary to repeat injections of flumazenil if a long-acting benzodiazepine was used.

Patients who receive flumazenil should be monitored continually, and life-support equipment should be readily available. If the patient has been taking a benzodiazepine for a long period, administration of flumazenil may precipitate a rapid withdrawal syndrome that necessitates supportive measures. Headache, dizziness, vertigo, nausea, and vomiting may be associated with use of flumazenil.

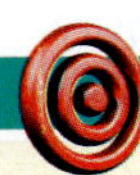

FOCUS POINTS

- Anxiety is a feeling of tension, nervousness, apprehension, or fear. Anxiolytic drugs, such as the benzodiazepines, depress the CNS to diminish these feelings.
- CNS depressants, such as sedatives, block the awareness of and reaction to environmental stimuli. They induce drowsiness, as do hypnotic drugs, which also depress the CNS and inhibit neuronal arousal.
- Hypnotics react with GABA inhibitory sites to depress the CNS. They can cause drowsiness, lethargy, and other CNS effects.

Barbiturates

The **barbiturates** were once the sedative/hypnotic drugs of choice. Not only is the likelihood of sedation and other adverse effects greater with these drugs than with newer sedative/hypnotic drugs, but the risk of addiction and dependence is also greater. For these reasons, newer anxiolytic drugs have replaced the barbiturates in most instances. Table 20.2 lists the currently available barbiturates, including common indications and specific information about each drug.

Therapeutic Actions and Indications

The barbiturates are general CNS depressants that inhibit neuronal impulse conduction in the ascending RAS, depress the cerebral cortex, alter cerebellar function, and depress motor output (see Figure 20.1). Thus, they can cause sedation, hypnosis, anesthesia, and, in extreme cases, coma. In general, barbiturates are indicated for relief of the signs and symptoms of anxiety, for sedation, insomnia, preanesthesia, and seizures. Parenteral forms, which reach peak levels faster and have a faster onset of action, may be used for treatment of acute manic reactions and many forms of seizures (see Chapter 23).

Pharmacokinetics

The barbiturates are absorbed well, reaching peak levels in 20 to 60 minutes. They are metabolized in the liver to varying degrees, depending on the drug, and excreted in the urine. The longer-acting barbiturates tend to be metabolized slower and excreted to a greater degree unchanged in the urine. The barbiturates are known to induce liver enzyme systems, increasing the metabolism of the barbiturate broken down by that system, as well as that of any other drug that may be metabolized by that enzyme system. Patients with hepatic or renal dysfunction require lower doses of the drug to avoid toxic effects and should be monitored closely. Barbiturates are lipid soluble; they readily cross the placenta and enter breast milk.

Contraindications and Cautions

Contraindications to barbiturates include allergy to any barbiturate and a previous history of addiction to sedative/hypnotic drugs *because the barbiturates are more addicting than most other anxiolytics.* Other contraindications are latent or manifest porphyria, *which may be exacerbated;* marked hepatic impairment or nephritis, *which may alter the metabolism and excretion of these drugs;* and respiratory distress or severe respiratory dysfunction, *which could be exacerbated by the CNS depression caused by these drugs.* Pregnancy is a contraindication *because of potential adverse effects on the fetus;* congenital abnormalities have been reported with barbiturate use.

Caution should be used in patients with acute or chronic pain *because barbiturates can cause paradoxical excitement, masking other symptoms;* with seizure disorders *because abrupt withdrawal of a barbiturate can precipitate status epilepticus;* and with chronic hepatic, cardiac, or respiratory diseases, *which could be exacerbated by the depressive effects of these drugs.* Care should be taken with lactating women *because of the potential for adverse effects on the infant.*

Adverse Effects

As previously stated, the adverse effects caused by barbiturates are more severe than those associated with other, newer sedatives/hypnotics. For this reason, barbiturates are no longer considered the mainstay for the treatment of anxiety.

CRITICAL THINKING SCENARIO 20-1

Benzodiazepines

THE SITUATION

P.P., a 43-year-old mother of three teenage sons, comes to the outpatient department for a routine physical examination. Results are unremarkable except for blood pressure of 145/90 mm Hg, pulse rate of 98 bpm, and apparent tension—she is jittery, avoids eye contact, and sometimes appears teary-eyed. She says that she is having some problems dealing with "life in general." Her sons present many stresses and her husband, who is busy with his career, has little time to deal with issues at home. When he *is* home, he is very demanding. In addition, she thinks she is beginning menopause and is having trouble coping with the idea of menopause as well as with some of the symptoms. Overall, she feels lonely and has no outlet for her anger, tension, or stress. A health care provider, who reassures P.P. that this problem is common in women of her age, prescribes the benzodiazepine diazepam (*Valium*) to help P.P. deal with her anxiety.

CRITICAL THINKING

What sort of crisis intervention would be most appropriate for P.P.?

What nursing interventions are helpful at this point?

What nondrug interventions might be helpful?

What other support systems could be used to help P.P. deal with all that is going on in her life?

Think about the overwhelming problems that P.P. has to deal with on a daily basis and how the anxiolytic effects of diazepam might change her approach to these problems. Could the problems actually get worse?

Develop a care plan for the long-term care of P.P.

DISCUSSION

Anxiolytics are useful for controlling the unpleasant signs and symptoms of anxiety. The diazepam prescribed for P.P. may provide some immediate relief, enabling her to survive the "crisis" period and plan changes in her life in general. However, the associated drowsiness and sedation may make coping with the problems in her life even more difficult. She should be taught the adverse effects of diazepam, the warning signs of serious adverse effects, and the health problems to report.

A follow-up evaluation should be scheduled. Additional meetings with the same health care provider are important for the long-term solution to P.P.'s anxiety. Her need for drug therapy should be re-evaluated once she can discover other support systems and develop other ways of coping. Although anxiolytic therapy may be beneficial initially, it will not solve the problems that are causing anxiety, and in this case, the causes for the anxiety are specific. The anxiolytic should be considered only as a short-term aid.

Unlike P.P., many patients in severe crisis do not consciously identify the many causes of stress, or stressors. However, P.P. has identified a list of factors that makes her life stressful. This facilitates the development of coping strategies. She may find the following support systems helpful:

- Referral to a counselor and involvement of the entire family in identifying problems and ways to deal with them.
- Support groups for women in various stages of life (e.g., entering menopause, mothers of children who are entering the teens). Just having the opportunity to discuss problems and explore ways of dealing with them helps many people.

NURSING CARE GUIDE FOR P.P.: DIAZEPAM

Assessment: History and Examination

Allergies to diazepam, psychoses, acute narrow angle glaucoma, acute alcohol intoxication, impaired liver or kidney function, pregnancy, breast-feeding, concurrent use of alcohol, omeprazole, cimetidine, disulfiram, oral contraceptives, theophylline, ranitidine

CV: blood pressure, pulse, perfusion

CNS: orientation, affect, reflexes, vision

Skin: color, lesions, texture

Respiratory: respiration, adventitious sounds

GI: abdominal examination, bowel sounds

Laboratory tests: hepatic and renal function tests, complete blood count

Nursing Diagnoses

Disturbed Thought Processes and Disturbed Sensory Perception (Visual, Kinesthetic) related to CNS effects

Risk for Injury related to CNS effects

Disturbed Sleep Patterns related to CNS effects

Deficient Knowledge regarding drug therapy

Benzodiazepines *(continued)*

Implementation

Provide comfort and safety measures, small meal, drug with food if GI upset occurs, bowel program as needed; taper dosage after long-term use; reduce dosage if other medications include narcotics; lower dose with renal or hepatic impairment.

Provide support and reassurance to deal with drug effects.

Provide patient teaching regarding drug, dosage, adverse effects, safety precautions and unusual symptoms to report.

Evaluation

Evaluate drug effects: relief of signs and symptoms of anxiety.

Monitor for adverse effects, particularly sedation, dizziness, insomnia, blood dyscrasia, GI upset, hepatic or renal dysfunction, cardiovascular effects.

Monitor for drug–drug interactions.

Evaluate effectiveness of patient teaching program.

Evaluate effectiveness of comfort and safety measures.

Patient Teaching for P.P.

☐ The drug that has been prescribed for you is called diazepam, or *Valium*. It belongs to a class of drugs called benzodiazepines, which are used to relieve tension and nervousness. Exactly how the drug works is not completely understood, but it does relax muscle spasms, relieve insomnia, and promote calm. Common side effects of this drug include:

- *Dizziness and drowsiness:* Avoid driving or performing hazardous or delicate tasks that require concentration if these effects occur.
- *Nausea, vomiting, and weight loss:* Small frequent meals may help to relieve nausea. If weight loss occurs, monitor the loss; if the loss is extensive, consult your health care provider. Do not take this drug with antacids.
- *Constipation or diarrhea:* These reactions usually pass with time. If they do not, consult with your health care provider for appropriate therapy.
- *Vision changes, slurred speech, unsteadiness:* These effects also subside with time. Take extra care in your activities for the first few days. If these reactions do not go away after 3 or 4 days, consult your health care provider.
- Report any of the following conditions to your health care provider: *rash, fever, sore throat, insomnia, depression, clumsiness, or nervousness.*

☐ Tell any doctor, nurse, or other health care provider involved in your care that you are taking this drug.

☐ Keep this drug and all medications safely away from children or pets.

☐ Avoid the use of over-the-counter medications or herbal therapies while you are taking this drug. If you think that you need one of these products, consult with your health care provider about the best choice because many of these products can interfere with your medication.

☐ Avoid alcohol while you are taking this drug. Combining alcohol and a benzodiazepine can cause serious problems.

☐ If you have been taking this drug for a prolonged time, do not stop taking it suddenly. Your body will need time to adjust to the loss of the drug, and the dosage will need to be reduced gradually to prevent serious problems. When discontinuing use of this drug, tell your health care provider if the following occurs: trembling, muscle cramps, sweating, irritability, confusion, or seizures.

In addition, the development of physical tolerance and psychological dependence is more likely with the barbiturates than with other anxiolytics.

The most common adverse effects are related to general CNS depression. CNS effects may include drowsiness, somnolence, lethargy, ataxia, vertigo, a feeling of a "hangover," thinking abnormalities, paradoxical excitement, anxiety, and hallucinations. GI signs and symptoms such as nausea, vomiting, constipation, diarrhea, and epigastric pain may occur. Associated cardiovascular effects may include bradycardia, hypotension (particularly with IV administration), and syncope. Serious hypoventilation may occur, and respiratory depression and laryngospasm may also result, particularly with IV administration. Hypersensitivity reactions, including rash, serum sickness, and Stevens–Johnson syndrome, which is sometimes fatal, may also occur.

Clinically Important Drug–Drug Interactions

Increased CNS depression results if these agents are taken with other CNS depressants, including alcohol, antihista-

Table 20.2 DRUGS IN FOCUS

Barbiturates Used as Anxiolytic–Hypnotics*

Drug Name	Dosage/Route	Usual Indications
amobarbital (*Amytal sodium*)	Adult: 65–500 mg IM or IV; reduce dosage with older patients Pediatric: (6–12 yr): 65–500 mg IM or IV; monitor very closely	Sedative–hypnotic; convulsions; manic reactions **Onset:** 15–60 min **Duration:** 3–8 h **Special considerations:** Monitor carefully if administered by IV
butabarbital (*Butisol*)	Adult: 15–30 mg PO t.i.d. to q.i.d.; 50–100 mg PO at bedtime for sedation; reduce dosage in elderly Pediatric: 7.5–30 mg PO based on age and weight	Short-term sedative–hypnotic **Onset:** 45–60 min **Duration:** 6–8 h **Special considerations:** Taper gradually after long-term use; use caution in children, may produce aggressiveness, excitability
mephobarbital (*Mebaral*)	Adult: 32–100 mg PO t.i.d. to q.i.d.; 400–600 mg/day PO for seizures; reduce dosage in elderly patients Pediatric: 16–32 mg PO t.i.d. to q.i.d.; 16–64 mg PO t.i.d. to q.i.d. for seizures	Anxiolytic; antiepileptic **Onset:** 30–60 min **Duration:** 10–16 h **Special considerations:** Taper gradually after long-term use; use caution in children, may produce aggressiveness, excitability
pentobarbital (*Nembutal*)	Adult: 20 mg PO t.i.d. to q.i.d.; 100 mg at bedtime for insomnia; 120–200 mg PR; 150–200 mg IM or 100 mg IV; reduce dosage in elderly patients Pediatric: 2–6 mg/kg/day; adjust dosage based on age and weight	Sedative–hypnotic; preanesthetic **Onset:** 10–15 min **Duration:** 2–4 h **Special considerations:** Taper gradually after long-term use; give IV slowly; monitor injection sites
P phenobarbital (*Luminal*)	Adult: 30–120 mg/day PO, IM, or IV; reduce dosage in elderly patients Pediatric: 1–3 mg/kg IV or IM	Sedative–hypnotic; control of seizures; preanesthetic **Onset:** 10–60 min **Duration:** 4–16 h **Special considerations:** Taper gradually after long-term use; give IV slowly; monitor injection sites
secobarbital (*Seconal*)	Adult: 100–300 mg PO; reduce dosage in elderly patients Pediatric: 2–6 mg/kg PO	Preanesthetic sedation; convulsive seizures of tetanus **Onset:** rapid **Duration:** 1–4 h **Special considerations:** Taper gradually after long-term use

*Onset of action and duration are important in selecting the correct drug for a particular use.

mines, and other tranquilizers. If other CNS depressants are used, dosage adjustments are necessary.

There often is an altered response to phenytoin if it is combined with barbiturates; evaluate the patient frequently if this combination cannot be avoided. If barbiturates are combined with monoamine oxidase (MAO) inhibitors, increased serum levels and effects occur. If the older sedatives/hypnotics are combined with MAO inhibitors, patients should be monitored closely and necessary dosage adjustments made.

In addition, because of an enzyme-induction effect of barbiturates in the liver, the following drugs may not be as effective as desired: oral anticoagulants, digoxin, tricyclic antidepressants (TCAs), corticosteroids, oral contraceptives, estrogens, acetaminophen, metronidazole, phenmetrazine, carbamazepine, beta-blockers, griseofulvin, phenylbutazones, theophyllines, quinidine, and doxycycline. If these agents are given in combination with barbiturates, patients should be monitored closely; frequent dosage adjustments may be necessary to achieve the desired therapeutic effect.

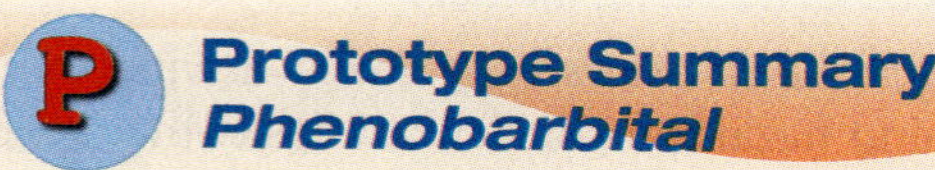

Indications: Sedation, short-term treatment of insomnia, long-term treatment of tonic–clonic seizures and cortical focal seizures, emergency control of certain acute convulsive episodes, preanesthetic

Actions: Inhibits conduction in the ascending RAS; depresses the cerebral cortex; alters cerebellar function; depresses motor output; can produce excitation, sedation, hypnosis, anesthesia, and deep coma; and has anticonvulsant activity

Pharmacokinetics:

Route	Peak	Onset	Duration
Oral	15 min	30–60 min	10–16 h
IM, Sub-Q		10–30 min	4–6 h
IV	up to 15 min	5 min	4–6 h

$T_{1/2}$: 79 hours; metabolized in the liver, excreted in urine

Adverse effects: Somnolence, agitation, confusion, hyperkinesias, ataxia, vertigo, CNS depression, hallucinations, bradycardia, hypotension, syncope, nausea, vomiting, constipation, diarrhea, hypoventilation, apnea, withdrawal syndrome, rash, Stevens–Johnson syndrome

Nursing Considerations for Patients Receiving Barbiturates

Assessment: History and Examination

Screen for the following, *which could be contraindications or cautions for the use of the drug:* any known allergies to barbiturates or a history of addiction to sedative/hypnotic drugs; impaired hepatic or renal function *that could alter the metabolism and excretion of the drug;* cardiac dysfunction or respiratory dysfunction; seizure disorders; acute or chronic pain disorders; and pregnancy or lactation.

Include screening *for baseline status before beginning therapy and for the occurrence of any potential adverse effects*. Assess the following: temperature and weight; blood pressure and pulse, including perfusion; skin color and lesions; affect, orientation, and reflexes; respiratory rate and adventitious sounds; and bowel sounds.

Nursing Diagnoses

The patient receiving a barbiturate may have the following nursing diagnoses related to drug therapy:

- Disturbed Thought Processes and Disturbed Sensory Perception (Visual, Auditory, Kinesthetic, Tactile) related to CNS effects
- Risk for Injury related to CNS effects
- Impaired Gas Exchange related to respiratory depression
- Deficient Knowledge regarding drug therapy

Implementation With Rationale

- Do not administer these drugs intra-arterially *because serious arteriospasm and gangrene could occur*. Monitor injection sites carefully *for local reactions*.
- Do not mix IV drugs in solution with any other drugs *to avoid potential drug–drug interactions*.
- Give parenteral forms only if oral forms are not feasible or available, and switch to oral forms as soon as possible *to avoid serious reactions or adverse effects*.
- Give IV medications slowly *because rapid administration may cause cardiac problems*.
- Provide standby life-support facilities *in case of severe respiratory depression or hypersensitivity reactions*.
- Taper dosage gradually after long-term therapy, especially in patients with epilepsy. Acute withdrawal *may precipitate seizures or cause withdrawal syndrome in these patients*.
- Provide comfort measures *to help patients tolerate drug effects,* including small, frequent meals; access to bathroom facilities; bowel program as needed; consuming food with the drug if GI upset is severe; and environmental control, safety precautions, orientation, and appropriate skin care as needed.
- Provide thorough patient teaching, including drug name, prescribed dosage, measures for avoidance of adverse effects, and warning signs that may indicate possible problems. Instruct patients about the need for periodic monitoring and evaluation *to enhance patient knowledge about drug therapy and to promote compliance*.
- Offer support and encouragement *to help the patient cope with the diagnosis and the drug regimen*.

Evaluation

- Monitor patient response to the drug (alleviation of signs and symptoms of anxiety, sleep, sedation, reduction in seizure activity).
- Monitor for adverse effects (sedation, hypotension, cardiac arrhythmias, hepatic or renal dysfunction, skin reactions, dependence).
- Evaluate effectiveness of teaching plan (patient can give the drug name, dosage, possible adverse effects to watch for, specific measures to help avoid adverse effects, and the importance of continued follow-up).
- Monitor effectiveness of comfort measures and compliance with regimen.

Other Anxiolytic and Hypnotic Drugs

Other drugs are used to treat anxiety or to produce hypnosis that do not fall into either the benzodiazepine or the barbiturate group. See Table 20.3 for a summary of the other anxiolytic–hypnotic drugs. Such medications include the following:

- Paraldehyde (*Paral*), a very old drug, is still used orally and rectally to sedate patients with delirium tremens or

Table 20.3 DRUGS IN FOCUS

Other Anxiolytic–Hypnotic Drugs

Drug Name	Usual Indications
buspirone (*BuSpar*)	Oral drug for anxiety disorders; unlabeled use; signs and symptoms of premenstrual syndrome **Special considerations:** May cause dry mouth, headache
chloral hydrate (*Aquachloral*)	Administered PO or PR for nocturnal sedation, preoperative sedation **Special considerations:** Withdraw gradually over 2 wk in patients maintained for weeks or months
dexmedetomidine (*Precedex*)	IV drug used for newly intubated and mechanically ventilated patients in the ICU **Special considerations:** Do not use longer than 24 h; monitor patient continually
diphenhydramine (*Benadryl*)	Oral, IM, or IV for sleep aid, motion sickness, allergic rhinitis **Special considerations:** Antihistamine, drying effects common Oral drug for short-term treatment of insomnia (up to 1 wk)
eszopiclone (*Lunesta*)	Oral drug for the treatment of insomnia **Special considerations:** Tablet must be swallowed whole; patient must remain in bed for 8 h
meprobamate (*Miltown*)	Oral drug used for the short-term management of anxiety disorders **Special considerations:** Supervise dose in patients who are addiction prone; withdraw gradually over 2 wk if patient has been maintained on the drug for weeks or months
paraldehyde (*Paral*)	Given PO or PR for sedation in acute psychiatric excitement and acute alcoholic withdrawal **Special considerations:** Dilute before use; use food to improve taste; avoid contact with plastic; keep away from heat or flame; discard any unused portion
promethazine (*Phenergan*)	Oral, IM, or IV use to decrease the need for postoperative pain relief and for preoperative sedation **Special considerations:** An antihistamine; monitor injection sites carefully
ramelteon (*Rozerem*)	Oral drug for the treatment of insomnia characterized by difficulty falling asleep **Special considerations:** Take 30 min before bed; allow 8 h for sleep; monitor for depression and suicidal ideation
zaleplon (*Sonata*)	Oral drug for the short-term treatment of insomnia **Special considerations:** Must remain in bed for 4 h after taking drug
zolpidem (*Ambien*)	Oral drug for short-term treatment of insomnia **Special considerations:** Dispense least amount possible to depressed and/or suicidal patients; withdraw gradually if used for prolonged period

psychiatric conditions characterized by extreme excitement. It is rapidly absorbed and metabolized in the liver. Excretion of paraldehyde can occur unchanged through the lungs, or the metabolites can be found in the urine. Paraldehyde has a distinctive odor. It cannot be stored in plastic containers or dispensed with a plastic spoon or syringe.

- Meprobamate (*Miltown*) is an older drug that is used to manage acute anxiety for up to 4 months. It works in the limbic system and thalamus and has some anticonvulsant properties and central nervous system muscle relaxing effects. It is rapidly absorbed and is metabolized in the liver and excreted in urine.
- Chloral hydrate (*Aquachloral*) is frequently used to produce nocturnal sedation or preoperative sedation. Its mechanism of action is unknown. It is rapidly absorbed from the GI tract and metabolized in the liver and kidney for excretion in the bile and urine.
- Zaleplon (*Sonata*) and zolpidem (*Ambien*) both of which cause sedation, are used for the short-term treatment of insomnia. They are thought to work by affecting serotonin levels in the sleep center near the RAS. Patients should be going to bed and able to stay there for 4 to 8 hours when taking these drugs. They are all metabolized in the liver and excreted in the urine. Caution should be used in patients with hepatic or renal impairment. Elderly patients are especially sensitive to these drugs; they should receive a lower dose and should be monitored carefully.
- Dexmedetomidine (*Precedex*) is given intravenously at a starting dose of 1 mcg/kg over 10 minutes and then a controlled infusion for up to 24 hours. It is used for sedation of newly intubated and mechanically ventilated patients in an ICU.
- Eszopiclone (*Lunesta*) is a new agent used to treat insomnia. It is thought to react with GABA sites near benzodiazepine receptors. It is rapidly absorbed, metabolized in the urine, and excreted in the urine. The patient should take this drug just before bed and should allow 8 hours for sleep.
- Antihistamines (promethazine [*Phenergan*], diphenhydramine [*Benadryl*]) can be very sedating in some people. They are used as preoperative medications and postoperatively to decrease the need for narcotics. Patients need to be monitored for thickened respiratory secretions and breathing difficulties, a problem that can cause concern after anesthesia.
- Buspirone (*BuSpar*), a newer antianxiety agent, has no sedative, anticonvulsant, or muscle-relaxant properties,

and its mechanism of action is unknown. However, it reduces the signs and symptoms of anxiety without many of the CNS effects and severe adverse effects associated with other anxiolytic drugs. It is rapidly absorbed from the GI tract, metabolized in the liver, and excreted in urine. Caution should be used in patients with hepatic or renal impairment and in elderly patients.

- Ramelteon (*Rozerem*), introduced in 2005, is the first of a new class of sedatives/hypnotics, the melatonin receptor agonists. This drug stimulates melatonin receptors, which are thought to be involved in the maintenance of circadian rhythm and the sleep–wake cycle. Ramelteon is used for the treatment of insomnia characterized by difficulty with sleep onset. It is rapidly absorbed with peak levels in 30 to 90 minutes. It is metabolized in the liver and excreted in the feces and urine. It should be administered 30 minutes before bed. Patients should be monitored for depression and suicidal ideation.

WEB LINKS

Health care providers and patients may want to consult the following Internet sources: http://www.anxiety-panic.com Information on anxiety and anxiety-related disorders.

http://www.adaa.org Information on research, treatment, and support groups related to anxiety and anxiety-related disorders.

http://www.nimh.nih.gov Information on education programs related to anxiety and anxiety-related disorders.

http://mhsource.com Patient-oriented and professional information on issues related to mental health.

Points to Remember

- Anxiety is a sense of tension, nervousness, apprehension, or fear in response to an actual or an unknown stimulus. In the extreme, anxiety may produce physiological manifestations and may interfere with activities of daily life.
- Anxiolytics, or minor tranquilizers, are drugs used to treat anxiety by depressing the CNS. When given at higher doses, these drugs may be sedatives or hypnotics.
- Sedatives block the awareness of and reaction to environmental stimuli, resulting in associated CNS depression that may cause drowsiness, lethargy, and other effects. This action can be beneficial when a patient is very excited or afraid.
- Hypnotics further depress the CNS, particularly the RAS, to inhibit neuronal arousal and induce sleep.
- Benzodiazepines are a group of drugs used as anxiolytics. They react with GABA inhibitory sites to depress the CNS. They can cause drowsiness, lethargy, and other CNS effects.
- Barbiturates are an older class of drugs used as anxiolytics, sedatives, and hypnotics. Because they are associated with potentially serious adverse effects and interact with many other drugs, they are less desirable than the benzodiazepines or other anxiolytics.
- Buspirone, a newer anxiolytic drug, does not cause sedation or muscle relaxation. Because of the absence of CNS effects, it is much preferred in certain circumstances (e.g., when a person must drive, go to work, or maintain alertness).

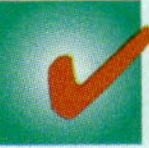

CHECK YOUR UNDERSTANDING

Answers to the questions in this chapter may be found in the Answer Key in the back of the book.

Multiple Choice

Select the best answer to the following.

1. Drugs that are used to alter a patient's response to the environment are called
   a. hypnotics.
   b. sedatives.
   c. antiepileptics.
   d. anxiolytics.

2. The benzodiazepines are the most frequently used anxiolytic drugs because
   a. they are anxiolytic at doses much lower than those needed for sedation or hypnosis.
   b. they can also be stimulating.
   c. they are more likely to cause physical dependence than older anxiolytic drugs.
   d. they do not affect any neurotransmitters.

3. Barbiturates cause liver enzyme induction, which could lead to
   a. rapid metabolism and loss of effectiveness of other drugs metabolized by those enzymes.
   b. increased bile production.
   c. CNS depression.
   d. the need to periodically lower the barbiturate dose to avoid toxicity.

4. A person who could benefit from an anxiolytic drug for short-term treatment of insomnia would *not* be prescribed

a. zolpidem.
b. chloral hydrate.
c. buspirone.
d. meprobamate.

5. Anxiolytic drugs block the awareness of and reaction to the environment. This effect would *not* be beneficial
   a. to relieve extreme fear.
   b. to moderate anxiety related to unknown causes.
   c. in treating a patient who must drive a vehicle for a living.
   d. in treating a patient who is experiencing a stress reaction.

6. Mr. Jones is the chief executive officer of a large company and has been experiencing acute anxiety attacks. His physical examination was normal, and he was diagnosed with anxiety. Considering his occupation and his need to be alert and present to large groups on a regular basis, the following anxiolytic would be a drug of choice for Mr. Jones:
   a. phenobarbital
   b. diazepam
   c. clorazepate
   d. buspirone

7. The benzodiazepines react with
   a. GABA receptor sites in the RAS to cause inhibition of neural arousal.
   b. norepinephrine receptor sites in the sympathetic nervous system.
   c. acetylcholine receptor sites in the parasympathetic nervous system.
   d. monoamine oxidase to increase norepinephrine breakdown.

8. A pediatric patient is prescribed phenobarbital preoperatively to relieve anxiety and produce sedation. After giving the injection, you should assess the patient for
   a. acute Stevens–Johnson syndrome.
   b. bone marrow depression.
   c. paradoxical excitement.
   d. withdrawal syndrome.

Multiple Response

Select all that apply.

1. In assessing a client who is experiencing anxiety, the nurse would expect to find which of the following?
   a. Rapid breathing
   b. Rapid heart rate
   c. Fear and apprehension
   d. Constricted pupils
   e. Decreased abdominal sounds
   f. Hypotension

2. Your client has a long history of anxiety and has always responded well to diazepam. She has just learned that she is pregnant and feels very anxious. She would like a prescription for diazepam to get her through her early anxiety. What rationale would the nurse use in explaining why this is not recommended?
   a. This drug is known to cause a predictable syndrome of birth defects, including cleft lip and pyloric stenosis.
   b. Babies born to mothers taking benzodiazepines may progress through a neonatal withdrawal syndrome.
   c. Cardiac defects and small brain development may occur if this drug is taken in the first trimester.
   d. This drug almost always causes loss of the pregnancy.
   e. The hormones the body produces during pregnancy will make you unresponsive to diazepam.
   f. This drug could have adverse effects on your baby; we should explore nondrug measures to help you deal with the anxiety.

Fill in the Blanks

1. ________________ is a feeling of tension, nervousness, apprehension, or fear that usually involves unpleasant reactions to a stimulus, which is actual or unknown.

2. Mild anxiety may serve as a stimulus or ____________ in some situations.

3. ________________ are drugs that can calm patients and make them unaware of their environment.

4. Drugs that can cause sleep are called ______________.

5. Anxiolytics can prevent feelings of ________________ or ________________.

6. Patients who are restless, nervous, irritable, or overreacting to stimuli could benefit from ______________.

7. Hypnosis or sleep can be caused by drugs that ________________ the central nervous system (CNS).

8. ________________ are the most frequently used anxiolytic drugs.

Matching

Match the generic name of these commonly used anxiolytic drugs with the associated brand name.

1. ______________________ clonazepam
2. ______________________ lorazepam
3. ______________________ temazepam
4. ______________________ alprazolam

5. ______________________ oxazepam
6. ______________________ triazolam
7. ______________________ diazepam
8. ______________________ chlordiazepoxide
9. ______________________ flurazepam
10. ______________________ clorazepate

A. *Restoril*
B. *Xanax*
C. *Klonopin*
D. *Valium*
E. *Ativan*
F. *Librium*
G. *Serax*
H. *Halcion*
I. *Tranxene*
J. *Dalmane*

Bibliography and References

Bailey, K. (1998). *Psychotropic drug facts.* Philadelphia: Lippincott-Raven.

Drug facts and comparisons. (2006). St. Louis: Facts and Comparisons.

Gilman, A., Hardman, J. G., & Limbird, L. E. (Eds.). (2006). *Goodman and Gilman's the pharmacological basis of therapeutics* (11th ed.). New York: McGraw-Hill.

Karch, A. M. (2006). *2007 Lippincott's nursing drug guide.* Philadelphia: Lippincott Williams & Wilkins.

Porth, C. M. (2005). *Pathophysiology: Concepts of altered health states* (7th ed.). Philadelphia: Lippincott Williams & Wilkins.

Professional's guide to patient drug facts. (2006). St. Louis: Facts and Comparisons.

CHAPTER 21

Antidepressant Agents

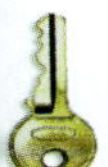

KEY TERMS

affect

biogenic amines

depression

monoamine oxidase (MAO) inhibitor

selective serotonin reuptake inhibitor (SSRI)

tricyclic antidepressant (TCA)

tyramine

LEARNING OBJECTIVES

Upon completion of this chapter, you will be able to:

1. Describe the biogenic theory of depression.
2. Describe the therapeutic actions, indications, pharmacokinetics, contraindications, most common adverse reactions, and important drug–drug interactions associated with each class of antidepressant: TCAs, MAO inhibitors, SSRIs, and miscellaneous agents.
3. Discuss the use of antidepressants across the lifespan.
4. Compare and contrast the prototype drugs for each class of antidepressant with the other drugs in that class and with drugs in the other classes of antidepressants.
5. Outline the nursing considerations and teaching needs for patients receiving each class of antidepressant.

TRICYCLIC ANTI-DEPRESSANTS

amitriptyline
amoxapine
clomipramine
desipramine
doxepin
P imipramine
maprotiline
nortriptyline
protriptyline
trimipramine

MONOAMINE OXIDASE INHIBITORS

isocarboxazid
P phenelzine
tranylcypromine

SELECTIVE SEROTONIN REUPTAKE INHIBITORS

citalopram
duloxetine
escitalopram
P fluoxetine
fluvoxamine
paroxetine
sertraline

OTHER ANTI-DEPRESSANTS

bupropion
mirtazapine
nefazodone
trazodone
venlafaxine

When you ask people how they feel, they may say "pretty good" or "not so great." People's responses are usually appropriate to what is happening in their lives, and they describe themselves as being in a good mood or a bad mood. Some days are better than others.

Affect is a term that is used to refer to people's feelings in response to their environment, whether positive and pleasant or negative and unpleasant. All people experience different affective states at various times in their lives. These states of mind, which change in particular situations, usually do not last very long and do not often involve extremes of happiness or depression. If a person's mood goes far beyond the usual, normal "ups and downs," he or she is said to have an affective disorder.

Depression and Antidepressants

Depression, a very common affective disorder, strikes millions of people every year. In **depression**, feelings of sadness are much more severe and long-lasting than the suspected precipitating event, and the mood of affected individuals is much more intense. The depression may not even be traceable to a specific event or stressor (i.e., there are no external causes). Patients who are depressed may have little energy, sleep disturbances, a lack of appetite, limited libido, and inability to perform activities of daily living. They may describe overwhelming feelings of sadness, despair, hopelessness, and disorganization.

In many cases, the depression is never diagnosed, and the patient is treated for physical manifestations of the underlying disease, such as fatigue, malaise, obesity, anorexia, or alcoholism and drug dependence. Clinical depression is an actual disorder that can interfere with a person's family life, job, and social interactions. Left untreated, it can produce multiple physical problems that can lead to further depression or, in extreme cases, even suicide.

Biogenic Amine Theory of Depression

Research on development of the drugs known to be effective in relieving depression led to formulation of the current hypothesis regarding the cause of depression. Scientists have theorized that depression results from a deficiency of norepinephrine (NE), dopamine, or serotonin (5HT), which are all **biogenic amines**, in key areas of the brain. Both NE and 5HT are released throughout the brain by neurons that react with multiple receptors to regulate arousal, alertness, attention, moods, appetite, and sensory processing. Deficiencies of these neurotransmitters may develop for three known reasons. First, monoamine oxidase (MAO) may break them down to be recycled or restored in the neuron. Second, rapid fire of the neurons may lead to their depletion. Third, the number or sensitivity of postsynaptic receptors may increase, thus depleting neurotransmitter levels.

Depression also may occur as a result of other, yet unknown causes. This condition may be a syndrome that reflects either activity or lack of activity in a number of sites in the brain, including the arousal center (reticular activating system, or RAS), the limbic system, and basal ganglia.

Drug Therapy

Today, the use of agents that alter the concentration of neurotransmitters in the brain is the most effective means of treating depression with drugs. The antidepressant drugs used today counteract the effects of neurotransmitter deficiencies in three ways. First, they may inhibit the effects of MAO, leading to increased NE or 5HT in the synaptic cleft. Second, they may block reuptake by the releasing nerve, leading to increased neurotransmitter levels in the synaptic cleft. Third, they may regulate receptor sites and breakdown of neurotransmitters, leading to an accumulation of neurotransmitter in the synaptic cleft.

Antidepressants may be classified into three groups: the tricyclic antidepressants (TCAs), the MAOIs, and the selective serotonin reuptake inhibitors (SSRIs). Other drugs that are used as antidepressants similarly increase the synaptic cleft concentrations of these neurotransmitters (Figure 21.1). For information on how antidepressants affect people from young to old, see Box 21.1.

Tricyclic Antidepressants

The **tricyclic antidepressants (TCAs)**, including the amines, secondary amines, and tetracyclics, all reduce the reuptake of 5HT and NE into nerves. Because all TCAs are similarly effective, the choice of TCA depends on individual response to the drug and tolerance of adverse effects. A patient who does not respond to one TCA may respond to another drug from this class. Table 21.1 lists the currently available TCAs, including the specific type and the occurrence of sedation and other adverse effects.

Therapeutic Actions and Indications

The TCAs inhibit presynaptic reuptake of the neurotransmitters NE and 5HT, which leads to an accumulation of these neurotransmitters in the synaptic cleft and increased stimulation of the postsynaptic receptors. The exact mechanism of action in decreasing depression is not known but is thought to be related to the accumulation of NE and 5HT in certain areas of the brain.

TCAs are indicated for the relief of symptoms of depression. The sedative effects of these drugs may make them more effective in patients whose depression is characterized by anxiety and sleep disturbances. They are effective for treat-

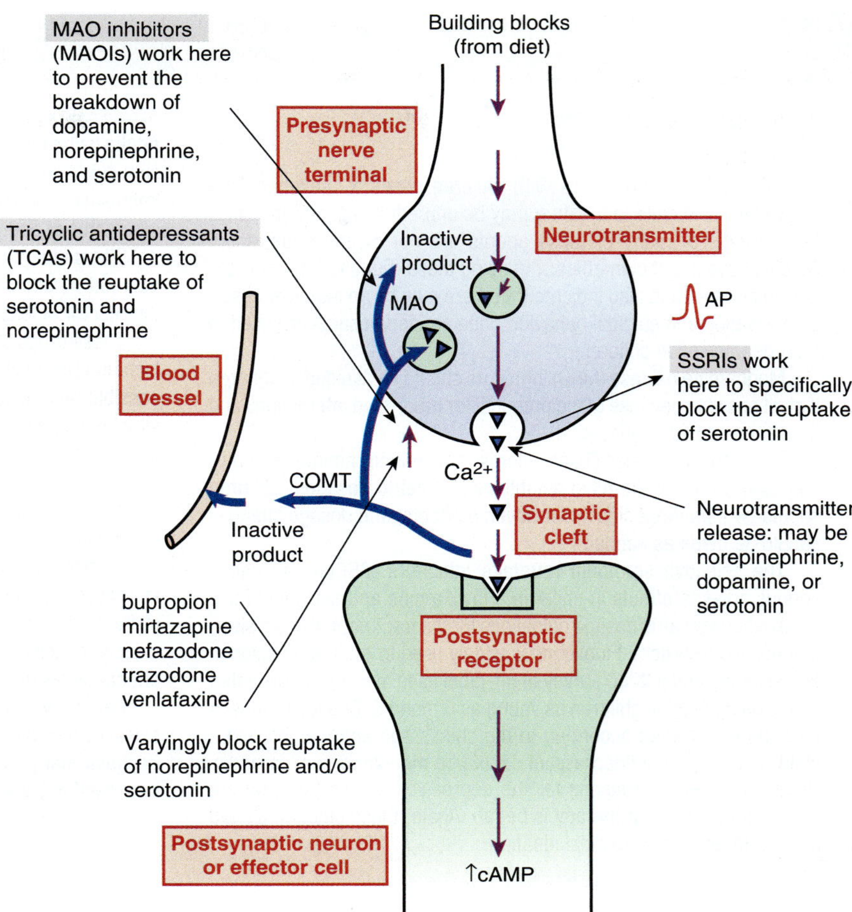

FIGURE 21.1 Sites of action for the antidepressants: Monoamine oxidase inhibitors (MAOIs), tricyclic antidepressants (TCAs), selective serotonin reuptake inhibitors (SSRIs), and other agents. cAMP, cyclic adenosine monophosphate; COMT, catecholamine-O-methyltransferase.

ing enuresis in children older than 6 years. Some of these drugs are being investigated for the treatment of chronic, intractable pain. In addition, the TCAs are anticholinergic. Clomipramine is now also approved for use in the treatment of obsessive–compulsive disorders (OCDs).

Pharmacokinetics

The TCAs are well absorbed from the gastrointestinal (GI) tract, reaching peak levels in 2 to 4 hours. They are highly bound to plasma proteins and are lipid soluble; this allows them to be distributed widely in the tissues, including the brain. TCAs are metabolized in the liver and excreted in the urine, with relatively long half-lives, ranging from 8 to 46 hours. Patients with liver impairment need a lower dose of the drug to avoid toxic levels. The TCAs cross the placenta and enter breast milk. They should not be used during pregnancy or lactation unless the benefit to the mother clearly outweighs the potential risk to the neonate.

Contraindications and Cautions

One contraindication to the use of TCAs is the presence of allergy to any of the drugs in this class. Other contraindications include recent myocardial infarction *because of the potential occurrence of reinfarction or extension of the infarct with the cardiac effects of the drug;* myelography within the previous 24 hours or in the next 48 hours; and concurrent use of an MAOI *because of the potential for serious adverse effects or toxic reactions.* In addition, pregnancy and lactation are contraindications *because of the potential for adverse effects in the fetus and neonate.*

Caution should be used with TCAs in patients with preexisting cardiovascular (CV) disorders *because of the cardiac stimulatory effects of the drug* and with *any condition that would be exacerbated by the anticholinergic effects,* such as angle-closure glaucoma, urinary retention, prostate hypertrophy, or GI or genitourinary (GU) surgery. Care should also be taken with psychiatric patients, *who may exhibit a worsening of psychoses or paranoia,* and with manic–depressive patients, *who may shift to a manic stage.* In addition, caution is necessary in patients with a history of seizures *because the seizure threshold may be decreased secondary to stimulation of the receptor sites* and in elderly patients. The presence of hepatic or renal disease, *which could interfere with metabolism and excretion of these drugs and lead to toxic levels,* also necessitates caution.

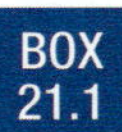

BOX 21.1 **DRUG THERAPY ACROSS THE LIFESPAN**

Antidepressant Agents

CHILDREN

Use of antidepressant drugs with children poses a challenge. The response of the child to the drug may be unpredictable, and the long-term effects of many of these agents are not clearly understood. Studies have not shown efficacy in using these drugs to treat depression in children and also indicate that there may be an increase in suicidal ideation and suicidal behavior when antidepressants are used to treat depression in children.

Monoamine oxidase (MAO) inhibitors should be avoided in children if at all possible because of the potential for drug–food interactions and the serious adverse effects.

Of the tricyclic drugs (TCAs), clomipramine, imipramine, nortriptyline, and trimipramine have established pediatric dosages. Children should be monitored closely for adverse effects, and dosage changes should be made as needed.

The selective serotonin reuptake inhibitors (SSRIs) can cause serious adverse effects in children. Fluvoxamine and sertraline have established pediatric dosage guidelines for the treatment of obsessive–compulsive disorders. Fluoxetine is widely used to treat depression in adolescents, and a 2000 survey of off-label uses of drugs showed that it was being used in children as young as 6 months. Dosage regimens must be established according to the child's age and weight, and a child receiving an antidepressant should be monitored very carefully. Underlying medical reasons for the depression should be ruled out before antidepressant therapy is begun. Again, these children should be monitored for any suicidal ideation.

ADULTS

Adults using these drugs should have medical causes for their depression ruled out before therapy is begun. Thyroid disease, hormonal imbalance, and cardiovascular disorders can all lead to the signs and symptoms of depression.

The patient needs to understand that the effects of drug therapy may not be seen for 4 weeks and that it is important to continue the therapy for at least that long.

These drugs should be used very cautiously during pregnancy and lactation because of the potential for adverse effects on the fetus and possible neurological effects on the baby. Use should be reserved for situations in which the benefits to the mother far outweigh the potential risks to the neonate.

OLDER ADULTS

Older patients may be more susceptible to the adverse effects of these drugs, from unanticipated central nervous system (CNS) effects to increased sedation, dizziness, and even hallucinations. Dosages of all of these drugs need to be reduced and the patient monitored very closely for toxic effects. Safety measures should be provided if CNS effects do occur.

Patients with hepatic or renal impairment should be monitored very closely while taking these drugs. Decreased dosages may be needed. Because many older patients also have renal or hepatic impairment, they need to be screened carefully.

Adverse Effects

The adverse effects of TCAs are associated with the effects of the drugs on the central nervous system (CNS) and on the peripheral nervous system. Sedation, sleep disturbances, fatigue, hallucinations, disorientation, visual disturbances, difficulty in concentrating, weakness, ataxia, and tremors may occur.

Use of TCAs may lead to GI anticholinergic effects, such as dry mouth, constipation, nausea, vomiting, anorexia, increased salivation, cramps, and diarrhea. Resultant GU effects may include urinary retention and hesitancy, loss of libido, and changes in sexual functioning. CV effects such as orthostatic hypotension, hypertension, arrhythmias, myocardial infarction, angina, palpitations, and stroke may also pose problems. Miscellaneous reported effects include alopecia, weight gain or loss, flushing, chills, and nasal congestion.

These adverse effects may be intolerable to some patients, who then stop taking the particular TCA. Abrupt cessation of all TCAs causes a withdrawal syndrome characterized by nausea, headache, vertigo, malaise, and nightmares.

Clinically Important Drug–Drug Interactions

If TCAs are given with cimetidine, fluoxetine, or ranitidine, an increase in TCA levels results, with an increase in both therapeutic and adverse effects, especially anticholinergic conditions. Patients should be monitored closely, and appropriate dosage reductions should be made.

Other drug combinations may also pose problems. The combination of TCAs and oral anticoagulants leads to higher serum levels of the anticoagulants and increased risk of bleeding. Blood tests should be done frequently, and appropriate dosage adjustments in the oral anticoagulant should be made.

If TCAs are combined with sympathomimetics or clonidine, the risk of arrhythmias and hypertension is increased. This combination should be avoided, especially in patients with underlying cardiovascular disease.

The combination of TCAs with MAOIs leads to a risk of severe hyperpyretic crisis with severe convulsions, hypertensive episodes, and death. This combination should be avoided. Although TCAs and MAOIs have been used together in selected patients who do not respond to a single agent, the risk of severe adverse effects is very high.

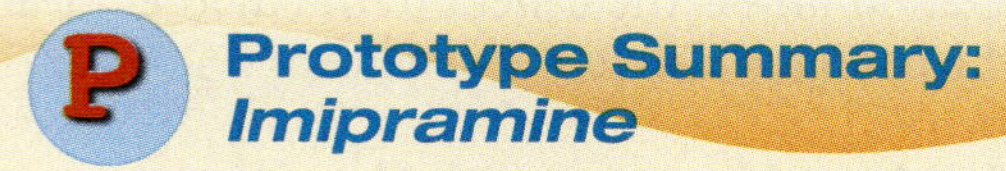

Prototype Summary: *Imipramine*

Indications: Relief of symptoms of depression; enuresis in children older than 6 years; unlabeled consideration—control of chronic pain

Table 21.1 Tricyclic Antidepressants: Most Common Side Effects

Drug Name	Type	Common Side Effects: Sedation	Anticholinergic	Hypotension	Cardiovascular	Usual Dosage
amitriptyline (*generic*)	Amine	++++	++++	++++	++	75–150 mg/day PO
amoxapine (*Asendin*)	Amine	+	+	++	++	50–100 mg PO b.i.d. to t.i.d.
clomipramine (*Anafranil*)	Amine	+++	+++	+++	+++	Adult: 25–50 mg PO q.i.d. Pediatric: 25 mg PO q.i.d. to a maximum of 3 mg/kg/day
desipramine (*Norpramin*)	Secondary amine	+	+	++	++	100–200 mg/day PO
doxepin (*Sinequan*)	Amine	+++	+++	++	++	25–50 mg PO t.i.d.
P imipramine (*Tofranil*)	Amine	++	++	+++	++	Adult: 50–200 mg/day PO Pediatric: 30–40 mg/day PO Enuresis: 25 mg/day 1 h before bed
maprotiline (*generic*)	Tetracyclic	++	+	++	++	75–150 mg/day PO; reduce dosage in elderly patients
nortriptyline (*Aventyl, Pamelor*)	Secondary amine	+	+	+	+	Adult: 25–50 mg PO t.i.d. to q.i.d. Pediatric: 30–50 mg/day PO in divided doses Geriatric: 30–50 mg/day PO in divided doses
protriptyline (*Vivactil*)	Secondary amine	+	+++	+	+	15–40 mg/day PO in three or four divided doses; 5 mg PO t.i.d. for elderly patients
trimipramine (*Surmontil*)	Amine	+++	++	++	++	Adult: 75–150 mg/day PO Pediatric: 50 mg/day PO Geriatric: 50–100 mg/day PO

++++ = marked effects; +++ = moderate effects; ++ = mild effects; + = negligible effects.

Actions: Inhibits presynaptic reuptake of norepinephrine and serotonin; anticholinergic at CNS and peripheral receptors; sedating

Pharmacokinetics:

Route	Onset	Peak
Oral	Varies	2–4 h

$T_{1/2}$: 8–16 hours, metabolized in the liver, excretion in the urine

Adverse effects: sedation, anticholinergic effects, confusion, anxiety, orthostatic hypotension, dry mouth, constipation, urinary retention, rash, bone marrow depression

Nursing Considerations for Patients Receiving Tricyclic Antidepressants

Assessment: History and Examination

Screen for the following, *which could be contraindications or cautions for the use of the drug:* any known allergies to these drugs; impaired liver or kidney function, *which could alter metabolism and excretion of the drug;* glaucoma, benign prostatic hypertrophy, cardiac dysfunction, GI obstruction, surgery, or recent myocardial infarction, *all of which could be exacerbated by the effects of the drug;* and pregnancy or lactation. Find out whether the patient has a history of seizure disorders or a history of psychiatric problems or myelography within the past 24 hours or in the next 48 hours, or is taking an MAOI.

Include screening *for baseline status before beginning therapy and for any potential adverse effects.* Assess the following: temperature and weight; skin color and lesions; affect, orientation, and reflexes; vision; blood pressure, including orthostatic blood pressure; pulse and perfusion; respiratory rate and adventitious sounds; and bowel sounds on abdominal examination. Obtain an electrocardiogram, as well as renal and liver function tests.

Nursing Diagnoses

The patient receiving a TCA may have the following nursing diagnoses related to drug therapy:

- Acute Pain related to anticholinergic effects, headache, CNS effects

- Decreased Cardiac Output related to CV effects
- Disturbed Thought Processes and Disturbed Sensory Perception (Visual, Auditory, Kinesthetic, Tactile, or Olfactory) related to CNS effects
- Risk for Injury related to CNS effects
- Deficient Knowledge regarding drug therapy

Implementation With Rationale

- Limit drug access if the patient is suicidal *because of the potential for overdose.*
- Maintain initial dosage for 4 to 8 weeks *to evaluate the therapeutic effect.*
- Give parenteral forms of the drug only if oral forms are not feasible or available; switch to an oral form, *which is less toxic and associated with fewer adverse effects,* as soon as possible.
- Give the major portion of the dose at bedtime if drowsiness and anticholinergic effects are severe *to decrease the risk of patient injury. Elderly patients may not be able to tolerate larger doses.*
- Reduce the dosage if minor adverse effects occur, and discontinue the drug slowly if major or potentially life-threatening adverse effects occur *to ensure patient safety.*
- Provide comfort measures *to help the patient tolerate drug effects.* These measures may include voiding before dosing, instituting a bowel program as needed, taking food with the drug if GI upset is severe, and environmental control (lighting, temperature, stimuli).
- Provide thorough patient teaching, including drug name, prescribed dosage, measures for avoidance of adverse effects, and warning signs that may indicate possible problems. Instruct patients about the need for periodic monitoring and evaluation *to enhance patient knowledge about drug therapy and to promote compliance.*
- Offer support and encouragement *to help patients cope with the diagnosis and the drug regimen.*

Evaluation

- Monitor patient response to the drug (alleviation of signs and symptoms of depression).
- Monitor for adverse effects (sedation, anticholinergic effects, hypotension, cardiac arrhythmias).
- Evaluate effectiveness of teaching plan (patient can give the drug name, dosage, possible adverse effects to watch for, specific measures to help avoid adverse effects, and importance of continued follow-up).
- Monitor the effectiveness of comfort measures and compliance with the regimen.

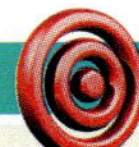

FOCUS POINTS

- Affect is the expression of an emotional response.
- Depression is an affective disorder characterized by inappropriate sadness, despair, and hopelessness.
- According to the biogenic amine theory, depression is caused by a brain deficiency of the biogenic amines: norepinephrine (NE), serotonin (5HT), and dopamine. Antidepressant drugs, such as TCAs, MAOIs, and SSRIs, raise the level of the biogenic amines.

Monoamine Oxidase Inhibitors

At one time, MAOIs were used more often, but now they are used rarely because they require a specific dietary regimen to prevent toxicity. Safer drugs that are usually just as effective have replaced them. Agents still in use include the following:

- Isocarboxazid (*Marplan*) at one time became unavailable because it was infrequently used but reappeared in 1998 when researchers found that some patients who did not respond to the newer, safer antidepressants could respond to this drug.
- Phenelzine (*Nardil*) is also reserved for use in patients who do not respond to other antidepressants or who cannot take other antidepressants for some reason.
- Tranylcypromine (*Parnate*) is used for adult outpatients with reactive depression. This agent is also associated with potentially fatal drug–food interactions.

The choice of an MAOI depends on the prescriber's experience and individual response. A patient who does not respond to one MAOI may respond to another.

Therapeutic Actions and Indications

The **monoamine oxidase (MAO) inhibitors** irreversibly inhibit MAO, an enzyme found in nerves and other tissues (including the liver), that breaks down the biogenic amines NE, dopamine, and 5HT. This allows these amines to accumulate in the synaptic cleft and in neuronal storage vesicles, causing increased stimulation of the postsynaptic receptors and, it is thought, relief of depression. The MAOIs are generally indicated for treatment of the signs and symptoms of depression in patients who cannot tolerate or do not respond to other, safer antidepressants (Table 21.2).

Pharmacokinetics

The MAOIs are well absorbed from the GI tract, reaching peak levels in 2 to 3 hours. They are metabolized in the liver

Table 21.2 DRUGS IN FOCUS

Monoamine Oxidase Inhibitors

Drug Name	Dosage/Route	Usual Indications
isocarboxazid (*Marplan*)	10 mg PO b.i.d., may reach a maximum of 40 mg/day	Depression not responsive to other agents
P phenelzine (*Nardil*)	15 mg PO t.i.d.; maintenance 15 mg/day PO	Depression not responsive to other agents
tranylcypromine (*Parnate*)	30 mg/day PO in divided doses; maximum 60 mg/day	Adult reactive depression

primarily by acetylation and are excreted in the urine. Patients with liver or renal impairment and those known as "slow acetylators" may require lowered doses to avoid exaggerated effects of the drugs. The MAOIs cross the placenta and enter breast milk. Avoid use during pregnancy and lactation unless the benefit to the mother clearly outweighs the potential risk to the neonate.

Contraindications and Cautions

Contraindications to the use of MAOIs include allergy to any of these antidepressants; pheochromocytoma *because the sudden increases in NE levels could result in severe hypertension and CV emergencies;* CV disease, including hypertension, coronary artery disease, angina, and congestive heart failure, *which could be exacerbated by increased NE levels;* and known abnormal CNS vessels or defects *because the potential increase in blood pressure and vasoconstriction associated with higher NE levels could precipitate a stroke.* A history of headaches may also be a contraindication.

Other contraindications include renal or hepatic impairment, *which could alter the metabolism and excretion of these drugs and lead to toxic levels,* and myelography within the past 24 hours or in the next 48 hours *because of the risk of severe reaction to the dye used in myelography.*

In addition, caution should be used with psychiatric patients, *who could be overstimulated or shift to a manic phase as a result of the stimulation associated with MAOIs,* and in patients with seizure disorders or hyperthyroidism, *both of which could be exacerbated by the stimulation of these drugs.* Care should also be taken with patients who are soon to undergo elective surgery *because of the potential for unexpected effects with NE accumulation during the stress reaction,* and with female patients who are pregnant or breast-feeding *because of potential adverse effects on the fetus and neonate.*

Adverse Effects

The MAOIs are associated with more adverse effects, more of which are fatal, than most other antidepressants. The effects relate to the accumulation of NE in the synaptic cleft. Dizziness, excitement, nervousness, mania, hyperreflexia, tremors, confusion, insomnia, agitation, and blurred vision may occur.

MAOIs can cause liver toxicity. Other GI effects can include nausea, vomiting, diarrhea or constipation, anorexia, weight gain, dry mouth, and abdominal pain. Urinary retention, dysuria, incontinence, and changes in sexual function may also occur. Cardiovascular effects can include orthostatic hypotension, arrhythmias, palpitations, angina, and the potentially fatal hypertensive crisis. This last condition is characterized by occipital headache, palpitations, neck stiffness, nausea, vomiting, sweating, dilated pupils, photophobia, tachycardia, and chest pain. It may progress to intracranial bleeding and fatal stroke.

Clinically Important Drug–Drug Interactions

Drug interactions of MAOIs with other antidepressants include hypertensive crisis, coma, and severe convulsions with TCAs, and a potentially life-threatening serotonin syndrome with SSRIs. A period of 6 weeks should elapse after stopping an SSRI before beginning therapy with an MAOI.

If MAOIs are given with other sympathomimetic drugs (e.g., methyldopa, guanethidine), sympathomimetic effects increase. Combinations with insulin or oral antidiabetic agents result in additive hypoglycemic effects. Patients who receive these combinations must be monitored closely, and appropriate dosage adjustments should be made.

Clinically Important Drug–Food Interactions

Tyramine and other pressor amines that are found in food, which are normally broken down by MAO enzymes in the GI tract, may be absorbed in high concentrations in the presence of MAOIs, resulting in increased blood pressure. The hypertensive crisis is often associated with eating foods that contain tyramine. In addition, tyramine causes the release of stored NE from nerve terminals, which further contributes to high blood pressure. Patients who take MAOIs should avoid the tyramine-containing foods listed in Table 21.3.

Table 21.3 Tyramine-Containing Foods

Foods High in Tyramine	Foods With Moderate Amounts of Tyramine	Foods With Low Amounts of Tyramine
Aged cheeses: cheddar cheese, blue cheese, Swiss cheese, Camembert Aged or fermented meats, fish or poultry: chicken paté, beef liver paté, caviar Brewer's yeast Fava beans Red wines: Chianti, burgundy, sherry, vermouth Smoked or pickled meats, fish or poultry: herring, sausage, corned beef, salami, pepperoni	Meat extracts: consommé, bouillon Pasteurized light and pale beer Avocados	Distilled liquors: vodka, gin, Scotch, rye Cheeses: American, mozzarella, cottage cheese, cream cheese Chocolate Fruits: figs, raisins, grapes, pineapple, oranges Sour cream Soy sauce Yogurt

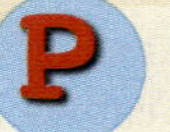

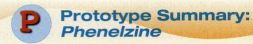

Prototype Summary: Phenelzine

Indications: Treatment of patients with depression who are unresponsive to other antidepressive therapy or in whom other antidepressive therapy is contraindicated

Actions: Irreversibly inhibits MAO, allowing norepinephrine, serotonin, and dopamine to accumulate in the synaptic cleft; this accumulation is thought to be responsible for the clinical effects

Pharmacokinetics:

Route	Onset	Duration
Oral	Slow	48–96 h

$T_{1/2}$: Unknown, metabolized in the liver, excreted in the urine

Adverse effects: Dizziness, vertigo, headache, overactivity, hyperreflexia, tremors, mania, weakness, drowsiness, fatigue, sweating, orthostatic hypotension, constipation, diarrhea, dry mouth, edema, anorexia, potential for hypertensive crisis

Nursing Considerations for Patients Receiving Monoamine Oxidase Inhibitors

Assessment: History and Examination

Screen for the following, *which could be contraindications or cautions for use of the drug:* any known allergies to these drugs; impaired liver or kidney function *that could alter the metabolism and excretion of the drug;* cardiac dysfunction; GI or GU obstruction; surgery, including elective surgery; seizure disorders; psychiatric conditions; and occurrence of myelography within the past 24 hours or in the next 48 hours. Find out whether female patients are pregnant or breast-feeding.

Include screening *for baseline status before beginning therapy and for any potential adverse effects.* Assess the following: temperature and weight; skin color and lesions; affect, orientation, and reflexes; vision; blood pressure, including orthostatic blood pressure; pulse and perfusion; respiratory rate and adventitious sounds; and bowel sounds on abdominal examination. Obtain an electrocardiogram and renal and liver function tests.

Nursing Diagnoses

The patient receiving an MAOI may have the following nursing diagnoses related to drug therapy:

- Acute Pain related to sympathomimetic effects, headache, CNS effects
- Decreased Cardiac Output related to CV effects
- Disturbed Thought Processes and Disturbed Sensory Perception (Visual, Kinesthetic) related to CNS effects
- Risk for Injury related to CNS effects
- Deficient Knowledge regarding drug therapy

Implementation With Rationale

- Limit drug access to potentially suicidal patients *to decrease the risk of overdose.*
- Monitor the patient for 2 to 4 weeks *to ascertain onset of full therapeutic effect.*
- Monitor blood pressure and orthostatic blood pressure carefully *to arrange for a slower increase in dosage as needed for patients who show a tendency toward hypotension.*

- Monitor liver function before and periodically during therapy and *arrange to discontinue the drug at the first sign of liver toxicity.*
- Discontinue the drug and monitor the patient carefully at any complaint of severe headache *to decrease the risk of severe hypertension and cerebrovascular effects.*
- Have phentolamine or another adrenergic blocker on standby *as treatment in case of hypertensive crisis.*
- Provide comfort measures *to help the patient tolerate drug effects.* These include voiding before dosing, instituting a bowel program as needed, taking food with the drug if GI upset is severe, and environmental control (lighting, temperature, decreased stimulation).
- Provide a list of potential drug–food interactions that can cause severe toxicity *to decrease the risk of a serious drug–food interaction.* Provide a diet that is low in tyramine-containing foods.
- Provide thorough patient teaching, including drug name, prescribed dosage, measures for avoidance of adverse effects, and warning signs that may indicate possible problems. Instruct patients about the need for periodic monitoring and evaluation *to enhance patient knowledge about drug therapy and to promote compliance.*
- Offer support and encouragement *to help patients cope with the disease and the drug regimen.*

Evaluation

- Monitor patient response to the drug (alleviation of signs and symptoms of depression).
- Monitor for adverse effects (sedation, sympathomimetic effects, hypotension, cardiac arrhythmias, GI disturbances, hypertensive crisis).
- Evaluate the effectiveness of the teaching plan (patient can give the drug name, dosage, possible adverse effects to watch for, specific measures to help avoid adverse effects, importance of continued follow-up, and importance of avoiding foods high in tyramine).
- Monitor the effectiveness of comfort measures and compliance with the regimen.

Selective Serotonin Reuptake Inhibitors

Selective serotonin reuptake inhibitors (SSRIs), the newest group of antidepressant drugs, specifically block the reuptake of 5HT, with little to no known effect on NE. Because SSRIs do not have the many adverse effects associated with TCAs and MAOIs, they are a better choice for many patients. SSRIs include the following agents:

- Fluoxetine (*Prozac*), the first SSRI, has been successfully used to treat depression, obsessive compulsive disorders (OCDs), bulimia, panic disorders, and premenstrual dysphoric disorder (PMDD). It is being investigated for use in the treatment of other psychiatric disorders, including obesity, alcoholism, chronic pain, and various neuropathies.

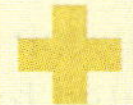

FOCUS ON **PATIENT SAFETY**

Patients who see more than one health care provider often assume that all of the health care providers discuss their case and treatment. This is not always the case, and it falls to the patient to remember to mention drugs that have been ordered by other health care providers. Caution must be used with fluoxetine—known as *Prozac* for depression but also known as *Sarafem* when used for PMDD. *Prozac* and *Sarafem* are trade names for the same drug, and a patient could inadvertently be prescribed both of these drugs—*Prozac* from the primary care provider and *Sarafem* from the gynecologist. If the patient has not received detailed teaching about these drugs, she could inadvertently be taking twice the recommended dose.

- Fluvoxamine (*Luvox*), which is under investigation for the treatment of depression, bulimia, panic disorder, and social phobia, is currently indicated only for the treatment of OCDs.
- Paroxetine (*Paxil*) is indicated for the treatment of depression, panic disorders, posttraumatic stress reaction, social anxiety disorders, general anxiety disorders, PMDD, and OCDs. It is being investigated for the treatment of chronic headache, diabetic neuropathy, and hot flashes.
- Sertraline (*Zoloft*) is used to treat depression and OCDs, posttraumatic stress disorders, PMDD, social anxiety disorder, and panic disorders.
- Citalopram (*Celexa*) is indicated only for the treatment of depression, but has been used to treat panic disorder, PMDD, OCDs, social phobias, trichotillomania, and posttraumatic stress disorders.
- Escitalopram (*Lexapro*) is an isomer of citalopram that is approved for the treatment of major depressive disorder and maintenance of patients with major depressive disorder and generalized anxiety disorder. It is being studied for use in panic disorders.
- Duloxetine (*Cymbalta*), the newest SSRI, may block NE reuptake. It is indicated for the treatment of major depressive disorder and management of neuropathic pain associated with diabetic peripheral neuropathy. It is being studied for treatment of fibromyalgia and stress incontinence.

With the SSRIs, a period of up to 4 weeks is necessary for realization of the full therapeutic effect. Patients may respond well to one SSRI and yet show little or no response to another one. The choice of drug depends on the indications and individual response. Box 21.2 provides more information.

Therapeutic Actions and Indications

As previously stated, SSRIs more specifically block the reuptake of 5HT, with little known effect on NE. This action increases the levels of 5HT in the synaptic cleft and may contribute to the antidepressant and other effects attributed to these drugs.

SSRIs are indicated for the treatment of depression, OCDs, panic attacks, bulimia, PMDD, posttraumatic stress disorders, social phobias, and social anxiety disorders (Table 21.4). Ongoing investigations are focusing on the use of these antidepressant drugs in the treatment of other psychiatric disorders.

Pharmacokinetics

The SSRIs are well absorbed from the GI tract, metabolized in the liver, and excreted in the urine and feces. The half-life varies widely with the drug being used. The SSRIs have been associated with congenital abnormalities in animal studies and should be used during pregnancy only if the benefits to the mother clearly outweigh the potential risks to the fetus. The SSRIs enter breast milk and can cause adverse effects in

BOX 21.2 CULTURAL CONSIDERATIONS FOR DRUG THERAPY

The Popularity of Prozac

A rise in the diagnosis of depression began in the 1990s, with that decade's fast-paced lifestyle, high-stress jobs, explosion of information, and rapid change. Many people who have high expectations of both themselves and others are overworked and overstimulated to a point at which they become clinically depressed.

There is now a selection of relatively safe and nontoxic drugs that can be used to treat depression—the selective serotonin reuptake inhibitors (SSRIs). For several years, the SSRIs remained in the top-selling category of prescription drugs. Fluoxetine (*Prozac*), in particular, has been the subject of numerous talk shows, books, and movies. In many ways, *Prozac* was the "in" drug of the 1990s. This societal phenomenon put pressure on health care providers to prescribe a drug even if it was not appropriate to a given patient's situation. In some instances, patients just wanted the drug that helped their friend. They may not have been willing to listen to their health care provider or to take the time to be properly diagnosed; they just wanted an SSRI. *Prozac* is not the solution to everyone's problem, and it is often difficult to explain this fact to a patient. It also may be hard to get the patient to understand that this drug is not a quick fix; it takes 4 to 6 weeks to achieve full therapeutic effectiveness. Fortunately, the SSRIs have the least adverse effects of the antidepressants, and such fads usually pass in a few years.

It is important to remember the powerful effects of the media on health care-seeking behavior. As more and more drugs are advertised in magazines and on television, patients are becoming aware of options and "cures" that they might like to try. Patient education is a tricky yet important part of any health care intervention and an extremely important aspect of health care in our society.

Table 21.4 DRUGS IN FOCUS

Selective Serotonin Reuptake Inhibitors

Name	Usual Dosage	Usual Indication
citalopram (*Celexa*)	20 mg/day PO b.i.d., up to 40 mg/day may be needed	Treatment of depression in adults
duloxetine (*Cymbalta*)	20 mg PO b.i.d., up to 60 mg/day if needed	Treatment of depression and neuropathic pain associated with diabetic neuropathy
escitalopram (*Lexapro*)	10 mg/day PO as a single dose; 10–20 mg/day PO maintenance	Treatment of major depressive disorder and maintenance of patients with major depressive disorder
P fluoxetine (*Prozac; Sarafem*)	20 mg/day PO in the AM; do not exceed 60 mg/day; reduce dosage with hepatic impairment; also available in a 90-mg, once-a-week formulation	Treatment of depression, bulimia, obsessive-compulsive disorders (OCDs), panic disorders, premenstrual dysphoric disorder (PMDD) in adults
fluvoxamine (*Luvox*)	Adult: 50 mg PO at bedtime to a maximum of 300 mg/day; reduce dosage with hepatic impairment Pediatric (8–17 yr): 25 mg PO at bedtime; do not exceed 250 mg/day	Treatment of OCDs
paroxetine (*Paxil*)	10–20 mg/day PO; do not exceed 50 mg/day; or 62.5 mg/day controlled-release tablets; reduce dosage in hepatic, renal dysfunction and with the elderly	Treatment of depression, OCDs, PMDD, and various panic disorders in adults
sertraline (*Zoloft*)	Adult: 25–50 mg/day PO; reduce dosage with hepatic dysfunction OCD Pediatric: 25–50 mg/day PO based on age and severity of OCD	Treatment of depression, OCDs, social anxiety disorder, post-traumatic stress disorder, panic disorders, PMDD

the baby, so a different method of feeding the baby should be selected if an SSRI is required by the mother. Recent studies have linked the incidence of suicidal ideation and suicide attempts to the use of these drugs in pediatric patients.

Contraindications and Cautions

The SSRIs are contraindicated in the presence of allergy to any of these drugs and during pregnancy and lactation *because of the potential for serious adverse effects on the neonate.* Caution should be used in patients with impaired renal or hepatic function *that could alter the metabolism and excretion of the drug, leading to toxic effects,* or with diabetes, *which could be exacerbated by the stimulating effects of these drugs.*

Adverse Effects

The adverse effects associated with SSRIs, which are related to the effects of increased 5HT levels, include CNS effects such as headache, drowsiness, dizziness, insomnia, anxiety, tremor, agitation, and seizures. GI effects such as nausea, vomiting, diarrhea, dry mouth, anorexia, constipation, and changes in taste often occur, as do GU effects, including painful menstruation, cystitis, sexual dysfunction, urgency, and impotence. Respiratory changes may include cough, dyspnea, upper respiratory infections, and pharyngitis. Other reported effects are sweating, rash, fever, and pruritus. Box 21.3 provides information about ongoing research into adverse effects in young people.

Clinically Important Drug–Drug Interactions

Because of the risk of serotonin syndrome if SSRIs are used with MAOIs, this combination should be avoided, and at least 2 to 4 weeks should be allowed between use of the two types of drugs if switching from one to the other. In addition, the use of SSRIs with TCAs results in increased therapeutic and toxic effects. If these combinations are used, patients should be monitored closely, and appropriate dosage adjustments should be made. For more information see Box 21.4.

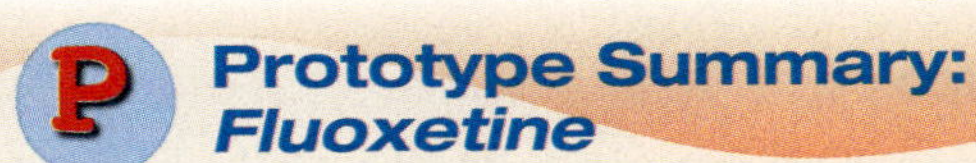

Prototype Summary: *Fluoxetine*

Indications: Treatment of depression, OCDs, bulimia, PMDD, panic disorders; unlabeled uses include chronic pain, alcoholism, neuropathies, obesity

Actions: Inhibits CNS neuronal reuptake of serotonin with little effect on norepinephrine and little affinity for cholinergic, histaminic, or alpha-adrenergic sites

BOX 21.3 FOCUS ON THE **EVIDENCE**

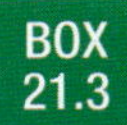

Childhood Suicide and Antidepressants

The FDA issued a talk paper in late spring 2003 after reports from the British press cited an increase in suicidal behavior in children being treated with paroxetine (*Paxil*). The FDA compiled a review of reports for eight different antidepressant drugs—citalopram, fluoxetine, fluvoxamine, mirtazapine, nefazodone, paroxetine, sertraline and venlafaxine—that were being studied for use in pediatric populations.

The data from these studies did not clearly establish a link between increased suicidal ideation and the use of these antidepressants, but the data also did not establish effectiveness in major depressive disorder in children for any of the drugs, except fluoxetine. Many journals and news reports have discussed an increase in suicide attempts and completed suicides in pediatric patients being treated with antidepressants. Many anecdotal reports have been submitted to Medwatch reporting the same events. The FDA points out, however, that these reports are hard to interpret and, without a control group, it is difficult to know if these effects are also seen in this age group of children even when they are not being treated with antidepressants. In 20 placebo-controlled studies involving these eight drugs and more than 4100 pediatric patients, there were no reports of completed suicides.

In fall 2004, the FDA issued an advisory to all prescribers noting the studies that have been done and concluding that there is not enough evidence at this point that suicidal ideation is inherent to many major depressive disorders. All of these drugs should be used with caution and prescriptions written in the smallest quantity feasible, parents should be educated about the warning signs of suicide. Continued research is being carried out to study the actual cause and effect. The FDA has issued guidelines based on a review of all studies. See www.fda.gov; click on "Antidepressants."

BOX 21.4 HERBAL AND ALTERNATIVE THERAPIES

Patients being treated with SSRIs are at an increased risk of developing a severe reaction, including serotonin syndrome, as well as an increased sensitivity to light if they are also taking St. John's wort. Because this herbal therapy is often used to self-treat depression, it is important to forewarn any patient who is taking an SSRI not to combine it with taking St. John's wort.

Also caution patients that there is an increased risk of seizures if evening primrose is used with antidepressants, and patients should be cautioned against this combination. Interactions have also been reported when antidepressants are combined with ginkgo, ginseng, and valerian. Patients should be cautioned against using these herbs while taking antidepressants.

Pharmacokinetics:

Route	Onset	Peak
Oral	Slow	6–8 h

$T_{1/2}$: 2–4 weeks, metabolized in the liver, excreted in the urine and feces

Adverse effects: Headache, nervousness, insomnia, drowsiness, anxiety, tremor, dizziness, sweating, rash, nausea, vomiting, diarrhea, dry mouth, anorexia, sexual dysfunction, upper respiratory infections, weight loss, fever

Nursing Considerations for Patients Receiving Selective Serotonin Reuptake Inhibitors

Assessment: History and Examination

Screen for the following conditions, *which could be contraindications or cautions for use of the drug:* any known allergies to SSRIs; impaired liver or kidney function, *which could alter metabolism and excretion of the drug;* and diabetes mellitus. Find out whether female patients are pregnant or breast-feeding.

Include *screening for baseline status before beginning therapy and for any potential adverse effects.* Assess for the following: temperature and weight; skin color and lesions; affect, orientation, and reflexes; vision; blood pressure and pulse; respiratory rate and adventitious sounds; and bowel sounds on abdominal examination. Obtain renal and liver function tests (Critical Thinking Scenario 21-1).

Nursing Diagnoses

The patient receiving an SSRI may have the following nursing diagnoses related to drug therapy:

- Acute Pain related to GI, GU, CNS effects
- Disturbed Thought Processes and Disturbed Sensory Perception (Kinesthetic, Tactile) related to CNS effects
- Imbalanced Nutrition related to GI effects
- Deficient Knowledge regarding drug therapy

Implementation With Rationale

- Arrange for lower dosage in elderly patients and in those with renal or hepatic impairment *because of the potential for severe adverse effects.*
- Monitor patient for up to 4 weeks *to ascertain onset of full therapeutic effect before adjusting dosage.*
- Establish suicide precautions for severely depressed patients and limit the quantity of the drug dispensed *to decrease the risk of overdose.*
- Administer the drug once a day in the morning *to achieve optimal therapeutic effects.* If the dosage is increased or if the patient is having severe GI effects, the dosage can be divided.

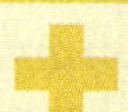

FOCUS ON PATIENT SAFETY

When administering medications, confusion about similar drug names may present a hazard, for example with *Celexa* (citalopram), *Celebrex* (celecoxib), *Xanax* (alprazolam), and *Cerebyx* (fosphenytoin). Use caution. Serious adverse effects have been reported as well as important loss of therapeutic effects when the wrong drug is given. If any of these drugs is ordered for your patient, make sure you know the indication for the drug, as well as the generic name of the prescribed drug.

- Suggest that patients use barrier contraceptives *to prevent pregnancy while taking this drug because serious fetal abnormalities can occur.*
- Provide comfort measures *to help patients tolerate drug effects.* These may include voiding before dosing, instituting a bowel program as needed, taking food with the drug if GI upset is severe, or environmental control (lighting, temperature, stimuli).
- Provide thorough patient teaching, including the drug name, prescribed dosage, measures for avoidance of adverse effects, and warning signs that may indicate possible problems. Instruct patients about the need for periodic monitoring and evaluation *to enhance patient knowledge about drug therapy and to promote compliance.*
- Offer support and encouragement *to help patients cope with the disease and the drug regimen.*

Evaluation

- Monitor patient response to the drug (alleviation of signs and symptoms of depression, OCD, bulimia, panic disorder).
- Monitor for adverse effects (sedation, dizziness, GI upset, respiratory dysfunction, GU problems, skin rash).
- Evaluate effectiveness of the teaching plan (patient can give the drug name, dosage, possible adverse effects to watch for, specific measures to help avoid

CRITICAL THINKING SCENARIO 21-1

Selective Serotonin Reuptake Inhibitors

The Situation

D.J., a 46-year-old married woman, complains of weight gain, malaise, fatigue, sleeping during the day, loss of interest in daily activities, and bouts of crying for no apparent reason. On examination, she weighs 8 pounds more than the standard weight for her height; all other findings are within normal limits. In conversation with a nurse, D.J. says that in the past 10 months, several events have occurred. She lost both of her parents, her only child graduated from high school and went away to college, her nephew died of renal failure, her one sister learned she had metastatic breast cancer, and she lost her job as a day care provider when the client family moved out of town. In addition, the family cat of 17 years was diagnosed with terminal leukemia. D.J. is prescribed fluoxetine (*Prozac*) and is given an appointment with a counselor.

Critical Thinking

What nursing interventions are appropriate at this time? What sort of crisis intervention would be most appropriate? *Balance the benefits of pointing out all of the losses and points of grief that you detect in D.J.'s story with the risks of upsetting her strained coping mechanisms.* What can D.J. expect to experience as a result of the SSRI therapy? How can you help D.J. cope during the lengthy period it takes to reach therapeutic effects? What other future interventions should be planned with D.J.?

Discussion

Many patients in severe crisis do not consciously identify the many things that are causing them stress. They have developed coping mechanisms to help them survive and cope with their day-to-day activities. However, D.J. seems to have reached her limit, and she exhibits many of the signs and symptoms of depression. However, it is important to make sure that she does not have some underlying medical condition that could be contributing to her complaints. Because of her age, she may also be perimenopausal, which could account for some of her problems.

It is hoped that the fluoxetine, an SSRI, will enable D.J. to regain her ability to cope and her normal affect. The drug should give her brain a chance to reach a new biochemical balance. Before she begins taking the fluoxetine, she should receive a written sheet listing the pertinent drug information, adverse effects to watch for, warning signs to report, and a telephone number to call in case she has questions later or just needs to talk. The written information is especially important because she may not remember drug-related discussions or instructions clearly.

Once the SSRI reaches therapeutic levels, which can take as long as 4 weeks, D.J. may start to feel like her "old self" and may be strong enough to begin dealing with all her grief. She may recover from her need for the SSRI over time, and use of the medication can then be discontinued.

Nursing Care Guide for D.J.: Fluoxetine

Assessment: History and Examination

Allergies to fluoxetine or any other antidepressant SSRI; renal or hepatic dysfunction; pregnancy or lactation; diabetes

Concurrent use of TCAs, cyproheptadine, lithium, MAO inhibitors, benzodiazepines, alcohol, other SSRIs

CV: blood pressure, pulse

CNS: orientation, affect, reflexes, vision

Skin: color, lesions, texture

Respiratory: respiration, adventitious sounds

GI: abdominal examination, bowel sounds

Laboratory tests: hepatic and renal function tests

Nursing Diagnoses

Acute Pain related to GI, GU, CNS effects

Disturbed Thought Processes related to CNS effects

Imbalanced Nutrition related to GI effects

Deficient Knowledge regarding drug therapy

Implementation

Administer drug in morning; divide doses if GI upset occurs.

Provide comfort, safety measures; small meals; void before dosing; side rails; pain medication as needed; suggest barrier contraceptive; limit dosage with potentially suicidal patients; lower dose with renal or hepatic impairment.

(continued)

Selective Serotonin Reuptake Inhibitors *(continued)*

Provide support and reassurance to help D.J. deal with drug effects (4-week delay in full effectiveness).

Provide patient teaching regarding drug dosage, adverse effect conditions to report, and the need to use barrier contraceptives.

Evaluation

Evaluate drug effects: relief of signs and symptoms of depression.

Monitor for adverse effects: sedation, dizziness, insomnia; respiratory dysfunction; GI upset; GU problems; rash.

Monitor for drug–drug interactions.

Evaluate effectiveness of patient teaching program.

Evaluate effectiveness of comfort and safety measures.

Patient Teaching for D.J.

☐ The drug that has been prescribed is called a selective serotonin reuptake inhibitor or SSRI. SSRIs change the concentration of serotonin in specific areas of the brain. An increase in serotonin level is believed to relieve depression.

☐ The drug should be taken once a day in the morning. If your dosage has been increased or if your are having stomach upset, the dose may be divided.

☐ It may take as long as 4 weeks before you feel the full effects of this drug. Continue to take the drug every day during that time so that the concentration of the drug in your body eventually reaches effective levels.

☐ Common side effects of SSRIs include the following:

- *Dizziness, drowsiness, nervousness, and insomnia:* If these effects occur, avoid driving or performing hazardous or delicate tasks that require concentration.
- *Nausea, vomiting and weight loss:* Small frequent meals may help. Monitor your weight loss; if it becomes excessive, consult your health care provider.
- *Sexual dysfunction and flu-like symptoms:* These effects may be temporary. Consult with your health care provider if these conditions become bothersome.
- Report any of the following conditions to your health care provider: *rash mania, seizures, and severe weight loss.*

☐ Tell your doctors, nurses, and other health care providers that you are taking this drug. Keep this drug and all medications out of the reach of children and pets. Do not take this drug during pregnancy because severe fetal abnormalities could occur. The use of barrier contraceptives is recommended while you are taking this drug. If you think that you are pregnant or would like to become pregnant, consult with your health care provider.

adverse effects, importance of continued follow-up, and importance of avoiding pregnancy).

- Monitor the effectiveness of comfort measures and compliance with the regimen.

Other Antidepressants

Some other effective antidepressants do not fit into any of the three groups that have been discussed in this chapter. These drugs have varying effects on NE, 5HT, and dopamine. Although it is not known how their actions are related to clinical efficacy, these agents may be most effective in treating depression in patients who do not respond to other antidepressants (Table 21.5). They may even be used before MAOIs or TCAs, which have many more adverse effects. Other antidepressants include the following:

- Bupropion (*Wellbutrin, Zyban*), which weakly blocks reuptake of NE, 5HT, and dopamine, is effective in the treatment of depression. At lower doses, this drug is effective in smoking cessation. It is well absorbed from the GI tract, metabolized in the liver, and excreted in the urine. There are no adequate studies done in pregnancy, and the drug should be used during pregnancy only if the benefits to the mother clearly outweigh the potential risks to the fetus. Bupropion does enter breast milk and should not be used by nursing mothers. The drug is available in a sustained-release formulation as well as an extended release formula, which some patients find to be more convenient.

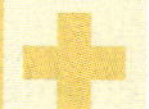

FOCUS ON PATIENT SAFETY

A situation similar to that posed by *Prozac* and *Sarafem* (described earlier) may occur with drugs by the trade name of *Wellbutrin* and *Zyban*, both of which are bupropion. *Wellbutrin* could be prescribed

Table 21.5 DRUGS IN FOCUS

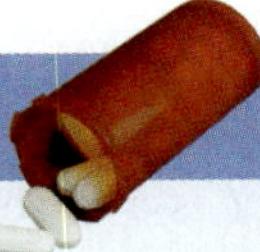

Other Antidepressants

Name	Usual Dosage	Usual Indication
bupropion (*Wellbutrin, Wellbutrin SR, Wellbutrin XL, Zyban*)	300 mg/day PO given in three doses; or 150 mg PO b.i.d. in sustained-release form or 150–300 mg/day as a single dose of extended-release form	Treatment of depression in adults, smoking cessation
mirtazapine (*Remeron*)	15 mg/day PO, may be increased to a maximum of 45 mg/day; reduce dosage in elderly and those with renal or hepatic dysfunction	Treatment of depression in adults
nefazodone (*generic*)	100 mg PO b.i.d., to a maximum of 600 mg/day; reduce dosage in elderly	Treatment of depression in adults
trazodone (*Desyrel*)	150 mg/day PO in divided doses; up to 600 mg/day, reduce dosage with the elderly Pediatric: 1.5–2 mg/kg/day PO in divided doses; do not exceed 6 mg/kg/day	Treatment of depression in adults and children 6–18 yr
venlafaxine (*Effexor, Effexor XR*)	75 mg/day PO in divided doses, to 375 mg/day; 75 mg/day PO sustained-release formulation to a maximum 225 mg/day; reduce dosage with hepatic and renal impairment	Treatment and prevention of depression in generalized anxiety disorder; social anxiety disorder

for a patient with depression and *Zyban* could be prescribed for the same patient by another health care provider to help the patient stop smoking. In such a case, the patient could inadvertently overdose on bupropion. It is very important that the patient knows the generic name as well as the brand name of the drug being ordered. Giving it to the patient in writing, with an explanation to share this information with all health care providers, could prevent serious medication errors from happening.

- Mirtazapine (*Remeron*) is used to treat depression. How its many anticholinergic effects relate to its antidepressive effects is not known. It is rapidly absorbed from the GI tract, extensively metabolized in the liver, and excreted in the urine. Mirtazapine has a half-life of 20 to 40 hours. Little is known about its effects in pregnancy and lactation, and it should be used during those times only if the benefit to the mother clearly outweighs the potential risk to the neonate.
- Nefazodone (*generic*), which is given twice daily, is effective in the treatment of some cases of depression. It has a short half-life of 2 to 4 hours. It is well absorbed from the GI tract, metabolized in the liver, and excreted in the urine. It has been associated with severe liver toxicity in some patients. Little is known about its effects in pregnancy and breast-feeding, and it should be used during those times only if the benefit to the mother clearly outweighs the potential risk to the fetus or neonate.
- Trazodone (*Desyrel*), which blocks 5HT and some 5HT precursor reuptake, is effective in some forms of depression but has many CNS effects associated with its use. It is readily absorbed from the GI tract, extensively metabolized in the liver, and excreted in urine and feces. Trazodone caused fetal abnormalities in animal studies and crosses into breast milk. It should be used during pregnancy and lactation only if the benefits to the mother clearly outweigh the potential risks to the fetus.
- Venlafaxine (*Effexor*) has fewer adverse CNS effects and is known to mildly block reuptake of NE, 5HT, and dopamine. It is very effective in treating some cases of depression, and its popularity has increased with the introduction of an extended-release form that does away with the multiple daily doses that are required with the regular form. It reportedly has good effects in decreasing addictive behaviors. Venlafaxine is readily absorbed from the GI tract, extensively metabolized in the liver, and excreted in urine. Adequate studies have not been done in pregnancy and lactation, and it should be used during those times only if the benefit to the mother clearly outweighs the potential risk to the neonate.

WEB LINKS

Health care providers and patients may want to consult the following Internet sources:

http://www.depression.com Information on depression including diagnosis, research, treatment.

http://www.depressionalliance.org Information on depression, signs and symptoms, community resources, support groups.

http://www.nimh.nih.gov/publicat/depressionmenu.cfm Information on women and depression.

http://teachhealth.com Information on education programs related to depression, stress, drug therapy, and so forth for patients and health professionals.

http://nimh.nih.gov Patient-oriented and professional information on issues related to mental health.

Points to Remember

- *Affect* is a term that refers to the feelings that people experience when they respond emotionally.
- Depression is an affective disorder characterized by overwhelming sadness, despair, and hopelessness that is inappropriate with respect to the event or events that precipitated the depression. Depression is a very common problem; it is associated with many physical manifestations and is often misdiagnosed. It could be that depression is caused by a series of events that are not yet understood.
- The biogenic amine theory states that depression is caused by a deficiency of the biogenic amines—norepinephrine (NE), serotonin (5HT), and dopamine—in certain key areas of the brain.
- Antidepressant drugs—TCAs, MAOIs, and SSRIs—increase the concentrations of the biogenic amines in the brain.
- Selection of an antidepressant depends on individual drug response and tolerance of associated adverse effects. The adverse effects of TCAs are sedating and anticholinergic; those of MAOIs are CNS related and sympathomimetic. The adverse effects of SSRIs are fewer, but they do cause CNS changes.
- Other antidepressants with unknown mechanisms of action are also effective in treating depression.

CHECK YOUR UNDERSTANDING

Answers to the questions in this chapter may be found in the Answer Key in the back of the book.

Multiple Choice

Select the best answer to the following.

1. The biogenic amine theory of depression states that depression is a result of
   a. an unpleasant childhood.
   b. GABA inhibition.
   c. deficiency of NE, dopamine, or 5HT in key areas of the brain.
   d. blockages within the limbic system, which controls emotions and affect.

2. When teaching a patient receiving tricyclic antidepressants (TCAs), it is important to remember that they are associated with many anticholinergic adverse effects. Teaching about these drugs should include anticipation of
   a. increased libido and increased appetite.
   b. polyuria and polydipsia.
   c. urinary retention, arrhythmias, and constipation.
   d. hearing changes, cataracts, and nightmares.

3. Adverse effects may limit the usefulness of TCAs with some patients. Nursing interventions that could alleviate some of the unpleasant aspects of these adverse effects include
   a. always administering the drug when the patient has an empty stomach.
   b. reminding the patient not to void before taking the drug.
   c. increasing the dosage to override the adverse effects.
   d. taking the major portion of the dose at bedtime to avoid experiencing drowsiness and the unpleasant anticholinergic effects.

4. You might question an order for an MAOI as a first step in the treatment of depression, remembering that these drugs are reserved for use in cases in which there has been no response to other agents because
   a. MAOIs can cause hair loss.
   b. MAOIs are associated with potentially serious drug–food interactions.
   c. MAOIs are mostly recommended for use in surgical patients.
   d. MAOIs are more expensive than other agents.

5. Your patient is being treated for depression and is started on a regimen of *Prozac* (fluoxetine). She calls you 10 days after the drug therapy has started to report that nothing has changed and she wants to try a different drug. You should
   a. try sertraline (*Zoloft*) because some patients respond to one SSRI and not another.
   b. ask her to try a few days without the drug to see whether there is any difference.
   c. add an MAOI to her drug regimen to get an increased antidepressant effect.
   d. encourage her to keep taking the drug as prescribed because it usually takes up to 4 weeks to see the full antidepressant effect.

6. The drug of choice for a patient with a documented obsessive–compulsive disorder who is also suffering from depression and occasional panic disorder would be
   a. *Celexa.*
   b. *Paxil.*
   c. *Luvox.*
   d. *Prozac.*

7. Venlafaxine (*Effexor*) is a relatively new antidepressant that might be very effective for use in patients who

a. have proven to be responsive to other antidepressants.
b. can tolerate multiple side effects.
c. are reliable at taking multiple daily dosings.
d. have not responded to other antidepressants and would benefit from once-a-day dosing.

8. Depression is an affective disorder that is
a. always precipitated by a specific event.
b. most common in patients with head injuries.
c. characterized by overwhelming sadness, despair, and hopelessness.
d. very evident and easy to diagnose in the clinical setting.

Multiple Response

Select all that apply.

1. Depression is a very common affective disorder that strikes many people. In assessing a client who might be suffering from depression, the nurse would expect to find which of the following?
a. Lack of energy
b. Hyperactivity
c. Sleep disturbances
d. Libido problems
e. Confusion
f. Decreased reflexes

2. A client reports that he thinks he is taking an antidepressant, but he is not sure. In reviewing his medication history, which of the following drugs would be considered antidepressants?
a. Tetracyclic drugs
b. Cholinergics
c. SSRIs
d. MAOIs
e. ARBs
f. Benzodiazepines

Word Scramble

Unscramble the following letters to form the names of commonly used antidepressants.

1. porbpnuio ______________________________

2. otlinuexfe ______________________________

3. mamicoprline ______________________________

4. flaxivenaen ______________________________

5. zipneehlne ______________________________

6. tnexopraei ______________________________

7. pimiminrae ______________________________

Fill in the Blank

1. The biogenic amines linked to depression include ____________, ____________, and ____________.

2. The MAOIs block the ____________ of norepinephrine, leading to an accumulation of that neurotransmitter in the ____________.

3. The SSRIs block the ____________ of serotonin, leading to an increase in that neurotransmitter near the receptor sites.

4. The tricyclic antidepressants are believed to reduce the reuptake of ____________ and ____________ in all nerves that produce those neurotransmitters.

5. Because of a risk of increased blood pressure, patients taking MAOIs should avoid foods high in ________________.

6. Fluoxetine, one of the first SSRIs approved for use in depression, is also approved for use in women with ________________.

7. ____________, used as an antidepressant, is also used to aid in smoking cessation.

8. Some of the drawbacks of tricyclic antidepressant therapy are the many ____________________ effects associated with the drugs, including dry mouth, urinary retention, and constipation.

Bibliography and References

Bailey, K. (1998). *Psychotropic drug facts.* Philadelphia: Lippincott-Raven.
Drug facts and comparisons. (2006). St. Louis: Facts and Comparisons.
Gilman, A., Hardman, J. G., & Limbird, L. E. (Eds.) (2006). *Goodman and Gilman's the pharmacological basis of therapeutics* (11th ed.). New York: McGraw-Hill.
Karch, A. M. (2006). *2007 Lippincott's nursing drug guide.* Philadelphia: Lippincott Williams & Wilkins.
Porth, C. M. (2005). *Pathophysiology: Concepts of altered health states* (7th ed.). Philadelphia: Lippincott Williams & Wilkins.
Professional's guide to patient drug facts. (2006). St. Louis: Facts and Comparisons.
Reports of suicidality in pediatric patients being treated with antidepressants for major depressive disorder. October 27, 2003, FDA Center for Drug Evaluation and Research: www.fda.gov/cder/drug/advisory.

CHAPTER 22

Psychotherapeutic Agents

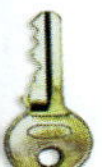

KEY TERMS

antipsychotic

attention-deficit disorder

major tranquilizer

mania

narcolepsy

neuroleptic

schizophrenia

LEARNING OBJECTIVES

Upon completion of this chapter, you will be able to:

1. Define the term psychotherapeutic agent and list conditions that the psychotherapeutic agents are used to treat.
2. Describe the therapeutic actions, indications, pharmacokinetics, contraindications, most common adverse reactions and important drug–drug interactions associated with each class of psychotherapeutic agent: typical antipsychotics, atypical antipsychotics, antimanics, central nervous system stimulants.
3. Discuss the use of psychotherapeutic agents across the lifespan.
4. Compare and contrast the prototype drugs for each class of psychotherapeutic agent with other drugs in that class and with drugs in the other classes of psychotherapeutic agents.
5. Outline the nursing considerations and teaching needs for patients receiving each class of psychotherapeutic agents.

ANTIPSYCHOTIC/NEUROLEPTIC DRUGS

Typical Antipsychotics

P chlorpromazine
fluphenazine
haloperidol
loxapine
molindone
perphenazine
pimozide
prochlorperazine
thioridazine
thiothixene
trifluoperazine

Atypical Antipsychotics

aripiprazole
P clozapine
olanzapine
quetiapine
risperidone
ziprasidone

ANTIMANIC DRUG

lithium

CENTRAL NERVOUS SYSTEM STIMULANTS

dexmethylphenidate
dextroamphetamine
P methylphenidate
modafinil
pemoline

The drugs discussed in this chapter are used to treat psychoses—perceptual and behavioral disorders. These psychotherapeutic drugs are targeted at thought processes rather than affective states. Although these drugs do not cure any of these disorders, they do help patients function in a more acceptable manner and carry on activities of daily living. These drugs are used in both adults and children (Box 22.1).

Mental Disorders and Their Classification

Mental disorders are now thought to be caused by some inherent dysfunction within the brain that leads to abnormal thought processes and responses. Most theories attribute these disorders to some sort of chemical imbalance in specific areas within the brain. Diagnosis of a mental disorder is often based on distinguishing characteristics described in the *Diagnostic and Statistical Manual of Mental Disorders,* 4th edition, text revision (*DSM-IV-TR*). Because no diagnostic laboratory tests are available, patient assessment and response must be carefully evaluated to determine the basis of a particular problem. Selected disorders are discussed here.

Schizophrenia, the most common type of psychosis, can be very debilitating and prevents affected individuals from functioning in society. Characteristics of schizophrenia include hallucinations, paranoia, delusions, speech abnormalities, and affective problems. This disorder, which seems to have a very strong genetic association, may reflect a fundamental biochemical abnormality.

Mania, with its associated bipolar illness (i.e., manic-depressive illness), is characterized by periods of extreme overactivity and excitement. Bipolar illness involves extremes of depression followed by hyperactivity and excitement. This condition may reflect a biochemical imbalance followed by overcompensation on the part of neurons and their inability to re-establish stability.

Narcolepsy is characterized by daytime sleepiness and sudden periods of loss of wakefulness. This disorder may reflect problems with stimulation of the brain by the reticular activating system (RAS) or problems with response to that stimulation.

Attention-deficit disorders involve various conditions characterized by an inability to concentrate on one activity for longer than a few minutes and a state of hyperkinesis. These conditions are usually diagnosed in school-aged children but can occur in adults.

BOX 22.1 **DRUG THERAPY ACROSS THE LIFESPAN**

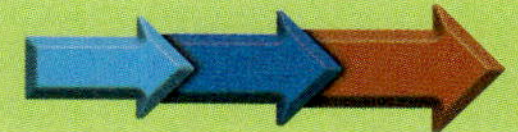

Psychotherapeutic Agents

CHILDREN

Many of these agents are used in children, often in combination with other central nervous system (CNS) drugs in an attempt to control symptoms and behavior. Long-term effects of many of these agents are not known, and parents should be informed of this fact.

Of the antipsychotics, chlorpromazine, haloperidol, pimozide, prochlorperazine, thioridazine, and trifluoperazine are the only ones with established pediatric regimens. The dose is often higher than that required for adults. The child should be monitored carefully for adverse effects and developmental progress.

Lithium does not have a recommended pediatric dose, and the drug should not ordinarily be used in children. If it is used, the dosage should be carefully calculated from the child's age and weight, and the child should be monitored very closely for renal, CNS, cardiovascular, and endocrine function.

The CNS stimulants are often used in children to manage various attention-deficit disorders. Caution should be used with extended-release preparations, because they differ markedly in timing and effectiveness. The child should be assessed carefully and challenged periodically for the necessity of continuing the drug.

ADULTS

Adults using these drugs should be under regular care and should be monitored regularly for adverse effects. The QTc interval should be evaluated before thioridazine, ziprasidone, or mesoridazine is prescribed and periodically during use.

Patients receiving lithium should be encouraged to maintain hydration and salt intake. They need to understand the importance of periodic monitoring of serum lithium levels.

These drugs should be used very cautiously during pregnancy and lactation because of the potential for adverse effects on the fetus or neonate. A woman maintained on one of these drugs needs to be counseled about the risk to the fetus versus the risk of returning symptoms if the drug is stopped. Use should be reserved for situations in which the benefits to the mother far outweigh the potential risks to the neonate. Women of childbearing age who need to take lithium should be advised to use barrier contraceptives while taking the drug because of the potential for serious congenital abnormalities.

OLDER ADULTS

Older patients may be more susceptible to the adverse effects of these drugs. Dosages of all of these drugs need to be reduced and patients monitored very closely for toxic effects and to provide safety measures if CNS effects do occur.

Patients with renal impairment should be monitored very closely while taking lithium. Decreased dosages may be needed. Because many older patients may also have renal impairment, they need to be screened carefully. They should be urged to maintain hydration and salt intake, which can be a challenge with some older patients.

Prolongation of the QTc interval, associated with use of thioridazine, ziprasidone, or mesoridazine, may be a concern in elderly patients with coronary disease. Careful screening and monitoring should be done if these drugs are needed for such patients.

Antipsychotic/ Neuroleptic Drugs

The **antipsychotic** drugs, which are essentially dopamine receptor blockers, are used to treat disorders that involve thought processes. Because of their associated neurological adverse effects, these medications are also called **neuroleptic** agents. At one time, these drugs were known as **major tranquilizers**. However, that name is no longer used because the primary action of these drugs is not sedation but a change in neuron stimulation and response (Figure 22.1).

Table 22.1 lists the antipsychotics in use today and gives information about their relative potencies and associated adverse effects. Any of these drugs may be effective in a particular patient; the selection of a specific drug depends on the desired potency and patient tolerance of the associated adverse effects. A patient who does not respond to one drug may react successfully to another agent. (Responses may also vary because of cultural issues [Box 22.2].) To determine the best therapeutic regimen for a particular patient, it may be necessary to try more than one drug.

Antipsychotics are classified as either typical or atypical. The classic, typical antipsychotics are primarily dopamine receptor blockers (which may be referred to as phenothiazines) that cause several adverse effects associated with dopamine blockade, including hypotension, anticholinergic effects, and extrapyramidal side effects (EPS). Newer, atypical antipsychotics block both dopamine receptors and serotonin receptors. This dual action may help alleviate some of the unpleasant neurological effects and depression associated with the typical antipsychotics.

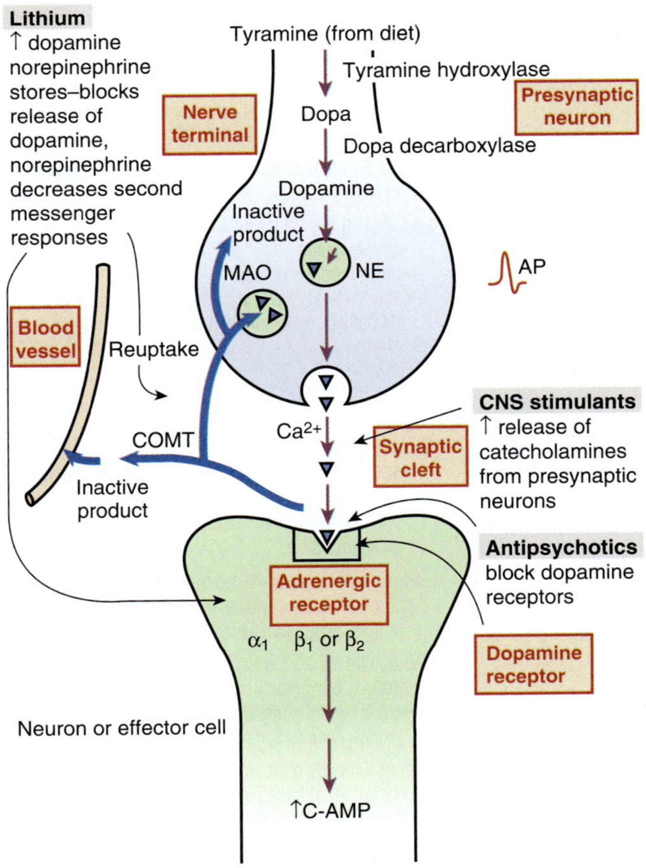

FIGURE 22.1 Sites of action of the drugs used to treat mental disorders: antipsychotics, central nervous system stimulants, lithium.

Therapeutic Actions and Indications

It is not understood which of the several actions of antipsychotics corrects the manifestations of schizophrenia. The typical antipsychotic drugs block dopamine receptors, preventing the stimulation of the postsynaptic neurons by dopamine. They also depress the RAS, limiting the stimuli coming into the brain, and they have anticholinergic, antihistamine, and alpha-adrenergic blocking effects, all related to the blocking of the dopamine receptor sites. Atypical antipsychotics block both dopamine and serotonin receptors. The antipsychotics are indicated for schizophrenia and for manifestations of other psychotic disorders, including hyperactivity, combative behavior, agitation in the elderly, and severe behavioral problems in children (short-term control).

Pharmacokinetics

The antipsychotics are erratically absorbed from the gastrointestinal (GI) tract, depending on the drug and the preparation of the drug. Intramuscular doses provide four to five times the active dose as oral doses, requiring caution if switching between routes. The antipsychotics are widely distributed in the tissues and are often stored in the tissues, being released for up to 6 months after the drug is stopped. They are metabolized in the liver and excreted through the bile and urine. Children tend to metabolize these drugs faster than do adults, and elderly patients tend to metabolize them more slowly. The antipsychotics cross the placenta and enter breast milk. They should not be used during pregnancy or lactation unless the benefit to the mother clearly outweighs the potential risk to the fetus or neonate.

Contraindications and Cautions

Antipsychotic drugs are contraindicated in the presence of underlying diseases *that could be exacerbated by the dopamine-blocking effects of these drugs.* They are also contraindicated in the following conditions, *which can be exacerbated by the drugs:* central nervous system (CNS) depression, circulatory collapse, Parkinson's disease, coronary disease, severe hypotension, bone marrow suppression, and blood dyscrasias. Prolongation of the QTc interval is a contraindication to the use of mesoridazine, thioridazine, and ziprasidone, all of which can further prolong the QTc interval, *leading to increased risk of serious cardiac arrhythmias.*

Table 22.1 Antipsychotics/Neuroleptics, Indicating Side Effects Most Frequently Associated With Each Drug

Drug Name	Potency	Common Side Effects: *Sedation*	*Anticholinergic*	*Hypotension*	*Extrapyramidal*	Usual Dosage
Typical Antipsychotics						
chlorpromazine (*Thorazine*)	Low	++++	+++	+++	++	Adult: 25 mg IM for acute episode, may be repeated; switch to 25–50 mg PO t.i.d. Pediatric: 0.5–1 mg/kg q4–8h PO, IM, or PR
fluphenazine (*Prolixin*)	High	+	+	+	++++	Adult: 0.5–10 mg/day PO in divided doses; 1.25–10 mg/day IM in divided doses Geriatric: 1–2.5 mg/day PO, adjust dose based on response
haloperidol (*Haldol*)	High	+	+/–	+	++++	Adult: 0.5–2 mg PO t.i.d. or 2–5 mg IM, may be repeated in 1 h, 4–8 h more common Geriatric: reduce dosage Pediatric (3–12 yr): 0.5 mg/day PO; 0.05–0.075 mg/kg/day PO for Tourette's syndrome and behavioral syndromes
loxapine (*Loxitane*)	Medium	+++	++	++	+++	Adult: 20–60 mg/day PO; 12.5–50 mg IM or IV for acute states
molindone (*Moban*)	Medium	+	++	+/–	+	Adult: initially 50–75 mg/day PO, maintenance at 5–25 mg PO t.i.d. to q.i.d.
perphenazine (*Trilafon*)	Medium	++	+	++	+++	Adult: 4–8 mg PO t.i.d. or 5–10 mg IM q6h; switch to oral as soon as possible Geriatric: one-half to one-third of adult dose
pimozide (*Orap*)	High	+	+	++	+++	Adult: 1–2 mg/day PO in divided doses Pediatric (>12 yr): 0.05 mg/kg PO at bedtime; do not exceed 10 mg/day
prochlorperazine (*Compazine*)	Low	+	++	+	+++	Adult: 5–10 mg PO t.i.d. to q.i.d.; 10–20 mg IM for acute states Geriatric: reduce dosage Pediatric: 2.5 mg PO t.i.d.; 0.03 mg/kg IM for acute states; 20–25 mg/day PR
thioridazine (*generic*)	Low	++++	+++	+++	+	Adult: 50–100 mg PO t.i.d., monitor QTc intervals Pediatric: up to 3 mg/kg/day PO
thiothixene (*Navane*)	High	+	+	+	++++	Adult: 2 mg PO t.i.d.; up to a maximum 60 mg/day in severe cases
trifluoperazine (*generic*)	High	+	+	+	++++	Adult: 2–5 mg PO b.i.d.; 1–2 mg IM q4–6h in severe cases Geriatric: reduce dosage Pediatric (6–12 yr): 1 mg PO daily or b.i.d.: 1 mg IM daily or b.i.d. for severe cases
Atypical Antipsychotics						
aripiprazole (*Abilify*)	Medium	+	+	++	+	Adult: 10–15 mg/day PO
clozapine (*Clozaril*)	Low	++++	++	+++	+/–	Adult: initially 25 mg PO b.i.d. to t.i.d.; up to 500 mg/day; available only through the *Clozaril* Patient Management System, which monitors WBC and compliance issues, only 1-wk supply given at a time
olanzapine (*Zyprexa, Zyprexa Zydis*)	High	++++	++	+++	+	Adult: 5–10 mg/day PO, up to 20 mg/day PO for bipolar mania; available in disintegrating tablets, which can be taken without swallowing
quetiapine (*Seroquel*)	Medium	++++	++	++	+/–	Adult: initially 25 mg PO b.i.d., up to 300–400 mg/day Geriatric: hepatic impairment or hypotensives; reduce dosage and titrate very slowly
risperidone (*Risperdal*)	High	+++	+	++	++	Adult: 1 mg PO b.i.d. up to 8 mg/day Geriatric: renal impaired hypotensives; 0.5 mg PO b.i.d. initially, titrate slowly
ziprasidone (*Geodon*)	Medium	+++	++	+	+	Adult: 20–80 mg PO b.i.d.; rapid control of as stated behavior: 10–20 mg IM, maximum dose 40 mg/day IM; monitor QTc intervals

Each + indicates increased incidence of that adverse effect.

BOX 22.2 CULTURAL CONSIDERATIONS FOR DRUG THERAPY

Antipsychotic Drugs

The ways in which patients in certain cultural groups respond to antipsychotic drugs—either physiologically or emotionally—may vary. Therefore, when a pharmacological regimen is incorporated into overall patient care, health care providers must consider and respect an individual patient's cultural beliefs and needs.

- African Americans respond more rapidly to antipsychotic medications and have a greater risk for development of disfiguring adverse effects, such as tardive dyskinesia. Consequently, these patients should be started off at the lowest possible dose and monitored closely. African Americans also display a higher red blood cell plasma lithium ratio than Caucasians do, and they report more adverse effects from lithium therapy. These patients should be monitored closely because they have a higher potential for lithium toxicity at standard therapeutic ranges.
- Patients in Asian countries, such as India, Turkey, Malaysia, China, Japan, and Indonesia, receive lower doses of neuroleptics and lithium to achieve the same therapeutic response as seen in patients in the United States. This may be related to these individuals' lower body mass as well as metabolic differences, and it may have implications for dosing protocols for patients in these ethnic groups who undergo therapy in the United States.
- Arab American patients metabolize antipsychotic medications more slowly than Asian Americans do and may require lower doses to achieve the same therapeutic effects as in Caucasians.
- Individuals in some cultures use herbs and other folk remedies, and the use of herbs may interfere with the metabolism of Western medications. The nurse should carefully assess for herbal use and be aware of potential interactions.

Caution should be used in the presence of medical conditions *that could be exacerbated by the anticholinergic effects of the drugs,* such as glaucoma, peptic ulcer, and urinary or intestinal obstruction. In addition, care should be taken in patients with seizure disorders *because the threshold for seizures could be lowered;* in those with thyrotoxicosis *because of the possibility of severe neurosensitivity;* and in active alcoholism *because of potentiation of the CNS depression.*

Other situations that warrant caution include myelography within the last 24 hours or scheduled within the next 48 hours *because severe neuron reaction to the dye used in these tests can occur,* and pregnancy or lactation *because of the potential of adverse effects on the fetus or neonate.* Because children are more apt to develop dystonia from the drugs, *which could confuse the diagnosis of Reye's syndrome,* caution should be used with children younger than 12 years of age who have a CNS infection or chickenpox. *The use of antipsychotics may result in bone marrow suppression, leading to blood dyscrasias,* so care should be taken with patients who are immunosuppressed and those who have cancer.

Adverse Effects

The adverse effects associated with the antipsychotic drugs are related to their dopamine-blocking, anticholinergic, antihistamine, and alpha-adrenergic activities. The most common CNS effects are sedation, weakness, tremor, drowsiness, and extrapyramidal effects—pseudoparkinsonism, dystonia, akathisia, tardive dyskinesia, and potentially irreversible neuroleptic malignant syndrome (Figure 22.2). Anticholinergic effects include dry mouth, nasal congestion, flushing, constipation, urinary retention, sexual impotence, glaucoma, blurred vision, and photophobia. Cardiovascular (CV) effects, which are probably related to the dopamine-blocking effects, include hypotension, orthostatic hypotension, cardiac arrhythmias, congestive heart failure, and pulmonary edema. Several of these agents (thioridazine, mesoridazine, ziprasidone) are associated with prolongation of the QTc interval, which could lead to serious or even fatal cardiac arrhythmias. Patients receiving these drugs should have a baseline and periodic electrocardiogram (ECG) during therapy. In late 2003, the U.S. Food and Drug Administration (FDA) required that all of the atypical antipsychotics include warnings that there is a risk for the development of diabetes mellitus when these drugs are used. Consequently, when patients are maintained on any of the atypical antipsychotics, they should be monitored regularly for the signs and symptoms of diabetes mellitus. In 2005, the FDA issued a public health advisory regarding the use of antipsychotics. Postmarketing studies showed that when these drugs were used to control behavioral symptoms of dementia in older adults, the patients being treated experienced increased cardiovascular events and death. None of these drugs is approved for this use, but it was common practice in many settings to use them, off-label, to establish behavioral control of patients with dementia. The manufacturers of all of these drugs sent out "Dear Health Care Provider" letters to remind health care providers that this is not an approved use and to alert them of the risk for death if they used the drug in this way. The FDA also requested that a black-box warning be placed on the prescribing information of the antipsychotic drugs, outlining this safety information.

Respiratory effects such as laryngospasm, dyspnea, and bronchospasm may also occur. The phenothiazines (chlorpromazine, fluphenazine, prochlorperazine, promethazine, and thioridazine) often turn the urine pink to reddish-brown as a result of their excretion. Although this effect may cause great patient concern, it has no clinical significance. In addition, bone marrow suppression is a possibility with some antipsychotic agents.

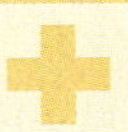

FOCUS ON PATIENT SAFETY

Name confusion has been reported between chlorpromazine (an antipsychotic) and chlorpropamide (an antidiabetic agent). Serious adverse effects have occurred. Manufacturers of these two drugs have been working to make the labels of the drugs very distinctive

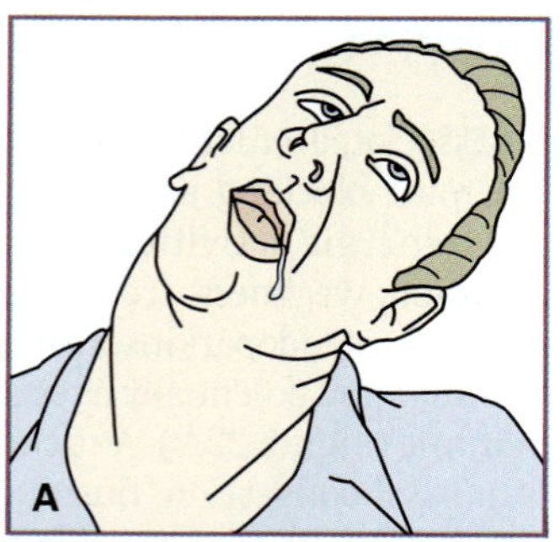

A. Dystonia—spasms of the tongue, neck, back, and legs. Spasms may cause unnatural positioning of the neck, abnormal eye movements, excessive salivation.

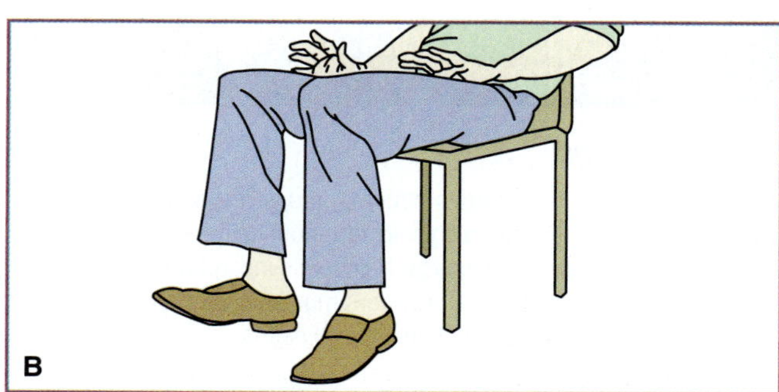

B. Akathisia—continuous restlessness, inability to sit still. Constant moving, foot tapping, hand movements may be seen.

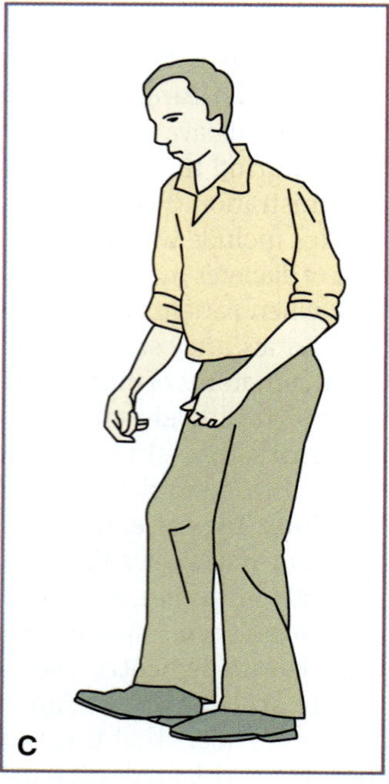

C. Pseudoparkinsonism—muscle tremors, cogwheel rigidity, drooling, shuffling gait, slow movements.

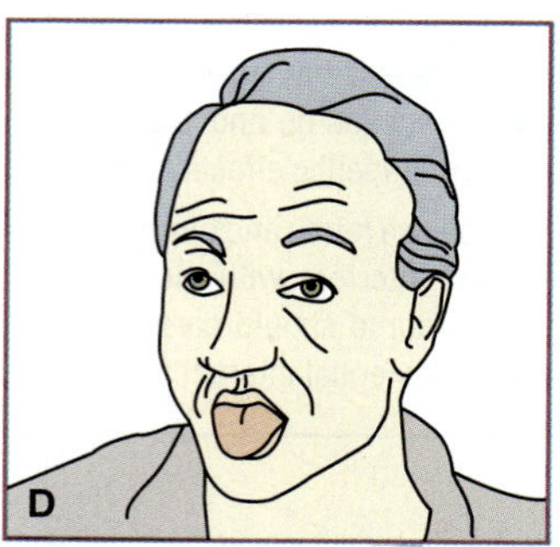

D. Tardive dyskinesia—abnormal muscle movements such as lip smacking, tongue darting, chewing movements, slow and aimless arm and leg movements.

FIGURE 22.2 Common neurological effects of antipsychotic drugs.

to help alleviate some of these errors. If your patient is prescribed chlorpromazine, make sure the patient is aware of the name of the drug, its intended use, and what it should look like.

Clinically Important Drug–Drug Interactions

Because the combination of antipsychotics with beta-blockers may lead to an increase in the effect of both drugs, this combination should be avoided if possible. Antipsychotic-alcohol combinations result in an increased risk of CNS depression, and antipsychotic–anticholinergic combinations lead to increased anticholinergic effects, so dosage adjustments are necessary. Patients who take either of these combinations should be monitored closely for adverse effects, and supportive measures should be provided. Patients should not take mesoridazine, thioridazine, or ziprasidone with any other drug that is associated with prolongation of the QTc interval. See Box 22.3 for a potential drug–herb interaction.

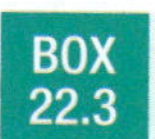

BOX 22.3 HERBAL AND ALTERNATIVE THERAPIES

Evening Primrose

Patients with schizophrenia should be advised to avoid the use of evening primrose. This herb has been associated with increased symptoms and CNS hyperexcitability.

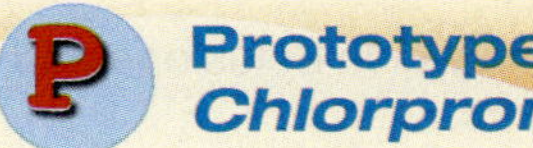

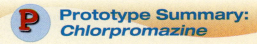

Prototype Summary: *Chlorpromazine*

Indications: Management of manifestations of psychotic disorders; relief of preoperative restlessness; adjunctive treatment of tetanus; acute intermittent porphyria; severe behavioral problems in children; control of hiccups, nausea, and vomiting

Actions: Blocks postsynaptic dopamine receptors in the brain; depresses those parts of the brain involved in wakefulness and emesis; anticholinergic; antihistaminic; alpha-adrenergic blocking

Pharmacokinetics:

Route	Onset	Peak	Duration
Oral	30–60 min	2–4 h	4–6 h
IM	10–15 min	15–20 min	4–6 h

$T_{1/2}$: 2 hours, then 30 hours; metabolized in the liver, excreted in the urine

Adverse effects: Drowsiness, insomnia, vertigo, extrapyramidal symptoms, orthostatic hypotension, photophobia, blurred vision, dry mouth, nausea, vomiting, anorexia, urinary retention, photosensitivity

Prototype Summary: *Clozapine*

Indications: Management of severely ill schizophrenics who are unresponsive to standard drugs; reduction of risk of recurrent suicidal behavior in patients with schizophrenia or schizoaffective disorder

Actions: Blocks dopamine and serotonin receptors; depresses the RAS; anticholinergic; antihistaminic; alpha-adrenergic blocking

Pharmacokinetics:

Route	Onset	Peak	Duration
Oral	Varies	1–6 h	Weeks

$T_{1/2}$: 4–12 hours; metabolized in the liver, excreted in the urine and feces

Adverse effects: Drowsiness, sedation, seizures, dizziness, syncope, headache, tachycardia, nausea, vomiting, fever, neuroleptic malignant syndrome

Nursing Considerations for Patients Receiving Antipsychotic/Neuroleptic Drugs

Assessment: History and Examination

Screen for the following conditions, *which could be contraindications or cautions for the use of the drug:* any known allergies to these drugs, severe CNS depression, circulatory collapse, coronary disease including prolonged QTc interval, brain damage, severe hypotension, glaucoma, respiratory depression, urinary or intestinal obstruction, thyrotoxicosis, seizure disorder, bone marrow suppression, pregnancy or lactation, and myelography within the past 24 hours or scheduled in the next 48 hours. In children younger than 12 years of age, screen for CNS infections.

Include screening *for baseline status before beginning therapy and for any potential adverse effects.* Assess the following: temperature; skin color and lesions; CNS orientation, affect, reflexes, and bilateral grip strength; bowel sounds and reported output; pulse, auscultation, and blood pressure, including orthostatic blood pressure; respiration rate and adventitious sounds; and urinary output. Obtain liver and renal function tests, thyroid function tests, ECG if appropriate, and complete blood count (CBC).

Nursing Diagnoses

The patient receiving antipsychotics may have the following nursing diagnoses related to drug therapy:

- Impaired Physical Mobility related to extrapyramidal effects
- Decreased Cardiac Output related to hypotensive effects
- Risk for Injury related to CNS effects and sedation
- Impaired Urinary Elimination related to anticholinergic effects
- Deficient Knowledge regarding drug therapy

Implementation With Rationale

- Do not allow the patient to crush or chew sustained-release capsules, *which will decrease their absorption and effectiveness.*
- If the patient receives parenteral forms, keep the patient recumbent for 30 minutes *to reduce the risk of orthostatic hypotension.*
- Consider warning the patient or the patient's guardians about the risk of development of tardive dyskinesias with continued use *so they are prepared for that neurological change.*

- Monitor CBC *to arrange to discontinue the drug at signs of bone marrow suppression.*
- Arrange for gradual dose reduction after long-term use. *Abrupt withdrawal has been associated with gastritis, nausea, vomiting, dizziness, arrhythmias, and insomnia.*
- Provide positioning of legs and arms *to decrease the discomfort of dyskinesias.*
- Provide sugarless candy and ice chips *to increase secretions* and frequent mouth care *to prevent dry mouth from becoming a problem.*
- Encourage the patient to void before taking a dose *if urinary hesitancy or retention is a problem.*
- Provide safety measures such as siderails and assistance with ambulation if CNS effects or orthostatic hypotension occurs *to prevent patient injury.*
- Provide for vision examinations *to determine ocular changes and arrange appropriate dosage change.*
- Provide thorough patient teaching, including drug name, prescribed dosage, measures for avoidance of adverse effects, warning signs that may indicate possible problems, and the need for monitoring and evaluation *to enhance patient knowledge about drug therapy and to promote compliance.* (Refer to Critical Thinking Scenario 22-1.) Warn patients that urine may have a pink to reddish-brown color.
- Offer support and encouragement *to help patients cope with their drug regimen.*

Evaluation

- Monitor patient response to the drug (decrease in signs and symptoms of psychotic disorder).
- Monitor for adverse effects (sedation, anticholinergic effects, hypotension, extrapyramidal effects, bone marrow suppression).
- Evaluate effectiveness of teaching plan (patient can give the drug name and dosage, possible adverse effects to watch for, specific measures to prevent adverse effects, and warning signs to report).
- Monitor the effectiveness of comfort measures and compliance with the regimen (see Critical Thinking Scenario 22-1).

FOCUS POINTS

- Mental disorders are thought process disorders possibly cased by brain dysfunction. A psychosis is a thought disorder, and schizophrenia is the most common psychosis in which delusions and hallucinations are hallmarks.
- Antipsychotic drugs are dopamine-receptor blockers that are effective in helping people to organize thought patterns and to respond appropriately to stimuli.
- Antipsychotics can cause hypotension, anticholinergic effects, sedation, and extrapyramidal effects, including parkinsonism, ataxia, and tremors.

Antimanic Drugs

Mania, the opposite of depression, occurs in individuals with bipolar disorder, who experience a period of depression followed by a period of mania. The cause of mania is not understood, but it is thought to be an overstimulation of certain neurons in the brain. The mainstay for treatment of mania is lithium (Table 22.2).

Lithium salts (*Lithane, Lithotabs*) are taken orally for the management of manic episodes and prevention of future episodes. These very toxic drugs can cause severe CNS, renal, and pulmonary problems that may lead to death. Despite the potential for serious adverse effects, lithium is used with caution because it is consistently effective in the treatment of mania. The therapeutically effective serum level is 0.6 to 1.2 mEq/L.

In 2003, the FDA approved the use of lamotrigine (*Lamictal*), an antiepileptic agent, for the long-term maintenance of bipolar disorder. Studies have found that lamotrigine use decreases the occurrence of acute mood episodes. Lamotrigine is discussed in Chapter 23. Also approved was the use of olanzapine (*Zyprexa*), aripiprazole (*Abilify*), and ziprasidone (*Geodon*), atypical antipsychotics, for the short-term management of acute manic episodes of bipolar disorder in combination with lithium and valproate. Quetiapine (*Seroquel*), also an atypical antipsychotic, was also approved as an adjunct or as monotherapy for the treatment of manic episodes associated with bipolar disorder. These new approvals were the first advances since the 1970s in the treatment of bipolar disorder.

Therapeutic Actions and Indications

Lithium functions in several ways. It alters sodium transport in nerve and muscle cells; inhibits the release of norepinephrine and dopamine, but not serotonin, from stimulated neurons; increases the intraneuronal stores of norepinephrine and dopamine slightly; and decreases intraneuronal content of second messengers. This last mode of action may allow it to selectively modulate the responsiveness of hyperactive neurons that might contribute to the manic state. Although

CRITICAL THINKING SCENARIO 22-1

Antipsychotic Drugs

The Situation

B.A., a 36-year-old, single, professional woman, was diagnosed with chronic schizophrenia when she was a senior in high school. Her condition has been well controlled with chlorpromazine (*Thorazine*), and she is able to maintain steady employment, live in her own home, and carry on a fairly active social life. At her last evaluation, she appeared to be developing bone marrow suppression, and her physician decided to try to taper the drug dosage. As the dosage was being lowered, B.A. became withdrawn and listless, missed several days of work, and canceled most of her social engagements. Afraid of interacting with people, she stayed in bed most of the time. She reported having thoughts of death and paranoid ideation about her neighbors that she was beginning to think might be true.

Critical Thinking

What nursing interventions are appropriate at this time?

What supportive measures might be useful to help B.A. cope with this crisis and allow her to function normally again?

What happens to brain chemistry after long-term therapy with phenothiazines?

What drug options should be tried?

Are there any other options that might be useful?

Discussion

Schizophrenia is not a disorder that can be resolved simply with proper counseling. B.A., an educated woman with a long history of taking phenothiazines, realizes the necessity of drug therapy to correct the chemical imbalance in her brain. She may need a high-potency antipsychotic to return her to the level of functioning she had reached before experiencing this setback. Her knowledge of her individual responses can be used to help select an appropriate drug and dosage. Her experiences may also facilitate her care planning and new drug regimen.

B.A. will need support to cope with problems at work—from her inability to go in to work, to coping with feelings about not meeting her social obligations, to finding the motivation to get up and become active again. She might do well with behavior modification techniques that give her some control over her activities and allow her to use her knowledge and experience with her own situation to her advantage in forming a new medical regimen. She may need support in explaining her problem to her employer and her social contacts in ways that will help her avoid the prejudice associated with mental illness and will allow her every opportunity to return to her regular routine as soon as she can.

Because it may take several months to find the drug or drugs that will bring B.A. back to a point of stabilization, it is important to have a consistent, reliable health care team in place to support her through this stabilization period. She should have a reliable contact person to call when she has questions and when she needs support.

Nursing Care Guide for B.A.: Antipsychotic/Neuroleptic Drugs

Assessment: History and Examination

Allergies to any of these drugs; CNS depression; CV disease; pregnancy or lactation; myelography; glaucoma; hypotension; thyrotoxicosis; seizures

Concurrent use of anticholinergics, barbiturate anesthetics, alcohol, meperidine, beta blockers, epinephrine, norepinephrine, guanethidine

CV: blood pressure, pulse, orthostatic blood pressure

CNS: orientation, affect, reflexes, vision

Skin: color, lesions, texture

Respiratory: respiration, adventitious sounds

GI: abdominal examination, bowel sounds

Laboratory tests: thyroid, liver and renal function tests, CBC

Nursing Diagnoses

Impaired Physical Mobility related to extrapyramidal effects

Risk for Injury related to CNS effects

Decreased Cardiac Output related to CV effects

Impaired Urinary Elimination related to anticholinergic effects

Deficient Knowledge regarding drug therapy

(continued)

Antipsychotic Drugs *(continued)*

Implementation

Give drug in evening; do not allow patient to chew or crush sustained-release capsules.

Provide comfort and safety measures: void before dosing; raise siderails; provide sugarless lozenges, mouth care; institute safety measures if CNS effects occur; position patient to relieve dyskinesia discomfort; taper dosage after long-term therapy.

Provide support and reassurance to help patient cope with drug effects.

Teach patient about drug, dosage, adverse effects, conditions to report, and precautions.

Evaluation

Evaluate drug effects: relief of signs and symptoms of psychotic disorders.

Monitor for adverse effects: sedation, dizziness, insomnia; anticholinergic effects; extrapyramidal effects; bone marrow suppression; skin rash.

Monitor for drug–drug interactions as listed.

Evaluate effectiveness of patient teaching program.

Evaluate effectiveness of comfort and safety measures.

Patient Teaching for B.A.

- ☐ The drugs that are useful for treating schizophrenia are called antipsychotic or neuroleptic drugs. These drugs affect the activities of certain chemicals in your brain and are used to treat certain mental disorders.
- ☐ Drugs in this group should be taken exactly as prescribed. Because these drugs affect many body systems, it is important that you have medical checkups regularly.
- ☐ Common effects of these drugs include:
  - *Dizziness, drowsiness, and fainting:* Avoid driving or performing hazardous tasks or delicate tasks that require concentration if these occur. Change position slowly. The dizziness usually passes after 1 to 2 weeks of drug use.
  - *Pink or reddish urine (with phenothiazines):* These drugs sometimes cause urine to change color. Do not be alarmed by this change; it does not mean that your urine contains blood.
  - *Sensitivity to light:* Bright light might hurt your eyes and sunlight might burn your skin more easily. Wear sunglasses and protective clothing when you must be out in the sun.
  - *Constipation:* Consult with your health care provider if this becomes a problem.
  - Report any of the following conditions to your health care provider: *sore throat, fever, rash, tremors, weakness, and vision changes.*
- ☐ Tell any doctor, nurse, or other health care provider that you are taking this drug.
- ☐ Keep this drug and all medications out of the reach of children.
- ☐ Avoid the use of alcohol or other depressants while you are taking this drug. You also may want to limit your use of caffeine if you feel very tense or cannot sleep.
- ☐ Avoid the use of over-the-counter drugs while you are on this drug. Many of them contain ingredients that could interfere with the effectiveness of your drug. If you feel that you need one of these preparations, consult with your health care provider about the most appropriate choice.
- ☐ Take this drug exactly as prescribed. If you run out of medicine or find that you cannot take your drug for any reason, consult your health care provider. After this drug has been used for a period of time, additional adverse effects may occur if it is suddenly stopped. This drug dosage will need to be tapered over time.

the biochemical actions of lithium are known, the exact mechanism of action in decreasing the manifestations of mania are not understood.

Lithium is indicated for the treatment of manic episodes of manic-depressive or bipolar illness and for maintenance therapy to prevent or diminish the frequency and intensity of future manic episodes. This agent is currently being investigated for the improvement of neutrophil counts in patients with cancer chemotherapy-induced neutropenia and as prophylaxis of cluster headaches and migraine headaches.

Pharmacokinetics

Lithium is readily absorbed from the GI tract, reaching peak levels in 30 minutes to 3 hours. It follows the same distribution pattern in the body as water. It slowly crosses the blood–brain barrier. Lithium is excreted from the kidney, although about 80% is reabsorbed. During periods of sodium depletion or dehydration, the kidney reabsorbs more lithium into the serum, often leading to toxic levels. Therefore, patients must be encouraged to maintain hydration while taking this

Table 22.2 DRUGS IN FOCUS

Antimanic Drugs

Drug Name	Dosage/Route	Usual Indications
aripiprazole (*Abilify*)	30 mg/day PO	Treatment of acute manic and mixed episodes of bipolar disorders
lamotrigine (*Lamictal*)	25 mg/day PO	Long-term maintenance of bipolar disorders
lithium (*Lithotabs, Lithobid*)	600 mg PO t.i.d. for acute episodes; 300 mg PO t.i.d. to q.i.d. for maintenance; reduce dosage with elderly patients	Treatment of manic episodes of manic-depressive illness; maintenance therapy to prevent or diminish the frequency and intensity of future manic episodes; not recommended for children <12 yr
olanzapine (*Zyprexa, Zyprexa Zydis*)	10 mg/day PO; range 5–20 mg/day	Short-term management of acute manic episodes associated with bipolar disorder, in combination with lithium or valproate
quetiapine (*Seroquel*)	50 mg PO b.i.d., titrate to a maximum 800 mg/day	Adjunct or monotherapy for the treatment of manic episodes associated with bipolar disorder
ziprasidone (*Geodon*)	40 mg PO b.i.d. with food	Treatment of acute manic and mixed episodes of bipolar disorders

drug. Lithium crosses the placenta and has been associated with congenital abnormalities. Women of childbearing age should be advised to use birth control while taking this drug. It also enters breast milk and can cause toxic effects in the baby. Breastfeeding should be discontinued while using lithium.

Contraindications and Cautions

Lithium is contraindicated in the presence of hypersensitivity to lithium. In addition, it is contraindicated in the following conditions: significant renal or cardiac disease *that could be exacerbated by the toxic effects of the drug;* a history of leukemia; metabolic disorders, including sodium depletion; dehydration; and diuretic use *because lithium depletes sodium reabsorption, and severe hyponatremia may occur.* (Hyponatremia leads to lithium retention and toxicity.) Pregnancy and lactation are also contraindications *because of the potential for adverse effects on the fetus or neonate.* Caution should be used in any condition *that could alter sodium levels,* such as protracted diarrhea or excessive sweating; with suicidal or impulsive patients; and in patients who have infection with fever, *which could be exacerbated by the toxic effects of the drug.*

Adverse Effects

The adverse effects associated with lithium are directly related to serum levels of the drug.

- *Serum levels of less than 1.5 mEq/L:* CNS problems, including lethargy, slurred speech, muscle weakness, and fine tremor; polyuria, which relates to renal toxicity; and beginning of gastric toxicity, with nausea, vomiting, and diarrhea
- *Serum levels of 1.5 to 2 mEq/L:* Intensification of all of the above reactions, with ECG changes
- *Serum levels of 2 to 2.5 mEq/L:* Possible progression of CNS effects to ataxia, clonic movements, hyperreflexia, and seizures; possible CV effects such as severe ECG changes and hypotension; large output of dilute urine secondary to renal toxicity; fatalities secondary to pulmonary toxicity
- *Serum levels greater than 2.5 mEq/L:* Complex multi-organ toxicity, with a significant risk of death

Clinically Important Drug–Drug Interactions

Some drug–drug combinations should be avoided. A lithium–haloperidol combination may result in an encephalopathic syndrome, consisting of weakness, lethargy, confusion, tremors, extrapyramidal symptoms, leukocytosis, and irreversible brain damage.

If lithium is given with carbamazepine increased CNS toxicity may occur, and a lithium–iodide salt combination results in an increased risk of hypothyroidism. Patients who receive either of these combinations should be monitored carefully. In addition, a thiazide diuretic–lithium combination increases the risk of lithium toxicity because of the loss of sodium and increased retention of lithium. If this combination is used, the dosage of lithium should be decreased and the patient should be monitored closely.

In the following instances, the serum lithium level should be monitored closely and appropriate dosage adjustments made. With the combination of lithium and some urine-alkalinizing drugs, including antacids and tromethamine, there is a possibility of decreased effectiveness of

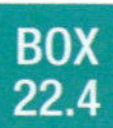

BOX 22.4 HERBAL AND ALTERNATIVE THERAPIES

Psyllium

Patients being treated with lithium should be encouraged not to use the herbal therapy psyllium, which is used to treat constipation and to lower cholesterol levels. If combined with lithium, the absorption of the lithium may be blocked and the patient will not receive therapeutic levels. If the patient feels a need for a drug to relieve constipation, or is concerned about cholesterol levels, he or she should be encouraged to discuss alternative measures with the health care provider.

lithium. If lithium is combined with indomethacin or with some nonsteroidal anti-inflammatory drugs, higher plasma levels of lithium occur. See Box 22.4 for a common drug–herbal therapy interaction.

Nursing Considerations for Patients Receiving an Antimanic Drug

Assessment: History and Examination

Screen for the following conditions, *which could be contraindications or cautions for the use of the drug:* any known allergies to lithium; renal or CV disease; dehydration; sodium depletion, use of diuretics, protracted sweating, or diarrhea; suicidal or impulsive patients with severe depression; pregnancy or lactation; and infection with fever.

Include screening *for baseline status before beginning therapy and for any potential adverse effects.* Assess the following: temperature; skin color and lesions; CNS orientation, affect, and reflexes; bowel sounds and reported output; pulse, auscultation, and blood pressure, including orthostatic blood pressure; respiration rate and adventitious sounds; and urinary output. Obtain liver and renal function tests, thyroid function tests, CBC, and baseline ECG, and obtain serum lithium levels as appropriate.

Nursing Diagnoses

The patient receiving lithium may have the following nursing diagnoses related to drug therapy:

- Acute Pain related to GI, CNS, and vision effects
- Risk for Injury related to CNS effects
- Impaired Urinary Elimination related to renal toxic effects
- Disturbed Thought Processes related to CNS effects
- Deficient Knowledge regarding drug therapy

Implementation With Rationale

- Give the drug cautiously, with daily monitoring of serum lithium levels, to patients with significant renal or CV disease, dehydration, or debilitation, as well as those taking diuretics, *to monitor for toxic levels and to arrange for appropriate dosage adjustment.*
- Give the drug with food or milk *to alleviate GI irritation if GI upset is severe.*
- Arrange to decrease dose after acute manic episodes. *Lithium tolerance is greatest during acute episodes and decreases when the acute episode is over.*
- Ensure that the patient maintains adequate intake of salt and fluid *to decrease toxicity.*
- Monitor the patient's clinical status closely, especially during the initial stages of therapy, *to provide appropriate supportive management as needed.*
- Arrange for small frequent meals, sugarless lozenges to suck, and frequent mouth care, *to increase secretions and decrease discomfort as needed.*
- Provide safety measures such as siderails and assistance with ambulation if CNS effects occur *to prevent patient injury.*
- Provide thorough patient teaching, including drug name, prescribed dosage, measures for avoidance of adverse effects, warning signs that may indicate possible problems, and the need to avoid pregnancy while taking lithium *to enhance patient knowledge about drug therapy and to promote compliance.*
- Offer support and encouragement *to help the patient cope with the drug regimen.*

Evaluation

- Monitor patient response to the drug (decreased manifestations and frequency of manic episodes).
- Monitor for adverse effects (CV toxicity, renal toxicity, GI upset, respiratory complications).
- Evaluate the effectiveness of the teaching plan (patient can give the drug name and dosage and describe the possible adverse effects to watch for, specific measures to help avoid adverse effects, warning signs to report, and the need to avoid pregnancy).
- Monitor the effectiveness of comfort measures and compliance with the regimen.

Central Nervous System Stimulants

CNS stimulants are used clinically to treat both attention-deficit disorders and narcolepsy. Paradoxically, these drugs calm hyperkinetic children and help them focus on one

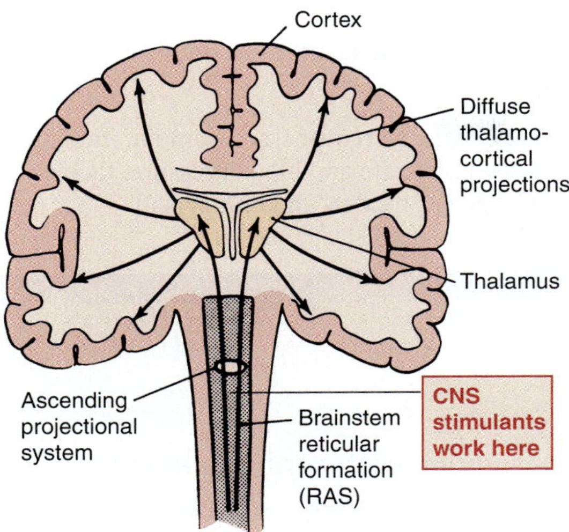

FIGURE 22.3 Site of action of the central nervous system (CNS) stimulants in the reticular activating system (RAS).

activity for a longer period. They also redirect and excite the arousal stimuli from the RAS (Figure 22.3; see also Figure 22.1). The CNS stimulants that are used to treat attention-deficit disorder and narcolepsy include the following drugs (Table 22.3).

- Methylphenidate (*Ritalin, Concerta*) is commonly used for the treatment of attention-deficit disorders and other behavioral syndromes associated with hyperactivity, as well as narcolepsy. It is now available in various forms allowing for dosing one, two, or three times a day.
- Dexmethylphenidate (*Focalin*), approved in late 2001, is an isomer of methylphenidate and is used in lower doses than methylphenidate. It is approved only for treatment of attention-deficit hyperactivity disorder in patients 6 years of age and older.
- Dextroamphetamine (*Dexedrine*), an oral drug, is also used as short-term adjunctive therapy for exogenous obesity.
- Modafinil (*Provigil*), a newer drug, is approved for use in treating narcolepsy, for improving wakefulness with shift work sleep disorder, and for improving wakefulness in people with obstructive sleep apnea/hypopneas syndrome. It is not associated with many of the systemic stimulatory effects of some of the other CNS stimulants.

Therapeutic Actions and Indications

The CNS stimulants act as cortical and RAS stimulants, possibly by increasing the release of catecholamines from presynaptic neurons, leading to an increase in stimulation of the postsynaptic neurons. The paradoxical effect of calming hyperexcitability through CNS stimulation seen in attention-deficit syndrome is believed to be related to increased stimulation of an immature RAS, which leads to the ability to be more selective in response to incoming stimuli.

The CNS stimulants are indicated for the treatment of attention-deficit syndromes, including behavioral syndromes characterized by hyperactivity and distractibility, as well as narcolepsy and improvement of wakefulness in people with various sleep disorders.

Pharmacokinetics

These drugs are rapidly absorbed from the GI tract, reaching peak levels in 2 to 4 hours. They are metabolized in the liver and excreted in the urine, with half-lives ranging from 2 to 15 hours, depending on the drug. Safety for use during pregnancy and lactation has not been established; during those periods, these drugs should be used only if the benefit to the mother clearly outweighs the potential risk to the fetus or neonate.

Table 22.3 DRUGS IN FOCUS

Central Nervous System Stimulants

Drug Name	Dosage/Route	Usual Indications
dexmethylphenidate (*Focalin*)	2.5–5 mg PO b.i.d.; do not exceed 10 mg PO b.i.d.	Treatment of attention-deficit hyperactivity disorder in patients age ≥6 yr
dextroamphetamine (*Dexedrine*)	Narcolepsy: 5–60 mg/day PO in divided doses Attention-deficit disorders: 2.5–5 mg/day PO taken in the morning Obesity: 5–30 mg/day PO (not recommended for children <12 yr)	Narcolepsy, attention-deficit disorders, behavioral syndromes, exogenous obesity
P methylphenidate (*Ritalin, Concerta*)	Adult: 10–60 mg/day PO in divided doses depending on preparation Pediatric: 5 mg PO b.i.d.; increase gradually, do not exceed 60 mg/day	Narcolepsy, attention-deficit disorders, behavioral syndromes
modafinil (*Provigil*)	200 mg/day PO as a single dose; reduce dosage with hepatic impairment and in the elderly	Narcolepsy in adults, improving wakefulness in various sleep disorders

Contraindications and Cautions

The CNS stimulants are contraindicated in the presence of known allergy to the drug. Other contraindications include the following conditions: marked anxiety, agitation, or tension and severe fatigue or glaucoma, *which could be exacerbated by the CNS stimulation caused by these drugs;* cardiac disease, *which could be aggravated by the stimulatory effects of these drugs;* and pregnancy and lactation *because of the potential for adverse effects on the fetus or neonate.*

Caution should be used in patients with a history of seizures, *which could be potentiated by the CNS stimulation;* with a history of drug dependence, including alcoholism, *because these drugs may result in physical and psychological dependence;* and with hypertension, *which could be exacerbated by the stimulatory effects of these drugs.*

Adverse Effects

The adverse effects associated with these drugs are related to the CNS stimulation they cause. CNS effects can include nervousness, insomnia, dizziness, headache, blurred vision, and difficulty with accommodation. GI effects such as anorexia, nausea, and weight loss may occur. CV effects can include hypertension, arrhythmias, and angina. Skin rashes are a common reaction to some of these drugs. Physical and psychological dependence may also develop. Because CNS stimulants have this effect, the drugs are controlled substances.

Clinically Important Drug–Drug Interactions

The combination of a CNS stimulant with a monoamine oxidase (MAO) inhibitor leads to an increased risk of adverse effects and increased toxicity and should be avoided if possible. Likewise, the combination of a CNS stimulant with guanethidine, which results in a decrease in antihypertensive effects, should be avoided.

In addition, the combination of CNS stimulants with tricyclic antidepressants or phenytoin leads to a risk of increased drug levels. Patients who receive such a combination should be monitored for toxicity.

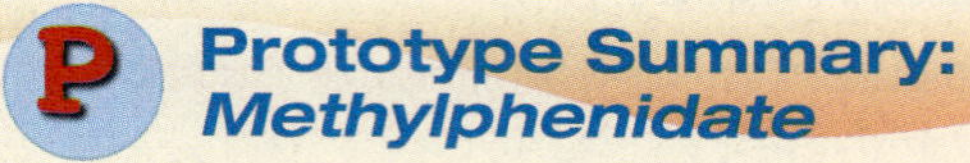

Prototype Summary: Methylphenidate

Indications: Narcolepsy and attention-deficit disorder

Actions: Mild cortical stimulant with CNS actions similar to those of amphetamines

Pharmacokinetics:

Route	Onset	Peak	Duration
Oral	Varies	1–3 h	4–6 h

$T_{1/2}$: 1–3 hours; metabolized in the liver; excreted in the urine

Adverse effects: Nervousness, insomnia, increased or decreased pulse rate and blood pressure, tachycardia, loss of appetite, nausea, abdominal pain

Nursing Considerations for Patients Receiving Central Nervous System Stimulants

Assessment: History and Examination

Screen for the following conditions, *which could be contraindications or cautions for the use of the drug:* any known allergies to the drug; glaucoma, anxiety, tension, fatigue, or seizure disorder; cardiac disease and hypertension; pregnancy or lactation; a history of leukemia; and history of drug dependency, including alcoholism.

Include screening *for baseline status before beginning therapy and for any potential adverse effects.* Assess the following: temperature; skin color and lesions; CNS orientation, affect, and reflexes; ophthalmic examination; bowel sounds and reported output; pulse, auscultation, and blood pressure, including orthostatic blood pressure; respiration rate and adventitious sounds; and urinary output. Obtain a CBC.

Nursing Diagnoses

The patient receiving CNS stimulants may have the following nursing diagnoses related to drug therapy:

- Disturbed Thought Processes related to CNS effects of the drug
- Decreased Cardiac Output related to CV effects of the drug
- Risk for Injury related to CNS and visual effects of the drug
- Deficient Knowledge regarding drug therapy

Implementation With Rationale

- Ensure proper diagnosis of behavioral syndromes and narcolepsy *because these drugs should not be used until underlying medical causes of the problem are ruled out.*
- Arrange to interrupt the drug periodically in children who are receiving the drug for behavioral syndromes *to determine whether symptoms recur and therapy should be continued.*
- Arrange to dispense the least amount of drug possible *to minimize the risk of overdose and abuse.*

- Administer the drug before 6 PM *to reduce the incidence of insomnia.*
- Monitor weight, CBC, and ECG *to ensure early detection of adverse effects and proper interventions.*
- Consult with the school nurse or counselor *to ensure comprehensive care of school-aged children receiving CNS stimulants* (Box 22.5).
- Provide safety measures such as siderails and assistance with ambulation if CNS effects occur *to prevent patient injury.*
- Provide thorough patient teaching, including drug name, prescribed dosage, measures for avoidance of adverse effects, warning signs that may indicate possible problems, and the need for monitoring and evaluation *to enhance patient knowledge about drug therapy and to promote compliance.* Offer support and encouragement to help the patient cope with the drug regimen.

Evaluation

- Monitor patient response to the drug (decrease in manifestations of behavioral syndromes, decrease in daytime sleep and narcolepsy).
- Monitor for adverse effects (CNS stimulation, CV effects, rash, physical or psychological dependence, GI dysfunction).
- Evaluate the effectiveness of the teaching plan (patient can give the drug name and dosage, name possible adverse effects to watch for and specific measures to help avoid adverse effects, and describe the need for follow-up and evaluation).
- Monitor the effectiveness of comfort measures and compliance with the regimen.

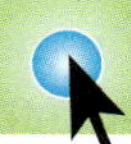

WEB LINKS

Health care providers and patients may want to consult the following Internet sources:

http://www.uic.edu/depts/cnr Information on sleep disorders research and treatment.

http://www.psychiatry24×7.com Information on education programs, research, and other information related to mental illness.

http://www.mhsource.com Information on mental health resources, support groups, and related information.

http://aap.org Information on mental health-related issues in the child and adolescent.

http://www.adhdnews.com Information about specific diagnoses, treatment, and support groups for attention-deficit hyperactivity disorder (ADHD).

http://mentalhelp.net Information on mental health-related issues, treatments, and community issues.

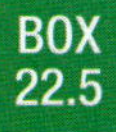

BOX 22.5 FOCUS ON THE **EVIDENCE**

School Nursing and Ritalin Administration

In the past several years, the number of school children receiving diagnoses of attention-deficit disorder or minimal brain dysfunction and being prescribed methylphenidate (*Ritalin*) has increased dramatically. Because this drug needs to be given two or three times each day, it has become the responsibility of the school nurse to dispense the drug during the day. Some school nurses reportedly spend between 50% and 70% of their time administering these drugs and completing the necessary paperwork. In 2000–2001, several long-acting formulations of methylphenidate became available.

Concerta, available in an extended-release tablet in 18- and 36-mg strengths, is now also available in a 54-mg strength. This form is suggested for every-12-hours dosing. *Metadate CD* is approved as a 20-mg extended-release capsule that is suggested as a once-daily treatment for children with attention deficit disorder. *Ritalin SR* is another extended-release formulation that is designed to be given every 8 hours. These extended-release forms are not interchangeable, and the instructions that come with the drug that is prescribed should be checked carefully. The advantage of these extended-release forms is expected to be a decrease in the number of students who must see the nurse for medication during the school day and, perhaps, a decrease in the stigma that may be associated with needing this drug.

The school nurse has additional responsibilities besides administering the drug. The school nurse is responsible for assessing children's response to the drug and for coordinating the teacher's and health care providers' input into each individual case, including the incidence of adverse effects and the appropriateness of the drug therapy. The nurse should

- Ensure that the proper diagnosis is made before supporting the use of the drug.
- Constantly evaluate and work with the primary health care provider to regularly challenge children without the drug to see whether the drug is doing what is expected or whether the child is maturing and no longer needs the drug therapy.

The school nurse needs to be prepared to be an advocate for the best therapeutic intervention for a particular child. Because long-term methylphenidate therapy is associated with many adverse effects, use of the drug should not be taken lightly. A federal review of the *Ritalin* issues facing the country today can be found at http://commdocs.house.gov/committees/edu/hedcew6-109.000/hedcew6-109.htm

Points to Remember

- Mental disorders are disorders of thought processes that may be caused by some inherent dysfunction within the brain. Psychoses are thought disorders.
- Schizophrenia, the most common psychosis, is characterized by delusions, hallucinations, and inappropriate responses to stimuli.
- Mania is a state of hyperexcitability, one extreme of bipolar disorder.
- An attention-deficit disorder is a behavioral syndrome characterized by hyperactivity and a short attention span.
- Narcolepsy is a disorder characterized by daytime sleepiness and sudden loss of wakefulness.
- Antipsychotics are dopamine-receptor blockers. Side effects include hypotension, anticholinergic effects, sedation, and extrapyramidal effects, including parkinsonism, ataxia, and tremors.
- Lithium, a membrane stabilizer, is the only effective antimanic drug. Because it is a very toxic salt, serum levels must be carefully monitored to prevent severe toxicity.
- CNS stimulants, which stimulate cortical levels and the RAS to increase RAS activity, are used to treat attention-deficit disorders and narcolepsy. These drugs improve concentration and the ability to filter and focus incoming stimuli.

CHECK YOUR UNDERSTANDING

Answers to the questions in this chapter may be found in the Answer Key in the back of the book.

Multiple Choice

Select the best answer to the following.

1. Mental disorders are now thought to be caused by some inherent dysfunction within the brain that leads to abnormal thought processes and responses. They include
   a. depression.
   b. anxiety.
   c. seizures.
   d. schizophrenia.

2. Antipsychotic drugs are basically
   a. serotonin reuptake inhibitors.
   b. norepinephrine blockers.
   c. dopamine receptor blockers.
   d. acetylcholine stimulators.

3. Adverse effects associated with antipsychotic drugs are related to the drugs' effects on receptor sites and can include
   a. insomnia and hypertension.
   b. dry mouth, hypotension, and glaucoma.
   c. diarrhea and excessive urination.
   d. increased sexual drive and improved concentration.

4. Lithium toxicity can be dangerous. Patient assessment to evaluate for appropriate lithium levels would look for
   a. serum lithium levels greater than 3 mEq/L.
   b. serum lithium levels greater than 4 mEq/L.
   c. serum lithium levels less than 1.5 mEq/L.
   d. undetectable serum lithium levels.

5. Your patient, a 6-year-old boy, is starting a regimen of *Ritalin* (methylphenidate) to control an attention-deficit disorder. Family teaching should include which of the following?
   a. This drug can be shared with other family members who might seem to need it.
   b. This drug may cause insomnia, weight loss, and GI upset.
   c. Do not alert the school nurse to the fact that this drug is being taken because the child could have problems later on.
   d. This drug should not be stopped for any reason for several years.

6. Antipsychotic drugs are also known as neuroleptic drugs because
   a. they cause numerous neurological effects.
   b. they frequently cause epilepsy.
   c. they are also minor tranquilizers.
   d. they are the only drugs known to directly affect nerves.

7. Attention-deficit disorders (the inability to concentrate or focus on an activity) and narcolepsy (sudden episodes of sleep) are both most effectively treated with the use of
   a. neuroinhibitors.
   b. dopamine receptor blockers.
   c. major tranquilizers.
   d. CNS stimulants.

8. Haloperidol (*Haldol*) is a potent antipsychotic that is associated with
   a. severe extrapyramidal effects.
   b. severe sedation.
   c. severe hypotension.
   d. severe anticholinergic effects.

Multiple Response

Select all that apply.

1. Before administering lithium to a client, the nurse should check for the concomitant use of which of the following drugs, which could cause serious adverse effects?
   a. Ibuprofen
   b. Haloperidol
   c. Thiazide diuretics
   d. Antacids
   e. Ketoconazole
   f. Theophylline

2. Dyskinesias are a common side effect of antipsychotic drugs. Nursing interventions for the patient receiving antipsychotic drugs should include which of the following?
   a. Positioning to decrease discomfort of dyskinesias
   b. Implementing safety measures to prevent injury
   c. Encouraging the patient to chew tablets to prevent choking
   d. Careful teaching to alert the patient and family about this adverse effect
   e. Applying ice to the joints to prevent damage
   f. Pureeing all food to decrease the risk of aspiration

Matching

Match the following words with the appropriate definition.

1. ______________________ schizophrenia
2. ______________________ narcolepsy
3. ______________________ attention-deficit disorder
4. ______________________ neuroleptic
5. ______________________ major tranquilizer
6. ______________________ mania
7. ______________________ antipsychotic

A. A state of hyperexcitability
B. A behavioral syndrome characterized by an inability to concentrate
C. A mental disorder characterized by daytime sleepiness and sudden periods of loss of wakefulness
D. A name once used to describe antipsychotic drugs
E. A drug used to treat a disorder of the thought processes; a dopamine receptor blocker
F. A psychotic disorder characterized by delusions, hallucinations, and thought and speech disturbances
G. An antipsychotic drug, so named because of the numerous neurological adverse effects caused by these drugs

Web Exercise

Your patient has received a diagnosis of seasonal affective disorder (SAD). She does not want to take any medication, although her signs and symptoms are nearly incapacitating. Help your patient investigate alternative treatment plans for SAD. Go to http://www.mhsource.com to get started.

Bibliography and References

American Psychiatric Association. (2004). *DSM-IV-TR* (4th ed., text revision). Washington, DC: Author.

Bailey, K. (1998). *Psychotropic drug facts.* Philadelphia: Lippincott-Raven.

Drug facts and comparisons. (2006). St. Louis: Facts and Comparisons.

Gilman, A., Hardman, J. G., & Limbird, L. E. (Eds.). (2006). *Goodman and Gilman's the pharmacological basis of therapeutics* (11th ed.). New York: McGraw-Hill.

Karch, A. M. (2006). *2007 Lippincott's nursing drug guide.* Philadelphia: Lippincott Williams & Wilkins.

Porth, C. M. (2005). *Pathophysiology: Concepts of altered health states* (7th ed.). Philadelphia: Lippincott Williams & Wilkins.

Professional's guide to patient drug facts. (2006). St. Louis: Facts and Comparisons.

CHAPTER 23

Antiepileptic Agents

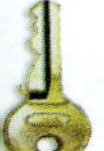

KEY TERMS

absence seizure
antiepileptic
convulsion
epilepsy
focal seizure
generalized seizure
grand mal seizure
partial seizure
petit mal seizure
seizure
status epilepticus
tonic–clonic seizure

LEARNING OBJECTIVES

Upon completion of this chapter, you will be able to:

1. Define the terms generalized seizure, tonic–clonic seizure, absence seizure, partial seizure, and status epilepticus.
2. Describe the therapeutic actions, indications, pharmacokinetics, contraindications, most common adverse reactions, and important drug–drug interactions associated with each class of antiepileptic agents: hydantoins, barbiturates, benzodiazepines, succinimides, and agents for partial seizures.
3. Discuss the use of antiepileptic drugs across the lifespan.
4. Compare and contrast the prototype drugs for each class of antiepileptic drug with the other drugs in that class and with drugs from the other classes.
5. Outline the nursing considerations and teaching needs for patients receiving each class of antiepileptic agents.

DRUGS FOR TREATING TONIC–CLONIC (GRAND MAL) SEIZURES

Hydantoins

ethotoin
fosphenytoin
mephenytoin
P phenytoin

Barbiturates and Barbiturate-like Drugs

mephobarbital
P phenobarbital
primidone

Benzodiazepines

clonazepam
P diazepam

DRUGS FOR TREATING ABSENCE (PETIT MAL) SEIZURES

Succinimides

P ethosuximide
methsuximide

Other Drugs for Absence (Petit Mal) Seizures

acetazolamide
P valproic acid
zonisamide

DRUGS FOR TREATING PARTIAL (FOCAL) SEIZURES

P carbamazepine
clorazepate
felbamate
gabapentin
lamotrigine
levetiracetam
oxcarbazepine
pregabalin
tiagabine
topiramate

Epilepsy, the most prevalent of the neurological disorders, is not a single disease but a collection of different syndromes. All of these conditions are characterized by the same feature: sudden discharge of excessive electrical energy from nerve cells located within the brain, which leads to a seizure. In some cases, this release stimulates motor nerves, resulting in convulsions, with tonic–clonic muscle contractions that have the potential to cause injury, tics, or spasms. Other discharges may stimulate autonomic or sensory nerves and cause very different effects, such as a barely perceptible, temporary lapse in consciousness or a sympathetic reaction. Because epilepsy involves a loss of control, it can be very frightening to patients when they're first diagnosed (Box 23.1).

The treatment of epilepsy varies widely, depending on the exact problem and its manifestations. The drugs that are used to manage epilepsy are called **antiepileptics** (Box 23.2). These agents are sometimes referred to as anticonvulsants, but because not all types of epilepsy involve **convulsions**, this term is not generally applicable. The drug of choice for any given situation depends on the type of epilepsy and patient tolerance for associated adverse effects (Table 23.1 and Box 23.3).

BOX 23.1 FOCUS ON **CLINICAL SKILLS**

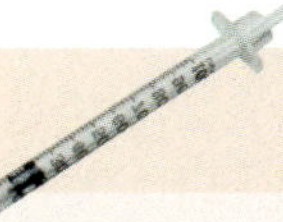

Teaching and Counseling Patients With Epilepsy

Epilepsy, with its stigma, is frightening to people who know little about the disease. This condition has long been associated with some sort of brain dysfunction or possession by the devil or evil spirits. In some eras, exorcism was the first choice of treatment for a person with a seizure disorder. A person who receives a diagnosis of epilepsy must deal with this stigma as well as the significance of the diagnosis. What does having epilepsy mean? Individuals who are newly diagnosed with epilepsy must consider restrictions on their independence as well as the prospect of chronic therapy for control of this problem.

In our society, the ability to be readily mobile—to drive to appointments, work, or religious obligations—is very important to many people. Most states require physicians to report new diagnoses of epilepsy. In most cases, the driving privileges of affected individuals are revoked, at least temporarily. The conditions for recovering the license vary with the diagnosis and the laws of each state.

The person who is newly diagnosed with epilepsy has to cope not only with the stigma of epilepsy, but also with the loss of a driver's license. The nurse may be in the best position to help the patient adjust to both of these problems through patient education and referrals to community resources. Thorough patient teaching should include the following:

- Explanations of old stigmas
- Ways in which people may react to the diagnosis
- Ways in which patients can educate family, friends, and employers about the realities of the condition and its treatment
- Actions to take if a seizure happens so that no injuries occur and no panic develops
- Information about the availability of public transportation
- The importance of encouraging patients with epilepsy to carry or wear a MedicAlert identification, to alert any emergency caregivers to their condition and to what drugs they are taking if they are not able to speak for themselves.
- Contact information regarding other community support services

Many communities have epilepsy support groups that can supply information on valuable resources as well as updated facts about the laws in each area. While patients are first adjusting to epilepsy and its implications, it may help to put them in contact with such organizations. The local chapter of the Epilepsy Foundation of America may be able to offer support groups, lists of resources, and support. Individuals with epilepsy should have several options for getting around without feeling that they are being a burden or an imposition.

Nature of Epilepsy

The form that a particular seizure takes depends on the location of the cells that initiate the electrical discharge and the neural pathways that are stimulated by the initial volley of electrical impulses. For the most part, epilepsy seems to be caused by abnormal neurons that are very sensitive to stimulation or over-respond for some reason. They do not appear to be different from other neurons in any other way. **Seizures** caused by these abnormal cells are called primary seizures because no underlying cause can be identified. In some cases, however, outside factors—head injury, drug overdose, environmental exposure, and so on—may precipitate seizures. Such seizures are often referred to as secondary seizures.

Classification of Seizures

Correct diagnosis of seizure type is very important for determining the correct medication to prevent future seizures while causing the fewest problems and adverse effects. Seizures may be grouped into two main types, and they are further classified within these two categories.

Generalized Seizures

Generalized seizures begin in one area of the brain and rapidly spread throughout both hemispheres of the brain. Patients who have a generalized seizure usually experience a loss of consciousness resulting from this massive electrical activity throughout the brain.

Generalized seizures are further classified into the following five types:

1. **Tonic–clonic seizures**, formerly known as **grand mal seizures**, involve dramatic tonic–clonic muscle contractions, loss of consciousness, and a recovery period characterized by confusion and exhaustion.
2. **Absence seizures**, formerly known as **petit mal seizures**, involve abrupt, brief (3- to 5-second) periods of loss of consciousness. Absence seizures occur commonly in children and frequently disappear at puberty.

BOX 23.2 DRUG THERAPY ACROSS THE LIFESPAN

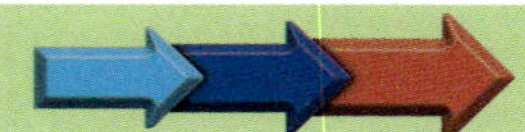

Antiepileptic Agents

CHILDREN

Antiepileptic drugs can have an impact on a child's learning and social development. Children may also be more sensitive to the sedating effects of some of these drugs. Children should be monitored very closely and often require a switch to a different agent or dosage adjustments based on their response.

Newborns (1 to 10 days of age) respond best to intramuscular phenobarbital if an antiepileptic is needed.

Older children (2 months to 6 years of age) absorb and metabolize many of these drugs more quickly than adults do and require a larger dosage per kilogram to maintain therapeutic levels. Careful calculation of drug dosage using both weight and age are important in helping the child to receive the best therapeutic effect with the least toxicity. After the age of 10 to 14 years, many of these drugs can be given in the standard adult dose.

Parents of children receiving these drugs should receive consistent support and education about the seizure disorder and the medications being used to treat it. Many communities have local support groups that can offer lots of educational materials and support programs. It is a very frightening experience to watch your child have a tonic–clonic seizure, and parents should be supported with this in mind.

ADULTS

Adults using these drugs should be under regular care and should be monitored regularly for adverse effects. They should be encouraged to carry or wear a Medic-Alert identification to alert emergency personnel that antiepileptic drugs are being taken. Adults also need education and support to deal with the old stigma of seizures as well as the lifestyle changes and drug effects that they may need to cope with.

Most of these drugs have been associated with fetal abnormalities in animal studies. Some of them are clearly associated with predictable congenital effects in humans. Women of childbearing age should be encouraged to use contraceptives while taking these drugs. If a pregnancy does occur, or if a woman taking one of these drugs desires to become pregnant, the importance of the drug to the mother should be weighed against the potential risk to the fetus. Stopping an antiepileptic can precipitate seizures that could cause anoxia and its related problems for the mother and the baby. Women who are nursing should be encouraged to find another way of feeding the baby to avoid the sedating and central nervous system effects that the drugs can have on the infant.

OLDER ADULTS

Older patients may be more susceptible to the adverse effects of these drugs. Dosages of all of these drugs may need to be reduced, and the patient should be monitored very closely for toxic effects and to provide safety measures if central nervous system effects do occur.

Patients with renal or hepatic impairment should be monitored very closely. Baseline renal and liver function tests should be done and dosages adjusted as appropriate. Serum levels of the drug should be monitored closely in such cases to prevent serious adverse effects.

The older patient should also be encouraged to wear or carry a Medic-Alert identification in case there is an emergency and the patient is not able to communicate information about the drug or disorder.

3. Myoclonic seizures involve short, sporadic periods of muscle contractions that last for several minutes. They are relatively rare and are often secondary seizures.
4. Febrile seizures are related to very high fevers and usually involve convulsions. Febrile seizures most frequently occur in children; they are usually self-limited and do not reappear.
5. **Status epilepticus**, potentially the most dangerous of seizure conditions, is a state in which seizures rapidly recur again and again.

Partial Seizures

Partial seizures, also called **focal seizures**, involve one area of the brain and do not spread throughout the entire organ. The presenting symptoms depend on exactly where the excessive electrical discharge is occurring in the brain. Partial seizures can be further classified as follows:

- Simple partial seizures occur in a single area of the brain and may involve a single muscle movement or sensory alteration.
- Complex partial seizures involve complex sensory changes such as hallucinations, mental distortion, changes in personality, loss of consciousness, and loss of social inhibitions. Motor changes may include involuntary urination, chewing motions, diarrhea, and so on. The onset of complex partial seizures usually occurs by the late teens.

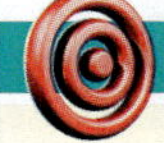

FOCUS POINTS

- Epilepsy is characterized by seizures that result from sudden discharge of excessive electrical energy from nerve cells in the brain.

  There are two types of seizures: generalized (tonic–clonic, absence, myoclonic, febrile, or rapid recurring) and partial, or focal (simple or complex).

Drugs for Treating Tonic–Clonic (Grand Mal) Seizures

Various drugs are used to treat tonic–clonic (grand mal) seizures. Drugs that are used to treat generalized seizures stabilize the nerve membranes by blocking channels in the

Table 23.1 Drugs Used to Treat Various Types of Seizures

Drug	Type of Seizure						
	Tonic–clonic	*Absence*	*Myoclonic*	*Febrile*	*Status Epilepticus*	*Simple Partial*	*Complex Partial*
Mephobarbital	0	0	—	—	—	—	—
Phenobarbital	0	—	—	X	0	0	—
Primidone	0	—	—	0	—	0	0
Clonazepam	—	0	X	—	—	—	—
Diazepam	0	—	—	—	X	—	—
Ethotoin	X	—	—	—	—	—	—
Fosphenytoin	—	—	—	—	X	—	—
Mephenytoin	0	—	0	—	—	0	0
Phenytoin	X	—	—	—	X	X	X
Ethosuximide	—	X	—	—	—	—	—
Methsuximide	—	0	—	—	—	—	—
Acetazolamide	0	—	—	—	—	—	—
Valproic acid	—	0	X	—	—	—	0
Zonisamide	—	0	—	—	—	—	—
Carbamazepine	X	—	—	—	—	X	X
Clorazepate	—	—	—	—	—	0	0
Felbamate	—	—	—	—	—	0	0
Gabapentin	—	—	—	—	—	0	0
Lamotrigine	—	—	—	—	—	0	0
Levetiracetam	—	—	—	—	—	0	0
Oxcarbazepine	—	—	—	—	—	0	0
Pregabalin	—	—	—	—	—	0	0
Tiagabine	—	0	—	—	—	0	0
Topiramate	—	—	—	—	—	0	0

X, primary treatment, a drug of choice; 0, adjunctive therapy or used when unresponsive to other treatments; —, not a use.

BOX 23.3 CULTURAL CONSIDERATIONS FOR DRUG THERAPY

Altered Metabolism of Antiepileptic Drugs

Because of differences in liver enzyme functioning among Arab Americans and Asian Americans, patients in these ethnic groups may not metabolize antiepileptic drugs in the same way as patients in other ethnic groups. They may require not only lower doses to achieve the same therapeutic effects, but also frequent dose adjustment.

Nurses need to be aware that the therapeutic range for patients in these ethnic groups may differ from standard norms and that these patients may be more apt to show adverse or toxic reactions to antiepileptic drugs at lower doses. As with all medications, the lowest possible dose should be used. Serum drug levels should be closely monitored and titrated carefully and slowly to achieve the maximum benefits with the fewest adverse effects.

cell membrane or altering receptor sites. Because they work generally on the central nervous system (CNS), sedation and other CNS effects often result. In particular, the drugs that are indicated for tonic–clonic seizures (the hydantoins, the barbiturates, and the barbiturate-like drugs [Table 23.2]) affect the entire brain and reduce the chance of sudden electrical outburst. Associated adverse effects are often related to total brain stabilization (Figure 23.1).

Hydantoins

The hydantoins stabilize nerve membranes and limit the spread of excitability from the initiating focus (see Figure 23.1), possibly by promoting the exit of sodium ions from the cell, returning the cell to a stable resting membrane potential. Because hydantoins are generally less sedating than many other antiepileptics, they may be the drugs of choice for patients who are not willing to tolerate sedation

Table 23.2 DRUGS IN FOCUS

Drugs for Treating Tonic–Clonic (Grand Mal) Seizures

Drug Name	Dosage/Route	Usual Indications
Hydantoins		
ethotoin (*Peganone*)	Adult: 2–3 g/day PO in four to six divided doses Pediatric: 500 mg to 1 g/day PO; consider age and weight	Tonic–clonic (grand mal) and psychomotor seizures
fosphenytoin (*Cerebyx*)	Adult: loading dose, 15–20 mg phenytoin equivalent (PE) per kilogram IV given as 100–150 mg PE per minute; maintenance, 4–6 mg PE per kilogram per day; reduce dosage with renal or hepatic impairment	Short-term control of status epilepticus, prevention of seizures after neurosurgery
mephenytoin (*Mesantoin*)	Adult: 200–600 mg/day PO Pediatric: 100–400 mg/day PO	Tonic–clonic (grand mal), psychomotor, and partial (focal) seizures
P phenytoin (*Dilantin*)	Adult: 100 mg PO t.i.d., up to 300–400 mg/day; 10–15 mg/kg IV Pediatric: 5–8 mg/kg/day PO; 5–10 mg/kg IV in divided doses	Tonic–clonic (grand mal) seizures, status epilepticus prevention, and treatment of seizures after neurosurgery
Barbiturates and Barbiturate-Like Drugs		
mephobarbital (*Mebaral*)	Adult: 400–600 mg/day PO; decrease dosage and monitor elderly patients and debilitated patients closely Pediatric (≤5 yr): 16–32 mg PO t.i.d. to q.i.d. Pediatric (>5 yr): 32–64 mg PO t.i.d. to q.i.d.	Sedative/hypnotic, tonic–clonic (grand mal) and absence (petit mal) seizures
P phenobarbital (*Solfoton, Luminal*)	Adult: 60–100 mg/day PO; 200–320 mg IM or IV for acute episodes, may be repeated in 6 h; reduce dosage with elderly and with renal or hepatic impairment Pediatric: 3–6 mg/kg/day PO; four to six mg/kg/day IM or IV; 15–20 mg/kg IV over 10–15 min for status epilepticus	Sedative–hypnotic, tonic–clonic (grand mal) seizures, status epilepticus, cortical focal seizures, simple partial seizures
primidone (*Mysoline*)	Adult: 250 mg PO five to six times per day Pediatric (>8 yr): 250 mg PO five to six times per day Pediatric (<8 yr): 125–250 mg PO t.i.d.	Tonic–clonic (grand mal), partial, and refractory seizures
Benzodiazepines		
clonazepam (*Klonopin*)	Adult: initially 1.5 mg/day PO in three divided doses, up to a maximum 20 mg/day Pediatric (>10 yr): 0.01–0.03 mg/kg/day PO initially, then up to 0.1–0.2 mg/kg/day PO	Absence (petit mal) and myoclonic seizures
P diazepam (*Valium*)	Adult: 2–10 mg PO b.i.d. to q.i.d.; or 0.2 mg/kg PR, may repeat in 4–12 h; 2–20 mg IM or IV Geriatric or debilitated patients: 2–2.5 mg PO daily to b.i.d.; or 2–5 mg IM or IV Pediatric: 1–2.5 mg PO t.i.d. to q.i.d.; or 0.3–0.5 mg/kg PR with a repeat in 4–12 h if needed; 0.25 mg/kg IV over 3 min, may repeat in 15–30 min for up to three doses	Relieving tension, anxiety; muscle spasm; short-term treatment of severe convulsions, status epilepticus

and drowsiness. They do have significant adverse effects (e.g., severe liver toxicity). In many situations, less toxic drugs (e.g., the benzodiazepines) have replaced them.

The hydantoins include the following agents:

- Phenytoin (*Dilantin*), the prototype hydantoin, is used in the treatment of tonic–clonic seizures and status epilepticus, as well as in the prevention and treatment of seizures after neurosurgery. It is available in oral and parenteral forms. It is well absorbed from the gastrointestinal (GI) tract, metabolized in the liver, and excreted in the urine. Patients with hepatic impairment are at risk for increased toxicity from the drug. Therapeutic serum levels range from 10 to 20 mcg/mL.
- Ethotoin (*Peganone*) is used to control tonic–clonic and myoclonic seizures. It is also well absorbed from the GI tract, metabolized in the liver, and excreted in the urine. The therapeutic serum levels of ethotoin are from 15 to 50 mcg/mL.
- Fosphenytoin (*Cerebyx*) is used for short-term control of status epilepticus and to prevent seizures after neurosurgery. It is given intramuscularly or intravenously. Fosphenytoin is metabolized in the liver and excreted in the urine. The therapeutic phenytoin serum levels peak about 10 to 20 minutes after the infusion, and the patient must be monitored closely for cardiovascular reactions during this period. Patients with hepatic and/or renal

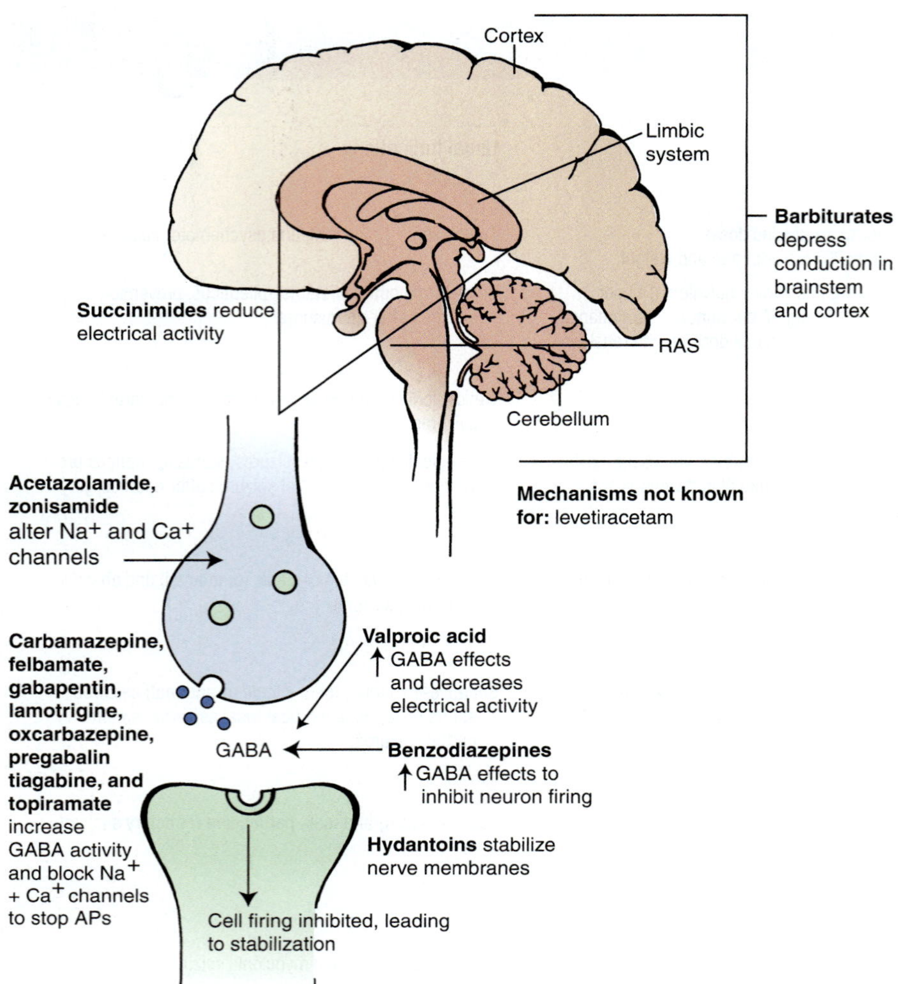

FIGURE 23.1 Sites of action of drugs used to treat various types of epilepsy. APs, action potentials; GABA, gamma-aminobutyric acid; RAS, reticular activating system.

impairment are at increased risk for toxic effects because of alterations in metabolism and excretion of the drug. Such patients should be monitored closely, and the dosage should be reduced accordingly.

- Mephenytoin (*Mesantoin*) is used for the treatment of tonic–clonic, myoclonic, and partial (focal) seizures in patients who do not respond to less toxic antiepileptic agents. This drug has been associated with severe hepatic toxicity, bone marrow suppression, and often unacceptable dermatological reactions. Mephenytoin is well absorbed from the GI tract and metabolized in the liver with bile secretion. The therapeutic serum level has not been established. Patients with hepatic impairment should be monitored very closely.

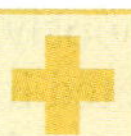

FOCUS ON **PATIENT SAFETY**

Be aware that name confusion has been reported between *Cerebyx* (fosphenytoin), *Celebrex* (celecoxib, a nonsteroidal anti-inflammatory agent), *Celexa* (citalopram, an SSRI antidepressant), and *Xanax* (alprazolam, an antianxiety drug). Because these drugs have sound-alike, look-alike names, if your patient is prescribed any of these drugs, make sure you know what the drug is being used for and that the patient is getting the correct prescribed drug.

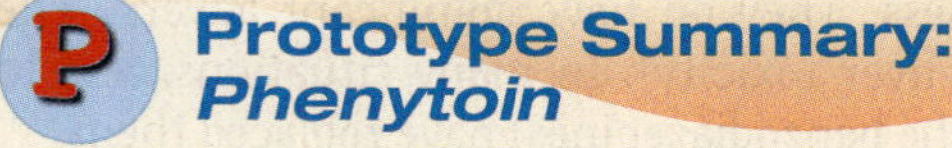

Prototype Summary: *Phenytoin*

Indications: Control of tonic–clonic and psychomotor seizures; prevention of seizures during neurosurgery; control of status epilepticus

Actions: Stabilizes neuronal membranes and prevents hyperexcitability caused by excessive stimulation; limits the spread of seizure activity from an active focus; has cardiac antiarrhythmic effects similar to those of lidocaine

Pharmacokinetics:

Route	Onset	Peak	Duration
Oral	Slow	2–12 h	6–12 h
IV	1–2 h	Rapid	12–24 h

$T_{1/2}$: 6–24 hours; metabolized in the liver, excreted in the urine

Adverse effects: Nystagmus, ataxia, dysarthria, slurred speech, mental confusion, dizziness, fatigue, tremor, headache, dermatitis, Stevens–Johnson syndrome, nausea, gingival hyperplasia, liver damage, hematopoietic complications, sometimes fatal

Barbiturates and Barbiturate-like Drugs

The barbiturates and barbiturate-type drugs inhibit impulse conduction in the ascending reticular activating system (RAS), depress the cerebral cortex, alter cerebellar function, and depress motor nerve output; because they depress nerve function, they can produce sedation, hypnosis, anesthesia, and deep coma. The degree of depression is dose related. At doses below those needed to cause hypnosis, these drugs block seizure activity.

- Phenobarbital (*Solfoton, Luminal*), which is available in oral and parenteral forms, is used for the emergency control of status epilepticus and acute seizures associated with eclampsia, tetanus, and other conditions. In addition, it is used orally for the long-term management of tonic–clonic and cortical focal seizures and can be very effective in the treatment of simple partial seizures. It is well absorbed from the GI tract, metabolized in the liver, and excreted in the urine. This drug has very low lipid solubility, giving it a slow onset and a very long duration of activity. The therapeutic serum level range is 15 to 40 mcg/mL.
- Primidone (*Mysoline*), which is structurally very similar to phenobarbital, is an alternative choice in the treatment of tonic–clonic or partial seizures. It tends to have a longer half-life than phenobarbital and is available only in an oral form. Primidone may be combined with other agents to treat seizures that cannot be controlled by any other antiepileptic. It is well absorbed from the GI tract, metabolized in the liver to phenobarbital metabolites, and excreted in the urine. The therapeutic serum levels are 5 to 12 mcg/mL.
- Mephobarbital (*Mebaral*) is used for the treatment of tonic–clonic and absence seizures and is also used as an anxiolytic/hypnotic agent. It is well absorbed from the GI tract, metabolized in the liver, and excreted in the urine. It has a long half-life of 11 to 67 hours. It is commonly associated with CNS and GI effects. Its cardiovascular effects (hypotension, bradycardia, circulatory collapse) and respiratory effects (apnea, hypoventilation) make it less desirable than many of the other antiepileptic agents.

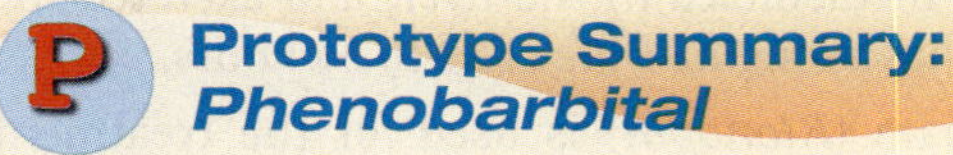

Prototype Summary: Phenobarbital

Indications: Long-term treatment of generalized tonic–clonic and cortical focal seizures; emergency control of certain acute convulsive episodes (status epilepticus, tetanus, eclampsia, meningitis); anticonvulsant treatment of generalized tonic–clonic seizures and focal seizures (parenteral); sedative; preanesthetic; short-term treatment of insomnia

Actions: General CNS depressant; inhibits impulse conduction in the ascending RAS; depresses the cerebral cortex; alters cerebellar function; depresses motor output; and can produce excitation, sedation, hypnosis, anesthesia, and deep coma

Pharmacokinetics:

Route	Onset	Duration
Oral	30–60 min	10–16 h
IM, Sub-Q	10–30 min	4–6 h
IV	5 min	4–6 h

$T_{1/2}$: 79 hours; metabolized in the liver, excreted in the urine

Adverse effects: Somnolence, insomnia, vertigo, nightmares, lethargy, nervousness, hallucinations, insomnia, anxiety, dizziness, bradycardia, hypotension, syncope, nausea, vomiting, constipation, diarrhea, hypoventilation, respiratory depression, tissue necrosis at injection site, withdrawal syndrome

Benzodiazepines

The benzodiazepines may potentiate the effects of gamma-aminobutyric acid (GABA), an inhibitory neurotransmitter that stabilizes nerve cell membranes. These drugs, which appear to act primarily in the limbic system and the RAS, also cause muscle relaxation and relieve anxiety without affecting cortical functioning substantially. In general, these drugs have limited toxicity and are well tolerated by most people. (See Chapter 20 for use of benzodiazepines as sedatives and anxiolytics.) The benzodiazepines described here are used as antiepileptics.

- Diazepam (*Valium*), the prototype benzodiazepine, is useful in relieving tension, anxiety, and muscle spasm. Available in oral, rectal, and parenteral forms, it is used to treat severe convulsions and status epilepticus, alcohol withdrawal, and tetanus; is given to relieve preoperative anxiety; and is being studied for use in the treatment of panic attacks. Diazepam is not used for long-term management of epilepsy. Diazepam is well absorbed from the GI tract, metabolized in the liver, and excreted in the urine. It has a long half-life of 20 to 50 hours.

- Clonazepam (*Klonopin*) is used for the treatment of absence (petit mal) seizures and myoclonic seizures. Patients who do not respond to succinimides may respond to this drug. Clonazepam may lose its effectiveness within 3 months (affected patients may respond to dosage adjustment). Clonazepam is being studied for use in the treatment of panic attacks, restless leg movements during sleep, hyperkinetic dysarthria, acute manic episodes, multifocal tic disorders, neuralgias, and as an adjunct in the treatment of schizophrenia. It is now available in an orally disintegrating tablet, making it a good choice for patients who have difficulty swallowing capsules or tablets. It is well absorbed from the GI tract, metabolized in the liver, and excreted in the urine. Clonazepam also has a long half-life of 18 to 50 hours.

P Prototype Summary: *Diazepam*

Indications: Management of anxiety disorders; acute alcohol withdrawal; muscle relaxant; treatment of tetanus; adjunct in status epilepticus and severe recurrent convulsive seizures; preoperative relief of anxiety and tension; management of epilepsy in patients who require intermittent use to control bouts of increased seizure activity

Actions: Acts in the limbic system and reticular formation; potentiates the effects of GABA; has little effect on cortical function

Pharmacokinetics:

Route	Onset	Peak	Duration
Oral	30–60 min	1–2 h	3 h
IM	15–30 min	30–45 min	3 h
IV	1–5 min	30 min	15–60 min
Rectal	Rapid	1.5 h	3 h

$T_{1/2}$: 20–80 hours; metabolized in the liver, excreted in the urine

Adverse effects: Drowsiness, sedation, depression, lethargy, apathy, fatigue, disorientation, bradycardia, tachycardia, paradoxical excitatory reactions, constipation, diarrhea, incontinence, urinary retention, drug dependence with withdrawal syndrome

Therapeutic Actions and Indications

In general, the hydantoins, barbiturates, and benzodiazepines all stabilize nerve membranes throughout the CNS to decrease excitability and hyperexcitability to stimulation. By decreasing conduction through nerve pathways, they reduce the tonic–clonic, muscular, and emotional responses to stimulation. Both hydantoins and barbiturates stabilize the nerve membrane directly by influencing ionic channels in the cell membrane. Specifically, phenobarbital depresses conduction in the lower brainstem and the cerebral cortex and depresses motor conduction. Benzodiazepines decrease excitability and conduction (see Figure 23.1).

Several drugs in these three groups are indicated for tonic–clonic seizures and status epilepticus, for prevention of seizures that occur after neurosurgery, and for adjunctive therapy for other seizure disorders or sedation and muscle relaxation (varies with drug). For specifics on these drugs, see Chapter 20.

Contraindications and Cautions

Hydantoins, barbiturates, and benzodiazepines are generally contraindicated in the presence of allergy to any of these drugs. Many of these agents *are associated with specific birth defects* and should not be used in pregnancy unless the risk of seizures outweighs the potential risk to the fetus. In such cases, the mother should be informed of the potential risks. The risk of taking a woman with a seizure disorder off of an antiepileptic drug that has stabilized her condition may be greater than the risk of the drug to the fetus. Discontinuing the drug could result in status epilepticus, which has a high risk of hypoxia for the mother and the fetus. Research has not been able to show the effects of even a minor seizure during pregnancy on the fetus, making it important to prevent seizures during pregnancy if at all possible. Women of child-bearing age should be urged to use barrier contraceptives while taking these drugs. If a pregnancy does occur, the woman should receive educational materials and counseling. Other contraindications include lactation, *because these drugs cross into breast milk and may cause adverse effects on the neonate,* and coma, depression, or psychoses, *which could be exacerbated by the generalized CNS depression.*

Caution should be used with elderly or debilitated patients *who may respond adversely to the CNS depression* and with patients who have impaired renal or liver function *that may interfere with drug metabolism and excretion.*

Adverse Effects

The most common adverse effects associated with drugs in all three groups—hydantoins, barbiturates, and benzodiazepines—relate to CNS depression and its effects on body function: depression, confusion, drowsiness, lethargy,

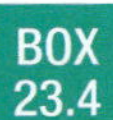

BOX 23.4 HERBAL AND ALTERNATIVE THERAPIES

Patients being treated for epilepsy should be advised not to use the herb evening primrose because it increases the risk of having seizures. Patients being treated with barbiturates or phenytoin should be advised not to use ginkgo, which could cause serious adverse effects.

fatigue, constipation, dry mouth, anorexia, cardiac arrhythmias and changes in blood pressure, urinary retention, and loss of libido.

Specific adverse effects with the hydantoins include severe liver toxicity, bone marrow suppression, gingival hyperplasia, and potentially serious dermatological reactions (e.g., hirsutism, coarsening of facial skin), all of which are directly related to cellular toxicity.

In addition, benzodiazepines and phenobarbital may be associated with physical dependence and withdrawal syndrome. Phenobarbital has also been linked to severe dermatological reactions and the development of drug tolerance related to changes in drug metabolism over time.

Clinically Important Drug–Drug Interactions

Because the risk of CNS depression is increased when any of the drugs in these three groups are taken with alcohol, patients should be advised not to drink alcohol while they are taking these agents. In addition, the individual drugs are associated with a wide variety of drug–drug interactions. Therefore, a drug reference should be reviewed carefully before any drug is added or withdrawn from a therapeutic regimen that involves any of these agents. Box 23.4 discusses a hazardous drug–herbal therapy interaction of which patients taking antiepileptic medication should be aware.

Nursing Considerations for Patients Receiving Hydantoins

See Chapter 20 for nursing considerations for patients receiving barbiturates or benzodiazepines.

Assessment: History and Examination

Screen for the following conditions, *which may be cautions or contraindications to the use of the drug:* any known allergies to these drugs; cardiac arrhythmias, hypotension, diabetes, coma, psychoses; pregnancy and lactation; and renal or hepatic dysfunction. Obtain a description of seizures, including onset, aura, duration, and recovery.

Include screening *for baseline status before beginning therapy and for any potential adverse effects.* Assess the following: skin color and lesions; temperature; CNS orientation, affect, reflexes, and bilateral grip strength; bowel sounds and reported output; pulse, auscultation, and blood pressure; urinary output; and electroencephalogram (EEG) if appropriate. Assess liver and renal function tests.

Nursing Diagnoses

The patient receiving hydantoins may have the following nursing diagnoses related to drug therapy:

- Acute Pain related to GI, CNS, and genitourinary effects
- Disturbed Thought Processes related to CNS effects
- Risk for Injury related to CNS effects
- Impaired Skin Integrity related to dermatological effects
- Deficient Knowledge regarding drug therapy

Implementation With Rationale

- Discontinue the drug at any sign of hypersensitivity reaction, liver dysfunction, or severe skin rash, *to limit reaction and prevent potentially serious reactions.*
- Administer the drug with food *to alleviate GI irritation if GI upset is a problem.*
- Monitor for adverse effects and provide appropriate supportive care as needed *to help the patient cope with these effects.*
- Monitor for drug–drug interactions *to arrange to adjust dosages appropriately if any drug is added or withdrawn from the drug regimen.*
- Arrange for counseling for women of childbearing age who are taking these drugs. *Because these drugs have the potential to cause serious damage to the fetus,* women should understand the risk of birth defects and use barrier contraceptives to avoid pregnancy.
- Provide thorough patient teaching, including drug name and prescribed dosage, as well as measures for avoidance of adverse effects, warning signs that may indicate possible problems, and the need for monitoring and evaluation *to enhance patient knowledge about drug therapy and to promote compliance.* (See Critical Thinking Scenario 23-1.)
- Suggest the wearing or carrying of a MedicAlert bracelet *to alert emergency workers and health care providers about the use of an antiepileptic drug.*

CRITICAL THINKING SCENARIO 23-1

Antiepileptic Drugs

The Situation

J.M., an athletic, 18-year-old high school senior, suffered his first seizure during math class. He seemed attentive and alert, and then he suddenly slumped to the floor and suffered a full tonic–clonic (grand mal) seizure. The other students were frightened and did not know what to do. Fortunately, the teacher was familiar with seizures and quickly reacted to protect J.M. from hurting himself and to explain what was happening.

J.M. was diagnosed with idiopathic generalized epilepsy with tonic–clonic (grand mal) seizures. The combination of phenytoin and phenobarbital that he began taking made him quite drowsy during the day. These drugs were unable to control the seizures, and he suffered three more seizures in the next month—one at school and two at home. J.M. is now undergoing re-evaluation for possible drug adjustment and counseling.

Critical Thinking

What teaching implications should be considered when meeting with J.M.? *Consider his age and the setting of his first seizure.*

What problems might J.M. encounter in school and in athletics related to the diagnosis and the prescribed medication? *Consider measures that may help him avoid some of the unpleasant side effects related to this particular drug therapy. Driving a car may be a central social focus in the life of a high school senior.*

What problems can be anticipated and confronted before they occur concerning laws that forbid individuals with newly diagnosed epilepsy from driving?

Develop a teaching protocol for J.M. How will you involve the entire family in the teaching plan?

Discussion

On their first meeting, it is important for the nurse to establish a trusting relationship with J.M. and his family. J.M., who is at a sensitive stage of development, requires a great deal of support and encouragement to cope with the diagnosis of epilepsy and the need for drug therapy. He may need to ventilate his feelings and concerns and discuss how he can re-enter school without worrying about having a seizure in class. The nurse should implement a thorough drug teaching program, including a description of warning signs to watch for that should be reported to a health care professional. J.M. should be encouraged to take the following preventive measures:

- Have frequent oral hygiene to protect the gums.
- Avoid operating dangerous machinery or performing tasks that require alertness while drowsy and confused.
- Pace activities as much as possible to help deal with any fatigue and malaise.
- Take the drugs with meals if gastrointestinal upset is a problem.

This information should be given to both J.M. and his family in written form for future reference, along with the name of a health care professional and a telephone number to call with questions or comments. The importance of continuous medication to suppress the seizures should be stressed. The adverse effects of many of these drugs make it difficult for some patients to remain compliant with their drug regimen.

After the discussion with J.M., the nurse should meet with his family members, who also need support and encouragement to deal with his diagnosis and its implications. They need to know what seizures are, how the prescribed antiepileptic drugs affect the seizures, what they can do when seizures occur, and complete information about the drugs he must take and their anticipated drug effects. In addition, it is important to work with family members to determine whether any particular thing precipitated the seizures. In other words, was there any warning or aura? This may help with adjustment of drug dosages or avoidance of certain situations or stimuli that precipitate seizures. Family members should be encouraged to report and record any seizure activity that occurs.

Most states do not permit individuals with newly diagnosed epilepsy to drive, and states have varying regulations about the return of the driver's license after a seizure-free interval. If driving makes up a major part of J.M.'s social activities, this news may be even more unacceptable than his diagnosis. J.M. and his family should be counseled and helped to devise other ways of getting places and coping with this restriction. J.M. may be interested in referral to a support group for teens with similar problems, where he can share ideas, support, and frustrations.

J.M.'s condition is a chronic one that will require continual drug therapy and evaluation. He will need periodic reteaching and should have the opportunity to ask additional questions and to ventilate his feelings. J.M. should be encouraged to wear or carry a MedicAlert tag so that

Antiepileptic Drugs *(continued)*

emergency medical personnel are aware of his diagnosis and the medications he is taking.

Nursing Care Guide for J.M.: Antiepileptic Agents

Assessment: History and Examination

Allergies to any of these drugs; hypotension; arrhythmias; bone marrow suppression; coma; psychoses; pregnancy or lactation; hepatic or renal dysfunction

Concurrent use of valproic acid, cimetidine, disulfiram, isoniazid, phenacemide, sulfonamides, diazoxide, folic acid, rifampin, sucralfate, theophylline, primidone, acetaminophen

CV: blood pressure, pulse, peripheral perfusion

CNS: orientation, reflexes, affect, strength, EEG

Skin: color, lesions, texture, temperature

GI: abdominal evaluation, bowel sounds

Respiratory: respiration, adventitious sounds

Laboratory tests: CBC, liver and renal function tests

Nursing Diagnoses

Acute Pain related to GI, CNS, and GU effects

Risk for Injury related to CNS effects

Disturbed Thought Processes related to CNS effects

Deficient Knowledge regarding drug therapy

Impaired Skin Integrity related to dermatological effects

Implementation

Discontinue drug at first sign of liver dysfunction or skin rash.

Provide comfort and safety measures: positioning; give with meals; skin care.

Provide support and reassurance to cope with diagnosis, restrictions, and drug effects.

Provide patient teaching regarding drug name, dosage, side effects, symptoms to report, and the need to wear MedicAlert information; other drugs to avoid.

Evaluation

Evaluate drug effects: decrease in incidence and frequency of seizures; serum drug levels within therapeutic range.

Monitor for adverse effects: CNS effects (multiple); bone marrow suppression; rash, skin changes; GI effects—nausea, anorexia; arrhythmias.

Monitor for drug–drug interactions: increased depression with CNS depressants, alcohol; drugs as listed.

Evaluate effectiveness of patient teaching program.

Evaluate effectiveness of comfort/safety measures.

Patient Teaching for J.M.

- ☐ The drugs that are being evaluated for you are called antiepileptic agents. They are used to stabilize abnormal cells in the brain that have been firing excessively and causing seizures.
- ☐ The timing of these doses is very important. To be effective, this drug must be taken regularly.
- ☐ Do not stop taking this drug suddenly. If for any reason you are unable to continue taking the drug, notify your health care provider at once. This drug must be slowly withdrawn when its use is discontinued.
- ☐ Common effects of these drugs include:
  - *Fatigue, weakness, and drowsiness:* Try to space activities evenly throughout the day and allow rest periods to avoid these effects. Take safety precautions and avoid driving or operating dangerous machinery if these conditions occur.
  - *Headaches and difficulty sleeping:* These usually disappear as your body adjusts to the drug. If they persist and become too uncomfortable, consult with your health care provider.
  - *Gastrointestinal upset, loss of appetite, and diarrhea or constipation:* Taking the drug with food or eating small, frequent meals may help alleviate this problem.
  - Report any of the following conditions to your health care provider: *skin rash, severe nausea and vomiting, impaired coordination, yellowing of the eyes or skin, fever, sore throat, personality changes, and unusual bleeding or bruising.*
- ☐ It is advisable to wear or carry a Medic-Alert warning so that any person who takes care of you in an emergency will know that you are taking this drug.
- ☐ Tell any doctor, nurse, or other health care provider involved in your care that you are taking this drug.
- ☐ Keep this drug and all medications out of the reach of children.
- ☐ Do not take any other drug, including over-the-counter medications and alcohol, without consulting with your health care provider. Many of these preparations interact with the drug and could cause adverse effects.
- ☐ Report and record any seizure activity that you have while you are taking this drug.
- ☐ Take this drug exactly as prescribed. Regular medical follow-up, which may include blood tests, will be necessary to evaluate the effects of this drug on your body.

- Offer support and encouragement *to help the patient cope with the drug regimen.*

Evaluation

- Monitor patient response to the drug (decrease in incidence or absence of seizures; serum drug levels within the therapeutic range).
- Monitor for adverse effects (CNS changes, GI depression, urinary retention, arrhythmias, blood pressure changes, liver toxicity, bone marrow suppression, severe dermatological reactions).
- Evaluate effectiveness of teaching plan (patient can give the drug name and dosage and name possible adverse effects to watch for, and specific measures to prevent adverse effects; patient is aware of the risk of birth defects and the need to carry information about the diagnosis and use of this drug).
- Monitor the effectiveness of comfort measures and compliance with the regimen.

FOCUS POINTS

- Drugs used to treat tonic–clonic seizures include the barbiturates, the hydantoins, and the benzodiazepines.
- All of these drugs stabilize nerve membranes throughout the CNS to decrease excitability and hyperexcitability to stimulation.
- Adverse effects associated with these drugs reflect the CNS depression—lethargy, somnolence, fatigue, dry mouth, constipation, and dizziness. Serious liver, bone marrow, and dermatological problems can occur with specific drugs.

Drugs for Treating Absence (Petit Mal) Seizures

Absence or petit mal seizures involve a brief, sudden, and self-limited loss of consciousness. The patient may just stare into space or may exhibit rapid blinking, which could last 3 to 5 seconds. Many people are not aware that a seizure is happening. This type of seizure frequently occurs in children, starting at about 3 years of age, and usually disappears by puberty.

Succinimides

The drugs that are most frequently used to treat these seizures are different from the drugs used to treat or prevent tonic–clonic seizures. The succinimides and drugs that modulate the inhibitory neurotransmitter GABA are most frequently used. The succinimides include the following agents (see also Table 23.3):

- Ethosuximide (*Zarontin*) is the drug of choice for treating absence seizures. It has relatively few adverse effects compared with many other antiepileptic drugs. Ethosuximide is available for oral use. The established therapeutic serum level for ethosuximide is 40 to 100 mcg/mL.
- Methsuximide (*Celontin*), another oral drug, is used to treat absence seizures that are resistant to other drugs. It has been associated with bone marrow suppression.

Therapeutic Actions and Indications

Although the exact mechanism of action is not understood, the succinimides suppress the abnormal electrical activity in the brain that is associated with absence seizures. The action may be related to activity in inhibitory neural pathways in the brain (see Figure 23.1).

Ethosuximide and methsuximide are indicated for the control of absence seizures. Ethosuximide should be tried first; methsuximide should be reserved for the treatment of seizures that are refractory to other agents because it is associated with more severe adverse effects.

Table 23.3 DRUGS IN FOCUS

Drugs for Treating Absence (Petit Mal) Seizures–Succinimides

Drug Name	Dosage/Route	Usual Indications
P ethosuximide (*Zarontin*)	Adult and pediatric >6 yr: 500 mg/day PO Pediatric (3–6 yr): 250 mg/day PO, increase cautiously as needed	Drug of choice for absence (petit mal) seizures
methsuximide (*Celontin*)	Adult: 300 mg/day PO, up to 1.2 g/day Pediatric: determine dosage by age and weight considerations	Treatment of absence (petit mal) seizures refractory to other agents

Pharmacokinetics

The succinimides are readily absorbed from the GI tract, reaching peak levels in 1 to 7 hours, depending on the drug. They are metabolized in the liver and excreted in the urine. The half-life of ethosuximide is 30 hours in children and 60 hours in adults; the half-life of methsuximide is 2.6 to 4 hours. These drugs cross the placenta and enter breast milk. Use during pregnancy should be discussed with the woman because of the potential for adverse effects on the fetus. Another method of feeding the baby should be used if one of these drugs is needed during lactation.

Contraindications and Cautions

The succinimides are contraindicated in the presence of allergy to any of these drugs. Caution should be used with succinimides in the following conditions: renal or hepatic disease, *which could interfere with the metabolism and excretion of these drugs and lead to toxic levels;* pregnancy and lactation *because of the potential of adverse effects on the fetus or neonate;* and intermittent porphyria, *which could be exacerbated by the adverse effects of these drugs.*

Adverse Effects

Many of the adverse effects associated with the succinimides are related to their depressing effects in the CNS, including depression, drowsiness, fatigue, ataxia, insomnia, headache, and blurred vision. GI depression with nausea, vomiting, anorexia, weight loss, GI pain, and constipation or diarrhea may also occur. Bone marrow suppression, including potentially fatal pancytopenia, and dermatological reactions such as pruritus, urticaria, alopecia, and Stevens–Johnson syndrome may occur as a result of direct chemical irritation of the skin and bone marrow.

Clinically Important Drug–Drug Interactions

Use of succinimides with primidone may cause a decrease in serum levels of primidone. Patients should be monitored and appropriate dosage adjustments made if these two agents are used together.

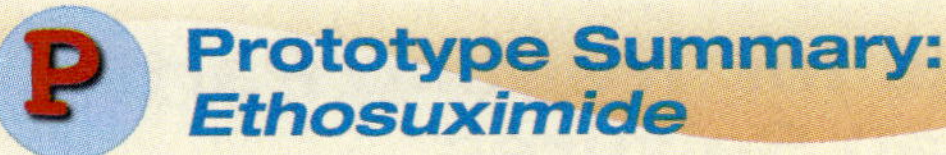

Prototype Summary: *Ethosuximide*

Indications: Control of absence seizures

Actions: May act in inhibitory neuronal systems; suppresses the EEG pattern associated with absence seizures; reduces frequency of attacks

Pharmacokinetics:

Route	Peak
Oral	3–7 h

$T_{1/2}$: 30 hours (children), 60 hours (adults); metabolized in the liver, excreted in the urine and bile

Adverse effects: Drowsiness, ataxia, dizziness, irritability, nervousness, headache, blurred vision, pruritus, Stevens–Johnson syndrome, nausea, vomiting, epigastric pain, anorexia, diarrhea, pancytopenia

Nursing Considerations for Patients Receiving Succinimides

Assessment: History and Examination

Screen for the following conditions, *which could be cautions or contraindications to use of the drug:* any known allergies to these drugs; pregnancy or lactation; renal or hepatic dysfunction; and intermittent porphyria.

Include screening *for baseline status before beginning therapy and for any potential adverse effects.* Assess the following: temperature; skin color and lesions; CNS orientation, affect, reflexes, and bilateral grip strength; EEG if appropriate; bowel sounds and reported output; pulse, auscultation, and blood pressure; and urinary output. Check liver and renal function tests.

Nursing Diagnoses

The patient receiving succinimides may have the following nursing diagnoses related to drug therapy:

- Acute Pain related to GI, CNS, and dermatological effects
- Disturbed Thought Processes related to CNS effects
- Risk for Infection related to bone marrow suppression
- Impaired Skin Integrity related to dermatological effects
- Deficient Knowledge regarding drug therapy

Implementation With Rationale

- Administer the drug with food *to alleviate GI irritation if GI upset is a problem.*
- Monitor complete blood count (CBC) before and periodically during therapy *to detect bone marrow suppression early and provide appropriate interventions.*
- Discontinue the drug if skin rash, bone marrow suppression, or unusual depression or personality changes occur *to prevent the development of more serious adverse effects.*
- Discontinue the drug slowly, and never withdraw the drug quickly *because rapid withdrawal may precipitate absence seizures.*

- Arrange for counseling for women of childbearing age who are taking these drugs. *Because these drugs have the potential to cause serious damage to the fetus,* women should understand the risk of birth defects and use barrier contraceptives to avoid pregnancy.
- Evaluate for therapeutic blood levels (40 to 100 mcg/mL) for ethosuximide *to ensure the most appropriate dosage of the drug.*
- Provide thorough patient teaching, including the drug name and prescribed dosage, as well as measures for avoidance of adverse effects, warning signs that may indicate possible problems, and the need for monitoring and evaluation *to enhance patient knowledge about drug therapy and to promote compliance.*
- Suggest the wearing or carrying of a MedicAlert bracelet *to alert emergency workers and health care providers about the use of an antiepileptic drug.*
- Offer support and encouragement *to help the patient cope with the drug regimen.*

Evaluation

- Monitor patient response to the drug (decrease in incidence or absence of seizures; serum drug level within therapeutic range).
- Monitor for adverse effects (CNS changes, GI depression, arrhythmias, blood pressure changes, bone marrow suppression, severe dermatological reactions).
- Evaluate the effectiveness of the teaching plan (patient can give the drug name and dosage and name possible adverse effects to watch for and specific measures to prevent adverse effects; patient is aware of the risk of birth defects and the need to carry information about the diagnosis and use of this drug).
- Monitor the effectiveness of comfort measures and compliance with the regimen.

Other Drugs for Treating Absence (Petit Mal) Seizures

Three other drugs that are used in the treatment of absence seizures do not fit into a specific drug class (Table 23.4).

One such drug is valproic acid (*Depakene*), which reduces abnormal electrical activity in the brain and may also increase GABA activity at inhibitory receptors. This agent is the drug of choice for the treatment of myoclonic seizures. Because it is sometimes associated with hepatic toxicity and because other agents may have fewer adverse effects, valproic acid is a second-choice drug for the treatment of absence seizures. It is also effective in mania, migraine headaches, and partial seizures. It is readily absorbed from the GI tract, reaching peak levels in 1 to 4 hours. It is metabolized in the liver and excreted in the urine with a half-life of 6 to 16 hours. Valproic acid crosses the placenta and enters breast milk; it should not be used during pregnancy or lactation unless the benefit clearly outweighs the risk to the fetus or neonate.

Acetazolamide (*Diamox*) is a sulfonamide drug that is especially effective for treatment of absence seizures in children. It is also used to treat open-angle and secondary glaucoma, as prophylaxis and treatment of acute mountain sickness, and to decrease edema associated with congestive heart failure and drug use. It is readily absorbed from the GI tract and is excreted unchanged in the urine with a half-life of 2.5 to 6 hours. It is known to cross the placenta and enter breast milk and should not be used during pregnancy or lactation unless the benefit clearly outweighs the risk to the fetus or neonate.

Another sulfonamide, zonisamide (*Zonegran*), is a newer agent that inhibits voltage-sensitive sodium and calcium channels, thus stabilizing nerve cell membranes and modulating calcium-dependent presynaptic release of excitatory neurotransmitters. It is used as an adjunct to other drugs for the treatment of absence seizures. Zonisamide is well absorbed from the GI tract, reaching peak levels in 2 to 6 hours. It is primarily excreted unchanged in the urine, with a half-life of 63 hours. It crosses the placenta and has been shown to be teratogenic in animal studies. Women of childbearing age should be advised to use contraception while taking this drug. It is not known whether zonisamide enters breast milk, but because of the potential for serious adverse effects on the baby, it should not be used during lactation. When it is discontinued, zonisamide should be tapered over 2 weeks because of a risk of precipitating seizures. Patients who take this drug should be very well hydrated; there is a risk of renal calculi development.

Drugs for Treating Partial (Focal) Seizures

Focal seizures, or partial seizures, are so called because they involve only part of the brain and usually originate from one site or focus. The presenting symptoms depend on exactly where in the brain the excessive electrical discharge is occurring. Partial seizures can be simple, involving only a single muscle or reaction, or complex, involving a series of reactions or emotional changes.

Drugs used in the treatment of partial seizures include the following (Table 23.5).

- Carbamazepine (*Tegretol, Atretol,* and others) is often the drug of choice for treatment of partial seizures. Chemically related to the tricyclic antidepressants, it has also been used in the treatment of tonic–clonic seizures,

Table 23.4 DRUGS IN FOCUS

Other Drugs for Treating Absence (Petit Mal) Seizures

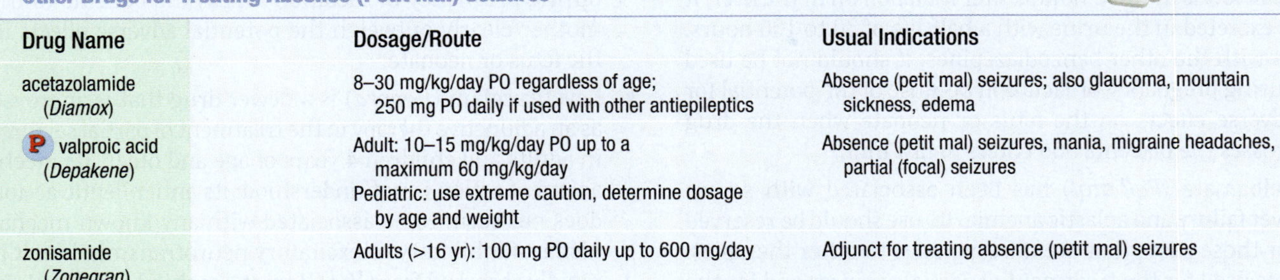

Drug Name	Dosage/Route	Usual Indications
acetazolamide (*Diamox*)	8–30 mg/kg/day PO regardless of age; 250 mg PO daily if used with other antiepileptics	Absence (petit mal) seizures; also glaucoma, mountain sickness, edema
P valproic acid (*Depakene*)	Adult: 10–15 mg/kg/day PO up to a maximum 60 mg/kg/day Pediatric: use extreme caution, determine dosage by age and weight	Absence (petit mal) seizures, mania, migraine headaches, partial (focal) seizures
zonisamide (*Zonegran*)	Adults (>16 yr): 100 mg PO daily up to 600 mg/day	Adjunct for treating absence (petit mal) seizures

trigeminal neuralgia, and bipolar disorder. It has the ability to inhibit polysynaptic responses and to block sodium channels to prevent the formation of repetitive action potentials in the abnormal focus. Carbamazepine is absorbed from the GI tract and metabolized in the liver by the cytochrome P450 system. It is excreted in the urine. Carbamazepine can cause fetal harm and should not be used during pregnancy. Women of childbearing age should be advised to use contraception. It also enters breast milk and can cause serious adverse effects in the baby. If the drug is needed during lactation, another method of feeding the baby should be used.

Table 23.5 DRUGS IN FOCUS

Drugs for Treating Partial (Focal) Seizures

Drug Name	Dosage/Route	Usual Indications
P carbamazepine (*Tegretol, Atretol*)	Adult: 800–1200 mg/day PO in divided doses q6–8h Pediatric (>12 yr): adult doses, do not exceed 1000 mg/day Pediatric (6–12 yr): 20–30 mg/kg/day PO in divided doses t.i.d. to q.i.d. Pediatric (<6 yr): 35 mg/kg/day PO	Drug of choice for partial (focal) seizures; tonic–clonic (grand mal) seizures, trigeminal neuralgia; bipolar disorder
clorazepate (*Tranxene, Gen-Xene*)	Adult: 7.5 mg PO t.i.d., up to 90 mg/day Pediatric (9–12 yr): 7.5 mg PO b.i.d., up to 60 mg/day	Adjunct for partial seizures, anxiety, alcohol withdrawal
felbamate (*Felbatol*)	Adult and children >14 yr: 2600 mg/day PO Pediatric (2–14 yr): 15 mg/kg/day PO in divided doses three to four times per day	Monotherapy or adjunctive therapy for partial seizures; adjunctive therapy for Lennox–Gastaut syndrome in children
gabapentin (*Neurontin*)	Adult: 900–1800 mg/day PO in divided doses t.i.d. Pediatric (3–12 yr): 10–15 mg/kg/day PO in divided doses	Adjunct in treating partial seizures; treatment of post-herpetic pain
lamotrigine (*Lamictal*)	Adult: 300–500 mg/day PO in divided doses b.i.d. Pediatric (2–12 yr): 1–5 mg/kg/day PO in divided doses b.i.d. Pediatric (>12 yr): 100–400 mg/day PO in divided doses b.i.d.	Adjunct in treating partial seizures; adjunct for Lennox–Gastaut syndrome in children; long-term treatment of bipolar disorders
levetiracetam (*Keppra*)	Adult: 500 mg PO b.i.d. up to 3000 mg/day Pediatric (4–16 yr): 10 mg/kg PO b.i.d. to a maximum of 1500–3000 mg/day	Adjunctive treatment of partial seizures in adults
oxcarbazepine (*Trileptal*)	Adult: 600 mg PO b.i.d. Pediatric (4–16 yr): 8–10 mg/kg/day PO	Monotherapy or adjunctive therapy of partial seizures in adults and children 4–16 yr of age
pregabalin (*Lyrica*)	150–600 mg/day PO in divided doses *Neuropathic pain:* 100 mg PO t.i.d. *Postherpetic neuralgia:* 75–150 mg PO t.i.d.	Adjunctive treatment of partial seizures; management of neuropathic pain associated with diabetic peripheral neuropathy and postherpetic neuralgia
tiagabine (*Gabitril*)	Adult: 4 mg PO daily up to 56 mg/day in two to four divided doses Pediatric (12–18 yr): 4 mg PO daily up to a maximum 32 mg/day in two to four divided doses	Adjunct in treating partial seizures
topiramate (*Topamax*)	Adult: 400 mg PO daily in two divided doses; reduce dosage in renal impairment Pediatric (2–16 yr): 5–9 mg/kg/day PO in two divided doses	Adjunct in treating partial seizures in adults

- Clorazepate (*Tranxene, Gen-Xene,* and others), a benzodiazepine that is indicated for anxiety and alcohol withdrawal, is also used as adjunctive therapy for partial seizures. It is rapidly absorbed from the GI tract, reaching peak levels in 1 to 2 hours. After metabolism in the liver, it is excreted in the urine with a half-life of 30 to 100 hours. As with the other benzodiazepines, it should not be used during pregnancy or lactation because of the potential for adverse effects on the fetus or neonate when the drug crosses the placenta and enters breast milk.
- Felbamate (*Felbatol*) has been associated with severe liver failure and aplastic anemia. Its use should be reserved for those cases that are unresponsive to other therapies. It is used for the treatment of partial seizures and for the seizures associated with Lennox–Gastaut syndrome in children. Felbamate is absorbed well from the GI tract and is primarily excreted unchanged in the urine with a half-life of 20 to 23 hours. There are no clear studies about the effects of the drug during pregnancy and lactation. Therefore, it should not be used during pregnancy or lactation unless the benefits to the mother clearly outweigh potential adverse effects in the fetus or neonate.
- Gabapentin (*Neurontin*), is used as adjunctive therapy in the treatment of partial seizures in adults and children ages 3 to 12 years and for the treatment of post-herpetic neuralgia. It has orphan drug status for the treatment of amyotrophic lateral sclerosis. It is also being studied for the treatment of tremors associated with multiple sclerosis, for neuropathic pain, for bipolar disorder, and for migraine prophylaxis. Gabapentin is well absorbed from the GI tract and widely distributed in the body. It is excreted unchanged in the urine with a half-life of 5 to 7 hours. Patients with renal dysfunction are at higher risk for toxic effects of the drug and need a lower dosage. Gabapentin crosses the placenta and enters breast milk. It was found to be toxic to the fetus in animal studies. Use during pregnancy and lactation should be reserved for those situations in which the benefit to the mother clearly outweighs the potential risk to the fetus or neonate.
- Lamotrigine (*Lamictal*) is also used as adjunctive therapy or monotherapy in the treatment of partial seizures and in the treatment of the seizures associated with Lennox–Gastaut syndrome in adults and children 2 years of age and older; in 2003 it was approved for long-term treatment of bipolar disorder. It is being studied for use in tonic–clonic seizures, absence seizures, myoclonic seizures, and drug-resistant seizures of multiple types. It may inhibit voltage-sensitive sodium and calcium channels, stabilize nerve cell membranes, and modulate calcium-dependent presynaptic release of excitatory neurotransmitters. Lamotrigine is rapidly absorbed from the GI tract, metabolized in the liver, and primarily excreted in the urine. The half-life of lamotrigine is approximately 25 hours. It has been associated with very serious to life-threatening rashes, and the drug should be discontinued at the first sign of any rash. There are no clear studies about the effects of the drug during pregnancy or lactation, although it was shown to be toxic to the fetus in animal studies. It should not be used during pregnancy or lactation unless the benefits to the mother clearly outweigh the potential adverse effects in the fetus or neonate.
- Levetiracetam (*Keppra*) is a newer drug that is approved as an adjunctive therapy in the treatment of partial seizures in adults and children 4 years of age and older. Its mechanism of action is not understood; its antiepileptic action does not seem to be associated with any known mechanisms of inhibitory or excitatory neurotransmission. It is rapidly absorbed from the GI tract, reaching peak levels in 1 hour. It goes through very little metabolism, with most of the drug being excreted unchanged in the urine with a half-life of 6 to 8 hours. Patients with renal dysfunction are more likely to experience toxic effects of the drug, and the dosage for these patients needs to be decreased accordingly. There are no clear studies about the effects of the drug during pregnancy or lactation, although it was shown to be toxic to the fetus in animal studies. It should not be used during pregnancy or lactation unless the benefits to the mother clearly outweigh the potential adverse effects in the fetus or neonate.

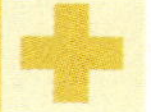

FOCUS ON **PATIENT SAFETY**

Be aware that name confusion has been reported between *Keppra* (levetiracetam) and *Kaletra* (lopinavir/ritonavir), an HIV antiviral combination drug. Both drugs come in a liquid form, and confusion has been reported in the administration of the two drugs, causing serious adverse effects. Use extreme caution.

- Oxcarbazepine (*Trileptal*) was approved in 2000 for the treatment of partial seizures in adults and children 4 to 16 years of age as monotherapy or in combination with other antiepileptics. It is being studied as an alternate treatment of bipolar disease. The exact mechanism of antiseizure activity is not known. It does inhibit voltage-sensitive sodium channels, stabilizing hyperexcited nerve cell membranes. It also increases potassium conductance and modulates calcium-dependent presynaptic release of excitatory neurotransmitters. Any or all of these effects may be responsible for the antiseizure effects of the drug. Oxcarbazepine is completely absorbed from the GI tract and extensively metabolized in the liver. It is excreted in the urine with a half-life of 2 and then 9 hours. Oxcarbazepine is teratogenic in animal studies and should not be used during pregnancy. It is found in breast milk; if the drug is needed during lactation, another method of feeding the baby should be used.
- Pregabalin (*Lyrica*) was introduced in the United States in 2005. This drug has a high binding affinity for voltage-

gated calcium channels in the cerebrovascular system. It seems to modulate the calcium function in these neurons, leading to a decreased release of neurotransmitters into the synaptic cleft and a decrease in cell activity. It is approved for the adjunctive treatment of adults with partial-onset seizures and for the management of neuropathic pain associated with diabetic peripheral neuropathy and postherpetic neuralgia. It is being studied for the management of fibromyalgia. Pregabalin is rapidly absorbed orally, reaching peak levels in 1.5 hours. It is not metabolized, but is eliminated unchanged in the urine with a half-life of 6.3 hours. It is not known if this drug crosses the placenta or enters breast milk. Because of the potential for adverse effects on the neonate, this drug should be used during pregnancy and lactation only if the benefits to the mother clearly outweigh any potential effects on the neonate. Men considering fathering a child should be advised that in animal studies, males receiving this drug had decreased fertility and associated birth defects in offspring. The adverse effects most commonly seen with this drug are related to CNS depression—tremor, dizziness, somnolence, and visual changes. This drug does have a controlled substance rating as Category V. It can cause feelings of well-being and euphoria. Because of this, its use should be limited in patients who have a history of abuse of medications or alcohol.

- Tiagabine (*Gabitril*) is used as adjunctive therapy in the treatment of partial seizures in adults and in children 12 to 18 years of age. It has also been associated with serious skin rash. It binds to GABA reuptake receptors, causing an increase in GABA levels in the brain. Because GABA is an inhibitory neurotransmitter, the result is a stabilizing of nerve membranes and a decrease in excessive activity. Tiagabine is rapidly absorbed from the GI tract, reaching peak levels in 45 minutes. It is metabolized in the liver by the cytochrome P450 system. It is excreted in the urine with a half-life of 4 to 7 hours. There are no clear studies about the effects of the drug during pregnancy or lactation, although it was shown to be toxic to the fetus in animal studies. It should not be used during pregnancy or lactation unless the benefits to the mother clearly outweigh the potential adverse effects in the fetus or neonate.
- Topiramate (*Topamax*) is a newer drug that is used as adjunctive therapy for partial seizures in adults and children 2 to 16 years of age. It is also approved for treatment of tonic–clonic seizures, for prevention of migraine headaches, and as adjunct therapy in Lennox–Gastaut syndrome. It is being studied for use in cluster headaches, infantile spasms, alcohol dependence, bulimia nervosa, and weight loss. Topiramate is rapidly absorbed from the GI tract, reaching peak levels in 2 hours. It is widely distributed and excreted unchanged in the urine. Patients with renal impairment should receive a reduced dosage of the drug. It has been associated with marked CNS depression. It may interfere with sodium channels, causing a stabilizing of nerve membranes, and it also may increase GABA activity. There are no clear studies about the effects of the drug during pregnancy or lactation, although it was shown to be toxic to the fetus in animal studies. It should not be used during pregnancy or lactation unless the benefits to the mother clearly outweigh the potential adverse effects in the fetus or neonate.

Therapeutic Actions and Indications

The drugs used to control partial seizures stabilize nerve membranes in two ways—either directly, by altering sodium and calcium channels, or indirectly, by increasing the activity of GABA, an inhibitory neurotransmitter, and thereby decreasing excessive activity (see Figure 23.1). Each of these drugs has a slightly different mechanism of action, as noted earlier.

These drugs are indicated for the treatment of partial seizures. Carbamazepine, oxcarbazepine, and felbamate are used as monotherapy, and the other drugs are used as adjunctive therapy.

Contraindications and Cautions

Contraindications to the drugs used to control partial seizures include the following conditions: presence of any known allergy to the drug; bone marrow suppression, *which could be exacerbated by the drug effects;* and severe hepatic dysfunction, *which could be exacerbated and could interfere with the metabolism of the drugs.*

Caution should be used in the following situations: in pregnancy or lactation *because of the potential adverse effects on the fetus or neonate;* with renal or hepatic dysfunction, *which could alter the metabolism and excretion of the drugs;* and with renal stones, *which could be exacerbated by the effects of some of these agents.*

Adverse Effects

The most frequently occurring adverse effects associated with the drugs used for partial seizures relate to the CNS depression that results. The following conditions may occur: drowsiness, fatigue, weakness, confusion, headache, and insomnia; GI depression, with nausea, vomiting, and anorexia; and upper respiratory infections. These antiepileptics can also be directly toxic to the liver and the bone marrow, causing dysfunction. The exact effects of each drug vary.

Clinically Important Drug–Drug Interactions

If any of these drugs are taken with other CNS depressants or alcohol, a potential for increased CNS depression exists.

Patients should be cautioned to avoid alcohol while taking drugs for partial seizures or to take extreme precautions if such combinations cannot be avoided.

In addition, numerous drug–drug interactions are associated with carbamazepine. A drug reference should be consulted whenever a drug is added or withdrawn from a carbamazepine-containing regimen. Dosage adjustments may be necessary.

Prototype Summary: Carbamazepine

Indications: Treatment of refractory seizure disorders, including partial seizures with complex patterns; tonic–clonic seizures; mixed seizures; trigeminal neuralgia

Actions: Inhibits polysynaptic responses and blocks post-tetanic potentiations; mechanism of action is not understood; related to the tricyclic antidepressants

Pharmacokinetics:

Route	Onset	Peak
Oral	Slow	4–5 h
ER oral	Slow	3–12 h

$T_{1/2}$: 25–65 hours, then 12–17 hours; metabolized in the liver, excreted in the urine and feces

Adverse effects: Drowsiness, ataxia, dizziness, nausea, vomiting, CV complications, hepatitis, hematological disorders, Stevens–Johnson syndrome

Nursing Considerations for Patients Receiving Drugs to Treat Partial (Focal) Seizures

Assessment: History and Examination

Screen for the following conditions, *which could be cautions or contraindications for the use of the drug:* any known allergies to these drugs; pregnancy or lactation; bone marrow suppression; hepatic dysfunction; renal dysfunction; and renal stones.

Include screening *for baseline status before beginning therapy and for any potential adverse effects.* Assess the following: temperature; skin color and lesions; CNS orientation, affect, reflexes, and bilateral grip strength; EEG; pulse and blood pressure; respiration and adventitious sounds; and bowel sounds and reported output. Check liver and renal function tests, urinalysis, and CBC with differential.

Nursing Diagnoses

The patient taking a drug to treat partial seizures may have the following nursing diagnoses related to drug therapy:

- Acute Pain related to GI and CNS effects
- Disturbed Thought Processes related to CNS effects
- Risk for Injury related to CNS and bone marrow effects
- Deficient Knowledge regarding drug therapy

Implementation With Rationale

- Administer the drug with food *to alleviate GI irritation if GI upset is a problem.*
- Monitor CBC before and periodically during therapy *to detect and prevent serious bone marrow suppression.*
- Discontinue the drug if skin rash, bone marrow suppression, unusual depression, or personality changes occur *to prevent further serious adverse effects.*
- Discontinue the drug slowly and never withdraw the drug quickly *because rapid withdrawal may precipitate seizures.*
- Arrange for counseling for women of childbearing age who are taking these drugs. *Because these drugs have the potential to cause serious damage to the fetus,* women should understand the risk of birth defects and use barrier contraceptives to avoid pregnancy.
- Evaluate for therapeutic blood levels of carbamazepine (4 to 12 mcg/mL) *to ensure that the most effective dosage is being used.*
- Provide thorough patient teaching, including drug name and prescribed dosage, as well as measures for avoidance of adverse effects, warning signs that may indicate possible problems, and the need for monitoring and evaluation, *to enhance patient knowledge about drug therapy and to promote compliance.*
- Suggest that the patient wear or carry a Medic-Alert bracelet *to alert emergency workers and health care providers about the use of an antiepileptic drug.*
- Offer support and encouragement *to help the patient cope with the drug regimen.*

Evaluation

- Monitor patient response to the drug (decrease in incidence or absence of seizures).

- Monitor for adverse effects (CNS changes, GI depression, bone marrow suppression, severe dermatological reactions, liver toxicity, renal stones).
- Evaluate effectiveness of teaching plan (patient can give the drug name and dosage and name possible adverse effects to watch for, and specific measures to prevent adverse effects; patient is aware of the risk of birth defects and the need to carry information about the diagnosis and use of this drug).

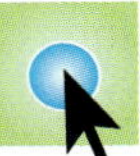

WEB LINKS

Health care providers and patients may want to consult the following Internet sources:

http://www.aesnet.org Information on epilepsy, including support groups, research, and treatment.

http://www.ninds.nih.gov Information on education programs, research, and other information related to seizure disorders.

http://www.efa.org Information about epilepsy research, treatment, and laws.

Points to Remember

- Epilepsy is a collection of different syndromes, all of which have the same characteristic: a sudden discharge of excessive electrical energy from nerve cells located within the brain. This event is called a seizure.
- Seizures can be divided into two groups: generalized and partial (focal).
- Generalized seizures can be further classified as tonic–clonic (grand mal); absence (petit mal); myoclonic; febrile; and rapidly recurrent (status epilepticus).
- Partial (focal) seizures can be further classified as simple or complex.
- Drug treatment depends on the type of seizure that the patient has experienced and the toxicity associated with the available agents.
- Drug treatment is directed at stabilizing the overexcited nerve membranes and/or increasing the effectiveness of GABA, an inhibitory neurotransmitter.
- Adverse effects associated with antiepileptics (e.g., insomnia, fatigue, confusion, GI depression, bradycardia) reflect the CNS depression caused by the drugs.
- Patients being treated with an antiepileptic should be advised to wear or carry a Medic-Alert notification to alert emergency medical professionals to their epilepsy and their use of antiepileptic drugs.

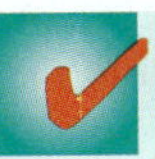

CHECK YOUR UNDERSTANDING

Answers to the questions in this chapter may be found in the Answer Key in the back of the book.

Multiple Choice

Select the best answer to the following.

1. Epilepsy is
   a. always characterized by grand mal seizures.
   b. only a genetic problem.
   c. the most prevalent neurological disorder.
   d. the name given to one brain disorder.

2. Generalized seizures could include all of the following except
   a. petit mal seizures.
   b. febrile seizures.
   c. grand mal seizures.
   d. complex seizures.

3. Patients who are maintained on an antiepileptic drug should be encouraged to
   a. give up their driver's license.
   b. wear or carry a MedicAlert notice.
   c. take antihistamines to help dry up secretions.
   d. keep the diagnosis a secret to avoid prejudice.

4. Drugs that are commonly used to treat grand mal seizures include
   a. barbiturates, benzodiazepines, and hydantoins.
   b. barbiturates, antihistamines, and local anesthetics.
   c. hydantoins, phenobarbital, and phensuximide.
   d. benzodiazepines, phensuximide, and valproic acid.

5. The drug of choice for the treatment of absence seizures is
   a. valproic acid.
   b. methsuximide.
   c. phensuximide.
   d. ethosuximide.

6. Focal or partial seizures
   a. start at one point and spread quickly throughout the brain.

b. are best treated with benzodiazepines.
c. involve only part of the brain.
d. are easily diagnosed and recognized.

7. One drug that is used alone in the treatment of partial seizures is
a. carbamazepine.
b. topiramate.
c. lamotrigine.
d. gabapentin.

8. Treatment of epilepsy is directed at
a. blocking the transmission of nerve impulses into the brain.
b. stabilizing overexcited nerve membranes and/or increasing the inhibitory neurotransmitter GABA.
c. blocking peripheral nerve terminals.
d. thickening the meninges to damp brain electrical activity.

Multiple Response

Select all that apply.

1. A client has been stabilized on phenytoin (*Dilantin*) for several years and has not experienced a grand mal seizure in more than 3 years. The client decides to stop the drug because it no longer seems to be needed. In counseling the client, the nurse should include which of the following points?
a. He will always need this drug.
b. This drug needs to be slowly tapered to avoid potentially serious adverse effects.
c. He is probably correct and the drug is not needed.
d. The drug should not be stopped until appropriate blood tests are done.
e. Stopping the drug suddenly could precipitate seizures because the nerves will be more sensitive.
f. His insurance company won't cover any problems that might occur if he stops the drug without physician approval.

2. The most common adverse effects associated with antiepileptic therapy reflect the depression of the CNS. In assessing a client on antiepileptic therapy, the nurse would monitor the patient for which of the following?
a. Hypertension
b. Insomnia
c. Confusion
d. GI depression
e. Increased salivation
f. Tachycardia

Fill in the Blanks

1. ____________________, the most prevalent of the neurologic disorders, is a collection of different syndromes, all characterized by a sudden discharge of excessive electrical energy from nerve cells located within the brain.

2. Sudden discharge of excessive electrical energy in the brain leads to a(n) ____________________.

3. If motor nerves are stimulated by this sudden discharge of electrical energy, a ______________ may occur with tonic–clonic muscle contractions.

4. Epilepsy is managed using a class of drugs called ____________________.

5. Tonic–clonic seizures, formerly known as ____________________, involve dramatic tonic–clonic muscle contractions, loss of consciousness, and a recovery period that is characterized by confusion and exhaustion.

6. A petit mal seizure, now called a(n) ______________, involves abrupt, brief (3–5 seconds) periods of loss of consciousness.

7. Seizures that involve short, sporadic periods of muscle contractions that last for several minutes are called ____________________.

8. Seizures that are related to very high fevers and usually involve convulsions are called ______________.

9. The most dangerous of seizure conditions is a state in which seizures rapidly recur again and again, which is referred to as ____________________.

10. Partial or ____________________ seizures involve one area of the brain and do not spread throughout the entire brain.

Web Exercise

Your patient is a teenage girl who has just received a diagnosis of epilepsy. Go to the internet and find information for the patient, her family and her school. Start with information on epilepsy, including support groups, research, and treatment at http://www.aesnet.org. Use links provided on this site to prepare a teaching plan for the entire family.

Bibliography and References

Bailey, K. (1998). *Psychotropic drug facts.* Philadelphia: Lippincott-Raven.
Drug facts and comparisons. (2006). St. Louis: Facts and Comparisons.
Gilman, A., Hardman, J. G., & Limbird, L. E. (Eds.). (2006). *Goodman and Gilman's the pharmacological basis of therapeutics* (11th ed.). New York: McGraw-Hill.
Karch, A. M. (2006). *2007 Lippincott nursing drug guide.* Philadelphia: Lippincott Williams & Wilkins.
Porth, C. M. (2005). *Pathophysiology: Concepts of altered health states* (7th ed.). Philadelphia: Lippincott Williams & Wilkins.
Professional's guide to patient drug facts. (2006). St. Louis: Facts and Comparisons.

CHAPTER 24

Antiparkinsonism Agents

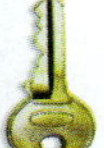

KEY TERMS

anticholinergic
bradykinesia
corpus striatum
dopaminergic
Parkinson's disease
substantia nigra

LEARNING OBJECTIVES

Upon completion of this chapter, you will be able to:

1. Describe the current theory of the cause of Parkinson's disease and correlate this with the clinical presentation of the disease.
2. Describe the therapeutic actions, indications, pharmacokinetics, contraindications, most common adverse reactions, and important drug–drug interactions associated with the anticholinergics, dopaminergics, and adjunctive therapies used to treat Parkinson's disease.
3. Discuss the use of antiparkinsonism drugs across the lifespan.
4. Compare and contrast the prototype drugs for each class of antiparkinsonism agents with the other drugs in that class and with drugs from the other classes used to treat the disease.
5. Outline the nursing considerations and teaching needs for patients receiving each class of antiparkinsonism agents.

ANTICHOLINERGICS

benztropine
P biperiden
diphenhydramine
procyclidine
trihexyphenidyl

DOPAMINERGICS

amantadine
apomorphine
bromocriptine
carbidopa–levodopa
P levodopa
pergolide
pramipexole
ropinirole

ADJUNCTIVE AGENTS

entacapone
selegiline
tolcapone

In the 1990s, several prominent figures—former heavyweight boxing champion Muhammad Ali, former U.S. Attorney General Janet Reno, and actor Michael J. Fox—revealed that they had **Parkinson's disease**, a progressive, chronic neurologic disorder. In general, Parkinson's disease may develop in people of any age (Box 24.1), but it usually affects those who are past middle age and entering their 60s or even older. Therefore, the occurrence of Parkinson's disease in these leading individuals who at the time of diagnosis were relatively young people is that much more interesting. The cause of the condition is not known.

At this time, there is no cure for Parkinson's disease. Therapy is aimed at management of signs and symptoms to provide optimal functioning for as long as possible.

Parkinson's Disease and Parkinsonism

Lack of coordination is characteristic of Parkinson's disease or parkinsonism. Rhythmic tremors develop, insidiously at first. In some muscle groups, these tremors lead to rigidity, and in others, weakness. Affected patients may have trouble maintaining position or posture, and they may develop the condition known as **bradykinesia**, marked by difficulties in performing intentional movements and extreme slowness or sluggishness.

As Parkinson's disease progresses, walking becomes a problem; a shuffling gait is a hallmark of the condition. In addition, patients may drool, and their speech may be slow and slurred. As the cranial nerves are affected, they may develop a masklike expression. Parkinson's disease does not affect the higher levels of the cerebral cortex, so a very alert and intelligent person may be trapped in a progressively degenerating body. Parkinsonism is a term used to describe the Parkinson's disease–like extrapyramidal symptoms that are adverse effects associated with particular drugs or brain injuries.

Causal Theories

Although the cause of Parkinson's disease is not known, it is known that the signs and symptoms of the disease relate to damage to neurons in the basal ganglia of the brain (Figure 24.1). Theories about the cause of the degeneration range from viral infection, blows to the head, brain infection, atherosclerosis, and exposure to certain drugs and environmental factors.

BOX 24.1 DRUG THERAPY ACROSS THE LIFESPAN

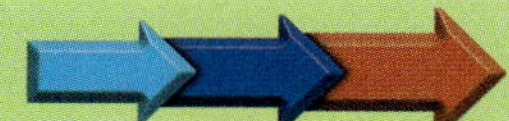

Antiparkinsonism Agents

CHILDREN

The safety and effectiveness of most of these drugs has not been established in children. The incidence of Parkinson's disease in children is very small. Children do, however, experience parkinsonian symptoms as a result of drug effects.

If a child needs an antiparkinsonian drug, diphenhydramine is the drug of choice. If further relief is needed and another drug is tried, careful dosage calculations should be done based on age and weight, and the child should be monitored very closely for adverse effects.

ADULTS

The eventual dependence and lack of control that accompany Parkinson's disease are devastating to all patients and their families but may be particularly overwhelming to individuals in their prime of life who value high degrees of autonomy, self-determination, and independence. Although these characteristics are not associated with any particular ethnic group, they are valued more highly among certain cultures than others. For example, Latinos—who traditionally have strong extended family ties—may not have the same problems adjusting to a chronic, debilitating illness in a relative as members of other ethnic groups. It is important for the nurse to assess all families with sensitivity to determine what convictions they hold and plan nursing care accordingly.

Adults diagnosed with Parkinson's disease require extensive teaching and support and help coping with the disease as well as with the effects of the drugs.

With the increasing interest in herbal and alternative therapies, it is important to stress the need to inform the health care provider about any other treatment being used. Vitamin B_6 can pose a serious problem for patients who are taking some of these drugs.

Women of childbearing age should be advised to use contraception when they are on these drugs. If a pregnancy does occur, or is desired, they need counseling about the potential for adverse effects. Women who are nursing should be encouraged to find another method of feeding the baby because of the potential for adverse drug effects on the baby.

OLDER ADULTS

Although Parkinson's disease may affect individuals of any age, gender, or nationality, the frequency of the disease increases with age. This debilitating condition, which affects more men than women, may be one of many chronic problems associated with aging.

The drugs that are used to manage Parkinson's disease are associated with more adverse effects in older people with long-term problems. Both anticholinergic and dopaminergic drugs aggravate glaucoma, benign prostatic hypertrophy, constipation, cardiac problems, and chronic obstructive pulmonary diseases. Special precautions and frequent follow-up visits are necessary for older patients with Parkinson's disease, and their drug dosages may need to be adjusted frequently to avoid serious problems. In many cases, other agents are given to counteract the effects of these drugs, and patients then have complicated drug regimens with many associated adverse effects and problems. Consequently, it is essential for these patients to have extensive written drug-teaching protocols.

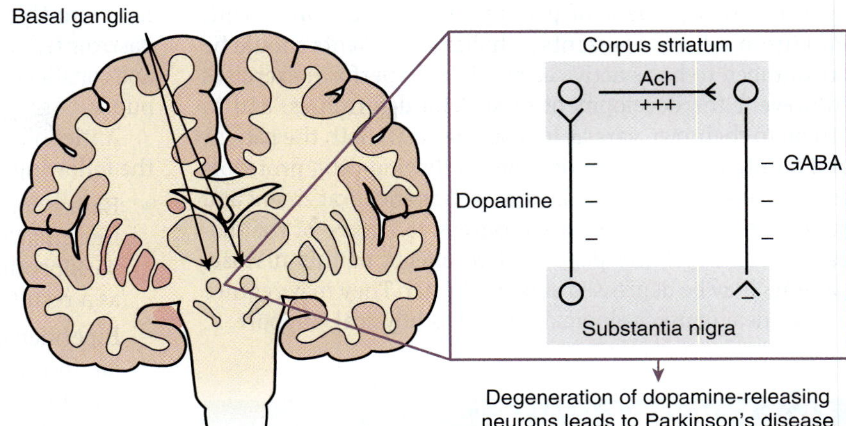

FIGURE 24.1 Schematic representation of the degeneration of neurons that leads to Parkinson's disease. Cells in the corpus striatum send impulses to the substantia nigra using GABA to inhibit activity. In turn, the substantia nigra sends impulses to the corpus striatum, using dopamine, to inhibit activity. Cortical areas use acetylcholine (Ach) to stimulate intentional movements.

Even though the actual cause is not known, the mechanism that causes the signs and symptoms of Parkinson's disease is understood. In a part of the brain called the **substantia nigra**, a dopamine-rich area, nerve cell bodies begin to degenerate. This process results in a reduction of the number of impulses sent to the **corpus striatum** in the basal ganglia. This area of the brain, in conjunction with the substantia nigra, helps maintain muscle tone not related to any particular movement. The corpus striatum is connected to the substantia nigra by a series of neurons that use the inhibitory neurotransmitter gamma-aminobutyric acid (GABA). The substantia nigra sends nerve impulses back into the corpus stratum using the inhibitory neurotransmitter dopamine. The two areas then mutually inhibit activity in a balanced manner.

Higher neurons from the cerebral cortex secrete acetylcholine in the area of the corpus striatum as an excitatory neurotransmitter to coordinate intentional movements of the body. When there is a decrease in dopamine in the area, it causes a chemical imbalance in this area of the brain that allows the cholinergic or excitatory cells to dominate. This affects the functioning of the basal ganglia and of the cortical and cerebellar components of the extrapyramidal motor system. The extrapyramidal system is one that provides coordination for unconscious muscle movements, including those that control position, posture, and movement. The result of this imbalance in the motor system is apparent as the manifestations of Parkinson's disease (see Figure 24.1).

Drug Therapy

At this time, there is no treatment that arrests the neuron degeneration of Parkinson's disease and the eventual decline in patient function. Surgical procedures involving the basal ganglia have been tried with varying success at prolonging the degeneration caused by this disease. Drug therapy remains the primary treatment (Figure 24.2).

Today, therapy is aimed at restoring the balance between the declining levels of dopamine, which has an inhibitory effect on the neurons in the basal ganglia, and the now-dominant cholinergic neurons, which are excitatory. This may help reduce the signs and symptoms of parkinsonism and restore normal function for a time.

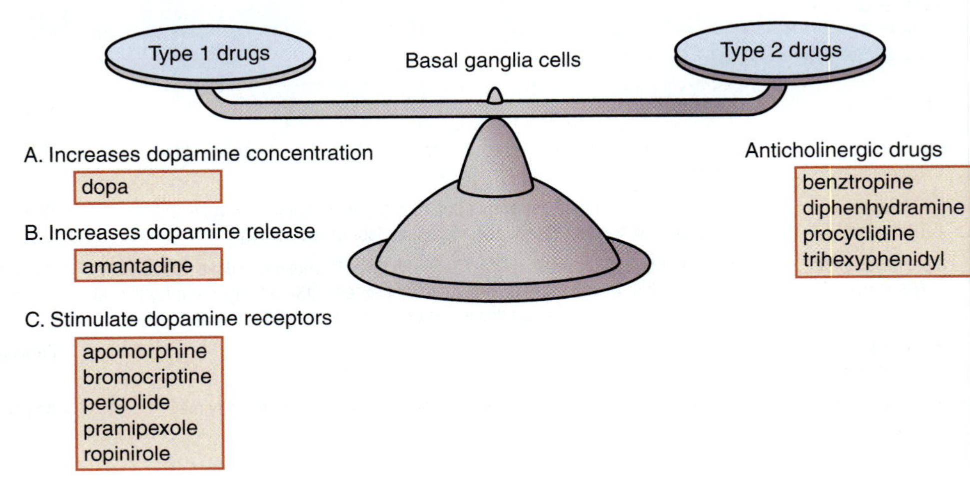

FIGURE 24.2 Drug therapy in treating Parkinson's disease is aimed at achieving a balance between the stimulating cholinergic effects and the inhibitory effects of dopamine in the basal ganglia. Type 1 drugs affect dopamine and are inhibitory. Type 2 drugs block cholinergic effects, preventing stimulation.

Total management of patient care in individuals with Parkinson's disease presents a challenge. Patients should be encouraged to be as active as possible, to perform exercises to prevent the development of skeletal deformities, and to attend to their own care as long as they can. Both the patient and family need instruction about following drug protocols and monitoring adverse effects, as well as encouragement and support for coping with the progressive nature of the disease. Because of the degenerative effects of this disease, patients may be depressed and emotional. They may require a great deal of psychological, as well as physical, support.

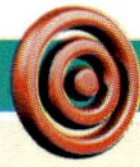

FOCUS POINTS

- Parkinson's disease is a progressive nervous system disease characterized by tremors, changes in posture and gait, and a masklike facial expression.
- The loss of dopamine-secreting cells is thought to be responsible for Parkinson's disease.

Anticholinergics

Anticholinergics are drugs that oppose the effects of acetylcholine at receptor sites in the substantia nigra and the corpus striatum, thus helping restore chemical balance in the area. At this time, the anticholinergics used to treat parkinsonism are synthetic drugs that have been developed to have a greater affinity for cholinergic receptor sites in the central nervous system (CNS) than for those in the peripheral nervous system. However, they still block, to some extent, the cholinergic receptors that are responsible for stimulation of the parasympathetic nervous system's postganglionic effectors and are associated with the adverse effects resulting from this blockage (see Chapter 33), including slowed gastrointestinal (GI) motility and secretions with dry mouth and constipation, urinary retention, blurred vision, and dilated pupils.

Anticholinergics used to treat Parkinson's disease include the following (also see Table 24.1):

- Benztropine (*Cogentin*) is available in oral and intramuscular/intravenous forms. This agent is used to treat parkinsonism and Parkinson-like symptoms that occur as a result of drug effects of phenothiazines.
- Biperiden (*Akineton*) is available in oral and intramuscular forms. This medication is used for the adjunctive treatment of parkinsonism and to treat the drug-induced parkinsonism associated with phenothiazine use.
- Diphenhydramine (*Benadryl*), also used for many other purposes, is often used in combination with other agents to treat Parkinson's disease. This agent is indicated for the treatment of parkinsonism, including drug-induced disease, especially in elderly patients who cannot tolerate more potent drugs and in patients at the early stages of disease.
- Procyclidine (*Kemadrin*) is available only in oral form. This agent is used for the treatment of any type of parkinsonism. In severe cases, it is combined with other drugs, and it is often the drug of choice to control the excessive salivation that occurs with the use of neuroleptic medication.
- Trihexyphenidyl (*Artane*) is used as adjunct therapy with levodopa. It can be used alone for the control of drug-induced extrapyramidal disorders.

Therapeutic Actions and Indications

The anticholinergics block the action of acetylcholine in the CNS to help normalize the acetylcholine–dopamine imbalance. As a result, these drugs reduce the degree of rigidity and,

Table 24.1 DRUGS IN FOCUS

Anticholinergic Antiparkinsonism Drugs

Drug Name	Dosage/Route	Usual Indications
benztropine (*Cogentin*)	0.5–6 mg/day PO may be needed; 1–2 mg IM or IV; reduce dosage in older patients	Parkinsonism, drug-induced parkinsonism
(P) biperiden (*Akineton*)	2 mg PO t.i.d. to q.i.d. to a maximum of 16 mg/day; 2 mg IM or IV, repeated in ½ hour as needed, do not give more than four doses per day	Parkinsonism, drug-induced parkinsonism
diphenhydramine (*Benadryl*)	Adult: 25–50 mg PO t.i.d. to q.i.d.; 10–50 mg IM or IV, maximum dose 400 mg/day Pediatric: 12.5–25 mg PO t.i.d. to q.i.d; do not exceed 300 mg/day; 5 mg/kg/day IM or IV divided into four equal doses; maximum daily dose 300 mg	Parkinsonism, particularly in the elderly or those with mild forms
procyclidine (*Kemadrin*)	2.5–5 mg PO t.i.d.	Parkinsonism; control of excessive salivation
trihexyphenidyl (*Artane*)	1–2 mg PO daily initially, titrate up to 6–10 mg/day; up to 15 mg/day may be needed	Adjunct to levodopa in treatment of parkinsonism

to a lesser extent, the tremors associated with Parkinson's disease. The peripheral anticholinergic effects that sometimes occur with the use of these drugs help alleviate some of the other adverse effects associated with Parkinson's disease, including drooling.

Anticholinergic drugs are indicated for the treatment of parkinsonism, whether idiopathic, atherosclerotic, or post-encephalitic, and for the relief of symptoms of extrapyramidal disorders associated with the use of some drugs, including phenothiazines. Although these drugs are not as effective as levodopa in the treatment of advancing cases of the disease, they may be useful as adjunctive therapy and for patients who no longer respond to levodopa.

Pharmacokinetics

The anticholinergic drugs are variably absorbed from the GI tract, reaching peak levels in 1 to 4 hours. They are metabolized in the liver and excreted by cellular pathways. All of them cross the placenta and enter breast milk. They should be used during pregnancy and lactation only if the benefit to the mother clearly outweighs the potential risk to the fetus or neonate. The safety and efficacy for use in children have not been established.

Contraindications and Cautions

Anticholinergics are contraindicated in the presence of allergy to any of these agents. In addition, they are contraindicated in narrow-angle glaucoma, GI obstruction, genitourinary (GU) obstruction, and prostatic hypertrophy, *all of which could be exacerbated by the peripheral anticholinergic effects of these drugs,* and in myasthenia gravis, *which could be exacerbated by the blocking of acetylcholine receptor sites at neuromuscular synapses.*

Caution should be used in the following conditions: tachycardia and other dysrhythmias; hypertension or hypotension *because the blocking of the parasympathetic system may cause a dominance of sympathetic stimulatory activity;* hepatic dysfunction, *which could interfere with the metabolism of the drugs and lead to toxic levels;* lactation *because the drugs cross into breast milk and may cause adverse effects in infants;* and pregnancy *because these drugs do cross the placenta.* In addition, these agents should be used with caution in individuals who work in hot environments *because reflex sweating may be blocked. These people are at risk for heat prostration.*

Adverse Effects

The use of anticholinergics for parkinsonism is associated with CNS effects that relate to the blocking of central acetylcholine receptors, such as disorientation, confusion, and memory loss. Agitation, nervousness, delirium, dizziness, light-headedness, and weakness may also occur.

Anticipated peripheral anticholinergic effects include dry mouth, nausea, vomiting, paralytic ileus, and constipation related to decreased GI secretions and motility. In addition, other adverse effects may occur, including the following: tachycardia, palpitations, and hypotension related to the blocking of the suppressive cardiac effects of the parasympathetic nervous system; urinary retention and hesitancy related to a blocking of bladder muscle activity and sphincter relaxation; blurred vision and photophobia related to pupil dilation and blocking of lens accommodation; and flushing and reduced sweating related to a blocking of the cholinergic sites that stimulate sweating and blood vessel dilation in the skin.

Clinically Important Drug–Drug Interactions

When these anticholinergic drugs are used with other drugs that have anticholinergic properties, including the tricyclic antidepressants and the phenothiazines, there is a risk of potentially fatal paralytic ileus and an increased risk of toxic psychoses. If such combinations must be given, patients should be monitored closely. Dosage adjustments should be made, and supportive measures should be taken. In addition, when antipsychotic drugs are combined with anticholinergics, there is a risk for decreased therapeutic effect of the antipsychotics, possibly because of a central antagonism of the two agents.

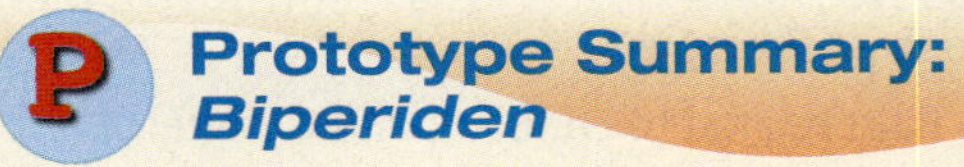

Prototype Summary: *Biperiden*

Indications: Adjunctive therapy of parkinsonism; relief of symptoms of extrapyramidal disorders that accompany phenothiazine therapy

Actions: Acts as an anticholinergic, principally in the CNS, returning balance to the basal ganglia and reducing the severity of rigidity, akinesia, and tremors; peripheral anticholinergic effects help to reduce drooling and other secondary effects of parkinsonism

Pharmacokinetics:

Route	Onset	Peak	Duration
Oral	1 h	1–1.5 h	6–12 h
IM	15 min	Unknown	Unknown

$T_{1/2}$: 18.4–24.3 hours; metabolized in the liver

Adverse effects: Disorientation, confusion, memory loss, nervousness, light-headedness, dizziness, depression, blurred vision, mydriasis, dry mouth, constipation, urinary retention, urinary hesitation, flushing, decreased sweating

Nursing Considerations for Patients Receiving Anticholinergic Antiparkinsonism Drugs

Assessment: History and Examination

Screen for the following conditions, *which could be contraindications or cautions to the use of the drug:* any known allergies to these drugs; GI depression or obstruction; urinary hesitancy or obstruction; benign prostatic hypertrophy; cardiac arrhythmias or hypotension; glaucoma; myasthenia gravis; pregnancy or lactation; hepatic dysfunction; and exposure to a hot environment.

Include screening *to determine baseline status before beginning therapy and to monitor for potential adverse effects.* Assess the following: temperature; skin color and lesions; CNS orientation, affect, reflexes, bilateral grip strength, and spasticity evaluation; respiration and adventitious sounds; pulse, blood pressure, and cardiac output; bowel sounds and reported output; urinary output and bladder palpation; and liver and renal function tests.

Nursing Diagnoses

The patient taking an anticholinergic antiparkinsonism drug may have the following nursing diagnoses related to drug therapy:

- Acute Pain related to GI, CNS, and GU effects
- Disturbed Thought Processes related to CNS effects
- Risk for Injury related to CNS effects
- Deficient Knowledge regarding drug therapy

Implementation With Rationale

- Arrange to decrease dosage or discontinue the drug *if dry mouth becomes so severe that swallowing becomes difficult.* Provide sugarless lozenges to suck and frequent mouth care to help with this problem.
- Give the drug with caution and arrange for a decrease in dosage in hot weather or with exposure to hot environments *because patients are at increased risk for heat prostration because of decreased ability to sweat.*
- Give the drug with meals if GI upset is a problem, before meals if dry mouth is a problem, and after meals if drooling occurs and the drug causes nausea *to facilitate compliance with drug therapy.*
- Monitor bowel function and institute a bowel program *if constipation is severe.*
- Ensure that the patient voids before taking the drug *if urinary retention is a problem.*
- Establish safety precautions if CNS or vision changes occur *to prevent patient injury.*
- Provide thorough patient teaching about topics such as the drug name and prescribed dosage, measures to help avoid adverse effects, warning signs that may indicate problems, and the need for periodic monitoring and evaluation *to enhance patient knowledge about drug therapy and to promote compliance.*
- Offer support and encouragement *to help the patient cope with the disease and drug regimen.*

Evaluation

- Monitor patient response to the drug (improvement in signs and symptoms of parkinsonism).
- Monitor for adverse effects (CNS changes, urinary retention, GI depression, tachycardia, decreased sweating, flushing).
- Evaluate the effectiveness of the teaching plan (patient can give the drug name and dosage, name possible adverse effects to watch for and specific measures to prevent adverse effects, and discuss the importance of continued follow-up).
- Monitor the effectiveness of comfort measures and compliance with the regimen.

Dopaminergics

Dopaminergics, drugs that increase the effects of dopamine at receptor sites, have been proven to be even more effective than anticholinergics in the treatment of parkinsonism. Dopamine itself does not cross the blood–brain barrier; other drugs that act like dopamine or increase dopamine concentrations indirectly must be used to increase dopamine levels in the brain. These drugs are effective as long as enough intact neurons remain in the substantia nigra to respond to increased levels of dopamine. After the neural degeneration has progressed beyond a certain point, patients no longer respond to these drugs.

Levodopa (*Dopar*) is the mainstay of treatment for parkinsonism (see Critical Thinking Scenario 24-1). This precursor of dopamine crosses the blood-brain barrier, where it is converted to dopamine. In this way, it acts like a replacement therapy. Levodopa is almost always given in combination form with carbidopa as a fixed-combination drug (*Sinemet*). In this combination form, carbidopa inhibits the enzyme dopa decarboxylase in the periphery, diminishing the metabolism of levodopa in the GI tract and in peripheral tissues and leading to higher levels crossing the blood–brain barrier. Because the carbidopa decreases the amount

CRITICAL THINKING SCENARIO 24-1

Effects of Vitamin B_6 Intake on Levodopa Levels

The Situation

S.S., a 58-year-old man with well-controlled Parkinson's disease presents with severe nausea, anorexia, fainting spells, and heart palpitation. He has been maintained on levodopa for the Parkinson's disease and he claims to have followed his drug regimen religiously.

According to S.S. the only change in his lifestyle has been the addition of several health foods and vitamins. His daughter, who recently returned from her freshman year in college, has begun a new health regimen, including natural foods and plenty of supplemental vitamins. She was so enthusiastic about her new approach that everyone in the family agreed to give this diet a try.

Critical Thinking

Based on S.S.'s signs and symptoms, what has probably occurred?

In Parkinson's disease, is it possible to differentiate a deterioration of illness from a toxic reaction to a drug?

What nursing implications should be considered when teaching S.S. and his family about the effects of vitamin B_6 on levodopa levels?

In what ways can the daughter cope with her role in this crisis?

Develop a new care plan for S.S. that involves all family members and that includes drug teaching.

Discussion

The presenting symptoms reflect an increase in Parkinson symptoms, as well as an increase in peripheral dopamine reactions (e.g., palpitations, fainting, anorexia, nausea). It is necessary to determine whether the problem involves a further degeneration in the neurons in the substantia nigra or the particular medication that S.S. has been taking. In many patients, responsiveness to levodopa is lost as neural degeneration continues.

The explanation of the new lifestyle—full of grains, natural foods, and vitamins—alerted a nurse to the possibility of excessive vitamin B_6 intake. In reviewing the vitamin bottles and some of the food packages supplied by S.S., it seemed that too much vitamin B_6, which speeds the conversion of levodopa to dopamine before it can cross the blood–brain barrier, might be the reason parkinsonism recurred.

The status of S.S.'s Parkinson's disease should be evaluated, and then he can be restarted on levodopa. The smallest dose possible should be used to begin, with slow increases following to achieve the maximum benefit with the fewest side effects. It would be wise to consider combining the drug with carbidopa to prevent some of the patient's recent problems.

In addition, S.S. should receive thorough drug teaching in written form for future reference. The need to avoid vitamin B_6 should be emphasized. The entire family should be involved in an explanation of what happened and how this situation can be avoided in the future. Because the daughter may feel guilty about her role, she should have the opportunity to discuss her feelings and explore the positive impact of healthy food on nutrition and quality of life. This situation can serve as a good teaching example for staff, as well as presenting them with an opportunity to review drug therapy in Parkinson's disease and the risks and benefits of more extreme diets.

Nursing Care Guide for S.S.: Levodopa

Assessment: History and Examination

Allergies to levodopa; COPD; dysrhythmias, hypotension, hepatic or renal dysfunction; psychoses; peptic ulcer; glaucoma

Concurrent use of MAOIs, phenytoin, pyridoxine, papaverine, or TCAs

Focus physical examination on

CV: blood pressure, pulse rate, peripheral perfusion, ECG results

CNS: orientation, affect, reflexes, grip strength

Renal: output, bladder palpation

GI: abdominal examination, bowel sounds

Respiratory: respiration, adventitious sounds

Laboratory tests: renal and liver function tests, CBC

Nursing Diagnoses

Acute Pain related to GI, GU, and CNS effects

Risk for Injury related to CNS effects

Disturbed Thought Processes related to CNS effects

Deficient Knowledge regarding drug therapy

(continued)

Effects of Vitamin B_6 Intake on Levodopa Levels *(continued)*

Implementation

Ensure safe and appropriate administration of drug.

Provide comfort and safety: slow positioning changes; assess orientation, provide pain medication as needed; give drug with food; administer with carbidopa; have patient void before each dose.

Provide support and reassurance to deal with disease and drug effects.

Instruct the patient regarding drug dosage, effects, and adverse symptoms to report.

Evaluation

Evaluate drug effects: relief of signs and symptoms of Parkinson's disease

Monitor for adverse effects: CNS effects; renal changes, urinary retention; GI effects (constipation); increased sweating or flushing.

Monitor for drug–drug interactions: hypertensive crisis with MAOIs, decreased effects with vitamin B_6 or phenytoin.

Evaluate effectiveness of patient teaching program.

Evaluate effectiveness of comfort and safety measures.

Patient Teaching for S.S.

- ☐ The drug that has been prescribed is called levodopa. It increases the levels of dopamine in the central areas of the brain and helps to reduce the signs and symptoms of Parkinson's disease.
- ☐ Often, this drug is combined with carbidopa, which allows the correct levels of levodopa to reach the brain.
- ☐ People who take this drug must have their individual dosage needs adjusted over time. Common effects of this drug include:
  - *Fatigue, weakness, and drowsiness:* Try to space activities evenly through the day; allow rest periods to avoid these side effects. Take safety precautions and avoid driving or operating dangerous machinery if these conditions occur.
  - *Dizziness, fainting:* Change position slowly to avoid dizzy spells.
  - *Increased sweating, darkened urine:* This is a normal reaction. Avoid very hot environments.
  - *Headaches, difficulty sleeping:* These usually pass as the body adjusts to the drug. If they become too uncomfortable and persist, consult with your health care provider.
  - Report any of the following to your health care provider: *uncontrolled movements of any body part, chest pain or palpitations, depression or mood changes, difficulty in voiding, or severe or persistent nausea and vomiting.*
- ☐ Be aware that vitamin B_6 interferes with the effects of levodopa. If you feel that you need a vitamin product, consult with your health care provider about using an agent that does not contain vitamin B_6.
- ☐ Avoid eating large quantities of health foods that contain vitamin B_6, such as grains and brans. If you are taking a carbidopa–levodopa combination, these precautions are not as important.
- ☐ Tell any doctor, nurse, or other health care provider involved in your care that you are taking this drug.
- ☐ Keep this drug and all medications out of the reach of children.
- ☐ Do not overexert yourself when you begin to feel better. Pace yourself.
- ☐ Take this drug exactly as directed and schedule regular medical checkups to evaluate the effects of this drug.

of levodopa needed to reach a therapeutic level in the brain, the dosage of levodopa can be decreased, which reduces the incidence of adverse side effects.

Carbidopa is not the only agent that is used primarily to improve the effectiveness of levodopa therapy (see Box 24.1). Other dopaminergics that are used in the treatment of parkinsonism include the following (also see Table 24.2):

- Amantadine (*Symmetrel*) is an antiviral drug that also seems to increase the release of dopamine. This drug can be effective as long as there is a possibility of more dopamine release.
- Bromocriptine (*Parlodel*) acts as a direct dopamine agonist on dopamine receptor sites in the substantia nigra. Because this drug does not depend on cells in the area to biotransform it or to increase release of already produced dopamine, it may be effective longer than levodopa or amantadine.
- Pergolide (*Permax*) is used as an adjunct to carbidopa–levodopa therapy. It directly stimulates postsynaptic dopamine receptors in the substantia nigra, an effect that also may lead to inhibition of prolactin secretion and a rise in growth hormone levels.

Table 24.2 DRUGS IN FOCUS

Dopaminergic Antiparkinsonism Drugs

Drug Name	Dosage/Route	Usual Indications
amantadine (*Symmetrel*)	100 mg PO b.i.d.; up to 400 mg/day has been used	Antiviral; idiopathic and drug-induced parkinsonism in adults
apomorphine (*Apokyn*)	2–6 mg Sub-Q t.i.d.; given with trimethobenzamide: 300 mg PO t.i.d.	Intermittent treatment of hypomobility "off" episodes of advanced Parkinson's disease
bromocriptine (*Parlodel*)	1.25 mg PO b.i.d.; titrate up to 10–40 mg/day	Idiopathic Parkinson's disease; may be beneficial in later stages when response to levodopa decreases
P levodopa (*Dopar*)	0.5–1 g/day PO in two divided doses; titrate up to 8 g/day; most often given in combination with carbidopa as *Sinemet:* 25 mg carbidopa/100 mg levodopa PO t.i.d.	Idiopathic Parkinson's disease
pergolide (*Permax*)	0.05 mg/day PO for 2 days, then slowly titrate to 3 mg/day	Adjunct with carbidopa–levodopa for idiopathic Parkinson's disease
pramipexole (*Mirapex*)	0.125 mg PO t.i.d., titrate up to 1.5 mg PO t.i.d.	Idiopathic Parkinson's disease
ropinirole (*Requip*)	0.25 mg PO t.i.d.; titrate up to maximum dose of 24 mg/day	Idiopathic Parkinson's disease in early stages and in later stages combined with levodopa; restless legs syndrome

- Pramipexole (*Mirapex*) directly stimulates dopamine receptors in the substantia nigra. It may be effective after levodopa effects have weakened.
- Ropinirole (*Requip*) is a newer drug that directly stimulates dopamine receptors. It has proved useful in both early and later stages of Parkinson's disease in conjunction with levodopa, when the effects of levodopa are no longer sufficient to provide symptomatic relief. It is also approved for the treatment of restless legs syndrome. A number of adjuncts are also used in levodopa therapy (Boxes 24.2 and 24.3).

BOX 24.2 Current Combination Therapy

A fixed-combination tablet became available in 2003 for patients who were at a point in their Parkinson's disease where they required the addition of the adjunct drug entacapone. This fixed combination tablet contains carbidopa, levodopa, and entacapone. The tablet comes in three strengths:

50 mg levodopa, 12.5 mg carbidopa, 200 mg entacapone: *Stalevo 50*

100 mg levodopa, 25 mg carbidopa, 200 mg entacapone: *Stalevo 100*

150 mg levodopa, 37.5 mg carbidopa, 200 mg entacapone: *Stalevo 150*

The patient should be stabilized on each drug separately before switching to the correct preparation of the fixed-combination product. The usual dose is one tablet every 3–8 hours. This combination reduces the number of tablets the patient needs to swallow each day.

- Apomorphine (*Apokyn*) is the newest adjunctive therapy for Parkinson's disease. It directly binds with postsynaptic dopamine receptors. Apomorphine is approved for intermittent treatment of hypomobility "off" episodes caused by the end-of-dose wearing off and unpredictable on-off episodes seen in advanced Parkinson's disease. Apomorphine is given subcutaneously with an antiemetic; there is a risk of hypotension and prolonged QT interval with this drug, so the patient must be monitored closely.

Therapeutic Actions and Indications

The dopaminergics work by increasing the levels of dopamine in the substantia nigra or directly stimulating the dopamine receptors in that area. This action helps restore the balance between the inhibitory and stimulating neurons. The dopaminergics are indicated for the relief of the signs and symptoms of idiopathic Parkinson's disease. Amantadine, which is also used as an antiviral agent, may be effective in treating drug-induced Parkinson's disease as well.

After degeneration has progressed to the extent that the nerves are damaged or gone, these drugs are no longer effective. These drugs control Parkinson's disease only as long as functioning dopamine receptors remain in the substantia nigra.

Pharmacokinetics

The dopaminergics are generally well absorbed from the GI tract and widely distributed in the body. Apomorphine must be given subcutaneously. The dopaminergics are metabolized

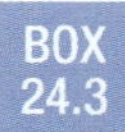

BOX 24.3 Adjuncts to Levodopa Therapy

Entacapone (*Comtan*) is used with carbidopa–levodopa to increase the plasma concentration and duration of action of levodopa. It does this by inhibiting catecholamine-*O*-methyl transferase (COMT), a naturally occurring enzyme that eliminates catecholamines, including dopamine. It is given with the carbidopa–levodopa at a dose of 200 mg PO, with a maximum of eight doses a day. It is readily absorbed from the gastrointestinal (GI) tract, metabolized in the liver, and excreted in urine and feces. Women of childbearing age should be encouraged to use barrier contraceptives while taking this drug, which crosses the placenta and could have adverse effects on the fetus.

Tolcapone (*Tasmar*) works in a similar way with carbidopa–levodopa to further increase plasma levels of levodopa. Tolcapone also blocks the enzyme COMT, which is responsible for the breakdown of dopamine. Because this drug has been associated with fulminant and potentially fatal liver damage, it is contraindicated in the presence of liver disease. Tolcapone is reserved for use in later stages of Parkinson's disease, when carbidopa–levodopa is losing its effectiveness. It undergoes hepatic metabolism after GI absorption and is excreted in the urine and feces. It is given in doses of 100 or 200 mg PO t.i.d., up to a maximum of 600 mg/day. Women of childbearing age should be encouraged to use barrier contraceptives while taking this drug, which crosses the placenta and could have adverse effects on the fetus.

Selegiline (*Carbex, Eldepryl*) is used with carbidopa–levodopa after patients have shown signs of deteriorating response to this treatment. Its mechanism of action is not understood. It does irreversibly inhibit monoamine oxidase (MAO), which has an important role in the breakdown of catecholamines, including dopamine. The maximum daily dose of the drug is 10 mg, and the dose of levodopa needs to be reduced when this drug is started. It is well absorbed from the GI tract, extensively metabolized in the liver, and excreted in urine. It is not known whether this drug crosses the placenta, but it should be used in pregnancy only if the benefits to the mother clearly outweigh any potential risks to the fetus. Because of the risk of MAO inhibitor–induced hypertensive effects, patients should be urged to immediately report severe headache and any other unusual symptoms that they have not experienced before.

in the liver and peripheral cells and excreted in the urine. They cross the placenta, but there are no adequate studies of use of these drugs in pregnancy. They should be used during pregnancy only if the benefits to the mother clearly outweigh the potential risks to the fetus. Dopaminergics enter breast milk and should not be used during lactation because of the potential for adverse effects in the baby.

Contraindications and Cautions

The dopaminergics are contraindicated in the presence of any known allergy to the drug or drug components. They are also contraindicated in the following conditions: angle-closure glaucoma, *which could be exacerbated by these drugs;* history or presence of suspicious skin lesions with levodopa *because this drug has been associated with the development of melanoma;* and lactation *because of potential adverse effects on the baby.*

Caution should be *used with any condition that could be exacerbated by dopamine receptor stimulation,* such as cardiovascular disease, including myocardial infarction, arrhythmias, and hypertension; bronchial asthma; history of peptic ulcers; urinary tract obstruction; and psychiatric disorders. Care should also be taken in pregnancy *because these drugs cross the placenta and could adversely affect the fetus,* and in renal and hepatic disease, *which could interfere with the metabolism and excretion of the drug.*

Adverse Effects

The adverse effects associated with the dopaminergics usually result from stimulation of dopamine receptors. CNS effects may include anxiety, nervousness, headache, malaise, fatigue, confusion, mental changes, blurred vision, muscle twitching, and ataxia. Peripheral effects may include anorexia, nausea, vomiting, dysphagia, and constipation or diarrhea; cardiac arrhythmias, hypotension, and palpitations; bizarre breathing patterns; urinary retention; and flushing, increased sweating, and hot flashes. Bone marrow depression and hepatic dysfunction have also been reported.

Clinically Important Drug–Drug Interactions

If dopaminergics are combined with monoamine oxidase inhibitors (MAOIs), therapeutic effects increase and a risk of hypertensive crisis exists. The MAOI should be stopped 14 days before beginning therapy with a dopaminergic.

The combination of levodopa with vitamin B_6 or with phenytoin may lead to decreased efficacy. Reduced effectiveness may also result if dopaminergics are combined with dopamine antagonists. In addition, patients who take dopaminergics should be cautioned to avoid over-the-counter vitamins; if such medications are used, the patient should be monitored closely because a decrease in effectiveness can result.

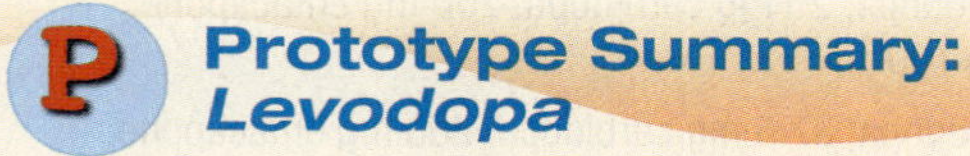

Prototype Summary: Levodopa

Indications: Treatment of parkinsonism

Actions: Precursor of dopamine, which is deficient in parkinsonism; crosses the blood–brain barrier, where it is converted to dopamine and acts as a replacement neurotransmitter; effective for 2–5 years in relieving the symptoms of Parkinson's disease

Pharmacokinetics:

Route	Onset	Peak	Duration
Oral	Varies	0.5–2 h	5 h

$T_{1/2}$: 1–3 hours; metabolized in the liver, excreted in the urine

Adverse effects: Adventitious movements, ataxia, increased hand tremor, dizziness, numbness, weakness, agitation, anxiety, anorexia, nausea, dry mouth, dysphagia, urinary retention, flushing, cardiac irregularities

Nursing Considerations for Patients Receiving Dopaminergic Antiparkinsonism Drugs

Assessment: History and Examination

Screen for the following conditions, *which could be contraindications or cautions for the use of the drug:* any known allergies to these drugs or drug components; GI depression or obstruction; urinary hesitancy or obstruction; cardiac arrhythmias or hypertension; glaucoma; respiratory disease; pregnancy or lactation; and renal or hepatic dysfunction. With levodopa, check for skin lesions or history of melanoma. With apomorphine, check for history of prolonged QT interval.

Include screening *to determine baseline status before beginning therapy and to monitor for any potential adverse effects.* Assess the following: temperature; skin color and lesions; CNS orientation, affect, reflexes, bilateral grip strength, and spasticity; vision; respiration and adventitious sounds; pulse, blood pressure, and cardiac output; bowel sounds and reported output; and urinary output and bladder palpation. Check liver and renal function tests and complete blood count (CBC) with differential. Establish baseline electrocardiogram if apomorphine is used.

Nursing Diagnoses

The patient taking a dopaminergic antiparkinsonism drug may have the following nursing diagnoses related to drug therapy:

- Acute Pain related to GI, CNS, and GU effects
- Disturbed Thought Processes related to CNS effects
- Risk for Injury related to CNS effects and incidence of orthostatic hypertension
- Deficient Knowledge regarding drug therapy

Implementation With Rationale

- Arrange to decrease dosage of the drug if therapy has been interrupted for any reason *to prevent acute peripheral dopaminergic effects.*
- Evaluate disease progress and signs and symptoms periodically and record *for reference of disease progress and drug response.*
- Give the drug with meals *to alleviate GI irritation if GI upset is a problem.*
- Monitor bowel function and institute a bowel program *if constipation is severe.*
- Ensure that the patient voids before taking the drug *if urinary retention is a problem.*
- Establish safety precautions if CNS or vision changes occur *to prevent patient injury.*
- Monitor hepatic, renal, and hematological tests periodically during therapy *to detect early signs of dysfunction and consider re-evaluation of drug therapy.*
- Provide support services and comfort measures as needed *to improve patient compliance.*
- Provide thorough patient teaching about topics such as the drug name and prescribed dosage, measures to help avoid adverse effects, warning signs that may indicate problems, and the need for periodic monitoring and evaluation *to enhance patient knowledge about drug therapy and to promote compliance.*
- Offer encouragement *to help the patient cope with the disease and drug regimen.*

Evaluation

- Monitor patient response to the drug (improvement in signs and symptoms of parkinsonism).
- Monitor for adverse effects (CNS changes, urinary retention, GI depression, tachycardia, increased sweating, flushing).
- Evaluate the effectiveness of the teaching plan (patient can give the drug name and dosage, name possible adverse effects to watch for and specific measures to prevent adverse effects, and discuss the importance of continued follow-up).
- Monitor the effectiveness of comfort measures and compliance with the regimen.

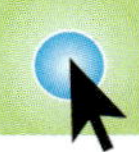

WEB LINKS

Health care providers and patients may want to consult the following Internet sources: Information on parkinsonism, ataxia, and related disorders, including support groups, research, and treatment:

http://www.ataxia.org Information on education programs, research, and other information related to parkinsonism.

http://www.ninds.nih.gov Information on neurosciences, including current research and theories.
http://www.neuroguide.com Information on support services and aids for activities of daily living.
http://www.accessunlimited.com/links.html

Points to Remember

- Parkinson's disease is a progressive, chronic neurological disorder for which there is no cure.
- Signs and symptoms of Parkinson's disease include tremor, changes in posture and gait, slow and deliberate movements (bradykinesia), and eventually drooling and changes in speech.
- Loss of dopamine-secreting neurons in the substantia nigra is characteristic of Parkinson's disease. Destruction of dopamine-secreting cells leads to an imbalance between excitatory cholinergic cells and inhibitory dopaminergic cells.
- Drug therapy for Parkinson's disease is aimed at restoring the dopamine–acetylcholine balance. The signs and symptoms of the disease can be managed until the degeneration of neurons is so extensive that a therapeutic response no longer occurs.
- Anticholinergic drugs are used to block the excitatory cholinergic receptors, and dopaminergic drugs are used to increase dopamine levels or to directly stimulate dopamine receptors.
- Many adverse effects are associated with the drugs used for treating Parkinson's disease, including CNS changes, anticholinergic (atropine-like) effects, and dopamine stimulation in the peripheral nervous system.

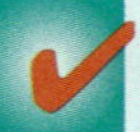

CHECK YOUR UNDERSTANDING

Answers to the questions in this chapter may be found in the Answer Key in the back of the book.

Multiple Choice

Select the best answer to the following.

1. Parkinson's disease is a progressive, chronic neurological disorder that is usually
   a. associated with severe head injury.
   b. associated with chronic diseases.
   c. associated with old age.
   d. known to affect people of all ages with no known cause.

2. Parkinson's disease reflects an imbalance between inhibitory and stimulating activity of nerves in the
   a. reticular activating system.
   b. cerebellum.
   c. basal ganglia.
   d. limbic system.

3. The main, underlying problem with Parkinson's disease seems to be a decrease in the neurotransmitter
   a. acetylcholine.
   b. norepinephrine.
   c. dopamine.
   d. serotonin.

4. Anticholinergic drugs are effective in early Parkinson's disease. They act
   a. to block the stimulating effects of acetylcholine in the brain to bring activity back into balance.
   b. to block the signs and symptoms of the disease, making it more acceptable.
   c. to inhibit dopamine effects in the brain.
   d. to increase the effectiveness of GABA.

5. A patient receiving an anticholinergic drug for Parkinson's disease is planning a winter trip to Tahiti. The temperature in Tahiti is 70 degrees warmer than at home. What precautions should the patient be urged to take?
   a. Take the drug with plenty of water to stay hydrated.
   b. Reduce dosage and take extreme precautions because you are at increased risk for heat stroke because of the anticholinergic effects of the drug.
   c. Wear sunglasses and use sunscreen because of photophobia that will develop.
   d. Avoid drinking the water.

6. Replacing dopamine in the brain would seem to be the best treatment for Parkinson's disease. This is difficult because dopamine
   a. is broken down in gastric acid.
   b. is not available in drug form.
   c. cannot cross the blood–brain barrier.
   d. is used up in the periphery before it can reach the brain.

7. A patient taking levodopa and over-the-counter megavitamins might experience
   a. cure from Parkinson's disease.
   b. return of parkinsonism symptoms and increased blood pressure, pulse, respirations, sweating, and feeling of tension.
   c. improved health and well-being.
   d. a resistance to viral infections.

8. A patient who has been diagnosed with Parkinson's disease for many years and whose symptoms were controlled using *Sinemet* has started to exhibit increasing signs of Parkinson's disease. Possible treatment might include
   a. increased exercise program.
   b. addition of pergolide to the drug regimen.
   c. combination therapy with an anticholinergic or other dopaminergic drug.
   d. changes in diet to eliminate vitamin B_6.

Multiple Response

Select all that apply.

1. A client asks the nurse to explain parkinsonism to him. Which of the following possible causes of parkinsonism might be included in the explanation?
   a. Adverse effect of drug therapy
   b. Head injury
   c. Viral infection
   d. Dementia
   e. Bacterial infection
   f. Birth defect

2. No therapy is available that will stop the loss of neurons and the eventual decline of function in clients with Parkinson's disease. As a result, nursing care should involve which of the following interventions?
   a. Regular exercises to slow loss of function
   b. Support and education as drugs fail and new therapy is needed
   c. Community and family support networking
   d. Discontinuation of drug therapy to test for a cure
   e. Special vitamin therapy to slow the loss of the neurons
   f. Explanations of the adjunctive drug therapy that may be used

Word Scramble

Unscramble the following letters to form the names of commonly used antiparkinsonism drugs.

1. poolaved ____________________
2. yopclicdinre ____________________
3. gloierped ____________________
4. pedrinibe ____________________
5. tanmadaeni ____________________
6. poorinirel ____________________
7. zoptrebnine ____________________
8. inebtripcorom ____________________

Web Exercise

M.J. was diagnosed with Parkinson's disease at the age of 42, when tremors began to interfere with his job as a watch repairman. His disease was well controlled with carbidopa–levodopa (*Sinemet*) for 7 years, but now the disease is progressing rapidly. You are trying to work with the family to prepare them for what is to come and to help them to make the most of M.J.'s abilities while they struggle with his prognosis. Go to http://www.ninds.nih.gov and find information that will be helpful for this family.

Bibliography and References

Bailey, K. (1998). *Psychotropic drug facts.* Philadelphia: Lippincott-Raven.

Drug facts and comparisons. (2006). St. Louis: Facts and Comparisons.

Gilman, A., Hardman, J. G., & Limbird, L. E. (Eds.). (2006). *Goodman and Gilman's the pharmacological basis of therapeutics* (11th ed.). New York: McGraw-Hill.

Karch, A. M. (2006). *2007 Lippincott's nursing drug guide.* Philadelphia: Lippincott Williams & Wilkins.

Porth, C. M. (2005). *Pathophysiology: Concepts of altered health states* (7th ed.). Philadelphia: Lippincott Williams & Wilkins.

Professional's guide to patient drug facts. (2006). St. Louis: Facts and Comparisons.

CHAPTER 25

Muscle Relaxants

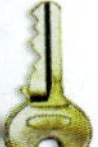

KEY TERMS

basal ganglia
cerebellum
extrapyramidal tract
hypertonia
interneuron
pyramidal tract
spasticity

LEARNING OBJECTIVES

Upon completion of this chapter, you will be able to:

1. Describe a spinal reflex and discuss the pathophysiology of muscle spasm and muscle spasticity.
2. Describe the therapeutic actions, indications, pharmacokinetics, contraindications, most common adverse reactions, and important drug–drug interactions associated with the centrally acting and the direct-acting skeletal muscle relaxants.
3. Discuss the use of muscle relaxants across the lifespan.
4. Compare and contrast the prototype drugs baclofen and dantrolene with other muscle relaxants in their classes.
5. Outline the nursing considerations, including important teaching points, for patients receiving an anesthetic.

CENTRALLY ACTING SKELETAL MUSCLE RELAXANTS

P baclofen
carisoprodol
chlorphenesin
chlorzoxazone
cyclobenzaprine
metaxalone
methocarbamol
orphenadrine
tizanidine

DIRECT-ACTING SKELETAL MUSCLE RELAXANTS

botulinum toxin type A
botulinum toxin type B
P dantrolene

Many injuries and accidents result in local damage to muscles or the skeletal anchors of muscles. These injuries may lead to muscle spasm and pain, which may be of long duration and may interfere with normal functioning. Damage to central nervous system (CNS) neurons may cause a permanent state of muscle **spasticity** as a result of loss of nerves that help maintain balance in controlling muscle activity.

Neuron damage, whether temporary or permanent, may be treated with skeletal muscle relaxants. Most skeletal muscle relaxants work in the brain and spinal cord, where they interfere with the cycle of muscle spasm and pain. However, the botulinum toxins and dantrolene enter muscle fibers directly. See Box 25.1 for how these muscle relaxants work in various age groups.

Nerves and Movement

Posture, balance, and movement are the result of a constantly fluctuating sequence of muscle contraction and relaxation. The nerves that regulate these actions are the spinal motor neurons. These neurons are influenced by higher-level brain activity in the **cerebellum** and **basal ganglia**, which provide coordination of contractions, and in the cerebral cortex, which allows conscious thought to regulate movement.

Spinal Reflexes

The spinal reflexes are the simplest nerve pathways that monitor movement and posture (Figure 25.1). Spinal reflexes can be simple, involving an incoming sensory neuron and an outgoing motor neuron, or more complex, involving **interneurons** that communicate with the related centers in the brain. Simple reflex arcs involve sensory receptors in the periphery and spinal motor nerves. Such reflex arcs make up what is known as the spindle gamma loop system; they respond to stretch receptors on muscle fibers to cause a muscle fiber contraction that relieves the stretch. In this system, nerves from stretch receptors form a synapse with gamma nerves in the spinal cord, which send an impulse to the stretched muscle fibers to stimulate their contraction. These reflexes are responsible for maintaining muscle tone and keeping an upright position against the pull of gravity. Other spinal reflexes may involve synapses with interneurons within the spinal cord, which adjust movement and response based on information from higher brain centers and coordinate movement and position.

Brain Control

Many areas within the brain influence the spinal motor nerves. Areas of the brainstem, the basal ganglia, and the cerebellum

BOX 25.1 DRUG THERAPY ACROSS THE LIFESPAN

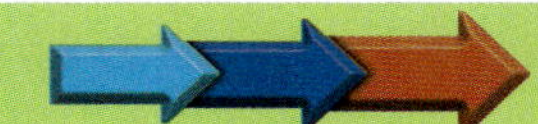

Skeletal Muscle Relaxants

CHILDREN

The safety and effectiveness of most of these drugs have not been established in children. If a child older than 12 years of age requires a skeletal muscle relaxant after an injury, metaxalone has an established pediatric dosage. Other agents have been used, with adjustments to the adult dosage based on the child's age and weight.

Baclofen is often used to relieve the muscle spasticity associated with cerebral palsy. A caregiver needs intensive education in the use of the intrathecal infusion pump and how to monitor the child for therapeutic as well as adverse effects.

Methocarbamol is the drug of choice if a child needs to be treated for tetanus.

Dantrolene is used to treat upper motor neuron spasticity in children. The dosage is based on body weight and increases over time. The child should be screened regularly for central nervous system (CNS) and gastrointestinal (including hepatic) toxicity.

ADULTS

Adults being treated for acute musculoskeletal pain should be cautioned to avoid driving and to take safety precautions against injury because of the related CNS effects, including dizziness and drowsiness.

Adults complaining of muscle spasm pain that may be related to anxiety often respond very effectively to diazepam, which is a muscle relaxant and anxiolytic.

Women of childbearing age should be advised to use contraception when they are taking these drugs. If a pregnancy does occur, or is desired, they need counseling about the potential for adverse effects. Women who are nursing should be encouraged to find another method of feeding the baby because of the potential for adverse drug effects on the baby.

Premenopausal women are also at increased risk for the hepatotoxicity associated with dantrolene and should be monitored very closely for any change in hepatic function and given written information about the prodrome syndrome that often occurs with the hepatic toxicity.

OLDER ADULTS

Older patients are more likely to experience the adverse effects associated with these drugs—CNS, gastrointestinal, and cardiovascular. Because older patients often also have renal or hepatic impairment, they are also more likely to have toxic levels of the drug related to changes in metabolism and excretion.

Carisoprodol is the centrally acting skeletal muscle relaxant of choice for older patients and for those with hepatic or renal impairment.

If dantrolene is required for an older patient, lower doses and more frequent monitoring are needed to assess for potential cardiac, respiratory, and liver toxicity.

Older women who are receiving hormone replacement therapy are at the same risk for development of hepatotoxicity as premenopausal women and should be monitored accordingly.

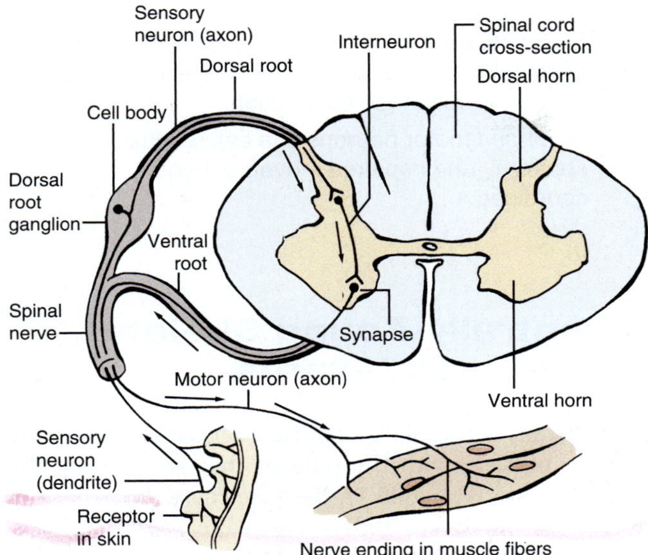

FIGURE 25.1 Reflex arc showing the pathway of impulses.

modulate spinal motor nerve activity and help coordinate activity among various muscle groups, thereby allowing coordinated movement and control of body muscle motions. Nerve areas within the cerebral cortex allow conscious, or intentional, movement. Nerves within the cortex send signals down the spinal cord, where they cross to the opposite side of the spinal cord before sending out nerve impulses to cause muscle contraction. In this way, each side of the cortex controls muscle movement on the opposite side of the body.

Different fibers control different types of movements. These fibers that control precise, intentional movement make up the **pyramidal tract** within the CNS. The **extrapyramidal tract** is composed of cells from the cerebral cortex as well as from several subcortical areas, including the basal ganglia and the cerebellum. This tract modulates or coordinates unconsciously controlled muscle activity, and it allows the body to make automatic adjustments in posture or position and balance. The extrapyramidal tract controls lower-level, or crude, movements.

Neuromuscular Abnormalities

All of the areas mentioned work together to allow for a free flow of impulses into and out of the CNS to coordinate posture, balance, and movement. When injuries, diseases, and toxins affect the normal flow of information into and out of the CNS motor pathways, many clinical signs and symptoms may develop, ranging from simple muscle spasms to spasticity, or sustained muscle spasm, and paralysis.

Muscle Spasm

Muscle spasms often result from injury to the musculoskeletal system—for example, overstretching a muscle, wrenching a joint, or tearing a tendon or ligament. These injuries can cause violent and painful involuntary muscle contractions. It is thought that these spasms are caused by the flood of sensory impulses coming to the spinal cord from the injured area. These impulses can be passed through interneurons to spinal motor nerves, which stimulate an intense muscle contraction. The contraction cuts off blood flow to the muscle fibers in the injured area, causing lactic acid to accumulate, resulting in pain. The new flood of sensory impulses caused by the pain may lead to further muscle contraction, and a vicious cycle may develop (Box 25.2).

Muscle Spasticity

Muscle spasticity is the result of damage to neurons within the CNS, rather than injury to peripheral structures. Because the spasticity is caused by nerve damage in the CNS, it is a permanent condition. Spasticity may result from an increase in excitatory influences or a decrease in inhibitory influences within the CNS. The interruption in the balance among all of these higher influences within the CNS may

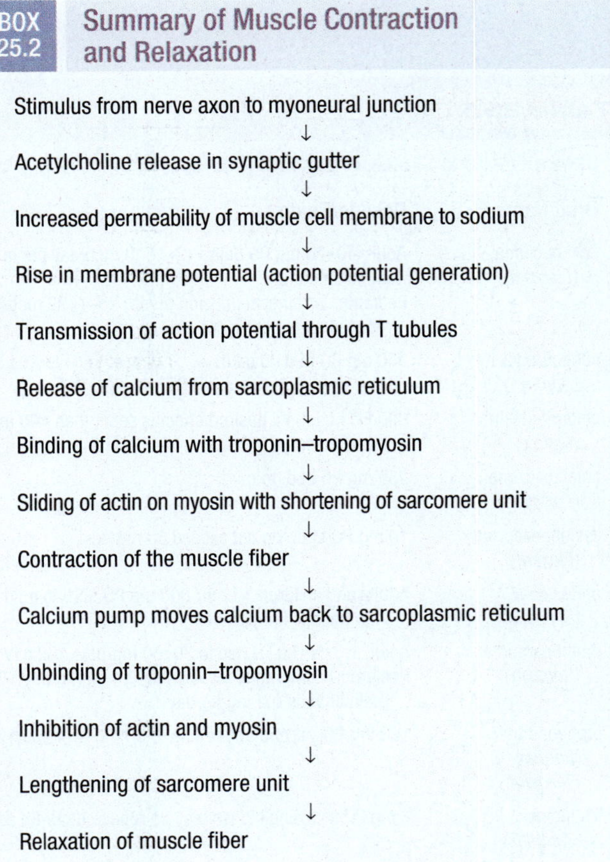

BOX 25.2 Summary of Muscle Contraction and Relaxation

Stimulus from nerve axon to myoneural junction
↓
Acetylcholine release in synaptic gutter
↓
Increased permeability of muscle cell membrane to sodium
↓
Rise in membrane potential (action potential generation)
↓
Transmission of action potential through T tubules
↓
Release of calcium from sarcoplasmic reticulum
↓
Binding of calcium with troponin–tropomyosin
↓
Sliding of actin on myosin with shortening of sarcomere unit
↓
Contraction of the muscle fiber
↓
Calcium pump moves calcium back to sarcoplasmic reticulum
↓
Unbinding of troponin–tropomyosin
↓
Inhibition of actin and myosin
↓
Lengthening of sarcomere unit
↓
Relaxation of muscle fiber

lead to excessive stimulation of muscles, or **hypertonia**, in opposing muscle groups at the same time, a condition that may cause contractures and permanent structural changes. This control imbalance also results in a loss of coordinated muscle activity.

For example, the signs and symptoms of cerebral palsy and paraplegia are related to the disruption in the nervous control of the muscles. The exact presentation of any chronic neurological disorder depends on the specific nerve centers and tracts that are damaged and how the control imbalance is manifested.

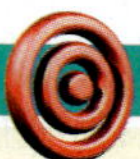

FOCUS POINTS

- Movement and muscle control are regulated by spinal reflexes and the upper CNS.
- Spinal reflexes can be simple, involving an incoming sensory neuron and an outgoing motor neuron, or more complex, involving interneurons that communicate with the related centers in the brain.
- The pyramidal tract in the cerebellum coordinates intentional muscle movement, and the extrapyramidal tract in the cerebellum and basal ganglia coordinates involuntary muscle activity.
- Muscle or skeletal damage may send a multitude of stimuli to the spinal cord and result in muscle spasms or extended contraction.
- Damaged motor neurons can cause muscle spasticity and impaired movement and coordination.

Centrally Acting Skeletal Muscle Relaxants

The centrally acting skeletal muscle relaxants work in the CNS to interfere with the reflexes that are causing the muscle spasm (Table 25.1). Because these drugs lyse or destroy spasm, they are often referred to as spasmolytics. They work in the upper levels of the CNS, so possible depression must be anticipated with their use. These drugs include

- Baclofen (*Lioresal*), which is used for the treatment of muscle spasticity associated with neuromuscular diseases such as multiple sclerosis, muscle rigidity, and spinal cord injuries. This agent, which is available in oral and intrathecal forms, can be administered via a delivery pump for the treatment of central spasticity.

Table 25.1 DRUGS IN FOCUS

Centrally Acting Skeletal Muscle Relaxants

Drug Name	Dosage/Route	Usual Indications
P baclofen (*Lioresal*)	Adult: 40–80 mg PO daily, 12–1500 mcg/day per intrathecal infusion pump Pediatric: intrathecal infusion pump, 24–1199 mcg/day—base dosage on patient response	Muscle spasticity, spinal cord injuries
carisoprodol (*Soma*)	350 mg PO t.i.d. to q.i.d.	Relief of discomfort of acute musculoskeletal conditions in adults
chlorphenesin (*Malate*)	800 PO t.i.d. until desired effect is seen; then 400 mg PO q.i.d. may be sufficient	Relief of discomfort of acute musculoskeletal conditions
chlorzoxazone (*Paraflex*)	250 mg PO t.i.d. to q.i.d.	Relief of discomfort of acute musculoskeletal conditions in adults
cyclobenzaprine (*Flexeril*)	10 mg PO t.i.d., do not exceed 60 mg/day	Relief of discomfort of acute musculoskeletal conditions in adults
metaxalone (*Skelaxin*)	Adults and children >12 yr: 800 mg PO t.i.d. to q.i.d.; reduce dosage with hepatic impairment	Relief of discomfort of acute musculoskeletal conditions
methocarbamol (*Robaxin*)	Adult: 1.5 g PO q.i.d., up to 30–60 mg/day; 1–2 g IV or IM for tetanus Pediatric: 15 mg/kg IV for tetanus; 0.4 mg/kg/day PO initially; maintenance 0.2 mg/kg/day	Relief of discomfort of acute musculoskeletal conditions in adults; tetanus
orphenadrine (*Banflex, Flexoject*)	100 mg PO, AM and at bedtime or 60 mg IV or IM q12h	Relief of discomfort of acute musculoskeletal conditions in adults; quinidine-induced leg cramps (100 mg PO at bedtime)
tizanidine (*Zanaflex*)	8 mg PO as a single dose may be repeated q6–8h as needed	Relief of discomfort of acute musculoskeletal conditions in adults

- Carisoprodol (*Soma*), which is indicated for the relief of discomfort associated with musculoskeletal pain. It may be safer than the other spasmolytics in older patients and in those with renal or hepatic dysfunction.
- Chlorphenesin (*Maolate*), which has the same indication as carisoprodol but a longer duration of action.
- Chlorzoxazone (*Paraflex*), which is also indicated for the relief of discomfort associated with musculoskeletal pain.
- Cyclobenzaprine (*Flexeril*), which is recommended for the relief of discomfort associated with painful, acute musculoskeletal conditions. This agent, available only in an oral form, is associated with few adverse effects.
- Metaxalone (*Skelaxin*), which is recommended as an adjunct for the relief of discomfort associated with acute, painful musculoskeletal conditions. Caution must be used with this drug in patients with any hepatic impairment. This is one of the few skeletal muscle relaxants with an established pediatric dose for children older than 12 years.
- Methocarbamol (*Robaxin*), which is used to relieve the same conditions as cyclobenzaprine and also to alleviate signs and symptoms of tetanus. It is available in oral and parenteral forms.
- Orphenadrine (*Banflex, Flexoject*), another parenteral drug, which is available for the relief of acute, painful musculoskeletal conditions. This agent is also being tried for the relief of quinidine-resistant leg cramps.
- Tizanidine (*Zanaflex*), which is approved for the acute and intermittent management of increased muscle tone associated with spasticity. It has been associated with liver toxicity and should be used with caution if a patient has hepatic dysfunction. It is also associated with hypotension in some patients.

Diazepam (*Valium*), a drug widely used as an anxiety agent (see Chapter 20), also has been shown to be an effective centrally acting skeletal muscle relaxant. It may be advantageous in situations in which anxiety may precipitate the muscle spasm.

Other measures in addition to these drugs should be used to alleviate muscle spasm and pain. Such modalities as rest of the affected muscle, heat applications to increase blood flow to the area to remove the pain-causing chemicals, physical therapy to return the muscle to normal tone and activity, and anti-inflammatory agents (including nonsteroidal anti-inflammatory drugs [NSAIDs]) if the underlying problem is related to injury or inflammation may help (Box 25.3).

Therapeutic Actions and Indications

Although the exact mechanism of action of these skeletal muscle relaxants is not known, it is thought to involve action in the upper or spinal interneurons. Tizanidine is an alpha-adrenergic agonist and is thought to increase inhibition of presynaptic motor neurons in the CNS. The primary indication for the use of centrally acting skeletal muscle agents is the relief of discomfort associated with acute, painful musculoskeletal conditions as an adjunct to rest, physical therapy, and other measures.

Pharmacokinetics

Most of these agents are rapidly absorbed and metabolized in the liver. Baclofen is not metabolized, but like the other skeletal muscle relaxants, it is excreted in the urine. No good studies exist regarding the effects of these agents during pregnancy and lactation; therefore, use should be limited to those situations in which the benefit to the mother clearly outweighs any potential risk to the fetus or neonate.

Contraindications and Cautions

Centrally acting skeletal muscle relaxants are contraindicated in the presence of any known allergy to any of these

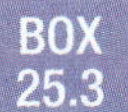

Fixed-Combination Skeletal Muscle Relaxants

Some products are available that combine a centrally acting muscle relaxant with an anti-inflammatory or analgesic agent. These products tend to facilitate relief of the discomfort associated with acute painful musculoskeletal conditions. They should be used as adjuncts to rest, physical therapy, and other measures.

Drug Name	Composition	Dosage
Soma Compound	200 mg carisoprodol/325 mg aspirin	1–2 tablets PO q.i.d.
Soma Compound with codeine	200 mg carisoprodol/325 mg aspirin/16 mg codeine	1–2 tablets PO q.i.d
Flexaphen[a]	250 mg chlorzoxazone/300 mg acetaminophen	2 capsules PO q.i.d.
Lobac[a]	200 mg salicylamide/20 mg phenyltoloxamine/300 mg acetaminophen	2 capsules PO q.i.d.
Norgesic[a]	25 mg orphenadrine/385 mg aspirin/30 mg caffeine	1–2 tablets PO t.i.d. to q.i.d.
Norgesic Forte[a]	50 mg orphenadrine/770 mg aspirin/60 mg caffeine	1 tablet PO t.i.d. to q.i.d.

[a] Rated by the U.S. Food and Drug Administration as "possibly effective" for this indication.

drugs and with skeletal muscle spasms resulting from rheumatic disorders. In addition, baclofen should not be used to treat any spasticity that contributes to locomotion, upright position, or increased function. *Blocking this spasticity results in loss of these functions.*

All centrally acting skeletal muscle relaxants should be used cautiously in the following circumstances: with a history of epilepsy *because the CNS depression and imbalance caused by these drugs may exacerbate the seizure disorder;* with cardiac dysfunction *because muscle function may be depressed;* with any condition marked by muscle weakness *that the drugs could make much worse;* and with hepatic or renal dysfunction, *which could interfere with the metabolism and excretion of the drugs, leading to toxic levels.* These agents should be used with caution in pregnancy or lactation *because of adverse effects to the fetus or neonate.*

Adverse Effects

The most frequently seen adverse effects associated with these drugs relate to the associated CNS depression: drowsiness, fatigue, weakness, confusion, headache, and insomnia. Gastrointestinal (GI) disturbances, which may be linked to CNS depression of the parasympathetic reflexes, include nausea, dry mouth, anorexia, and constipation. In addition, hypotension and arrhythmias may occur, again as a result of depression of normal reflex arcs. Urinary frequency, enuresis, and feelings of urinary urgency reportedly may occur. Chlorzoxazone may discolor the urine, becoming orange to purple-red when metabolized and excreted. Patients should be warned about this effect to prevent any fears of blood in the urine.

Clinically Important Drug–Drug Interactions

If any of the centrally acting skeletal muscle relaxants are taken with other CNS depressants or alcohol, CNS depression may increase. Patients should be cautioned to avoid alcohol while taking these muscle relaxants; if this combination cannot be avoided, they should take extreme precautions.

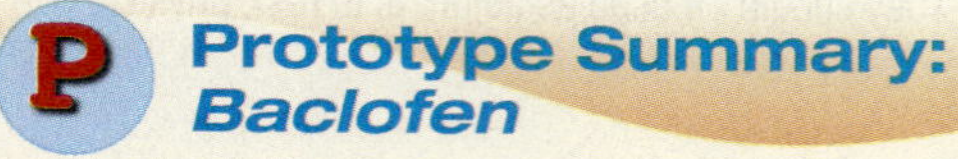

Prototype Summary: Baclofen

Indications: Alleviation of signs and symptoms of spasticity; may be of use in spinal cord injuries or spinal cord diseases

Actions: GABA analog; exact mechanism of action is not understood; inhibits monosynaptic and polysynaptic spinal reflexes; CNS depressant

Pharmacokinetics:

Route	Onset	Peak	Duration
Oral	1 h	2 h	4–8 h
Intrathecal	30–60 min	4 h	4–8 h

$T_{1/2}$: 3–4 hours; not metabolized; excreted in the urine

Adverse effects: Transient drowsiness, dizziness, weakness, fatigue, constipation, headache, insomnia, hypotension, nausea, urinary frequency

Nursing Considerations for Patients Receiving Centrally Acting Skeletal Muscle Relaxants

Assessment: History and Examination

Screen for the following conditions, *which could be cautions or contraindications for the use of the drug:* any known allergies to these drugs; cardiac depression, epilepsy, muscle weakness, rheumatic disorder; pregnancy or lactation; and renal or hepatic dysfunction.

Include screening *for baseline status before beginning therapy and for any potential adverse effects.* Assess the following: temperature; skin color and lesions; CNS orientation, affect, reflexes, bilateral grip strength, and spasticity evaluation; bowel sounds and reported output; and liver and renal function tests.

Nursing Diagnoses

The patient who is receiving a centrally acting skeletal muscle relaxant may have the following nursing diagnoses related to drug therapy:

- Acute Pain related to GI and CNS effects
- Disturbed Thought Processes related to CNS effects
- Risk for Injury related to CNS effects
- Deficient Knowledge regarding drug therapy

Implementation With Rationale

- Provide additional measures to relieve discomfort—heat, rest for the muscle, NSAIDs, positioning—*to augment the effects of the drug at relieving the musculoskeletal discomfort.*
- Discontinue the drug at any sign of hypersensitivity reaction or liver dysfunction *to prevent severe toxicity.*
- If using baclofen, taper drug slowly over 1 to 2 weeks *to prevent the development of psychoses and hal-*

lucinations. Use baclofen cautiously in patients whose spasticity contributes to mobility, posture, or balance *to prevent loss of this function.*

- If the patient is receiving baclofen through a delivery pump, the patient should understand the pump, the reason for frequent monitoring, and how to adjust the dose and program the unit *to enhance patient knowledge and promote compliance.*
- Monitor respiratory status *to evaluate adverse effects and arrange for appropriate dosage adjustment or discontinuation of the drug.*
- Provide thorough patient teaching, including drug name, prescribed dosage, measures for avoidance of adverse effects, warning signs that may indicate possible problems, and the need for monitoring and evaluation *to enhance patient knowledge about drug therapy and to promote compliance.*
- Offer support and encouragement *to help the patient cope with the drug regimen.*

Evaluation

- Monitor patient response to the drug (improvement in muscle spasm and relief of pain; improvement in muscle spasticity).
- Monitor for adverse effects (CNS changes, GI depression, urinary urgency).
- Evaluate the effectiveness of the teaching plan (patient can give the drug name and dosage, name possible adverse effects to watch for and specific measures to prevent adverse effects, and describe, if necessary, proper intrathecal administration).
- Monitor the effectiveness of comfort measures and compliance with the regimen.

Direct-Acting Skeletal Muscle Relaxants

One drug is currently available for use in treating (general) spasticity that directly affects peripheral muscle contraction. This drug, dantrolene (*Dantrium*), has become important in the management of spasticity associated with neuromuscular diseases such as cerebral palsy (see Critical Thinking Scenario 25-1), multiple sclerosis, muscular dystrophy, polio, tetanus, quadriplegia, and amyotrophic lateral sclerosis (ALS). This agent is not used for the treatment of muscle spasms associated with musculoskeletal injury or rheumatic disorders. The botulinum toxins A and B bind directly to the receptor sites of motor nerve terminals and inhibit the release of acetylcholine, leading to local muscle paralysis. These two drugs are injected locally and used for specific muscle groups. (See Table 25.2 for more about these drugs.)

Therapeutic Actions and Indications

Dantrolene acts within skeletal muscle fibers, interfering with the release of calcium from the muscle tubules (Figure 25.2; see Box 25.2). This action prevents the fibers from contracting. Dantrolene does not interfere with neuromuscular transmissions, and it does not affect the surface membrane of skeletal muscle.

Dantrolene is indicated for the control of spasticity resulting from upper motor neuron disorders, including spinal cord injury, myasthenia gravis, muscular dystrophy, and cerebral palsy (oral form). Continued long-term use is justified as long as the drug reduces painful and disabling spasticity. Long-term use results in a decrease of the amount and intensity of required nursing care.

Dantrolene is also indicated for the prevention of malignant hyperthermia, a state of intense muscle contraction and resulting hyperpyrexia. Malignant hyperthermia may occur as an adverse reaction to certain neuromuscular junction blockers that are used to induce paralysis during surgery. (This occurs more often with succinylcholine than with other neuromuscular junction blockers; see Chapter 28.) Dantrolene is used orally as preoperative prophylaxis in susceptible patients who must undergo anesthesia and after acute episodes to prevent recurrence. The agent is also used parenterally to treat malignant hyperthermia crisis.

Botulinum toxin type B (*Myobloc*) is a direct-acting skeletal muscle relaxant that is approved for the reduction of the severity of abnormal head position and neck pain associated with cervical dystonia. An injection of 5000 to 10,000 units is given IM into the affected muscles, causing muscle relaxation and relieving the tight spasm that can distort head position and cause pain.

In April 2002, the FDA approved botulinum toxin type A (*Botox Cosmetic*), a similar drug, to improve the appearance of glabellar lines (frown lines) between the eyebrows. Four units of the drug are injected between the eyebrows, relaxing the muscles and relieving the appearance of lines. The injection needs to be repeated every 3 months. Adverse effects associated with this use include headache, respiratory infections, flu-like syndrome, and droopy eyelids in severe cases. Pain, redness, and muscle weakness were also reported. The reactions tended to be temporary, but there have been reports of reactions that lasted several months. The FDA strongly reminds providers that this is a prescription drug and should be used only under close medical supervision, and not injected at trendy "Botox parties." In 2004, this drug was also approved for treatment of cervical dystonia, strabismus, and blepharospasm associated with dystonia in patients 12 years of age or older, and for treatment of severe primary axillary hyperhidrosis (sweating) when injected into the axillary area.

(text continues on page 408)

CRITICAL THINKING SCENARIO 25-1

Skeletal Muscle Relaxants for Cerebral Palsy

The Situation

L.G. is 26 years old. He was diagnosed with cerebral palsy shortly after his birth. He lives in the community in a group home with six other affected people. Two adult caregivers provide supervision. In the past few months, L.G.'s spasticity has progressed severely, making it impossible for him to carry on his daily activities without extensive assistance.

Following a clinical evaluation, his health care team suggests trying a course of dantrolene therapy. After learning about the risks of dantrolene-related hepatic dysfunction, L.G. decides that the benefits of dantrolene therapy are more important to him than the risks of hepatotoxicity. The health care team proceeds with a complete physical examination, including liver enzyme analysis. Therapy begins and a clinic staff member schedules L.G. for a visit by a public health nurse in 4 days.

Critical Thinking

What basic principles must be included in the nursing care plan for L.G. for the visiting nurses? *Think about the importance of including the adult caregivers in any teaching or evaluation programs. Consider specific problems that could develop that L.G. would be unable to handle on his own.*

What therapeutic goals might the nurse set with L.G. and his caregiver? How might these be evaluated?

What additional drug-related information should be posted in the group home and reviewed with L.G. and his caregivers?

Discussion

In the first visit to the home, the nurse needs to establish a relationship with L.G. and his caregivers. They should all realize that drug therapy, and other measures, are needed to help L.G. attain his full potential and make use of his existing assets. Step-by-step therapeutic goals should be established and written down for future reference. Small reachable goals, such as partially dressing himself, walking to the table for meals, and managing parts of his daily hygiene routine are best at the beginning. Written goals provide a good basis for future evaluation when drug therapy is stopped briefly to determine its therapeutic effectiveness. It also helps L.G. to see progress and improvement.

In addition, the nurse should perform a complete examination to obtain baseline data. The patient should be asked about any noticeable changes or problems since starting the drug. If improvement appears to have occurred, the dosage may be slowly increased until the optimal level of functioning has been achieved. The nurse is in a position to evaluate this and report it to the primary caregiver.

While in the home, the nurse can also evaluate resources and environmental limitations and suggest improvements (e.g., use of leg braces). L.G. and his caregivers should receive a drug teaching card that includes a telephone number to call with questions or concerns; warning signs of liver disease; and a list of findings to report. The nurse should discuss anticipated appointments for liver function tests to ensure that L.G. can keep the appointments. The health care team should work closely with L.G. to maximize his involvement in his care and to minimize unnecessary problems and confusion. Because the treatment involves a long-term commitment, a good working relationship among all members of the health care team is important to ensure continuity of care and optimal results.

Nursing Care Guide for L.G.: Muscle Relaxants

Assessment: History and Examination

Concentrate the health history on allergies to any skeletal muscle relaxants, respiratory depression, muscle weakness, hepatic or renal dysfunction, and concurrent use of verapamil or alcohol.

Focus the physical examination on the following:

CV: blood pressure pulse rate, peripheral perfusion, ECG

CNS: orientation, affect, reflexes, gip strength

Skin: color, lesions, texture, temperature

GI: abdominal examination, bowel sounds

Respiratory: respiration, adventitious sounds

Laboratory tests: renal and hepatic function

Nursing Diagnoses

Acute Pain related to GI, GU, and CNS effects

Risk for Injury related to CNS effects

Disturbed Thought Processes related to CNS effects

Deficient Knowledge regarding drug therapy

Skeletal Muscle Relaxants for Cerebral Palsy *(continued)*

Implementation

Discontinue drug at first sign of liver dysfunction.

Provide comfort and safety measures: positioning, orientation, safety measures, pain medication as needed.

Provide support and reassurance to help L.G. deal with spasticity and drug effects.

Teach L.G. about drug, dosage, drug effects and symptoms of reportable serious adverse effects.

Evaluation

Evaluate drug effects: relief of spasticity, improved daily function.

Monitor for adverse effects: multiple CNS effects, respiratory depression, rash, skin changes, GI problems (diarrhea, hepatotoxicity), urinary urgency or weakness.

Monitor for drug–drug interactions: myocardial suppression with verapamil or alcohol.

Evaluate effectiveness of patient teaching program.

PATIENT TEACHING FOR L.G.

- ☐ The drug prescribed for you is a direct-acting skeletal muscle relaxant called dantrolene (*Dantrium*). This drug makes spastic muscles relax. Because this drug may cause liver damage, it is important that you have regular medical check-ups.
- ☐ Common side effects of skeletal muscle relaxants, such as dantrolene, include:
  - *Fatigue, weakness, and drowsiness:* Try to pace activities evenly throughout the day and allow rest periods to avoid discouraging side effects. If they become too severe, consult your health care provider.
  - *Dizziness and fainting:* Change position slowly to avoid dizzy spells. If these effects should occur, avoid activities that require coordination and concentration.
  - *Diarrhea:* Be sure to be near bathroom facilities if this occurs. This effect usually subsides after a few weeks.
  - Report any of the following to your health care provider: *fever, chills, rash, itching, changes in the color of your urine or stool, or a yellowish tint to the eyes or skin.*
- ☐ Keep this drug and all medications out of the reach of children.
- ☐ Do not overexert yourself when you begin to feel better. Pace yourself.
- ☐ Take this drug exactly as directed and schedule regular medical checkups to evaluate the effects of this drug on your body.

Table 25.2 DRUGS IN FOCUS

Direct-Acting Skeletal Muscle Relaxants

Drug Name	Dosage/Route	Usual Indications
P dantrolene (*Dantrium*)	Adult: initially 25 mg PO; increase based on spinal cord injuries; prevention and management of response to a maximum 400 mg/day for spasticity Prevention of malignant hyperthermia: 4–8 mg/kg/day PO for 1–2 d before surgery, or 2.5 mg/kg IV over 1 h, given 1 h before surgery; postcrisis, 4–8 mg/kg/day PO for 1–3 days Pediatric: initially 0.5 mg/kg/day PO b.i.d., titrate to a maximum 100 mg PO q.i.d. for spasticity; for malignant hyperthermia, follow adult dosage	Upper motor neuron-associated muscle spasticity; malignant hyperthermia
botulinum toxin type A (*Botox Cosmetic*)	Adult: 20 units (0.5 mL solution) injected as divided doses of 0.1 mL into each of five sites (two in each corrugator muscle, and one in the procerus muscle) repeated every 3–4 mo; local injection associated with particular disorder—see manufacturer's guidelines	Improvement of appearance in glabellar lines associated with corrugator or procerus muscle activity in adults; treatment of cervical dystonia; treatment of severe primary axillary hyperhydrosis; treatment of strabismus and blepharospasm associated with dystonia
botulinum toxin type B (*Myobloc*)	2500–5000 units IM injected locally into affected muscles	Reduction of severity of abnormal head position and neck pain associated with cervical dystonia

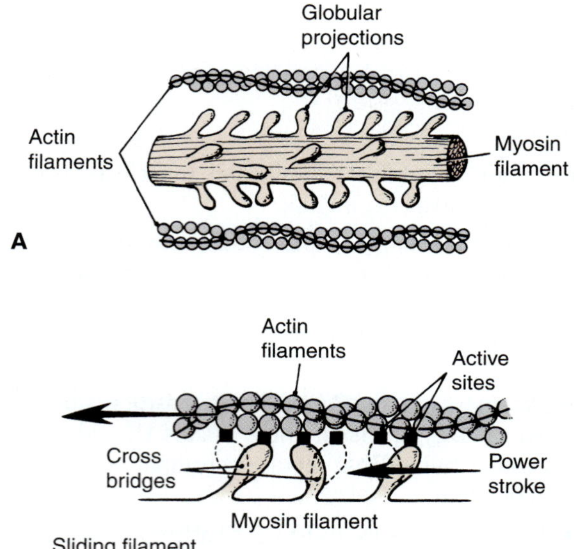

FIGURE 25.2 Sliding filament mechanism of muscle contraction. **(A)** The relationship between the myosin filament and the actin filament projections. **(B)** The bridges formed by the myosin filament along successive sites on the actin filaments, as outlined in Box 25.2.

Pharmacokinetics

Dantrolene is slowly absorbed from the GI tract. It is metabolized in the liver with a half-life of 4 to 8 hours. Excretion is through the urine. Dantrolene crosses the placenta and was found to be embryotoxic in animal studies. Use should be reserved for those situations in which the benefit to the mother clearly outweighs the risk to the fetus. Dantrolene enters breast milk and is contraindicated for use during lactation. Safety for use in children younger than 5 years of age has not been established; because the long-term effects are not known, careful consideration should be given to use of the drug in children. The botulinum toxins are not generally absorbed systemically.

Contraindications and Cautions

Dantrolene is contraindicated in the presence of any known allergy to the drug. It is also contraindicated in the following conditions: spasticity that contributes to locomotion, upright position, or increased function, *which would be lost if that spasticity were blocked;* active hepatic disease, *which might interfere with metabolism of the drug and because of known liver toxicity;* and lactation *because the drug may cross into breast milk and cause adverse effects in the infant.* The botulinum toxins are contraindicated in the presence of allergy to any component of the drug or with active infection at the site of the injection *because injecting the drug could aggravate the infection.*

Caution should be used with dantrolene in the following circumstances: in women and in all patients older than 35 years *because of increased risk of potentially fatal hepatocellular disease* (Box 25.4); in patients with a history of liver disease or previous dysfunction, *which could make the liver more susceptible to cellular toxicity;* in those with respiratory depression, *which could be exacerbated by muscular weakness;* in those with cardiac disease *because cardiac muscle depression may be a risk;* and during pregnancy *because of the potential for adverse effects on the fetus.* Caution should be used with the botulinum toxins with any peripheral neuropathic disease; with neuromuscular disorders, *which could be exacerbated by the effects of the drug;* with pregnancy and lactation; and with any known cardiovascular disease.

Adverse Effects

The most frequently seen adverse effects associated with dantrolene relate to drug-caused CNS depression: drowsiness, fatigue, weakness, confusion, headache and insomnia, and visual disturbances. GI disturbances may be linked to direct irritation or to alterations in smooth muscle function caused by the drug-induced calcium effects. Such adverse GI effects may include GI irritation, diarrhea, constipation, and abdominal cramps. Dantrolene may also cause direct hepatocellular damage and hepatitis that can be fatal. Urinary frequency, enuresis, and feelings of urinary urgency reportedly occur, and crystalline urine with pain or burning on urination may result. In addition, several unusual adverse effects may occur, including acne, abnormal hair growth, rashes, photosensitivity, abnormal sweating, chills, and myalgia.

The botulinum toxins have been associated with anaphylactic reactions; with headache, dizziness, muscle pain and paralysis; and with redness and edema at the injection site.

BOX 25.4 Gender Considerations: Understanding the Risks of Liver Damage With Dantrolene

Dantrolene (*Dantrium*) is associated with potentially fatal hepatocellular injury. When liver damage begins to occur, patients often experience a prodrome, or warning syndrome, which includes anorexia, nausea, and fatigue. The incidence of such hepatic injury is greater in women and in patients older than 35 years of age.

In women, a combination of dantrolene and estrogen seems to affect the liver, thus posing a greater risk. Women of all ages may be at increased risk, because those entering menopause may be taking hormone replacement therapy. Patients older than 35 years of age are at increasing risk of liver injury because of the changing integrity of the liver cells that comes with age and exposure to toxins over time.

If a particular woman needs dantrolene for relief of spasticity, she should not be taking any estrogens (e.g., birth control pills, hormone replacement therapy), and she should be monitored closely for any sign of liver dysfunction. For safer relief of spasticity in these patients, baclofen may be helpful.

Clinically Important Drug–Drug Interactions

If dantrolene is combined with estrogens, the incidence of hepatocellular toxicity is apparently increased. If possible, this combination should be avoided. If the botulinum toxins are used with other drugs that interfere with neuromuscular transmission—neuromuscular junction (NMJ) blockers, lincosamides, quinidine, magnesium sulfate, anticholinesterases, succinylcholine, or polymyxin—or with aminoglycosides, there is a risk of additive effects. If any of these must be given in combination, extreme caution should be used.

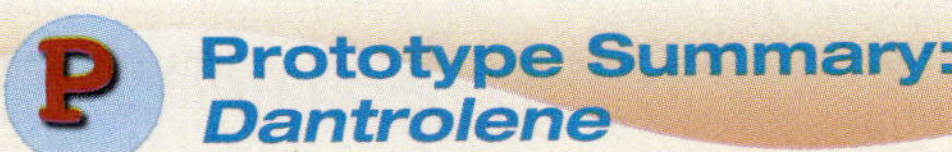

Prototype Summary: Dantrolene

Indications: Control of clinical spasticity resulting from upper motor neuron disorders; preoperatively to prevent or attenuate the development of malignant hyperthermia in susceptible patients; IV for management of fulminant malignant hyperthermia

Actions: Interferes with the release of calcium from the sarcoplasmic reticulum within skeletal muscles, preventing muscle contraction; does not interfere with neuromuscular transmission

Pharmacokinetics:

Route	Onset	Peak	Duration
Oral	Slow	4–6 h	8–10 h
IV	Rapid	5 h	6–8 h

$T_{1/2}$: 9 hours (oral), 4–8 hours (IV); excreted in the urine

Adverse effects: Drowsiness, dizziness, weakness, fatigue, diarrhea, hepatitis, myalgia, tachycardia, transient blood pressure changes, rash, urinary frequency

Nursing Considerations for Patients Receiving a Direct-Acting Skeletal Muscle Relaxant

Assessment: History and Examination

Screen for the following conditions, *which could be cautions or contraindications for the use of the drug:* any known allergies to these drugs; cardiac depression; epilepsy; muscle weakness; respiratory depression; pregnancy and lactation; and renal or hepatic dysfunction.

Include screening *for baseline status before beginning therapy and for any potential adverse effects.* Assess the following: temperature; skin color and lesions; CNS orientation, affect, reflexes, bilateral grip strength, and spasticity; respiration and adventitious sounds; pulse, electrocardiogram (ECG), and cardiac output; bowel sounds and reported output; and liver and renal function tests.

Nursing Diagnoses

The patient taking a direct-acting skeletal muscle relaxant may have the following nursing diagnoses related to drug therapy:

- Acute Pain related to GI and CNS effects
- Disturbed Thought Processes related to CNS effects
- Risk for Injury related to CNS effects
- Deficient Knowledge regarding drug therapy

Implementation With Rationale

- Discontinue the drug at any sign of liver dysfunction. *Early diagnosis of liver damage may prevent permanent dysfunction. Arrange for the drug to be discontinued if signs of liver damage appear.* A prodrome, with nausea, anorexia, and fatigue, is present in 60% of patients with evidence of hepatic injury.
- Monitor intravenous access sites for potential extravasation *because the drug is alkaline and very irritating to tissues.*
- Institute other supportive measures (e.g., ventilation, anticonvulsants as needed, cooling blankets) for the treatment of malignant hyperthermia *to support the patient through the reaction.*
- Periodically discontinue the drug for 2 to 4 days *to monitor therapeutic effectiveness.* A clinical impression of exacerbation of spasticity indicates a positive therapeutic effect and justifies continued use of the drug.
- Establish a therapeutic goal before beginning oral therapy (e.g., to gain or enhance the ability to engage in a therapeutic exercise program; to use braces; to accomplish transfer maneuvers) *to promote patient compliance and a sense of success with therapy.*
- Discontinue the drug if diarrhea becomes severe *to prevent dehydration and electrolyte imbalance.* The drug may be restarted at a lower dose.
- Provide thorough patient teaching, including drug name, prescribed dosage, measures for avoidance of adverse effects, warning signs that may indicate possible problems, and the need for monitoring and evaluation *to enhance patient knowledge about drug therapy and to promote compliance.*

- Offer support and encouragement to help the patient cope with the drug regimen.

Evaluation

- Monitor patient response to the drug (improvement in spasticity, improvement in movement and activities).
- Monitor for adverse effects (CNS changes, diarrhea, liver toxicity, urinary urgency).
- Evaluate the effectiveness of the teaching plan (patient can give the drug name and dosage, possible adverse effects to watch for and specific measures to prevent adverse effects, and therapeutic goals).
- Monitor the effectiveness of comfort measures and compliance with the regimen.

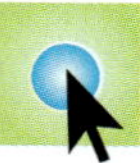

WEB LINKS

Health care providers and patients may want to consult the following Internet sources:

http://www.ahc.umn.edu/ahc_content/colleges/medschool/departments/neurology/wellstonemuscular_dystrophy_center/ Information on muscle physiology and muscle disorders and diseases.

http://www.mhaus.org Information on malignant hyperthermia.

http://www.ucp.org Information for patients and health care professionals about cerebral palsy research and treatment.

http://www.spinalcord.org Patient information regarding cerebral palsy.

Points to Remember

- Movement and control of muscles is regulated by spinal reflexes and influences from upper-level central nervous system areas, including the basal ganglia, cerebellum, and cerebral cortex.
- Upper-level controls of muscle activity include the pyramidal tract in the cerebellum, which regulates coordination of intentional muscle movement, and the extrapyramidal tract in the cerebellum and basal ganglia, which coordinates crude movements related to unconscious muscle activity.
- Damage to a muscle or anchoring skeletal structure may result in the arrival of a flood of impulses to the spinal cord. Such overstimulation may lead to a muscle spasm or a state of increased contraction.
- Damage to motor neurons can cause muscle spasticity, with a lack of coordination between muscle groups and loss of coordinated activity, including the ability to perform intentional tasks and maintain posture, position, and locomotion.
- Centrally acting skeletal muscle relaxants are used to relieve the effects of muscle spasm. Dantrolene, a direct-acting skeletal muscle relaxant, is used to control spasticity and prevent malignant hyperthermia.
- The botulinum toxin type B is used to reduce the severity of abnormal head position and neck pain associated with cervical dystonia. Botulinum toxin type A is used to improve the appearance of moderate to severe glabellar lines and to treat cervical dystonia, severe primary axillary hyperhidrosis, and strabismus and blepharospasm associated with dystonia.

CHECK YOUR UNDERSTANDING

Answers to the questions in this chapter may be found in the Answer Key in the back of the book.

Multiple Choice

Select the best answer to the following.

1. A muscle spasm often results from
   a. damage to the basal ganglia.
   b. central nervous system damage.
   c. injury to the musculoskeletal system.
   d. chemical imbalance within the CNS.

2. Muscle spasticity is the result of
   a. direct damage to a muscle cell.
   b. overstretching of a muscle.
   c. tearing of a ligament.
   d. damage to neurons within the CNS.

3. Signs and symptoms of tetanus, which includes severe muscle spasm, are best treated with
   a. baclofen.
   b. diazepam.
   c. carisoprodol.
   d. methocarbamol.

4. The drug of choice for a patient experiencing severe muscle spasms and pain precipitated by anxiety would be
   a. methocarbamol.
   b. baclofen.
   c. diazepam.
   d. carisoprodol.

5. Dantrolene (*Dantrium*) differs from the other skeletal muscle relaxants because
   a. it acts in the highest levels of the CNS.
   b. it is used to treat muscle spasms as well as muscle spasticity.
   c. it cannot be used to treat neuromuscular disorders.
   d. it acts directly within the skeletal muscle fiber and not within the CNS.

6. The use of neuromuscular junction blockers may sometimes cause a condition known as malignant hyperthermia. The drug of choice for prevention or treatment of this condition is
   a. baclofen.
   b. diazepam.
   c. dantrolene.
   d. methocarbamol.

7. Dantrolene is associated with potentially fatal cellular damage. If your patient's condition is being managed with dantrolene, the patient should
   a. have repeated CBCs during therapy.
   b. have renal function tests done monthly.
   c. be monitored for signs of liver damage and have liver function tests done regularly.
   d. have a thorough eye examination before and periodically during therapy.

Multiple Response

Select all that apply.

1. Spasmolytics or centrally acting muscle relaxants block the reflexes in the central nervous system that lead to spasm. While a patient is taking one of these drugs, which of the following interventions should be implemented?
   a. Rest for the affected muscle
   b. Heat to the affected area
   c. Ice packs to the affected area
   d. Use of anti-inflammatory agents
   e. Body temperature check every 2 hours to watch for malignant hyperthermia
   f. Positioning to decrease pain and spasm

2. Muscle relaxants would be used in which of the following circumstances?
   a. To treat spasticity related to spinal cord injury
   b. To treat spasticity that contributes to locomotion, upright position, or increase in function
   c. To treat spasticity that is related to toxins, such as tetanus
   d. To treat spasticity that is a result of neuromuscular degeneration
   e. To reduce the severity of head position associated with cervical dystonia
   f. To reduce the appearance of frown lines (glabellar lines)

Matching

Match the following words with the appropriate definitions.

1. ______________________ spasticity
2. ______________________ hypertonia
3. ______________________ hypotonia
4. ______________________ basal ganglia
5. ______________________ intraneurons
6. ______________________ pyramidal tract
7. ______________________ extrapyramidal tract
8. ______________________ cerebellum

A. Neurons that communicate between other neurons
B. Fibers within the central nervous system (CNS) that control precise, intentional movement
C. Sustained contractions of muscles
D. Lower portion of the brain associated with coordination of muscle movements and voluntary muscle movement
E. State of excessive muscle response and activity
F. Lower area of the brain associated with coordination of unconscious muscle movements
G. Cells that coordinate unconsciously controlled muscle activity
H. State of limited or absent muscle response and activity

True or False

Indicate whether the following statements are true (T) or false (F).

_____ 1. The nerves that affect movement, position, and posture are the spinal sensory neurons.

_____ 2. The basal ganglia and the cerebellum modulate spinal motor nerve activity and help coordinate activity between various muscle groups.

_____ 3. Fibers that control precise, intentional movement make up the extrapyramidal tract.

_____ 4. The pyramidal tract modulates or coordinates unconsciously controlled muscle activity and allows the body to make automatic adjustments in posture, position, and balance.

_____ 5. Muscle spasticity is the result of damage to neurons within the CNS, rather than injury to peripheral structures.

_____ 6. Excessive stimulation of muscles is referred to as hypotonia.

_____ 7. Centrally acting skeletal muscle relaxants work in the CNS to interfere with the reflexes that are causing the muscle spasm.

_____ 8. Dantrolene acts within skeletal muscle fibers, interfering with the release of potassium from the muscle tubules, to prevent the fibers from contracting.

_____ 9. The primary indication for the use of centrally acting skeletal muscle agents is the relief of discomfort associated with acute, painful musculoskeletal conditions.

_____ 10. Centrally acting muscle relaxants should be used as an adjunct to rest, physical therapy, and other measures.

Bibliography and References

Drug facts and comparisons. (2006). St. Louis: Facts and Comparisons.

Gilman, A., Hardman, J. G., & Limbird, L. E. (Eds.). (2006). *Goodman and Gilman's the pharmacological basis of therapeutics* (11th ed.). New York: McGraw-Hill.

Karch, A. M. (2006). *2007 Lippincott's nursing drug guide.* Philadelphia: Lippincott Williams & Wilkins.

Porth, C. M. (2005). *Pathophysiology: Concepts of altered health states* (7th ed.). Philadelphia: Lippincott Williams & Wilkins.

Professional's guide to patient drug facts. (2006). St. Louis: Facts and Comparisons.

CHAPTER 26

Narcotics and Antimigraine Agents

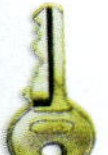

KEY TERMS

A fibers
A-delta and C fibers
ergot derivatives
gate control theory
migraine headache
narcotics
narcotic agonists
narcotic agonists-antagonists
narcotic antagonists
opioid receptors
spinothalamic tracts
triptan

LEARNING OBJECTIVES

Upon completion of this chapter, you will be able to:

1. Outline the gate theory of pain and explain therapeutic ways to block pain using the gate theory.
2. Describe the therapeutic actions, indications, pharmacokinetics, contraindications, most common adverse reactions, and important drug–drug interactions associated with narcotics and antimigraine drugs.
3. Discuss the use of narcotics and antimigraine drugs across the lifespan.
4. Compare and contrast the prototype drugs morphine, pentazocine, naloxone, ergotamine, and sumatriptan with other drugs in their respective classes.
5. Outline the nursing considerations, including important teaching points, for patients receiving a narcotic or an antimigraine drug.

NARCOTICS

Narcotic Agonists

codeine
fentanyl
hydrocodone
hydromorphone
levorphanol
meperidine
methadone
P morphine
opium
oxycodone
oxymorphone
propoxyphene
remifentanil
sufentanil

Narcotic Agonists-Antagonists

buprenorphine
butorphanol
nalbuphine
P pentazocine

Narcotic Antagonists

nalmefene
P naloxone
naltrexone

ANTIMIGRAINE DRUGS

Ergot Derivatives

dihydroergotamine
P ergotamine

Triptans

almotriptan
eletriptan
frovatriptan
naratriptan
rizatriptan
P sumatriptan
zolmitriptan

Pain, by definition, is a sensory and emotional experience associated with actual or potential tissue damage. The perception of pain is part of the clinical presentation in many disorders and is one of the hardest sensations for patients to cope with during the course of a disease or dysfunction. The drugs involved in the management of severe pain, whether acute or chronic, are discussed in this chapter. These agents all work in the central nervous system (CNS)—the brain and the spinal cord—to alter the way that pain impulses arriving from peripheral nerves are processed. These agents can change the perception and tolerance of pain. Two major types of drugs are considered here: the narcotics, the opium derivatives that are used to treat many types of pain, and the antimigraine drugs, which are reserved for the treatment of **migraine headaches**, a type of severe headache. These drugs are used with patients of all ages (Box 26.1).

Pain Perception

Pain occurs whenever tissues are damaged. The injury to cells releases many chemicals, including kinins and prostaglandins, which stimulate specific sensory nerves (Figure 26.1). Two small-diameter sensory nerves, called the **A-delta and C fibers**, respond to stimulation by generating nerve impulses that produce pain sensations. Pain impulses from the skin, subcutaneous tissues, muscles, and deep visceral structures are conducted to the dorsal, or posterior, horn of the spinal cord on these fibers. In the spinal cord, these nerves form synapses with spinal cord nerves that then send impulses to the brain.

In addition, large-diameter sensory nerves enter the dorsal horn of the spinal cord. These so-called **A fibers** do not transmit pain impulses; instead, they transmit sensations associated with touch and temperature. The A fibers, which are larger and conduct impulses more rapidly than do the smaller fibers, can actually block the ability of the smaller fibers to transmit their signals to the secondary neurons in the spinal cord. The dorsal horn, therefore, can be both excitatory and inhibitory with pain impulses that are transmitted from the periphery.

The impulses reaching the dorsal horn are transmitted upward toward the brain by a number of specific ascending nerve pathways. These pathways run from the spinal cord into the thalamus, where they form synapses with various nerve cells that transmit the information to the cerebral cortex, along the **spinothalamic tracts**. According to the **gate control theory**, the transmission of these impulses can be modulated all along these tracts (Figure 26.2). All along the spinal cord, the interneurons can act as "gates" by blocking

BOX 26.1 DRUG THERAPY ACROSS THE LIFESPAN

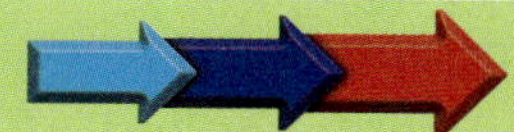

Narcotics and Antimigraine Agents

CHILDREN

The safety and effectiveness of many of these drugs have not been established in children. If a narcotic is used, the dosage should be calculated very carefully and the child should be monitored closely for the adverse effects associated with narcotic use.

Narcotics that have an established pediatric dose include codeine, fentanyl (but not transdermal fentanyl), hydrocodone, meperidine, and morphine. Narcotics that are not recommended for children are levorphanol, oxymorphone, oxycodone, and propoxyphene.

Methadone is not recommended as an analgesic. If a child older than 13 years of age requires a narcotic agonist-antagonist, buprenorphine is the drug of choice. Naloxone is the drug of choice for reversal of narcotic effects and narcotic overdose in children.

None of the drugs used to treat migraines are recommended for use in children. The ergot derivatives can have many adverse effects in children, and the triptans do not have the clinical experience to recommend them for use in children.

ADULTS

Adults being treated for acute pain should be reassured that the risk of addiction to a narcotic during treatment is remote. They should be encouraged to ask for pain medication before the pain is acute, to get better coverage for their pain. Many institutions allow patients to self-regulate intravenous drips to control their own pain postoperatively. Adults requesting treatment for migraine headaches should be carefully evaluated before one of the antimigraine drugs is used to ensure that the headache being treated is of the type that can benefit from these drugs.

The narcotics are contraindicated or should only be used with caution during pregnancy because of the potential for adverse effects on the fetus. These drugs enter breast milk and can cause opioid effects in the baby, so caution should be used during lactation. Morphine, meperidine, and oxymorphone are often used for analgesia during labor. The mother should be monitored closely for adverse reactions and, if the drug is used over a prolonged labor, the newborn infant should be monitored for opioid effects.

The ergots and the statins are contraindicated during pregnancy because of the potential for adverse effects in the mother and fetus. Women of childbearing age should be advised to use contraception while they are taking these drugs. Women who are nursing should be encouraged to find another method of feeding the baby because of the potential for adverse drug effects on the baby.

OLDER ADULTS

Elderly patients should be specifically asked whether they require pain medication. Because many older patients can recall a time when nurses were able to spend more time with patients, they may tend to believe that the nurse will meet their needs.

Older patients are more likely to experience the adverse effects associated with these drugs, including central nervous system, gastrointestinal, and cardiovascular effects. Because older patients often have renal or hepatic impairment, they are also more likely to have toxic levels of the drug related to changes in metabolism and excretion. The older patient should have safety measures in effect—siderails, call light, assistance to ambulate—when receiving one of these drugs in the hospital setting.

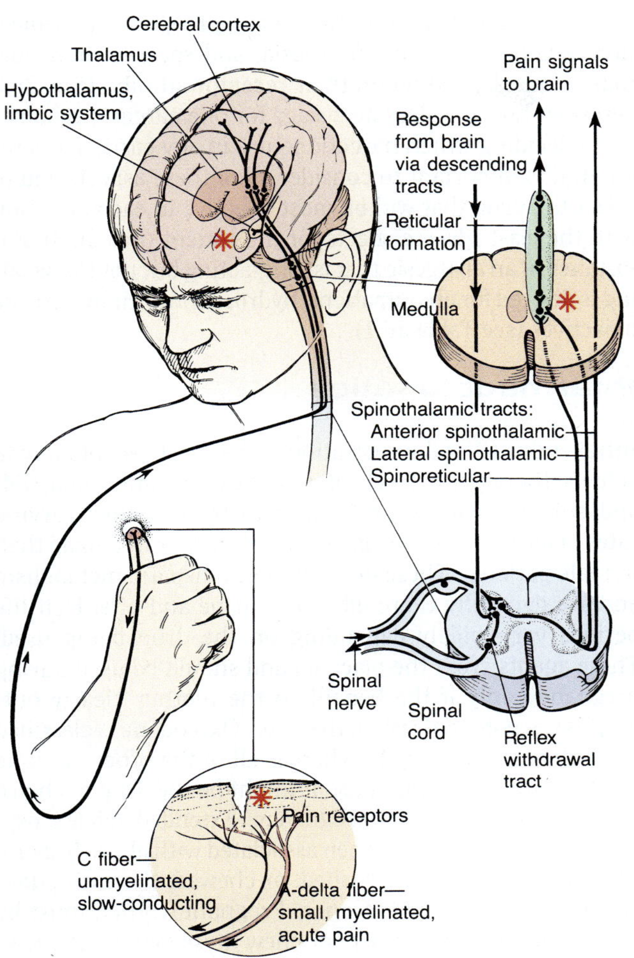

FIGURE 26.1 Neural pathways of pain.

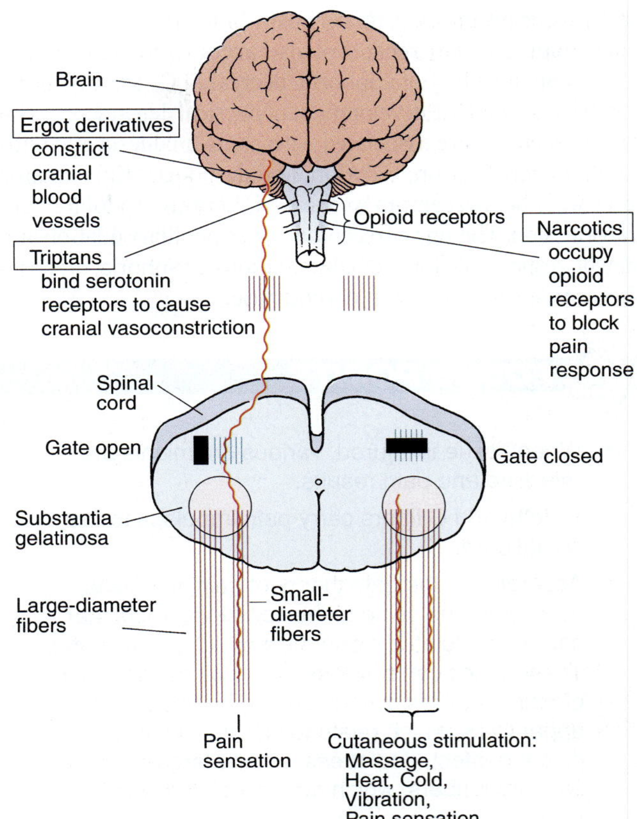

FIGURE 26.2 Gate control theory of pain. Narcotics occupy opioid receptors to block pain response. Ergot derivatives constrict cranial blood vessels, and triptans bind serotonin receptors to cause cranial vasoconstriction.

the ascending transmission of pain impulses. It is thought that the gates can be closed by stimulation of the larger A fibers and by descending impulses coming down the spinal cord from higher levels in such areas as the cerebral cortex, the limbic system, and the reticular activating system.

The inhibitory influence of the higher brain centers on the transmission of pain impulses helps explain much of the mystery associated with pain. Several factors, including learned experiences, cultural expectations, individual tolerance, and the placebo effect, can activate the descending inhibitory nerves from the upper central nervous system. Pain management usually involves the use of drugs, but it may also incorporate these other factors. The placebo effect, stress reduction, acupuncture, and back rubs (which stimulate the A fibers) all can play an important role in the effective management of pain.

Narcotics

The **narcotics**, or opioids, were first derived from the opium plant. Although most narcotics are now synthetically prepared, their chemical structure resembles that of the original plant alkaloids. All drugs in this class are similar in that they occupy specific opioid receptors in the CNS.

Opioid Receptors

Opioid receptors respond to naturally occurring peptins, the endorphins and the enkephalins. These receptors are found in the CNS, on nerves in the periphery, and on cells in the gastrointestinal (GI) tract. In the brainstem, opioid receptors help control blood pressure, pupil diameter, GI secretions, and the chemoreceptor trigger zone (CTZ) that regulates nausea and vomiting, cough, and respiration. In the spinal cord and thalamus, these receptors help integrate and relate incoming information about pain. In the hypothalamus, they may interrelate the endocrine and neural response to pain. In the limbic system, the receptors incorporate emotional aspects of pain and response to pain. At peripheral nerve sites, the opioids may block the release of neurotransmitters that are related to pain and inflammation.

The narcotic drugs that are used vary with the type of opioid receptors with which they react. This accounts for a change in pain relief, as well as a variation in the side effects that can be anticipated. Four types of opioid receptors have been identified: mu (μ), kappa (κ), beta (β), and sigma (ϵ).

The mu-receptors are primarily pain-blocking receptors. Besides analgesia, mu-receptors also account for respiratory depression, a feeling of euphoria, decreased GI activity, pupil constriction, and the development of physical dependence. The kappa-receptors are associated with some analgesia and with pupillary constriction, sedation, and dysphoria. Enkephalins react with beta-receptors in the periphery to modulate pain transmission. The sigma-receptors cause pupillary dilation and may be responsible for the hallucinations, dysphoria, and psychoses that can occur with narcotic use.

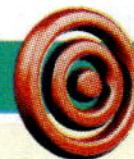

FOCUS POINTS

- When tissue is injured, various chemicals are released and pain results.
- A-delta and C fibers carry pain impulses to the spinal cord.
- According to the gate theory of pain, impulses travel from the spine to the cortex via tracts that can be modulated along the way at specific gates. These gates can be closed to block transmission of pain impulses by descending nerves from the upper CNS, which relate to emotion, culture, placebo effect, and stress, and by large-diameter sensory A fibers, which are associated with touch.
- Endogenous endorphins and enkephalins react with opioid receptors to regulate transmission of pain.
- Narcotics are derived from the opium plant; they bind to opioid receptors to relieve pain and promote feelings of well-being or euphoria.

Narcotic Agonists

The **narcotic agonists** are drugs that react with the opioid receptors throughout the body to cause analgesia, sedation, or euphoria. Anticipated effects other than analgesia are mediated by the types of opioid receptors affected by each drug. Because of the potential for the development of physical dependence while taking these drugs, the narcotic agonists are classified as controlled substances. The degree of control is determined by the relative ability of each drug to cause physical dependence. The available narcotic agonists are listed in Table 26.1.

Therapeutic Actions and Indications

The narcotic agonists act at specific opioid receptor sites in the CNS to produce analgesia, sedation, and a sense of well-being. They are used as antitussives and as adjuncts to general anesthesia to produce rapid analgesia, sedation, and respiratory depression. Indications for narcotic agonists include relief of severe acute or chronic pain, preoperative medication, analgesia during anesthesia, and specific individual indications depending on their receptor affinity. (Box 26.2 describes how to calculate dosage for one narcotic agonist.)

In deciding which narcotic to use in any particular situation, it is important to consider all of these aspects and to select the drug that will be most effective in each situation with the least adverse effects for the patient (Box 26.3). For instance, if an analgesic that is long-acting but not too sedating is desired for an outpatient, hydrocodone might fit those objectives (see Table 26.1).

Pharmacokinetics

Intravenous (IV) administration is the most reliable way to achieve therapeutic levels of narcotics. Intramuscular (IM) and subcutaneous (Sub-Q) administration offer varying rates of absorption, and absorption is slower in female than in male patients. These drugs undergo hepatic metabolism and are generally excreted in the urine and bile. Half-life periods vary widely depending on the drug being used. These agents cross the placenta and should be used during pregnancy only if the benefit to the mother clearly outweighs the potential risk to the fetus. Oxycodone is classified as pregnancy category B, whereas all of the other narcotic agonists are in category C, so it might be the drug of choice if one is needed during pregnancy. Extended release oxycodone (*OxyContin*) has been associated with abuse because when the tablet is cut, crushed, or chewed, the entire dose of the drug is released at once. Pregnant women must be cautioned not to cut, crush, or chew these tablets. The narcotics are known to enter breast milk, but there are no documented adverse effects on the baby. Many sources recommend waiting 4 to 6 hours after receiving a narcotic to feed the baby.

Contraindications and Cautions

The narcotic agonists are contraindicated in the following conditions: presence of any known allergy to any narcotic agonist; pregnancy, labor, or lactation *because of potential adverse effects on the fetus or neonate, including respiratory depression;* diarrhea caused by poisons *because depression of GI activity could lead to increased absorption and toxicity;* and after biliary surgery or surgical anastomoses *because of the adverse effects associated with GI depression and narcotics.*

Caution should be used in patients with respiratory dysfunction, *which could be exacerbated by the respiratory depression caused by these drugs;* recent GI or genitourinary (GU) surgery; acute abdomen or ulcerative colitis, *which could become worse with the depressive effects of the narcotics;* head injuries, alcoholism, delirium tremens, or cerebral vascular disease, *which could be exacerbated by the CNS effects of the drugs;* and liver or renal dysfunction, *which could alter the metabolism and excretion of the drugs.*

Table 26.1 DRUGS IN FOCUS

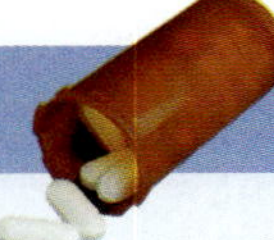

Narcotic Agonists

Drug Name	Dosage/Route	Usual Indications
codeine	Adult: 15–60 mg PO, IM, IV, or Sub-Q q4–6h; 10–20 mg PO q4–6h for cough Pediatric: 0.5 mg/kg PO, IM, or Sub-Q q4–6h; 2.5–10 mg PO q4–6h for cough	Relief of mild to moderate pain; coughing induced by mechanical or chemical irritation of the respiratory tract
fentanyl (*Duragesic*)	Adult: 0.05–0.1 mg IM, 30–60 min before surgery; 0.002 mg/kg IV or IM during surgery; 0.05–0.1 mg postoperatively; 5 mcg/kg transmucosal; for transdermal patch, calculate the previous day's narcotics need and use table to convert to patch strength Pediatric (>2 yr): 2–3 mcg/kg IM or IV; base transmucosal dose on weight and do not exceed 400 mcg	For analgesia before, during, and after surgery; transdermal patch for management of chronic pain
hydrocodone (*Hycodan*)	Adult: 5–10 mg PO q4h in combination products for pain: 5–10 mg PO q4–6h for cough Pediatric (2–12 yr): 1.25–5 mg PO q4–6h	Relief of cough; relief of moderate pain in combination products
hydromorphone (*Dilaudid*)	2–4 mg PO q4–6h or 3 mg PR q6–8h or 1–4 mg Sub-Q or IM q4–6h	Relief of moderate to severe pain in adults
levorphanol (*Levo-Dromoran*)	1 mg IV by slow injection or 1–2 mg IM or Sub-Q q6–8h or 2 mg PO q6–8h	Management of moderate to severe pain in adults; post-operative pain in adults
meperidine (*Demerol*)	Adult: 50–150 mg PO IM, or Sub-Q q3–4h; during labor, 100 mg IM or Sub-Q q1–3h Pediatric: 1–1.8 mg/kg IM, Sub-Q, or PO q3–4h	Relief of moderate to severe pain, preoperative analgesia and support of anesthesia, and obstetrical analgesia
methadone (*Dolophine*)	2.5–10 mg IM, Sub-Q, or PO q3–4h for pain; 15–20 mg PO for withdrawal, then 20 mg PO q4–8h for maintenance treatment	Relief of severe pain; detoxification and temporary maintenance treatment of narcotic addiction in adults
P morphine (*Roxanol, Astramorph*)	Adult: 10–20 mg solution PO or 15–30 mg tablets PO q4h or 10 mg Sub-Q or IM q4h *or* 2–10 mg/70 kg IV over 4–5 min or 10–20 mg PR q4h Pediatric: 0.1–0.2 mg/kg IM or Sub-Q q4h	Relief of moderate to severe chronic and acute pain; preoperatively and postoperatively and during labor
opium (*Paregoric*)	Adult: 0.6 mL liquid PO q.i.d. or 5–10 mL camphorated tincture one to four times per day PO Pediatric: 0.005–0.02 mg/kg PO q3–4h *or* 0.25–0.5 mL/kg PO q1–4h of camphorated tincture	Treatment of diarrhea, relief of moderate pain
oxycodone (*OxyContin*)	10–30 mg PO q4h as needed	Relief of moderate to severe pain in adults
oxymorphone (*Numorphan*)	0.5 mg IV initially; 1–1.5 mg IM or Sub-Q q4–6h as needed; 0.5–1 mg IM for labor; 5 mg PR q4–6h	Relief of moderate to severe pain in adults; preoperative medication; obstetrical analgesia
propoxyphene (*Darvon, Darvon-N*)	65 mg PO q4h as needed; *Darvon N*—100 mg PO q4h as needed	Relief of mild to moderate pain in adults **Special considerations:** limit use in suicidal or addiction-prone patients
remifentanil (*Ultiva*)	Adult and children >2 yr: dosage determined by general anesthetic being used	Analgesic for use during general anesthesia **Special considerations:** must be under the direct supervision of anesthesia practitioner
sufentanil (*Sufenta*)	Adult: 1–2 mcg/kg IV with general anesthesia Pediatric: 10–25 mcg/kg IV	Analgesic for use during general anesthesia; used as an epidural agent in labor and delivery **Special considerations:** must be under the direct supervision of anesthesia practitioner

Adverse Effects

The most frequently seen adverse effects associated with narcotic agonists relate to their effects on various opioid receptors. Respiratory depression with apnea, cardiac arrest, and shock may result from narcotic-caused CNS respiratory depression. Orthostatic hypotension is commonly seen with some narcotics. Such GI effects as nausea, vomiting, constipation, and biliary spasm may occur as a result of CTZ stimulation and negative effects on GI motility. Neurological effects such as light-headedness, dizziness, psychoses, anxiety, fear, hallucinations, pupil constriction, and impaired mental processes may occur as a result of the stimulation of CNS opioid receptors in the cerebrum, limbic system, and hypothalamus. GU effects, including ureteral spasm, urinary retention, hesitancy, and loss of libido, may be related to

BOX 26.2 FOCUS ON **CALCULATIONS**

You are taking care of a 4-year-old child after surgery. An order has been written for 1.5 mg/kg meperidine IM q3–4h as needed. The child is waking up and crying, so you decide to start the pain medication. The meperidine is available as 10 or 50 mg/mL. You note that the child weighs 20 kg. How much meperidine would you inject?

$$20 \text{ kg} \times 1.5 \text{ mg/kg} = 30 \text{ mg needed}$$

You could give 3 mL of the 10-mg/mL preparation:

$$(x \text{ mL}/30 \text{ mg} = 1 \text{ mL}/10 \text{ mg};\ x = 3)$$

Or you could give 0.6 mL of the 50-mg/mL preparation:

$$(x \text{ mL}/30 \text{ mg} = 1 \text{ mL}/50 \text{ mg};\ x = 0.6 \text{ mL})$$

In this case, you might prefer to give the child the smaller volume, using 0.6 mL of the 50-mg/mL solution to deliver the 30 mg of meperidine.

direct receptor stimulation or to CNS activation of sympathetic pathways. In addition, sweating and dependence (both physical and psychological) are possible, more so with some agents than with others.

Clinically Important Drug–Drug Interactions

When narcotic agonists are given with the barbiturate general anesthetics, or with some phenothiazines and monoamine oxidase inhibitors (MAOIs), the likelihood of respiratory depression, hypotension, and sedation or coma is increased. If these drug combinations cannot be avoided, patients should be monitored closely and appropriate supportive measures taken.

BOX 26.3 CULTURAL CONSIDERATIONS FOR DRUG THERAPY

Differences in Responses to Narcotic Therapy

Because of physical and cultural differences among various ethnic groups, patients from certain groups respond differently to particular medications. Nurses should keep in mind that patients in some ethnic groups are genetically predisposed to metabolize medications differently. For example, Arab Americans may not achieve the same pain relief from narcotics as patients in other ethnic groups; their inborn differences in metabolism may require larger doses to achieve therapeutic effects.

Some African American patients seem to have a decreased sensitivity to the pain-relieving qualities of some narcotics, although the reason for this is unknown. Moreover, increasing the dosage of these medications may not increase the level of pain relief and actually may be toxic. In such cases, another class of medication might be used to "boost" the pain-relieving qualities of the narcotic.

Among some immigrant and first-generation Asian Americans, it may not be socially acceptable to show strong emotion, such as that associated with pain. The sensitive nurse will frequently ask such patients if they are comfortable or require additional medication.

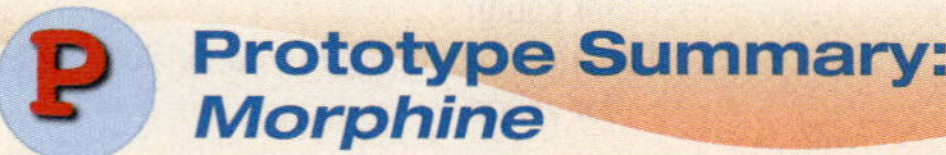

Indications: Relief of moderate to severe acute or chronic pain; preoperative medication; component of Brompton's cocktail for severe chronic pain; intraspinal to reduce intractable pain

Actions: Acts as an agonist at specific opioid receptors in the CNS to produce analgesia, euphoria, and sedation

Pharmacokinetics:

Route	Onset	Peak	Duration
Oral	Varies	60 min	5–7 h
TPR	Rapid	20–60 min	5–7 h
Sub-Q	Rapid	50–90 min	5–7 h
IM	Rapid	30–60 min	5–6 h
IV	Immediate	20 min	5–6 h

$T_{1/2}$: 1.5–2 hours; metabolized in the liver, excreted in the urine and bile

Adverse effects: Light-headedness, dizziness, sedation, nausea, vomiting, dry mouth, constipation, ureteral spasm, respiratory depression, apnea, circulatory depression, respiratory arrest, shock, cardiac arrest

Nursing Considerations for Patients Receiving Narcotic Agonists

Assessment: History and Examination

Screen for the following conditions, *which could be cautions or contraindications for the use of the drug:* any known allergies to these drugs; pregnancy; respiratory dysfunction; GI or biliary surgery; psychoses; convulsive disorders; diarrhea caused by toxins; alcoholism or delirium tremens; and renal or hepatic dysfunction.

Include screening *for baseline status before beginning therapy and for any potential adverse effects.* Assess the following: CNS orientation, affect, reflexes, pupil size; respiration and adventitious sounds; pulse, blood pressure, and cardiac output; bowel sounds and reported output; bladder palpation and voiding pattern.

Check liver and renal function tests, as well as electroencephalogram (EEG) and electrocardiogram (ECG) as appropriate.

Nursing Diagnoses

The patient receiving a narcotic agonist may have the following nursing diagnoses related to drug therapy:

- Acute Pain related to GI, CNS, and GU effects
- Disturbed Sensory Perception (Visual, Auditory, and Kinesthetic) related to CNS effects
- Impaired Gas Exchange related to respiratory depression
- Constipation related to GI effects
- Deficient Knowledge regarding drug therapy

Implementation With Rationale

- Provide a narcotic antagonist and equipment for assisted ventilation on standby during IV administration *to support the patient in case severe reaction occurs.*
- Monitor injection sites for irritation and extravasation *to provide appropriate supportive care if needed.*
- Monitor timing of analgesic doses. *Prompt administration may provide a more acceptable level of analgesia and lead to quicker resolution of the pain.*
- Use extreme caution when injecting a narcotic into any body area that is chilled or has poor perfusion or shock *because absorption may be delayed. After repeated doses, an excessive amount is absorbed all at once.*
- Use additional measures for relief of pain, such as back rubs, stress reduction, hot packs, and ice packs *to increase the effectiveness of the narcotic and reduce pain.*
- Reassure patients that the risk of addiction is minimal. *Most patients who receive narcotics for medical reasons do not develop dependency syndromes.*
- Provide thorough patient teaching, including drug name and prescribed dosage, measures for avoidance of adverse effects, warning signs that may indicate possible problems, and the need for monitoring and evaluation, *to enhance patient knowledge about drug therapy and to promote compliance.* (See Critical Thinking Scenario 26-1.)
- Offer support and encouragement *to help the patient cope with the drug regimen.*

Evaluation

- Monitor patient response to the drug (relief of pain, cough suppression, sedation).
- Monitor for adverse effects (CNS changes, GI depression, respiratory depression, constipation).
- Evaluate the effectiveness of the teaching plan (patient can give the drug name and dosage and describe possible adverse effects to watch for, specific measures to prevent adverse effects, and warning signs to report).
- Monitor the effectiveness of comfort measures and compliance with the regimen.

Narcotic Agonists-Antagonists

The **narcotic agonists-antagonists** stimulate certain opioid receptors but block other such receptors. These drugs, which have less abuse potential than the pure narcotic agonists, all have about the same analgesic effect as morphine. Like morphine, they may cause sedation, respiratory depression, and constipation. They have also been associated with more psychotic-like reactions, and they may even induce a withdrawal syndrome in patients who have been taking narcotics for a long period.

Available narcotic agonists-antagonists include the following (Table 26.2):

- Buprenorphine (*Buprenex*) is recommended for treatment of mild to moderate pain; it is available for use in IM and IV forms.
- Butorphanol (*Stadol, Stadol NS*) is used as a preoperative medication to relieve moderate to severe pain. This drug is formulated in IM and IV preparations and as a nasal spray. It is effective in the treatment of migraine headaches, with fewer peripheral adverse effects than many of the traditional antimigraine drugs.
- Nalbuphine (*Nubain*) is used to treat moderate to severe pain, as an adjunct for general anesthesia, and to relieve pain during labor and delivery. This drug, which is formulated in Sub-Q, IM, and IV preparations, should not be given to patients who are allergic to sulfites.
- Pentazocine (*Talwin*) is also available in an oral form, making it the preferred drug for patients who will be switched from parenteral to oral forms after surgery or labor. This drug has been abused in combination with tripelennamine ("Ts and Blues") because of the hallucinogenic, euphoric effect of the two drugs, with potentially fatal complications.

Therapeutic Actions and Indications

The narcotic agonists-antagonists act at specific opioid receptor sites in the CNS to produce analgesia, sedation, euphoria, and hallucinations. In addition, they block opioid receptors

CRITICAL THINKING SCENARIO 26-1

Using Morphine to Relieve Pain

The Situation

L.M., a 25-year-old businessman, was in a car crash and suffered a fractured pelvis, a fractured left tibia, a fractured right humerus, and multiple contusions and abrasions. For the first 2 days after surgery to reduce the fractures, L.M. was heavily sedated. As healing progressed, he was given IM injections of morphine every 4 hours as needed for pain. L.M. requested medication every 2 to 3 hours and became very agitated by the end of the prescribed 4 hours. L.M.'s physician decided to switch him to meperidine given IM every 3 hours for 2 days and then to oral dosage in an attempt to wean him from the narcotics.

Critical Thinking

What basic principles must be included in the nursing care plan for this patient? *Think about the difficult position the floor nurse is in when L.M. begins demanding pain relief before the prescribed time limit.*

What implications will L.M.'s agitation have on the way that the staff responds to him and on other patients in the area?

What other nursing measures could be used to help relieve pain and make the narcotic more effective?

What plans could the health team make with L.M. to give him more control over his situation and increase the chances that the pain relief will be effective?

Discussion

In assessing L.M.'s response to drug therapy, you suspect that the morphine was not providing the desired therapeutic effect. Numerous research studies have shown that, in general, the dosage of narcotics prescribed for acute pain relief provides inadequate analgesic coverage. It could be that the dose of morphine ordered for L.M. was just not sufficient to relieve his pain. This patient has many causes of acute pain and will heal more quickly if the pain is managed better. He has requested more drugs because the dosage is too small or the intervals between doses are too long to effectively relieve his pain. Intravenous morphine could be added to complement his pain management. Other measures may be successful in helping the morphine relieve the pain. Back rubs, environmental controls to decrease excessive stimuli (e.g., noise, lighting, temperature, interruptions), and stress reduction may all be useful.

L.M. may be very anxious about his injuries, and the opportunity to vent his feelings and concerns may alleviate some of the tension associated with pain. He may fear that if he does not request the medication early, he will not get it by the prescribed time. The nursing staff can work on this concern and figure out a way to reassure him that the medication will be delivered on time. Changing from morphine to meperidine may improve the analgesic effects, partly because of a placebo reaction that may occur when he is told that this drug will be more effective and partly because people respond differently to different narcotics.

The health care team should try to discuss the concerns with L.M., including the concern about the physical dependence. L.M. is a businessman and may respond positively to having some input into his care; he may even offer suggestions as to how he could cope better and adjust to his situation. Cortical impulses can close gates as effectively as descending inhibitory pathways, and stimulation of the cortical pathways through patient education and active involvement should be considered an important aspect of pain relief. Because L.M.'s injuries are extensive, a long-term approach should be taken to his care. The sooner that L.M. can be involved, the better the situation will be for everyone involved.

Nursing Care Guide for L.M.: Narcotics

Assessment: History and Examination

Assess history of allergies to any narcotic drug, respiratory depression, GI or biliary surgery, hepatic or renal dysfunction, alcoholism, convulsive disorders.

Focus the physical examination on the following:

CV: blood pressure, pulse rate, peripheral perfusion, ECG

CNS: orientation, affect, reflexes, grip strength

Skin: color, lesions, texture, temperature

GI: abdominal examination, bowel sounds

Respiratory: respiration, adventitious sounds

Laboratory tests: renal and liver function tests

Nursing Diagnoses

Acute Pain related to GI, CNS, GU effects

Disturbed Sensory Perceptions (Visual, Auditory, Kinesthetic) related to CNS effects

Using Morphine to Relieve Pain *(continued)*

Impaired Gas Exchange related to respiratory depression

Deficient Knowledge regarding drug therapy

Constipation

Implementation

Provide a narcotic antagonist, facilities for assisted ventilation during IV administration.

Provide comfort and safety measures: orientation, accurate timing of doses, monitoring for extravasation, and additional measures for pain relief to increase effects.

Provide support and reassurance to deal with drug effects, addiction potential.

Provide patient teaching about the drug, dosage, drug effects, and symptoms of serious reactions to report.

Evaluation

Evaluate drug effects: relief of pain, sedation.

Monitor for adverse effects: CNS effects (multiple), respiratory depression, rash, skin changes, GI depression, constipation.

Monitor drug–drug interactions: increased respiratory depression, sedation, coma with barbiturate anesthetics, monoamine oxidase inhibitors, phenothiazines.

Evaluate effectiveness of patient teaching program.

Evaluate effectiveness of comfort and safety measures.

Patient Teaching for L.M.

☐ A narcotic is used to relieve pain. Do not hesitate to take this drug if you feel uncomfortable. Remember that it is important to use the drug before the pain becomes severe and thus more difficult to treat.

☐ Common effects of these drugs include:

- *Constipation:* Your health care provider will suggest appropriate measures to alleviate this common problem.
- *Dizziness, drowsiness, and visual changes:* If any of these occur, avoid driving, operating complex machinery, or performing delicate tasks. If these effects occur in the hospital, the siderails on the bed may be raised for your own protection.
- *Nausea and loss of appetite:* Taking the drug with food may help. Lying quietly until these sensations pass may also help alleviate this problem.
- Report any of the following to your health care provider: *severe nausea or vomiting, skin rash, or shortness of breath or difficulty breathing.*

☐ Avoid the use of alcohol, antihistamines, and other over-the-counter drugs while taking this drug. Many of these drugs could interact with this narcotic.

☐ Tell any doctor, nurse, dentist, or other health care provider involved in your care that you are taking this drug.

☐ Keep this drug and all medications out of the reach of children.

☐ Do not take any leftover medication for other disorders, and do not let anyone else take your medication.

☐ Take this drug exactly as prescribed. Regular medical follow-up is necessary to evaluate the effects of this drug on your body.

that may be stimulated by other narcotics. These drugs have three functions: (1) relief of moderate to severe pain, (2) adjuncts to general anesthesia, and (3) relief of pain during labor and delivery.

Pharmacokinetics

These drugs are readily absorbed after IM administration and reach rapid peak levels when given intravenously. They are metabolized in the liver and are excreted in urine or feces. They are known to cross the placenta, but no adequate studies are available regarding their effects during pregnancy. They should be used during pregnancy only if the benefit to the mother clearly outweighs the risk to the fetus. They are used to relieve pain during labor, which provides a short-term exposure to the fetus. They are known to enter breast milk and should be used with caution during lactation because of the potential for adverse effects on the baby.

Contraindications and Cautions

Narcotic agonists-antagonists are contraindicated in the presence of any known allergy to any narcotic agonist-antagonist and during pregnancy and lactation *because of potential adverse effects on the neonate, including respiratory depression.* (However, these drugs may be used to relieve pain during labor and delivery.)

Caution should be used in cases of physical dependence on a narcotic *because a withdrawal syndrome may be precipitated;* the narcotic antagonistic properties can block the analgesic effect and intensify the pain. Narcotic agonists-antagonists may be desirable for relieving chronic pain in

Table 26.2 DRUGS IN FOCUS

Narcotic Agonists-Antagonists

Drug Name	Dosage/Route	Usual Indications
buprenorphine (*Buprenex*)	Adults and children >13 yr: 0.3 mg IM or slow IV q6h as needed	Mild to moderate pain
butorphanol (*Stadol*)	Adult: 0.5–2 mg IV q3–4h or 1–4 mg IM q3–4h; 1 mg nasal spray, repeated in 60–90 min, then in 3–4 h as needed Geriatric: use one-half of the adult dose at twice the usual interval Pediatric: not recommended for children <18 yr	Preoperative medication, moderate to severe pain, migraine headache
nalbuphine (*Nubain*)	10 mg/70 kg IM, Sub-Q, or IV q3–6h as needed; do not exceed 160 mg/day	Labor and delivery, adjunct to general anesthesia, moderate to severe pain in adults
P pentazocine (*Talwin*)	Adults and children >12 yr: 30 mg IM, Sub-Q, or IV q3–4h as needed *or* 50 mg PO q3–4h as needed; do not exceed 360 mg/day; 30 mg IM most common for labor	Moderate to severe pain, labor and delivery, postpartum pain, adjunct to general anesthesia

patients who are susceptible to narcotic dependence, but extreme care must be used if patients are switched directly from a narcotic agonist to one of these drugs.

Caution should also be exercised in the following conditions: chronic obstructive pulmonary disease or other respiratory dysfunction, *which could be exacerbated by respiratory depression;* acute myocardial infarction (MI), documented coronary artery disease (CAD), or *hypertension that could be exacerbated by cardiac stimulatory effects of these drugs;* and renal or hepatic dysfunction *that could interfere with the metabolism and excretion of the drug.*

Pentazocine also may cause cardiac stimulation including arrhythmias, hypertension, and increased myocardial oxygen consumption, which could lead to angina, MI, or congestive heart failure; *therefore, care must be taken in patients with known heart disease.*

Adverse Effects

The most frequently seen adverse effects associated with narcotic agonists-antagonists relate to their effects on various opioid receptors. Respiratory depression with apnea and suppression of the cough reflex is associated with the respiratory depression caused by the narcotics. Nausea, vomiting, constipation, and biliary spasm may occur as a result of CTZ stimulation and the negative effects on GI motility. Light-headedness, dizziness, psychoses, anxiety, fear, hallucinations, and impaired mental processes may occur as a result of the stimulation of CNS opioid receptors in the cerebrum, limbic system, and hypothalamus. GU effects, including ureteral spasm, urinary retention, hesitancy, and loss of libido, may be related to direct receptor stimulation or to CNS activation of sympathetic pathways. Although sweating and dependence, both physical and psychological, are possible, their occurrence is considered less likely than with narcotic agonists.

Clinically Important Drug–Drug Interactions

When narcotic agonists-antagonists, like narcotic agonists, are given with barbiturate general anesthetics, the likelihood of respiratory depression, hypotension, and sedation or coma increases. If this combination cannot be avoided, patients should be monitored closely and appropriate supportive measures taken.

Use of narcotic agonists-antagonists in patients who have previously received narcotics puts these patients at risk. When such a sequence of drugs is used, patients require support and monitoring.

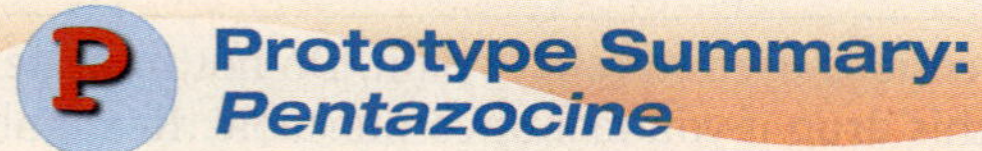

Prototype Summary: *Pentazocine*

Indications: Relief of moderate to severe pain; preanesthetic medication and a supplement to surgical anesthesia

Actions: An agonist at specific opioid receptors in the CNS, producing analgesia and sedation; an agonist at sigma opioid receptors, causing dysphoria and hallucinations; acts at mu-receptors to antagonize the analgesia and euphoria

Pharmacokinetics:

Route	Onset	Peak	Duration
Oral, IM, Sub-Q	15–30 min	1–3 h	3 h
IV	2–3 min	15 min	3 h

$T_{1/2}$: 2–3 hours; metabolized in the liver, excreted in the urine and bile

Adverse effects: Light-headedness, dizziness, sedation, euphoria, nausea, vomiting, constipation, tachycardia, palpitations, sweating, ureteral spasm, physical dependence

Nursing Considerations for Patients Receiving Narcotic Agonists-Antagonists

Assessment: History and Examination

Screen for the following conditions, *which could be cautions or contraindications for the use of the drug:* any known allergies to these drugs or to sulfites if using nalbuphine; pregnancy or lactation; respiratory dysfunction; MI or CAD; and renal or hepatic dysfunction.

Include screening *for baseline status before beginning therapy and for any potential adverse effects.* Assess the following: CNS orientation, affect, reflexes, and pupil size; respiration and adventitious sounds; pulse, blood pressure, and cardiac output; bowel sounds and reported output; and liver and renal function tests, as well as ECG.

Nursing Diagnoses

The patient receiving a narcotic agonist-antagonist may have the following nursing diagnoses related to drug therapy:

- Acute Pain related to GI and CNS effects
- Disturbed Sensory Perception (Visual, Auditory, Kinesthetic) related to CNS effects
- Impaired Gas Exchange related to respiratory depression
- Deficient Knowledge regarding drug therapy

Implementation With Rationale

- Provide a narcotic antagonist and equipment for assisted ventilation on standby during IV administration *to provide patient support in case of severe reaction.*
- Monitor injection sites for irritation and extravasation *to provide appropriate supportive care if needed.*
- Monitor timing of analgesic doses. *Prompt administration may provide a more acceptable level of analgesia and lead to quicker resolution of the pain.*
- Use extreme caution when injecting these drugs into any body area that is chilled or has poor perfusion or shock *because absorption may be delayed, and after repeated doses an excessive amount is absorbed all at once.*
- Use additional measures to relieve pain (e.g., back rubs, stress reduction, hot packs, ice packs) *to increase the effectiveness of the narcotic being given and reduce pain.*
- Institute comfort and safety measures, such as siderails and assistance with ambulation *to ensure patient safety;* bowel program as needed *to treat constipation;* environmental controls *to decrease stimulation;* and small, frequent meals *to relieve GI distress if GI upset is severe.*
- Reassure patients that the risk of addiction is minimal. *Most patients who receive these drugs for medical reasons do not develop dependency syndromes.*
- Provide thorough patient teaching, including drug name and prescribed dosage, as well as measures for avoidance of adverse effects, warning signs that may indicate possible problems, and the need for monitoring and evaluation *to enhance patient knowledge about drug therapy and to promote compliance.* (See Critical Thinking Scenario 26-1.)
- Offer support and encouragement *to help the patient cope with the drug regimen.*

Evaluation

- Monitor patient response to the drug (relief of pain, sedation).
- Monitor for adverse effects (CNS changes, GI depression, respiratory depression, arrhythmias, hypertension).
- Evaluate the effectiveness of the teaching plan (patient can give the drug name and dosage and describe possible adverse effects to watch for, specific measures to prevent adverse effects, and warning signs to report).
- Monitor the effectiveness of comfort measures and compliance with the regimen.

Narcotic Antagonists

The **narcotic antagonists** are drugs that bind strongly to opioid receptors, but they do not activate the receptors. These agents are useful in blocking unwanted adverse effects associated with narcotics, such as respiratory depression, and they play a role in the treatment of narcotic overdose. These drugs do not have an appreciable effect in most people, but individuals who are addicted to narcotics experience the signs and symptoms of withdrawal when rapidly receiving these drugs. The narcotic antagonists in use today include the following (Table 26.3):

- Nalmefene (*Revex*) can be given by the IV, IM, or Sub-Q route to reverse the effects of narcotics and to manage known or suspected narcotic overdose.
- Naloxone (*Narcan*) is used IV, IM, or Sub-Q to reverse adverse effects of narcotics and to diagnose suspected acute narcotic overdose.
- Naltrexone (*ReVia*) is used orally in the management of alcohol or narcotic dependence as part of a comprehensive treatment program.

Therapeutic Actions and Indications

The narcotic antagonists block opioid receptors and reverse the effects of opioids, including respiratory depression, sedation, psychomimetic effects, and hypotension. Their effects are seen in people who have been using narcotics or are dependent on narcotics.

These agents are indicated for reversal of the adverse effects of narcotic use, including respiratory depression and sedation, and for treatment of narcotic overdose. Naloxone is used to diagnose narcotic overdose (the naloxone challenge), and naltrexone is used as part of a comprehensive program to treat narcotic and/or alcoholic dependence.

Pharmacokinetics

These agents are well absorbed after injection and are widely distributed in the body. They undergo hepatic metabolism and are excreted primarily in the urine. There are no well-controlled studies during pregnancy, so they should be used during pregnancy only if the benefit to the mother clearly outweighs any potential risk to the fetus. They enter breast milk and should be used with caution during lactation because of the potential adverse effects on the baby.

Contraindications and Cautions

Narcotic antagonists are contraindicated in the presence of any known allergy to any narcotic antagonist. Caution should be used in the following circumstances: during pregnancy and lactation *because of potential adverse effects on the fetus and neonate;* with narcotic addiction *because of the precipitation of a withdrawal syndrome;* and with cardiovascular (CV) disease *which could be exacerbated by the reversal of the depressive effects of narcotics.*

Adverse Effects

The most frequently seen adverse effects associated with these drugs relate to the blocking effects of the opioid receptors. The most common effect is an acute narcotic abstinence syndrome that is characterized by nausea, vomiting, sweating, tachycardia, hypertension, tremulousness, and feelings of anxiety. CNS excitement and reversal of analgesia are especially common after surgery. CV effects related to the reversal of the opioid depression can include tachycardia, blood pressure changes, dysrhythmias, and pulmonary edema.

Drug–Drug Interactions

To reverse the effects of buprenorphine, butorphanol, nalbuphine, pentazocine, or propoxyphene, larger doses of narcotic antagonists may be needed.

Table 26.3 DRUGS IN FOCUS

Narcotic Antagonists

Drug Name	Dosage/Route	Usual Indications
nalmefene (*Revex*)	Adult: for reversal of postoperative opioid depression, 0.25 mcg/kg IV q2–5 min until desired reversal is obtained; for management of overdose, 0.5 mg/70 kg IV, then 1 mg IV 2–5 min later; reduce dosage in renal and hepatic disease	Reversal of opioid effects, management of narcotic overdose
P naloxone (*Narcan*)	Adult: for overdose, 0.4–2 mg IV, may repeat at 2–3 min intervals; for reversal of opioid effects, 0.1–0.2 mg IV, may repeat at 2–3 min intervals Pediatric: for overdose, 0.01 mg/kg IV, repeat as needed; for reversal of opioid effects, 0.005–0.01 mg IV at 2–3 min intervals	Diagnosis of narcotic overdose, reversal of opioid effects
naltrexone (*ReVia*)	Adult: 50 mg/day PO	Adjunct treatment of alcohol or narcotic dependence in adults

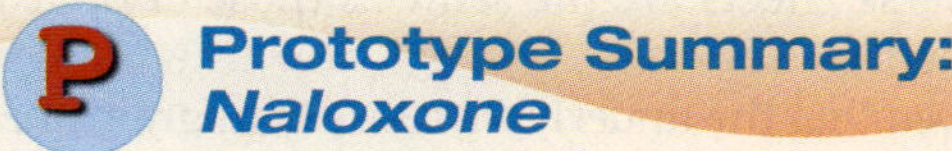

Prototype Summary: Naloxone

Indications: Complete or partial reversal of narcotic depression; diagnosis of suspected opioid overdose

Actions: Pure narcotic antagonist; reverses the effects of the opioids, including respiratory depression, sedation, and hypotension

Pharmacokinetics:

Route	Peak	Onset	Duration
IV	Unknown	2 min	4–6 h
IM, Sub-Q	Unknown	3–5 min	4–6 h

$T_{1/2}$: 30–81 min; metabolized in the liver, excreted in the urine

Adverse effects: Acute narcotic abstinence syndrome (nausea, vomiting, sweating, tachycardia, fall in blood pressure), hypotension, hypertension, pulmonary edema

Nursing Considerations for Patients Receiving Narcotic Antagonists

Assessment: History and Examination

Screen for the following conditions, *which could be cautions or contraindications to the use of the drug:* any known allergies to these drugs; pregnancy and lactation; MI or CAD; and narcotic addiction.

Include screening *for baseline status before beginning therapy and for any potential adverse effects.* Assess the following: CNS orientation, affect, reflexes, and pupil size; respiration and adventitious sounds; pulse, blood pressure, and cardiac output; and ECG.

Nursing Diagnoses

The patient receiving a narcotic antagonist may have the following nursing diagnoses related to drug therapy:

- Acute Pain related to withdrawal and CV effects
- Decreased Cardiac Output related to CV effects
- Deficient Knowledge regarding drug therapy

Implementation With Rationale

- Maintain open airway and provide artificial ventilation and cardiac massage as needed *to support the patient.* Administer vasopressors as needed *to manage narcotic overdose.*
- Administer naloxone challenge before giving naltrexone *because of the serious risk of acute withdrawal.*
- Monitor the patient continually, *adjusting the dosage as needed, during treatment of acute overdose.*
- Provide comfort and safety measures *to help the patient cope with the withdrawal syndrome.*
- Ensure that patients receiving naltrexone have been narcotic free for 7 to 10 days *to prevent severe withdrawal syndrome.* Check urine opioid levels if there is any question.
- If the patient is receiving naltrexone as part of a comprehensive narcotic or alcohol withdrawal program, the patient should be advised to wear or carry a Medic-Alert warning *so that medical personnel know how to treat the patient in an emergency.*
- Institute comfort and safety measures, such as siderails and assistance with ambulation *to ensure patient safety;* institute bowel program as needed *for treatment of constipation;* use environmental controls *to decrease stimulation;* and provide, small frequent meals *to relieve GI irritation if GI upset is severe.*
- Provide thorough patient teaching, including drug name and prescribed dosage, as well as measures for avoidance of adverse effects, warning signs that may indicate possible problems, and the need for monitoring and evaluation *to enhance patient knowledge about drug therapy and to promote compliance.* (See Critical Thinking Scenario 26-1.)
- Offer support and encouragement *to help the patient cope with the drug regimen.*

Evaluation

- Monitor patient response to the drug (reversal of opioid effects, treatment of alcohol dependence).
- Monitor for adverse effects (CV changes, arrhythmias, hypertension).
- Evaluate the effectiveness of the teaching plan (patient can give the drug name and dosage and describe possible adverse effects to watch for, specific measures to prevent adverse effects, and warning signs to report).
- Monitor the effectiveness of comfort measures and compliance with the regimen.

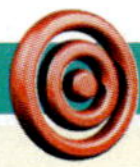

FOCUS POINTS

- Narcotic agonists react with opioid receptor sites to stimulate their activity; whereas narcotic agonists-antagonists react with some opioid receptor sites to stimulate activity and block other opioid receptor sites.
- Narcotic antagonists are used to treat narcotic overdose or to reverse unacceptable adverse effects.

Migraine Headaches

The term *migraine headache* is used to describe several different syndromes, all of which include severe, throbbing headaches on one side of the head. This pain can be so severe that it can cause widespread disturbance, affecting GI and CNS function, including mood and personality changes.

Migraine headaches should be distinguished from cluster headaches and tension headaches (Box 26.4). Cluster headaches usually begin during sleep and involve sharp, steady eye pain that lasts 15 to 90 minutes with sweating, flushing, tearing, and nasal congestion. Tension headaches, which usually occur at times of stress, feel like a dull band of pain around the entire head and last from 30 minutes to 1 week. They are accompanied by anorexia, fatigue, and a mild intolerance to light or sound.

There are at least two types of migraine headaches. Common migraines, which occur without an aura, cause severe, unilateral, pulsating pain that is frequently accompanied by nausea, vomiting, and sensitivity to light and sound. Such migraine headaches are often aggravated by physical activity. Classic migraines are usually preceded by an aura, or a sensation involving sensory or motor disturbances, that usually occurs about one-half hour before the pain begins. The pain and adverse effects are the same as those of the common migraine.

It is believed that the underlying cause of migraine headaches is arterial dilation. Headaches accompanied by an aura are associated with a hypoperfusion of the brain during the aura stage, followed by reflex arterial dilation and a hyperperfusion. The underlying cause and continued state of arterial dilation are not clearly understood, but they may be related to the release of bradykinins, serotonin, or a response to other hormones and chemicals.

For many years, the one standard treatment for migraine headaches was acute analgesia, often involving a narcotic, together with control of lighting and sound and the use of ergot derivatives. In the late 1990s, a new class of drugs, the triptans, was found to be extremely effective in treating migraine headaches without the adverse effects associated with ergot derivative use.

BOX 26.4 Gender Considerations: Headache Distribution

Headaches are distributed in the general population in a definite gender-related pattern. For example:

- Migraine headaches are three times more likely to occur in women than men.
- Cluster headaches are more likely to occur in men than in women.
- Tension headaches are more likely to occur in women than in men.

There is some speculation that the female predisposition to migraine headaches may be related to the vascular sensitivity to hormones. Some women can directly plot migraine occurrence to periods of fluctuations in their menstrual cycle. The introduction of the triptan class of antimigraine drugs has been beneficial for many of these women.

Ergot Derivatives

The **ergot derivatives** cause constriction of cranial blood vessels and decrease the pulsation of cranial arteries. As a result, they reduce the hyperperfusion of the basilar artery vascular bed. Because these agents are associated with many systemic adverse effects, their usefulness is limited in some patients.

Available ergot derivatives include the following (Table 26.4):

- Dihydroergotamine (*Migranal*) can be used in the IM or IV form or as a nasal spray to provide rapid relief from migraine headache. This agent is the drug of choice if the oral route of administration is not possible. In 2003, the parenteral form was approved for the treatment of cluster headaches.
- Ergotamine (generic), the prototype drug in this class, was the mainstay of migraine headache treatment before the triptans became available. This agent is administered sublingually for rapid absorption. *Cafergot,* the very popular oral form, combines ergotamine with caffeine to increase its absorption from the GI tract.

Therapeutic Actions and Indications

The ergot derivatives block alpha-adrenergic and serotonin receptor sites in the brain to cause a constriction of cranial vessels, a decrease in cranial artery pulsation, and a decrease in the hyperperfusion of the basilar artery bed. These drugs are indicated for the prevention or abortion of migraine or vascular headaches.

Pharmacokinetics

The ergot derivatives are rapidly absorbed from many routes, with an onset of action ranging from 15 to 30 minutes. They are metabolized in the liver and primarily excreted in the bile. These drugs cannot be used during pregnancy because they

Table 26.4 DRUGS IN FOCUS

Antimigraine Ergots

Drug Name	Dosage/Route	Usual Indications
dihydroergotamine (*Migranal, D.H.E. 45*)	One spray (0.5 mg) in each nostril, may repeat in 15 min for a total of four sprays or 1 mg IM at first sign of headache, repeat in 1 h for a total of 3 mg or 2 mg IV, do not exceed 6 mg/wk	Rapid treatment of acute attacks of migraines in adults
P ergotamine (*generic*)	One tablet sublingually at the first sign of headache, repeat at 30-min intervals for a total of three tablets; *or* one inhalation at first sign of headache, repeat in 5 min to a total of six inhalations per day	Prevention and abortion of migraine attacks in adults

cause serious adverse effects on the fetus and can have oxytocic effects on the mother. They are excreted in breast milk and can cause vomiting and diarrhea in the baby, so they should be used with extreme caution in nursing mothers.

Contraindications and Cautions

Ergot derivatives are contraindicated in the following circumstances: presence of allergy to ergot preparations; CAD, hypertension, or peripheral vascular disease, *which could be exacerbated by the CV effects of these drugs;* impaired liver function, *which could alter the metabolism and excretion of these drugs;* and pregnancy or lactation *because of the potential for adverse effects on the fetus and neonate.* Ergotism (vomiting, diarrhea, seizures) has been reported in affected infants.

Caution should be used in two instances: with pruritus, *which could become worse with drug-induced vascular constriction,* and with malnutrition *because ergot derivatives stimulate the CTZ and can cause severe GI reactions, possibly worsening malnutrition.*

Adverse Effects

The adverse effects of ergot derivatives can be related to the drug-induced vascular constriction. CNS effects include numbness, tingling of extremities, and muscle pain; CV effects such as pulselessness, weakness, chest pain, arrhythmias, localized edema and itching, and MI may also occur. In addition, the direct stimulation of the CTZ can cause GI upset, nausea, vomiting, and diarrhea. Ergotism, a syndrome associated with the use of these drugs, causes nausea, vomiting, severe thirst, hypoperfusion, chest pain, blood pressure changes, confusion, drug dependency (with prolonged use), and a drug withdrawal syndrome.

Clinically Important Drug–Drug Interactions

If these drugs are combined with beta-blockers, the risk of peripheral ischemia and gangrene is increased. Such combinations should be avoided.

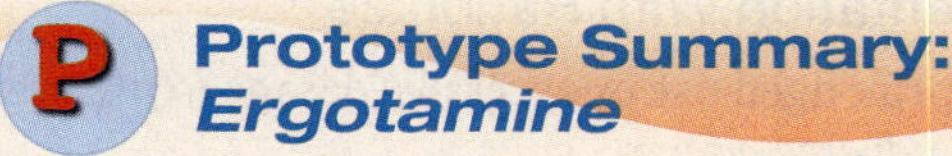

Prototype Summary: Ergotamine

Indications: Prevention or abortion of vascular headaches

Actions: Constricts cranial blood vessels, decreases pulsation of cranial arteries, and decreases hyperfusion of basilar artery vascular bed; mechanism of action is not understood

Pharmacokinetics:

Route	Onset	Peak
Sublingual	Rapid	0.5–3 h

$T_{1/2}$: 2.7 hours, then 21 hours; metabolized in the liver, excreted in the feces

Adverse effects: Numbness, tingling in the fingers and toes, muscle pain in the extremities, pulselessness or weakness in the legs, precordial distress, tachycardia, bradycardia, ergotism (nausea, vomiting, diarrhea, severe thirst, hypoperfusion, chest pain, confusion)

Nursing Considerations for Patients Receiving Ergot Derivatives

Assessment: History and Examination

Screen for the following conditions, *which could be cautions or contraindications to the use of the drug:* any known allergies to ergot derivatives; pregnancy or lactation; MI, CAD, or hypertension; impaired renal or hepatic function; pruritus; and malnutrition.

Include screening *for baseline status before beginning therapy and for any potential adverse effects.* Assess the following: temperature; skin color and lesions; CNS orientation, affect, and reflexes; respiration and adventitious sounds; pulse, blood pressure, and cardiac output; ECG and liver and renal function tests.

Nursing Diagnoses

The patient receiving an ergot derivative may have the following nursing diagnoses related to drug therapy:

- Acute Pain related to GI and vasoconstrictive effects
- Decreased Cardiac Output related to CV effects
- High Risk for Injury related to loss of peripheral sensation
- Deficient Knowledge regarding drug therapy

Implementation With Rationale

- Avoid prolonged use or excessive dosage *to prevent severe adverse effects.*
- Arrange for the use of atropine or phenothiazines if nausea and vomiting are severe *because these are the appropriate drugs to relieve nausea and vomiting.*
- Provide comfort and safety measures, such as environmental controls and stress reduction, *for the prevention of headache and to provide additional pain relief as needed.*
- Assess extremities carefully *to ensure that no decubitus ulcer or gangrene is present when using drugs that cause peripheral vasoconstriction, which could further aggravate these conditions.*
- Provide supportive measures *to ensure patient safety if acute overdose should occur.*
- Provide thorough patient teaching, including drug name and prescribed dosage, as well as measures for avoidance of adverse effects, warning signs that may indicate possible problems, and the need for monitoring and evaluation, *to enhance patient knowledge about drug therapy and to promote compliance.*
- Offer support and encouragement *to help the patient cope with the drug regimen.*

Evaluation

- Monitor patient response to the drug (prevention or abortion of migraine headaches).
- Monitor for adverse effects (CV changes, arrhythmias, hypertension, peripheral vasoconstriction).
- Evaluate the effectiveness of the teaching plan (patient can give the drug name and dosage and describe possible adverse effects to watch for, specific measures to prevent adverse effects, and warning signs to report).
- Monitor the effectiveness of comfort measures and compliance with the regimen.

Triptans

The **triptans** are a new class of drugs that cause cranial vascular constriction and relief of migraine headache pain in many patients. These drugs are not associated with all of the vascular and GI effects of the ergot derivatives. The triptan of choice for a particular patient depends on personal experience and other pre-existing medical conditions. A patient may have a poor response to one triptan and respond well to another.

Available triptans include the following (also see Table 26.5):

- Sumatriptan (*Imitrex*), the first drug of this class, is used for the treatment of acute migraine attacks. It can be given orally, subcutaneously, or by nasal spray; when given by the Sub-Q route, it has proved very effective against cluster headaches. It is not recommended for use in elderly patients because they are more susceptible to the adverse effects of the drug, including decreased hepatic function, increased risk of hypertension, and increased risk of coronary artery disease.
- Naratriptan (*Amerge*) is used orally only for the treatment of acute migraines. It has been associated with severe birth defects and is not recommended for patients with severe renal or hepatic dysfunction.
- Rizatriptan (*Maxalt*) is used orally for the treatment of acute migraine attacks with or without aura. This drug is also available as an oral fast-dissolving tablet. Because this agent seems to have more angina-related effects, it is not recommended for patients with a history of CAD. It has also been shown to cause fetal abnormalities in animal studies and should not be used during pregnancy.
- Zolmitriptan (*Zomig*) is used orally only for the treatment of acute migraine; it is also available in an orally disintegrating tablet, making it useful if swallowing is difficult.
- Almotriptan (*Axert*) is approved for the treatment of acute migraine with or without aura in adults. This drug, released in 2001, is reported to have fewer side effects than the other triptans, but long-term use studies are not available.
- Frovatriptan (*Frova*) was approved in late 2001 and has the advantage of a long half-life. It is used orally as a treatment of acute migraines with or without aura. Although long-term studies are not available, it is thought that the longer half-life of this drug will prevent the rebound headaches that may be seen with other triptans.
- Eletriptan (*Relpax*) was approved in 2003. It is only available as an oral agent and is used for the treatment of acute migraine with or without aura.

Therapeutic Actions and Indications

The triptans bind to selective serotonin receptor sites to cause vasoconstriction of cranial vessels, relieving the signs and symptoms of migraine headache. They are indicated for

Table 26.5 DRUGS IN FOCUS

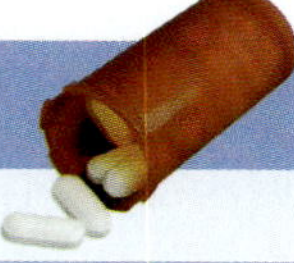

Antimigraine Triptans

Drug Name	Dosage/Route	Usual Indications
almotriptan (*Axert*)	6.25–12.5 mg PO at onset of aura or symptoms	Acute migraines in adults
eletriptan (*Relpax*)	20–40 mg PO; may repeat in 2 h if needed; do not exceed 80 mg/day	Acute migraines in adults
frovatriptan (*Frova*)	2.5 mg PO as a single dose at first sign of headache; may repeat in 2 h; do not exceed three doses in 24 h	Acute migraines in adults
naratriptan (*Amerge*)	1–2.5 mg PO with fluid; may repeat in 4 h if needed	Acute migraines in adults
rizatriptan (*Maxalt; Maxalt MLT*)	5–10 mg PO; may repeat in 2 h; do not exceed 30 mg/day	Acute migraines in adults; orally disintegrating tablet may be useful with difficulty swallowing
P sumatriptan (*Imitrex*)	50–100 mg PO at first sign of headache, may repeat in 2 h, do not exceed 200 mg/day; *or* 6 mg Sub-Q; *or* 5, 10, or 20 mg by nasal spray in one nostril, may repeat in 2 h, do not exceed 40 mg/day	Acute migraines, cluster headaches in adults
zolmitriptan (*Zomig, Zomig ZMT*)	2.5 mg PO; may repeat in 2 h; do not exceed 10 mg/day	Acute migraines in adults

the treatment of acute migraine and are not used for prevention of migraines. Sumatriptan injection is also indicated for the treatment of cluster headaches.

Pharmacokinetics

The triptans are rapidly absorbed from many sites; they are metabolized in the liver (sumatriptan by monoamine oxidase) and are primarily excreted in the urine. They cross the placenta and have been shown to be toxic to the fetus in animal studies. They should be used in pregnancy only if the benefit to the mother clearly outweighs any potential risks to the fetus. They have also been shown to enter breast milk and should be used with caution during lactation. The safety and efficacy of use in children have not been established.

Contraindications and Cautions

Triptans are contraindicated with any of the following conditions: allergy to any triptan; pregnancy *because of the possibility of severe adverse effects on the fetus;* and active CAD, *which could be exacerbated by the vessel-constricting effects of these drugs.* These drugs should be used with caution in elderly patients *because of the possibility of underlying vascular disease;* in patients with risk factors for CAD; in lactating women *because of the possibility of adverse effects on the infant;* and in patients with renal or hepatic dysfunction, *which could alter the metabolism and excretion of the drug.*

Adverse Effects

The adverse effects associated with the triptans are related to the vasoconstrictive effects of the drugs. CNS effects may include numbness, tingling, burning sensation, feelings of coldness or strangeness, dizziness, weakness, myalgia, and vertigo. GI effects such as dysphagia and abdominal discomfort may occur. CV effects can be severe and include blood pressure alterations and tightness or pressure in the chest.

Clinically Important Drug–Drug Interactions

Combining triptans with ergot-containing drugs results in a risk of prolonged vasoactive reactions.

There is a risk of severe adverse effects if these drugs are used within 2 weeks after discontinuation of an MAO inhibitor *because of the increased vasoconstrictive effects that occur.* If triptans are to be given, it should be clear that the patient has not received an MAO inhibitor in more than 2 weeks.

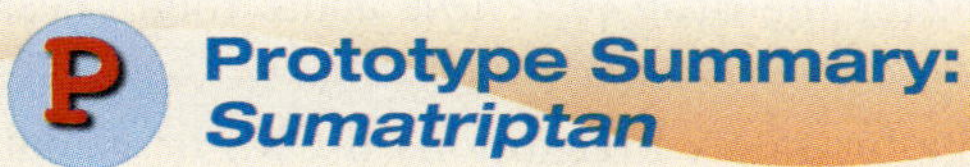

P Prototype Summary: Sumatriptan

Indications: Treatment of acute migraine; treatment of cluster headaches (Sub-Q route)

Actions: Binds to serotonin receptors to cause vasoconstrictive effects on cranial blood vessels

Pharmacokinetics:

Route	Onset	Peak	Duration
Nasal spray	Varies	5–20 min	Unknown
Oral	1–1.5 hr	2–4 h	Up to 24 h
Sub-Q	Rapid	1–5 h	Up to 24 h

$T_{1/2}$: 115 min; metabolized in the liver, excreted in the urine

Adverse effects: Dizziness, vertigo, weakness, myalgia, blood pressure alterations, tightness or pressure in the chest, injection site discomfort, tingling, burning sensations, numbness

Nursing Considerations for Patients Receiving Triptans

Assessment: History and Examination

Screen for the following conditions, *which could be cautions or contraindications for the use of the drug:* any known allergies to triptans; pregnancy; MI, CAD, or hypertension; and hepatic or renal dysfunction.

Include screening *for baseline status before beginning therapy and for any potential adverse effects.* Assess the following: temperature; skin color and lesions; CNS orientation, affect, and reflexes; respiration and adventitious sounds; pulse, blood pressure, and cardiac output; ECG and liver and renal function tests.

Nursing Diagnoses

The patient receiving a triptan may have the following nursing diagnoses related to drug therapy:

- Acute Pain related to CV and vasoconstrictive effects
- Decreased Cardiac Output related to CV effects
- Disturbed Sensory Perception (Visual, Auditory, Kinesthetic, and Tactile) related to CNS effects
- Deficient Knowledge regarding drug therapy

Implementation With Rationale

- Administer the drug to relieve acute migraines; *these drugs are not used for prevention.*
- Arrange for safety precautions if CNS or visual changes occur *to prevent patient injury.*
- Provide comfort and safety measures, such as environmental controls and stress reduction, *for the relief of headache.* Provide additional pain relief as needed.
- Monitor the blood pressure of any patient with a history of CAD, and discontinue the drug if any sign of angina or prolonged hypertension occurs *to prevent severe vascular effects.*
- Provide thorough patient teaching, including drug name and prescribed dosage, as well as measures for avoidance of adverse effects, warning signs that may indicate possible problems, and the need for monitoring and evaluation, *to enhance patient knowledge about drug therapy and to promote compliance.*
- Offer support and encouragement *to help the patient cope with the drug regimen.*

Evaluation

- Monitor patient response to the drug (relief of acute migraine headaches).
- Monitor for adverse effects (CV changes, arrhythmias, hypertension, CNS changes).
- Evaluate the effectiveness of the teaching plan (patient can give the drug name and dosage and describe possible adverse effects to watch for, specific measures to prevent adverse effects, and warning signs to report).
- Monitor the effectiveness of comfort measures and compliance with the regimen.

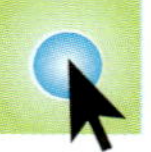

WEB LINKS

Health care providers and patients may want to consult the following Internet sources:

http://www.ampainsoc.org Information on pain, physiology, and management.

http://www.aapainmanage.org Information on education programs, research, and other topics related to pain management.

http://www.mayohealth.org Information on chronic pain and the use of narcotics.

http://health.nih.gov/result.asp?disease_id=303 Information on migraines—support groups, treatment, and research.

http://www.geocities.com/HotSprings/Spa/7379/migraine.html Information for patients and families on migraine headaches—understanding them, treatments, and support groups.

Points to Remember

- Pain occurs any time that tissue is injured and various chemicals are released. The pain impulses are carried to the spinal cord by small-diameter A-delta and C fibers, which form synapses with interneurons in the dorsal horn of the spinal cord.
- Opioid receptors, which are found throughout various tissues in the body, react with endogenous endorphins

and enkephalins to modulate the transmission of pain impulses.

- Narcotics, derived from the opium plant, react with opioid receptors to relieve pain. In addition, they lead to constipation, respiratory depression, sedation, and suppression of the cough reflex, and they stimulate feelings of well-being or euphoria.
- Because narcotics are associated with the development of physical dependence, they are controlled substances.
- The effectiveness and adverse effects associated with specific narcotics are associated with their particular affinity for various types of opioid receptors.
- Narcotic agonists react with opioid receptor sites to stimulate their activity.
- Narcotic agonists-antagonists react with some opioid receptor sites to stimulate activity and block other opioid receptor sites. These drugs are not as addictive as pure narcotic agonists.
- Narcotic antagonists, which work to reverse the effects of narcotics, are used to treat narcotic overdose or to reverse unacceptable adverse effects.
- Migraine headaches are severe, throbbing headaches on one side of the head that may be associated with an aura or warning syndrome. These headaches are thought to be caused by arterial dilation and hyperperfusion of the brain vessels.
- Treatment of migraines may involve either ergot derivatives or triptans. Ergot derivatives cause vasoconstriction and are associated with sometimes severe systemic vasoconstrictive effects, whereas triptans, a new class of selective serotonin receptor blockers, cause CNS vasoconstriction but are not associated with as many adverse systemic effects.

CHECK YOUR UNDERSTANDING

Answers to the questions in this chapter may be found in the Answer Key in the back of the book.

Multiple Choice

Select the best answer to the following.

1. According to the gate control theory, pain
   a. is caused by gates in the CNS.
   b. can be blocked or intensified by the opening or closing of gates in the CNS.
   c. is caused by gates in peripheral nerve sensors.
   d. cannot be affected by learned experiences.

2. Opioid receptors are found throughout the body
   a. only in people who have become addicted to opiates.
   b. in increasing numbers with chronic pain conditions.
   c. and incorporate pain perception and blocking.
   d. and cause endorphin release.

3. Most narcotics are controlled substances because
   a. they are very expensive.
   b. they can cause respiratory depression.
   c. they can be addictive.
   d. they can be used only in a hospital setting.

4. Injecting a narcotic into an area of the body that is chilled can be dangerous because
   a. an abscess will form.
   b. the injection will be very painful.
   c. absorption may be delayed and an excessive amount absorbed all at once.
   d. narcotics are inactivated in cold temperatures.

5. Proper administration of an ordered narcotic
   a. can lead to addiction.
   b. should be done promptly to prevent increased pain and the need for larger doses.
   c. would include holding the drug as long as possible until the patient really needs it.
   d. should rely on the patient's request for medication.

6. Migraine headaches
   a. occur during sleep and involve sweating and eye pain.
   b. occur with stress and feel like a dull band around the entire head.
   c. often occur when drinking coffee.
   d. are throbbing headaches on one side of the head.

7. The triptans are a class of drugs that bind to selective serotonin receptor sites and cause
   a. cranial vascular dilation.
   b. cranial vascular constriction.
   c. depression.
   d. nausea and vomiting.

8. The only triptan that has been approved for use in treating cluster headaches as well as migraines is
   a. naratriptan.
   b. rizatriptan.
   c. sumatriptan.
   d. zolmitriptan.

Multiple Response

Select all that apply.

1. Narcotics are drugs that react with opioid receptors throughout the body. The use of these drugs is associated with which of the following?
   a. Hypnosis
   b. Sedation
   c. Analgesia
   d. Euphoria
   e. Orthostatic hypotension
   f. Increased salivation

2. A narcotic would be the analgesic of choice in which of the following?
   a. A patient with severe postoperative pain
   b. A patient with severe chronic obstructive pulmonary disease and difficulty breathing
   c. A patient with severe, chronic pain
   d. A patient with ulcerative colitis
   e. A patient with recent biliary surgery
   f. A cancer patient with severe bone pain

Matching

Match the generic name of these commonly used narcotic agonists with the associated brand name.

1. ____________________ fentanyl
2. ____________________ hydrocodone
3. ____________________ hydromorphone
4. ____________________ levorphanol
5. ____________________ meperidine
6. ____________________ methadone
7. ____________________ morphine
8. ____________________ oxycodone
9. ____________________ propoxyphene

A. Darvon
B. Dolophine
C. Demerol
D. Dilaudid
E. OxyContin
F. Hycodan
G. Duragesic
H. Roxanol
I. Levo-Dromoran

Definitions

Define the following terms.

1. A fibers ____________________

____

2. A-delta and C fibers ____________________

____

3. gate control theory ____________________

____

4. migraine headache ____________________

____

5. narcotics ____________________

____

6. narcotic agonists ____________________

____

7. narcotic agonists-antagonists ____________________

____

8. narcotic antagonists ____________________

____

9. opioid receptors ____________________

____

10. triptan ____________________

____

Bibliography and References

Drug facts and comparisons. (2006). St. Louis: Facts and Comparisons.

Gilman, A., Hardman, J. G., & Limbird, L. E. (Eds.). (2006). *Goodman and Gilman's the pharmacological basis of therapeutics* (11th ed.). New York: McGraw-Hill.

Karch, A. M. (2006). *2007 Lippincott's nursing drug guide.* Philadelphia: Lippincott Williams & Wilkins.

Porth, C. M. (2005). *Pathophysiology: Concepts of altered health states* (7th ed.). Philadelphia: Lippincott Williams & Wilkins.

Professional's guide to patient drug facts. (2006). St. Louis: Facts and Comparisons.

CHAPTER 27

General and Local Anesthetic Agents

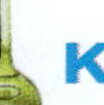

KEY TERMS

amnesia
analgesia
balanced anesthesia
general anesthetic
induction
local anesthetic
plasma esterase
unconsciousness
volatile liquid

LEARNING OBJECTIVES

Upon completion of this chapter, you will be able to:

1. Describe the concept of balanced anesthesia.
2. Describe the therapeutic actions, indications, pharmacokinetics, contraindications, most common adverse reactions, and important drug–drug interactions associated with general, regional, and local anesthetics.
3. Outline the preoperative and postoperative needs of a patient undergoing anesthesia.
4. Compare and contrast the prototype drugs thiopental, midazolam, nitrous oxide, halothane, benzocaine, and lidocaine with other drugs in their respective classes.
5. Outline the nursing considerations, including important teaching points, for patients receiving anesthetics.

GENERAL ANESTHETICS

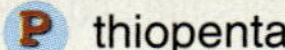

Barbiturates

methohexital
P thiopental

Nonbarbiturate General Anesthetics

droperidol
etomidate
ketamine
P midazolam
propofol

Gases

cyclopropane
ethylene
nitrous oxide

Volatile Liquids

desflurane
enflurane
P halothane
isoflurane
sevoflurane

LOCAL ANESTHETICS

Esters

benzocaine
chloroprocaine
procaine
tetracaine

Amides

bupivacaine
dibucaine
levobupivacaine
P lidocaine
mepivacaine
prilocaine
ropivacaine

Other

pramoxine

Anesthetics are drugs that are used to cause complete or partial loss of sensation. The anesthetics can be subdivided into general and local anesthetics depending on their site of action. **General anesthetics** are central nervous system (CNS) depressants used to produce loss of pain sensation and consciousness. **Local anesthetics** are drugs used to cause loss of pain sensation and feeling in a designated area of the body without the systemic effects associated with severe CNS depression. This chapter discusses various general and local anesthetics. (See Box 27.1 for information on using anesthetics with various age groups.)

General Anesthetics

When administering general anesthetics, several different drugs are combined to achieve the following goals: **analgesia**, or loss of pain perception; **unconsciousness**, or loss of awareness of one's surroundings; and **amnesia**, or inability to recall what took place. General anesthetics also block the body's reflexes. Blockage of autonomic reflexes prevents involuntary reflexes from responding to injury to the body that might compromise a patient's cardiac, respiratory, gastrointestinal (GI), and immune status. Blockage of muscle reflexes prevents jerking movements that might interfere with the success of the surgical procedure.

Risk Factors Associated With General Anesthetics

Use of general anesthetics involves a widespread CNS depression, which is not without risks. Several factors must be taken into consideration before the use of general anesthesia, which usually involves a series of drugs aimed at achieving the best effect with the fewest side effects. Because of the wide systemic effects of general anesthetics, patients should be evaluated for potential risks. When anesthetic drugs are selected, the following factors are kept in mind so that the potential risk to each particular patient is minimized:

- *CNS factors:* Underlying neurological disease (e.g., epilepsy, stroke, myasthenia gravis) that presents a risk for abnormal reaction to the CNS-depressing and muscle-relaxing effects of these drugs.
- *Cardiovascular factors:* Underlying vascular disease, coronary artery disease, or hypotension, which put patients at

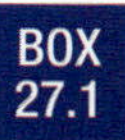

DRUG THERAPY ACROSS THE LIFESPAN

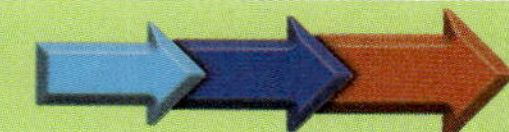

Anesthetic Agents

CHILDREN

Children are at greater risk for complications after anesthesia—laryngospasm, bronchospasm, aspiration, and even death. They require very careful monitoring and support, and the anesthetist needs to be very skilled at calculating dosage and balance during the procedure. Propofol is widely used for diagnostic tests and short procedures in children older than 3 years of age because of its rapid onset and metabolism and generally smooth recovery. Halothane is widely used for children, especially those with respiratory dysfunction, because it tends to dilate bronchi. It cannot be used with any increase in intracranial pressure, which it increases. Sevoflurane has a minimal impact on intracranial pressure and allows a very rapid induction and recovery with minimal sympathetic reaction. It is still quite expensive, however, which may limit its use. The dosage of anesthetics may need to be higher in children, and that factor will be considered by the anesthetist.

Nursing care after general anesthesia should include support and reassurance; assessment of the child for any skin breakdown related to immobility, and safety precautions until full recovery has occurred.

Local anesthetics are used in children in much the same way that they are used in adults.

Bupivacaine, levobupivacaine, and tetracaine do not have established doses for children younger than 12 years of age. Benzocaine should not be used in children younger than 1 year of age.

When topically applying a local anesthetic, it is important to remember that there is greater risk of systemic absorption and toxicity with infants.

Tight diapers can act like occlusive dressings and increase systemic absorption. Children need to be cautioned not to bite themselves when receiving dental anesthesia.

ADULTS

Adults require a considerable amount of teaching and support when receiving anesthetics, including what will happen, what they will feel, how it will feel when they recover, and the approximate time to recovery.

Adults should be monitored closely until fully recovered from general anesthetics and should be cautioned to prevent injury when receiving local anesthetics. It is important to remember to reassure and talk to adults who may be aware of their surroundings yet unable to speak.

Most of the general anesthetics are not recommended for use during pregnancy because of the potential risk to the fetus. Short-onset and local anesthetics are frequently used at delivery. Use of a regional or other local anesthetic is usually preferred if surgery is needed during pregnancy. During lactation, it is recommended that the mother wait 4 to 6 hours to feed the baby after the anesthetic is used.

OLDER ADULTS

Older patients are more likely to experience the adverse effects associated with these drugs, including central nervous system, cardiovascular, and dermatological effects. Thinner skin and the possibility of decreased perfusion to the skin makes them especially susceptible to skin breakdown during immobility. Because older patients often also have renal or hepatic impairment, they are also more likely to have toxic levels of the drug related to changes in metabolism and excretion. The older patient should have safety measures in effect, such as siderails, a call light, and assistance to ambulate; special efforts to provide skin care to prevent skin breakdown are especially important with older skin. The older patient may require longer monitoring and regular orienting and reassuring. After general anesthesia, it is very important to promote vigorous pulmonary toilet to decrease the risk of pneumonia.

risk for severe reactions to anesthesia, such as hypotension and shock, dysrhythmias, and ischemia.

- *Respiratory factors:* Obstructive pulmonary disease (e.g., asthma, chronic obstructive pulmonary disease, bronchitis), which can complicate the delivery of gas anesthetics as well as the intubation and mechanical ventilation that must be used in most cases of general anesthesia.
- *Renal and hepatic function:* Conditions that interfere with the metabolism and excretion of anesthetics (e.g., acute renal failure, hepatitis) and could result in prolonged anesthesia and the need for continued support during recovery. Toxic reactions to the accumulation of abnormally high levels of anesthetic agents may even occur.

Balanced Anesthesia

With the wide variety of drugs available, the anesthesiologist has the opportunity to try to balance the therapeutic effects needed with the potential for adverse effects by ordering a variety of anesthetic drugs. **Balanced anesthesia** is the use of a combination of drugs, each with a specific effect, to achieve analgesia, muscle relaxation, unconsciousness, and amnesia, rather than the use of a single drug. Balanced anesthesia commonly involves the following agents:

- *Preoperative medications,* which may include the use of anticholinergics that decrease secretions to facilitate intubation and prevent bradycardia associated with neural depression.
- *Sedative–hypnotics* to relax the patient, facilitate amnesia, and decrease sympathetic stimulation.
- *Antiemetics* to decrease the nausea and vomiting associated with GI depression.
- *Antihistamines* to decrease the chance of allergic reaction and to help dry up secretions.
- *Narcotics* to aid analgesia and sedation.

Many of these drugs are given before the anesthetic to facilitate the process, and some are maintained during surgery to aid the anesthetic, allowing therapeutic effects at lower doses. For example, patients may receive a neuromuscular junction (NMJ) blocker and a rapid-acting intravenous anesthetic to induce anesthesia, and then a gas anesthetic to balance it during the procedure and allow easier recovery. Careful selection of appropriate anesthetic agents, along with monitoring and support of the patient, helps to alleviate many problems.

Administration of General Anesthetics

Anesthesia is delivered by a physician or nurse anesthetist trained in the delivery of these potent drugs with equipment for intubation, mechanical ventilation, and full life support. During the delivery of anesthesia, the patient can go through predictable stages, referred to as the depth of anesthesia. These stages are as follows:

Stage 1, the analgesia stage, refers to the loss of pain sensation, with the patient still conscious and able to communicate.

Stage 2, the excitement stage, is a period of excitement and often combative behavior, with many signs of sympathetic stimulation (e.g., tachycardia, increased respirations, blood pressure changes).

Stage 3, surgical anesthesia, involves relaxation of skeletal muscles, return of regular respirations, and progressive loss of eye reflexes and pupil dilation. Surgery can be safely performed in stage 3.

Stage 4, medullary paralysis, is very deep CNS depression with loss of respiratory and vasomotor center stimuli, in which death can occur rapidly.

Induction

Induction is the period from the beginning of anesthesia until stage 3, or surgical anesthesia is reached. The danger period for many patients during induction is stage 2 because of the systemic stimulation that occurs. Many times a rapid-acting anesthetic is used to move quickly through this phase and into stage 3. NMJ blockers may be used during induction to facilitate intubation, which is necessary to support the patient with mechanical ventilation during anesthesia.

Maintenance

Maintenance is the period from stage 3 until the surgical procedure is complete. A slower, more predictable anesthetic, such as a gas anesthetic, may be used to maintain the anesthesia once the patient is in stage 3.

Recovery

Recovery is the period from discontinuation of the anesthetic until the patient has regained consciousness, movement, and the ability to communicate. During recovery, the patient must be continuously monitored to provide life support as needed and to monitor for any adverse effects of the drugs being used.

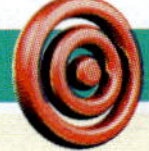

FOCUS POINTS

- General anesthetics relieve pain, block muscle reflexes, and produce analgesia, amnesia, and unconsciousness.
- In patients with underlying CNS, cardiovascular, or respiratory diseases, general anesthetics may cause harm by producing widespread CNS depression.
- Induction of anesthesia is the period ranging from administration of the anesthetic to the point of surgical anesthesia.
- Balanced anesthesia involves giving a variety of drugs rather than a single drug to achieve analgesia, muscle relaxation, unconsciousness, and amnesia.

Types of General Anesthetics

Several different types of drugs are used as general anesthetics. These include barbiturate and nonbarbiturate anesthetics, volatile liquids, and gas anesthetics (Table 27.1).

Barbiturate Anesthetics

The barbiturate anesthetics are intravenous drugs used to induce rapid anesthesia, which is then maintained with an inhaled drug. They include the following:

- Thiopental (*Pentothal*) is probably the most widely used of the intravenous anesthetics. This agent has a very rapid onset of action and an ultrashort recovery period. Because it has no analgesic properties, the patient may need additional analgesics after surgery.
- Methohexital (*Brevital*) has a rapid onset of action and a recovery period that is even more ultrashort. This agent cannot come in contact with silicone (rubber stoppers and disposable syringes often contain silicone) because it will cause an immediate breakdown of the silicone. As a result, it poses special problems, and special precautions must be taken. Like thiopental, methohexital also lacks analgesic properties, and the patient may require postoperative analgesics. Because of its rapid onset, this drug can cause respiratory depression and apnea, so it should not be used until the anesthesiologist and staff are ready and equipped for intubation and respiratory support.

Prototype Summary: *Thiopental*

Indications: Induction of anesthesia, maintenance of anesthesia; induction of a hypnotic state

Actions: Depresses the CNS to produce hypnosis and anesthesia without analgesia

Pharmacokinetics:

Route	Onset	Duration
IV	1 min	20–30 min

$T_{1/2}$: 3–8 hours; metabolized in the liver, excreted in the urine

Adverse effects: Emergence delirium, headache, restlessness, anxiety, cardiovascular depression, respiratory depression, apnea, salivation, hiccups, skin rashes

Nonbarbiturate Anesthetics

The other drugs used for intravenous administration in anesthesia are nonbarbiturates with a wide variety of effects. Such anesthetics include the following:

- Midazolam (*generic*) is the prototype nonbarbiturate anesthetic. This agent has a rapid onset but does not reach peak effectiveness for 30 to 60 minutes. It is more likely to cause nausea and vomiting than are some of the other anesthetics. It is a very potent amnesiac.
- Droperidol (*Inapsine*) has a rapid onset of action and an ultrashort recovery period. It should be used with caution in patients with renal or hepatic failure. During the recovery period, this agent may cause hypotension, chills, hallucinations, and drowsiness.
- Etomidate (*Amidate*) has an ultrashort onset and a rapid recovery period. This agent is sometimes used for sedation of patients on ventilators. During the recovery phase, many patients experience myoclonic and tonic movements as well as nausea and vomiting. Etomidate is not recommended for use in children younger than 10 years of age.
- Ketamine (*Ketalar*) has a rapid onset of action and a very slow recovery period (45 minutes). This agent has been associated with a bizarre state of unconsciousness in which the patient appears to be awake but is unconscious and cannot feel pain. This drug, which causes sympathetic stimulation with increase in blood pressure and heart rate, may be helpful in situations when cardiac depression is dangerous. Ketamine crosses the blood–brain barrier and can cause hallucinations, dreams, and psychotic episodes.
- Propofol (*Diprivan*) is a very short-acting anesthetic with a rapid onset of action, and often is used for short procedures. It often causes local burning on injection. It can cause bradycardia, hypotension, and in extreme cases, pulmonary edema.

Prototype Summary: *Midazolam*

Indications: Sedation, anxiolysis, and amnesia before diagnostic, therapeutic, or endoscopic procedures; induction of anesthesia; continuous sedation of intubated patients

Actions: Acts mainly at the limbic system and RAS; potentiates the effects of GABA; has little effect on cortical function; exact mechanism of action is not understood

Pharmacokinetics:

Route	Onset	Peak	Duration
Oral	30–60 min	12 h	2–6 h
IM	15 min	30 min	2–6 h
IV	3–5 min	<30 min	2–6 h

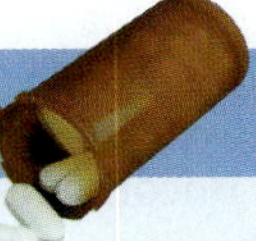

Table 27.1 DRUGS IN FOCUS

General Anesthetics

Drug	Onset	Recovery	Analgesia	Systems Alert[a] *CV*	*Resp*	*CNS*	*GI*	*Renal*	*Hepatic*
Barbiturates									
methohexital (*Brevital*)	rapid	ultra, ultrashort	none	—	+++	—	—	—	—
P thiopental (*Pentothal*)	rapid	ultrashort	none	—	—	—	—	—	—
Nonbarbiturate Anesthetics									
droperidol (*Inapsine*)	3–10 min	2–4 h	—	++	—	+	—	+	+
etomidate (*Amidate*)	1 min	3–5 min	—	—	—	+	++	—	—
ketamine (*Ketalar*)	rapid	45 min	+	++	—	+++	—	—	—
P midazolam (*generic*)	15 min	rapid	+	—	+++	—	++	—	—
propofol (*Diprivan*)	rapid	rapid	+	++	+	++	—	—	—
Gases									
cyclopropane (orange)	1–2 min	rapid	—	—	—	++	++	—	—
ethylene (red)	rapid	rapid	—	—	—	+	+	—	—
nitrous oxide (blue)	1–2 min	rapid	++++	+++	+	+	—	—	—
Volatile Liquids									
desflurane (*Suprane*)	rapid	rapid	+	—	++++	—	—	—	—
enflurane (*Ethrane*)	rapid	rapid	+	+	+	—	—	++	—
P halothane (*Fluothane*)	rapid	rapid	+	++	—	—	+	—	+++
isoflurane (*generic*)	rapid	rapid	+	++	+	—	+	—	—
sevoflurane (*Ultane*)	rapid	rapid	+	—	++	—	—	—	—

[a]Systems alert indicates physiological systems with anticipated adverse effects to these drugs. When drugs are selected, the patient's condition and potential for serious problems with these adverse effects should be considered.

—, no effect; +, mild effect, ++, moderate effect; +++, strong effect; ++++, powerful effect

$T_{1/2}$: 1.8–6.8 hours; metabolized in the liver, excreted in the urine

Adverse effects: Transient drowsiness, sedation, drowsiness, lethargy, apathy, fatigue, disorientation, restlessness, constipation, diarrhea, incontinence, urinary retention, bradycardia, tachycardia, phlebitis at IV injection site

Anesthetic Gases

Like all inhaled anesthetics, anesthetic gases enter the bronchi and alveoli, rapidly pass into the capillary system (because gases flow from areas of higher concentration to areas of lower concentration), and are transported to the heart to be pumped throughout the body. These gases have a very high affinity for fatty tissue, including the lipid membrane of the nerves in the CNS. The gases pass quickly into the brain and cause severe CNS depression. Once the patient is in stage 3 of anesthesia, the anesthetist regulates the amount of gas that is delivered to ensure that it is sufficient to keep the patient unconscious but not enough to cause severe depression. This is done by decreasing the concentration of the gas that is flowing into the bronchi, creating a concentration gradient that results in the movement of gas in the opposite direction—out of the tissues and back to expired air. Anesthetic gases include the following:

- Nitrous oxide (blue cylinder) is the prototype anesthetic gas. Although this agent is a very potent analgesic, it is the weakest of the gas anesthetics and the least toxic. It moves so quickly in and out of the body that it can actually increase the volume of closed body compartments such as sinuses. Because nitrous oxide is such a potent analgesic with rapid onset and recovery, it is often used for dental surgery. Nitrous oxide is usually combined with other agents for anesthetic use. It can block the reuptake of oxygen after surgery and cause hypoxia. Because of this reaction, it is always given in combination with oxygen. Susceptible patients should be monitored for signs of hypoxia, chest pain, and stroke.
- Cyclopropane (orange cylinder) has a rapid onset of action and a rapid recovery. This agent is not a good analgesic, and the patient may experience pain, headache, nausea, vomiting, and delirium during the recovery phase.
- Ethylene (red cylinder) is less toxic than most of the other gas anesthetics. However, its use can leave the patient with a headache and a very unpleasant taste in the mouth. This agent has a rapid onset of action and a rapid recovery.

Volatile Liquids

Inhaled anesthetics are either gases or **volatile liquids** that are unstable at room temperature and release gases. These gases are then inhaled by the patient, so these volatile liquids act like gas anesthetics.

Most of the volatile liquids in use today are halogenated hydrocarbons such as the following:

- Halothane (*Fluothane*) is the prototype of the volatile liquids. It has a rapid onset of action and rapid recovery. It is associated with vomiting, bradycardia, and hypotension and has an increased risk of causing hepatic toxicity. Halothane is metabolized in the liver to toxic hydrocarbons and bromide; therefore, it can contribute to hepatic toxicity. Its recovery syndrome is characterized by fever, anorexia, nausea, vomiting, and eventual hepatitis, which can progress to fatal hepatic necrosis. Although this syndrome is rare, halothane is not used more frequently than every 3 weeks to reduce patient risk.
- Desflurane (*Suprane*) has a rapid onset and rapid recovery. This agent is associated with a collection of respiratory reactions, including cough, increased secretions, and laryngospasm. Therefore, it should be avoided in patients with respiratory problems and in those with increased sensitivity. In addition, its use is not recommended for induction in pediatric patients.
- Enflurane (*Ethrane*) has a rapid onset and a rapid recovery. Because this agent is associated with renal toxicity, cardiac arrhythmias, and respiratory depression, it is not to be used for patients with known cardiac or respiratory disease or with renal dysfunction.
- Isoflurane (generic) has a rapid onset and recovery. It can cause muscle relaxation. Isoflurane is associated with hypotension, hypercapnia, muscle soreness, and a bad taste in the mouth, but it does not cause cardiac arrhythmias or respiratory irritation as do some other volatile liquids.
- Sevoflurane (*Ultane*) is the newest of the volatile liquids. This agent has a very rapid onset of action and a very rapid clearance. Because of this, adverse effects are thought to be minimal.

P Prototype Summary: Halothane

Indications: Induction and maintenance of general anesthesia

Actions: Depresses the CNS, causing anesthesia; relaxes muscles; sensitizes the myocardium to the effects of norepinephrine and epinephrine

Pharmacokinetics:

Route	Onset	Peak	Duration
Inhaled	Rapid	Rapid	End of inhalation

$T_{1/2}$: Unknown; metabolized in the liver, excreted in the urine

Adverse effects: Transient drowsiness, sedation, drowsiness, lethargy, apathy, fatigue, disorientation, restlessness, constipation, diarrhea, incontinence, urinary retention, bradycardia, tachycardia, hypoxia, acidosis, apnea, arrhythmias, hepatic injury

Overview of General Anesthetics

Therapeutic Actions and Indications

The mechanism of action of the general anesthetics is not understood (Figure 27.1). It is known, however, that depression of the reticular activating system and the cerebral cortex occurs. General anesthetics are indicated for producing sedation, hypnosis, anesthesia, amnesia, and unconsciousness to allow performance of painful surgical procedures.

Pharmacokinetics

The general anesthetics tend to be lipid soluble and therefore are distributed widely throughout the body, including

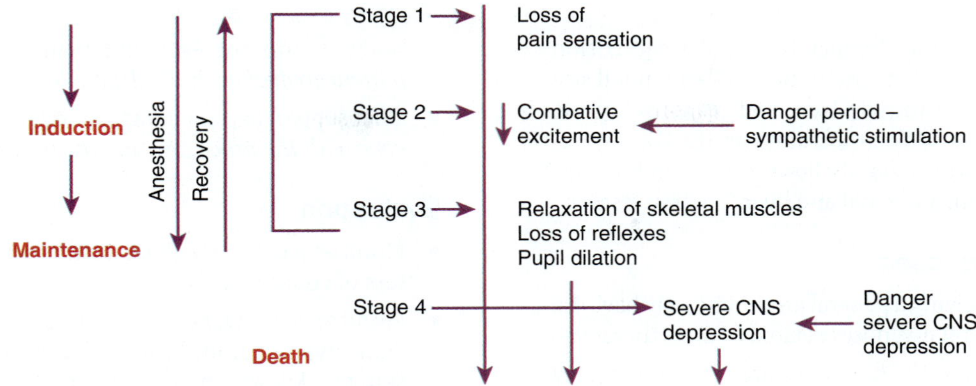

FIGURE 27.1 Stages of general anesthesia.

the CNS. They are generally metabolized in the liver, necessitating caution with patients who have hepatic dysfunction. Because they cross the placenta, they should be used during pregnancy only if they are clearly needed and the benefit to the mother outweighs any potential risk to the fetus. Women who are nursing should wait 4 to 6 hours after recovery from the anesthetic before nursing the baby.

Contraindications and Cautions

General anesthetics are contraindicated with status asthmaticus *because of the difficulty in providing ventilatory support to these patients and the risk of exacerbation of the problem with CNS depression.* These agents are also contraindicated when there is an absence of suitable veins for intravenous administration, *which could be dangerous if life support measures became necessary and intravenous delivery of life-saving drugs is essential.*

Caution should be used in cases of severe cardiovascular disease, hypotension, or shock; conditions in which hypnotic effects may be prolonged or potentiated with increased intracranial pressure; and myasthenia gravis—*all of which could be exacerbated by the depressive effects of these drugs and may necessitate extra support and prolonged monitoring during surgery.* Droperidol should be used with caution in patients with renal or hepatic failure.

Adverse Effects

The adverse effects associated with general anesthetics are often associated with the depressive effects of these drugs and may include the following conditions: circulatory depression; hypotension; shock; decreased cardiac output; arrhythmias; respiratory depression, including apnea, laryngospasm, bronchospasm, hiccups, and coughing; headache; nausea and vomiting; prolonged somnolence; and in some cases delirium. The halogenated hydrocarbons may cause malignant hyperthermia, with extreme muscle rigidity, severe hyperpyrexia, acidosis, and in some cases death. If this condition occurs, it is treated with dantrolene. In addition, there is also always a risk of skin breakdown secondary to immobility when patients receive general anesthetics.

Clinically Important Drug–Drug Interactions

Several potentially dangerous drug–drug interactions have been reported with the general anesthetics. If ketamine and halothane are used in combination, severe cardiac depression with hypotension and bradycardia may occur. If these agents must be used together, the patient should be monitored closely. Ketamine may also potentiate the muscular blocking of NMJ blockers, and the patient may require prolonged periods of respiratory support.

Combinations of barbiturate anesthetics and narcotics may produce apnea more commonly than occurs with other analgesics. The nonbarbiturate anesthetic midazolam is associated with increased toxicity and length of recovery when used in combination with inhaled anesthetics, other CNS depressants, narcotics, propofol, or thiopental. If any of these agents are used in combination, careful balancing of drug doses is necessary.

Table 27.1 lists the general anesthetics commonly used today. They are used only under the direct supervision of an anesthesia practitioner who delivers the drug and monitors the drug effects.

Nursing Considerations for Patients Receiving General Anesthetics

Assessment: History and Examination

Screen for the following conditions, *which could be contraindications or cautions for the use of the drug:* any known allergies to general anesthetics; impaired liver or kidney function; myasthenia gravis; personal or family history of malignant hyperthermia; and cardiac or respiratory disease.

Include screening *for baseline status before beginning therapy and for any potential adverse effects.*

Assess the following: temperature and weight; skin color and lesions; affect, orientation, reflexes, pupil size and reaction, and muscle tone and response; pulse, blood pressure, and electrocardiogram (ECG); respiration and adventitious sounds; bowel sounds and abdominal examination; and renal and liver function tests.

Nursing Diagnoses

The patient receiving a general anesthetic may have the following nursing diagnoses related to drug therapy:

- Impaired Gas Exchange related to respiratory depression
- Impaired Skin Integrity related to immobility
- Disturbed Thought Processes and Disturbed Sensory Perception related to CNS depression
- Deficient Knowledge regarding drug therapy

Implementation With Rationale

- The drug must be administered by trained personnel (usually an anesthesiologist) *because of the potential risks associated with its use.*
- Have equipment on standby to maintain airway and provide mechanical ventilation *when patient is not able to maintain respiration because of CNS depression.*
- Monitor temperature *for prompt detection and treatment of malignant hyperthermia.* Maintain dantrolene on standby.
- Monitor pulse, respiration, blood pressure, ECG, and cardiac output continually during administration. In addition, monitor temperature and reflexes. *Dosage adjustment may be needed to alleviate potential problems and to maximize overall benefit with the least toxicity.*
- Monitor the patient until the recovery phase is complete and the patient is conscious and able to move and communicate *to ensure patient safety.*
- Provide comfort measures *to help the patient tolerate drug effects.* Provide pain relief as appropriate, along with reassurance and support *to deal with the effects of anesthesia and loss of control;* skin care and turning *to prevent skin breakdown;* and supportive care *for conditions such as hypotension and bronchospasm.*
- Provide thorough patient teaching preoperatively, *realizing that most patients who receive the drug will be unconscious or will be receiving teaching about a particular procedure.*
- Information about the anesthetic (e.g., what to expect, rate of onset, time to recovery) should be incorporated into the teaching plan *to prepare the patient to deal with the drug effects.*
- Offer support and encouragement *to help the patient cope with the procedure and the drugs being used.*

Evaluation

- Monitor patient response to the drug (analgesia, loss of consciousness).
- Monitor for adverse effects (respiratory depression, hypotension, bronchospasm, GI slowdown, skin breakdown, malignant hyperthermia).
- Evaluate the effectiveness of the teaching plan (patient can relate anticipated effects of the drug and the recovery process).
- Monitor the effectiveness of comfort measures and compliance with the regimen.

Local Anesthetics

Local anesthetics are drugs that cause a loss of sensation in limited areas of the body. They are used primarily to prevent the patient from feeling pain for varying periods of time after they have been administered in the peripheral nervous system. In increasing concentrations, local anesthetics can also cause loss of the following sensations (in this sequence): temperature, touch, proprioception (position sense), and skeletal muscle tone. If these other aspects of nerve function are progressively lost, recovery occurs in the reverse order of the loss.

The local anesthetics are very powerful nerve blockers, and it is very important that their effects be limited to a particular area of the body. They should not be absorbed systemically. Systemic absorption could produce toxic effects on the nervous system and the heart (e.g., severe CNS depression, cardiac arrhythmias). Local anesthetics are either esters or amides. The esters are broken down immediately in the plasma by enzymes known as **plasma esterases**. The amides are metabolized more slowly in the liver, and serum levels of these drugs can increase and lead to toxicity.

Modes of Administration

The way in which a local anesthetic is administered helps increase its effectiveness by delivering it directly to the area that is causing or will cause the pain, thereby decreasing systemic absorption and related toxic effects (Figure 27.2). There are five types of local anesthetic administration: topical, infiltration, field block, nerve block, and intravenous regional anesthesia.

Topical Administration

Topical anesthesia involves applying a cream, lotion, ointment, or drop of a local anesthetic to traumatized skin to

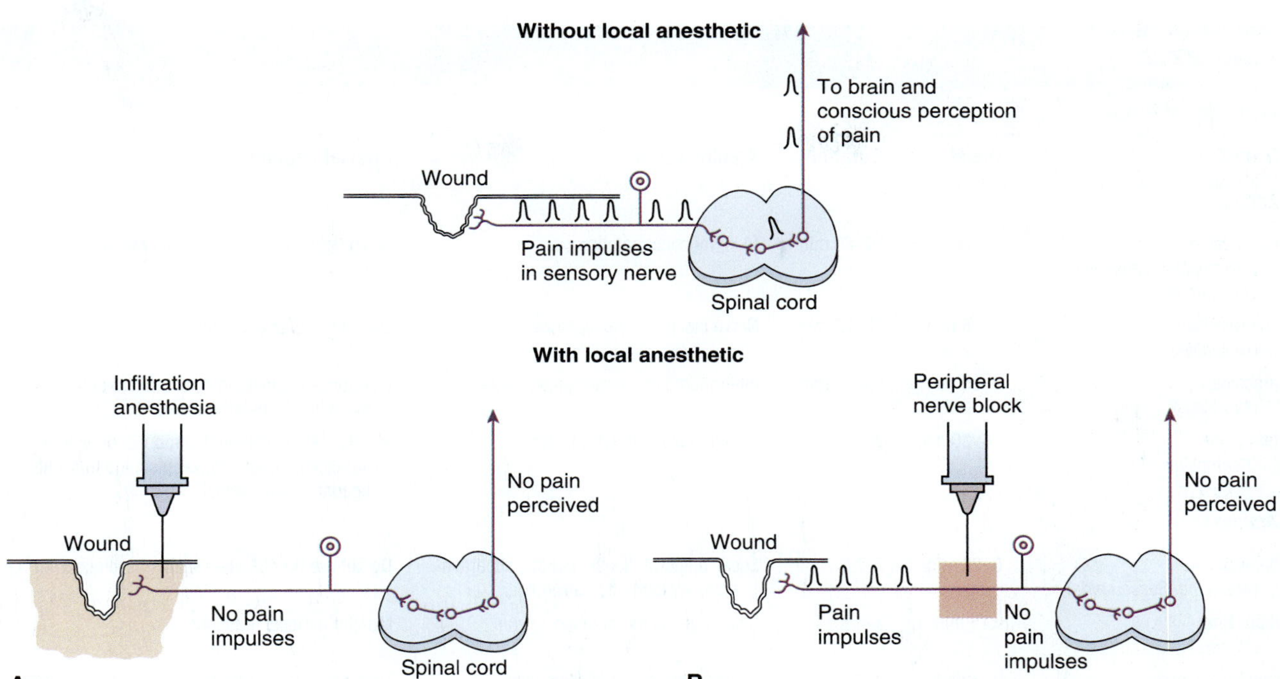

FIGURE 27.2 Mechanism of action of local anesthetics. *Top:* An injury produces pain impulses (action potentials) that are conducted and transmitted in an area of the brain in which pain is perceived. **(A)** Conduction of the pain impulse has been blocked by infiltration anesthetics at the site of the injury. **(B)** A nerve block at some distance from the injury. Local anesthetics block the movement of sodium into the nerve and prevent nerve depolarization, stopping the transmission of the pain impulse.

relieve pain. It can also involve applying these to the mucous membranes in the eye, nose, throat, mouth, urethra, anus, or rectum to relieve pain or to anesthetize the area to facilitate a medical procedure. Although systemic absorption is rare with topical application, it can occur if there is damage or breakdown of the tissues in the area.

Infiltration

Infiltration anesthesia involves injecting the anesthetic directly into the tissues to be treated (e.g., sutured, drilled, cut). This injection brings the anesthetic into contact with the nerve endings in the area and prevents them from transmitting nerve impulses to the brain.

Field Block

Field block anesthesia involves injecting the anesthetic all around the area that will be affected by the operation. This is more intense than infiltration anesthesia because the anesthetic agent comes in contact with all of the nerve endings surrounding the area. This type of block is often used for tooth extractions.

Nerve Block

Nerve block anesthesia involves injecting the anesthetic at some point along the nerve or nerves that run to and from the region in which the loss of pain sensation or muscle paralysis is desired. These blocks are performed not in the surgical field, but at some distance from the field; they involve a greater area with potential for more adverse effects. Several types of nerve blocks are possible. A peripheral nerve block blocks the sensory and motor aspects of a particular nerve for relief of pain or for diagnostic purposes. With a central nerve block, the anesthetic is injected into the roots of the nerves in the spinal cord. In epidural anesthesia, the drug is injected into the space where the nerves emerge from the spinal cord. A caudal block involves injection into the sacral canal, below the epidural area.

Intravenous Regional Anesthesia

Intravenous regional anesthesia involves carefully draining all of the blood from the patient's arm or leg, securing a tourniquet to prevent the anesthetic from entering the general circulation, and then injecting the anesthetic into the vein of the arm or leg. This technique is used for very specific surgical procedures.

Characteristics of Local Anesthetics

Several agents may be used as local anesthetics. The agent of choice depends on the method of administration, the length of time for which the area is to be anesthetized, and consideration of potential adverse effects. The different local anesthetics are listed in Table 27.2.

Table 27.2 DRUGS IN FOCUS

Local Anesthetics

Drug	Onset	Duration	Administration	Special Cautions
Esters				
benzocaine (*Dermoplast, Lanacane, Unguentine*)	1 min	30–60 min	Skin, mucous membranes	Avoid tight bandages with skin preparation
chloroprocaine (*Nesacaine*)	6–15 min	15–75 min	Nerve block, caudal, epidural	Do not use with subarachnoid administration
procaine (*Novocain*)	2–25 min	15–75 min	Infiltration, peripheral, spinal, dental	Monitor skin condition if immobile; keep supine to avoid headache after spinal
tetracaine (*Pontocaine*)	15–30 min	2–25 h	Spinal, prolonged spinal, skin	Monitor skin condition if immobile; provide reassurance if prolonged; keep supine to avoid headache after spinal
Amides				
bupivacaine (*Marcaine, Sensorcaine*)	5–20 min	2–7 h	Local, epidural, dental, caudal, subarachnoid, sympathetic, retrobulbar	Do not use Bier Block—deaths have occurred
dibucaine (*Nupercainal*)	<15 min	3–4 h	Skin, mucous membranes	Monitor for local reactions
levobupivacaine (*Chirocaine*)	5–20 min	2–7 h	Regional block, OB, postop pain	Less cardiac and CNS toxicity than bupivacaine, suggests safer use in some patients
P lidocaine (*Dilocaine, Solarcaine, Xylocaine, Lidoderm, Octocaine*)	5–15 min	30–90 min	Caudal, epidural, spinal cervical, dental, skin, mucous membrane, topical patch	Short acting, preferred for short procedures; danger if absorbed systemically
mepivacaine (*Carbocaine, Isocaine, Polocaine*)	3–15 min	45–90 min	Nerve block, OB, cervical, epidural, dental, local infiltration	Caution with renal impairment
prilocaine (*Cilanest*)	1–15 min	0.5–3 h	Nerve block, dental	Advise patients not to bite themselves
ropivacaine (*Naropin*)	1–5 min	2–6 h	Nerve block, epidural, caudal	Avoid rapid infusion; offers good pain management postop and OB
Other				
pramoxine (*Tronothane, PrameGel, Itch-X, Prax*)	3–5 min	<60 min	Skin, mucous membranes	Do not cover with tight bandages; protect patient from injury

Therapeutic Actions and Indications

Local anesthetics work by causing a temporary interruption in the production and conduction of nerve impulses. They affect the permeability of nerve membranes to sodium ions, which normally infuse into the cell in response to stimulation. By preventing the sodium ions from entering the nerve, they stop the nerve from depolarizing. A particular section of the nerve cannot be stimulated, and nerve impulses directed toward that section are lost when they reach that area. Local anesthetics are indicated for infiltration anesthesia, peripheral nerve block, spinal anesthesia, and the relief of local pain. See Box 27.2 for a discussion of a new topical anesthetic dermal patch.

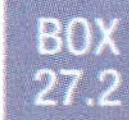

Combination Local Anesthetic

In 2005, the U.S. Food and Drug Administration approved a local anesthetic product that combines lidocaine and tetracaine in a dermal patch. This drug, called *Synera*, was approved for use on intact skin to provide local dermal anesthesia when doing venipunctures or inserting IV cannulae, or for superficial dermatological procedures that could cause discomfort for the patient. When using it for venipunctures or inserting an IV, one patch is applied 20 to 30 minutes before the procedure. If a superficial dermatological procedure is being performed, one patch is applied to the area 30 minutes before the procedure. The patch must be removed if the patient is undergoing a magnetic resonance imaging scan to prevent burning related to the dermal patch. The site should be monitored for any local irritation.

Pharmacokinetics

The ester local anesthetics are broken down immediately in the plasma by enzymes known as plasma esterases. The amide local anesthetics are metabolized more slowly in the liver, and serum levels of these drugs can increase and lead to toxicity. They should be used during pregnancy and lactation only if the benefit outweighs any potential risk to the fetus or neonate that could occur if the drug is inadvertently absorbed systemically.

Contraindications and Cautions

The local anesthetics are contraindicated with any of the following conditions: history of allergy to any one of these agents or to parabens; heart block, *which could be greatly exacerbated with systemic absorption;* shock, *which could alter the local delivery and absorption of these drugs;* and decreased plasma esterases, *which could result in toxic levels of the ester-type local anesthetics.*

Adverse Effects

The adverse effects of these drugs may be related to their local blocking of sensation (e.g., skin breakdown, self-injury, biting oneself). Other problematic effects are associated with the route of administration and the amount of drug that is absorbed systemically. These effects are related to the blockade of nerve depolarization throughout the system. Effects that may occur include CNS effects such as headache, restlessness, anxiety, dizziness, tremors, blurred vision, and backache; GI effects such as nausea and vomiting; cardiovascular effects such as peripheral vasodilation, myocardial depression, arrhythmias, and blood pressure changes, all of which may lead to fatal cardiac arrest; and respiratory arrest.

Clinically Important Drug–Drug Interactions

When local anesthetics and succinylcholine are given concurrently, increased and prolonged neuromuscular blockade occurs. There is also less risk of systemic absorption and increased local effects if these drugs are combined with epinephrine.

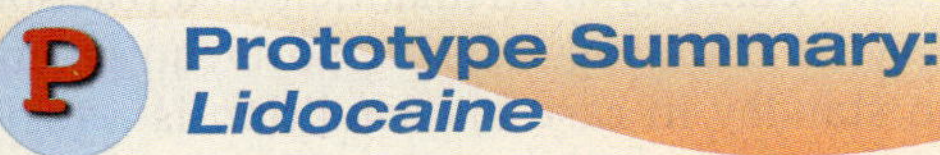

Prototype Summary: *Lidocaine*

Indications: Infiltration anesthesia, peripheral and sympathetic nerve blocks, central nerve blocks, spinal and caudal anesthesia, topical anesthetic for skin or mucous membrane disorders

Actions: Blocks the generation and conduction of action potentials in sensory nerves by reducing sodium permeability, reducing the height and rate of rise of the action potential, increasing the excitation threshold, and slowing conduction velocity

Pharmacokinetics:

Route	Onset	Peak	Duration
IM	5–10 min	5–15 min	2 h
Topical	Not generally absorbed systemically		

$T_{1/2}$: 10 min, then 1.5–3 hours; metabolized in the liver, excreted in the urine

Adverse effects: Headache, backache, hypotension, urinary retention, urinary incontinence, pruritus, seizures; when locally applied: burning, stinging, swelling, tenderness

Nursing Considerations for Patients Receiving Local Anesthetics

Assessment: History and Examination

Screen for the following conditions, *which could be cautions or contraindications to the use of the drug:* any known allergies to these drugs or to parabens; impaired liver function; low plasma esterases; heart block; shock; and pregnancy or lactation.

Include screening *for baseline status before beginning therapy and for any potential adverse effects.* Assess the following: body temperature and weight; skin color and lesions; affect, orientation, reflexes, pupil size and reaction, and muscle tone and response; pulse, blood pressure, and ECG; respiration and adventitious sounds; and liver function tests and plasma esterases (if appropriate).

Nursing Diagnoses

The patient receiving a local anesthetic may have the following nursing diagnoses related to drug therapy:

- Disturbed Sensory Perception (Kinesthetic, Tactile) related to anesthetic effect
- Impaired Skin Integrity related to immobility
- Risk for Injury related to loss of sensation and mobility
- Deficient Knowledge regarding drug therapy

Implementation With Rationale

- Have equipment on standby *to maintain airway and provide mechanical ventilation if needed.*
- Ensure that drugs for managing hypotension, cardiac arrest, and CNS alterations are on standby *in case of severe reaction and toxicity.*
- Ensure that patients receiving spinal anesthesia are well hydrated and remain lying down for up to 12 hours after the anesthesia *to minimize headache.*
- Establish safety precautions *to prevent skin breakdown and injury during the time that the patient has a loss of sensation and/or mobility.*
- Provide comfort measures *to help the patient tolerate drug effects.* Provide pain relief as appropriate; reassurance and support *to deal with the effects of anesthesia and loss of control;* skin care and turning *to prevent skin breakdown;* and supportive care for hypotension *to prevent shock or serious hypoxia.*
- Provide thorough patient teaching *to explain what to expect, safety precautions that will be needed, and when to expect return of function.*
- Offer support and encouragement *to help the patient cope with the procedure and drugs being used.*

Evaluation

- Monitor patient response to the drug (loss of feeling in designated area).
- Monitor for adverse effects (respiratory depression, blood pressure changes, arrhythmias, GI upset, skin breakdown, injury, CNS alterations).
- Evaluate the effectiveness of the teaching plan (patient can relate the anticipated effects of the drug and the recovery process) (see Critical Thinking Scenario 27-1).

CRITICAL THINKING SCENARIO 27-1

Local Anesthesia

The Situation

A.M., a 32-year-old male athlete with a history of asthma (which could indicate pulmonary dysfunction) was admitted to the hospital for an inguinal hernia repair. At the patient's request, the surgeon elected to use a local anesthetic employing spinal anesthesia. Because the extent of the repair was unknown (A.M. had undergone two previous repairs), levobupivacaine, a long-acting anesthetic, was selected. He remained alert (BP 120/64, P 62, R 10) and stable throughout the procedure. Two hours after the conclusion of the procedure, A.M. appeared agitated (BP 154/68, P 88, R 12). Although he did not complain of discomfort, he did state that he still had no feeling and had only limited movement of his legs.

Critical Thinking

What safety precautions need to be taken?

What nursing interventions should be done at this point?

How could the patient be reassured? *Think about the anxiety level of the patient—an athlete who elected to have local anesthesia may have a problem with control and feel somewhat invincible. Consider the anxiety that loss of mobility and sensation in the legs may cause in a person who makes his living as an athlete.*

In addition, consider the expected duration of action of levobupivacaine and the rate of return of function.

Discussion

Levobupivacaine is a long-acting anesthetic with effects that may persist for several hours. The timing of the drug's effects should be explained to A.M., and he should be monitored for a period of time to determine whether his agitated state and slightly elevated vital signs are a result of anxiety or an unanticipated reaction to the surgery or the drug. Life-support equipment should be on standby in case his condition is a toxic drug reaction or some unanticipated problem occurring after surgery.

The nurse is in the best position to perform the following interventions: explaining the effects of the drug and the anticipated recovery schedule; keeping the patient

Local Anesthesia *(continued)*

as flat as possible to decrease the headache usually associated with spinal anesthesia; encouraging the patient to turn from side to side periodically to allow skin care to be performed and to alleviate the risk of pressure sore development; and staying with the patient as much as possible to reassure him, to answer questions, and to encourage him to talk about his feelings and reaction.

If the agitated state is caused by a stress reaction, the patient should return to normal; comfort measures, teaching, and reassurance should be provided. An elevated systolic pressure with a normal diastolic pressure often is an indication of a sympathetic stress response. An athlete is more likely than most people to suffer great anxiety and fear if his legs become numb and he is unable to move them. Teaching and comfort measures may be all that is needed to relieve the anxiety and ensure a good recovery.

Nursing Care Guide for A.M.: Local Anesthesia

Assessment: History and Examination

Assess for allergies to local anesthetics or to parabens, cardiac disorders, vascular problems, hepatic dysfunction; also assess for concurrent use of succinylcholine

Focus physical examination on the following:

CV: blood pressure, pulse, peripheral perfusion, ECG

CNS: orientation, affect, reflexes, vision

Skin: color, lesions, texture, sweating

Respiratory: respiration, adventitious sounds

Laboratory tests: liver function tests, plasma esterases

Nursing Diagnoses

Disturbed Sensory Perception (Kinesthetic, Tactile) related to anesthesia

Impaired Skin Integrity related to immobility

Risk for Injury related to loss of sensation, and mobility

Deficient Knowledge regarding drug therapy

Implementation

Administer drug under strict supervision.

Provide comfort and safety measures: positioning, skin care, siderails, pain medication as needed, maintain airway, ventilate patient, antidotes on standby.

Provide support and reassurance to deal with loss of sensation and mobility.

Provide patient teaching about procedure being performed and what to expect.

Provide life support as needed.

Evaluation

Evaluate drug effects: loss of sensation, loss of movement.

Monitor for adverse effects: cardiovascular effects (BP changes, arrhythmias), respiratory depression, GI upset, CNS alterations, skin breakdown, anxiety, and fear.

Monitor for drug–drug interactions as indicated for each drug.

Evaluate effectiveness of patient teaching program and comfort and safety measures.

Constantly monitor vital signs and muscular function and sensation as it returns.

Patient Teaching for A.M.

Teaching about local anesthetics is usually incorporated into the overall teaching plan about the procedure that the patient will undergo. Things to highlight with the patient would include:

☐ Discussion of the overall procedure:
- What it will feel like (any numbness, tingling, inability to move, pressure, pain, choking?)
- Any anticipated discomfort
- How long it will last
- Concerns during the procedure: report any discomfort and ask any questions as they arise

☐ Discussion of the recovery:
- How long it will take
- Feelings to expect: tingling, numbness, pressure, itching
- Pain that will be felt as the anesthesia wears off
- Measures to reduce pain in the area
- Signs and symptoms to report (e.g., pain along a nerve route, palpitations, feeling faint, disorientation)

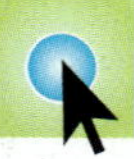

WEB LINKS

Health care providers and patients may want to consult the following Internet sources:

http://www.anesthesia-analgesia.org Information on anesthesia—physiology and research.

http://www.pain.com Information on regional anesthesia.

http://www.anesthesiologyonline.com Information for patients about types of anesthesia, research, and teaching protocols.

Points to Remember

- General anesthetics are drugs used to produce pain relief, analgesia, amnesia, and unconsciousness and to block muscle reflexes that could interfere with a surgical procedure or put the patient at risk for harm.
- The use of general anesthetics involves a widespread CNS depression that could be harmful, especially in patients with underlying CNS, cardiovascular, or respiratory diseases.
- Anesthesia proceeds through predictable stages from loss of sensation to total CNS depression and death.
- Induction of anesthesia is the period of time from the beginning of anesthesia administration until the patient reaches surgical anesthesia.
- Balanced anesthesia involves giving a variety of drugs, including anticholinergics, rapid intravenous anesthetics, inhaled anesthetics, NMJ blockers, and narcotics.
- Patients receiving general anesthetics should be monitored for any adverse effects and to provide reassurance and safety precautions until the recovery of sensation, mobility, and ability to communicate.
- Local anesthetics block the depolarization of nerve membranes, preventing the transmission of pain sensations and motor stimuli.
- Local anesthetics are administered to deliver the drug directly to the desired area and to prevent systemic absorption, which could lead to serious interruption of nerve impulses and response.
- Ester-type local anesthetics are immediately destroyed by plasma esterases. Amide local anesthetics are destroyed in the liver and have a greater risk of accumulation and systemic toxicity.
- Nursing care of patients receiving anesthetics should include safety precautions to prevent injury and skin breakdown; support and reassurance to deal with the loss of sensation and mobility; and patient teaching regarding what to expect to decrease stress and anxiety.

CHECK YOUR UNDERSTANDING

Answers to the questions in this chapter may be found in the Answer Key in the back of the book.

Multiple Choice

Select the best answer to the following.

1. The most dangerous period for many patients undergoing general anesthesia is during
   a. stage 1, when communication becomes difficult.
   b. stage 2, when systemic stimulation occurs.
   c. stage 3, when skeletal muscles relax.
   d. there is no real danger during general anesthesia.
2. Recovery after a general anesthetic refers to the period of time
   a. from the beginning of the anesthesia until the patient is ready for surgery.
   b. during the surgery when anesthesia is maintained at a certain level.
   c. from the discontinuation of the anesthetic until the patient has regained consciousness, movement, and the ability to communicate.
   d. when the patient is in the most danger of CNS depression.
3. While a patient is receiving a general anesthetic, he or she must be continually monitored because
   a. the patient has no pain sensation.
   b. generalized CNS depression affects all body functions and could cause problems for patients with CNS, CV, or respiratory disorders.
   c. the patient cannot move.
   d. the patient cannot communicate.
4. Because of the risks to the patient, general anesthetics are administered
   a. under the watchful eye of a nursing supervisor.
   b. only by graduate nurses.

c. only by trained personnel (usually an anesthesiologist).
d. by surgeons.

5. Local anesthetics are used to block feeling in specific body areas. If given in increasing concentrations, local anesthetics can cause loss, in order, of the following:
   a. temperature sensation, touch sensation, proprioception, and skeletal muscle tone.
   b. touch sensation, skeletal muscle tone, temperature sensation, and proprioception.
   c. proprioception, skeletal muscle tone, touch sensation, and temperature sensation.
   d. skeletal muscle tone, touch sensation, temperature sensation, and proprioception.

Multiple Response

Select all that apply.

1. Comfort measures that are important for a patient receiving a local anesthetic would include which of the following?
   a. Skin care and turning
   b. Reassurance over loss of control and sensation
   c. Use of antihypertensive agents
   d. Use of analgesics as needed
   e. Ice applied to the area involved
   f. Safety precautions to prevent injury

2. A nurse would anticipate the use of general anesthetics for which of the following reasons?
   a. To produce analgesia
   b. To produce amnesia
   c. To activate the reticular activating system
   d. To block muscle reflexes
   e. To cause unconsciousness
   f. To prevent nausea

3. Balanced anesthesia combines different classes of drugs to achieve the best effects with the fewest adverse effects. Balanced anesthesia usually involves the use of which of the following?
   a. Anticholinergics
   b. Narcotics
   c. Sedative/hypnotics
   d. Adrenergic beta-blockers
   e. Dantrolene
   f. Neuromuscular blocking agents

Fill in the Blanks

1. General anesthetics are drugs used to produce ____________, ____________, ____________, and ____________ and to block muscle reflexes that could interfere with a surgical procedure or put the patient at risk for harm.

2. Anesthesia proceeds through predictable stages from ____________ to total central nervous system (CNS) depression and ____________.

3. ____________ is the time from the beginning of anesthesia administration until the patient reaches surgical anesthesia.

4. ____________ involves giving a variety of drugs, including anticholinergics, rapid intravenous (IV) anesthetics, inhaled anesthetics, neuromuscular junction (NMJ) blockers, and narcotics.

5. Local anesthetics block the ____________, preventing the transmission of pain sensations and motor stimuli.

6. The use of general anesthetics involves a widespread ____________ that could be harmful, especially in patients with underlying CNS, cardiovascular (CV), or respiratory diseases.

7. Patients receiving general anesthetics should be monitored for any adverse effects, offered reassurance, and provided with safety precautions until the recovery of ____________, ____________, and ____________.

8. The adverse effects of local anesthetics may be related to their local blocking of sensation; such effects may include ____________, ____________, and ____________.

Web Exercise

Your patient wants information about the various types of anesthesia that are used and how they would affect the body and recovery. You can find information for patients about types of anesthesia at http://www.anesthesiologyonline.com/. Search this site for appropriate teaching protocols and prepare a comparison of the types and actions for the patient to review with you.

Bibliography and References

Drug facts and comparisons. (2006). St. Louis: Facts and Comparisons.

Gilman, A., Hardman, J. G., & Limbird, L. E. (Eds.). (2006). *Goodman and Gilman's the pharmacological basis of therapeutics* (11th ed.). New York: McGraw-Hill.

Karch, A. M. (2006). *2007 Lippincott's nursing drug guide.* Philadelphia: Lippincott Williams & Wilkins.

Porth, C. M. (2005). *Pathophysiology: Concepts of altered health states* (7th ed.). Philadelphia: Lippincott Williams & Wilkins.

Professional's guide to patient drug facts. (2006). St. Louis: Facts and Comparisons.

CHAPTER 28

Neuromuscular Junction Blocking Agents

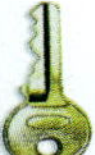

KEY TERMS

acetylcholine receptor site
depolarizing
malignant hyperthermia
nondepolarizing
paralysis
sarcomere
sliding filament theory

LEARNING OBJECTIVES

Upon completion of this chapter, you will be able to:

1. Draw and label a neuromuscular junction.
2. Describe the therapeutic actions, indications, pharmacokinetics, contraindications, most common adverse reactions, and important drug–drug interactions associated with the depolarizing and nondepolarizing neuromuscular junction blockers.
3. Discuss the use of neuromuscular junction blockers across the lifespan.
4. Compare and contrast the prototype drugs tubocurarine and succinylcholine with other neuromuscular junction blockers.
5. Outline the nursing considerations, including important teaching points, for patients receiving a neuromuscular junction blocker.

NONDEPOLARIZING NEUROMUSCULAR BLOCKERS

atracurium
cisatracurium
mivacurium
pancuronium
rocuronium
P tubocurarine
vecuronium

DEPOLARIZING NEUROMUSCULAR BLOCKER

P succinylcholine

Drugs that affect the neuromuscular junction (NMJ), the NMJ blockers, can be divided into two groups. One group, the **nondepolarizing** NMJs, includes those agents that act as antagonists to acetylcholine (ACh) at the NMJ and prevent depolarization of muscle cells. The other group, the **depolarizing** NMJs (of which there is one drug), act as an ACh agonist at the junction, causing stimulation of the muscle cell and then preventing it from repolarizing. Both of these types of drugs are used to cause **paralysis**, or loss of muscular function, for performance of surgical procedures or facilitation of mechanical ventilation. (See Box 28.1 for information about using NMJ blockers with various age groups.)

The Neuromuscular Junction

The NMJ blockers affect the normal functioning of muscles by interfering with the normal processes that occur at the junction of nerve and muscle cell. The functional unit of a muscle, called a **sarcomere**, is made up of light and dark filaments formed by actin and myosin molecules arranged in orderly stacks that give the sarcomere a striated or striped appearance (Figure 28.1). Normal muscle function involves the arrival of a nerve impulse at the motor nerve terminal, followed by the release of ACh into the synaptic cleft. At the **acetylcholine receptor site** on the effector side of the synapse, the ACh interacts with the nicotinic cholinergic receptors, causing depolarization of the muscle membrane. This depolarization allows the release of calcium ions, stored in tubules, into the cell. The calcium binds to troponin, a chemical found throughout the sarcomere, and the binding of troponin causes the release of actin and myosin binding sites, allowing them to react with each other. ACh is broken down by acetylcholinesterase, freeing the receptor for further stimulation.

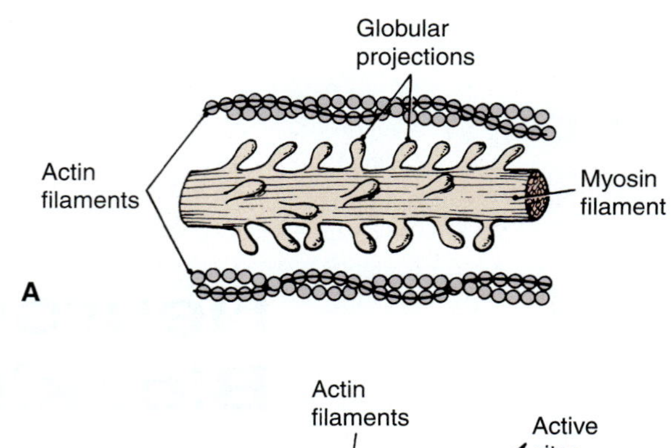

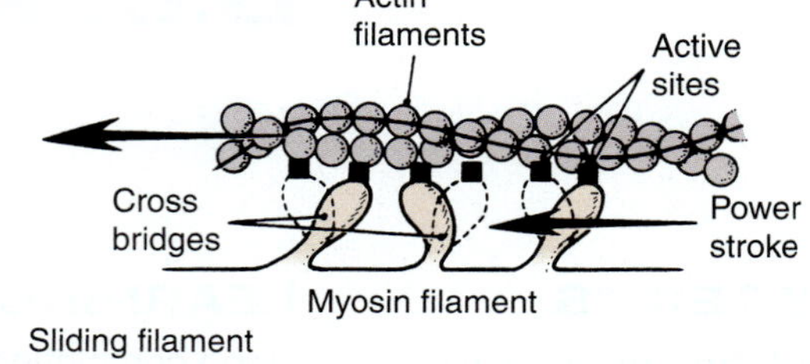

FIGURE 28.1 Sliding filament theory of muscle contraction.

The actin and myosin molecules react with each other again and again, sliding along the filament and making it shorter. This is a contraction of the muscle fiber according to the **sliding filament theory**. As the calcium is removed from the cell during repolarization of the muscle membrane, the troponin is freed and once again prevents the actin and myosin from reacting with each other. The muscle filament then relaxes or slides back to the resting position. Muscle tone results from a dynamic balance between excitatory and inhibitory impulses to the muscle. Muscle paralysis may occur when ACh cannot react with the cholinergic muscle receptor or when the muscle cells cannot repolarize to allow new stimulation and muscle contraction.

BOX 28.1 **DRUG THERAPY ACROSS THE LIFESPAN**

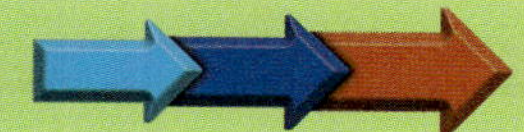

Neuromuscular Junction (NMJ) Blocking Agents

CHILDREN

Children require very careful monitoring and support after the use of NMJ blockers. These agents are used by anesthetists who are skilled in their use and with full support services available.

The nondepolarizing NMJs are preferable because of the lack of muscle contraction with its resultant discomfort on recovery. Succinylcholine is usually preferred when a very short-acting, rapid-onset blocker is needed (e.g., for intubation).

ADULTS

Adults need to be monitored closely for full return of muscle function. If succinylcholine is used, they need to be told that they will experience muscle pain and discomfort when the procedure is over.

The NMJs are used during pregnancy and lactation only if the benefit to the mother outweighs the potential risk to the fetus or neonate.

OLDER ADULTS

Because older patients often also have renal or hepatic impairment, they are more likely to have toxic levels of the drug related to changes in metabolism and excretion. The older patient should receive special efforts to provide skin care to prevent skin breakdown, which is more likely with older skin. The older patient may require longer monitoring and regular orienting and reassuring.

Nondepolarizing Neuromuscular Junction Blockers

The first nondepolarizing NMJ blocker to be discovered was curare, a poison used on the tips of arrows or spears by primitive hunters to paralyze their game. Animals died when their respiratory muscles became paralyzed. Because the poison was destroyed by the cooking process, or by gastric acid if the meat were eaten raw, it was safe for humans. Curare was first purified for clinical use as the NMJ blocker tubocurarine.

All nondepolarizing NMJ blockers are similar in structure to ACh and occupy the muscular cholinergic receptor site, preventing ACh from reacting with the receptor. These agents do not cause activation of muscle cells, and consequently muscle contraction does not occur. Because they are not broken down by acetylcholinesterase, their effect is more long-lasting than that of ACh. NMJ blockers are used when clinical situations require muscle paralysis.

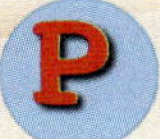

Prototype Summary: *Tubocurarine*

Indications: Adjunct to general anesthesia; to induce skeletal muscle relaxation; to reduce the intensity of muscle contractions in electroconvulsive therapy; to facilitate care of patients undergoing mechanical ventilation

Actions: Occupies the muscular cholinergic receptor site, preventing ACh from reacting with the receptor; does not cause activation of muscle cells; causes a flaccid paralysis

Pharmacokinetics:

Route	Onset	Duration
IV	6 min	25–90 min

$T_{1/2}$: <5 min, then 7–40 min, then 2–3 hours; metabolized in the tissues, excreted unchanged in the urine

Adverse effects: Respiratory depression, apnea, bronchospasm, cardiac arrhythmias

Depolarizing Neuromuscular Junction Blocker: Succinylcholine

Succinylcholine, a depolarizing NMJ blocker, attaches to the ACh receptor site on the muscle cell, depolarizing the muscle. This depolarization causes stimulation of the muscle and muscle contraction. Unlike ACh, succinylcholine is not broken down instantly, and the result is a prolonged contraction of the muscle, which cannot be restimulated. Eventually a gradual repolarization occurs as continually stimulated channels in the cell membrane close. Certain ethnic groups can have a genetic predisposition for lengthened paralysis (Box 28.2).

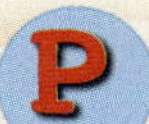

Prototype Summary: *Succinylcholine*

Indications: Adjunct to general anesthesia; to facilitate endotracheal intubation; to induce skeletal muscle relaxation during surgery or mechanical ventilation

Actions: Combines with ACh receptors at the motor endplate to produce depolarization; this inhibits neuromuscular transmission, causing a flaccid paralysis

Pharmacokinetics:

Route	Onset	Duration
IV	30–60 sec	4–6 min

$T_{1/2}$: 2–3 min; metabolized in the tissues, excreted unchanged in the urine

Adverse effects: Muscle pain, related to the contraction of the muscles as a first reaction; respiratory depression, apnea

BOX 28.2 CULTURAL CONSIDERATIONS FOR DRUG THERAPY

Succinylcholine and Paralysis

Succinylcholine is broken down in the body by cholinesterase, an enzyme found in the plasma. Several conditions may cause the body to produce less of this enzyme, including cirrhosis, metabolic disorders, carcinoma, burns, dehydration, malnutrition, hyperpyrexia, thyrotoxicosis, collagen diseases, and exposure to neurotoxic insecticides. If plasma cholinesterase levels are low, the serum levels of succinylcholine remain elevated, and the paralysis can last much longer than anticipated. These patients need support and ventilation for long periods after surgery.

There is also a genetic predisposition to low plasma cholinesterase levels. Patients should be asked whether they or any family member has a history of either low plasma cholinesterase levels or prolonged recovery from anesthetics. Alaskan Eskimos belong to such a genetic group, and they are especially likely to suffer prolonged paralysis and inability to breathe for several hours after succinylcholine has been used for surgery. If there is no other drug of choice for these patients, special care must be taken to monitor their response and ensure their breathing for an extended postoperative period.

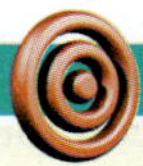

FOCUS POINTS

- The nerves and muscles communicate at the neuromuscular junction (NMJ) with acetylcholine (ACh) acting as the neurotransmitter.
- NMJ blockers prevent skeletal muscle function.
- Nondepolarizing NMJ blockers prevent ACh from exciting the muscle, and paralysis ensues because the muscle cannot respond.
- Depolarizing NMJ blockers cause muscle paralysis by acting like ACh. They excite (depolarize) the muscle and prevent repolarization and further stimulation.

Therapeutic Actions and Indications

All of the NMJ blockers are structurally similar to ACh and compete with ACh for muscle ACh receptor sites. They are hydrophilic, instead of lipophilic, so they do not readily cross the blood–brain barrier. The nondepolarizing NMJ blockers act by blocking the ACh receptor so that it cannot be stimulated. Depolarizing NMJ blockers prevent muscle movement by prohibiting the depolarization of the muscle membrane. The depolarizing NMJ blocker succinylcholine (*Anectine, Quelicin*) works by reacting with the ACh receptor and causing a prolonged depolarization, which causes first muscle contraction and then flaccid paralysis. Both effects cause muscles to stop responding to stimuli, and paralysis occurs. Clinically, muscle twitching occurs when the drug is first given and is followed by flaccid paralysis. Succinylcholine has a rapid onset and a short duration of action because it is broken down by cholinesterase in the plasma (Figure 28.2).

These drugs are indicated for any situation in which muscle paralysis is desired. The therapeutic uses of NMJ blocking are as follows:

- To serve as an adjunct to general anesthetics during surgery, when reflex muscle movement could interfere with the surgical procedure or the delivery of gas anesthesia.
- To facilitate mechanical intubation by preventing resistance to passing of the endotracheal tube and in situations in which patients "fight" or resist the respirator.
- To facilitate electroconvulsive therapy when intense skeletal muscle contractions as a result of electric shock could cause the patient broken bones or other injury.

Several NMJ blockers are available, with different times of onset and durations of activity. The drug of choice in any given situation is determined by the procedure being performed, including the estimated time involved (Figure 28.3).

Pharmacokinetics

In general, the NMJs are metabolized in the serum, although metabolism is dependent on the liver to produce the needed plasma cholinesterases. Patients with hepatic impairment may experience prolonged effects of the drugs. Most of the metabolites are excreted in the urine. Patients with renal impairment may be at risk for increased toxicity from the drugs. There are no well-controlled studies regarding the effects of these drugs during pregnancy, and they should be used during pregnancy only if they are clearly needed and the benefits outweigh the potential risks to the fetus. Succinylcholine is often used during cesarean sections, where it does cross the placenta, but accurate timing prevents serious effects on the fetus. Effects during lactation are not known.

Contraindications and Cautions

The NMJ blockers are contraindicated in the following conditions: known allergy to any of these drugs; myasthenia gravis *because blocking of the ACh cholinergic receptors aggravates the neuromuscular disease* (which results from destruction of the ACh receptor sites) *and increases the muscular effects* (see Chapter 32); renal or hepatic disease, *which could interfere with the metabolism or excretion of these drugs, leading to toxic effects;* and pregnancy (some of these drugs are used in cesarean sections, but the dose needs to be decreased to protect the fetus).

Caution should be used in patients with any family or personal history of **malignant hyperthermia**, a serious adverse effect associated with these drugs that is characterized by extreme muscle rigidity, severe hyperpyrexia, acidosis, and death in some cases, *because malignant hyperthermia can occur with the use of these drugs.* Caution should also be used in the following circumstances: pulmonary or cardiovascular dysfunction, *which could be made worse by the paralysis of the respiratory muscles and resulting changes in perfusion and respiratory function;* altered fluid and electrolyte imbalance, *which could affect membrane stability and muscular function;* some respiratory conditions *that could be made worse by the histamine release associated with some of these agents;* and lactation *because of the potential for adverse effects on the baby.*

In addition, succinylcholine should be used with caution in patients with fractures *because the muscle contractions it causes might lead to additional trauma;* in those with narrow-angle glaucoma or penetrating eye injuries *because intraocular pressure increases;* and in those with paraplegia or spinal cord injuries, *which could cause loss of potassium from the overstimulated cells and hyperkalemia.* Extreme caution should be taken in the presence of genetic or disease-related conditions causing low plasma cholinesterase levels, such as cirrhosis, metabolic disorders, carcinoma, burns, dehydration, malnutrition, hyperpyrexia, thyroid toxicosis, collagen diseases, and exposure to neurotoxic insecticides. *Low plasma cholinesterase levels may result in a very prolonged paralysis because succinylcholine is not broken down in the plasma and*

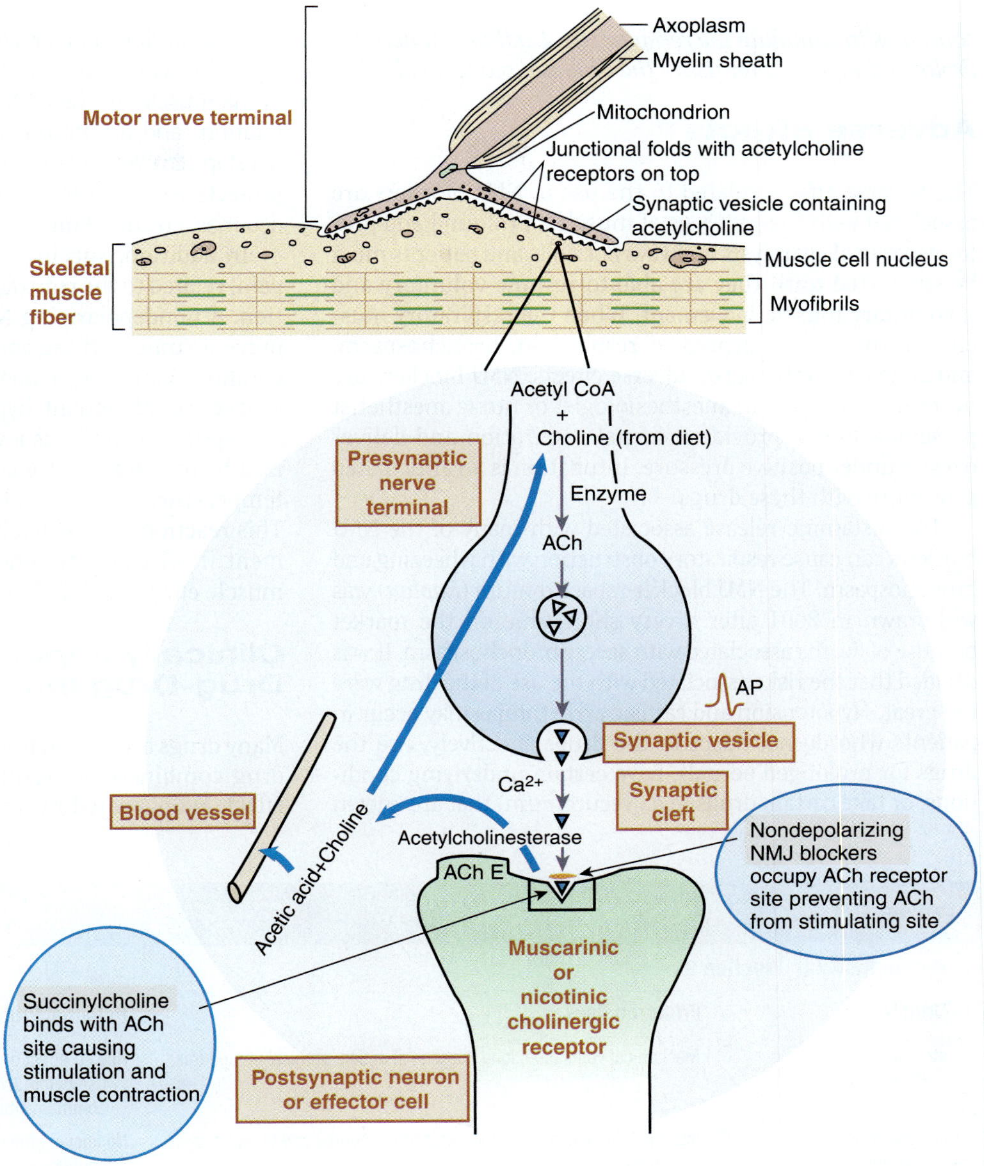

Axoplasm
Myelin sheath
Motor nerve terminal
Mitochondrion
Junctional folds with acetylcholine receptors on top
Synaptic vesicle containing acetylcholine
Skeletal muscle fiber
Muscle cell nucleus
Myofibrils
Acetyl CoA
+
Choline (from diet)
Presynaptic nerve terminal
Enzyme
ACh
AP
Synaptic vesicle
Ca2+
Synaptic cleft
Blood vessel
Acetic acid+Choline
Acetylcholinesterase
ACh E
Nondepolarizing NMJ blockers occupy ACh receptor site preventing ACh from stimulating site
Muscarinic or nicotinic cholinergic receptor
Succinylcholine binds with ACh site causing stimulation and muscle contraction
Postsynaptic neuron or effector cell

FIGURE 28.2 Sites of action of the neuromuscular junction (NMJ) blockers.

100
90
80
70
60
50
40
30
20
10
0
Minutes
atracurium
cisatracurium
mivacurium
pancuronium
rocuronium
tubocurarine
vecuronium
succinylcholine
Onset
Duration

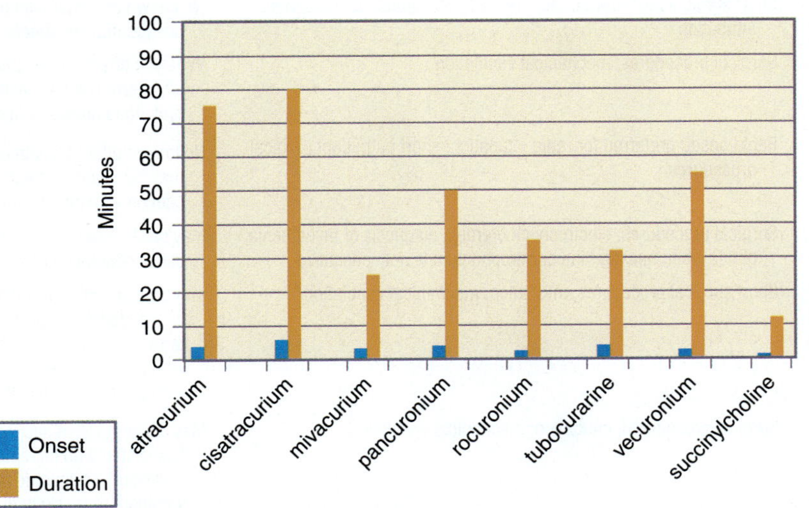

FIGURE 28.3 Onset and duration of NMJ blockers.

continues to stimulate the receptor site, leading to a need for prolonged support after use of the drug is discontinued.

Adverse Effects

The adverse effects related to the use of NMJ blockers are associated with the paralysis of muscles. Profound and prolonged muscle paralysis is always possible, and patients must be supported until they are able to resume voluntary and involuntary muscle movement. When the respiratory muscles are paralyzed, depressed respiration, bronchospasm, and apnea are anticipated adverse effects. NMJ blockers are never used without an anesthesiologist or nurse anesthetist present who can provide artificial respiration and deliver oxygen under positive pressure. Intubation is an anticipated procedure with these drugs.

The histamine release associated with many of the NMJ blockers can cause respiratory obstruction with wheezing and bronchospasm. The NMJ blocker rapacuronium (*Raplon*) was withdrawn in 2001 after a very short time on the market because of deaths associated with severe bronchospasm. It was decided that the risks associated with the use of the drug were too great. Hypotension and cardiac arrhythmias may occur in patients who do not adapt to the drugs effectively, use the drugs for prolonged periods, have certain underlying conditions, or take certain drugs (e.g., vecuronium) that are known to affect cardiovascular receptors. Prolonged drug use may also result in gastrointestinal (GI) dysfunction related to paralysis of the muscles in the GI tract; constipation, vomiting, regurgitation, and aspiration may occur. Decubitus ulcers may develop because the patient loses reflex muscle movement that protects the body from pressure sores. Hyperkalemia may occur as a result of muscle membrane alterations.

In addition, succinylcholine is associated with muscle pain, related to the contraction of the muscles as a first reaction. A nondepolarizing NMJ blocker may be given first to prevent some of these contractions and the associated discomfort. Aspirin also alleviates much of this pain after the procedure. Malignant hyperthermia, which may occur in susceptible patients, is a very serious condition characterized by massive muscle contraction, sharply elevated body temperature, severe acidosis, and if uncontrolled, death. This reaction is most likely with succinylcholine, and treatment involves dantrolene (see Chapter 25) to inhibit the muscle effects of the NMJ blocker (Table 28.1).

Clinically Important Drug–Drug Interactions

Many drugs are known to react with the NMJ blockers. Some drug combinations result in an increased neuromuscular effect. Halogenated hydrocarbon anesthetics such as halo-

Table 28.1 DRUGS IN FOCUS

Neuromuscular Junction Blockers

Drug Name	Preferred Uses	Potential Problems
atracurium (*Tracrium*)	Mechanical ventilation; long duration of action; surgical procedures	Has no effect on pain perception or consciousness; do not use before induction of anesthesia; bradycardia is more common with this drug; reduce dose in renal failure
cisatracurium (*Nimbex*)	Intermediate action; used for surgical procedures and to facilitate intubation	No known effect on pain perception or consciousness; contains benzyl alcohol, avoid use in neonates
mivacurium (*Mivacron*)	Short surgical procedures; rapid recovery; facilitates endotracheal intubation	No known effect on pain perception or consciousness; dosage may be affected by renal or hepatic impairment
pancuronium (*Pavulon*)	Surgical procedures; mechanical ventilation	Vagalytic effect, associated with increased heart rate; long-term use for mechanical ventilation, monitor for prolonged adverse effects
rocuronium (*Zemuron*)	Rapid onset; preferred for rapid intubation; short outpatient surgical procedures	No known effect on pain perception or consciousness; may be associated with pulmonary hypertension; use caution with hepatic impairment
P tubocurarine (*generic*)	Surgical procedures; electroshock therapy; diagnosis of myasthenia gravis when neostigmine or edrophonium is not conclusive	May cause histamine release and increase secretions; may cause neuroganglia blockade and cause hypotension
vecuronium (*Norcuron*)	Short surgical procedures; intubation; mechanical ventilation	May contain benzyl alcohol; avoid use in neonates, can cause fatalities in premature infants; monitor with long-term use during ventilation; if response does not occur with first twitch test, discontinue, may be associated with permanent muscle damage
P succinylcholine (*Anectine, Quelicin*)	Surgical procedures; intubation; mechanical ventilation	May cause myalgia secondary to muscle contraction; associated with increased intraocular pressure; increased intragastric pressure, which may cause vomiting; more likely to cause malignant hyperthermia

thane cause a membrane-stabilizing effect, which greatly enhances the paralysis induced by the NMJ blockers. If these drugs are used together for a procedure, dosage adjustments are necessary, and patients should be monitored closely until they recover fully. A combination of NMJ blockers and aminoglycoside antibiotics (e.g., gentamicin) also leads to increased neuromuscular blockage. Patients who receive this drug combination require a lower dose of NMJ blocker and prolonged support and monitoring after the procedure.

Calcium channel blockers may also greatly increase the paralysis caused by NMJ blockers because of their effects on the calcium channels in the muscle. If the combination of NMJ blockers and calcium channel blockers cannot be avoided, the dose of the NMJ agent should be lowered and the patient should be monitored closely until complete recovery occurs.

If NMJ blockers are combined with cholinesterase inhibitors, the effectiveness of the NMJ blockers is decreased because of a buildup of ACh in the synaptic cleft.

Combination with xanthines (e.g., theophylline, aminophylline) could result in reversal of the neuromuscular blockage. Patients receiving this combination of drugs should be monitored very closely during the procedure for the potential of early arousal and return of muscle function.

Nursing Considerations for Patients Receiving Neuromuscular Junction Blockers

Assessment: History and Examination

Screen for the following conditions, *which could be cautions or contraindications to use of the drug:* any known allergies to these drugs; impaired liver or kidney function; myasthenia gravis; pregnancy or lactation; impaired cardiac or respiratory function; personal or family history of malignant hyperthermia; and fractures, narrow-angle glaucoma, or paraplegia.

Include screening *for baseline status before beginning therapy and for any potential adverse effects.* Assess the following: body temperature; skin color and lesions; affect, orientation, reflexes, pupil size and reactivity, and muscle tone and response; pulse, blood pressure, and electrocardiogram (ECG); respiration and adventitious sounds; bowel sounds and abdominal examination; renal and liver function tests and serum electrolytes.

Nursing Diagnoses

The patient receiving an NMJ blocker may have the following nursing diagnoses related to drug therapy:

- Impaired Gas Exchange related to depressed respirations
- Impaired Skin Integrity related to immobility
- Impaired Verbal Communication
- Fear related to paralysis
- Deficient Knowledge regarding drug therapy

Implementation With Rationale

- Administration of the drug should be performed by trained personnel (usually an anesthesiologist) *because of the potential for serious adverse effects and the need for immediate ventilatory support.*
- Supplies and equipment should be on standby *to maintain airway and provide mechanical ventilation.*
- Do not mix the drug with any alkaline solutions such as barbiturates *because a precipitate may form, making it inappropriate for use.*
- Test patient response and recovery periodically if the drug is being given over a long period to maintain mechanical ventilation. *Discontinue the drug if response does not occur or is greatly delayed.*
- Monitor patient temperature *for prompt detection and treatment of malignant hyperthermia.*
- Maintain dantrolene on standby *for treatment of malignant hyperthermia if it should occur.*
- Arrange for a small dose of a nondepolarizing NMJ blocker before the use of succinylcholine *to reduce the adverse effects associated with muscle contraction.*
- Maintain a cholinesterase inhibitor on standby *to overcome excessive neuromuscular blockade caused by nondepolarizing NMJ blockers.*
- Provide a peripheral nerve stimulator on standby *to assess the degree of neuromuscular blockade, if appropriate.*
- Provide comfort measures *to help the patient tolerate drug effects,* such as pain relief as appropriate; reassurance, support, and orientation *for conscious patients unable to move or communicate;* skin care and turning *to prevent skin breakdown;* and supportive care *for emergencies such as hypotension and bronchospasm.*
- Monitor patient response closely (blood pressure, temperature, pulse, respiration, reflexes) *and adjust dosage accordingly to ensure the greatest therapeutic effect with minimal risk of toxicity.*
- Incorporate information on this drug into a thorough preoperative patient teaching plan *because most patients who receive the drug will be receiving teaching about a particular procedure and will be unconscious when the drug is given.* (See Critical Thinking Scenario 28-1.)
- Offer support and encouragement *to help the patient cope with drug effects.*

CRITICAL THINKING SCENARIO 28-1

Using Succinylcholine in an Elderly Patient

The Situation

S.N., an 82-year-old white woman in very good health, has been admitted to the hospital for an exploratory laparotomy to evaluate a probable abdominal mass. On admission, health care practitioners learned that she had a history of mild hypertension that was well regulated by diuretic therapy. She received a baseline physical examination and preoperative instruction. On the morning of the surgery, it was noted that the anesthesiologist planned to give her a general anesthetic and succinylcholine to ensure muscle paralysis.

Critical Thinking

What nursing care plans should be made for S.N.? *Consider the patient's age and associated chronic problems that often occur with aging. Also consider the support that she has available and potential physical and emotional support that she might need before and after this procedure. Use of a neuromuscular junction (NMJ) blocker in the elderly presents some nursing challenges that may not be seen with younger patients.* What particular nursing care activities should be considered with S.N.?

Because S.N. has been maintained on long-term diuretic therapy, she is at special risk for electrolyte imbalance.

What, if any, complications could arise if S.N. has electrolyte disturbances before surgery?

Discussion

Before surgery, the preoperative teaching protocol should be reviewed with the patient. S.N. should be advised that she may experience back, neck, and throat pain after the procedure. Reassure her that this is normal and that aspirin will be made available to alleviate the discomfort. Review deep breathing and coughing; she may need encouragement to clear secretions from her lungs and ensure full inflation. This is usually easier to do if it is a familiar activity. S.N.'s serum electrolytes should be evaluated before surgery because potassium imbalance can cause unexpected effects with succinylcholine. Renal and hepatic function tests also should be performed to ensure that the dosage of the NMJ blocker is not excessive.

During the procedure, S.N.'s cardiac and respiratory status should be monitored carefully for any potential problems; such effects are more common in people with underlying physical problems. Because of S.N.'s age and potential circulatory problems, she should receive meticulous skin care and turning as soon as the procedure allows this kind of movement. She should be turned frequently during the recovery period, and her skin should be checked for any breakdown. Nursing personnel must be near the patient until she has regained muscle control and the ability to communicate. She should be evaluated for the need for pain medication and position adjustments.

S.N. will require additional teaching about her diagnosis and potential treatment. This should wait until she has regained full ability to communicate and is able to respond and participate in any discussion that may be held. At that time, she may require emotional support and encouragement. It may be necessary to contact available family or social service agencies regarding her physical and medical needs.

Nursing Care Guide for S.N.: Succinylcholine

Assessment: History and Examination

Assess allergies to the drug, and assess for history of COPD, cardiac disorders, myasthenia gravis, hepatic or renal dysfunction, fractures, glaucoma

Concurrent use of aminoglycosides, calcium channel blockers

Focus the physical examination on the following:

CV: Blood pressure, pulse rate, peripheral perfusion, and ECG

CNS: orientation, affect, reflexes, and vision

Skin: color, lesions, texture, and sweating

GU: urinary output, bladder tone

GI: abdominal examination

Respiratory: respirations, adventitious sounds

Nursing Diagnoses

Impaired Gas Exchange related to depressed respirations

Impaired Skin Integrity related to immobility

Deficient Knowledge regarding drug therapy

Impaired Verbal Communication, fear related to paralysis and inability to communicate

Using Succinylcholine in an Elderly Patient *(continued)*

Implementation

Provide comfort and safety measures: positioning, skin care, temperature control, pain medication as needed, maintain airway, ventilate patient, have antidotes on standby.

Provide support and reassurance to deal with paralysis and inability to communicate.

Provide patient teaching about procedure being performed and what to expect.

Assist with life support as needed.

Evaluation

Evaluate drug effects: muscle paralysis.

Monitor for adverse effects: CV effects (tachycardia, hypotension, respiratory distress, increased respiratory secretions), GI effects (constipation, nausea), skin breakdown, anxiety, fear.

Monitor for drug–drug interactions as indicated.

Evaluate effectiveness of patient teaching program and comfort and safety measures.

Constantly monitor vital signs and watch for return of normal muscular function.

Patient Teaching for S.N.

- ☐ Before the surgery is performed, you will be given a drug to paralyze your muscles called a neuromuscular blocking agent. It is important that your muscles do not move at this time because it could interfere with the procedure.
- ☐ Common effects of these drugs include complete paralysis:
  - You will not be able to move or to speak while you are receiving this drug.
  - You will not be able to breathe on your own, and you will receive assistance in breathing.
- ☐ This drug may not affect your level of consciousness, and it can be very frightening to be unable to communicate with anyone around you. Someone will be with you, will try to anticipate your needs, and will explain what is going on at all times.
- ☐ This drug may have no effect on your pain perception. Every effort will be made to make sure that you do not experience pain.
- ☐ You will be receiving succinylcholine; with this drug, you may experience back and throat pain related to muscle contractions that occur. You will be able to take aspirin to relieve this discomfort.
- ☐ Recovery of your muscle function may take 2 to 3 hours, and someone will be nearby at all times until you have recovered from the paralysis.

Evaluation

- Monitor patient response to the drug (adequate muscle paralysis).
- Monitor for adverse effects (respiratory depression, hypotension, bronchospasm, GI slowdown, skin breakdown, fear related to helplessness and inability to communicate).
- Evaluate the effectiveness of the teaching plan (patient can relate anticipated effects of the drug and the recovery process).
- Monitor the effectiveness of comfort measures and compliance with the regimen

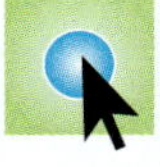

WEB LINKS

Health care providers and patients may want to consult the following Internet sources:

http://www.anesthesia.wisc.edu Information on cholinesterase deficiencies—research, diagnosis, and so on.

http://muscle.ucsd.edu/musintro/jump.shtml Information on the physiology of the NMJ, and the effects of blocking the junction.

http://www.sccm.org Information on paralysis of ventilator patients, particularly the use of pancuronium.

http://www.aana.com/patients/ Patient guides to general anesthetics, what to expect, and how they work.

Points to Remember

- The nerves communicate with muscles at a point called the neuromuscular junction (NMJ), using acetylcholine (ACh) as the neurotransmitter.
- NMJ blockers prevent skeletal muscle function.
- Nondepolarizing NMJ blockers prevent ACh from exciting the muscle, and paralysis ensues because the muscle is unable to respond.

- Depolarizing NMJ blockers cause muscle paralysis by acting like ACh and exciting the muscle (depolarization), preventing repolarization and further stimulation of that muscle cell.
- NMJ blockers are primarily used as adjuncts to general anesthesia, to facilitate endotracheal intubation, to facilitate mechanical ventilation, and to prevent injury during electroconvulsive therapy.
- Adverse effects of NMJ blockers, such as prolonged paralysis, inability to breathe, weakness, muscle pain and soreness, and effects of immobility, are related to muscle function blocking.
- Care of patients receiving NMJ blockers must include support and reassurance because communication is decreased with paralysis; vigilant maintenance of airways and respiration; prevention of skin breakdown; and monitoring for return of function.

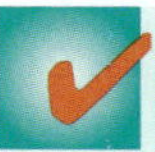

CHECK YOUR UNDERSTANDING

Answers to the questions in this chapter may be found in the Answer Key in the back of the book.

Multiple Choice

Select the best answer to the following.

1. Nondepolarizing NMJ blockers
   a. antagonize acetylcholine to prevent depolarization of muscle cells.
   b. act as agonists of acetylcholine and cause depolarization of muscle cells.
   c. prevent the repolarization of muscle cells.
   d. are associated with painful muscle contractions on administration.

2. Curare is used as a poison on arrow tips in some cultures. Curare
   a. is a depolarizing NMJ blocker.
   b. causes muscle paralysis in the brain, leading to respiratory arrest and death.
   c. is not affected by cooking.
   d. has no clinical use today.

3. Succinylcholine has a rapid onset of action and a short duration of activity because it
   a. does not bind well to receptor sites.
   b. rapidly crosses the blood–brain barrier and is lost.
   c. is broken down by acetylcholinesterase that is found in the plasma.
   d. is very unstable.

4. Whenever NMJ blockers are used, the patient
   a. must be in an intensive care unit.
   b. must be intubated to ensure continuation of respirations.
   c. will have no memory of any events.
   d. will have no adverse effects after the drug is stopped.

5. Malignant hyperthermia can occur with any NMJ blocker, but it most often occurs with succinylcholine. This disorder is treated with
   a. barbiturates.
   b. ice packs.
   c. dantrolene.
   d. diazepam.

6. Patient recovery from an NMJ blocker
   a. is predictable, based on the drug given.
   b. can be affected by genetic enzyme deficiency.
   c. can always be ensured because of the drug half-life.
   d. can be shortened by administration of oxygen.

7. When preparing NMJ blockers for administration, it is important that they
   a. are not mixed in with any alkaline solutions because a precipitate may form.
   b. are not exposed to light.
   c. are not mixed with any other drug.
   d. are not mixed with heparin.

Multiple Response

Select all that apply.

1. An NMJ blocker would be a drug of choice for which of the following?
   a. To facilitate endotracheal intubation
   b. To facilitate mechanical ventilation
   c. To prevent injury during electroconvulsive therapy
   d. To relieve pain during labor and delivery
   e. To treat myasthenia gravis
   f. To treat a patient with a history of malignant hyperthermia

Matching

Match the NMJ blocker with the appropriate brand name.

1. ____________________ atracurium
2. ____________________ cisatracurium

3. ______________________ mivacurium
4. ______________________ pancuronium
5. ______________________ rocuronium
6. ______________________ vecuronium

A. *Tracrium*
B. *Norcuron*
C. *Nimbex*
D. *Mivacron*
E. *Zemuron*
F. *Pavulon*

Web Exercise

Your patient is very concerned about the need for general anesthesia for his elective surgery. The patient has been very involved in his own health care and wants to feel that he is well informed before undergoing the procedure. Go to: http://www.vitacost.com/science/hn/Drug/Anesthetic_Major.htm and help the patient explore the effects and actions of general anesthetics, what to expect, how to be prepared, etc. Prepare a teaching sheet that could be used with other patients as well.

Bibliography and References

Drug facts and comparisons. (2006). St. Louis: Facts and Comparisons.

Gilman, A., Hardman, J. G., & Limbird, L. E. (Eds.). (2006). *Goodman and Gilman's the pharmacological basis of therapeutics* (11th ed.). New York: McGraw-Hill.

Karch, A. M. (2006). *2007 Lippincott's nursing drug guide.* Philadelphia: Lippincott Williams & Wilkins.

Porth, C. M. (2005). *Pathophysiology: Concepts of altered health states* (7th ed.). Philadelphia: Lippincott Williams & Wilkins.

Professional's guide to patient drug facts. (2006). St. Louis: Facts and Comparisons.

PART
V

Drugs Acting on the Autonomic Nervous System

CHAPTER 29

Introduction to the Autonomic Nervous System

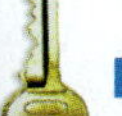

KEY TERMS

acetylcholinesterase
adrenergic receptors
alpha-receptor
autonomic nervous system
beta-receptor
cholinergic receptor
ganglia
monoamine oxidase (MAO)
muscarinic receptor
nicotinic receptor
parasympathetic nervous system
sympathetic nervous system

LEARNING OBJECTIVES

Upon completion of this chapter, you will be able to:

1. Describe how the autonomic nervous system differs anatomically from the rest of the nervous system.
2. Outline a sympathetic response and the clinical manifestation of this response.
3. Describe the alpha- and beta-receptors found within the sympathetic nervous system by sites and actions that follow the stimulation of each kind of receptor.
4. Outline the events that occur with stimulation of the parasympathetic nervous system.
5. Define the terms muscarinic receptor and nicotinic receptor, giving an example of each.

The **autonomic nervous system (ANS)** is sometimes called the involuntary or visceral nervous system because it mostly functions with little conscious awareness of its activity. Working closely with the endocrine system, the ANS helps to regulate and integrate the body's internal functions within a relatively narrow range of normal, on a minute-to-minute basis. The ANS integrates parts of the central nervous system (CNS) and peripheral nervous system to automatically react to changes in the internal and external environment (Figure 29.1).

General Functions

The main nerve centers for the ANS are located in the hypothalamus, the medulla, and the spinal cord. Nerve impulses that arise in peripheral structures are carried to these centers by afferent nerve fibers. These integrating centers in the CNS respond by sending out efferent impulses along the autonomic nerve pathways. These impulses adjust the functioning of various internal organs in ways that keep the body's internal environment constant, or homeostatic.

The ANS works to regulate blood pressure, heart rate, respiration, body temperature, water balance, urinary excretion, and digestive functions, among other things. The minute-to-minute control exerted by this system results from an interrelationship between opposing divisions of the autonomic system: the sympathetic and the parasympathetic divisions (Figure 29.2).

Divisions of the Autonomic Nervous System

Throughout the ANS, nerve impulses are carried from the CNS to the outlying organs by way of a two-neuron system. In most peripheral nervous system activities, the CNS nerve body sends an impulse directly to an effector organ or muscle. The ANS does not send impulses directly to the periphery. Instead, axons from CNS neurons end in **ganglia**, or groups of nerve bodies that are packed together, located outside the CNS. These ganglia receive information from the preganglionic neuron that started in the CNS and relay that information along postganglionic neurons. The postganglionic neurons transmit impulses to the neuroeffector cells—muscles, glands, and organs. The ANS is divided into two branches (sympathetic and parasympathetic) that differ in three basic ways: (1) the location of the originating cells in the CNS, (2) the location of the nerve ganglia, and (3) the preganglionic and postganglionic neurons (Table 29.1).

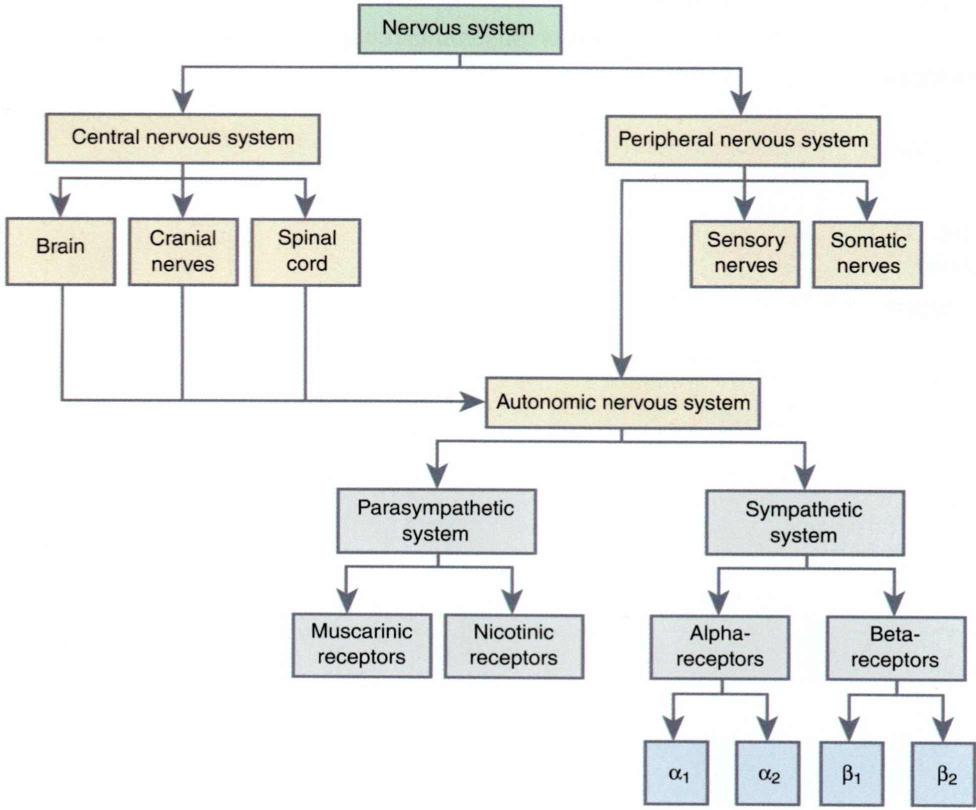

FIGURE 29.1 Organization of the nervous system.

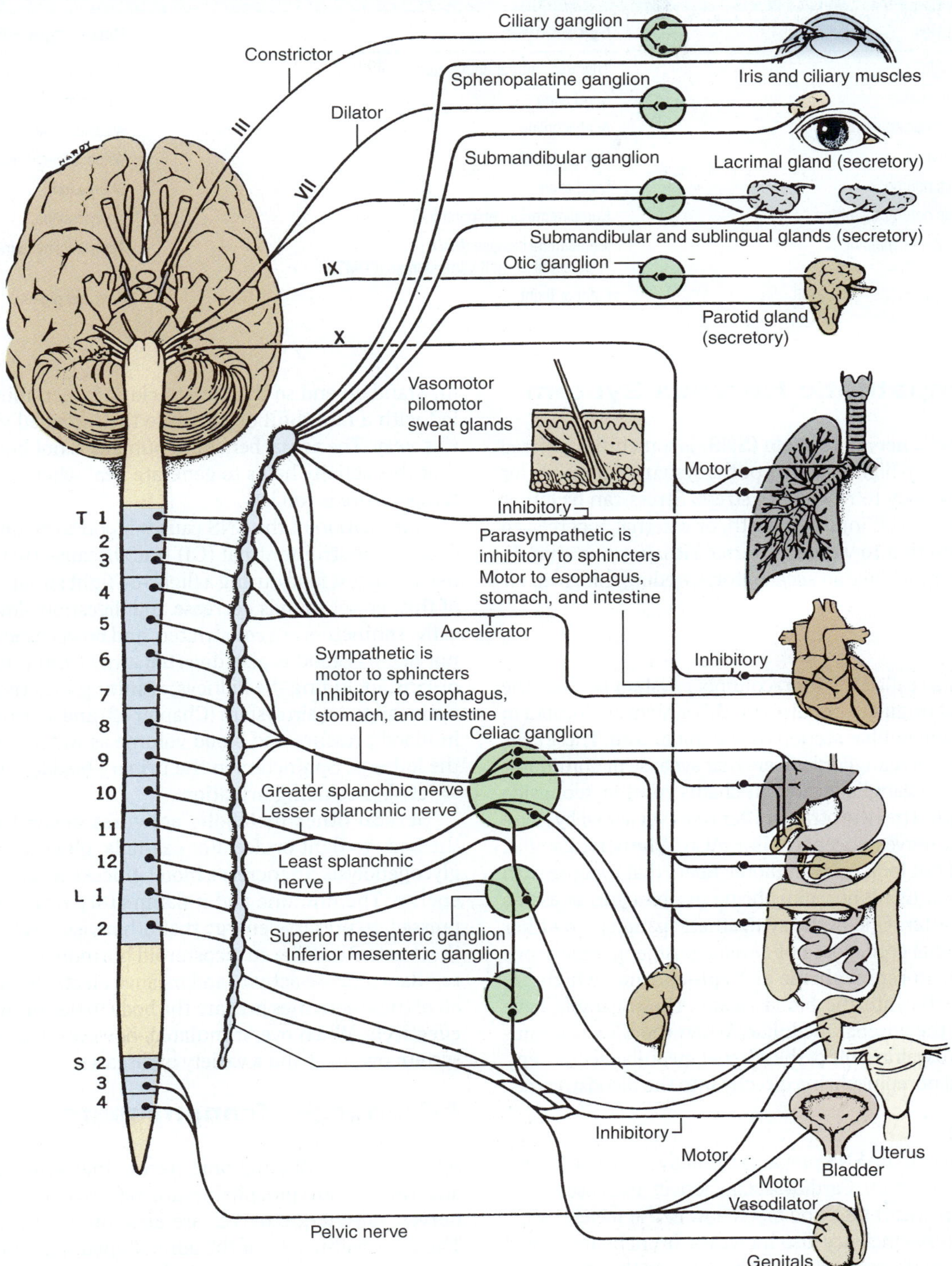

FIGURE 29.2 The autonomic nervous system. The parasympathetic, or craniosacral, division sends long preganglionic fibers that synapse with a second nerve cell in ganglia located close to or within the organs that are then innervated by short postganglionic fibers. The sympathetic, or thoracolumbar, division sends relatively short preganglionic fibers to the chains of paravertebral ganglia and to certain outlying ganglia. The second cell shown sends relatively long postganglionic fibers to the organs it innervates.

Table 29.1 Comparison of the Sympathetic and Parasympathetic Nervous Systems

Characteristic	Sympathetic	Parasympathetic
CNS nerve origin	Thoracic, lumbar spinal cord	Cranium, sacral spinal cord
Preganglionic neuron	Short axon	Long axon
Preganglionic neurotransmitter	Acetylcholine	Acetylcholine
Ganglia location	Next to spinal cord	Within or near effector organs
Postganglionic neuron	Long axon	Short axon
Postganglionic neurotransmitter	Norepinephrine, epinephrine	Acetylcholine
Neurotransmitter terminator	Monoamine oxidase (MAO), catechol-*O*-methyltransferase (COMT)	Acetylcholinesterase
General response	Fight or flight	Rest and digest

The Sympathetic Nervous System

The **sympathetic nervous system (SNS)** is sometimes referred to as the "fight-or-flight" system, or the system responsible for preparing the body to respond to stress. Stress can be either internal, such as cell injury or death, or external, a perceived or learned reaction to various external situations or stimuli. The SNS acts much like an accelerator, speeding things up for action.

Anatomy

The SNS is also called the thoracolumbar system because the CNS cells that originate impulses for this system are located in the thoracic and lumbar sections of the spinal cord. These cells send out short preganglionic fibers that synapse or communicate with nerve ganglia located in chains running alongside the spinal cord. The neurotransmitter that is released by these preganglionic nerves is acetylcholine (ACh). The nerve ganglia, in turn, send out long postganglionic fibers that synapse with neuroeffectors, using norepinephrine or epinephrine as the neurotransmitter. One of the sympathetic ganglia, on either side of the spinal cord, does not develop postganglionic axons but produces norepinephrine and epinephrine, which are secreted directly into the bloodstream. These ganglia have evolved into the adrenal medullae. When the SNS is stimulated, the chromaffin cells of the adrenal medullae secrete epinephrine and norepinephrine directly into the bloodstream.

Functions

When stimulated, the SNS prepares the body to flee or to turn and fight (Figure 29.3). Cardiovascular activity increases, as do blood pressure, heart rate, and blood flow to the skeletal muscles. Respiratory efficiency also increases; bronchi are dilated to allow more air to enter with each breath, and the respiratory rate increases. Pupils dilate to permit more light to enter the eye, to improve vision in darkened areas (which helps a person to see in order to fight or flee). Sweating increases to dissipate heat generated by the increased metabolic activity.

Piloerection (hair standing on end) also occurs. In lower animals, this important protection mechanism makes the fur stand on end so that an attacking larger animal is often left with a mouthful of fur while the intended victim scurries away. The actual benefit to humans is not known, except that this activity helps to generate heat when the core body temperature is too low.

Stimulation of the SNS causes blood to be diverted away from the gastrointestinal (GI) tract because there is no real need to digest food during a flight-or-fight situation. Because of this, bowel sounds decrease and digestion slows dramatically; sphincters are constricted, and bowel evacuation cannot occur. Blood is also diverted away from other internal organs, including the kidneys, resulting in activation of the renin–angiotensin system (Chapter 42) and a further increase in blood pressure and blood volume as water is retained by the kidneys. Sphincters in the urinary bladder are also constricted, precluding urination.

Several other metabolic activities occur that prepare the body to fight or flee. For example, glucose is formed by glycogenolysis, to increase blood glucose levels and provide energy. The immune and inflammatory reactions are suppressed, to preserve energy that otherwise might be used by these activities. The corticosteroid hormones are released to regulate glucose activity and balance electrolytes. Together, all of these activities prepare the body to flee or to fight more effectively. When overstimulated, however, they can lead to system overload and a variety of diseases.

Adrenergic Transmission

Sympathetic postganglionic nerves that synthesize, store, and release norepinephrine are referred to as adrenergic nerves. Adrenergic nerves are also found within the CNS. The chromaffin cells of the adrenal medulla also are adrenergic because they synthesize, store, and release norepinephrine as well as epinephrine.

Norepinephrine Synthesis and Storage

Norepinephrine belongs to a group of structurally related chemicals called catecholamines that also includes dopamine and epinephrine. Norepinephrine is made by the nerve cells

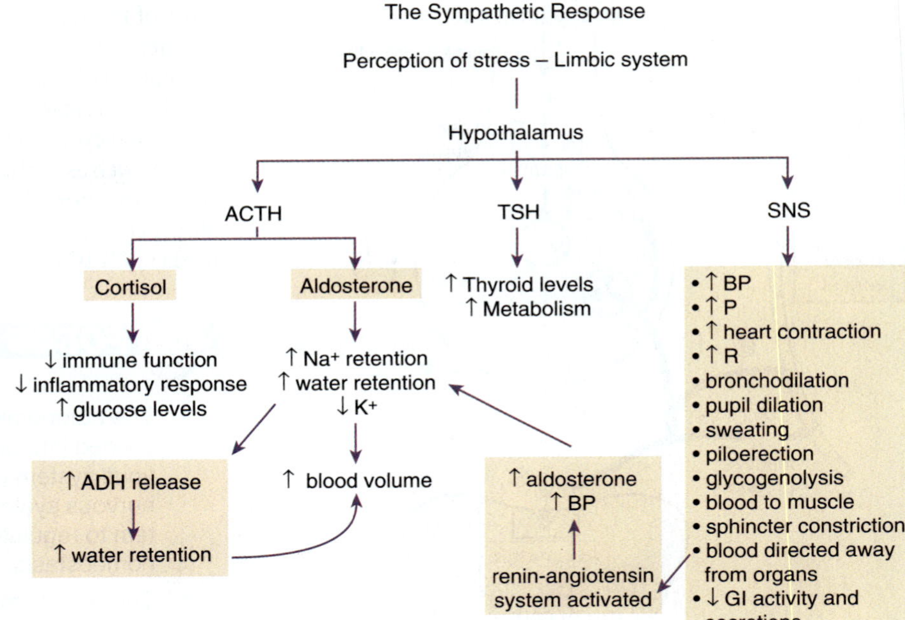

FIGURE 29.3 The "fight-or-flight" response: the sympathetic stress reaction. ACTH, adrenocorticotropic hormone; ADH, antidiuretic hormone; BP, blood pressure; GI, gastrointestinal; P, pulse; R, heart rate; SNS, sympathetic nervous system; TSH, thyroid stimulating hormone.

using tyrosine, which is obtained in the diet. Dihydroxyphenylalanine (dopa) is produced by a nerve, using tyrosine from the diet and other chemicals. With the help of the enzyme dopa decarboxylase, it is converted to dopamine, which in turn is converted to norepinephrine in adrenergic cells. The norepinephrine then is stored in granules or storage vesicles within the cell. These vesicles move down the nerve axon to the terminals of the axon, where they line up along the cell membrane. To be an adrenergic nerve, the nerve must contain all of the enzymes and building blocks necessary to produce norepinephrine (Figure 29.4).

Norepinephrine Release

When the nerve is stimulated, the action potential travels down the nerve axon and arrives at the axon terminal (see Chapter 19). The action potential then depolarizes the axon membrane. This action allows calcium into the nerve, causing the membrane to contract and the storage vesicles to fuse with the cell membrane, and then dump their load of norepinephrine into the synaptic gap or cleft. The norepinephrine travels across the very short gap to very specific adrenergic receptor sites on the effector cell on the other side of the synaptic gap.

Adrenergic Receptors

The receptor sites that react with neurotransmitters at adrenergic sites have been classified as **alpha-receptors** and **beta-receptors**; further classifications include alpha$_1$-, alpha$_2$-, beta$_1$-, and beta$_2$-receptors (Table 29.2). The distinction arises because different drugs that are known to affect the SNS may affect parts of the sympathetic response but not all of it. It is thought that receptors may respond to different concentrations of norepinephrine or different ratios of norepinephrine and epinephrine. **Adrenergic receptors** can be stimulated by the neurotransmitter released from the axon in the immediate vicinity, and they can be further stimulated by circulating norepinephrine and epinephrine secreted directly into the bloodstream by the adrenal medulla.

Alpha-Receptors

Alpha$_1$-receptors are found in blood vessels, in the iris, and in the urinary bladder. In blood vessels, they can cause vasoconstriction and increase peripheral resistance, thus raising blood pressure. In the iris, they cause pupil dilation. In the urinary bladder, they cause the increased closure of the internal sphincter.

Alpha$_2$-receptors are located on nerve membranes and act as modulators of norepinephrine release. When norepinephrine is released from a nerve ending, it crosses the synaptic cleft to react with its specific receptor site. Some of it also flows back to react with the alpha-receptor on the nerve membrane. This causes a reflex decrease in norepinephrine release. In this way, the alpha$_2$-receptor helps to prevent overstimulation of effector sites. These receptors are also found on the beta cells in the pancreas, where they help to moderate the insulin release stimulated by SNS activation.

Beta-Receptors

Beta$_1$-receptors are found in cardiac tissue, where they can stimulate increased myocardial activity and increased heart rate. They are also responsible for increased lipolysis or breakdown of fat for energy in peripheral tissues.

Beta$_2$-receptors are found in the smooth muscle in blood vessels, in the bronchi, in the periphery, and in uterine muscle. In blood vessels, beta$_2$ stimulation leads to vasodilation. Beta$_2$-receptors also cause dilation in the bronchi. In the

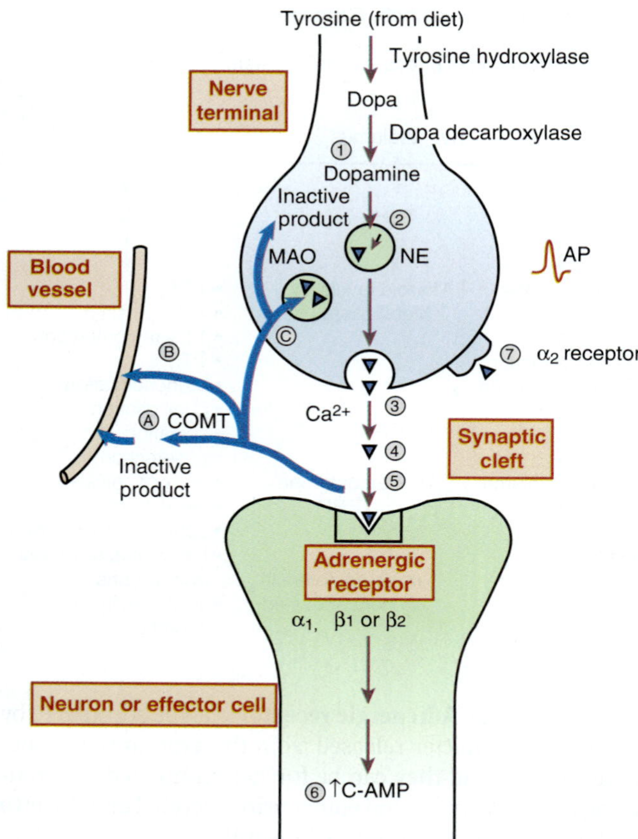

FIGURE 29.4 Sequence of events at an adrenergic synapse. *1.* Dopamine, a precursor of norepinephrine (NE), is synthesized from tyrosine in several steps. Metyrosine inhibits tyrosine hydroxylase; a drug given with dopa to parkinsonian patients inhibits dopa decarboxylase. *2.* Dopamine is taken into the storage vesicle and converted to NE. *3.* Release of neurotransmitter by action potential (AP) in presynaptic nerve. *4.* Diffusion of neurotransmitter across synaptic cleft. *5.* Combination of neurotransmitter with receptor. The events resulting from NE's occupying of receptor sites depend on the nature of the postsynaptic cell. *6.* Interaction of NE with many β-receptors leads to increased synthesis of cyclic adenosine monophosphate (C-AMP). *7.* Feedback control at α_2-receptor leads to decreased NE relapse from presynaptic neuron. An enzyme, catechol-*O*-methyl transferase (COMT), inactivates the NE (A), but the most important way in which the action of NE is terminated is by reuptake into the presynaptic neuron (C), where it may be reused or inactivated by another enzyme, monoamine oxidase (MAO). The neurotransmitter may also diffuse away from the synaptic cleft (B).

periphery, they can cause increased muscle and liver breakdown of glycogen and increased release of glucagon from the alpha cells of the pancreas. Stimulation of beta_2-receptors in the uterus results in relaxed uterine smooth muscle.

Termination of Transmission

Once norepinephrine has been released into the synaptic cleft, stimulation of the receptor site is terminated only when any extra norepinephrine, as well as the neurotransmitter that has reacted with the receptor site, is disposed of. Most of the free norepinephrine molecules are taken up by the nerve terminal that released them in a process called reuptake. This neurotransmitter is then repackaged into vesicles to be released later with nerve stimulation. This is an effective recycling effort by the nerve. Enzymes are also in the area, as well as in the liver, to metabolize or biotransform any remaining norepinephrine or any norepinephrine that is absorbed into circulation. These enzymes are **monoamine oxidase (MAO)** and catechol-*O*-methyl transferase (COMT).

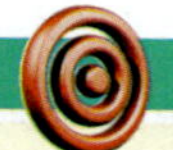

FOCUS POINTS

- The autonomic nervous system (ANS), which is divided into two branches—the sympathetic nervous system (SNS) and the parasympathetic nervous system—works with the endocrine system to regulate internal functioning and maintain homeostasis.
- The SNS is responsible for the fight-or-flight response.
- The SNS is composed of CNS cells arising in the thoracic or lumbar area of the spinal cord and long postganglionic axons that react with effector cells. The neurotransmitter used by the preganglionic cells is acetylcholine (ACh); the neurotransmitter used by the postganglionic cells is norepinephrine.
- Based on the effectors that they stimulate, SNS adrenergic receptors are classified as alpha_1-, alpha_2-, beta_1-, or beta_2-receptors.

The Parasympathetic Nervous System

In many areas, the **parasympathetic nervous system** works in opposition to the SNS. This allows the autonomic system to maintain a fine control over internal homeostasis. For instance, the SNS increases heart rate, and the parasympathetic system decreases it. Therefore, the ANS can influence heart rate by increasing or decreasing sympathetic activity or by increasing or decreasing parasympathetic activity. This is very much like controlling the speed of a car by moving between the accelerator and the brake or combining the two. Whereas the SNS is associated with the stress reaction and expenditure of energy, the parasympathetic system is associated with activities that help the body to store or conserve energy, a "rest-and-digest" response (Table 29.3).

Anatomy

The parasympathetic system is sometimes called the craniosacral system because the CNS neurons that originate parasympathetic impulses are found in the cranium (one of the most important being the vagus or tenth cranial nerve)

Table 29.2 Physiological Effects of Specific Receptor Sites in the Autonomic Nervous System

Sympathetic System	Parasympathetic System
Alpha$_1$-Receptors	Muscarinic receptors
Vasoconstriction	Pupil constriction
Increased peripheral resistance with increased blood pressure	Accommodation of the lens
Contracted piloerection muscles	Decreased heart rate
Pupil dilation	Increased GI motility
Thickened salivary secretions	Increased GI secretions
Closure of urinary bladder sphincter	Increased urinary bladder contraction
Male sexual emission	Male erection
Alpha$_2$-Receptors	Sweating
Negative feedback control of norepinephrine release from presynaptic neuron	Nicotinic receptors
Moderation of insulin release from the pancreas	Muscle contractions
Beta$_1$-Receptors	Release of norepinephrine from the adrenal medulla
Increased heart rate	Autonomic ganglia stimulation
Increased conduction through the atrioventricular node	
Increased myocardial contraction	
Lipolysis in peripheral tissues	
Beta$_2$-Receptors	
Vasodilation	
Bronchial dilation	
Increased breakdown of muscle and liver glycogen	
Release of glucagon from the pancreas	
Relaxation of uterine smooth muscle	
Decreased gastrointestinal (GI) muscle tone and activity	
Decreased GI secretions	
Relaxation of urinary bladder detrusor muscle	

Table 29.3 Effects of Autonomic Stimulation

Effector Site	Sympathetic Reaction	Parasympathetic Reaction
Eye structures		
Iris radial muscle	Contraction (pupil dilates)	—
Iris sphincter muscle	—	Contraction (pupil constricts)
Ciliary muscle	—	Contraction (lens accommodates for near vision)
Lacrimal glands	—	↑ Secretions
Heart	↑ Rate, contractility ↑ Atrioventricular conduction	↓ Rate ↓ Atrioventricular conduction
Blood vessels		
Skin, mucous membranes	Constriction	—
Skeletal muscle	Dilation	—
Bronchial muscle	Relaxation (dilation)	Constriction
Gastrointestinal system		
Muscle motility and tone	↓ Activity	↑ Activity
Sphincters	Contraction	Relaxation
Secretions	↓ Secretions	↑ Activity
Salivary glands	Thick secretions	Copious, watery secretions
Gallbladder	Relaxation	Contraction
Liver	Glyconeogenesis	—
Urinary bladder		
Detrusor muscle	Relaxation	Contraction
Trigone muscle and sphincter	Contraction	Relaxation
Sex organs		
Male	Emission	Erection (vascular dilation)
Female	Uterine relaxation	—
Skin structures		
Sweat glands	↑ Sweating	—
Piloerector muscles	Contracted (goosebumps)	—

—, no reaction or response.

and in the sacral area of the spinal cord (see Figure 29.1). It has long preganglionic axons that meet in ganglia located close to or within the organ that will be affected. The postganglionic axon is very short, going directly to the effector cell. The neurotransmitter used by both the preganglionic and postganglionic neurons is ACh.

Functions

Parasympathetic system stimulation results in the following actions:

- Increased motility and secretions in the GI tract to promote digestion and absorption of nutrients.
- Decreased heart rate and contractility to conserve energy and provide rest for the heart.
- Constriction of the bronchi, with increased secretions.
- Relaxation of the GI and urinary bladder sphincters, allowing evacuation of waste products.
- Pupillary constriction, which decreases the light entering the eye and decreases stimulation of the retina.

These activities are aimed at increasing digestion, absorption of nutrients, and building of essential proteins, as well as a general conservation of energy.

Cholinergic Transmission

Neurons that use ACh as their neurotransmitter are called cholinergic neurons. There are four basic kinds of cholinergic nerves:

1. All preganglionic nerves in the ANS, both sympathetic and parasympathetic
2. Postganglionic nerves of the parasympathetic system and a few SNS nerves, such as those that re-enter the spinal cord and cause general body reactions such as sweating
3. Motor nerves on skeletal muscles
4. Cholinergic nerves within the CNS

Acetylcholine Synthesis and Storage

ACh is an ester of acetic acid and an organic alcohol called choline. Cholinergic nerves use choline, obtained in the diet, to produce ACh. The last step in the production of the neurotransmitter involves choline acetyltransferase, an enzyme that is also produced within cholinergic nerves. Just like norepinephrine, the ACh is produced in the nerve and travels to the end of the axons, where it is packaged into vesicles. To be a cholinergic nerve, the nerve must contain all of the enzymes and building blocks necessary to produce ACh.

Acetylcholine Release

The vesicles full of ACh move to the nerve membrane; when an action potential reaches the nerve terminal, calcium entering the cell causes the membrane to contract and secrete the neurotransmitter into the synaptic cleft. The ACh travels across the synaptic cleft and reacts with very specific **cholinergic receptor** sites on the effector cell (Figure 29.5).

ACh receptors are found on organs and muscles. They have been classified as **muscarinic receptors** and **nicotinic receptors**. This classification is based on very early research of the ANS that used muscarine (a plant alkaloid from mushrooms) and nicotine (a plant alkaloid found in tobacco plants) to study the actions of the parasympathetic system.

Muscarinic Receptors

As the name implies, muscarinic receptors are receptors that can be stimulated by muscarine. They are found in visceral effector organs, in sweat glands, and in some vascular smooth muscle. Stimulation of muscarinic receptors causes pupil constriction, increased GI motility and secretions (including

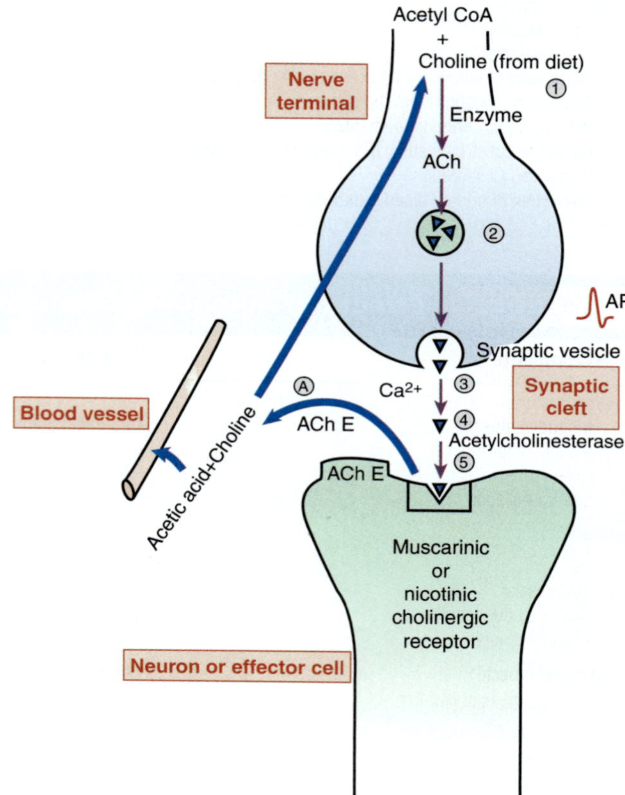

FIGURE 29.5 Sequence of events at a cholinergic synapse. *1.* Synthesis of acetylcholine (ACh) from choline (a substance in the diet) and a cofactor (the enzyme is choline acetyltransferase, CoA). *2.* Uptake of neurotransmitter into storage (synaptic) vesicle. *3.* Release of neurotransmitter by action potential (AP) in presynaptic nerve. *4.* Diffusion of neurotransmitter across synaptic cleft. *5.* Combination of neurotransmitter with receptor. The events resulting from ACh's occupying of receptor sites depend on the nature of the postsynaptic cell. ACh excites some cells and inhibits others. An enzyme, acetylcholinesterase (AChE), found in the tissues and on the postsynaptic cell, inactivates ACh (A). Some of the products diffuse into the circulation, but most of the choline formed is taken up and reused by the cholinergic neuron.

saliva), increased urinary bladder contraction, and a slowing of the heart rate.

Nicotinic Receptors

Nicotinic receptors are located in the CNS, the adrenal medulla, the autonomic ganglia, and the neuromuscular junction. Stimulation of nicotinic receptors causes muscle contractions, autonomic responses, and release of norepinephrine and epinephrine from the adrenal medulla.

Termination of Transmission

Once the effector cell has been stimulated by ACh, it is important to stop the stimulation and get rid of the ACh. The destruction of ACh is carried out by the enzyme **acetylcholinesterase**. This enzyme reacts with the ACh to form a chemically inactive compound. The breakdown of the released ACh is accomplished in a thousandth of a second and the receptor is vacated, allowing the effector membrane to repolarize and be ready for the next stimulation.

WEB LINKS

To explore the virtual ANS, consult the following Internet source: http://www.InnerBody.com

Points to Remember

- The autonomic nervous system (ANS) works with the endocrine system to regulate internal functioning and maintain homeostasis.
- The ANS is divided into two branches, the sympathetic nervous system (SNS) and the parasympathetic nervous system.
- The two branches of the ANS work in opposition to maintain minute-to-minute regulation of the internal environment and to allow rapid response to stress situations.
- The SNS, when stimulated, is responsible for the fight-or-flight response. It prepares the body for immediate reaction to stressors by increasing metabolism, diverting blood to big muscles, and increasing cardiac and respiratory function.
- The parasympathetic system, when stimulated, acts as a rest-and-digest response. It increases the digestion, absorption, and metabolism of nutrients and slows metabolism and function to save energy.
- The SNS is composed of CNS cells arising in the thoracic or lumbar area of the spinal cord, short preganglionic axons, ganglia located near the spinal cord, and long postganglionic axons that react with effector cells. The neurotransmitter used by the preganglionic cells is acetylcholine (ACh); the neurotransmitter used by the postganglionic cells is norepinephrine.
- One SNS ganglion on either side of the spinal cord does not develop postganglionic axons but instead secretes norepinephrine directly into the bloodstream to travel throughout the body to react with adrenergic receptor sites. These ganglia evolved into the adrenal medulla.
- The parasympathetic system comprises CNS cells that arise in the cranium and sacral region of the spinal cord, long preganglionic axons that secrete ACh, ganglia located very close to or within the effector tissue, and short postganglionic axons that also secrete ACh.
- Norepinephrine is made by adrenergic nerves using tyrosine from the diet. It is packaged in storage vesicles that align on the axon membrane and is secreted into the synaptic cleft when the nerve is stimulated. It reacts with specific receptor sites and is then broken down by MAO or COMT to relax the receptor site and recycle the building blocks of norepinephrine.
- ACh is made by choline from the diet and packaged into storage vesicles to be released by the cholinergic nerve into the synaptic cleft. ACh is broken down to an inactive form almost immediately by acetylcholinesterase.
- SNS adrenergic receptors are classified as being alpha$_1$-, alpha$_2$-, beta$_1$-, or beta$_2$-receptors based on the effectors that they stimulate.
- Parasympathetic system receptors are classified as muscarinic or nicotinic, depending on what response they have to these plant alkaloids.

CHECK YOUR UNDERSTANDING

Answers to the questions in this chapter may be found in the Answer Key in the back of the book.

Multiple Choice

Select the best answer to the following.

1. The autonomic nervous system functions to
   a. maintain balance and posture.
   b. maintain the special senses.
   c. regulate and integrate internal functions of the body.
   d. coordinate peripheral and central nerve pathways.

2. The autonomic nervous system differs from other systems in the CNS in that
   a. it uses only peripheral pathways.
   b. it affects organs and muscles by way of a two-neuron system.
   c. it uses a unique one-neuron system.
   d. it bypasses the CNS in all of its actions.

3. If you suspect that a person is very stressed and is experiencing a sympathetic stress reaction, you would expect to find
   a. increased bowel sounds and urinary output.
   b. constricted pupils and warm, flushed skin.
   c. slow heart rate and decreased systolic blood pressure.
   d. dilated pupils and elevated systolic blood pressure.

4. Stimulating only the beta_2-receptors in the sympathetic nervous system would result in
   a. increased heart rate.
   b. increased myocardial contraction.
   c. vasodilation and bronchial dilation.
   d. uterine contraction.

5. Once a postganglionic receptor site has been stimulated, the neurotransmitter must be broken down immediately. The sympathetic system breaks down postganglionic neurotransmitters by using
   a. liver enzymes and acetylcholinesterase.
   b. acetylcholinesterase and MAO.
   c. COMT and liver enzymes.
   d. MAO and COMT.

6. The parasympathetic nervous system, in most situations, opposes the actions of the sympathetic nervous system, allowing the autonomic nervous system to
   a. generally have no effect.
   b. maintain a fine control over internal homeostasis.
   c. promote digestion.
   d. respond to stress most effectively.

7. Cholinergic neurons, those using acetylcholine as their neurotransmitter, would *not* be found in
   a. motor nerves on skeletal muscles.
   b. preganglionic nerves in the sympathetic and parasympathetic systems.
   c. postganglionic nerves in the parasympathetic system.
   d. the adrenal medulla.

8. Stimulation of the parasympathetic nervous system would cause
   a. slower heart rate and increased GI secretions.
   b. faster heart rate and urinary retention.
   c. vasoconstriction and bronchial dilation.
   d. pupil dilation and muscle paralysis.

Multiple Response

Select all that apply.

1. The sympathetic nervous system
   a. is called the thoracolumbar system.
   b. is called the fight-or-flight system.
   c. is called the craniosacral system.
   d. uses acetylcholine as its sole neurotransmitter.
   e. uses epinephrine as its sole neurotransmitter.
   f. is active during a stress reaction.

2. The sympathetic system uses catecholamines at the postganglionic receptors. Which of the following are considered to be catecholamines?
   a. Dopamine
   b. Norepinephrine
   c. Acetylcholine
   d. Epinephrine
   e. Monoamine oxidase
   f. Serotonin

Matching

Match the following words with the appropriate definition.

1. ____________________ autonomic nervous system
2. ____________________ sympathetic nervous system
3. ____________________ parasympathetic nervous system
4. ____________________ ganglia
5. ____________________ adrenergic receptors
6. ____________________ cholinergic receptors
7. ____________________ alpha-receptors
8. ____________________ beta-receptors

9. ______________________ muscarinic receptors

10. ______________________ nicotinic receptors

11. ______________________ acetylcholinesterase

12. ______________________ monoamine oxidase (MAO)

A. Adrenergic receptors that are found in smooth muscles
B. Closely packed group of nerve cell bodies
C. Fight-or-flight response mediator
D. Enzyme that breaks down norepinephrine
E. Cholinergic receptors that also respond to stimulation by nicotine
F. Rest-and-digest response mediator
G. Receptor sites on effectors that respond to acetylcholine
H. Adrenergic receptors found in the heart, lungs, and vascular smooth muscle
I. Receptor sites on effectors that respond to norepinephrine
J. Cholinergic receptors that also respond to stimulation by muscarine
K. Portion of the central and peripheral nervous systems that, with the endocrine system, functions to maintain internal homeostasis
L. Enzyme that deactivates acetylcholine released from the nerve axon

Bibliography and References

Fox, S. (1991). *Perspectives on human biology.* Dubuque, IA: Wm. C. Brown.

Ganong, W. (2003). *Review of medical physiology* (21st ed.). Norwalk, CT: Appleton & Lange.

Gilman, A., Hardman, J. G., & Limbird, L. E. (Eds.). (2006). *Goodman and Gilman's the pharmacological basis of therapeutics* (11th ed.). New York: McGraw-Hill.

Guyton, A., & Hall, J. (2000). *Textbook of medical physiology* (10th ed.). Philadelphia: W. B. Saunders.

Porth, C. M. (2005). *Pathophysiology: Concepts of altered health states* (7th ed.). Philadelphia: Lippincott Williams & Wilkins.

CHAPTER 30

Adrenergic Agents

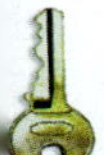

KEY TERMS

adrenergic agonist
alpha-agonist
beta-agonist
glycogenolysis
sympathomimetic

LEARNING OBJECTIVES

Upon completion of this chapter, you will be able to:

1. Describe two ways that sympathomimetic drugs act to produce effects at adrenergic receptors.
2. Describe the therapeutic actions, indications, pharmacokinetics, contraindications, most common adverse reactions, and important drug–drug interactions associated with adrenergic agents.
3. Discuss the use of adrenergic agents across the lifespan.
4. Compare and contrast the prototype drugs dopamine, phenylephrine, and isoproterenol with other adrenergic agents.
5. Outline the nursing considerations, including important teaching points, for patients receiving an adrenergic agent.

ALPHA- AND BETA-ADRENERGIC AGONISTS

dobutamine
P dopamine
ephedrine
epinephrine
metaraminol
norepinephrine

ALPHA-SPECIFIC ADRENERGIC AGONISTS

clonidine (alpha$_1$-specific)
midodrine
P phenylephrine

BETA-SPECIFIC ADRENERGIC AGONISTS

albuterol
bitolterol
isoetharine
P isoproterenol
levalbuterol
metaproterenol
pirbuterol
salmeterol
terbutaline

(ALSO SEE BETA-ADRENERGIC AGONISTS IN CHAPTER 55.)

Adrenergic agonists are also called **sympathomimetic** drugs because they mimic the effects of the sympathetic nervous system (SNS). The therapeutic and adverse effects associated with these drugs are related to their stimulation of adrenergic receptor sites. The use of adrenergic agonists varies from ophthalmic preparations for dilating pupils (Box 30.1) to systemic preparations used to support people who are in shock. They are used in patients of all ages (Box 30.2).

Adrenergic Agonists

The therapeutic and adverse effects associated with these drugs are related to their stimulation of adrenergic receptor sites (Figure 30.1). That stimulation can be either direct, by occupation of the adrenergic receptor, or indirect, by modulation of the release of neurotransmitters from the axon. Some drugs act in both ways.

BOX 30.1 FOCUS ON **CLINICAL SKILLS**

Administering Ophthalmic Medications

Some of the adrenergic agonists are applied in the eye; it is important to review the administration technique. First, wash hands thoroughly. Do not touch the dropper to the eye or to any other surfaces. Have the patient tilt his or her head back or lie down and stare upward. Gently grasp the lower eyelid and pull the eyelid away from the eyeball. Instill the prescribed number of drops into the pouch formed by the eyelid, and then release the lid slowly. Have the patient close the eye and look downward. Apply gentle pressure to the inside corner of the eye for 3–5 minutes to retard drainage. Do not rub the eyeball, and do not rinse the dropper. If more than one type of eyedrop is being used, wait 5 minutes before administering the next one.

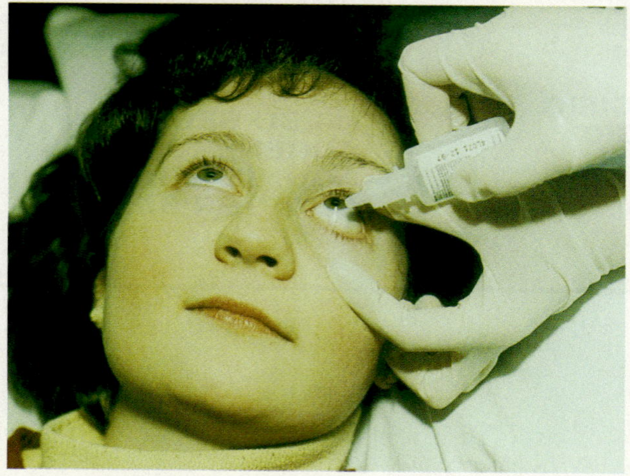

After gently exposing the lower conjunctival sac, the nurse administers an eyedrop (with permission from Taylor, C., Lillis, C., & LeMone, P. (2004). *Lippincott's photo atlas of medication administration.* Philadelphia: Lippincott Williams & Wilkins).

Alpha- and Beta-Adrenergic Agonists

Drugs that are generally sympathomimetic (that is, they stimulate all of the adrenergic receptors) are called **alpha-** and **beta-agonists** (Table 30.1). Some of these drugs are preparations of catecholamines.

Epinephrine (*Adrenalin, Sus-Phrine,* and others) is a naturally occurring catecholamine that interacts with both alpha- and beta-adrenergic receptors. It is used therapeutically in the treatment of shock, when increased blood pressure and heart contractility are essential; as one of the primary treatments for bronchospasm, by direct dilation of the bronchi; as an ophthalmic agent; and to produce a local vasoconstriction that prolongs the effects of local anesthetics.

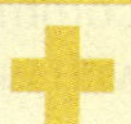

FOCUS ON **PATIENT SAFETY**

The herb ephedra has been in the headlines in recent years because people who were using the herb to promote weight loss have died suddenly. Several states have limited its sale within the state, and the U.S. Food and Drug Administration (FDA) is studying the herb—an isomer of epinephrine—and pushing for the authority to regulate the product. Patients should be taught about the potential danger of this product. Any patient who is at risk for serious reactions to the stimulatory effects of a sympathomimetic—patients with narrow-angle glaucoma, dehydration, cerebral or peripheral vascular disease, cardiac disease or arrhythmias, hypertension, renal dysfunction, thyroid disease, diabetes, prostatic disorders, pregnancy, or lactation—should receive direct teaching about the dangers of this product. To review the FDA warnings in preparing your teaching protocol, go to http://nccam.nih.gov/health/alerts/ephedra/consumer advisory.htm.

Norepinephrine (*Levophed*), another naturally occurring catecholamine, is not used as frequently as epinephrine. It is given intravenously to treat shock or during cardiac arrest to get sympathetic activity, but it has been replaced in recent years by dopamine.

Dopamine (*Intropin*) is the sympathomimetic of choice for the treatment of shock. It stimulates the heart and blood pressure but also causes a renal and splanchnic arteriole dilation that increases blood flow to the kidney, preventing the diminished renal blood supply and possible renal shutdown that can occur with epinephrine or norepinephrine.

Dobutamine (*Dobutrex*) is a synthetic catecholamine that has a slight preference for $beta_1$-receptor sites. It is used in the treatment of congestive heart failure because it can increase myocardial contractility without much change in rate and does not increase the oxygen demand of the

BOX 30.2 **DRUG THERAPY ACROSS THE LIFESPAN**

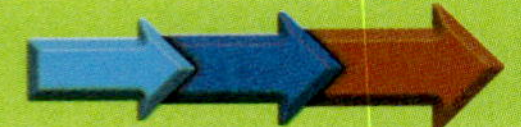

Adrenergic Agents

CHILDREN

Children are at greater risk for complications associated with the use of adrenergic agents, including tachycardia, hypertension, tachypnea, and gastrointestinal complications. The dosage for these agents needs to be calculated from the child's body weight and age. It is good practice to have a second person check the dosage calculation before administering the drug to avoid potential toxic effects. Children should be carefully monitored and supported during the use of these drugs.

Phenylephrine is often found in over-the-counter (OTC) allergy and cold preparations, and parents need to be instructed to be very careful with the use of these drugs—they should check the labels for ingredients, monitor the recommended dosage, and avoid combining drugs that contain similar ingredients.

ADULTS

Adults being treated with adrenergic agents for shock or shock-like states require constant monitoring and dosage adjustments based on their response. Patients who may be at increased risk for cardiac complications should be monitored very closely and started on a lower dose.

Adults using these agents for glaucoma or for seasonal rhinitis need to be cautioned about the use of OTC drugs and alternative therapies that might increase the drug effects and cause serious adverse effects.

Many of these drugs are used in emergency situations and may be used during pregnancy and lactation. In general, there are no adequate studies about their effects during pregnancy and lactation, and in those situations they should be used only if the benefit to the mother is greater than the risk to the fetus or neonate.

OLDER ADULTS

Older patients are more likely to experience the adverse effects associated with these drugs—central nervous system, cardiovascular, gastrointestinal, and respiratory. Because older patients often have renal or hepatic impairment, they are also more likely to have toxic levels of the drug related to changes in metabolism and excretion. Older patients should be started on lower doses of the drugs and should be monitored very closely for potentially serious arrhythmias or blood pressure changes.

They also should be cautioned about the use of OTC drugs and complementary therapies that could increase drug effects and cause serious adverse reactions.

cardiac muscle, an advantage over all of the other sympathomimetic drugs.

Ephedrine (*Pretz-D*) is a synthetically produced plant alkaloid that stimulates the release of norepinephrine from nerve endings and directly acts on adrenergic receptor sites. Although ephedrine was once used for everything from the treatment of shock to chronic management of asthma and allergic rhinitis, its use in many areas is declining because of the availability of less toxic drugs with more predictable onset and action. It is used as a nasal decongestant in a topical, nasal form.

Metaraminol (*Aramine*) is a synthetic agent that is very similar to norepinephrine. It is given as a single parenteral injection to prevent hypotension by increasing myocardial contractility and causing peripheral vasoconstriction. Its use is limited to situations in which dopamine or norepinephrine cannot be used.

Therapeutic Actions and Indications

The effects of the sympathomimetic drugs are mediated by the adrenergic receptors in target organs: heart rate increases with increased myocardial contractility, bronchi dilate and respirations increase in rate and depth, vasoconstriction occurs with increase in blood pressure, intraocular pressure decreases, **glycogenolysis** (breakdown of glucose stores so that the glucose can be used as energy) occurs throughout the body, pupils dilate, and sweating can increase (see Figure 30.1). These drugs are indicated for the treatment of hypotensive states or shock, bronchospasm, and some types of asthma. As noted earlier, dopamine has become the drug of choice for the treatment of shock and hypotensive states because it causes an increase in renal blood flow and does not cause the renal shutdown that has been associated with other agents. Ephedrine is also widely used as a local nasal drug for the treatment of seasonal rhinitis.

Pharmacokinetics

These drugs are generally absorbed rapidly after injection or passage through mucous membranes. They are metabolized in the liver and excreted in the urine. Because the sympathomimetic drugs stimulate the SNS, they should be used during pregnancy and lactation only if the benefits to the mother clearly outweigh any potential risks to the fetus or neonate.

Contraindications and Cautions

The alpha- and beta-agonists are contraindicated in patients with pheochromocytoma *because the systemic overload of catecholamines could be fatal;* with tachyarrhythmias or ventricular fibrillation *because the increased heart rate and oxygen consumption usually caused by these drugs could exacerbate these conditions;* with hypovolemia, *for which fluid replacement would be the treatment for the associated hypotension;* and with halogenated hydrocarbon general anesthetics, *which sensitize the myocardium to catecholamines and could cause serious cardiac effects.* Caution should be used with any kind of peripheral vascular disease (e.g., atherosclerosis, Raynaud's disease, diabetic endarteritis), *which could be exacerbated by systemic vasoconstriction.*

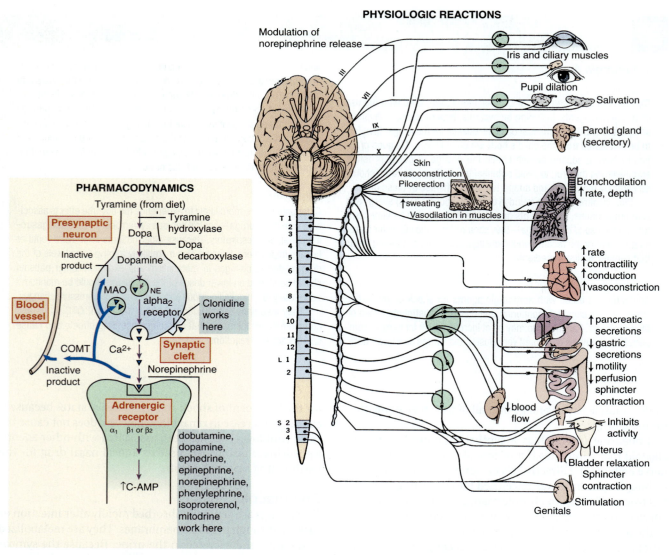

FIGURE 30.1 Pharmacodynamics of adrenergic agonists and associated physiologic reactions.

Adverse Effects

The adverse effects associated with the use of alpha- and beta-adrenergic agonists may be associated with the drugs' effects on the SNS: arrhythmias, hypertension, palpitations, angina, and dyspnea related to the effects on the heart and cardiovascular (CV) system; nausea and vomiting, related to the depressant effects on the gastrointestinal (GI) tract; and headache, sweating, and piloerection, related to the sympathetic stimulation.

Clinically Important Drug–Drug Interactions

Increased effects of tricyclic antidepressants and monoamine oxidase inhibitors (MAOIs) can occur because of the increased norepinephrine levels or increased receptor stimulation that occurs with both drugs. There is an increased risk of hypertension if alpha- and beta-adrenergic agonists are given with any other drugs that cause hypertension. (See also Box 30.3.)

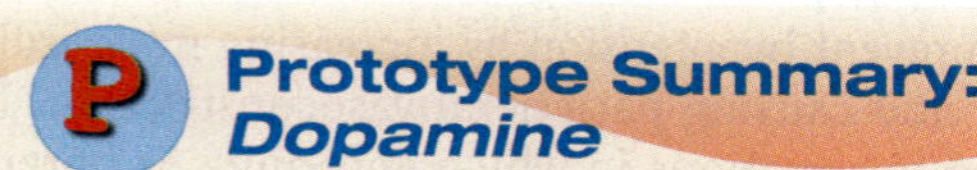

Prototype Summary: *Dopamine*

Indications: Correction of hemodynamic imbalances present in shock

Actions: Acts directly and by the release of norepinephrine from sympathetic nerve terminals; mediates dilation of vessels in the renal and splanchnic beds to maintain renal perfusion while stimulating the sympathetic response

Pharmacokinetics:

Route	Onset	Peak	Duration
IV	1–2 min	10 min	Length of infusion

Table 30.1 DRUGS IN FOCUS

Alpha- and Beta-Adrenergic Agonists

Drug Name	Dosage/Route	Usual Indications
dobutamine (*Dobutrex*)	2.5–10 mcg/kg/min IV with dosage adjusted based on patient response	Treatment of congestive heart failure
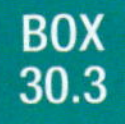 dopamine (*Intropin*)	Initially 5–10 mcg/kg/min IV with incremental increases up to 20–50 mcg/kg/min based on patient response	Treatment of shock
ephedrine (*Pretz-D*)	Adult: 25–50 mg IM, Sub-Q, or IV for acute treatment; 25–50 mg PO for asthma maintenance; instill solution in each nostril q4h for seasonal rhinitis Pediatric: 25–100 mg/m^2 IM or Sub-Q in four to six divided doses; 3 mg/kg/day in four to six divided doses PO, Sub-Q, or IV for bronchodilation; instill in each nostril q4h for seasonal rhinitis in children >6 yr	Treatment of signs and symptoms of seasonal rhinitis; hypotensive episodes
epinephrine (*Adrenalin, Sus-Phrine*)	Adult: 0.5–1.0 mg IV for acute treatment; 0.3–0.5 mg Sub-Q or IM for respiratory distress; may be used in nebulizer or as topical nasal drops Pediatric: 0.005–0.01 mg/kg IV, base dose on age, weight, and response; do not repeat more than q6h; topical nasal drops for children >6 yr as needed	Treatment of shock; to prolong effects of regional anesthetic
metaraminol (*Aramine*)	Adult: 2–10 mg Sub-Q or IM to prevent hypotension; 15–100 mg IV in 250–500 mL sodium chloride or dextrose solution to treat hypotension Pediatric: 0.01 mg/kg IV as a single dose	Treatment of shock if norepinephrine or dopamine cannot be used; prevention of hypotension with spinal anesthesia
norepinephrine (*Levophed*)	8–12 mcg base/min IV; base rate and dosage on patient response	Treatment of shock; cardiac arrest

$T_{1/2}$: 2 min; metabolized in the liver, excreted in the urine

Adverse effects: Tachycardia, ectopic beats, anginal pain, hypotension, dyspnea, nausea, vomiting, headache

BOX 30.3 HERBAL AND ALTERNATIVE THERAPIES

Patients being treated with adrenergic agonists who are also taking ma huang, guarana, or caffeine are at increased risk for overstimulation, including increased blood pressure, stroke, and death. Counsel patients to avoid these combinations.

Nursing Considerations for Patients Receiving Alpha- and Beta-Adrenergic Agonists

Assessment: History and Examination

Screen for the following conditions, *which could be cautions or contraindications to use of the drug:* any known allergies to these drugs; pheochromocytoma, tachyarrhythmias or ventricular fibrillation, or hypovolemia; general anesthesia with halogenated hydrocarbon anesthetics; and the presence of vascular disease, *which would require cautious use of the drug.*

Include screening *for baseline status before beginning therapy and for any potential adverse effects:* skin color and temperature; pulse, blood pressure, and electrocardiogram (ECG); respiration, adventitious sounds; urine output and electrolytes.

Nursing Diagnoses

The patient receiving an alpha- and beta-agonist may have the following nursing diagnoses related to drug therapy:

- Acute Pain related to CV and systemic effects
- Decreased Cardiac Output related to CV effects
- Ineffective Tissue Perfusion related to CV effects
- Deficient Knowledge regarding drug therapy

Implementation With Rationale

- Use extreme caution in calculating and preparing doses of these drugs *because even small errors could have serious effects.* Always dilute drug before use, if it is not prediluted *to prevent tissue irritation on injection.*

- Monitor patient response closely (blood pressure, ECG, urine output, cardiac output) and adjust dosage accordingly *to ensure the most benefit with the least amount of toxicity.*
- Maintain phentolamine on standby *in case extravasation occurs;* infiltration of the site with 10 mL saline containing 5 to 10 mg phentolamine is usually effective in saving the area.
- Provide thorough patient teaching, including measures to avoid adverse effects, warning signs of problems, and the need for monitoring and evaluation, *to enhance patient knowledge about drug therapy and to promote compliance.*
- Offer support and encouragement *to deal with the drug regimen.* (See Critical Thinking Scenario 30-1.)

Evaluation

- Monitor patient response to the drug (improvement in blood pressure, ocular pressure, bronchial airflow).
- Monitor for adverse effects (cardiovascular changes, decreased urine output, headache, GI upset).
- Evaluate the effectiveness of the teaching plan (patient can name the drug, dosage, adverse effects to watch for, specific measures to avoid adverse effects).
- Monitor the effectiveness of comfort measures and compliance with regimen.

FOCUS POINTS

- Adrenergic agonists (sympathomimetics) stimulate the adrenergic receptors in the SNS; sympathomimetic drugs stimulate the SNS.
- Alpha- and beta-adrenergic agonists stimulate all of the adrenergic receptors in the SNS. They induce a fight-or-flight response and are frequently used to treat shock.

Alpha-Specific Adrenergic Agonists

Alpha-specific adrenergic agonists, or alpha-agonists, are drugs that bind primarily to alpha-receptors, rather than to beta-receptors. Currently, three drugs are in this class (Table 30.2): phenylephrine (*Neo-Synephrine, Allerest, AK-Dilate,* and others), midodrine (*ProAmatine*), and clonidine (*Catapres*).

Phenylephrine, a potent vasoconstrictor with little or no effect on the heart or bronchi, is used in many combination cold and allergy products. Parenterally it is used to treat shock or shock-like states, to overcome paroxysmal supraventricular tachycardia, to prolong local anesthesia, and to maintain blood pressure during spinal anesthesia. Topically it is used to treat allergic rhinitis and to relieve the symptoms of otitis media. Ophthalmically it is used to dilate the pupils for eye examination, before surgery, or to relieve elevated eye pressure associated with glaucoma.

Midodrine is an oral drug that is used to treat orthostatic hypotension in patients who do not respond to traditional therapy. It activates alpha-adrenergic receptors, leading to peripheral vasoconstriction and an increase in vascular tone and blood pressure. This effect can cause a serious supine hypertension. Patients need to be monitored in the standing, sitting, and supine positions to determine whether this will be a problem.

Clonidine specifically stimulates CNS alpha$_2$-receptors. This leads to decreased sympathetic outflow from the CNS because the alpha$_2$-receptors moderate the release of norepinephrine from the nerve axon. Clonidine is used to treat essential hypertension as a step 2 drug, to treat chronic pain in cancer patients in combination with opiates and other drugs, and to ease withdrawal from opiates. Because of its centrally acting effects, clonidine is associated with many more CNS effects (bad dreams, sedation, drowsiness, fatigue, headache) than other sympathomimetics. Because it can also cause extreme hypotension, congestive heart failure, and bradycardia owing to its centrally mediated effects, it should be used carefully with any patient who is susceptible to such conditions. It is available in an oral and transdermal form and in injection form for epidural infusion to control pain.

Therapeutic Actions and Indications

The therapeutic effects of the alpha-specific adrenergic agonists come from the stimulation of alpha-receptors within the SNS (see Figure 30.1). The uses are varied, depending on the route of the drug and the drug being used. Clonidine is frequently used to treat essential hypertension. Phenylephrine is found in many cold and allergy products because it is so effective in constricting topical vessels and decreasing the swelling, signs, and symptoms of rhinitis. Midodrine is reserved for use in patients with orthostatic hypotension who do not respond to other therapies because it can cause supine hypertension.

Pharmacokinetics

These drugs are generally well absorbed and reach peak levels in a short period—20 to 45 minutes. They are widely distributed in the body, metabolized in the liver, and primarily excreted in the urine. There are no adequate studies about use during pregnancy and lactation, so use should be reserved for situations in which the benefit to the mother outweighs any potential risk to the fetus or neonate.

Contraindications and Cautions

The alpha-specific adrenergic agonists are contraindicated in the presence of allergy to the specific drug; severe hypertension or tachycardia *because of possible additive effects;*

CRITICAL THINKING SCENARIO 30-1

Adrenergic Agonist Toxicity

The Situation

M.C. is a 26-year-old man who has recently moved to the northeastern United States from New Mexico. He has been suffering from sinusitis, runny nose, and cold-like symptoms for 2 weeks. He appears at an outpatient clinic with complaints of headache, "jitters," inability to sleep, loss of appetite, and a feeling of impending doom. He states that he feels "on edge" and has not been productive in his job as a watch repairman and jewelry maker. According to his history, M.C. has been treated with several different drugs for nocturnal enuresis, a persisting childhood problem. Only ephedrine, which he has been taking for 2 years, has been successful. He has no other significant health problems. He denies any side effects from the use of ephedrine but does admit to self-medicating his nagging cold with over-the-counter (OTC) preparations—a nasal spray used four times a day and a combination decongestant–pain reliever. A physical examination reveals a pulse of 104, BP 154/86, R 16. The patient appears flushed and slightly diaphoretic.

Critical Thinking

What are the important nursing implications for M.C.? *Think about the problems that confront a patient in a new area seeking health care for the first time.*

What could be causing the problems that M.C. presents with? *The diagnosis of ephedrine overdose was eventually made based on the patient history of OTC drug use and the presenting signs and symptoms.*

Keeping in mind that this diagnosis means M.C. has an overstimulated sympathetic stress reaction; what other physical problems can be anticipated? *Overwhelming feelings of anxiety and stress are influencing M.C.'s response to work and health care.*

Given this fact, how may the nurse best deal with explaining the problem and how it could have happened—without making the patient feel uninformed or that the practice of his former health care provider is being questioned?

What treatment should be planned and what teaching points should be covered for M.C.?

Discussion

The first step in caring for M.C. is establishing a trusting relationship to help alleviate some of the anxiety he is feeling. Being in a new state and seeking health care in a new setting can be very stressful for patients under normal circumstances. In M.C.'s case, the sympathomimetic effects of the drugs that he has been taking make him feel even more anxious and jittery.

A careful patient history will help determine whether there are any underlying medical problems that could be exacerbated by these drug effects. A review of M.C.'s nocturnal enuresis and the treatments that have been tried will enhance understanding of his former health care and suggest possible implications for further study. This questioning will also reassure M.C. that he is an important member of the health team and that the information he has to offer is valued.

A careful review of the OTC drugs that M.C. has been using will be informative for the patient as well as for the health care providers who have not actually checked OTC drugs for those specific ingredients, but combining them to ease signs and symptoms often results in toxic levels and symptoms of overdose. M.C. will need a full teaching program about the effects of his ephedrine and which OTC drugs to avoid. The treatment for his current problems involves withdrawal of the OTC drugs; when these drug levels fall, the signs and symptoms will disappear. M.C. may also wish to avoid nicotine and caffeine, because these stimulants could increase his "jitters."

To build trust and ensure that the underlying cause of the problem was drug toxicity, M.C. should receive written patient instructions that highlight warning signs to report, including chest pain, palpitations, and difficulty voiding. He also should be given the health care provider's telephone number with instructions to call the next day and report on his health status. Finally, specimens of nasal discharge should be cultured and antibiotic treatment prescribed, if appropriate.

Nursing Care Guide for M.C.: Adrenergic Agonist Toxicity

Assessment: History and Examination

Assess the patient's history of drug allergies, cardiovascular dysfunction, pheochromocytoma, narrow-angle glaucoma, prostatic hypertrophy, thyroid disease, or diabetes, as well as concurrent use of MAOIs, tricyclic antidepressants, reserpine, ephedrine, or urinary alkalinizers.

Focus the physical examination on the following:

CV: Blood pressure, pulse rate, peripheral perfusion, and ECG

(continued)

Adrenergic Agonist Toxicity *(continued)*

CNS: orientation, affect, reflexes, peripheral sensation, and vision

Skin: color, temperature

GI: abdominal examination

GU: urine output, bladder percussion, prostate palpation

Respiratory: respiratory rate, adventitious sounds

Nursing Diagnoses

Decreased Cardiac Output related to CV effects

Acute Pain related to CV and systemic effects

Impaired Tissue Perfusion related to CV effects

Deficient Knowledge regarding drug therapy

Implementation

Ensure safe and appropriate administration of the drug.

Provide comfort and safety measures: temperature and lighting control, mouth care, and skin care.

Monitor blood pressure, pulse rate, and respiratory status throughout drug therapy.

Provide support and reassurance to deal with drug therapy and drug effects.

Provide patient teaching about drug name, dosage, side effects, precautions, and warning signs to report.

Evaluation

Evaluate drug effects: relief of enuresis.

Monitor for adverse effects: CV effects, dizziness, confusion, headache, rash, difficulty voiding, sweating, flushing, and pupillary dilation.

Monitor for drug–drug interactions as indicated.

Evaluate effectiveness of patient teaching program and comfort and safety measures.

Patient Teaching for M.C.

- ☐ The drug that you have been taking is ephedrine. It is called an adrenergic agonist (or a sympathomimetic drug). Ephedrine acts by mimicking the effects of the sympathetic nervous system, which is the part of your nervous system that is responsible for your response to fear or danger (this is called the "fight-or-flight" response). Because this drug triggers many effects in the body, you may experience some undesired adverse effects. It is crucial to discuss the effect of the drug with your health care provider and to try to make the effect as tolerable as possible.
- ☐ If the drug is in a solution, check it before each use. If the solution is pink, brown, or black, discard it.
- ☐ If you have diagnosed prostate problems, it might help to void before taking each dose of the drug.
- ☐ Some of the following adverse effects may occur:
  - *Restlessness or shaking:* If these occur, avoid driving, operating machinery, or performing delicate tasks.
  - *Flushing or sweating:* Avoid warm temperatures and heavy clothing; frequent washing with cool water may help.
  - *Heart palpitations:* If you feel your heart is beating too fast, or skipping beats, sit down for awhile and rest. If the feeling becomes too uncomfortable, notify your health care provider.
  - *Sensitivity to light:* Avoid glaring lights or wear sunglasses if in bright light. Be careful when moving between extremes of light because your vision may not adjust quickly.
  - Report any of the following to your health care provider: *difficulty voiding, chest pain, difficulty breathing, dizziness, headache, or changes in vision.*
- ☐ Do not stop taking this drug suddenly; make sure you have enough of your prescription. This drug dosage should be reduced gradually over 2 to 4 days when you are instructed to discontinue it by your health care provider.
- ☐ Avoid over-the-counter medications, including cold and allergy remedies and diet pills. If you feel that you need one of these, check with your health care provider first.
- ☐ Tell any health care provider who takes care of you that you are taking this drug.
- ☐ Keep this drug and all medication out of the reach of children. And do not share this drug with other people.

narrow-angle glaucoma, *which could be exacerbated by arterial constriction;* or pregnancy *because of potential adverse effects on the fetus.*

They should be used with caution in the presence of cardiovascular disease or vasomotor spasm *because these conditions could be aggravated by the vascular effects of the drug;* thyrotoxicosis or diabetes *because of the thyroid-stimulating and glucose-elevating effects of sympathetic stimulation;* lactation *because the drug may be passed to the infant and cause alpha-specific adrenergic stimulation;* or renal or hepatic impairment *which could interfere with metabolism and excretion of the drug.*

Therapeutic Actions and Indications

The therapeutic effects of isoproterenol are related to its stimulation of the beta-adrenergic receptors. Increased heart rate, conductivity, and contractility; bronchodilation; increased blood flow to skeletal muscles and splanchnic beds; and relaxation of the uterus are the drug's desired effects. Isoproterenol is indicated for the treatment of shock to increase cardiac activity; with cardiac arrest and certain ventricular arrhythmias to stimulate cardiac activity and conduction. It is especially effective in treating heart blocks in transplanted hearts.

Pharmacokinetics

Isoproterenol is rapidly distributed after injection; it is metabolized in the liver and excreted in the urine. The half-life is relatively short—less than 1 hour. Isoproterenol should be used during pregnancy and lactation only if the benefits to the mother clearly outweigh potential risks to the fetus or neonate.

Contraindications and Cautions

Isoproterenol is contraindicated in the presence of allergy to the drug or any components of the drug; with pulmonary hypertension; during anesthesia with halogenated hydrocarbons, *which sensitize the myocardium to catecholamines and could cause a severe reaction;* with eclampsia, uterine hemorrhage, and intrauterine death, *which could be complicated by uterine relaxation or increased blood pressure;* and during pregnancy and lactation *because of potential effects on the fetus or neonate.* Caution should be used with diabetes, thyroid disease, vasomotor problems, degenerative heart disease, or history of stroke, *all of which could be exacerbated by the sympathomimetic effects of the drug.*

Adverse Effects

Patients receiving this drug often experience adverse effects related to the stimulation of sympathetic adrenergic receptors. CNS effects include restlessness, anxiety, fear, tremor, fatigue, and headache. Cardiovascular effects can include tachycardia, angina, myocardial infarction, and palpitations. Pulmonary effects can be severe, ranging from difficulty breathing, coughing, and bronchospasm to severe pulmonary edema. GI upset, nausea, vomiting, and anorexia can occur as a result of the slowdown of the GI system by the SNS. Other anticipated effects can include sweating, pupil dilation, rash, and muscle cramps.

Clinically Important Drug–Drug Interactions

Increased sympathomimetic effects can be expected if this drug is taken with other sympathomimetic drugs. Decreased therapeutic effects can occur if this drug is combined with beta-adrenergic blockers.

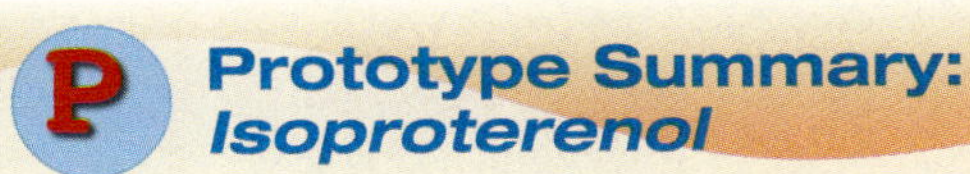

Prototype Summary: Isoproterenol

Indications: Management of bronchospasm during anesthesia; vasopressor during shock; adjunct in the management of cardiac standstill and arrest, as well as serious ventricular arrhythmias that require increased inotropic action.

Actions: Acts on beta-adrenergic receptors to produce increased heart rate, positive inotropic effect, bronchodilation, and vasodilation

Pharmacokinetics:

Route	Onset	Duration
IV	Immediate	1–2 min

$T_{1/2}$: Unknown; metabolized in the tissues

Adverse effects: Restlessness, apprehension, anxiety, fear, cardiac arrhythmias, tachycardia, nausea, vomiting, heartburn, respiratory difficulties, coughing, pulmonary edema, sweating, pallor

Nursing Considerations for Patients Receiving Beta-Specific Adrenergic Agonists

Assessment: History and Examination

Screen for the following conditions, *which could be cautions or contraindications to the use of the drug:* any known allergies to any drug or any components of the drug; pulmonary hypertension; anesthesia with halogenated hydrocarbons, *which sensitize the myocardium to catecholamines and could cause severe reaction;* eclampsia, uterine hemorrhage, and intrauterine death, *which could be complicated by uterine relaxation or increased blood pressure;* pregnancy and lactation *because of potential effects on the fetus or neonate;* diabetes, thyroid disease, vasomotor problems, degenerative heart disease, or history of stroke, *all of which could be exacerbated by the sympathomimetic effects of the drugs.*

Physical assessment should include screening *for baseline status before beginning therapy and for any potential adverse effects:* skin color and temperature; pulse, blood pressure, and ECG; respiration; adventitious sounds; and urine output and electrolytes.

Nursing Diagnoses

The patient receiving beta-agonists may have the following nursing diagnoses related to drug therapy:

- Acute Pain related to CV and systemic effects
- Decreased Cardiac Output related to CV effects

- Ineffective Tissue Perfusion related to CV effects
- Deficient Knowledge regarding drug therapy

Implementation With Rationale

- Monitor patient pulse and blood pressure carefully during administration *in order to arrange to discontinue the drug at any sign of pulmonary edema.*
- Maintain a beta-adrenergic blocker on standby when giving parenteral isoproterenol *in case severe reaction occurs.*
- Use minimal doses of isoproterenol needed to achieve desired effects *because drug tolerance can occur over time.*
- Arrange for supportive care and comfort measures, including rest and environmental control, *to relieve CNS effects;* provide headache medication and safety measures if CNS effects occur *to provide comfort and prevent injury;* avoid overhydration *to prevent pulmonary edema.*
- Provide thorough patient teaching, including the name of the drug, dosage, anticipated adverse effects, measures to avoid drug-related problems, warning signs of problems, and proper administration techniques, *to enhance patient knowledge about drug therapy and to promote compliance.*
- Offer support and encouragement *to help the patient deal with the drug regimen.*

Evaluation

- Monitor patient response to the drug (improvement in condition being treated, stabilization of blood pressure, prevention of preterm labor, cardiac stimulation).
- Monitor for adverse effects (GI upset, CNS changes, respiratory problems).
- Evaluate the effectiveness of the teaching plan (patient can name drug, dosage, adverse effects to watch for, specific measures to avoid adverse effects).
- Monitor the effectiveness of comfort measures and compliance to the regimen.

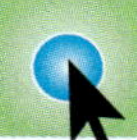

WEB LINKS

Health care providers and patients may want to consult the following Internet sources:

http://arbl.cvmbs.colostate.edu/hbooks/pathphys/endocrine/adrenal/medhormones.html Information on epinephrine and basic sympathomimetic effects.

http://www.ccmtutorials.com/cvs/clinshock/clinshock6.htm Information on the current treatment of shock.

http://www.aacn.org Information on the acute nursing care of patients in shock as well as research articles.

http://www.acc.org Information on cardiovascular research, treatments, and heart transplantation.

Points to Remember

- Adrenergic agonists are drugs used to stimulate the adrenergic receptors within the SNS. They are also called sympathomimetic drugs because they mimic the effects of the SNS.
- Sympathomimetic drugs are used when sympathetic stimulation is needed. The adverse effects associated with these drugs are usually also a result of sympathetic stimulation.
- Alpha- and beta-adrenergic agonists stimulate all of the adrenergic receptors in the SNS. They are used to induce a fight-or-flight response and are frequently used to treat shock.
- Alpha-specific adrenergic agonists stimulate only the alpha-receptors within the SNS. Clonidine stimulates alpha$_2$-receptors and is used to treat hypertension because its action blocks release of norepinephrine from nerve axons. Phenylephrine is used in many cold and allergy remedies because it is a powerful local vasoconstrictor. Midodrine is reserved for use in patients with orthostatic hypotension who do not respond to other therapies.
- Many of the beta$_2$-specific adrenergic agonists are used to manage and treat asthma, bronchospasm, and other obstructive pulmonary diseases.
- Isoproterenol, a beta-specific adrenergic agonist, is used to treat shock, cardiac standstill, and certain arrhythmias when used systemically; it is especially effective in the treatment of heart block in transplanted hearts.

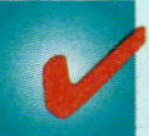

CHECK YOUR UNDERSTANDING

Answers to the questions in this chapter may be found in the Answer Key in the back of the book.

Multiple Choice

Select the best answer to the following.

1. Adrenergic drugs, because of their action in the body, are also called
   a. sympatholytic agents.
   b. cholinergic agents.
   c. sympathomimetic agents.
   d. anticholinergic agents.

2. The adrenergic agent of choice for treating the signs and symptoms of seasonal rhinitis would be
   a. norepinephrine.
   b. ephedrine.
   c. dobutamine.
   d. dopamine.

3. An adrenergic agent that is being used to treat shock is being given intravenously and it infiltrates. The nurse should
   a. watch the area for any signs of necrosis.
   b. notify the physician and decrease the rate of infusion.
   c. pull the IV and have phentolamine ready to infuse into the area.
   d. apply ice and elevate the arm.

4. Phenylephrine, an alpha-agonist, is found in many cold and allergy preparations. Adverse effects that should be watched for would include
   a. urinary retention and pupil constriction.
   b. hypotension and slow heart rate.
   c. cardiac arrhythmias and increased appetite.
   d. cardiac arrhythmias and difficulty urinating.

5. Adverse effects associated with adrenergic agents are related to the generalized stimulation of the sympathetic nervous system and could include
   a. slowed heart rate.
   b. constriction of the pupils.
   c. hypertension.
   d. increased GI secretions.

6. A patient has elected to take an over-the-counter cold preparation that contains phenylephrine. The patient should be advised not to take that drug if
   a. the patient has had thyroid or cardiovascular disease.
   b. the patient has a cough and runny nose.
   c. the patient has chronic obstructive pulmonary disease.
   d. the patient has hypotension.

Multiple Response

Select all that apply.

1. Isoproterenol is a pure beta-agonist. The nurse might expect to see it being used to treat which of the following conditions?
   a. Preterm labor
   b. Bronchospasm
   c. Cardiac standstill
   d. Shock
   e. Heart block in transplanted hearts
   f. Congestive heart failure

2. A nurse would question the order for an adrenergic agonist for a patient who is also receiving which of the following?
   a. Anticholinergic drugs
   b. Halogenated hydrocarbon anesthetics
   c. Beta-blockers
   d. Benzodiazepines
   e. MAO inhibitors
   f. Tricyclic antidepressants

Word Scramble

Unscramble the following letters to form the names of frequently used adrenergic agonists.

1. redhepnie ____________________
2. indocline ____________________
3. modanpie ____________________
4. torridine ____________________
5. aboutdimen ____________________
6. repronininehep ____________________
7. ratammnolie ____________________
8. yepphhnneeirl ____________________
9. nineppehire ____________________
10. pontlioreesor ____________________

Definitions

Define the following terms.

1. adrenergic agonist ______________________________
____
2. alpha-agonist ______________________________
____
3. beta-agonist ______________________________
____
4. glycogenolysis ______________________________
____
5. sympathomimetic ______________________________
____

Bibliography and References

Drug facts and comparisons. (2006). St. Louis: Facts and Comparisons.

Gilman, A., Hardman, J. G., & Limbird, L. E. (Eds.). (2006). *Goodman and Gilman's the pharmacological basis of therapeutics* (11th ed.). New York: McGraw-Hill.

Karch, A. M. (2006). *2007 Lippincott's nursing drug guide.* Philadelphia: Lippincott Williams & Wilkins.

Porth, C. M. (2005). *Pathophysiology: Concepts of altered health states* (7th ed.). Philadelphia: Lippincott Williams & Wilkins.

Professional's guide to patient drug facts. (2006). St. Louis: Facts and Comparisons.

CHAPTER 31

Adrenergic Blocking Agents

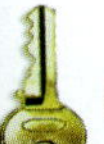

KEY TERMS

alpha$_1$-selective adrenergic blocking agents

beta-adrenergic blocking agents

beta$_1$-selective adrenergic blocking agents

bronchodilating effect

pheochromocytoma

specific adrenergic receptor sites

sympatholytic

LEARNING OBJECTIVES

Upon completion of this chapter, you will be able to:

1. Describe the effects of adrenergic receptors and correlate this with the clinical effects of adrenergic blocking.
2. Describe the therapeutic actions, indications, pharmacokinetics, contraindications, most common adverse reactions, and important drug–drug interactions associated with adrenergic blocking agents.
3. Discuss the use of adrenergic blocking agents across the lifespan.
4. Compare and contrast the prototype drugs labetalol, phentolamine, doxazosin, propranolol, and atenolol with other adrenergic blocking agents.
5. Outline the nursing considerations, including important teaching points, for patients receiving an adrenergic blocking agent.

ALPHA- AND BETA-ADRENERGIC BLOCKING AGENTS

amiodarone
bretylium
carvedilol
guanadrel
guanethidine
P labetalol

ALPHA-ADRENERGIC BLOCKING AGENTS

P phentolamine

ALPHA$_1$-SELECTIVE ADRENERGIC BLOCKING AGENTS

alfuzosin
P doxazosin
prazosin
tamsulosin
terazosin

BETA-ADRENERGIC BLOCKING AGENTS

carteolol
nadolol
penbutolol
pindolol
P propranolol
sotalol
timolol

BETA$_1$-SELECTIVE ADRENERGIC BLOCKING AGENTS

acebutolol
P atenolol
betaxolol
bisoprolol
esmolol
metoprolol

Adrenergic blocking agents are also called **sympatholytic** drugs because they lyse, or block, the effects of the sympathetic nervous system (SNS). The therapeutic and adverse effects associated with these drugs are related to their ability to react with **specific adrenergic receptor sites** without activating them. By occupying the adrenergic receptor site, they prevent norepinephrine released from the nerve terminal or from the adrenal medulla from activating the receptor, thus blocking the SNS effects.

Adrenergic Blockers

Both the therapeutic and the adverse effects associated with adrenergic blockers are related to their ability to prevent the signs and symptoms associated with SNS activation. The adrenergic blockers have varying degrees of specificity for the adrenergic receptor sites. For example, some can interact with all of the adrenergic sites (both alpha- and beta-receptors). Some are specific to alpha-receptors or even to just alpha$_1$-receptors. Some adrenergic blockers are specific to both beta$_1$- and beta$_2$-receptors, whereas others interact with just one type of beta-receptor, either beta$_1$- or beta$_2$-receptors. This specificity allows the clinician to select a drug that will have the desired therapeutic effects without the undesired effects that occur when the entire SNS is blocked. In general, however, the specificity of these drugs depends on the concentration of drug in the body. Most specificity is lost with higher serum drug levels (Figure 31.1).

The effects of the adrenergic blocking agents vary with the age of the patient. (See Box 31.1 for more information.)

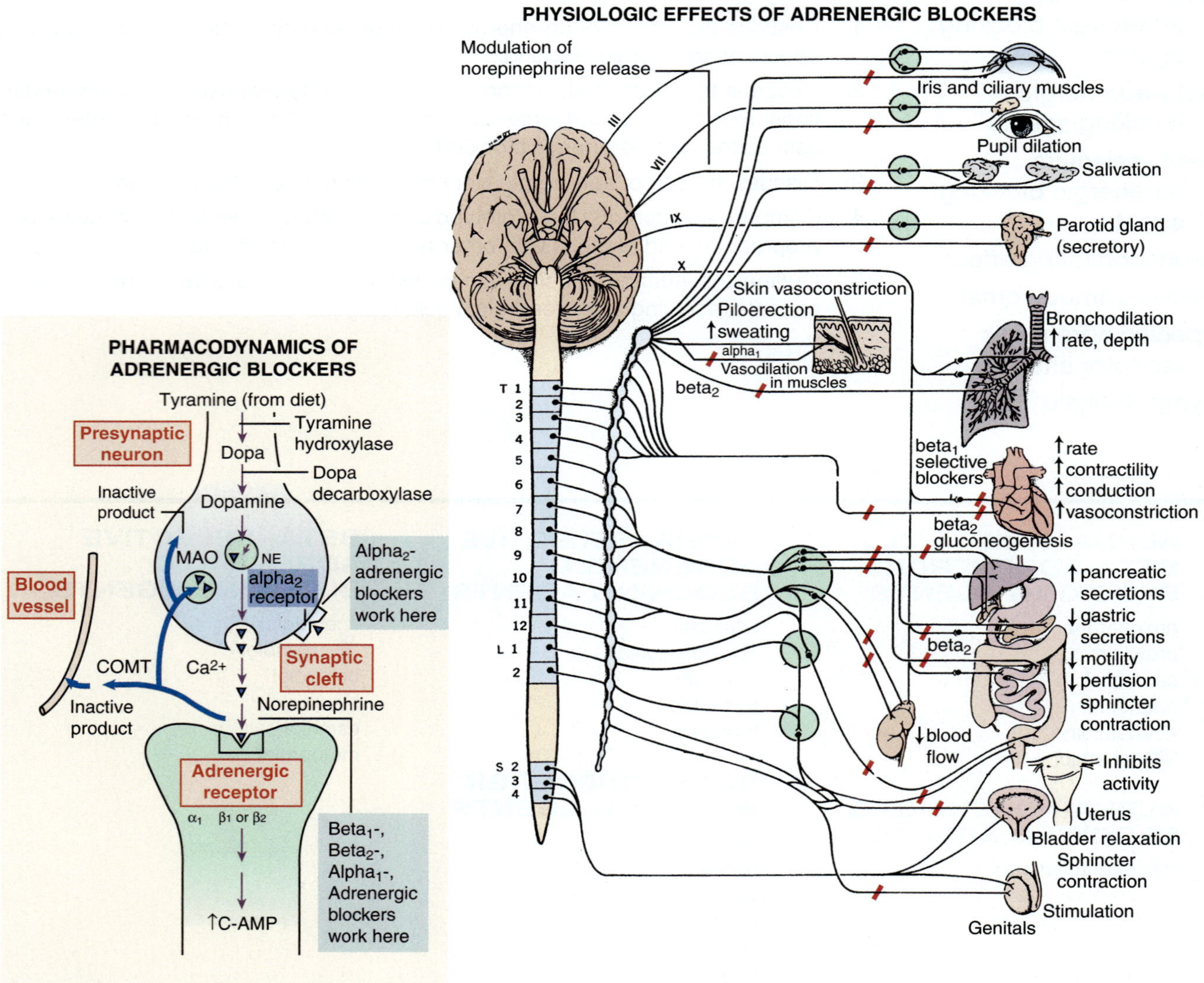

FIGURE 31.1 Site of action of adrenergic blockers and resultant physiologic responses. A bar indicates blocking of the effects indicated by those receptors.

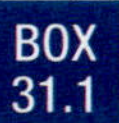

BOX 31.1 DRUG THERAPY ACROSS THE LIFESPAN

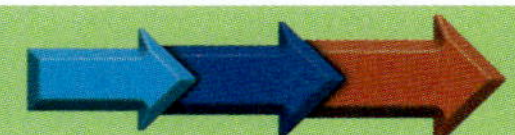

Adrenergic Blocking Agents

CHILDREN

Children are at greater risk for complications associated with the use of adrenergic blocking agents, including bradycardia, difficulty breathing, and changes in glucose metabolism. The safety and efficacy for use of these drugs has not been established for children younger than 18 years of age. If one of these drugs is used, the dosage for these agents needs to be calculated from the child's body weight and age. It is good practice to have a second person check the dosage calculation before administering the drug to avoid potential toxic effects. Three adrenergic blocking agents have established pediatric dosages, and they might be the drugs to consider when one is needed: guanethidine and prazosin, both used to treat hypertension, and phentolamine, which is used during surgery for pheochromocytoma. Children should be carefully monitored and supported during the use of these drugs.

ADULTS

Adults being treated with adrenergic blocking agents should be cautioned about the many adverse effects associated with the drugs. Patients with diabetes need to be re-educated about ways to monitor themselves for hyperglycemia and hypoglycemia, because the sympathetic reaction usually alerts patients that there is a problem with their glucose levels. Patients with severe thyroid disease are also at high risk when taking these drugs, and if one of them is needed, the patient should be monitored very closely. Propranolol and metoprolol are associated with more central nervous system (CNS) adverse effects than other adrenergic blockers, and patients who have CNS complications already or who develop CNS problems while taking an adrenergic blocker might do better with a different agent.

In general, there are no adequate studies about the effects of adrenergic blockers during pregnancy and lactation, and they should be used only in those situations in which the benefit to the mother is greater than the risk to the fetus or neonate. Adrenergic blockers can affect labor, and babies born to mothers taking these drugs may exhibit adverse cardiovascular, respiratory, and CNS effects. Many of these drugs were teratogenic in animal studies. Because of a similar risk of adverse reactions on the baby, nursing mothers should find another way to feed the baby if an adrenergic blocking drug is needed.

OLDER ADULTS

Older patients are more likely to experience the adverse effects associated with these drugs—CNS, cardiovascular, GI, and respiratory. Because older patients often also have renal or hepatic impairment, they are more likely to have toxic levels of the drug related to changes in metabolism and excretion. The older patient should be started on lower doses of the drugs and should be monitored very closely for potentially serious arrhythmias or blood pressure changes. Bisoprolol is often a drug of choice for older patients who require an adrenergic blocker for hypertension, because it is not associated with as many problems in the elderly and regular dosing profiles can be used.

These drugs can also be affected by various alternative or herbal remedies (Box 31.2.)

Alpha- and Beta-Adrenergic Blocking Agents

Drugs that block all adrenergic receptors are primarily used to treat cardiac-related conditions (Table 31.1). Amiodarone (*Cordarone*) and bretylium (*Bretylate* [CAN]), both alpha- and beta-adrenergic blockers, are only used as antiarrhythmics (see Chapter 45). Carvedilol (*Coreg*) is used as part of combination therapy in the treatment of hypertension and congestive heart failure (CHF). Guanadrel (*Hylorel*), an older drug, is used to treat hypertension that does not respond to thiazide diuretics. Guanethidine (*Ismelin*), another older drug, is used to treat hypertension and renal hypertension (high blood pressure caused by changes in renal blood flow or response). A newer drug, labetalol (*Normodyne, Trandate*), is used intravenously and orally to treat hypertension and can be used with diuretics. Labetalol has also been used to treat hypertension associated with pheochromocytoma and clonidine withdrawal.

BOX 31.2 HERBAL AND ALTERNATIVE THERAPIES

Patients who use alternative therapies as part of their daily regimen should be cautioned about potential increased adrenergic blocking effects if the following alternative therapies are combined with adrenergic blocking agents:

- *Ginseng, sage*—increased antihypertensive effects (risk of hypotension and increased central nervous system effects)
- *Xuan shen, nightshade*—slow heart rate (risk of severe bradycardia and reflex arrhythmias)
- *Celery, coriander, Di huang, fenugreek, goldenseal, Java plum, xuan seng*—lower blood glucose (increased risk of severe hypoglycemia)
- *Saw palmetto*—increased urinary tract complications

Patients who are prescribed an adrenergic blocking drug should be cautioned about the use of herbs, teas, and alternative medicines. If a patient feels that one of these agents is needed, the health care provider should be consulted and appropriate precautions should be taken to ensure that the patient is able to achieve the most therapeutic effects with the least adverse effects while taking the drug.

Table 31.1 DRUGS IN FOCUS

Alpha- and Beta-Adrenergic Blocking Agents

Drug Name	Dosage/Route	Usual Indications
amiodarone (*Cordarone*)	800–1600 mg/day PO, reduce to 400 mg/day for maintenance; 1000 mg IV over 24h; for maintenance 540 mg IV over 18h	Treatment of life-threatening ventricular arrhythmias
bretylium tosylate (*Bretylate* [CAN])	5–10 mg/kg IV over > 8 min; repeat ql–2h as needed	Treatment of life-threatening ventricular arrhythmias
carvedilol (*Coreg*)	6.25–12.5 mg PO b.i.d. for hypertension; 3.125–6.25 mg PO b.i.d. for congestive heart failure	Treatment of hypertension, congestive heart failure in adults
guanadrel (*Hylorel*)	20–75 mg PO in divided doses b.i.d.; reduce dosage with renal impairment	Treatment of hypertension in adults that does not respond to thiazide diuretics
guanethidine (*Ismelin*)	Adult: 25–50 mg PO daily; reduce dosage with renal impairment	Treatment of hypertension, renal hypertension
P labetalol (*Normodyne, Trandate*)	100 mg PO b.i.d. initially, maintenance 200–400 mg PO b.i.d.; 20 mg IV, slowly with additional doses given at 10-min intervals to a maximum dose of 300 mg for severe hypertension	Treatment of hypertension, pheochromocytoma, clonidine withdrawal, hypertension in adults

Therapeutic Actions and Indications

Adrenergic blocking agents competitively block the effects of norepinephrine at alpha- and beta-receptors throughout the SNS. This action prevents the signs and symptoms associated with a sympathetic stress reaction and results in lower blood pressure, slower pulse rate, and increased renal perfusion with decreased renin levels. These drugs are indicated to treat essential hypertension, alone or with diuretics.

Pharmacokinetics

These drugs are well absorbed and distributed throughout the body. They are metabolized in the liver and excreted in feces and urine. The half-life varies with the particular drug and preparation. There are no well-defined studies on the use of these drugs during pregnancy and lactation, so use should be reserved for those situations in which the benefit to the mother outweighs the potential risk to the neonate. The adrenergic blockers are not recommended for use in children younger than 18 years.

Contraindications and Cautions

The alpha- and beta-adrenergic blocking agents are contraindicated in patients with bradycardia or heart blocks, *which could be worsened by the slowed heart rate and conduction;* asthma, *which could be exacerbated by the loss of norepinephrine's* ***bronchodilating effect;*** shock or CHF, *which could become worse with the loss of the sympathetic reaction;* and pregnancy or lactation *because of the potential adverse effects on the fetus or neonate.*

These drugs should be used with caution in patients with diabetes *because the disorder could be aggravated by the blocked sympathetic response and because the usual signs and symptoms of hypoglycemia and hyperglycemia are lost when the SNS cannot respond.* Caution also should be used with bronchospasm, *which could progress to respiratory distress with the loss of norepinephrine's bronchodilating actions.*

Adverse Effects

The adverse effects associated with the use of alpha- and beta-adrenergic blocking agents are usually associated with the drug's effects on the SNS. These effects can include dizziness, paresthesias, insomnia, depression, fatigue, and vertigo, *which are related to the blocked effects of norepinephrine in the central nervous system* (CNS). Nausea, vomiting, diarrhea, anorexia, and flatulence are *associated with the loss of the balancing sympathetic effect on the gastrointestinal (GI) tract and increased parasympathetic dominance.* Cardiac arrhythmias, hypotension, CHF, pulmonary edema, and cerebrovascular accident, or stroke, are *related to the lack of stimulatory effects and loss of vascular tone in the cardiovascular (CV) system.* Bronchospasm, cough, rhinitis, and bronchial obstruction are *related to loss of the bronchodilating effects on the respiratory tract and vasodilation of the mucous membrane vessels.* Other effects reported include decreased exercise tolerance, hypoglycemia, and rash.

Clinically Important Drug–Drug Interactions

There is increased risk of excessive hypotension if any of these drugs are combined with enflurane, halothane, or isoflurane anesthetics. The effectiveness of diabetic agents is increased, leading to hypoglycemia when such agents are used with these drugs; patients should be monitored closely and dosage adjustments made as needed. In addition, carvedilol has been associated with potentially dangerous conduction system disturbances when combined with verapamil or diltiazem; if this combination is used, the patient should be monitored continuously.

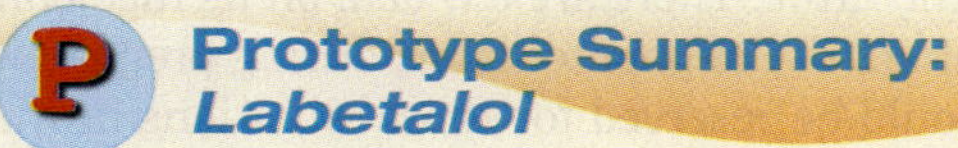

Prototype Summary: Labetalol

Indications: Hypertension, alone or in combination with other drugs; unlabeled uses—control of blood pressure in pheochromocytoma, clonidine withdrawal hypertension

Actions: Competitively blocks alpha- and beta-receptor sites in the SNS leading to lower blood pressure without reflex tachycardia and decreased renin levels

Pharmacokinetics:

Route	Onset	Peak	Duration
Oral	Varies	1–2 h	8–12 h
IV	Immediate	5 min	5.5 h

$T_{1/2}$: 6–8 hours, with hepatic metabolism and excretion in the urine

Adverse effects: Dizziness, vertigo, fatigue, gastric pain, flatulence, impotence, bronchospasm, dyspnea, cough, decreased exercise tolerance

Nursing Considerations for Patients Receiving Alpha- and Beta-Adrenergic Blocking Agents

Assessment: History and Examination

Screen for the following conditions, *which could be cautions or contraindications to use of the drug:* any known allergies to these drugs; presence of bradycardia or heart blocks, *which could be worsened by the slowing of heart rate and conduction;* asthma, *which could be exacerbated by the loss of the bronchodilating effect of norepinephrine;* shock or CHF, *which could become worse with the loss of the sympathetic reaction;* pregnancy or lactation *because of the potential adverse effects on the fetus or neonate;* diabetes, *which could be aggravated by the blocking of the sympathetic response and because the usual signs and symptoms of hypoglycemia and hyperglycemia are lost when the SNS cannot respond;* and bronchospasm, *which could progress to respiratory distress with the loss of the bronchodilating actions of norepinephrine.*

Include screening *for baseline status and any potential adverse effects:* skin color, temperature; pulse, blood pressure, cardiac output, electrocardiogram (ECG); respiration, adventitious sounds; and blood glucose levels and electrolytes.

Nursing Diagnoses

The patient receiving an alpha- or beta-adrenergic blocker may have the following nursing diagnoses related to drug therapy:

- Acute Pain related to CV and systemic effects
- Decreased Cardiac Output related to CV effects
- Ineffective Airway Clearance related to lack of bronchodilating effects
- Deficient Knowledge regarding drug therapy

Implementation With Rationale

- Do not discontinue abruptly after chronic therapy *because hypersensitivity to catecholamines may develop and the patient could have a severe reaction;* taper drug slowly over 2 weeks, monitoring patient.
- Consult with the physician about withdrawing the drug before surgery *because withdrawal is controversial; effects on the sympathetic system after surgery can cause problems.*
- Encourage the patient to adopt lifestyle changes, including diet, exercise, stopping smoking, and decreasing stress *to aid in lowering blood pressure.*
- Monitor for orthostatic hypotension and provide safety precautions if this occurs *to prevent injury to the patient.*
- Monitor for any sign of liver failure *in order to arrange to discontinue the drug if this occurs.* (This effect is more likely to happen with carvedilol.)
- Provide thorough patient teaching, including measures to avoid adverse effects, warning signs of problems, and the need for monitoring and evaluation *to enhance patient knowledge about drug therapy and to promote compliance.*
- Offer support and encouragement *to help the patient deal with the drug regimen.*

Evaluation

- Monitor patient response to the drug (improvement in blood pressure and CHF).
- Monitor for adverse effects (CV changes, headache, GI upset, bronchospasm, liver failure).
- Evaluate the effectiveness of the teaching plan (patient can name drug, dosage, adverse effects to watch for, specific measures to avoid adverse effects).
- Monitor the effectiveness of comfort measures and compliance with the regimen.

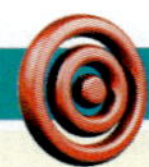

FOCUS POINTS

- Adrenergic blocking agents block the effects of the sympathetic nervous system (SNS).
- The alpha- and beta-adrenergic blocking agents lower blood pressure by blocking all of the receptor sites within the SNS.

Alpha-Adrenergic Blocking Agents

Some adrenergic blocking agents have a specific affinity for alpha-receptor sites. Their use is somewhat limited because of the development of even more specific and safer drugs.

Only one of these drugs, phentolamine, is still used (Table 31.2.) A **pheochromocytoma** is a tumor of the chromaffin cells of the adrenal medulla that periodically releases large amounts of norepinephrine and epinephrine into the system, with resultant severe hypertension and tachycardia. Phentolamine (*Regitine*) can be used to diagnose pheochromocytoma and to prevent severe hypertension reactions caused by manipulation of the pheochromocytoma before and during surgery. Phentolamine is most frequently used to prevent cell death and tissue sloughing after extravasation of intravenous norepinephrine or dopamine.

Therapeutic Actions and Indications

Phentolamine blocks the postsynaptic $alpha_1$-adrenergic receptors, decreasing sympathetic tone in the vasculature and causing vasodilation, which leads to a lowering of blood pressure. It also blocks presynaptic $alpha_2$-receptors, preventing the feedback control of norepinephrine release. The result is an increase in the reflex tachycardia that occurs when blood pressure is lowered. This drug is used to diagnose and manage episodes of pheochromocytoma. Phentolamine is also used to rescue cells injured by norepinephrine or dopamine extravasation; it causes vasodilation and a return of blood flow to the area.

Pharmacokinetics

Phentolamine is rapidly absorbed after injection and is excreted in the urine. There are few data on its metabolism and distribution. Use of phentolamine during pregnancy or lactation should be reserved for those situations in which the benefit to the mother outweighs any potential risk to the fetus or neonate.

Contraindications and Cautions

The alpha-adrenergic blocking agent is contraindicated in the presence of allergy to this or similar drugs and in the presence of coronary artery disease or myocardial infarction (MI) *because of the potential exacerbation of these conditions;* it should be used cautiously in pregnancy or lactation *because of the potential adverse effects on the fetus or neonate.*

Adverse Effects

Patients receiving this drug often experience extensions of the therapeutic effects, including hypotension, orthostatic hypotension, angina, MI, cerebrovascular accident, flushing, tachycardia, and arrhythmia—*all of which are related to vasodilation and decreased blood pressure.* Weakness and dizziness often occur *as a reaction to the hypotension.* Nausea, vomiting, and diarrhea may also occur.

Clinically Important Drug–Drug Interactions

Ephedrine and epinephrine may have decreased hypertensive and vasoconstrictive effects if they are taken concomitantly with phentolamine because these agents work in opposing ways in the body. Increased hypotension may occur if this drug is combined with alcohol, which is also a vasodilator.

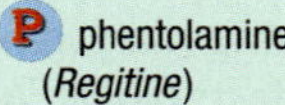

Table 31.2 DRUGS IN FOCUS

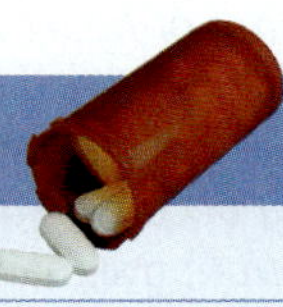

Alpha-Adrenergic Blocking Agents

Drug Name	Dosage/Route	Usual Indications
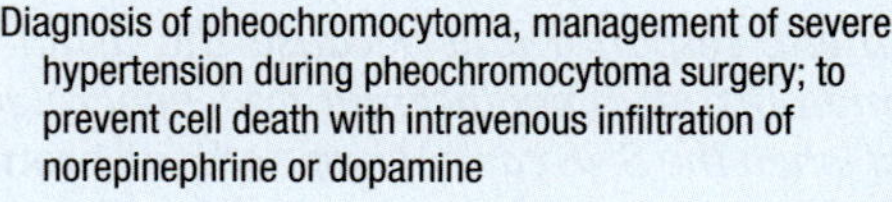 phentolamine (*Regitine*)	Adult: 5 mg IV or IM 1–2 h before surgery; 5–10 mg in 10 mL saline injected into area of extravasation within 12 h after extravasation Pediatric: 1 mg IM or IV 1–2 h before surgery; treat extravasation as in the adult	Diagnosis of pheochromocytoma, management of severe hypertension during pheochromocytoma surgery; to prevent cell death with intravenous infiltration of norepinephrine or dopamine

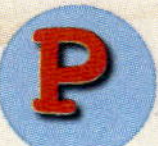

Prototype Summary: Phentolamine

Indications: Prevention or control of hypertensive episodes associated with pheochromocytoma; test for diagnosis of pheochromocytoma; prevention and treatment of dermal necrosis and sloughing associated with IV extravasation of norepinephrine or dopamine

Actions: Competitively blocks postsynaptic alpha$_1$- and presynaptic alpha$_2$-receptors, causing a vasodilation and lowering of blood pressure, accompanied by increased reflex tachycardia

Pharmacokinetics:

Route	Onset	Peak	Duration
IM	Rapid	20 min	30–45 min
IV	Immediate	2 min	15–30 min

$T_{1/2}$: Metabolism and excretion are unknown

Adverse effects: Acute and prolonged hypotensive episodes, MI, tachycardia, arrhythmias, nausea, flushing

Nursing Considerations for Patients Receiving Alpha-Adrenergic Blocking Agents

Assessment: History and Examination

Screen for the following conditions, *which could be cautions or contraindications to the use of the drug:* any known allergies to these drugs; presence of any cardiovascular diseases, *which may be contraindications to the use of these drugs;* and pregnancy or lactation, *which require caution for drug use.* Include screening *for baseline status and for any potential adverse effects:* assess orientation, affect, and reflexes to monitor for CNS changes related to drug therapy; blood pressure, pulse, ECG, peripheral perfusion, and cardiac output; and urine output.

Nursing Diagnoses

The patient receiving an alpha-adrenergic blocking agent may also have the following nursing diagnoses related to drug therapy:

- Risk for Injury related to CNS, CV effects of drug
- Decreased Cardiac Output related to blood pressure changes, arrhythmias, vasodilation
- Deficient Knowledge regarding drug therapy

Implementation With Rationale

- Monitor heart rate and blood pressure very carefully *in order to arrange to discontinue the drug if adverse reactions are severe;* provide supportive management if needed.
- Inject phentolamine directly into the area of extravasation of epinephrine or dopamine *to prevent local cell death.*
- Arrange for supportive care and comfort measures, such as rest, environmental control, and other measures, *to decrease CNS irritation;* provide headache medication *to alleviate patient discomfort;* arrange safety measures if CNS effects or orthostatic hypotension occur *to prevent patient injury.*
- Provide thorough patient teaching, including dosage, potential adverse effects, measures to avoid adverse effects, and warning signs of problems, *to enhance patient knowledge about drug therapy and to promote compliance.*
- Offer support and encouragement *to help the patient deal with the drug regimen.*

Evaluation

- Monitor patient response to the drug (improvement in signs and symptoms of pheochromocytoma, improvement in tissue condition after extravasation).
- Monitor for adverse effects (orthostatic hypotension, arrhythmias, CNS effects).
- Evaluate the effectiveness of the teaching plan (patient can name drug, dosage, adverse effects to watch for, specific measures to avoid adverse effects).
- Monitor the effectiveness of comfort measures and compliance to the regimen.

Alpha$_1$-Selective Adrenergic Blocking Agents

Alpha$_1$-selective adrenergic blocking agents (Table 31.3) are drugs that have a specific affinity for alpha$_1$-receptors. Doxazosin (*Cardura*) is used to treat hypertension and is also effective in the treatment of benign prostatic hyperplasia (BPH) (see Chapter 52). Prazosin (*Minipress*) is used to treat hypertension, alone or in combination with other drugs. Terazosin (*Hytrin*) is used to treat hypertension as well as BPH (see Chapter 52). Tamsulosin (*Flomax*) and alfuzosin (*Uroxatral*) are used only in the treatment of BPH and are discussed later in the book (see Chapter 52).

Table 31.3 DRUGS IN FOCUS

Alpha$_1$-Selective Adrenergic Blocking Agents

Drug Name	Dosage/Route	Usual Indications
alfuzosin (*Uroxatral*)	10 mg/day PO	Treatment of benign prostatic hyperplasia (BPH)
P doxazosin (*Cardura*)	1 mg/day PO up to 16 mg/day PO for hypertension; 1–8 mg PO/day for BPH	Treatment of hypertension and BPH
prazosin (*Minipress*)	Adult: 1 mg PO b.i.d. to t.i.d. with maintenance at 6–15 mg/day PO in divided doses Pediatric: 0.5–7 mg PO t.i.d.	Treatment of hypertension
tamsulosin (*Flomax*)	0.4–0.8 mg/day PO 30 min after the same meal each day	Treatment of BPH
terazosin (*Hytrin*)	1–5 mg/day PO, preferably at bedtime for hypertension; 10 mg/day PO for BPH	Treatment of hypertension and BPH

Therapeutic Actions and Indications

The therapeutic effects of the alpha$_1$-selective adrenergic blocking agents come from their ability to block the postsynaptic alpha$_1$-receptor sites. This causes a decrease in vascular tone and vasodilation, which leads to a fall in blood pressure. Because these drugs do not block the presynaptic alpha$_2$-receptor sites, the reflex tachycardia that accompanies a fall in blood pressure does not occur. These drugs can be used to treat BPH or hypertension, alone or as part of a combination therapy.

Pharmacokinetics

The alpha$_1$-selective adrenergic blocking agents are well absorbed and undergo extensive hepatic metabolism. *They therefore must be used with caution in patients with hepatic impairment.* They are excreted in the urine. Use during pregnancy and lactation should be limited to those situations in which the benefits to the mother outweigh the potential risks to the neonate *because these drugs cross the placenta and are known to enter breast milk.* Safety for use in children has not been established.

Contraindications and Cautions

The alpha$_1$-selective adrenergic blocking agents are contraindicated in the presence of allergy to any of these drugs and also with lactation *because the drugs cross into breast milk and could have adverse effects on the neonate.* They should be used cautiously in the presence of CHF or renal failure *because their blood pressure-lowering effects could exacerbate these conditions,* and with hepatic impairment, *which could alter the metabolism of these drugs.* Caution also should be used during pregnancy *because of the potential for adverse effects on the fetus.*

Adverse Effects

The adverse effects associated with the use of these drugs *are usually related to their effects of blocking the SNS.* CNS effects include dizziness, weakness, fatigue, drowsiness, and depression. Nausea, vomiting, abdominal pain, and diarrhea may occur *as a result of direct effects on the GI tract and sympathetic blocking.* Anticipated cardiovascular effects include arrhythmias, hypotension, edema, CHF, and angina. *The vasodilation caused by these drugs can also cause flushing, rhinitis, reddened eyes, nasal congestion, and priapism.*

Clinically Important Drug-Drug Interactions

Increased hypotensive effects may occur if these drugs are combined with any other vasodilating or antihypertensive drugs.

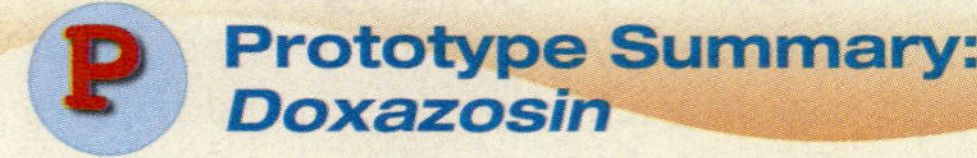

P Prototype Summary: *Doxazosin*

Indications: Treatment of mild to moderate hypertension as monotherapy or in combination with other antihypertensives; treatment of BPH

Actions: Reduces total peripheral resistance through alpha blockade; does not affect heart rate or cardiac output; increases high-density lipoproteins while lowering total cholesterol levels

Pharmacokinetics:

Route	Onset	Peak	Duration
Oral	Varies	2–3 h	Not known

$T_{1/2}$: 22 hours, with hepatic metabolism and excretion in the bile, feces, and urine

Adverse effects: Headache, fatigue, dizziness, postural dizziness, vertigo, tachycardia, edema, nausea, dyspepsia, diarrhea, sexual dysfunction

Nursing Considerations for Patients Receiving Alpha$_1$-Selective Adrenergic Blocking Agents

Assessment: History and Examination

Screen for the following conditions, *which could be cautions or contraindications to use of the drug:* any known allergies to either drug; pregnancy or lactation, *which could be contraindications or cautions for drug use;* and CHF or renal failure, *which could be exacerbated by drug use.*

Include screening *for baseline status and for any potential adverse effects:* assess orientation, affect, and reflexes *to monitor for CNS changes related to drug therapy;* blood pressure, pulse, ECG, peripheral perfusion, and cardiac output. Monitor cardiovascular effects as well as urinary output and renal function *to monitor effects on the renal system.*

Nursing Diagnoses

The patient receiving an alpha$_1$-selective adrenergic blocking agent may have the following nursing diagnoses related to drug therapy:

- Acute Pain related to headache, GI upset, flushing, nasal congestion
- Risk for Injury related to CNS, CV effects of drug
- Decreased Cardiac Output related to blood pressure changes, arrhythmias, vasodilation
- Deficient Knowledge regarding drug therapy

Implementation With Rationale

- Monitor blood pressure, pulse, rhythm, and cardiac output regularly *in order to arrange to adjust dosage or discontinue the drug if cardiovascular effects are severe.*
- Establish safety precautions if CNS effects or orthostatic hypotension occurs *to prevent patient injury.*
- Arrange for small, frequent meals if GI upset is severe *to relieve discomfort and maintain nutrition.*
- Arrange for supportive care and comfort measures (rest, environmental control, other measures) *to decrease CNS irritation;* provide headache medication *to alleviate patient discomfort;* arrange safety measures if CNS effects occur *to prevent patient injury.*
- Provide thorough patient teaching, including dosage, adverse effects to anticipate, measures to avoid adverse effects, and warning signs of problems *to enhance patient knowledge about drug therapy and to promote compliance.*
- Offer support and encouragement *to help the patient deal with the drug regimen.*

Evaluation

- Monitor patient response to the drug (lowering of blood pressure).
- Monitor for adverse effects (GI upset, CNS or cardiovascular changes).
- Evaluate the effectiveness of the teaching plan (patient can name drug, dosage, adverse effects to watch for, specific measures to avoid adverse effects).
- Monitor the effectiveness of comfort measures and compliance to the regimen.

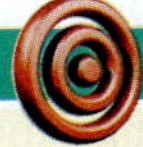

FOCUS POINTS

- Selective adrenergic blocking agents have specific affinity for alpha- or beta-receptors or for specific alpha$_1$-, beta$_1$-, or beta$_2$-receptor sites. Nonspecific alpha-adrenergic blocking agents are used to treat pheochromocytoma, a tumor of the adrenal medulla. A reflex tachycardia commonly occurs when the blood pressure falls.
- Alpha$_1$-selective adrenergic blocking agents decrease blood pressure by blocking the postsynaptic alpha$_1$-receptor sites, decreasing vascular tone, and promoting vasodilation.

Beta-Adrenergic Blocking Agents

The **beta-adrenergic blocking agents** are used to treat cardiovascular problems (hypertension, angina, migraine headaches) and to prevent reinfarction after MI (Table 31.4). These drugs are widely used today; in fact, propranolol (*Inderal*) was once the most prescribed drug in the country.

Propranolol has been approved for multiple uses, including treatment of hypertension, angina, idiopathic hypertrophic

Table 31.4 DRUGS IN FOCUS

Beta-Adrenergic Blocking Agents

Drug Name	Dosage/Route	Usual Indications
carteolol (*Cartrol*)	Initially 2.5 mg/day PO, titrate to 5–10 mg/day PO based on patient response; reduce dosage with renal impairment	Treatment of hypertension in adults
nadolol (*Corgard*)	Angina: 40–80 mg/day PO Hypertension: 40–80 mg/day PO, up to 320 mg/day may be needed; reduce dosage in renal impairment	Treatment of hypertension, management of angina in adults
penbutolol (*Levator*)	Initially 20 mg/day PO, titrate up to 40–80 mg/day PO based on patient response	Treatment of hypertension in adults
pindolol (*Visken*)	Initially 5 mg PO b.i.d., to a maximum of 60 mg/day PO	Treatment of hypertension in adults
P propranolol (*Inderal*)	Dosage varies widely based on indication; check your drug guide for specific information	Treatment of hypertension, angina, idiopathic hypertrophic subaortic stenosis, certain cardiac arrhythmias, pheochromocytoma; prophylaxis for migraine headache, prevention of stage fright
sotalol (*Betapace, Betapace AF*)	*Betapace:* 80 mg PO b.i.d., up to 320 mg PO b.i.d. may be needed *Betapace AF:* 80 mg/day PO based on QT interval and patient response, up to 120 mg b.i.d. may be needed Reduce dosage of both with renal impairment	Treatment of potentially life-threatening ventricular arrhythmias (*Betapace*); maintenance of normal sinus rhythm in patients with atrial fibrillation/flutter
timolol (*Blocadren, Timoptic*)	10 mg PO b.i.d., increases based on patient response; 1–2 gtt in affected eye(s) for glaucoma	Treatment of hypertension; prevention of reinfarction after myocardial infarction; prophylaxis for migraine; in ophthalmic form, reduction of intraocular pressure in open-angle glaucoma

subaortic stenosis (IHSS)-induced palpitations, angina and syncope, and certain cardiac arrhythmias induced by catecholamines or digoxin; prevention of reinfarction after MI; treatment of pheochromocytoma; prophylaxis for migraine headache (which may be caused by vasodilation and is relieved by vasoconstriction); prevention of stage fright (which is a sympathetic stress reaction to a particular situation); and treatment of essential tremors. It is very effective in blocking all of the beta-receptors in the SNS and was one of the first drugs of the class.

Since the introduction of propranolol, newer and more selective drugs have become available that are not associated with some of the adverse effects seen with total blockade of the SNS beta-receptors. Carteolol (*Cartrol*) is used for the treatment of hypertension, alone or in combination with other drugs. Penbutolol (*Levator*) and pindolol (*Visken*) are also used for the treatment of hypertension. The drug of choice would depend mostly on personal experience. Nadolol (*Corgard*) is used to treat hypertension and also for the chronic management of angina. It would be a drug of choice in an angina patient who is also hypertensive. Sotalol (*Betapace*) is reserved for use in the treatment of potentially life-threatening arrhythmias and is not recommended for any other use; *Betapace AF,* a newer preparation of the drug, is used in the treatment of atrial fibrillation. Timolol (*Blocadren, Timoptic*), a newer beta-adrenergic blocker, has several recommended uses, including treatment of hypertension, prevention of reinfarction after MI, prophylaxis for migraine, and in ophthalmic form, reduction of intraocular pressure in patients with open-angle glaucoma.

Therapeutic Actions and Indications

The therapeutic effects of these drugs are related to their competitive blocking of the beta-adrenergic receptors in the SNS. The blockade of the beta-receptors in the heart and in the juxtaglomerular apparatus of the nephron account for most of the therapeutic benefit of these drugs. Decreased heart rate, contractility, and excitability, as well as a membrane-stabilizing effect, lead to a decrease in arrhythmias, a decreased cardiac workload, and decreased oxygen consumption. The juxtaglomerular cells are not stimulated to release renin, which further decreases the blood pressure. These effects are useful in treating hypertension and chronic angina and can help to prevent reinfarction after an MI by decreasing cardiac workload and oxygen consumption.

Blocking of other SNS effects accounts for the use of propranolol to prevent stage fright. The decreased feelings of anxiety, decreased pulse and blood pressure, and decreased sweating and flushing help to alleviate situational anxiety. The mechanism of action in treating migraines is not clearly understood.

Timolol is used topically to reduce intraocular pressure through its relaxing effects on the eye muscles. Because it is applied topically, it is usually not absorbed systemically from this route.

Pharmacokinetics

These drugs are absorbed from the GI tract and undergo hepatic metabolism. Food has been found to increase the bioavailability of propranolol, although this effect was not found with other beta-adrenergic blocking agents. Absorption of sotalol is decreased by the presence of food. Propranolol also crosses the blood–brain barrier, but carteolol, nadolol, and sotalol do not, making them a better choice if CNS effects occur with propranolol. These drugs are excreted in the urine, *requiring caution in patients with renal impairment. Teratogenic effects have occurred in animal studies with all of these drugs except sotalol.* The use of any beta-adrenergic blocker during pregnancy should be reserved for situations in which the benefit to the mother outweighs the risk to the fetus. In general, they should not be used during lactation *because of the potential for adverse effects on the baby.* The safety and efficacy for use of these drugs in children have not been established.

Contraindications and Cautions

Beta-adrenergic blocking agents are contraindicated in the presence of allergy to any of these drugs or any components of the drug being used; with bradycardia or heart blocks, shock, or CHF, *which could be exacerbated by the cardiac-suppressing effects of these drugs;* with bronchospasm, chronic obstructive pulmonary disease (COPD), or acute asthma, *which could be made worse by the blocking of the sympathetic bronchodilation;* with pregnancy *because neonatal apnea, bradycardia, and hypoglycemia could occur;* and with lactation *because of the potential effects on the neonate, which could include slowed heart rate, hypotension, and hypoglycemia.* These drugs should be used cautiously in patients with diabetes and hypoglycemia *because of the blocking of the normal signs and symptoms of hypoglycemia and hyperglycemia;* with thyrotoxicosis *because of the adrenergic blocking effects on the thyroid gland;* or with hepatic dysfunction, *which could interfere with the metabolism of these drugs.*

Adverse Effects

Patients receiving these drugs often experience adverse effects *related to the blocking of the SNS's beta-receptors.* CNS effects include fatigue, dizziness, depression, paresthesias, sleep disturbances, memory loss, and disorientation. Cardiovascular effects can include bradycardia, heart block, CHF, hypotension, and peripheral vascular insufficiency. Pulmonary effects can range from difficulty breathing, coughing, and bronchospasm to severe pulmonary edema and bronchial obstruction. GI upset, nausea, vomiting, diarrhea, gastric pain, and even colitis can occur *as a result of unchecked parasympathetic activity and the blocking of the sympathetic receptors.* Genitourinary effects can include decreased libido, impotence, dysuria, and Peyronie's disease. Other effects that can occur include decreased exercise tolerance (patients often report that their "get up and go" is gone), hypoglycemia or hyperglycemia, and liver changes. (See Critical Thinking Scenario 31-1.)

Clinically Important Drug–Drug Interactions

A paradoxical hypertension occurs when beta-blockers are given with clonidine, and an increased rebound hypertension with clonidine withdrawal may also occur. It is best to avoid this combination.

A decreased antihypertensive effect occurs when beta-blockers are given with nonsteroidal anti-inflammatory drugs (NSAIDs); if this combination is used, the patient should be monitored closely, and dosage adjustment should be made to achieve the desired control of blood pressure.

An initial hypertensive episode followed by bradycardia may occur if these drugs are given with epinephrine. Another interaction is the possibility of peripheral ischemia if the beta-blockers are taken in combination with ergot alkaloids.

When these drugs are given with insulin or antidiabetic agents, there is a potential for change in blood glucose levels. The patient also will not display the usual signs and symptoms of hypoglycemia or hyperglycemia, which are caused by activation of the SNS. Because these effects are blocked, the patient will need new indications to alert him or her to potential problems. If this combination is used, the patient should monitor blood glucose levels frequently throughout the day and should be alert to new warnings about glucose imbalance.

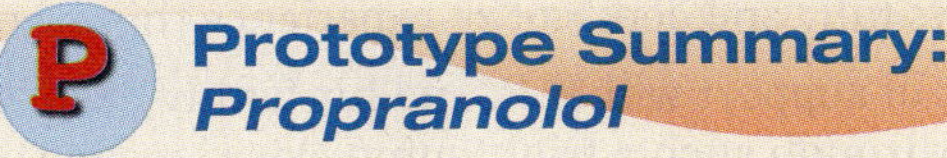

Indications: Treatment of hypertension, angina pectoris, IHSS, supraventricular tachycardia, tremor; prevention of reinfarction after MI; adjunctive therapy in pheochromocytoma; prophylaxis of migraine headache; management of situational anxiety

Actions: Competitively blocks beta-adrenergic receptors in the heart and juxtaglomerular apparatus; reduces vascular tone in the CNS

Pharmacokinetics:

Route	Onset	Peak	Duration
Oral	20–30 min	60–90 min	6–12 h
IV	Immediate	1 min	4–6 h

$T_{1/2}$: 3–5 hours with hepatic metabolism and excretion in the urine

Adverse effects: Allergic reaction, bradycardia, CHF, cardiac arrhythmias, cerebrovascular accident, pulmonary edema, gastric pain, flatulence, impotence, decreased exercise tolerance, bronchospasm

(text continues on page 502)

CRITICAL THINKING SCENARIO 31-1

Nonspecific Beta-Blockers (Propranolol)

The Situation

M.R., a 59-year-old man, had a diaphragmatic myocardial infarction (MI) last August. He recovered well and returned to work as a salesman within 8 weeks. Shortly after he resumed working, he began to suffer vague, pressure-type chest pains. His physician prescribed propranolol (*Inderal*) 10 mg q.i.d., and M.R. had no further problems until the following June, when acute respiratory distress developed while he was picnicking in a state park with his family. On the way to the emergency room, he suffered an apparent respiratory arrest. He was admitted to the hospital and placed in the respiratory intensive care unit. It was found that M.R. had a history of hay fever and allergic rhinitis during the pollen season but had never experienced such a severe reaction.

Critical Thinking

Why did M.R. have such a severe reaction? What appropriate measures should be taken to ensure that M.R. recovers fully and does not re-experience this event?

What sort of support will M.R. and his family need after going through such a frightening experience? Think about the children who may have witnessed the respiratory arrest and how they should be reassured, depending on their ages. *Think about the support M.R.'s wife may need and the fear that may now be associated with M.R.'s condition. M.R. has been taking propranolol for several months and needs to be weaned from it because the drug is somewhat responsible for the reaction that M.R. experienced.*

What kind of teaching program will need to be developed to help M.R. deal with his drugs, their effects, and his underlying cardiac problem?

Discussion

Propranolol, a nonspecific beta-blocker, was prescribed to decrease the workload and oxygen consumption required of M.R.'s heart and to prevent another MI. He did well on the drug until pollen season arrived. That is because propranolol, a nonspecific beta-blocker, prevented the compensatory bronchodilation that occurs when the sympathetic nervous system is stimulated. When the pollen reacted with M.R.'s airways, causing them to swell and become narrower, his swollen bronchial tubes were unable to allow air to flow through them. The result was bronchial constriction and respiratory distress that, in M.R.'s case, progressed to a respiratory arrest. Before he began taking propranolol, M.R. probably had been effectively compensating for the swelling of the bronchi through bronchodilation and had never experienced such a reaction. The propranolol needs to be weaned from M.R.'s system. M.R. should then be started on a specific beta-adrenergic blocker, which should decrease cardiac workload without interfering with reflex bronchodilation.

M.R. may want to discuss this frightening incident with his health care provider. He also may want to include his family in this discussion. It should be stressed that he did so well up to this point because he had not been exposed to pollen and therefore had not had the problem that brought him into the hospital this time. M.R. probably never reported the occurrence of hay fever to his health care provider when the drug was prescribed because it had never been a problem and probably did not seem significant to him. M.R. and his family should receive support and be encouraged to talk about what happened and how they reacted to it. It is normal to feel frightened and unsure when a loved one is in distress. A full teaching program, including information on M.R.'s heart disease and details about his new specific beta-adrenergic blocker, should be undertaken. M.R. should receive written information about the drug, including warning signs to watch for and adverse effects that may occur.

Nursing Care Guide for M.R.: Propranolol

Assessment: History and Examination

Review the patient's history for allergy to propranolol, CHF, shock, bradycardia, heart block, hypotension, COPD, thyroid disease, diabetes, respiratory impairment, concurrent use of: barbiturates, NSAIDs, piroxicam, sulindac, lidocaine, cimetidine, phenothiazines, clonidine, theophylline, and rifampin.

Focus the physical examination on the following:

CV: blood pressure, pulse, peripheral perfusion, ECG

CNS: orientation, affect, reflexes, vision

Skin: color, lesions, texture

GU: urinary output, sexual function

Nonspecific Beta-Blockers (Propranolol) *(continued)*

GI: abdominal, liver evaluation

Respiratory: respirations, adventitious sounds

Nursing Diagnoses

Decreased Cardiac Output related to CV effects

Acute Pain related to CNS, GI, systematic effects

Impaired Tissue Perfusion, related to CV effects

Deficient Knowledge regarding drug therapy

Implementation

Ensure safe and appropriate administration of drug.

Provide comfort and safety measures: assistance/siderails; temperature control; rest periods; mouth care; small, frequent meals.

Monitor blood pressure, pulse, and respiratory status throughout drug therapy.

Provide support and reassurance to deal with drug effects and discomfort, sexual dysfunction, and fatigue.

Provide patient teaching regarding drug name, dosage, side effects, precautions, and warning signs to report.

Evaluation

Evaluate drug effects: blood pressure within normal limit, decrease in anginal episodes, stabilized cardiac rhythm.

Monitor for adverse effects: CV effects: CHF, block; dizziness, confusion; sexual dysfunction; GI effects; hypoglycemia; respiratory problems.

Monitor for drug–drug interactions as indicated.

Evaluate effectiveness of patient teaching program.

Evaluate effectiveness of comfort and safety measures.

Patient Teaching for M.R.

☐ The drug that has been prescribed for you, propranolol, is a beta-adrenergic blocking agent. A beta-adrenergic blocking agent works to prevent certain stimulating activities that normally occur in the body in response to such factors as stress, injury, or excitement.

You should learn to take your own pulse and monitor it daily, writing the pulse rate on the calendar. Your current pulse rate is 82.

☐ Never discontinue this medication suddenly. If you find that your prescription is running low, notify your health care provider at once. This drug needs to be tapered over time to prevent severe reactions when its use is discontinued. Some of the following adverse effects may occur:

- *Fatigue, weakness*: Try to stagger your activities throughout the day to allow rest periods.
- *Dizziness, drowsiness*: If these should occur, take care to avoid driving, operating dangerous machinery, or doing delicate tasks. Change position slowly to avoid dizzy spells.
- *Change in sexual function*: Be assured that this is a drug effect and discuss it with your health care provider.
- *Nausea, diarrhea*: These gastrointestinal discomforts often diminish with time. If they become too uncomfortable or do not improve, talk to your health care provider.
- *Dreams, confusion*: These are drug effects. If they become too uncomfortable, discuss them with your health care provider.

☐ Report any of the following to your health care provider: very slow pulse, need to sleep on more pillows at night, difficulty breathing, swelling in the ankles or fingers, sudden weight gain, mental confusion or personality change, fever, or rash.

☐ Avoid over-the-counter medications, including cold and allergy remedies and diet pills. Many of these preparations contain drugs that could interfere with this medication. If you feel that you need one of these, check with your health care provider first.

☐ Tell any doctor, nurse, or other health care provider that you are taking these drugs, keep all medications out of the reach of children, and do not share these drugs with other people.

Nursing Considerations for Patients Receiving Beta-Adrenergic Blocking Agents

Assessment: History and Examination

Screen for the following conditions, *which could be cautions or contraindications to the use of the drug:* known allergy to any drug or to any components of the drug; bradycardia or heart blocks, shock, or CHF, *which could be exacerbated by the cardiac-suppressing effects of these drugs;* bronchospasm, COPD, or acute asthma, *which could be made worse by the blocking of the sympathetic bronchodilation;* pregnancy and lactation *because of the potential effects on the fetus or neonate;* diabetes or hypoglycemia; thyrotoxicosis; and hepatic dysfunction, *which could interfere with the metabolism of these drugs.*

Include screening *for baseline status and for any potential adverse effects:* skin color, temperature; pulse, blood pressure, ECG; respiration, adventitious sounds; abdominal examination, liver function tests, urine output, and electrolytes.

Nursing Diagnoses

The patient receiving beta-adrenergic blocking agents may have the following nursing diagnoses related to drug therapy:

- Acute Pain related to CNS, GI, and systemic effects
- Decreased Cardiac Output related to CV effects
- Ineffective Tissue Perfusion related to CV effects
- Deficient Knowledge regarding drug therapy

Implementation With Rationale

- Do not stop these drugs abruptly after chronic therapy but taper gradually over 2 weeks *because long-term use of these drugs can sensitize the myocardium to catecholamines, and severe reactions could occur.*
- Continuously monitor any patient receiving an intravenous form of these drugs *to avert serious complications caused by rapid sympathetic blockade.*
- Arrange for supportive care and comfort measures (rest, environmental control, other measures) *to relieve CNS effects;* institute safety measures if CNS effects occur *to prevent patient injury;* provide small, frequent meals and mouth care *to help relieve the discomfort of GI effects.*
- Provide thorough patient teaching, including name of the drug, dosage, anticipated adverse effects, measures to avoid drug-related problems, warning signs of problems, and proper administration techniques as needed *to enhance patient knowledge about drug therapy and to promote compliance.*
- Offer support and encouragement *to help the patient deal with the drug regimen.*

Evaluation

- Monitor patient response to the drug (lowering of blood pressure, decrease in anginal episodes, improvement in condition being treated).
- Monitor for adverse effects (GI upset, CNS changes, respiratory problems, CV effects, loss of libido, and impotence).
- Evaluate effectiveness of teaching plan (patient can name drug, dosage, adverse effects to watch for, specific measures to avoid adverse effects).
- Monitor the effectiveness of comfort measures and compliance with the regimen.

Beta$_1$-Selective Adrenergic Blocking Agents

Beta$_1$-selective adrenergic blocking agents have an advantage over the nonselective beta-blockers in some cases. Because they do not usually block beta$_2$-receptor sites, they do not block the sympathetic bronchodilation that is so important for patients with lung diseases or allergic rhinitis. Consequently, these drugs are preferred for patients who smoke or who have asthma, any other obstructive pulmonary disease, or seasonal or allergic rhinitis. These selective beta-blockers are also used for treating hypertension, angina, and some cardiac arrhythmias (Table 31.5).

Acebutolol (*Sectral*) is used for treating hypertension and premature ventricular contractions. Atenolol (*Tenormin*), which is more widely used, is prescribed to treat MI, chronic angina, and hypertension. Betaxolol (*Kerlone*) is used to treat hypertension; it is also available as an ophthalmic agent (*Betoptic*) to treat ocular hypertension and open-angle glaucoma. Bisoprolol (*Zebeta*) is reserved for use in treating hypertension. Esmolol (*Brevibloc*) is available as an intravenous agent for the treatment of supraventricular tachycardias (e.g., atrial flutter, atrial fibrillation) and non-compensatory tachycardia when the heart rate must be slowed. Metoprolol (*Lopressor, Toprol XL*) is used to treat hypertension and has an extended-release form that only needs to be taken once a day. It is also used to treat angina, to treat stable and symptomatic CHF, and to prevent reinfarction after MI. The beta$_1$-selective blocker of choice depends on the condition or combination of conditions being treated and personal experience with the drugs.

Table 31.5 DRUGS IN FOCUS

Beta$_1$-Selective Adrenergic Blocking Agents

Drug Name	Dosage/Route	Usual Indications
acebutolol (*Sectral*)	400 mg/day PO, up to 1200 mg/day may be used; decrease dosage with the elderly and with renal and hepatic impairment	Treatment of hypertension and premature ventricular contractions in adults
P atenolol (*Tenormin*)	Initially 50 mg/day PO, may increase to 100 mg/day; reduce dosage with renal impairment	Treatment of myocardial infarction (MI), chronic angina, hypertension in adults
betaxolol (*Kerlone, Betoptic*)	10–20 mg/day PO; reduce to 5 mg/day PO with the elderly; 1–2 gtts in affected eye(s) for glaucoma	Treatment of hypertension in adults; treatment of ocular hypertension, open-angle glaucoma
bisoprolol (*Zebeta*)	Initially 5 mg/day PO, up to 20 mg/day PO may be needed; reduce dosage with renal or hepatic impairment	Treatment of hypertension in adults
esmolol (*Brevibloc*)	50–200 mcg/kg/min IV with dosage based on patient response	Treatment of supraventricular tachycardias in adults
metoprolol (*Lopressor, Toprol XL*)	100–400 mg/day PO, based on patient response; XL preparation: 50–200 mg/day PO based on patient response	Treatment of hypertension, angina; prevention of reinfarction after MI; treatment of stable, symptomatic congestive heart failure (extended-release preparation only)

Therapeutic Actions and Indications

The therapeutic effects of these drugs are related to their ability to selectively block beta$_1$-receptors in the SNS. That selectivity occurs at therapeutic doses, but the selectivity is lost with doses higher than the recommended range. The blockade of the beta$_1$-receptors in the heart and in the juxtaglomerular apparatus account for most of the therapeutic benefit of these drugs. Decreased heart rate, contractility, and excitability, as well as a membrane-stabilizing effect, lead to a decrease in arrhythmias, decreased cardiac workload, and decreased oxygen consumption. The juxtaglomerular cells are not stimulated to release renin, which further decreases blood pressure. These effects are useful in treating hypertension and chronic angina and can help to prevent reinfarction after an MI by decreasing cardiac workload and oxygen consumption. At therapeutic doses, these drugs do not block the beta$_2$-receptors and therefore do not prevent sympathetic bronchodilation. These drugs are used to treat cardiac arrhythmias, hypertension, and angina; to prevent reinfarction after MI; and in ophthalmic form, to decrease intraocular pressure and to treat open-angle glaucoma. Metoprolol is also approved in the extended-release form for the treatment of stable, symptomatic CHF.

Pharmacokinetics

The beta$_1$-selective adrenergic blockers are absorbed from the GI tract. The bioavailability of metoprolol is increased if it is taken in the presence of food. These drugs are metabolized in the liver and excreted in the urine. Metoprolol readily crosses the blood–brain barrier and may cause more CNS effects than acebutolol and atenolol, which do not cross. *Because of the potential for adverse effects on the fetus and neonate,* these drugs should not be used during pregnancy and lactation unless the benefit to the mother outweighs the potential risk to the fetus or neonate. The safety and efficacy of the use of these drugs in children have not been established.

Contraindications and Cautions

The beta$_1$-selective adrenergic blockers are contraindicated in the presence of allergy to the drug or any components of the drug; with sinus bradycardia, heart block, cardiogenic shock, CHF, or hypotension, *all of which could be exacerbated by the cardiac-depressing and blood pressure-lowering effects of these drugs;* and with lactation *because of the potential adverse effects on the neonate.* They should be used with caution in patients with diabetes, thyroid disease, or COPD *because of the potential for adverse effects on these diseases with sympathetic blockade;* and in pregnancy *because of the potential for adverse effects on the fetus.*

Adverse Effects

Patients receiving these drugs often experience adverse effects related to the blocking of beta$_1$-receptors in the SNS. CNS effects include fatigue, dizziness, depression, paresthesias, sleep disturbances, memory loss, and disorientation. CV effects can include bradycardia, heart block, CHF, hypotension, and peripheral vascular insufficiency. Pulmonary effects ranging from rhinitis to bronchospasm and dyspnea can occur; these effects are not as likely to occur with these drugs as with the nonselective beta-blockers. GI upset, nausea, vomiting, diarrhea, gastric pain, and even colitis can occur as a result of unchecked parasympathetic activity and the blocking of the sympathetic receptors. Genitourinary effects can include decreased libido, impotence, dysuria, and Peyronie's disease. Other effects that can occur include decreased exercise tolerance (patients often report that their "get up and go" is gone), hypoglycemia or hyperglycemia, and liver changes that are reflected in increased concentrations of liver enzymes.

Clinically Important Drug–Drug Interactions

A decreased hypertensive effect occurs if these drugs are given with clonidine, NSAIDs, rifampin, or barbiturates. If such a combination is used, the patient should be monitored closely and dosage adjustment made.

There is an initial hypertensive episode followed by bradycardia if these drugs are given with epinephrine. Increased serum levels and increased toxicity of intravenous lidocaine will occur if it is given with these drugs.

An increased risk for postural hypotension occurs if these drugs are taken with prazosin. If this combination is used, the patient must be monitored closely and safety precautions taken.

The selective $beta_1$-blockers have increased effects if they are taken with verapamil, cimetidine, methimazole, or propylthiouracil. The patient should be monitored closely and appropriate dosage adjustment made.

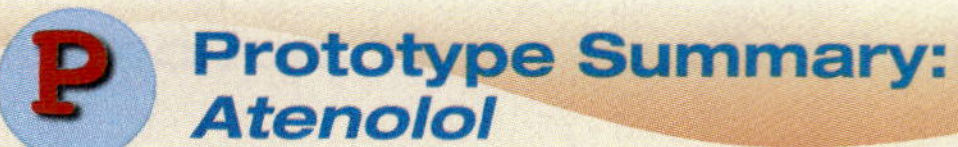

Prototype Summary: *Atenolol*

Indications: Treatment of angina pectoris, hypertension, myocardial infarction; unlabeled uses—prevention of migraine headaches, alcohol withdrawal syndrome, supraventricular tachycardias

Actions: Blocks $beta_1$-adrenergic receptors, decreasing the excitability of the heart, cardiac output, and oxygen consumption; decreases renin release, which lowers blood pressure

Pharmacokinetics:

Route	Onset	Peak	Duration
Oral	Varies	2–4 h	24 h
IV	Immediate	5 min	24 h

$T_{1/2}$: 6–7 hours, with excretion in the bile, feces, and urine

Adverse effects: Allergic reaction, dizziness, bradycardia, CHF, arrhythmias, gastric pain, flatulence, impotence, bronchospasm, decreased exercise tolerance

Nursing Considerations for Patients Receiving $Beta_1$-Selective Adrenergic Blocking Agents

Assessment: History and Examination

Screen for the following conditions, *which could be cautions or contraindications to the use of the drug:* known allergies to any drug or any components of the drug; bradycardia or heart blocks, shock, or CHF, *which could be exacerbated by the cardiac-suppressing effects of these drugs;* bronchospasm or COPD; pregnancy or lactation *because of the potential effects on the fetus or neonate;* diabetes or hypoglycemia; and thyrotoxicosis.

Include screening *for baseline status and for any potential adverse effects:* skin color, temperature; pulse, blood pressure, ECG; respiration, adventitious sounds; abdominal examination, urine output, and electrolytes.

Nursing Diagnoses

The patient receiving $beta_1$-adrenergic blockers may have the following nursing diagnoses related to drug therapy:

- Acute Pain related to CNS, GI, and systemic effects
- Decreased Cardiac Output related to cardiovascular effects
- Ineffective Tissue Perfusion related to cardiovascular effects
- Deficient Knowledge regarding drug therapy

Implementation With Rationale

- Do not stop these drugs abruptly after chronic therapy but taper gradually over 2 weeks *to prevent the possibility of severe reactions.* Long-term use of these drugs can sensitize the myocardium to catecholamines, *and severe reactions could occur.*
- Consult with the physician about discontinuing these drugs before surgery *because withdrawal of the drug before surgery when the patient has been maintained on the drug is controversial.*
- Give oral forms of the drug with food *to facilitate absorption.*
- Continuously monitor any patient receiving an intravenous form of these drugs *to detect severe reactions to sympathetic blockade and to ensure rapid response if these reactions occur.*
- Arrange for supportive care and comfort measures, including rest, environmental control, and other

measures, *to relieve CNS effects;* safety measures if CNS effects occur *to protect the patient from injury;* and small, frequent meals and mouth care *to relieve the discomfort of GI effects.*

- Provide thorough patient teaching, including the name of the drug, dosage, anticipated adverse effects, measures to avoid drug-related problems, and warning signs of problems, as well as proper administration, as needed *to enhance patient knowledge about drug therapy and to promote compliance.*
- Offer support and encouragement *to help the patient deal with the drug regimen.*

Evaluation

- Monitor patient response to the drug (lowered blood pressure, fewer anginal episodes, lowered intraocular pressure).
- Monitor for adverse effects (GI upset, CNS changes, cardiovascular effects, loss of libido and impotence, potential respiratory effects).
- Evaluate the effectiveness of the teaching plan (patient can name drug, dosage, adverse effects to watch for, specific measures to avoid adverse effects).
- Monitor the effectiveness of comfort measures and compliance with the regimen.

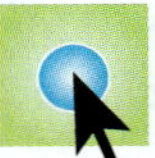

WEB LINKS

Health care providers and patients may want to consult the following Internet sources:

http://www.heartinfo.org/main Information on research, alternative methods of therapy, and pharmacology from the National Heart, Lung and Blood Institute.

http://amhrt.org Patient information, support groups, diet, exercise, and research information on hypertension and other cardiovascular diseases.

http://www.acc.org Information on cardiovascular research, treatments, hypertension, and arrhythmias.

Points to Remember

- Adrenergic blocking agents, or sympatholytic drugs, lyse or block the effects of the sympathetic nervous system (SNS).
- Both the therapeutic and the adverse effects associated with these drugs are related to their blocking of the normal responses of the SNS.
- The alpha- and beta-adrenergic blocking agents block all of the receptor sites within the SNS, which results in lower blood pressure, slower pulse, and increased renal perfusion with decreased renin levels. These drugs are indicated for the treatment of essential hypertension. They are associated with many adverse effects, including lack of bronchodilation, cardiac suppression, and diabetic reactions.
- Selective adrenergic blocking agents have been developed that, at therapeutic levels, have specific affinity for alpha- or beta-receptors or for specific alpha$_1$-, beta$_1$-, or beta$_2$-receptor sites. This specificity is lost at levels higher than the therapeutic range.
- Alpha-adrenergic drugs specifically block the alpha-receptors of the SNS. At therapeutic levels, they do not block beta-receptors.
- Nonspecific alpha-adrenergic blocking agents are used to treat pheochromocytoma, a tumor of the adrenal medulla.
- Alpha$_1$-selective adrenergic blocking agents block the post-synaptic alpha$_1$-receptor sites, causing a decrease in vascular tone and a vasodilation that leads to a fall in blood pressure without the reflex tachycardia that occurs when the presynaptic alpha$_2$-receptor sites are also blocked.
- Beta-blockers are drugs used to block the beta-receptors within the SNS. These drugs are used for a wide range of problems, including hypertension, stage fright, migraines, angina, and essential tremors.
- Blockade of all beta-receptors results in a loss of the reflex bronchodilation that occurs with sympathetic stimulation. This limits the use of these drugs in patients who smoke or have allergic or seasonal rhinitis, asthma, or COPD.
- Beta$_1$-selective adrenergic blocking agents do not block the beta$_1$-receptors that are responsible for bronchodilation and therefore are preferred in patients with respiratory problems.

CHECK YOUR UNDERSTANDING

Answers to the questions in this chapter may be found in the Answer Key in the back of the book.

Multiple Choice

Select the best answer to the following.

1. Adrenergic blocking drugs, because of their clinical effects, are also known as
   a. anticholinergics.
   b. sympathomimetics.
   c. parasympatholytics.
   d. sympatholytics.

2. You might give drugs that generally block all adrenergic receptor sites to treat
   a. signs and symptoms of allergic rhinitis.
   b. COPD.
   c. cardiac-related conditions.
   d. premature labor.

3. Phentolamine (*Regitine*), an alpha-adrenergic blocker, is most frequently used
   a. to prevent cell death after extravasation of intravenous dopamine or norepinephrine.
   b. to treat COPD.
   c. to treat hypertension.
   d. to block bronchoconstriction during acute asthma attacks.

4. You might administer an $alpha_1$-selective adrenergic blocking agent in the treatment of
   a. COPD.
   b. hypertension and BPH.
   c. erectile dysfunction.
   d. shock states and bronchospasm.

5. The beta-blocker of choice for a patient who is hypertensive and has angina would be
   a. nadolol.
   b. pindolol.
   c. timolol.
   d. carteolol.

6. You would question an order for $beta_1$-selective adrenergic blockers in the treatment of
   a. cardiac arrhythmias.
   b. hypertension.
   c. cardiogenic shock.
   d. open-angle glaucoma.

7. A smoker who is being treated for hypertension with a beta-blocker should be treated with a
   a. nonspecific beta-blocker.
   b. $beta_2$-specific beta-blocker.
   c. beta- and alpha-blockers.
   d. $beta_1$-specific blocker.

8. You would caution a patient who is taking an adrenergic blocker
   a. to avoid exposure to infection.
   b. to stop the drug if he/she experiences flu-like symptoms.
   c. never to stop the drug abruptly because it needs to be tapered slowly.
   d. to avoid exposure to the sun.

Multiple Response

Select all that apply.

1. A nurse would question an order for a beta-adrenergic blocker if the patient was also receiving what other drugs?
   a. Clonidine
   b. Ergot alkaloids
   c. Aspirin
   d. NSAIDs
   e. Triptans
   f. Epinephrine

2. The beta-adrenergic blocker propranolol is approved for a wide variety of uses. Which of the following would be approved indications?
   a. Migraine headaches
   b. Stage fright or situational anxiety
   c. Bronchospasm
   d. Reinfarction after an MI
   e. Erectile dysfunction
   f. Hypertension

Web Exercise

One of your male patients has received a diagnosis of essential hypertension. Because his father died at a young age of a heart attack, he is concerned about his risk for developing heart disease and asks you for more information. Go to the Internet and develop a teaching packet to address his concerns; http://www.fda.gov/hearthealth/ would be a good starting place.

True or False

Indicate whether the following statements are true (T) or false (F).

_____ 1. Adrenergic blocking agents are also called sympathomimetic drugs.

_____ 2. Drugs that block all adrenergic receptors are primarily used to treat cardiac-related conditions.

_____ 3. Adrenergic blocking agents competitively block the effects of norepinephrine at both alpha- and beta-receptors throughout the sympathetic nervous system (SNS), causing the signs and symptoms associated with a sympathetic stress reaction.

_____ 4. The adverse effects associated with adrenergic blocking agents of cardiac arrhythmias, hypotension, CHF, pulmonary edema, cerebral vascular accident, or stroke are related to the lack of stimulatory effects and loss of vascular tone in the cardiovascular system.

_____ 5. The therapeutic effects of the alpha$_1$-selective adrenergic blocking agents come from their ability to block the postsynaptic alpha$_1$-receptor sites. This causes a decrease in vascular tone and vasodilation, which leads to a fall in blood pressure.

_____ 6. The beta-adrenergic blocking agents are used to treat asthma and obstructive pulmonary diseases.

_____ 7. Propranolol is a widely prescribed drug that has been used to treat migraine headaches and stage fright (situational anxiety).

_____ 8. Beta-adrenergic blocking agents should not be stopped abruptly after chronic therapy but should be tapered gradually over 2 weeks.

Bibliography and References

Andrews, M., & Boyle, J. (2002). *Transcultural concepts in nursing care.* Philadelphia: Lippincott Williams & Wilkins.

Drug facts and comparisons. (2006). St. Louis: Facts and Comparisons.

Gilman, A., Hardman, J. G., & Limbird, L. E. (Eds.). (2006). *Goodman and Gilman's the pharmacological basis of therapeutics* (11th ed.). New York: McGraw-Hill.

Karch, A. M. (2006). *2007 Lippincott's nursing drug guide.* Philadelphia: Lippincott Williams & Wilkins.

The medical letter on drugs and therapeutics. (2006). New Rochelle, NY: Medical Letter.

Porth, C. M. (2005). *Pathophysiology: Concepts of altered health states* (7th ed.). Philadelphia: Lippincott Williams & Wilkins.

CHAPTER 32

Cholinergic Agents

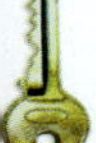

KEY TERMS

acetylcholinesterase
Alzheimer's disease
cholinergic
miosis
myasthenia gravis
nerve gas
parasympathomimetic

LEARNING OBJECTIVES

Upon completion of this chapter, you will be able to:

1. Describe the effects of cholinergic receptors and correlate this with the clinical effects of cholinergic drugs.
2. Describe the therapeutic actions, indications, pharmacokinetics, contraindications, most common adverse reactions, and important drug–drug interactions associated with the direct- and indirect-acting cholinergic agents.
3. Discuss the use of cholinergic agents across the lifespan.
4. Compare and contrast the prototype drugs bethanechol, donepezil, and pyridostigmine with other cholinergic agents.
5. Outline the nursing considerations, including important teaching points, for patients receiving a cholinergic agent.

DIRECT-ACTING CHOLINERGIC AGONISTS

P bethanechol
carbachol
cevimeline
pilocarpine

INDIRECT-ACTING CHOLINERGIC AGONISTS

ambenonium
P donepezil
edrophonium
galantamine
neostigmine
P pyridostigmine
rivastigmine
tacrine

REVERSING AGENT

pralidoxime

Cholinergic drugs are chemicals that act at the same site as the neurotransmitter acetylcholine (ACh). Because these sites are found extensively throughout the parasympathetic nervous system (PSNS), the stimulation of these sites produces a response similar to what is seen when the parasympathetic system is activated. As a result, these drugs are often called **parasympathomimetic** drugs because their action mimics the action of the parasympathetic nervous system. Because the action of these drugs cannot be limited to a specific site, their effects can be widespread throughout the body, and they are usually associated with many undesirable systemic effects.

Cholinergic Agonists

Cholinergic agonists are drugs that increase the activity of the ACh receptor sites throughout the body. These drugs work either directly or indirectly. Direct-acting cholinergic agonists occupy receptor sites for ACh on the membranes of the effector cells of the postganglionic cholinergic nerves, causing increased stimulation of the cholinergic receptor. In contrast, indirect-acting cholinergic agonists cause increased stimulation of the ACh receptor sites by reacting with the enzyme **acetylcholinesterase** and preventing it from breaking down the ACh that was released from the nerve. These drugs produce their effects indirectly by producing an increase in the level of ACh in the synaptic cleft, leading to increased stimulation of the cholinergic receptor site (Figure 32.1). The effects of these drugs differ across the lifespan, as discussed in Box 32.1.

Direct-Acting Cholinergic Agonists

The direct-acting cholinergic agonists are similar to ACh and react directly with receptor sites to cause the same reaction as ACh. These drugs tend to cause stimulation of the muscarinic receptors within the parasympathetic system.

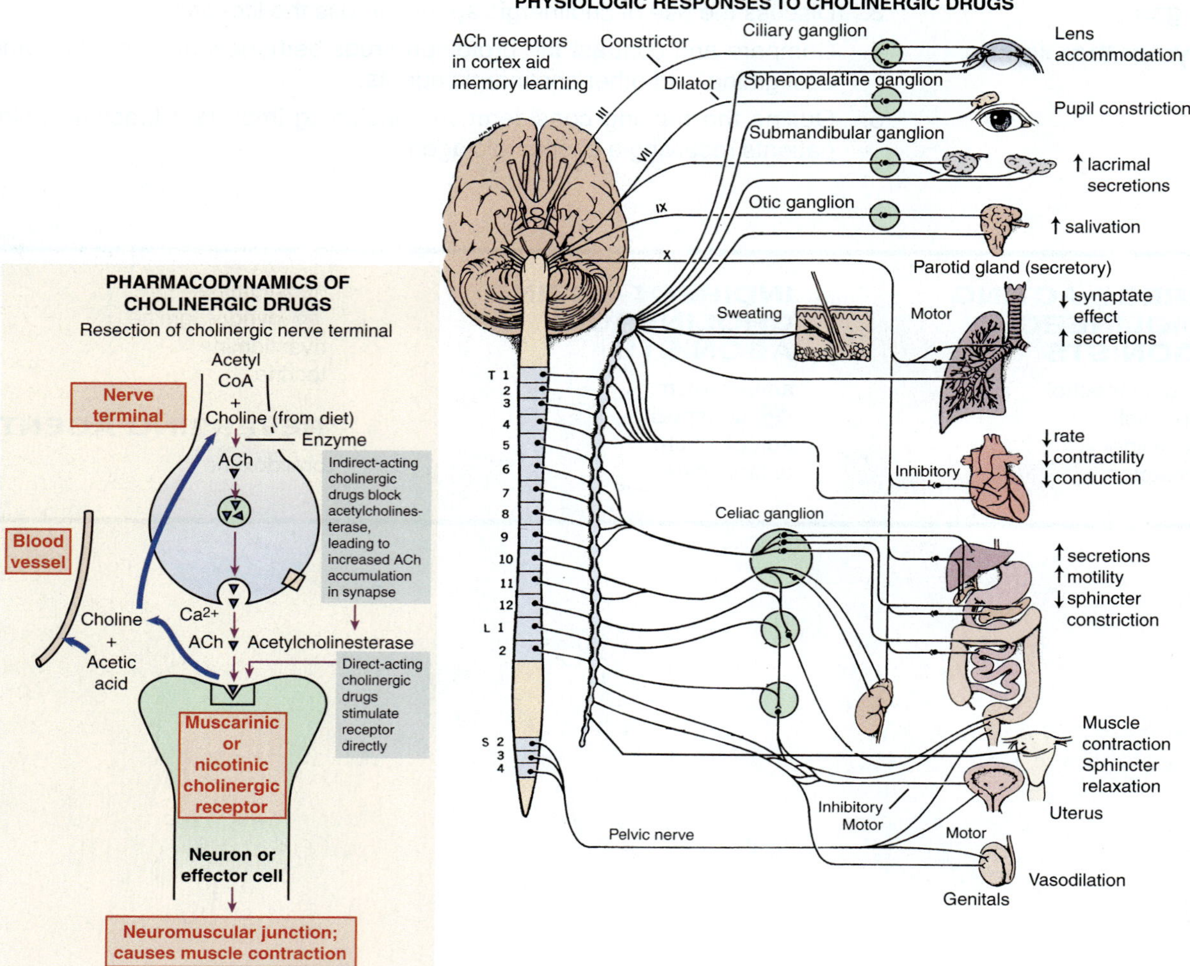

FIGURE 32.1 Pharmacodynamics of cholinergic drugs and associated physiologic responses.

BOX 32.1 **DRUG THERAPY ACROSS THE LIFESPAN**

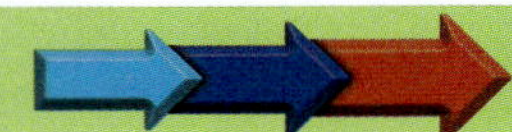

Cholinergic Agents

CHILDREN

Children may be more susceptible to the adverse effects associated with the cholinergic agents, including gastrointestinal (GI) upset, diarrhea, increased salivation that could lead to choking, and loss of bowel and bladder control, a problem that could cause stress in the child. Children should be monitored closely if these agents are used and should receive appropriate supportive care.

Bethanechol is approved for the treatment of neurogenic bladder in children older than 8 years of age. Neostigmine and pyridostigmine are used in the control of myasthenia gravis and for reversal of neuromuscular junction blocker effects in children. Care should be taken in determining the appropriate dose based on weight. Edrophonium is used for diagnosis of myasthenia gravis only.

ADULTS

Adults should be cautioned about the many adverse effects that can be anticipated when using a cholinergic agent. Flushing, increased sweating, increased salivation and GI upset, and urinary urgency often occur. The patient also needs to be aware that dizziness, drowsiness, and blurred vision may occur and that driving and operating dangerous machinery should be avoided.

In general, there are no adequate studies about the effects of these drugs during pregnancy and lactation. Therefore, the cholinergic agents should be used only in those situations in which the benefit to the mother is greater than the risk to the fetus or neonate. Nursing mothers who require one of these drugs should find another way to feed the baby.

OLDER ADULTS

Older patients are more likely to experience the adverse effects associated with these drugs—central nervous system, cardiovascular, GI, respiratory, and urinary. Because older patients often have renal or hepatic impairment, they are also more likely to have toxic levels of the drug related to changes in metabolism and excretion.

The older patient should be started on lower doses of the drugs and should be monitored very closely for potentially serious arrhythmias or hypotension. Safety precautions should be established if the drug causes dizziness or drowsiness. Special efforts may also be needed to help the patient maintain fluid intake and nutrition if the GI effects become uncomfortable. Taking the drug with food and offering the patient several small meals throughout the day may alleviate some of these problems.

They are used to increase bladder tone, urinary excretion, and GI secretions and as ophthalmic agents, which are not usually absorbed systemically. Their use today is infrequent; because they can cause widespread parasympathetic activity, the more specific and less toxic drugs that are now available are preferred.

The agent bethanechol (*Duvoid, Urecholine*) is available for use orally and subcutaneously to treat nonobstructive postoperative and postpartum urinary retention and to treat neurogenic bladder atony by directly increasing muscle tone and relaxing the sphincters. It has also been used to diagnose and treat reflux esophagitis. Although not indicated for use in children, this drug has been used orally in infants and children for the treatment of esophageal reflux. Cevimeline (*Evoxac*) is used to increase secretions and relieve the symptoms of dry mouth that are in seen in Sjögren's syndrome. It is approved for use in adults and is given three times a day, often with meals. The patient should be monitored for any swallowing difficulties because salivary secretions will increase and swallowing difficulties could result in aspiration. Adverse effects are associated with increased parasympathetic activation, and the patient needs to be monitored for dehydration, bradycardia, and discomfort associated with increased gastrointestinal (GI) activity. The drugs carbachol (*Miostat*) and pilocarpine (*Pilocar* and others) are available only as ophthalmic agents; they are used to induce **miosis**, or pupil constriction; to relieve the increased intraocular pressure of glaucoma; and to allow surgeons to perform certain surgical procedures (Table 32.1).

Therapeutic Actions and Indications

The direct-acting cholinergic agonists act at cholinergic receptors in the peripheral nervous system to mimic the effects of ACh and parasympathetic stimulation. These parasympathetic effects include slowed heart rate and decreased myocardial contractility, vasodilation, bronchoconstriction and increased secretions from bronchial mucus, increased GI activity and secretions, increase in bladder tone, relaxation of GI and bladder sphincters, and pupil constriction (see Figure 32.1).

The drugs of this type that are used systemically are bethanechol, which has an affinity for the cholinergic receptors in the urinary bladder, and cevimeline, which binds to muscarinic receptors throughout the system. Bethanechol increases the tone of the detrusor muscle of the bladder and relaxes the bladder sphincter to improve bladder emptying. Because this drug is not destroyed by acetylcholinesterase, the effects on the receptor site are longer than with stimulation by ACh. Cevimeline is used to increase secretions in the mouth and GI tract to relieve dry mouth associated with Sjögren's syndrome. Carbachol and pilocarpine are topical drugs that are not generally absorbed systemically, so they are not associated with severe adverse effects.

Pharmacokinetics

The direct-acting cholinergic agonists are generally well absorbed and have relatively short half-lives, ranging from

Table 32.1 DRUGS IN FOCUS

Direct-Acting Cholinergic Agonists

Drug Name	Dosage/Route	Usual Indications
P bethanechol (*Duvoid, Urecholine*)	10–50 mg PO b.i.d. to q.i.d.	Nonobstructive urinary retention, neurogenic bladder in adults and children >8 yr
carbachol (*Miostat*)	1–2 gtt in affected eye(s) as needed, up to three times a day	Glaucoma, miosis
cevimeline (*Evoxac*)	30 mg PO t.i.d.	Treatment of symptoms of dry mouth in patients with Sjögren's syndrome
pilocarpine (*Pilocar*)	1–2 gtt in affected eye(s) as needed, up to six times per day	Glaucoma, miosis

1 to 6 hours. The metabolism and excretion of these drugs is not known but is believed to occur at the synaptic level. It is not known whether these drugs cross the placenta or enter breast milk, but because of the potential for serious adverse effects on the fetus and neonate, they should not be used during pregnancy or lactation unless the benefit to the mother outweighs the potential risk to the neonate.

Contraindications and Cautions

These drugs are used sparingly *because of the potential undesirable systemic effects of parasympathetic stimulation.* They are contraindicated in the presence of any condition that would be exacerbated by parasympathetic effects. For example, bradycardia, hypotension, vasomotor instability, and coronary artery disease *could be made worse by the cardiac- and cardiovascular-suppressing effects of the parasympathetic system.* Peptic ulcer, intestinal obstruction, or recent GI surgery *could be negatively affected by the GI-stimulating effects of the peripheral nervous system.* Asthma *could be exacerbated by the increased parasympathetic effect, overriding the protective sympathetic bronchodilation.* Bladder obstruction or healing sites from recent bladder surgery *could be aggravated by the stimulatory effects on the bladder.* Epilepsy and parkinsonism *could be affected by the stimulation of ACh receptors in the brain.* Caution should be used during pregnancy and lactation *because of the potential adverse effects on the fetus or neonate.*

Adverse Effects

Patients should be cautioned about the potential adverse effects of these drugs. Even if the drug is being given as a topical ophthalmic agent, there is always a possibility that it will be absorbed. The adverse effects associated with these drugs are related to PSNS stimulation. GI effects can include nausea, vomiting, cramps, diarrhea, increased salivation, and involuntary defecation related to the increase in GI secretions and activity. Cardiovascular effects can include bradycardia, heart block, hypotension, and even cardiac arrest related to the cardiac-suppressing effects of the parasympathetic nervous system. Urinary tract effects can include a sense of urgency related to the stimulation of the bladder muscles and sphincter relaxation. Other effects may include flushing and increased sweating secondary to stimulation of the cholinergic receptors in the sympathetic nervous system.

Clinically Important Drug–Drug Interactions

There is an increased risk of cholinergic effects if these drugs are combined or given with acetylcholinesterase inhibitors. The patient should be monitored and appropriate dosage adjustments made.

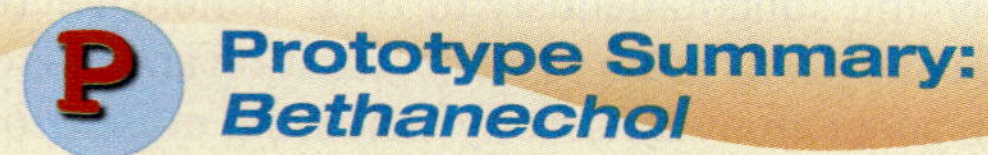

Indications: Acute postoperative or postpartum nonobstructive urinary retention; neurogenic atony of the bladder with retention

Actions: Acts directly on cholinergic receptors to mimic the effects of acetylcholine; increases tone of detrusor muscles and causes emptying of the bladder

Pharmacokinetics:

Route	Onset	Peak	Duration
Oral	30–90 min	60–90 min	1–6 h

$T_{1/2}$: Metabolism and excretion unknown; thought to be synaptic

Adverse effects: Abdominal discomfort, salivation, nausea, vomiting, sweating, flushing

Nursing Considerations for Patients Receiving Direct-Acting Cholinergic Agonists

Assessment: History and Examination

Screen for the following conditions, *which could be cautions or contraindications to use of the drug: known allergies to these drugs;* bradycardia, vasomotor instability, peptic ulcer, obstructive urinary or GI diseases; recent GI or genitourinary surgery; asthma; parkinsonism or epilepsy; and pregnancy or lactation, *all of which could be exacerbated or complicated by parasympathetic stimulation.*

Include screening *for baseline status before beginning therapy and for any potential adverse effects:* skin color, lesions, temperature; pulse, blood pressure, electrocardiogram (ECG); respiration, adventitious sounds; and urine output and bladder tone.

Nursing Diagnoses

The patient receiving a direct-acting cholinergic agonist may have the following nursing diagnoses related to drug therapy:

- Acute Pain related to GI effects
- Decreased Cardiac Output related to cardiovascular effects
- Impaired Urinary Elimination related to effects on the bladder
- Deficient Knowledge regarding drug therapy

Implementation With Rationale

- Ensure proper administration of ophthalmic preparations *to increase effectiveness of drug therapy.*
- Administer oral drug on an empty stomach *to decrease nausea and vomiting.*
- Monitor patient response closely, including blood pressure, ECG, urine output, and cardiac output, *and arrange to adjust dosage accordingly to ensure the most benefit with the least amount of toxicity.* Maintain atropine on standby *to reverse overdose or counteract severe reactions.*
- Provide safety precautions if the patient reports poor visual acuity in dim light *to prevent injury.*
- Provide thorough patient teaching, including measures to avoid adverse effects and warning signs of problems, as well as the need for monitoring and evaluation *to enhance patient knowledge about drug therapy and to promote compliance.*
- Offer support and encouragement *to help the patient deal with the drug regimen.*

Evaluation

- Monitor patient response to the drug (improvement in bladder function, miosis).
- Monitor for adverse effects (cardiovascular changes, GI stimulation, urinary urgency, respiratory distress).
- Evaluate the effectiveness of the teaching plan (patient can name drug, dosage, adverse effects to watch for, specific measures to avoid adverse effects, proper administration of ophthalmic drugs).
- Monitor the effectiveness of comfort and safety measures and compliance with the regimen.

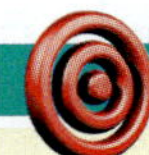

FOCUS POINTS

- Cholinergic drugs stimulate the parasympathetic nerves, some nerves in the brain, and the neuromuscular junction at the same site ACh does. They are used topically in the eye to produce miosis (pupillary constriction) and treat glaucoma. Systemically they are used to increase bladder tone (e.g., postpartum) and to increase secretions to relieve dry mouth associated with Sjögren's syndrome.

Indirect-Acting Cholinergic Agonists

The indirect-acting cholinergic agonists do not react directly with ACh receptor sites; instead, they react chemically with acetylcholinesterase (the enzyme responsible for the breakdown of ACh) in the synaptic cleft to prevent it from breaking down ACh. As a result, the ACh that is released from the presynaptic nerve remains in the area and accumulates, stimulating the ACh receptors. These drugs work at all ACh receptors, in the parasympathetic nervous system, in the central nervous system (CNS), and at the neuromuscular junction. All of these drugs bind reversibly to acetylcholinesterase, so their effects will pass with time. (Certain drugs, however, are irreversible acetylcholinesterase-inhibiting agents, requiring special considerations—see Boxes 32.2 and 32.3.) Table 32.2 provides information about each drug, its dosage, and indications for its use. The indirect-acting cholinergic agents fall into two main categories: (1) agents used to treat myasthenia gravis and (2) newer agents used to treat Alzheimer's disease.

Myasthenia Gravis Agents

Myasthenia gravis is a chronic muscular disease caused by a defect in neuromuscular transmission. It is thought to be

BOX 32.2 Pralidoxime: Antidote for Irreversible Acetylcholinesterase-Inhibiting Drugs

Pralidoxime *(Protopam Chloride),* the antidote for irreversible acetylcholinesterase-inhibiting drugs, is given intramuscularly or intravenously to reactivate the acetylcholinesterase that has been blocked by these drugs. Freeing up the acetylcholinesterase allows it to break down accumulated acetylcholine that has overstimulated acetylcholine receptor sites, causing paralysis.

Pralidoxime does not readily cross the blood–brain barrier, and it is most useful for treating peripheral drug effects. It reacts within minutes after injection and should be available for any patient receiving indirect-acting cholinergic agonists to treat myasthenia gravis. The patient and a significant other should understand when to use the drug and how to administer it.

Pralidoxime is also used with atropine (which does cross the blood–brain barrier and will block the effects of accumulated acetylcholine at central nervous system sites) to treat organophosphate pesticide poisonings and nerve gas exposure (see Box 32.3), both of which cause inactivation of acetylcholinesterase.

Adverse effects associated with the use of pralidoxime include dizziness, blurred vision, diplopia, headache, drowsiness, hyperventilation, and nausea. These effects are also seen with exposure to nerve gas and organophosphate pesticides, so it can be difficult to differentiate drug effects from the effects of the poisoning.

BOX 32.3 Nerve Gas: An Irreversible Acetylcholinesterase Inhibitor

Recent worldwide events and conflicts have made the potential use of **nerve gas** a major news story. Developed as a weapon, nerve gas is an irreversible acetylcholinesterase inhibitor. The drug is inhaled and quickly spreads throughout the body, where it permanently binds with acetylcholinesterase. This causes an accumulation of acetylcholine at nerve endings and a massive cholinergic response. The heart rate slows and becomes ineffective, pupils and bronchi constrict, the gastrointestinal tract increases activity and secretions, and muscles contract and remain that way. The muscle contraction soon freezes the diaphragm, causing breathing to stop. The bodies of people who are killed by nerve gas have a characteristic rigor of muscle contraction.

If nerve gas is expected, individuals who may be exposed are given intramuscular injections of atropine (to temporarily block cholinergic activity and to activate acetylcholine sites in the central nervous system) and pralidoxime (to free up the acetylcholinesterase to start breaking down acetylcholine). An autoinjection is provided to military personnel who may be at risk. The injector is used to give atropine and then pralidoxime. The injections are repeated in 15 minutes. If symptoms of nerve gas exposure exist after an additional 15 minutes, the injections are repeated. If symptoms still persist after a third set of injections, medical help should be sought.

Table 32.2 DRUGS IN FOCUS

Indirect-Acting Cholinergic Agonists

Drug Name	Dosage/Route	Usual Indications
ambenonium (*Mytelase*)	5–25 mg PO t.i.d. to q.i.d.	Myasthenia gravis in adults
P donepezil (*Aricept*)	5–10 mg PO daily at bedtime	Alzheimer's disease
edrophonium (*Tensilon, Enlon*)	Diagnosis: 2 mg IV over 15–30 sec, then 8 mg IV if response was seen or 10 mg IM, repeat with 2 mg IM in ½ hour to rule out false-negative results Antidote: 10 mg IV over 30–45 sec, repeat as needed, maximum dose—40 mg Pediatric (diagnosis only): 0.5–2 mg IV based on weight, or 2–5 mg IM	Myasthenia gravis diagnosis, antidote to neuromuscular junction blockers
galantamine (*Razadyne*)	4–12 mg PO b.i.d.; reduce dosage to 16 mg/day maximum with renal or hepatic impairment; available as an oral solution 4 mg/mL; range 16–32 mg/day	Alzheimer's disease
neostigmine (*Prostigmine*)	Adult: 0.5 mg Sub-Q or IM for control; 0.022 mg/kg IM for diagnosis; 0.5–2 mg IV as antidote, maximum dose 5 mg Pediatric: 0.01–0.04 mg/kg/dose IM, IV, or Sub-Q for control q2–3h; 0.04 mg/kg IM for diagnosis; 0.07–0.08 mg/kg IV, slowly, for antidote	Myasthenia gravis diagnosis and control, antidote to neuromuscular junction blockers
P pyridostigmine (*Regonol, Mestinon*)	Adult: average, 180–540 mg daily PO for myasthenia gravis; 0.1–0.25 mg/kg IV for antidote; 30 mg q8h starting several hours before exposure to nerve gas Pediatric: 7 mg/day PO in five or six divided doses for myasthenia gravis	Myasthenia gravis, antidote to neuromuscular junction blockers; increased survival after exposure to nerve gas
rivastigmine (*Exelon*)	1.5–6 mg PO b.i.d., based on patient response and tolerance	Alzheimer's disease
tacrine (*Cognex*)	10–40 mg PO q.i.d., based on patient response and tolerance	Alzheimer's disease

an autoimmune disease in which patients make antibodies to their ACh receptors. These antibodies cause gradual destruction of the ACh receptors, causing the patient to have fewer and fewer receptor sites available for stimulation. The disease is marked by progressive weakness and lack of muscle control with periodic acute episodes. The disease can progress to paralysis of the diaphragm, which prevents the patient from breathing and would prove fatal without intervention.

Drugs used to help patients with this progressive disease are acetylcholinesterase inhibitors. These drugs cause an accumulation of ACh in the synaptic cleft, providing a longer period of time for ACh to stimulate whatever receptors are still available.

Neostigmine (*Prostigmine*) is a synthetic drug that does not cross the blood–brain barrier but has a strong influence at the neuromuscular junction. It has a duration of action of 2 to 4 hours and therefore must be given every few hours, based on patient response, to maintain a therapeutic level. (See Critical Thinking Scenario 32-1.)

Pyridostigmine (*Regonol, Mestinon*), which has a longer duration of action than neostigmine (3 to 6 hours), is preferred in some cases for the management of myasthenia gravis because it does not need to be taken as frequently. It is available in oral and parenteral forms; the latter can be used if the patient is having trouble swallowing. It has recently been approved for military personnel to increase survival after exposure to particular **nerve gases**.

Ambenonium (*Mytelase*) is a newer drug that is similar to pyridostigmine in that it is taken only four times a day. Its main disadvantage is that it is available only in an oral preparation and cannot be used if the patient is unable to swallow tablets.

Edrophonium (*Tensilon, Enlon*) has a very short duration of action (10 to 20 minutes). Its primary use is as a diagnostic agent for myasthenia gravis, as discussed in Box 32.4. If a patient has a temporary reversal of symptoms after injection with edrophonium, it indicates a problem with the ACh neuromuscular receptors.

Alzheimer's Disease Drugs

Alzheimer's disease is a progressive disorder involving neural degeneration in the cortex that leads to a marked loss of memory and of the ability to carry on activities of daily living. Because of this, Alzheimer's disease can have very negative effects on family life (see Box 32.5). The cause of the disease is not yet known, but there is a progressive loss of ACh-producing neurons and their target neurons. Four cholinergic drugs are currently available to slow the progression of this disease: tacrine (*Cognex*), the first drug developed for the treatment of mild to moderate Alzheimer's dementia; galantamine (*Razadyne*), which is recommended for use with mild to moderate Alzheimer's dementia to delay progression of the disease and is available in tablet and oral solution forms; rivastigmine (*Exelon*), which is available in capsule and solution forms to help with patients who have swallowing difficulties; and donepezil (*Aricept*), which has once-a-day dosing. The once-a-day dosing offers a great advantage in a disease that affects memory and the patient's ability to remember to take pills throughout the day. In late 2003, an N-methyl-D-aspartate receptor antagonist, memantine, was also approved for use in the treatment of Alzheimer's disease (Box 32.6).

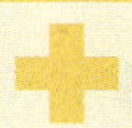

FOCUS ON **PATIENT SAFETY**

In 2005, as part of the continued effort to decrease medication errors, Ortho-McNeil, the makers of galantamine, announced that it was changing the name of its Alzheimer's drug from *Reminyl to Razadyne*. Many reports of name confusion between *Amaryl* (glimepiride; an antidiabetic agent) and *Reminyl,* some of which led to major problems involving glucose regulation and the occurrence of parasympathetic adverse effects when they were not anticipated, led to the decision to change the name.

Therapeutic Actions and Indications

All of the indirect-acting cholinergic agonists work by blocking acetylcholinesterase at the synaptic cleft. This blocking allows the accumulation of ACh released from the nerve endings and leads to increased and prolonged stimulation of ACh receptor sites at all of the postsynaptic cholinergic sites. These drugs can work to relieve the signs and symptoms of myasthenia gravis and increase muscle strength by accumulating ACh in the synaptic cleft at neuromuscular junctions.

The drugs preferred for use with myasthenia gravis are those that do not cross the blood–brain barrier. Drugs that do cross the blood–brain barrier and seem to affect mostly the cells in the cortex to increase ACh concentration are used in the treatment of mild to moderate Alzheimer's disease. Neostigmine and edrophonium, because of their rapid onset of action, are also used to reverse toxicity from nondepolarizing neuromuscular junction blocking drugs, which are used to paralyze muscles during surgery (see Chapter 28).

Pharmacokinetics

These drugs are well absorbed and distributed throughout the body. The drugs used to treat myasthenia gravis do not cross the blood–brain barrier, and their sites of metabolism and excretion are not known. The drugs used for Alzheimer's disease are metabolized in the liver by the cytochrome P450 system, so caution must be used with hepatic impairment and with many interacting drugs. They are excreted in the urine. Because there are no definitive studies on the effects of these drugs during pregnancy and lactation, they should be used during those times only if the benefit to the mother clearly outweighs the potential risks to the fetus or neonate.

CRITICAL THINKING SCENARIO 32-1

Cholinergic Agents for Distention

The Situation

A.J. has been returned to your unit after a lengthy abdominal surgery. She has not eaten since the previous evening but has no desire for the ice chips that have been offered. Her abdomen appears distended, and no bowel sounds are heard on auscultation. The harried house officer who is called decides that A.J. is probably suffering from either paralytic ileus or atonic bladder and orders an intramuscular injection of neostigmine (to reverse the effects of a neuromuscular junction blocker used during surgery) and several oral doses of bethanechol.

Critical Thinking

What could be responsible for A.J.'s symptoms? After abdominal surgery, it is not unusual to have some reflex intestinal atony because of the intestinal manipulation during surgery.

Do the ordered medications seem to be reasonable? What are the potential adverse effects to consider when giving two cholinergic drugs?

What are the potential complications from these drugs after gastrointestinal surgery? *Outline a care plan for A.J. considering her postoperative status, the potential problem she is encountering, the potential effects of the prescribed drug therapy, and the stress and anxiety she may be experiencing as a result of these complications.*

Do you think you would give the ordered medications? If not, what else should be done?

Discussion

The cholinergic drugs that have been ordered would produce some anticipated adverse effects related to their stimulation of the parasympathetic nervous system. These effects include increased bronchial secretions and bronchoconstriction, which could cause a problem in recovery from general anesthesia, requiring vigorous pulmonary toilet; increased gastric secretions and activity, which could cause major problems after abdominal surgery, including rupture or obstruction; hypotension and bradycardia, which could further complicate recovery from anesthesia and result in poor perfusion to the operative site; and increased tone and contractions of the bladder, which could cause some problems in the postoperative patient, depending on the site of the surgery and use of a catheter.

The most appropriate action in this case would be to question the drugs ordered and to refuse to give the medications until additional tests are done to evaluate the actual cause of the abdominal distention. An abdominal radiograph or ultrasound study would be helpful in determining the cause of the problem, which could just as easily be internal bleeding.

In the meantime, A.J. should receive support and comfort measures (e.g., positioning, medication). Baseline assessment should be done on all of those parameters most affected by anticholinergic drugs. If the cholinergic drugs are the most appropriate treatment in this case, baseline information will be in place to evaluate for any adverse effects of the drugs. If these drugs are used, very careful patient assessment will be necessary to ensure the safety of the patient in the postoperative phase and full recovery later.

Teaching plans should include the reason for the concerns, the reasons for additional tests, and the actions and anticipated side effects of the drugs, as well as supportive measures that will be taken to help A.J. cope with the therapy and recover fully.

Nursing Care Guide for A.J.: Cholinergic Agents for Distention

Assessment: History and Examination

Assess history of allergies to any of these drugs as well as history of coronary artery disease, hypotension, bradycardia, heart block, bowel or urinary obstruction, epilepsy, parkinsonism, recent GI or urinary surgery, and concurrent use of corticosteroids or succinylcholine.

Focus the physical examination on the following:

CV: Blood pressure, pulse rate, peripheral perfusion, ECG

CNS: orientation, affect, reflexes, vision

Skin: color, lesions, texture

GU: urinary output, bladder tone

GI: abdominal examination

Respiratory: respirations, adventitious sounds

Nursing Diagnoses

Decreased Cardiac Output related to CV effects

Acute Pain related to GI, systemic effects

Cholinergic Agents for Distention *(continued)*

Impaired Urinary Elimination related to GI effects

Deficient Knowledge regarding drug therapy

Implementation

Ensure safe and appropriate administration of drug.

Provide comfort and safety measures (e.g., physical assistance, raising siderails on the bed); temperature control; pain relief; small, frequent meals.

Monitor cardiac status and urine output throughout drug therapy.

Provide support and reassurance to deal with side effects, discomfort, and GI effects.

Provide patient teaching regarding drug name, dosage, side effects, precautions, and warning signs of serious adverse effects to report.

Evaluation

Evaluate drug effects: reversal of NMJ effects.

Monitor for adverse effects: CV effects—bradycardia, heart block, hypotension; urinary problems; GI effects; respiratory problems.

Monitor for drug–drug interactions.

Evaluate effectiveness of patient teaching program and comfort and safety measures.

Patient Teaching for A.J.

☐ The drug that was ordered for you is called neostigmine. It is called a cholinergic drug or a parasympathetic drug because it mimics the effects of the parasympathetic nervous system. Cholinergic drugs get this name because they act at certain nerve–nerve and nerve–muscle junctions in the body that are called cholinergic sites.

☐ Some of the following adverse effects may occur.

- *Nausea, excessive gas, diarrhea:* It is wise to be near bathroom facilities after taking your drug. If these symptoms become too severe, consult with your health care provider.
- *Flushing, sweating:* Staying in a cool environment and wearing lightweight clothing may help.
- *Urgency to void:* Maintaining access to a bathroom may relieve some of this discomfort.
- *Headache:* Aspirin or another headache medication (if not contraindicated in your particular case) will help to alleviate this pain.
- Report any of the following to your health care provider: *very slow pulse, light-headedness, fainting, excessive salivation, abdominal cramping or pain, weakness or confusion, blurring of vision.*

☐ Tell any doctor, nurse, or other health care provider involved in your care that you are taking these drugs.

Contraindications and Cautions

These drugs are contraindicated in the presence of allergy to any of these drugs; with bradycardia or intestinal or urinary tract obstruction, *which could be exacerbated by the stimulation of cholinergic receptors;* in pregnancy *because the uterus could be stimulated and labor induced;* and during lactation *because of the potential effects on the baby.*

Caution should be used with any condition that could be exacerbated by cholinergic stimulation. Although the effects of these drugs are generally more localized to the cortex and the neuromuscular junction, the possibility of parasympathetic effects should be considered carefully in patients with asthma, coronary disease, peptic ulcer, arrhythmias, epilepsy, or parkinsonism.

Adverse Effects

The adverse effects associated with these drugs are related to the stimulation of the parasympathetic nervous system. GI effects can include nausea, vomiting, cramps, diarrhea, increased salivation, and involuntary defecation related to the increase in GI secretions and activity caused by parasympathetic nervous system stimulation. Cardiovascular effects can include bradycardia, heart block, hypotension, and even cardiac arrest, related to the cardiac-suppressing effects of the parasympathetic nervous system. Urinary tract effects can include a sense of urgency related to stimulation of the bladder muscles and sphincter relaxation. Miosis and blurred vision, headaches, dizziness, and drowsiness can occur related to CNS cholinergic effects. Other effects may include flushing and increased sweating secondary to stimulation of the cholinergic receptors in the sympathetic nervous system.

Clinically Important Drug–Drug Interactions

There may be an increased risk of GI bleeding if these drugs are used with nonsteroidal anti-inflammatory drugs (NSAIDs)

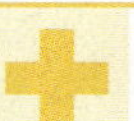

BOX 32.4 FOCUS ON **PATIENT SAFETY**

Myasthenic Crisis Versus Cholinergic Crisis

Myasthenia gravis is an autoimmune disease that runs an unpredictable course throughout the patient's life. Some patients have a very mild presentation (e.g., drooping eyelids) and go into remission with no further signs or symptoms for several years. Others have a more severe course, with progressive muscle weakness, confinement to a wheelchair, and so on. Many times, the disease goes through an intense phase called a myasthenic crisis, marked by extreme muscle weakness and respiratory difficulty.

Because of the variability of the disease and the tendency to have crises and periods of remission, management of the drug dosage for a patient with myasthenia gravis is a genuine nursing challenge. If a patient goes into remission, a smaller dosage will be needed. If a patient has a crisis, an increased dosage will be needed. To further complicate the clinical picture, the presentation of a cholinergic overdose or cholinergic crisis is similar to the presentation of a myasthenic crisis. The patient with a cholinergic crisis presents with progressive muscle weakness and respiratory difficulty as the accumulation of acetylcholine at the cholinergic receptor site leads to reduced impulse transmission and muscle weakness. This is a crisis when the respiratory muscles are involved.

For a myasthenic crisis, the correct treatment is increased cholinergic drug. However, treatment of a cholinergic crisis requires withdrawal of the drug. The patient's respiratory difficulty usually necessitates acute medical attention. At this point, the drug edrophonium can be used as a diagnostic agent to distinguish the two conditions. If the patient improves immediately after the edrophonium injection, the problem is a myasthenic crisis, which is improved by administration of the cholinergic drug. If the patient gets worse, the problem is probably a cholinergic crisis, and withdrawal of the patient's cholinergic drug along with intense medical support is indicated. Atropine helps to alleviate some of the parasympathetic reactions to the cholinergic drug. However, because atropine is not effective at the neuromuscular junction, only time will reverse the drug toxicity.

The patient and a significant other will need support, teaching, and encouragement to deal with the tricky regulation of the cholinergic medication throughout the course of the disease. Nurses in the acute care setting need to be mindful of the difficulty in distinguishing drug toxicity from the need for more drug—and be prepared to respond appropriately.

because of the combination of increased GI secretions and the GI mucosal erosion associated with the use of NSAIDs. If this combination is used, the patient should be monitored closely for any sign of GI bleeding. The effect of anticholinesterase drugs is decreased if they are taken in combination with any cholinergic drugs because these work in opposition to each other. Theophylline levels can be increased up to twofold if combined with tacrine; if that combination is used, the dosage of theophylline should be reduced accordingly and the patient monitored closely.

BOX 32.5 CULTURAL CONSIDERATIONS FOR DRUG THERAPY

Alzheimer's Disease

Alzheimer's disease was diagnosed increasingly in the 1990s. In the past, many people with Alzheimer's disease would have been diagnosed with senile dementia or dementia. This disease can affect individuals at any age, but it is seen mainly in elderly people and more often in men than in women. Currently, the only accurate way to diagnose Alzheimer's disease is at autopsy. However, many companies are working to develop a diagnostic test to permit pre-autopsy diagnosis.

Alzheimer's is a chronic, progressive disease on the brain's cortex. Eventually it results in memory loss so severe the patients may not remember how to perform basic activities of daily living and may not recognize close family members. Although Alzheimer's disease primarily strikes the elderly, it has a tremendous impact on family members of all ages. For example, adult children of Alzheimer's patients, many of whom are busy raising children of their own, may find themselves in the role of caregivers—in essence, becoming parents of their parent. This new role can put tremendous stress on individuals who are trying to struggle with work, family, and issues related to their parent's care.

When caring for an Alzheimer's patient and family, the nurse must remember that the patient's cultural background can affect how the family copes. For instance, those who tend to have solid extended families or who are part of communities that offer strong social support and interdependence may be better equipped to deal with caring for the patient as the disease progresses. In contrast, families that are more goal and achievement oriented and who value autonomy and independence may find themselves overwhelmed by the patient's needs and may require more support and referrals to community resources.

The nurse is in the best position to evaluate the family situation. By approaching each situation as unique and striving to incorporate cultural and social norms into the considerations for care, the nurse can help ease the family's burden while also maintaining the dignity of the patient and the family through this difficult experience.

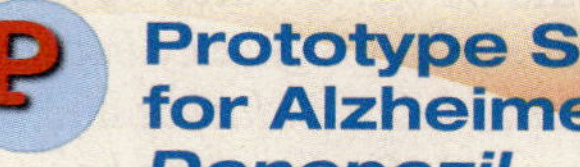

Prototype Summary for Alzheimer's Disease: Donepezil

Indications: Treatment of mild to moderate Alzheimer's disease

Actions: Reversible cholinesterase inhibitor that causes elevated acetylcholine levels in the cortex, which slows the neuronal degradation of Alzheimer's disease

Pharmacokinetics:

Route	Onset	Peak
Oral	Varies	2–4 h

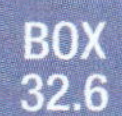

BOX 32.6 A New Drug for Treating Alzheimer's Disease

In late 2003, the FDA approved a new drug for treating Alzheimer's disease. The drug, memantine hydrochloride (*Namenda*), had been used in Europe for several years and had been reported to slow the memory loss of patients with moderate to severe dementia associated with Alzheimer's disease. Memantine has a low to moderate affinity for N-methyl-D-aspartate (NMDA) receptors with no effects on dopamine, GABA, histamine, glycine, or adrenergic receptor sites. It is thought that persistent activation of the CNS NMDA receptors contributes to the symptoms of Alzheimer's disease. By blocking these sites, it is thought that the symptoms are reduced or delayed.

The drug is available in a tablet form and an oral solution and is started at 5 mg/day PO, increasing by 5 mg/day at weekly intervals. The target dose is 20 mg/day given as 10 mg b.i.d. Dosage reduction should be considered in patients with renal impairment. Headache, dizziness, fatigue, confusion, and constipation are common adverse effects. The drug should not be taken with anything that alkalinizes the urine. Patients and family members need to understand that this drug is not a cure but may offer some extended time with mild symptoms. The long-term effects of this drug have not been studied in this country.

$T_{1/2}$: 70 hours; metabolism is in the liver and excretion is in the urine

Adverse effects: Insomnia, fatigue, rash, nausea, vomiting, diarrhea, dyspepsia, abdominal pain, muscle cramps

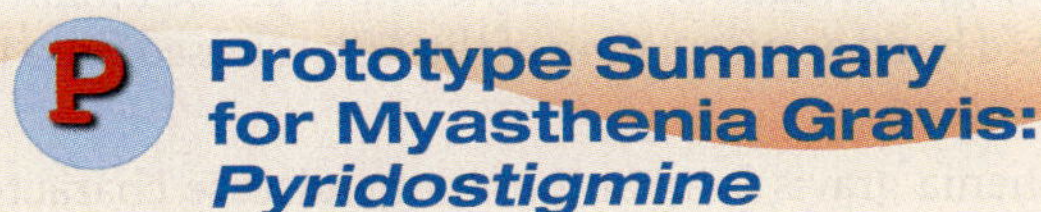

Prototype Summary for Myasthenia Gravis: *Pyridostigmine*

Indications: Treatment of myasthenia gravis, antidote for nondepolarizing neuromuscular junction blockers, increased survival in military personnel after exposure to nerve gas

Actions: Reversible cholinesterase inhibitor that increases the levels of acetylcholine, facilitating transmission at the neuromuscular junction

Pharmacokinetics:

Route	Onset	Duration
Oral	35–45 min	3–6 h
IM	15 min	3–6 h
IV	5 min	3–6 h

$T_{1/2}$: 1.9–3.7 hours; metabolism is in the liver and tissue, and excretion is in the urine

Adverse effects: Bradycardia, cardiac arrest, tearing, miosis, salivation, dysphagia, nausea, vomiting, increased bronchial secretions, urinary frequency, and incontinence

Nursing Considerations for Patients Receiving Indirect-Acting Cholinergic Agonists

Assessment: History and Examination

Screen for the following conditions, *which could be contraindications or cautions to use of the drug:* known allergies to any of these drugs; arrhythmias, coronary artery disease, hypotension, urogenital or GI obstruction, peptic ulcer, pregnancy, lactation, or recent GI or genitourinary surgery, *which could limit use of the drugs;* and regular use of NSAIDs, cholinergic drugs, or theophylline, *which could cause a drug–drug interaction.*

Include screening *for baseline status before beginning therapy and for any potential adverse effects:* assess orientation, affect, reflexes, ability to carry on activities of daily living (Alzheimer's drugs), and vision, *to monitor for CNS changes related to drug therapy;* blood pressure, pulse, ECG, peripheral perfusion, and cardiac output; urinary output, and renal and liver function tests *to monitor drug effects on the renal system and liver, which could change the metabolism and excretion of the drugs.*

Nursing Diagnoses

The patient receiving an indirect-acting cholinergic agonist may also have the following nursing diagnoses related to drug therapy:

- Disturbed Thought Processes related to CNS effects
- Acute Pain related to GI effects
- Decreased Cardiac Output related to blood pressure changes, arrhythmias, vasodilation
- Deficient Knowledge regarding drug therapy

Implementation With Rationale

- If the drug is given intravenously, administer it slowly, *to avoid severe cholinergic effects.*
- Maintain atropine sulfate on standby *as an antidote in case of overdose or severe cholinergic reaction.*
- Discontinue the drug if excessive salivation, diarrhea, emesis, or frequent urination becomes a problem *to decrease the risk of severe adverse reactions.*

- Administer the oral drug with meals *to decrease GI upset if it is a problem.*
- Mark the patient's chart and notify the surgeon if the patient is to undergo surgery *because prolonged muscle relaxation may occur if succinylcholine-type anesthetics are used.* The patient will require prolonged support and monitoring.
- Monitor the patient being treated for Alzheimer's disease for any progress, *because the drug is not a cure and only slows progression;* refer families to supportive services.
- The patient who is being treated for myasthenia gravis and a significant other should receive instruction in drug administration, warning signs of drug overdose, and signs and symptoms to report immediately *to enhance patient knowledge about drug therapy and to promote compliance.*
- Arrange for supportive care and comfort measures, including rest, environmental control, and other measures, *to decrease CNS irritation;* headache medication *to relieve pain;* safety measures if CNS effects occur *to prevent injury;* protective measures if CNS effects are severe *to prevent patient injury;* and small, frequent meals if GI upset is severe *to decrease discomfort and maintain nutrition.*
- Provide thorough patient teaching, including dosage and adverse effects to anticipate, measures to avoid adverse effects, and warning signs of problems, as well as proper administration for each route used *to enhance patient knowledge about drug therapy and to promote compliance.*
- Offer support and encouragement *to help the patient deal with the drug regimen.*

Evaluation

- Monitor patient response to the drug (improvement in condition being treated).
- Monitor for adverse effects (GI upset, CNS changes, cardiovascular changes, genitourinary changes).
- Evaluate the effectiveness of the teaching plan (patient can name drug, dosage, adverse effects to watch for, specific measures to avoid adverse effects, proper administration).
- Monitor the effectiveness of comfort measures and compliance to the regimen.

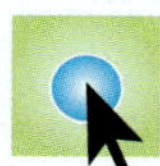

WEB LINKS

Health care providers and patients may want to consult the following Internet sources:

http://www.alzheimers.org Information on Alzheimer's disease research, conferences.

http://www.alz.org Information on resources, medical treatments, outreach programs, and local support groups involved with Alzheimer's disease.

http://www.myasthenia.org Information on current research on myasthenia gravis, treatments.

http://www.nlm.nih.gov/medlineplus/myastheniagravis.html Information on myasthenia gravis educational programs, local support groups, and resources.

http://www.emergency.com/nervgas.htm Information on nerve gas treatment protocols.

Points to Remember

- Cholinergic drugs are chemicals that act at the same site as the neurotransmitter acetylcholine (ACh), stimulating the parasympathetic nerves, some nerves in the brain, and the neuromuscular junction.
- Direct-acting cholinergic drugs react with the ACh receptor sites to cause cholinergic stimulation.
- Use of direct-acting cholinergic drugs is limited by the systemic effects of the drug. They are used to cause miosis and to treat glaucoma; one agent is available to treat neurogenic bladder and bladder atony postoperative or postpartum, and another agent is available to increase GI secretions and relieve the dry mouth of Sjögren's syndrome.
- Indirect-acting cholinergic drugs are acetylcholinesterase inhibitors. They block acetylcholinesterase to prevent it from breaking down ACh in the synaptic cleft.
- Cholinergic stimulation by acetylcholinesterase inhibitors is caused by an accumulation of the ACh released from the nerve ending.
- Myasthenia gravis is an autoimmune disease characterized by antibodies to the ACh receptors. This results in a loss of ACh receptors and eventual loss of response at the neuromuscular junction.
- Acetylcholinesterase inhibitors are used to treat myasthenia gravis because they are able to cause the accumulation of ACh in the synaptic cleft, prolonging stimulation of any ACh sites that remain.
- Alzheimer's disease is a progressive dementia characterized by a loss of ACh-producing neurons and ACh receptor sites in the neurocortex.
- Acetylcholinesterase inhibitors that cross the blood–brain barrier are used to manage Alzheimer's disease by increasing ACh levels in the brain and slowing the progression of the disease.
- Side effects associated with the use of these drugs are related to stimulation of the parasympathetic nervous system (bradycardia, hypotension, increased GI secretions and activity, increased bladder tone, relaxation of GI and

genitourinary sphincters, bronchoconstriction, pupil constriction) and may limit the usefulness of some of these drugs.

- Nerve gas is an irreversible acetylcholinesterase inhibitor that leads to toxic accumulations of ACh at cholinergic receptor sites and can cause parasympathetic crisis and muscle paralysis.
- Pralidoxime is an antidote for the irreversible acetylcholinesterase inhibitors; it frees the acetylcholinesterase that was inhibited.

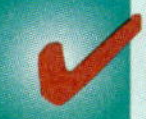

CHECK YOUR UNDERSTANDING

Answers to the questions in this chapter may be found in the Answer Key in the back of the book.

Multiple Choice

Select the best answer to the following.

1. Indirect-acting cholinergic agents
   a. react with acetylcholine receptor sites on the membranes of effector cells.
   b. react chemically with acetylcholinesterase to increase acetylcholine concentrations around effector cell receptor sites.
   c. are used to increase bladder tone and urinary excretion.
   d. should be given with food to decrease nausea.

2. Pilocarpine (*Pilocar*) is a frequently used drug in the clinical setting and would be indicated for the treatment of
   a. myasthenia gravis.
   b. neurogenic bladder.
   c. glaucoma.
   d. Alzheimer's disease.

3. Myasthenia gravis is treated with indirect-acting cholinergic agents that
   a. lead to accumulation of acetylcholine in the synaptic cleft and eventual stimulation of the muscle.
   b. block the GI effects of the disease.
   c. directly stimulate the remaining acetylcholine receptors.
   d. can be given only by injection.

4. The cholinergic drug of choice for a patient with myasthenia gravis who is no longer able to swallow would be
   a. tacrine.
   b. ambenonium.
   c. pyridostigmine.
   d. edrophonium.

5. Alzheimer's disease is marked by a progressive loss of memory and is associated with
   a. degeneration of dopamine-producing cells in the basal ganglia.
   b. loss of acetylcholine-producing neurons and their target neurons in the CNS.
   c. loss of acetylcholine receptor sites in the parasympathetic nervous system.
   d. increased levels of acetylcholinesterase in the CNS.

6. Donepezil (*Aricept*) would be the Alzheimer's disease drug of choice for a patient who
   a. cannot remember family members' names.
   b. is mildly inhibited and can still follow medical dosing regimens.
   c. is able to carry on normal activities of daily living.
   d. has memory problems and would benefit from once-a-day dosing.

7. Adverse effects associated with the use of cholinergic drugs would include
   a. constipation and insomnia.
   b. diarrhea and urinary urgency.
   c. tachycardia and hypertension.
   d. dry mouth and tachycardia.

8. Nerve gas is an irreversible acetylcholinesterase inhibitor that can cause muscle paralysis and death. An antidote to such an agent is
   a. atropine.
   b. propranolol.
   c. pralidoxime.
   d. neostigmine.

Multiple Response

Select all that apply.

1. A nurse is explaining myasthenia gravis to a family. Which of the following points would be included in the explanation?
   a. It is thought to be an autoimmune disease.
   b. It is associated with destruction of acetylcholine receptor sites.
   c. It is best treated with potent antibiotics.
   d. It is a chronic and progressive muscular disease.
   e. It is caused by demyelination of the nerve fiber.
   f. Once diagnosed, it has a 5-year survival rate.

2. A nurse would question an order for a cholinergic drug if the patient was also taking which of the following?
   a. Theophylline
   b. NSAIDs
   c. Cephalosporin
   d. Atropine
   e. Propranolol
   f. Memantine

Matching

Match the drug with its usual indication. (Some drugs may have more than one indication.)

1. ________________ pilocarpine
2. ________________ tacrine
3. ________________ neostigmine
4. ________________ ambenonium
5. ________________ pyridostigmine
6. ________________ edrophonium
7. ________________ rivastigmine
8. ________________ donepezil

A. Diagnosis of myasthenia gravis
B. Treatment of myasthenia gravis
C. Antidote for neuromuscular junction (NMJ) blockers
D. Glaucoma, miosis
E. Alzheimer's disease

Fill in the Blanks

1. Cholinergic drugs are chemicals that act at the same site as the neurotransmitter ________________.
2. Cholinergic drugs are often also called ________________ drugs because their action mimics the action of the parasympathetic nervous system.
3. ________________ cholinergic drugs act at acetylcholine receptor sites to cause the same reaction as acetylcholine would cause.
4. Cholinergic agents that prevent the breakdown of acetylcholine by blocking acetylcholinesterase are called ________________ cholinergic drugs.
5. ________________ is a progressive neurological condition that is marked by loss of the acetylcholine-producing neurons in the cerebral cortex.
6. ________________ ________________ is a chronic muscular disease that is caused by a defect in neuromuscular transmission; cholinergic drugs help patients with this disease.
7. Common adverse effects in the gastrointestinal (GI) tract seen with cholinergic drugs include ________________, ________________, ________________, and ________________.
8. Cardiovascular effects that are often seen with cholinergic drugs include ________________, ________________, and ________________.

Bibliography and References

Andrews, M., & Boyle, J. (2004). *Transcultural concepts in nursing care.* Philadelphia: Lippincott Williams & Wilkins.

Drug facts and comparisons. (2006). St. Louis: Facts and Comparisons.

Gilman, A., Hardman, J. G., & Limbird, L. E. (Eds.). (2006). *Goodman and Gilman's the pharmacological basis of therapeutics* (11th ed.). New York: McGraw-Hill.

Karch, A. M. (2006). *2007 Lippincott's nursing drug guide.* Philadelphia: Lippincott Williams & Wilkins.

The medical letter on drugs and therapeutics. (2006). New Rochelle, NY: Medical Letter.

Porth, C. M. (2005). *Pathophysiology: Concepts of altered health states* (7th ed.). Philadelphia: Lippincott Williams & Wilkins.

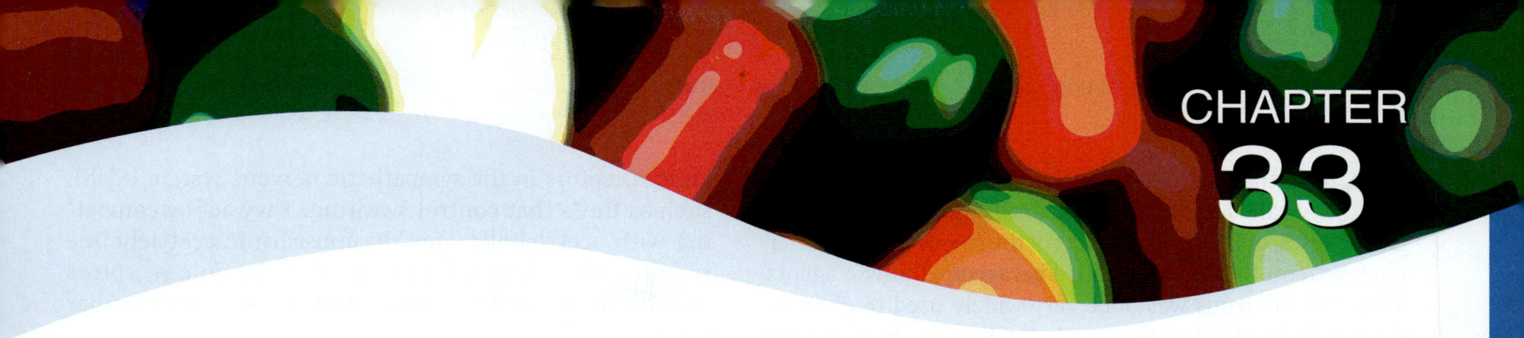

CHAPTER 33

Anticholinergic Agents

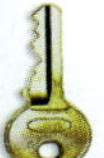

KEY TERMS

anticholinergic
belladonna
cycloplegia
mydriasis
parasympatholytic

LEARNING OBJECTIVES

Upon completion of the chapter, you will be able to:

1. Define anticholinergic agents.
2. Describe the therapeutic actions, indications, pharmacokinetics, contraindications, most common adverse reactions, and important drug–drug interactions of atropine.
3. Discuss the use of atropine across the lifespan.
4. Compare and contrast the prototype drug atropine with other anticholinergic agents.
5. Outline the nursing considerations, including important teaching points, for patients receiving anticholinergic agents.

ANTICHOLINERGIC AGENTS/ PARASYMPATHOLYTICS

P atropine
dicyclomine
flavoxate
glycopyrrolate
hyoscyamine
ipratropium
methscopolamine
propantheline
scopolamine
trospium

Drugs that are used to block the effects of acetylcholine are called **anticholinergic** drugs. Because this action lyses, or blocks, the effects of the parasympathetic nervous system, they are also called **parasympatholytic** agents. This class of drugs was once very widely used to decrease gastrointestinal (GI) activity and secretions in the treatment of ulcers and to decrease other parasympathetic activities to allow the sympathetic system to become more dominant. Today, more specific and less systemically toxic drugs are available for many of the conditions that would benefit from these effects, so this class of drugs is less commonly used. Atropine remains the only widely used anticholinergic drug. The use of anticholinergic agents with various age groups is discussed in Box 33.1.

Anticholinergics/ Parasympatholytics

Atropine (generic) has been used for many years and is derived from the plant **belladonna**. (Belladonna was once used by fashionable ladies of the European court to dilate their pupils in an effort to make them more innocent-looking and alluring.) The effect of anticholinergics with other herbal remedies is discussed in Box 33.2.

Both atropine and scopolamine (*Transderm-Scop* and generic) work by blocking only the muscarinic effectors in the parasympathetic nervous system and those few cholinergic receptors in the sympathetic nervous system (SNS), such as those that control sweating. They act by competing with acetylcholine for the muscarinic acetylcholine receptor sites. They do not block the nicotinic receptors and therefore have little or no effect at the neuromuscular junction.

Atropine is available for parenteral, oral, and topical use to block parasympathetic effects in a variety of situations (Table 33.1). Scopolamine is available in a transdermal form, as well as oral and parenteral forms (Box 33.3). Dicyclomine (*Antispas, Dibent,* and others) is an oral drug used to relax the GI tract in the treatment of hyperactive or irritable bowel. Glycopyrrolate (*Robinul*), available in oral and parenteral forms, can be used orally as an adjunct in the treatment of ulcers, although it is not a drug of choice. It is widely used systemically to decrease secretions before anesthesia or intubation and to protect the patient from the peripheral effects of cholinergic drugs used to reverse neuromuscular blockade. Propantheline (*Pro-Banthine*), an oral drug, was once widely used as an adjunct in the treatment of ulcers but now has been replaced, for the most part by the histamine-2 blockers. See Table 33.2 for a description of all the anticholinergic agents.

Flavoxate (see Chapter 52), ipratropium and trospium (see Chapter 55), and hyoscyamine and methscopolamine (see Chapter 58) are anticholinergic drugs with very specific indications that are discussed in relation to the systems they affect.

BOX 33.1 DRUG THERAPY ACROSS THE LIFESPAN

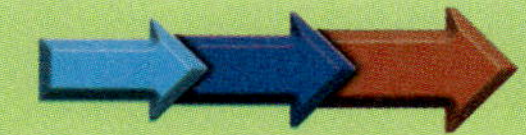

Anticholinergic Agents

CHILDREN

The anticholinergic agents are often used in children. Children are often more sensitive to the adverse effects of the drugs, including constipation, urinary retention, heat intolerance, and confusion. If a child is given one of these drugs, the child should be closely watched and monitored for adverse effects, and appropriate supportive measures should be instituted. Dicyclomine is not recommended for use in children.

ADULTS

Adults need to be made aware of the potential for adverse effects associated with the use of these drugs. They should be encouraged to void before taking the medication if urinary retention or hesitancy is a problem. They should be encouraged to drink plenty of fluids and to avoid hot temperatures, because heat intolerance can occur and it will be important to maintain hydration should this happen. Safety precautions may be needed if blurred vision and dizziness occur. The patient should be urged not to drive or perform tasks that require concentration and coordination.

These drugs should not be used during pregnancy, because they cross the placenta and could cause adverse effects on the fetus. If the benefit to the mother clearly outweighs the potential risk to the fetus, they should be used with caution. Nursing mothers should find another method of feeding the baby if an anticholinergic drug is needed because of the potential for serious adverse effects on the baby.

OLDER ADULTS

Older adults are more likely to experience the adverse effects associated with these drugs; dosage should be reduced, and the patient should be monitored very closely. Because older patients are more susceptible to heat intolerance owing to decreased body fluid and decreased sweating, extreme caution should be used when an anticholinergic drug is given. The patient should be urged to drink plenty of fluids and to avoid extremes of temperature on exertion in warm temperatures. Safety precautions may be needed if central nervous system effects are severe. The older adult is more likely to experience confusion, hallucinations, and psychotic syndromes when taking an anticholinergic drug. Older adults may also have renal impairment, making them more likely to have problems excreting these drugs. Further reduction in dosage may be needed in the older patient who also has renal dysfunction.

BOX 33.2 HERBAL AND ALTERNATIVE THERAPIES

The risk of anticholinergic effects can be exacerbated if anticholinergic agents are combined with burdock, rosemary, or turmeric used as herbal therapy. Advise patients who use herbal therapies to avoid these combinations.

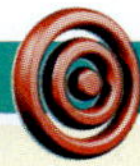

FOCUS POINTS

- At cholinergic receptor sites, anticholinergic drugs block the effects of acetylcholine. Because they block the effects of the parasympathetic nervous system, they are also known as parasympatholytic drugs.
- When the parasympathetic system is blocked, the pupils dilate, the heart rate rises, and GI activity and urinary bladder tone and function decrease.

BOX 33.3 FOCUS ON **CLINICAL SKILLS**

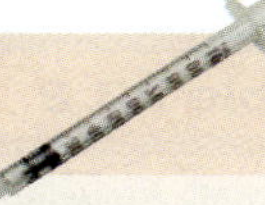

Applying Dermal Patch Delivery Systems

If a drug has been ordered to be given via a transdermal patch, review the proper technique for applying a transdermal patch. The patch should be applied to a clean, dry, intact and hairless area of the body. Do not shave an area of application—that could abrade the skin and lead to increased absorption. Hair may be clipped if necessary. Peel off the backing without touching the adhesive side of the patch. Place the patch at a new site each time to avoid skin irritation or degradation. Be sure to remove the old patch and clean the area when putting on a new transdermal patch. It is important to remember that many transdermal systems contain an aluminized barrier that could cause an electrical charge with arcing, smoke, and severe transdermal burns if a defibrillator is discharged over it. Remove any transdermal patches in the area if a defibrillator is to be used.

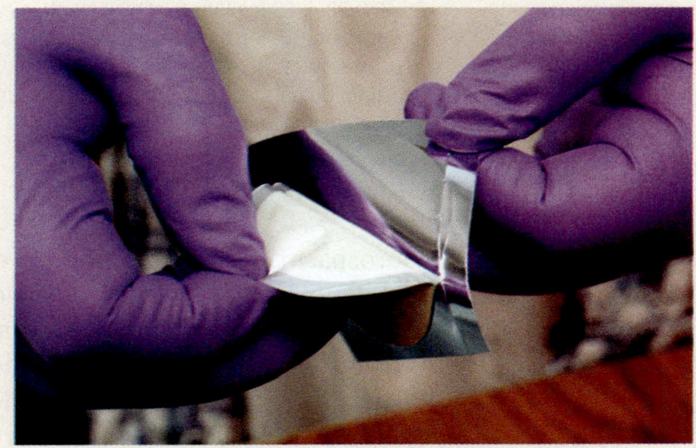

Carefully remove backing from patch without touching adhesive.

Therapeutic Actions and Indications

The anticholinergic drugs competitively block the acetylcholine receptors at the muscarinic cholinergic receptor sites that are responsible for mediating the effects of the parasympathetic postganglionic impulses (Figure 33.1). This means that atropine is used to depress salivation and bronchial secretions and to dilate the bronchi, but it can thicken respiratory secretions (causing obstruction of airways). Atropine also is used to inhibit vagal responses in the heart, to relax the GI and genitourinary tracts, to inhibit GI secretions, to cause **mydriasis** or relaxation of the pupil of the eye (also called a mydriatic effect [see Box 33.4]), and to cause **cycloplegia** or inhibition of the ability of the lens in the eye to accommodate to near vision (also called a cycloplegic effect). Anticholinergic drugs also are thought to block the effects of acetylcholine in the central nervous system (CNS).

Anticholinergic drugs can be used to decrease secretions before anesthesia; to treat parkinsonism; to restore cardiac rate and blood pressure after vagal stimulation during surgery; to relieve bradycardia caused by a hyperactive carotid

Table 33.1 Available Forms of Anticholinergic Drugs

	Available Forms					
Drug	*Oral*	*IM*	*IV*	*Sub-Q*	*Transdermal Patch*	*Ophthalmic*
atropine	×	×	×	×	—	×
dicyclomine	×	×	—	—	—	—
glycopyrrolate	×	×	×	×	—	—
propantheline	×	—	—	—	—	—
scopolamine	—	×	×	×	×	×

Table 33.2 DRUGS IN FOCUS

Anticholinergic Agents

Drug Name	Dosage/Route	Usual Indications
P atropine (*generic*)	0.4–0.6 mg IM, Sub-Q, or IV; use caution with older patients Pediatric: 0.1–0.4 mg IV, IM, or Sub-Q based on weight	Decrease secretions, bradycardia, pylorospasm, ureteral colic, relaxing of bladder, emotional lability with head injuries, antidote for cholinergic drugs, pupil dilation
dicyclomine (*Antispas, Dibent*)	160 mg/day PO in four divided doses; 80 mg/day IM in four divided doses—do not give IV	Irritable or hyperactive bowel in adults
glycopyrrolate (*Robinul*)	Adult: 1–2 mg PO b.i.d. to t.i.d. for ulcers; 0.004 mg/kg IM 30–60 min before surgery, then 0.1 mg IV during surgery Pediatric: 0.002–0.004 mg/kg IM 30–60 min before surgery, then 0.004 mg/kg IV during surgery	Decrease secretions, antidote for neuromuscular blockers
propantheline (*Pro-Banthine*)	Adult: 15 mg PO 30 min before meals and at bedtime Pediatric: as antisecretory agent, 1.5 mg/kg/day PO in divided doses t.i.d. to q.i.d. as antispasmodic, 2–3 mg/kg/day PO in divided doses q4–6h and at bedtime	Adjunctive therapy for ulcers; antisecretory, antispasmodic
scopolamine (*Transderm Scop*)	Adult: 0.32–0.65 mg Sub-Q or IM; 1–2 gtt in eye(s) for refraction; 1.5 mg transdermal every 3 days for motion sickness; use caution with older patients Pediatric: Do not use PO or transdermal system with children; 0.006 mg/kg Sub-Q, IM, or IV	Motion sickness, decrease secretions, obstetric amnesia, relief of urinary problems, adjunctive for ulcers, pupil dilation

sinus reflex; to relieve pylorospasm and hyperactive bowel; to relax biliary and ureteral colic; to relax bladder detrusor muscles and tighten sphincters (see Critical Thinking Scenario 33-1); to help to control crying or laughing episodes in patients with brain injuries; to relax uterine hypertonicity; to help in the management of peptic ulcer; to control rhinorrhea associated with hay fever; as an antidote for cholinergic drugs and for poisoning by certain mushrooms; and as an ophthalmic agent to cause mydriasis or cycloplegia in acute inflammatory conditions.

Scopolamine is also used to decrease the nausea and vomiting associated with motion sickness and has been used to induce obstetric amnesia and relax the mother. Other agents are used for specific indications, as noted earlier and summarized in Table 33.3.

Pharmacokinetics

The anticholinergics are well absorbed after administration. They are widely distributed throughout the body and cross the blood–brain barrier. Their half-lives vary with route and drug. They are excreted in the urine. These drugs should be used in pregnancy and lactation only if the benefit clearly outweighs the potential risk to the fetus or baby. Nursing mothers should find another way of feeding the baby if an anticholinergic drug is needed.

Contraindications and Cautions

Anticholinergics are contraindicated in the presence of known allergy to any of these drugs. They are also contraindicated with any condition that could be exacerbated by a blocking of the parasympathetic nervous system. These conditions include glaucoma *because of the possibility of increased pressure with pupil dilation;* stenosing peptic ulcer, intestinal atony, paralytic ileus, GI obstruction, severe ulcerative colitis, and toxic megacolon, *all of which could be intensified with a further slowing of GI activity;* prostatic hypertrophy and bladder obstruction, *which could be further compounded by a blocking of bladder muscle activity and a blocking of sphincter relaxation in the bladder;* cardiac arrhythmias, tachycardia, and myocardial ischemia, *which could be exacerbated by the increased sympathetic influence, including tachycardia and increased contractility that occurs when the parasympathetic nervous system is blocked;* impaired liver or kidney function, *which could alter the metabolism and excretion of the drug;* and myasthenia gravis, *which could worsen with further blocking of the cholinergic receptors.* (Low doses of atropine are sometimes used in myasthenia gravis to block unwanted GI and cardiovascular effects of the cholinergic drugs used to treat that condition.)

Caution should be used in patients who are breast-feeding *because of possible suppression of lactation;* hypertension *because of the possibility of additive hypertensive effects from the sympathetic system's dominance with parasympathetic nervous system blocking;* and spasticity and brain damage, *which could be exacerbated by cholinergic blockade within the CNS.*

Adverse Effects

The adverse effects associated with the use of anticholinergic drugs are caused by the systemic blockade of cholinergic

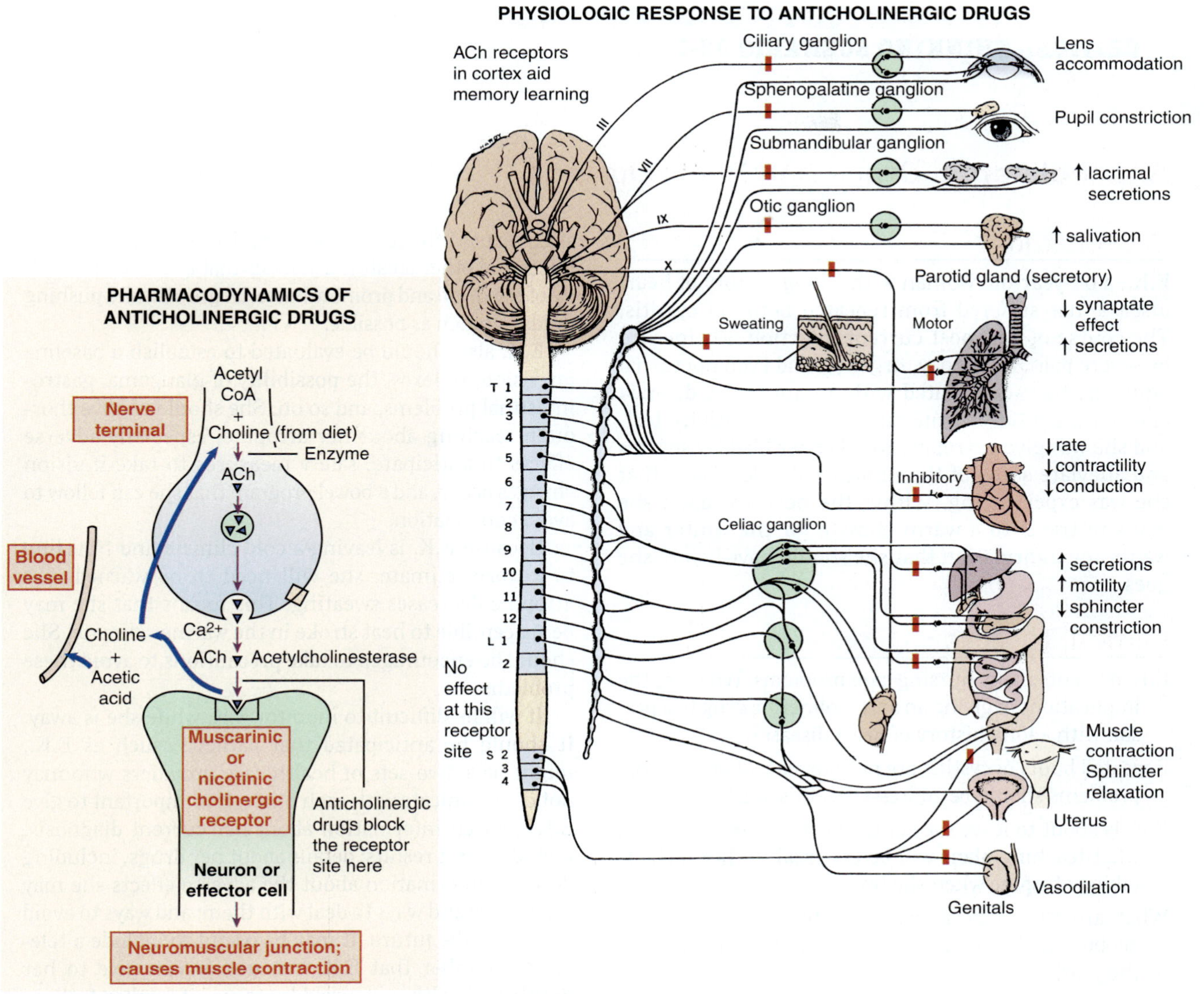

FIGURE 33.1 Pharmacodynamics of anticholinergic drugs and associated physiologic responses. A bar indicates blockade of that activity. For example, blocking the inhibitory effect on the heart will cause an increase in heart rate.

receptors. What are adverse effects in some cases may be the desired therapeutic effects in others. The intensity of adverse effects is related to drug dosage: The more of the drug in the system, the greater the systemic effects. These adverse effects could include the CNS effects of blurred vision, pupil dilation and resultant photophobia, cycloplegia, and increased intraocular pressure, all of which are related to the blocking of the parasympathetic effects in the eye.

Weakness, dizziness, insomnia, mental confusion, and excitement are effects related to the blocking of the cholinergic receptors within the CNS. Dry mouth results from the blocking of GI secretions. Altered taste perception, nausea, heartburn, constipation, bloated feelings, and paralytic ileus

(text continues on page 530)

BOX 33.4 CULTURAL CONSIDERATIONS FOR DRUG THERAPY

Mydriatic Effects

Nurses working in eye clinics or administering preoperative medications for eye surgery should be aware that mydriatics (including atropine) are much less effective in African Americans than in the general population. Increased dosage may be needed, and there may be a prolonged time to peak effect. This effect, although somewhat less pronounced, is seen in any individual with dark-pigmented eyes.

CRITICAL THINKING SCENARIO 33-1

Anticholinergic Drugs and Heart Disease

THE SITUATION

E.K., a 64-year-old woman with a long history of heart disease, has suffered from repeated bouts of cystitis. The course of her most current infection was marked by severe pain, frequency, urgency, and even nocturnal enuresis. She was treated with an antibiotic deemed appropriate after a urine culture and sensitivity test, and she was given atropine to relax her bladder spasms and alleviate some of the unpleasant side effects that she was experiencing. Within the next few days, she plans to travel to a warm climate for the winter and wants any information that she should have before she goes.

CRITICAL THINKING

E.K. presents many nursing care problems. What are the implications of giving an anticholinergic drug to a person with a long history of heart disease?

Repeated bouts of cystitis are not normal; what potential problems should be addressed in this area?

E.K. is about to leave for her winter home in the South; what teaching plans will be essential for her if she is taking atropine when she leaves?

What are the medical problems that can arise with people who live in different areas at different times of the year?

Considering her age, what written information should E.K. take with her as she travels?

DISCUSSION

E.K. is doing well with her cardiac problems at the moment, but she could develop problems as a result of the anticholinergic drug that has been prescribed. The anticipated adverse effect of tachycardia could tip the balance in a compensated heart, leading to congestive heart failure or oxygen delivery problems. She will need to be carefully evaluated for the status of her heart disease and potential problems.

E.K. should be further evaluated for the cause of her repeated bouts with cystitis. Does she have a structural problem, a dietary problem, or a simple hygiene problem? She should receive instruction on ways to avoid bladder infections, such as wiping only from front to back, voiding after sexual intercourse, avoiding baths, avoiding citrus juices and other alkaline ash foods that decrease the acidity of the urine and promote bacterial growth, and pushing fluids as much as possible.

E.K. also should be evaluated to establish a baseline for vision, reflexes, the possibility of glaucoma, gastrointestinal problems, and so on. She should receive thorough teaching about her atropine, especially adverse effects to anticipate, safety measures to take if vision changes occur, and a bowel program that she can follow to avoid constipation.

Because E.K. is leaving a cold climate and traveling to a warm climate, she will need to be warned that atropine decreases sweating. This means that she may be susceptible to heat stroke in the warmer climate. She should be encouraged to take precautions to avoid these problems.

It will be difficult to monitor E.K. while she is away. It should be anticipated that patients, such as E.K., might have two sets of health care providers who may not communicate with each other. It is important to give E.K. written information about her current diagnosis, including test results; details about her drugs, including dosages; information about the adverse effects she may experience and ways to deal with them; and ways to avoid cystitis in the future. It may be useful to include a telephone number that E.K. can use or can give to her Southern health care provider to use if further tests or follow-up is indicated.

NURSING CARE GUIDE FOR E.K.: HEART DISEASE

Assessment: History and Examination

Assess for a history of allergy to anticholinergic drugs, COPD, narrow-angle glaucoma, myasthenia gravis, bowel or urinary obstruction, tachycardia, and recent GI or urinary surgery.

Focus the physical examination on the following:

CV: blood pressure, pulse rate, peripheral perfusion, ECG
CNS: orientation, affect, reflexes, vision
Skin: color, lesions, texture, sweating
GU: urinary output, bladder tone
GI: abdominal exam
Respiratory: respiratory rate, adventitious sounds

Anticholinergic Drugs and Heart Disease *(continued)*

Nursing Diagnoses

Decreased Cardiac Output related to CV effects

Acute Pain related to GI, GU, CNS, CV effects

Constipation related to GI effects

Deficient Knowledge regarding drug therapy

Noncompliance related to adverse effects

Implementation

Ensure safe and appropriate administration of drug.

Provide comfort and safety measures, including assistance/siderails; temperature control; dark glasses; small, frequent meals; artificial saliva, fluids; sugarless lozenges, mouth care; bowel program.

Provide support and reassurance to deal with drug effects, discomfort, and GI effects.

Provide patient teaching regarding drug name, dosage, adverse effects, precautions, and warnings to report.

Monitor blood pressure and pulse rate and adjust dosage as needed.

Evaluation

Evaluate drug effects: pupil dilation, decrease in signs and symptoms being treated.

Monitor for adverse effects: CV effects—tachycardia, CHF; CNS—confusion, dreams; urinary retention; GI effects—constipation; visual blurring, photophobia.

Monitor for drug–drug interactions as indicated for each drug.

Evaluate effectiveness of patient teaching program and comfort and safety measures.

Patient Teaching for E.K.

- ☐ Parasympathetic blockers, parasympatholytics, or anticholinergics block or stop the actions of a group of nerves that are part of the parasympathetic nervous system. These drugs may decrease the activity of your GI tract, dilate your pupils, or speed up your heart.
- ☐ Some of the following adverse effects may occur:
  - *Dry mouth, difficulty swallowing:* Frequent mouth care will help to remove dried secretions and keep the mouth fresh. Sucking on sugarless candies will help to keep the mouth moist. Taking lots of fluids with meals (unless you are on fluid restriction) will help swallowing.
  - *Blurred vision, sensitivity to light:* If your vision is blurred, avoid driving, operating hazardous machinery, or doing close work that requires attention to details until your vision returns to normal. Dark glasses will help protect your eyes from the light.
  - *Retention of urine:* Take the drug just after you have emptied your bladder. Moderate your fluid intake while the drug's effects are the highest; if possible, take the drug before bedtime, when this effect will not be a problem.
  - *Constipation:* Include fluid and roughage in your diet, and follow any bowel regimen that you may have. Monitor your bowel movements so that appropriate laxatives can be taken if necessary.
  - *Flushing, intolerance to heat, decreased sweating:* This drug blocks sweating, which is your body's way of cooling off. This places you at increased risk for heat stroke. Avoid extremes of temperature, dress coolly on very warm days, and avoid exercise as much as possible.
  - Report any of the following to your health care provider: *eye pain, skin rash, fever, rapid heart beat, chest pain, difficulty breathing, agitation or mood changes, and impotence* (a dosage adjustment may help alleviate this problem).
- ☐ Avoid the use of over-the-counter medications, especially for sleep and nasal congestion; avoid antihistamines, diet pills, and cold capsules. These products may contain drugs that cause similar anticholinergic effects, which could cause a severe reaction. Consult with your health care provider if you feel that you need medication for symptomatic relief.
- ☐ Tell any doctor, nurse, or other health care provider involved in your care that you are taking these drugs.
- ☐ Keep this drug, and all medications, out of the reach of children. Do not share these drugs with other people.

Table 33.3 Effects of Parasympathetic Blockade and Associated Therapeutic Uses

Physiological Effect	Therapeutic Uses
Gastrointestinal	
Smooth muscle: blocks spasm, blocks peristalsis Secretory glands: decreases acid and digestive enzyme production	Decreases motility and secretory activity in peptic ulcer, gastritis, cardiospasm, pylorospasm, enteritis, diarrhea, hypertonic constipation
Urinary tract	
Decreases tone and motility in the ureters and fundus of the bladder; increases tone in the bladder sphincter	Increases bladder capacity in children with enuresis, spastic paraplegics; decreases urinary urgency and frequency in cystitis; antispasmodic in renal colic and to counteract bladder spasm caused by morphine
Biliary tract	
Relaxes smooth muscle, antispasmodic	Relief of biliary colic; counteracts spasms caused by narcotics
Bronchial muscle	
Weakly relaxes smooth muscle	Aerosol form may be used in asthma; may counteract bronchoconstriction caused by drugs
Cardiovascular system	
Increases heart rate (may decrease heart rate at very low doses); causes local vasodilation and flushing	Counteracts bradycardia caused by vagal stimulation, carotid sinus syndrome, surgical procedures; used to overcome heart blocks following MI; used to counteract hypotension caused by cholinergic drugs.
Ocular effects	
Pupil dilation, cycloplegia	Allows ophthalmological examination of the retina, optic disk; relaxes ocular muscles and decreases irritation in iridocyclitis, choroiditis
Secretions	
Reduces sweating, salivation, respiratory tract secretions	Preoperatively before inhalation anesthesia; reduces nasal secretions in rhinitis, hay fever; may be used to reduce excessive sweating in hyperhidrosis
Central nervous system	
Decreases extrapyramidal motor activity Atropine may cause excessive stimulation, psychosis, delirium, disorientation Scopolamine causes depression, drowsiness	Decreases tremor in parkinsonism; helps to prevent motion sickness; scopolamine may be in OTC sleep aids

are related to a slowing of GI activity. Tachycardia and palpitations are possible effects related to blocking of the parasympathetic effects on the heart. Urinary hesitancy and retention are related to the blocking of bladder muscle activity and relaxation of the sphincter. Decreased sweating and an increased predisposition to heat prostration are related to the inability to cool the body by sweating, a result of blocking of the sympathetic cholinergic receptors responsible for sweating. Suppression of lactation is related to anticholinergic effects in the breasts and in the CNS (see Table 33.3).

Clinically Important Drug–Drug Interactions

The incidence of anticholinergic effects increases if these drugs are combined with any other drugs with anticholinergic activity, including antihistamines, antiparkinsonism drugs, monoamine oxidase inhibitors (MAOIs), and tricyclic antidepressants (TCAs). If such combinations must be used, the patient should be monitored closely and dosage adjustments made. Patients should be advised to avoid over-the-counter products that contain these drugs. The effectiveness of phenothiazines decreases if they are combined with anticholinergic drugs, and the risk of paralytic ileus increases. This combination should be avoided.

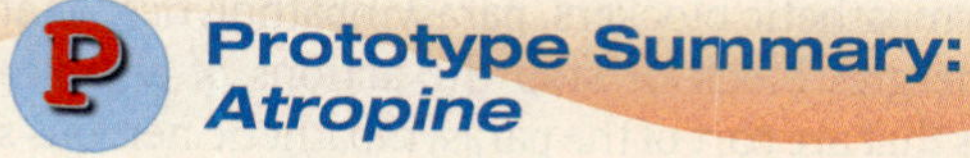

Prototype Summary: Atropine

Indications: To decrease secretions before surgery, treatment of parkinsonism, restoration of cardiac rate and arterial pressure following vagal stimulation, relief of bradycardia and syncope due to hyperactive carotid sinus reflex, relief of pylorospasm, relaxation of the spasm of biliary and ureteral colic and bronchospasm, control of crying and laughing episodes associated with brain lesions, relaxation of uterine hypertonicity, management of peptic ulcer, control of rhinorrhea associated with hay fever, antidote for cholinergic overdose and poisoning from various mushrooms

Actions: Competitively blocks acetylcholine muscarinic receptor sites, blocking the effects of the parasympathetic nervous system

Pharmacokinetics:

Route	Onset	Peak	Duration
IM	10–15 min	30 min	4 h
IV	Immediate	2–4 min	4 h
Sub-Q	Varies	1–2 h	4 h
Topical	5–10 min	30–40 min	7–14 days

$T_{1/2}$: 2.5 hours, with metabolism in the liver and excretion in the urine

Adverse effects: Blurred vision, mydriasis, cycloplegia, photophobia, palpitations, bradycardia, dry mouth, altered taste perception, urinary hesitancy and retention, decreased sweating, and predisposition to heat prostration (see Focus on Patient Safety for more information about atropine toxicity)

Nursing Considerations for Patients Receiving Anticholinergic Agents

Assessment: History and Examination

Screen for the following conditions, *which could be cautions or contraindications to use of the drug:* any known allergies to these drugs; glaucoma; stenosing peptic ulcer, intestinal atony, paralytic ileus, GI obstruction, severe ulcerative colitis, and toxic megacolon; prostatic hypertrophy and bladder obstruction; cardiac arrhythmias, tachycardia, and myocardial ischemia, *all of which could be exacerbated by parasympathetic blockade;* impaired liver or kidney function, *which could alter the metabolism and excretion of the drug;* myasthenia gravis, *which could become much worse with further blocking of the cholinergic receptors;* lactation, *because of possible suppression of lactation;* hypertension; and spasticity and brain damage, *which require cautious use of these drugs.*

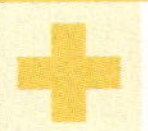

FOCUS ON **PATIENT SAFETY**

Atropine Toxicity

Atropine is used in a large variety of clinical settings to

- Decrease secretions, as a preoperative agent
- Treat parkinsonism (relieves tremor and rigidity)
- Restore cardiac rate and arterial pressure during general anesthesia when increased vagal stimulation causes a rapid parasympathetic response
- Relieve bradycardia and syncope with hyperreactive carotid sinus
- Relieve pylorospasm and hypertonic intestine
- Relax the spasm of biliary and ureteral colic and bronchospasm
- Relax the urinary bladder
- Control crying and laughing episodes in patients with brain lesions
- Treat closed head injuries that cause acetylcholine release
- Relax uterine hypertonicity
- Manage peptic ulcer
- Control rhinorrhea or acute rhinitis from hay fever
- Induce mydriasis for ophthalmic procedures

It also is used as an antidote to overdose with cholinergic drugs or cholinesterase inhibitors and as an antidote to poisoning with certain mushrooms.

Atropine can be a poison, causing severe toxicity. Because it is found in many natural products, including the belladonna plant, and may be present in herbal or alternative therapy products, atropine toxicity can occur inadvertently. Atropine toxicity should be considered whenever a patient receiving an anticholinergic drug presents with a sudden onset of bizarre mental and neurological symptoms. Toxicity is dose related and usually progresses as follows:

0.5 mg atropine—slight cardiac slowing, dryness of mouth, inhibition of sweating

1.0 mg atropine—definite mouth and throat dryness, thirst, rapid heart rate, pupil dilation

2.0 mg atropine—rapid heart rate, palpitations; marked mouth dryness; dilated pupils; some blurring of vision

5.0 mg atropine—all of the above and marked speech disturbances; difficulty swallowing; restlessness, fatigue, headache; dry and hot skin; difficulty voiding; reduced intestinal peristalsis

10.0 mg atropine—all of the above symptoms, more marked; pulse rapid and weak; iris nearly gone; vision blurred; skin flushed, hot, dry, and scarlet; ataxia; restlessness and excitement; hallucinations; delirium and coma

Treatment is as follows. If the poison was taken orally, immediate gastric lavage should be done to limit absorption. Physostigmine can be used as an antidote. A slow intravenous injection of 0.5 to 4 mg (depending on the size of the patient and the severity of the symptoms) usually reverses the delirium and coma of atropine toxicity. Physostigmine is metabolized rapidly, so the injection may need to be repeated every 1 to 2 hours until the atropine has been cleared from the system. Diazepam is the drug of choice if an anticonvulsant is needed. Cool baths and alcohol sponging may relieve the fever and hot skin. In extreme cases, respiratory support may be needed. It is important to remember that the half-life of atropine is 2.5 hours; at extremely high doses, several hours may be needed to clear the atropine from the body.

Include screening *for baseline status before beginning therapy and for any potential adverse effects:* skin color, lesions, temperature; affect, orientation, reflexes, pupil response; pulse, blood pressure, electrocardiogram; respiration, adventitious sounds; urine output, bladder tone; and bowel sounds and abdominal examination.

Nursing Diagnoses

The patient receiving anticholinergic drugs may have the following nursing diagnoses related to drug therapy:

- Acute Pain related to GI, CNS, genitourinary, and cardiovascular effects
- Decreased Cardiac Output related to cardiovascular effects
- Constipation, related to GI effects
- Noncompliance related to adverse drug effects
- Deficient Knowledge regarding drug therapy

Implementation With Rationale

- Ensure proper administration of the drug *to ensure effective use and decrease the risk of adverse effects.*
- Ensure adequate hydration and temperature control *to prevent hyperpyrexia.*
- Provide comfort measures *to help the patient tolerate drug effects:* sugarless lozenges to suck and frequent mouth care *to alleviate problems associated with dry mouth;* lighting control *to alleviate photophobia;* small and frequent meals *to alleviate GI discomfort;* bowel program *to alleviate constipation;* safety precautions *to prevent injury if CNS effects are severe;* analgesics *to relieve pain if headaches occur;* and voiding before taking medication, *if urinary retention is a problem* (commonly occurs with benign prostatic hyperplasia).
- Monitor patient response closely (blood pressure, electrocardiogram, urine output, cardiac output) *in order to arrange to adjust dosage accordingly to ensure benefit with the least amount of toxicity.*
- Provide thorough patient teaching, including measures to avoid adverse effects, warning signs of problems, and the need for monitoring and evaluation, *to enhance patient knowledge about drug therapy and to promote compliance.*
- Offer support and encouragement *to help the patient deal with the drug regimen.*

Evaluation

- Monitor patient response to the drug (improvement in disorder being treated).
- Monitor for adverse effects (cardiovascular changes, GI problems, CNS effects, urinary hesitancy and retention, pupil dilation and photophobia, decrease in sweating and heat intolerance).
- Evaluate the effectiveness of the teaching plan (patient can name drug, dosage, adverse effects to watch for, specific measures to avoid adverse effects, proper administration of ophthalmic drugs).
- Monitor the effectiveness of comfort measures and compliance with the regimen.

WEB LINK

Health care providers and patients may want to consult the following Internet source:

http://www.infoplease.com/ce5/CE003568.html Information on atropine and related anticholinergics.

Points to Remember

- Anticholinergic drugs block the effects of acetylcholine at cholinergic receptor sites.
- Anticholinergic drugs are also called parasympatholytic drugs because they block the effects of the parasympathetic nervous system.
- Blocking of the parasympathetic system causes an increase in heart rate, decrease in GI activity, decrease in urinary bladder tone and function, and pupil dilation and cycloplegia.
- These drugs also block cholinergic receptors in the CNS and sympathetic postganglionic cholinergic receptors, including those that cause sweating.
- Many systemic adverse effects are associated with the use of anticholinergic drugs; they are caused by the systemic cholinergic blocking effects that can also produce the desired therapeutic effect.
- Atropine is the most commonly used anticholinergic drug. It is indicated for a wide variety of conditions and is available in oral, parenteral, and topical forms.
- Patients receiving anticholinergic drugs must be monitored for dry mouth, difficulty swallowing, constipation, urinary retention, tachycardia, pupil dilation and photophobia, cycloplegia and blurring of vision, and heat intolerance caused by a decrease in sweating.

CHECK YOUR UNDERSTANDING

Answers to the questions in this chapter may be found in the Answer Key in the back of the book.

Multiple Choice

Select the best answer to the following.

1. Anticholinergic drugs are used
   a. to block the parasympathetic system to allow the sympathetic system to dominate.
   b. to block the parasympathetic system, which is commonly hyperactive.
   c. as the drugs of choice for treating ulcers.
   d. to stimulate GI activity.

2. Atropine and scopolamine work by blocking
   a. nicotinic receptors only.
   b. muscarinic and nicotinic receptors.
   c. muscarinic receptors only.
   d. adrenergic receptors to allow cholinergic receptors to dominate.

3. Sweating is blocked by anticholinergic agents, so nursing interventions for a patient receiving an anticholinergic should include
   a. covering the head at extremes of temperature.
   b. assuring hydration and temperature control.
   c. changing position slowly and protection from the sun.
   d. monitoring for difficulty swallowing.

4. Teaching patients who are taking anticholinergic drugs would *not* include
   a. encouraging the patient to void before dosing.
   b. a bowel program to deal with constipation.
   c. encouragement to suck sugarless lozenges to avoid the discomfort of dry mouth.
   d. exercise measures to increase the heart rate.

Multiple Response

Select all that apply.

1. A nurse would expect atropine to be used for which of the following?
   a. To depress salivation
   b. To dry up bronchial secretions
   c. To increase the heart rate
   d. To promote uterine contractions
   e. To treat myasthenia gravis
   f. To treat Alzheimer's disease

2. Remembering that anticholinergics block the effects of the parasympathetic nervous system, the nurse would question an order for an anticholinergic drug for patients with which of the following conditions?
   a. Ulcerative colitis
   b. Asthma
   c. Bradycardia
   d. Inner ear imbalance
   e. Glaucoma
   f. Prostatic hyperplasia

Fill in the Blanks

1. Anticholinergic drugs block the effects of ________________ at cholinergic receptor sites.

2. Anticholinergic drugs are also called ________________ drugs because they block the effects of the parasympathetic nervous system.

3. Blocking the parasympathetic system causes the following effects: ________________ in heart rate, ________________ in GI activity and in urinary bladder tone and function, pupil dilation, and cycloplegia.

4. These drugs also block cholinergic receptors in the CNS and those sympathetic postganglionic receptors that are cholinergic, including those that cause ________________.

5. ________________ is the prevention of accommodation of the lens for near vision.

6. Relaxation of the pupil of the eye is called a(n) ________________ effect.

7. ________________ is the most commonly used anticholinergic drug.

8. Patients receiving anticholinergic drugs must be monitored for problems related to eating because of the adverse effects of ________________ and ________________.

Web Exercise

Your patient has been ordered to report for military service in the Middle East. He calls to ask you to explain the nerve gas protocol to use in case of exposure to nerve gas. Go online and find the latest information about the use of atropine and other drugs for preventing paralysis when a soldier is exposed to nerve gas. Develop a brief teaching plan to explain how the drugs work and what signs and symptoms the user may experience.

Bibliography and References

Andrews, M., & Boyle, J. (2004). *Transcultural concepts in nursing care.* Philadelphia: Lippincott Williams & Wilkins.

Drug facts and comparisons. (2006). St. Louis: Facts and Comparisons.

Gilman, A., Hardman, J. G., & Limbird, L. E. (Eds.). (2006). *Goodman and Gilman's the pharmacological basis of therapeutics* (11th ed.). New York: McGraw-Hill.

Karch, A. M. (2006). *2007 Lippincott's nursing drug guide.* Philadelphia: Lippincott Williams & Wilkins.

The medical letter on drugs and therapeutics. (2006). New Rochelle, NY: Medical Letter.

Porth, C. M. (2005). *Pathophysiology: Concepts of altered health states* (7th ed.). Philadelphia: Lippincott Williams & Wilkins.

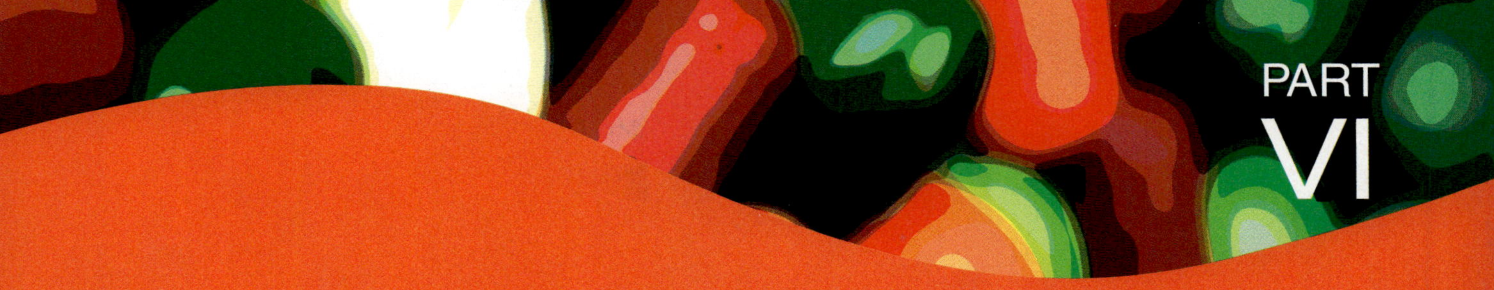

PART VI

Drugs Acting on the Endocrine System

CHAPTER 34

Introduction to the Endocrine System

KEY TERMS

anterior pituitary

diurnal rhythm

hormones

hypothalamic–pituitary axis (HPA)

hypothalamus

negative feedback system

neuroendocrine system

pituitary gland

posterior pituitary

releasing hormones or factors

LEARNING OBJECTIVES

Upon completion of this chapter, you will be able to:

1. Label a diagram showing the glands of the traditional endocrine system and list the hormones produced by each.
2. Describe two theories of hormone action.
3. Discuss the role of the hypothalamus as the master gland of the endocrine system, including influences on the actions of the hypothalamus.
4. Outline a negative feedback system within the endocrine system and explain the ways that this system controls hormone levels in the body.
5. Describe the hypothalamic–pituitary axis (HPA) and what would happen if a hormone level was altered within the HPA.

The nervous system and the endocrine system work together to maintain internal homeostasis and to integrate the body's response to the external environment. Their activities and functions are so closely related that it is probably more correct to refer to them as the **neuroendocrine system**. However, this section deals with drugs affecting the "traditional" endocrine system, which includes glands that secrete **hormones**, or chemical messengers, directly into the bloodstream to communicate within the body. (*Note:* Some organs function like endocrine glands, but they are not considered part of the traditional endocrine system.) Certain hormones that influence body functioning are not secreted by endocrine glands. For example, tissue hormones such as the prostaglandins are produced in various tissues and have effects at their local site. Neurotransmitters, such as norepinephrine and dopamine, also can be classified as hormones because they are secreted directly into the bloodstream for dispersion throughout the body. There also are many gastrointestinal (GI) hormones that are produced in GI cells and act locally. All of these hormones are addressed in the sections most related to their effects.*

Hormones

Hormones are chemicals that are produced in the body and that meet specific criteria. The following are characteristic of all hormones:

- They are produced in very small amounts.
- They are secreted directly into the bloodstream.
- They travel through the blood to specific receptor sites throughout the body.
- They act to increase or decrease the normal metabolic processes of cells when they react with their specific receptor sites.
- They are immediately broken down.

Hormones may react with specific receptor sites on a cell membrane to stimulate the nucleotide cyclic adenosine monophosphate (cAMP) within the cell to cause an effect. For example, when insulin reacts with an insulin receptor site, it activates intracellular enzymes that cause many effects, including changing the cell membrane's permeability to glucose. Hormones such as insulin that do not enter the cell act very quickly, often within seconds, to produce an effect.

* Gastrointestinal hormones are discussed in Part XI: Drugs Acting on the Gastrointestinal System. Neurotransmitters acting like hormones are discussed in Chapter 29: Introduction to the Autonomic Nervous System. The reproductive hormones are discussed in Chapter 39: Introduction to the Reproductive System. Hormones active in the inflammatory and immune responses are discussed in Part III: Drugs Acting on the Immune System. Specific traditional endocrine glands and hormones are discussed in Chapter 35 (hypothalamic and pituitary hormones), Chapter 36 (adrenocortical hormones), Chapter 37 (thyroid and parathyroid hormones), and Chapter 38 (pancreatic hormones).

Other hormones, such as estrogen, actually enter the cell and react with a receptor site inside the cell to change messenger RNA and affect the cell's function. These hormones take quite a while to produce an effect. The full effects of estrogen may not be seen for months to years, as evidenced by the changes that occur at puberty. Because the neuroendocrine system tightly regulates the body's processes within a narrow range of normal limits, overproduction or underproduction of any hormone can affect the body's activities and other hormones within the system.

The Hypothalamus

The **hypothalamus** is the coordinating center for the nervous and endocrine responses to internal and external stimuli. The hypothalamus constantly monitors the body's homeostasis by analyzing input from the periphery and the central nervous system (CNS) and coordinating responses through the autonomic, endocrine, and nervous systems. In effect, it is the "master gland" of the neuroendocrine system. This title was once given to the pituitary gland because of its many functions (see later discussion).

Situated at the base of the forebrain, the hypothalamus receives input from virtually all other areas of the brain, including the limbic system and the cerebral cortex. Because of its positioning, the hypothalamus is able to influence, and be influenced by, emotions and thoughts. The hypothalamus is located in an area of the brain that is poorly protected by the blood–brain barrier, so it is able to act as a sensor to various electrolytes, chemicals, and hormones that are in circulation and do not affect other areas of the brain. The hypothalamus has various neurocenters—areas specifically sensitive to certain stimuli—that regulate a number of body functions, including body temperature, thirst, hunger, water retention, sleep and waking, blood pressure, respiration, reproduction, and emotional reactions.

The hypothalamus maintains internal homeostasis by sensing blood chemistries and by stimulating or suppressing endocrine, autonomic, and CNS activity. In essence, it can turn the autonomic nervous system and its effects on or off. The hypothalamus also produces and secretes a number of **releasing hormones or factors** that stimulate the pituitary gland to stimulate or inhibit various endocrine glands throughout the body (Figure 34.1). These releasing hormones include growth hormone-releasing hormone (GHRH), thyrotropin-releasing hormone (TRH), gonadotropin-releasing hormone (GnRH), corticotropin-releasing hormone (CRH), and prolactin-releasing hormone (PRH). The hypothalamus also produces two inhibiting factors that act as regulators to shut off the production of hormones when levels become too high: growth hormone release-inhibiting factor (somatostatin) and prolactin-inhibiting factor (PIF) (Table 34.1). Recent research has indicated that PIF may actually be dopamine, a neurotransmitter. Patients who are taking dopamine-blocking drugs

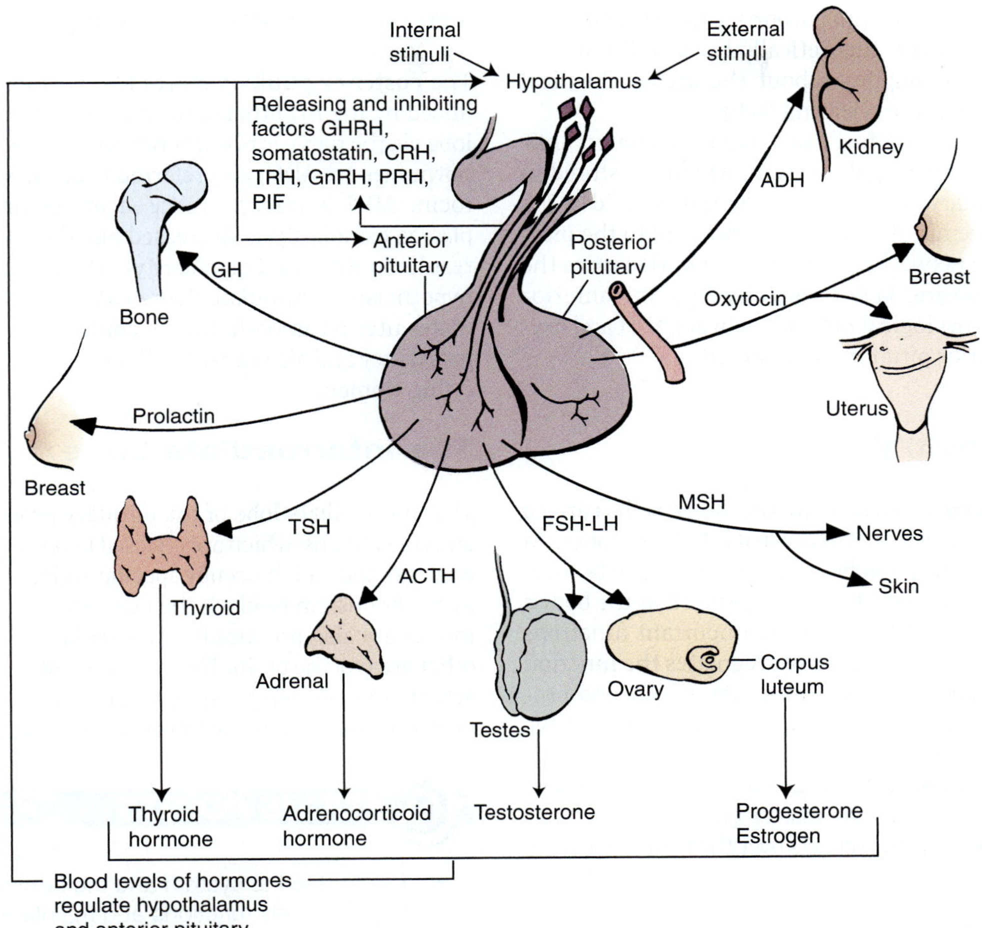

FIGURE 34.1 The traditional endocrine system.

Table 34.1 DRUGS IN FOCUS

Hypothalamic Releasing and Inhibiting Hormones and Associated Anterior Pituitary and Endocrine Gland Response

Hypothalamus Hormones	Anterior Pituitary Hormones	Target Organ Response
Stimulating Hormones		
CRH (corticotropin-releasing hormone)	ACTH (adrenocorticotropic hormone)	Adrenal corticosteroid hormones
TRH (thyroid-releasing hormone)	TSH (thyroid-stimulating hormone)	Thyroid hormone
GHRH (growth hormone–releasing hormone)	GH (growth hormone)	Cell growth
GnRH (gonadotropin-releasing hormone)	LH and FSH (luteinizing hormone, follicle-stimulating hormone)	Estrogen and progesterone (females), testosterone (males)
PRH (prolactin-releasing hormone)	Prolactin	Milk production
Inhibiting Hormones		
Somatostatin (growth hormone–inhibiting factor)		Stops release of GH
PIF (prolactin-inhibiting factors)		Stops release of prolactin

often develop galactorrhea (inappropriate milk production) and breast engorgement, theoretically because PIF also is blocked. Research is ongoing about the actual chemical structure of several of the releasing factors.

The hypothalamus produces two other hormones, antidiuretic hormone (ADH) and oxytocin, which are stored in the posterior pituitary to be released when stimulated by the hypothalamus. The hypothalamus is connected to the pituitary gland by two networks: A vascular network carries the hypothalamic releasing factors directly into the anterior pituitary, and a neurological network delivers ADH and oxytocin to the posterior pituitary to be stored.

The Pituitary

The **pituitary gland** is located in the bony sella turcica under a layer of dura mater. It is divided into three lobes: an anterior lobe, a posterior lobe, and an intermediate lobe. Traditionally, the anterior pituitary was known as the body's master gland because it has so many important functions and, through feedback mechanisms, regulates the function of many other endocrine glands. Also, its unique and protected position in the brain led early scientists to believe that it must be the chief control gland. However, as knowledge of the endocrine system has grown, scientists now designate the hypothalamus as the master gland because it has even greater direct regulatory effects over the neuroendocrine system.

The Anterior Pituitary

The **anterior pituitary** produces six major anterior pituitary hormones. These include growth hormone (GH), adrenocorticotropic hormone (ACTH), follicle-stimulating hormone (FSH), luteinizing hormone (LH), prolactin (PRL), and thyroid-stimulating hormone (TSH, also called thyrotropin) (see Figure 34.1). These hormones are essential for the regulation of growth, reproduction, and some metabolic processes. Deficiency or overproduction of these hormones disrupts this regulation.

The anterior pituitary hormones are released in a rhythmic manner into the bloodstream. Their secretion varies with time of day (often referred to as **diurnal rhythm**) or with physiological conditions such as exercise or sleep. Their release is affected by activity in the CNS; by hypothalamic hormones; by hormones of the peripheral endocrine glands; by certain diseases that can alter endocrine functioning; and by a variety of drugs, which can directly or indirectly upset the homeostasis in the body and cause an endocrine response.

The anterior pituitary also produces melanocyte-stimulating hormone (MSH) and lipotropins. MSH plays an important role in animals that use skin color changes as an adaptive mechanism. It also might be important for nerve growth and development in humans. Lipotropins stimulate fat mobilization but have not been clearly isolated in humans.

The Posterior Pituitary

The **posterior pituitary** stores two hormones that are produced by the hypothalamus and deposited in the posterior lobe via the nerve axons where they are produced. These two hormones are ADH, also referred to as vasopressin, and oxytocin. ADH is directly released in response to increased plasma osmolarity or decreased blood volume (which often results in increased osmolarity). The osmoreceptors in the hypothalamus stimulate the release of ADH. Oxytocin stimulates uterine smooth muscle contraction in late phases of pregnancy and also causes milk release or "let down" in lactating women.

The Intermediate Lobe

The intermediate lobe of the pituitary produces endorphins and enkephalins, which are released in response to severe pain or stress and which occupy specific endorphin-receptor sites in the brainstem to block the perception of pain. These hormones are also produced in tissues in the periphery and in other areas of the brain. They are released in response to overactivity of pain nerves, sympathetic stimulation, transcutaneous stimulation, guided imagery, and vigorous exercise.

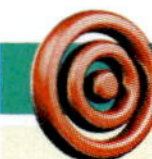

FOCUS POINTS

- The endocrine system and the nervous system regulate body functions and maintain homeostasis largely with the help of hormones, which are chemicals produced within the body. Hormones increase or decrease cellular activity.
- As the "master gland" of the neuroendocrine system, the hypothalamus helps regulate the central and autonomic nervous systems and the endocrine system to maintain homeostasis.
- The pituitary gland has three lobes: the anterior lobe produces stimulating hormones in response to hypothalamic stimulation; the posterior lobe stores ADH and oxytocin, which are two hormones produced by the hypothalamus; and the intermediate lobe produces endorphins and enkephalins to modulate pain perception.

Controls

Hypothalamic–Pituitary Axis

Because of its position in the brain, the hypothalamus is stimulated by many things, such as light, emotion, cerebral cortex activity, and a variety of chemical and hormonal stimuli. Together, the hypothalamus and the pituitary function closely to maintain endocrine activity along what is called the **hypothalamic–pituitary axis (HPA)** using a series of negative feedback systems.

Here is how a **negative feedback system** works. When the hypothalamus senses a need for a particular hormone, for example thyroid hormone, it secretes the releasing factor TRH directly into the anterior pituitary. In response to the TRH, the anterior pituitary secretes TSH, which in turn stimulates the thyroid gland to produce thyroid hormone. When the hypothalamus senses the rising levels of thyroid hormone, it stops secreting TRH, resulting in decreased TSH production and subsequent reduced thyroid hormone levels. The hypothalamus, sensing the falling thyroid hormone levels, secretes TRH again. The negative feedback system continues in this fashion, maintaining the levels of thyroid hormone within a relatively narrow range of normal (Figure 34.2).

It is thought that this feedback system is more complex than once believed. The hypothalamus probably also senses TRH and TSH levels and regulates TRH secretion within a narrow range, even if thyroid hormone is not produced. The anterior pituitary may also be sensitive to TSH levels and thyroid hormone, regulating its own production of TSH. This complex system provides backup controls and regulation if any part of the HPA fails. This system also can create complications, especially when there is a need to override or interact with the total system, as is the case with replacement therapy or treatment of endocrine disorders.

Two of the anterior pituitary hormones (i.e., growth hormone and prolactin) do not have a target organ and so cannot be regulated by the same type of feedback mechanism. Growth hormone release and prolactin release are directly inhibited by the hypothalamic inhibiting factors somatostatin and PIF, respectively. The hypothalamus may be stimulated to release inhibiting factors by increased circulating levels of hormones or by some mediating factor that is stimulated by these hormones. The HPA functions constantly to keep these particular hormones regulated.

Other Controls

Hormones other than stimulating hormones also are released in response to stimuli. For example, the endocrine pancreas produces and releases insulin, glucagon, and somatostatin from different cells in response to varying blood glucose levels. The parathyroid glands release parathormone in response to local calcium levels. The juxtaglomerular cells in the kidney release erythropoietin and renin in response to decreased pressure or decreased oxygenation of the blood flowing into the glomerulus. GI hormones are released in response to local stimuli in the area, such as acid, proteins, or calcium. The thyroid gland produces and secretes another hormone, called calcitonin, in direct response to serum calcium levels. Many different prostaglandins are released throughout the body in response to local stimuli in the tissues that produce them. Activation of the sympathetic nervous system directly causes release of ACTH and the adrenocorticoid hormones to prepare the body for fight or flight. Aldosterone, an adrenocorticoid hormone, is released in response to ACTH but also is released directly in response to high potassium levels.

As more is learned about the interactions of the nervous and endocrine systems, new ideas are being formed about how the body controls its intricate homeostasis. When administering any drug that affects the endocrine or nervous systems, it is important for the nurse to remember how closely related all of these activities are. Expected or unexpected adverse effects involving areas of the endocrine and nervous systems often occur.

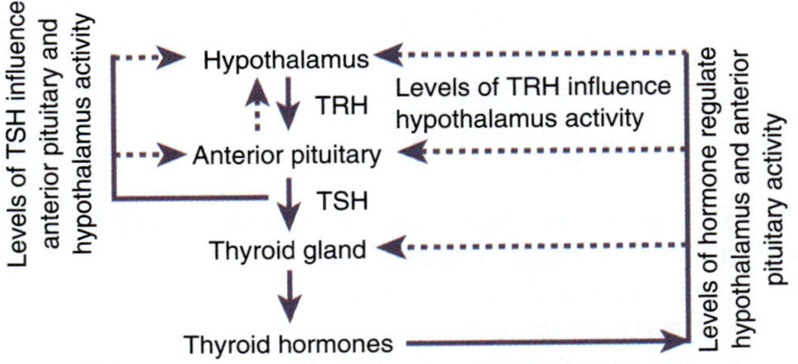

FIGURE 34.2 Negative feedback system. Thyroid hormone levels are regulated by a series of negative feedback systems influencing thyrotropin-releasing hormone (TRH), thyrotropin (TSH), and thyroid hormone levels.

WEB LINK

Students may want to explore up-to-date information from the following source:

http://www.innerbody.com/image/endoov.html Travel through the virtual endocrine system.

Points to Remember

- The endocrine system is a regulatory system that communicates through the use of hormones.
- Because the endocrine and nervous systems are tightly intertwined in the regulation of body homeostasis, they are often referred to as the neuroendocrine system.
- A hormone is a chemical that is produced within the body, is needed in only small amounts, travels to specific receptor sites to cause an increase or decrease in cellular activity, and is broken down immediately.
- The hypothalamus is the "master gland" of the neuroendocrine system. It helps regulate the central and autonomic nervous systems and the endocrine system to maintain homeostasis.
- The pituitary is made up of three lobes: anterior, posterior, and intermediate. The anterior lobe produces stimulating

hormones in response to hypothalamic stimulation. The posterior lobe stores two hormones produced by the hypothalamus, ADH and oxytocin. The intermediate lobe produces endorphins and enkephalins to modulate pain perception.

- The hypothalamus and pituitary operate by a series of negative feedback mechanisms called the hypothalamic–pituitary axis (HPA). The hypothalamus secretes releasing factors to cause the anterior pituitary to release stimulating hormones, which act with specific endocrine glands to cause the release of hormones or, in the case of growth hormone and prolactin, to stimulate cells directly. This stimulation shuts down the production of releasing factors, which leads to decreased stimulating factors and, subsequently, decreased hormone release.
- Growth hormone and prolactin are released by the anterior pituitary and directly influence cell activity. These hormones are regulated by the release of hypothalamic inhibiting factors in response to hormone levels or a cellular mediator.
- Some hormones are not influenced by the HPA and are released in response to direct, local stimulation.
- When any drug that affects either the endocrine or the nervous system is given, adverse effects may occur throughout both systems because they are closely interrelated.

CHECK YOUR UNDERSTANDING

Answers to the questions in this chapter may be found in the Answer Key in the back of the book.

Multiple Choice

Select the best answer to the following.

1. Aldosterone
   a. causes the loss of sodium and water from the renal tubules.
   b. is under direct hormonal control from the hypothalamus.
   c. is released into the bloodstream in response to angiotensin I.
   d. is released into the bloodstream in response to high potassium levels.

2. Antidiuretic hormone (ADH)
   a. is produced by the anterior pituitary.
   b. causes the retention of water by the kidneys.
   c. is released by the hypothalamus.
   d. causes the retention of sodium by the kidneys.

3. The endocrine glands
   a. form part of the communication system of the body.
   b. cannot be stimulated by hormones circulating in the blood.
   c. cannot be viewed as integrating centers of reflex arcs.
   d. are all controlled by the hypothalamus.

4. The hypothalamus maintains internal homeostasis and could be considered the master endocrine gland because
   a. it releases stimulating hormones that cause endocrine glands to produce their hormones.
   b. no hormone-releasing gland responds unless stimulated by the hypothalamus.
   c. it secretes releasing hormones that are an important part of the hypothalamic–pituitary axis that finely regulates the traditional endocrine system.
   d. it regulates temperature control and arousal, as well as hormone release.

5. The posterior lobe of the pituitary gland
   a. secretes a number of stimulating hormones.
   b. produces endorphins to modulate pain perception.
   c. has no function that has yet been identified.
   d. stores ADH and oxytocin, which are produced in the hypothalamus.

6. An example of a negative feedback system would be
   a. growth hormone control.
   b. prolactin control.
   c. melanocyte-stimulating hormone control.
   d. thyroid hormone control.

7. Internal body homeostasis and communication are regulated by
   a. the cardiovascular and respiratory systems.
   b. the nervous and cardiovascular systems.
   c. the endocrine and nervous systems.
   d. the endocrine and cardiovascular systems.

Multiple Response

Select all that apply.

1. Hormones exert their influence on human cells by influencing which of the following?
   a. Enzyme-controlled reactions
   b. Messenger RNA
   c. Lysosome activity
   d. Transcription RNA
   e. Cellular DNA
   f. Cyclic AMP activity

2. The specific criteria that define a hormone would include which of the following?
   a. It is produced in very small amounts.
   b. It is secreted directly into the bloodstream.
   c. It is slowly metabolized in the liver and lungs.
   d. It reacts with a very specific receptor set on a target cell.
   e. A mechanism is always available to immediately destroy it.
   f. It can change a cell's basic function.

3. Some endocrine glands do not respond to the hypothalamic–pituitary axis. These glands would include the
   a. thyroid gland.
   b. ovaries.
   c. parathyroid glands.
   d. adrenal cortex.
   e. endocrine pancreas.
   f. GI gastrin-secreting cells.

Matching

Match the anterior pituitary hormone with the endocrine response it elicits.

1. ______________________ adrenocorticotropic hormone (ACTH)
2. ______________________ growth hormone (GH)
3. ______________________ prolactin (PRL)
4. ______________________ thyroid-stimulating hormone (TSH)
5. ______________________ follicle-stimulating hormone (FSH)
6. ______________________ luteinizing hormone (LH)
7. ______________________ melanocyte-stimulating hormone (MSH)
8. ______________________ lipoproteins

A. Production of thyroid hormone
B. Stimulation of fat mobilization
C. Stimulation of ovulation
D. Release of cortisol, aldosterone
E. Nerve growth and development
F. Milk production in the mammary glands
G. Simulation of follicle development in the ovaries
H. Protein catabolism and cell growth

Word Scramble

Unscramble the following letters to form words associated with the endocrine system.

1. iittuprya dlang ______________________
2. nurliad yhhtmr ______________________
3. sleearngi ctasrof ______________________
4. nniusil ______________________
5. asumhatlpoyh ______________________
6. giveanet beefckad ______________________
7. smorenoh ______________________
8. torriesop iittuprya ______________________
9. canparse ______________________
10. potyhalamhci-ttipuayri sixa ______________________

Bibliography and References

Girard, J. (1991). *Endocrinology of puberty.* Farmington, CT: Karger.
Guyton, A., & Hall, J. (2000). *Textbook of medical physiology.* Philadelphia: W. B. Saunders.
Joseph, R. (1996). *Neuropsychiatry, neuropsychology and clinical neurosciences* (2nd ed.). Baltimore: Williams & Wilkins.
Karch, A. M. (2006). *2007 Lippincott's nursing drug guide.* Philadelphia: Lippincott Williams & Wilkins.
North, W. G., Moses, A. M., & Shafe, L. (Eds.). (1993). The neurohypophysis: A window on brain function. Proceedings of the 5th International Conference on Neurohypophysis, Hanover, New Hampshire, July 16–20, 1992. *Annals of the New York Academy of Sciences, 689,* 1–706.
Porth, C. (2005). *Pathophysiology: Concepts of altered health states* (7th ed.). Philadelphia: Lippincott Williams & Wilkins.

CHAPTER 35

Hypothalamic and Pituitary Agents

KEY TERMS

acromegaly
diabetes insipidus
dwarfism
gigantism
hypopituitarism

LEARNING OBJECTIVES

Upon completion of this chapter, you will be able to:

1. Describe the anatomical and physiological relationship between the hypothalamus and the pituitary gland and list the hormones produced by each.
2. Describe the therapeutic actions, indications, pharmacokinetics, contraindications, most common adverse reactions, and important drug–drug interactions associated with the hypothalamic and pituitary agents.
3. Discuss the use of hypothalamic and pituitary agents across the lifespan.
4. Compare and contrast the prototype drugs leuprolide, somatropin, bromocriptine mesylate, and vasopressin with other hypothalamic and pituitary agents.
5. Outline the nursing considerations, including important teaching points, for patients receiving a hypothalamic or pituitary agent.

HYPOTHALAMIC RELEASING HORMONES

abarelix
corticotropin-releasing hormone
ganirelix
gonadorelin
goserelin
histrelin
(P) leuprolide
nafarelin
sermorelin

ANTERIOR PITUITARY HORMONES

chorionic gonadotropin
corticotropin
cosyntropin
menotropins
(P) somatropin
somatropin rDNA origin
thyrotropin

GROWTH HORMONE ANTAGONISTS

(P) bromocriptine mesylate
octreotide acetate
pegvisomant

POSTERIOR PITUITARY HORMONES

desmopressin
(P) vasopressin

As described in Chapter 34, the endocrine system's main function is to maintain homeostasis. This is achieved through a complex balance of glandular activities that either stimulate or suppress hormone release. Too much or too little glandular activity disrupts the body's homeostasis, leading to various disorders and interfering with the normal functioning of other endocrine glands. The drugs presented in this chapter are those used to either replace or interact with the hormones or factors produced by the hypothalamus and pituitary. (See Box 35.1 for the use of these drugs in various age groups.)

Hypothalamic Releasing Factors

The hypothalamus uses a number of releasing hormones or factors to stimulate or inhibit the release of hormones from the anterior pituitary. These releasing hormones are growth hormone-releasing hormone (GHRH), thyrotropin-releasing hormone (TRH), gonadotropin-releasing hormone (GnRH), corticotropin-releasing hormone (CRH), and prolactin-releasing hormone (PRH). The hypothalamus also releases two inhibiting factors, somatostatin (growth hormone-inhibiting factor) and prolactin-inhibiting factor (PIF). These hormones are found in such minute quantities that their actual chemical structures have not been clearly identified. Not all of the hypothalamic hormones are used as pharmacological agents. A number of the hypothalamic releasing factors described here are used for diagnostic purposes only, and others are used primarily as antineoplastic agents.

CRH stimulates the release of adrenocorticotropic hormone (ACTH) from the anterior pituitary and is used to diagnose Cushing's disease (a condition characterized by hypersecretion of adrenocortical hormones in response to excessive ACTH release). It is being studied for the treatment of peritumoral brain edema.

Gonadorelin (*Factrel*) is a GnRH analog that is used for diagnostic purposes to check for anterior pituitary response and gonadotropin deficiency.

Goserelin (*Zoladex*) is an analog of GnRH. After an initial burst of follicle-stimulating hormone (FSH) and luteinizing hormone (LH) release, goserelin inhibits pituitary gonadotropin secretion with a resultant drop in the production of the sex hormones. This drug currently is used as an antineoplastic agent to treat prostatic cancers.

Histrelin (*Supprelin*), ganirelix (*Antagon*), and abarelix (*Plenaxis*) are GnRH agonists. With chronic use, histrelin inhibits gonadotropin secretion and decreases the levels of steroid sex hormones. It is used to treat precocious puberty in children. Ganirelix is used in fertility programs to inhibit premature LH surges in women undergoing controlled ovarian stimulation. Abarelix is used as palliative therapy in advanced prostate cancer for men who decline surgical castration and who are at risk for neurological compromise or ureteral or bladder obstruction due to metastases.

Leuprolide (*Lupron*) occupies pituitary GnRH receptor sites so that they no longer respond to GnRH. As a result, there is no stimulation for release of LH and FSH. This drug is used primarily as an antineoplastic agent to treat specific cancers. It is also used to treat endometriosis and precocious puberty that results from hypothalamic activity.

Nafarelin (*Synarel*), a potent agonist of GnRH, is used to decrease the production of gonadal hormones through repeated stimulation of their receptor sites. After about 4 weeks of therapy, gonadal hormone levels fall, and the cells

BOX 35.1 **DRUG THERAPY ACROSS THE LIFESPAN**

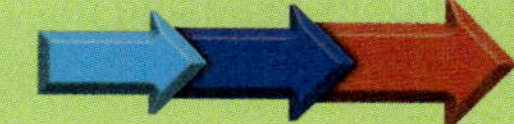

Hypothalamic and Pituitary Agents

CHILDREN

Children who receive any of the hypothalamic or pituitary agents need to be monitored closely for adverse effects associated with changes in overall endocrine function, particularly growth and development and metabolism. Periodic radiograph of the long bones as well as monitoring of blood sugar levels and electrolytes should be a standard part of the treatment plan. Children receiving growth hormone pose many challenges (see Box 35.2). Children who are using desmopressin for diabetes insipidus need to have the administration technique monitored and should have an adult responsible for the overall treatment protocol.

ADULTS

Adults also need frequent monitoring of electrolytes and blood sugar levels when receiving any of these agents. Adults using nasal forms of drugs to control diabetes insipidus should review the proper administration of the drug with the primary care provider periodically; inappropriate administration can lead to complications and lack of therapeutic effect. Adults receiving regular injections of these drugs should learn the proper storage, preparation, and administration of the drug, including rotation of injection sites.

These drugs should not be used during pregnancy or lactation unless the benefit to the mother clearly outweighs any risk to the fetus or neonate, because of the potential for severe adverse effects associated with the use of these drugs.

OLDER ADULTS

Older adults may be more susceptible to the imbalances associated with alterations in the endocrine system. They should be evaluated periodically during treatment for hydration and nutrition as well as for electrolyte balance. Proper administration technique should be reviewed, and nasal mucus membranes should be evaluated regularly, because older patients are more apt to develop dehydrated membranes and possibly ulcerations, leading to improper dosing of drugs delivered nasally.

they normally stimulate are quiet. This drug is used to treat endometriosis and precocious puberty.

Sermorelin (*Geref*) (GHRH) stimulates the production of growth hormone (GH) by the anterior pituitary. It is used for diagnostic purposes in short children to determine the presence of hypothalamic or pituitary dysfunction. It is also used to evaluate the therapeutic response in patients undergoing surgery or irradiation and to treat idiopathic growth hormone deficiency in children less than 8 years of age. It has orphan drug status with gonadotropin to induce ovulation and to treat cachexia associated with acquired immune deficiency syndrome (AIDS). All of the hypothalamic releasing factors are listed in Table 35.1.

Prototype Summary: *Leuprolide*

Indications: Treatment of advanced prostatic cancer, endometriosis, central precocious puberty, uterine leiomyomata

Actions: LHRH agonist that occupies pituitary gonadotropin-releasing hormone receptors and desensitizes them; causes an initial increase and then profound decrease in LH and FSH levels

Pharmacokinetics:

Route	Onset	Peak	Duration
IM depot	4 h	Variable	1, 2, 3, or 4 mo

$T_{1/2}$: 3 hours; metabolism and excretion unknown

Adverse effects: Dizziness, headache, pain, peripheral edema, myocardial infarction, nausea, vomiting, anorexia, constipation, urinary frequency, hematuria, hot flashes, increased sweating

Nursing Considerations for Patients Receiving Hypothalamic Releasing Factors

The specific nursing care of the patient who is receiving a hypothalamic releasing factor is related to the hormone (or hormones) that the drug is affecting (see Chapter 36 for adrenocorticoid hormones, Chapter 37 for thyroid hormones, and Chapters 40 and 41 for sex hormones). Drugs used for diagnostic purposes are

Table 35.1 DRUGS IN FOCUS

Hypothalamic Releasing Factors

Drug Name	Dosage/Route	Usual Indications
abarelix (*Plenaxis*)	100 mg IM, days 1, 15, and 29, and then q4wk	Treatment of advanced prostate cancer when other treatments are not acceptable or appropriate
ganirelix acetate (*Antagon*)	250 mcg Sub-Q on day 2 or 3 of the menstrual cycle	Inhibition of premature LH surge in women undergoing controlled ovarian overstimulation as part of a fertility program
gonadorelin (*Factrel*)	100 mg Sub-Q or IV on days 1–7 of the menstrual cycle	Evaluation of functional capacity and response of the gonadotropes of the anterior pituitary
corticotropin-releasing hormone (CRH) (*generic*)	10–25 units in 500 mL DSW infused over 8 h	Diagnosis of Cushing's disease
goserelin (*Zoladex*)	3.6 mg Sub-Q every 28 days or 10.8 mg Sub-Q every 3 mo	Treatment of prostatic cancers
histrelin (*Supprelin*)	10 mcg/kg/day Sub-Q	Treatment of precocious puberty in children
P leuprolide (*Lupron*)	Prostate cancer: 1 mg/day Sub-Q or various depot preparations: 3.75 mg IM endometriosis—once a month Precocious puberty: 5–10 mcg/kg/day Sub-Q	Treatment of specific cancers, endometriosis, and precocious puberty
nafarelin (*Synarel*)	400 mcg/day divided as one spray in left nostril AM or PM; one spray in right nostril AM or PM; Precocious puberty—1,600–1,800 mcg/day intranasally	Treatment of endometriosis and precocious puberty
sermorelin (*Geref*) (GHRH)	Idiopathic growth failure: 30 mcg/kg/day Sub-Q	Diagnosis of hypothalamic or pituitary dysfunction in short children; evaluation of response to surgery or irradiation; treatment of idiopathic growth failure; ovulation induction, AIDS-associated cachexia (orphan drug uses)

short lived; information about these agents should be included in any patient teaching about the diagnostic procedure. Nursing process guidelines for other agents can be found with the therapeutic drug class to which they belong (e.g., antineoplastic agents, Chapter 14).

Anterior Pituitary Hormones

Agents that affect pituitary function are used mainly to mimic or antagonize the effects of specific pituitary hormones. They may be used either as replacement therapy for conditions resulting from a hypoactive pituitary or for diagnostic purposes. The anterior pituitary hormones that are in use today include seven different drugs (Figure 35.1 and Table 35.2):

- Chorionic gonadotropin (*Chorex*) acts like LH and stimulates the production of testosterone and progesterone. It is used to treat hypogonadism in males, to induce ovulation in females with functioning ovaries, and to treat prepubertal cryptorchidism when there is no anatomical obstruction to testicular movement. (See Chapters 40 and 41 for nursing implications.)
- Corticotropin (*Acthar*), or ACTH, is used for diagnostic purposes to test adrenal function and responsiveness. Because it stimulates steroid release and anti-inflammatory effects, it also is used to treat various inflammatory disorders.
- Cosyntropin (*Cortrosyn*) is used to diagnose adrenal dysfunction. Because it has a rapid onset and a short duration of activity, it is not used for therapeutic purposes.
- Menotropins (*Pergonal*) is a purified preparation of gonadotropins. It is used as a fertility drug to stimulate ovu-

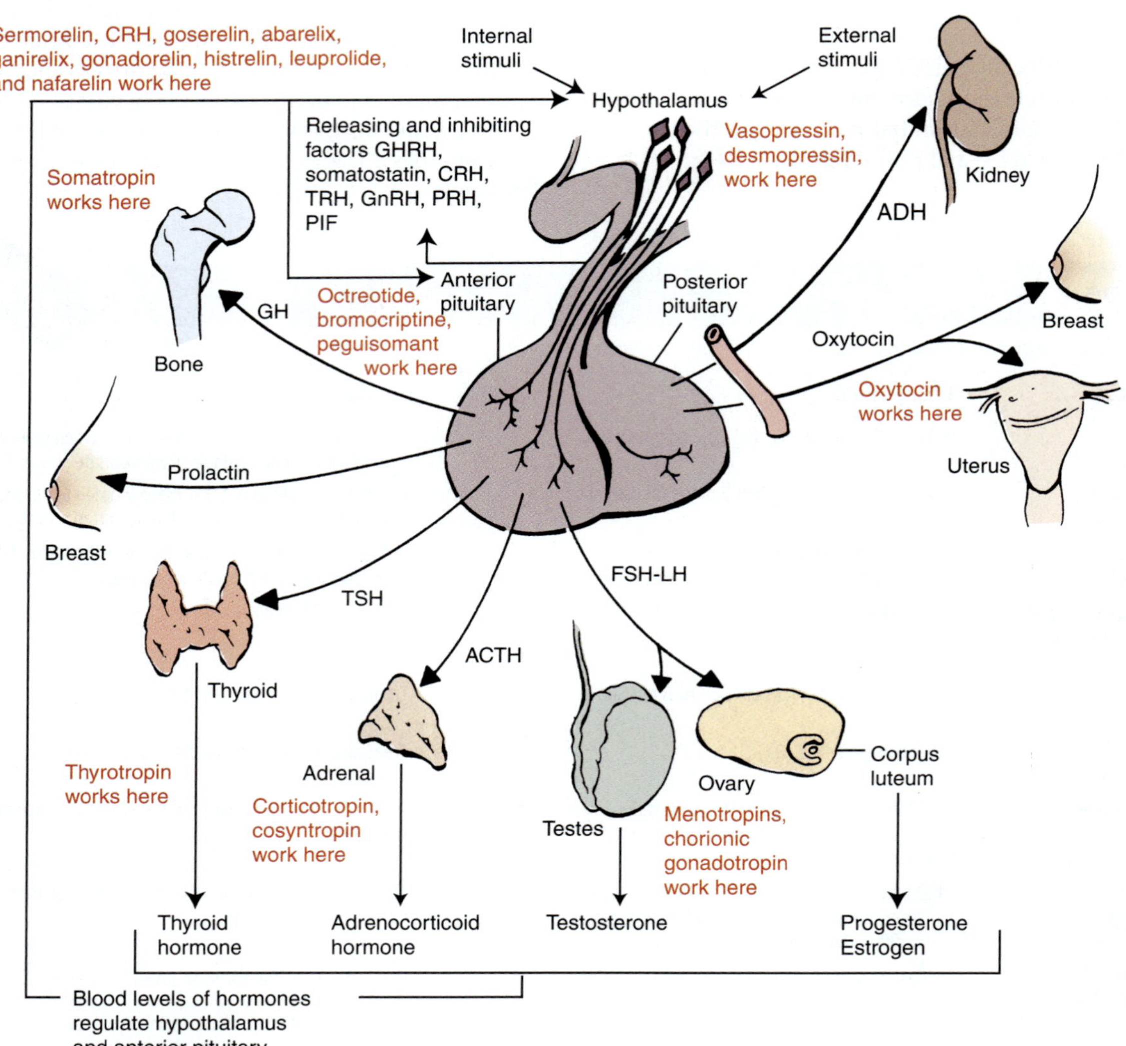

FIGURE 35.1 Sites of action of hypothalamic/pituitary agents.

Table 35.2 DRUGS IN FOCUS

Anterior Pituitary Hormones

Drug Name	Dosage/Route	Usual Indications
chorionic gonadotropin (*Chorex,* others)	Dosage varies with indication; 4,000–10,000 International Units IM one to three times per week is not unusual	Treatment of male hypogonadism, induction of ovulation, treatment of prepubertal cryptorchidism
corticotropin (*Acthar*)	Diagnosis: 10–25 units IV over 8 h Treatment: 20 International Units IM or Sub-Q q.i.d.	Diagnosis of adrenal function, treatment of various inflammatory disorders
cosyntropin (*Cortrasyn*)	0.25–0.75 mg IV or IM	Diagnosis of adrenal function
menotropins (*Pergonal*)	75 International Units FSH/75 IU LH/day IM for 9–12 days	Stimulation of ovulation and spermatogenesis
P somatropin (*Nutropin, Saizen, Humatrope*)	Dosage varies with each product, check manufacturer's instructions; must be given Sub-Q or IM	Treatment of children with growth failure
somatropin rDNA origin (*Zorbtive*)	0.1 mg/kg Sub-Q for 4 wk	Treatment of adults with short bowel syndrome
thyrotropin (*Thytropar*)	10 International Units IM for 1–3 days	Diagnosis of thyroid function

lation in women and spermatogenesis in men. (See Chapters 40 and 41 for nursing implications.)

- Somatropin (*Nutropin, Saizen, Genotropin, Serostim,* and others) is a GH that is produced with the use of recombinant DNA technology. It is used in the treatment of children with growth failure, girls with Turner's syndrome, wasting and cachexia associated with AIDS, and growth hormone deficiency in adults
- Somatropin rDNA origin (*Zorbtive*) is a new formulation of growth hormone used for as long as 4 weeks for the treatment of short bowel syndrome in adults to increase intestinal absorption of needed nutrients.
- Thyrotropin (*Thytropar*) is equivalent to TSH and is used as a diagnostic agent to evaluate thyroid function.

In clinical practice, the agent that is used purely as a replacement for anterior pituitary hormones is that acting as GH—somatropin.

Growth Hormone

GH is responsible for linear skeletal growth, the growth of internal organs, protein synthesis, and the stimulation of many other processes that are required for normal growth. **Hypopituitarism** is often seen as GH deficiency before any other signs and symptoms occur. Hypopituitarism may occur as a result of developmental abnormalities or congenital defects of the pituitary, circulatory disturbances (e.g., hemorrhage, infarction), acute or chronic inflammation of the pituitary, and pituitary tumors. GH deficiency in children results in short stature (**dwarfism**). Adults with somatropin deficiency syndrome (SDS) may have hypopituitarism as a result of pituitary tumors or trauma, or they may have been treated for GH deficiency as children, resulting in a shutdown of the pituitary production of somatotropin.

GH deficiency was once treated with GH injections extracted from the pituitary glands of cadavers. The supply of GH was therefore rather limited and costly (Box 35.2). Synthetic human GH is now available from recombinant DNA sources using genetic engineering. Synthetic GH is expensive, but it is thought to be safer than cadaver GH and is being used increasingly to treat GH deficiencies. Somatropin is the only GH replacement drug in use today (see Figure 35.1). Box 35.3 discusses an alternate treatment for growth failure.

Therapeutic Actions and Indications

As noted, somatropin is a hormone of recombinant DNA origin that is equivalent to human GH. Somatropin is indicated for the treatment of growth failure due to lack of GH or to chronic renal failure, for long-term treatment of growth failure in children born small for gestational age who do not achieve catch-up growth by 2 years of age, and for the treatment of short stature associated with Turner's syndrome. It is also approved to increase protein production and growth in various AIDS-related states. Box 35.4 discusses a new delivery system for somatropin.

Pharmacokinetics

Somatropin is injected and reaches peak levels within 7 hours. It is widely distributed in the body and localizes in highly

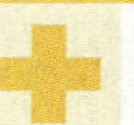

BOX 35.2 FOCUS ON **PATIENT SAFETY**

Growth Hormone Therapy

In the past, growth hormone therapy was expensive and unsafe. The use of cadaver pituitaries resulted in unreliable hormone levels and, in many cases, hypersensitivity reactions to the proteins found in the drug. With the advent of genetic engineering and the development of safer, more reliable forms of growth hormone, there has been a surge in use of the drug to treat children with short stature. Even so, the drug is still costly and not without adverse effects.

Growth hormone can be used to treat growth failure caused either by lack of growth hormone or by renal failure. It also can help children with normal growth hormone levels who are just genetically small. Before the drug is prescribed, the child must undergo screening procedures and specific testing (including radiographs and blood tests) and must display a willingness to have regular injections. The child taking this drug will need to have pretherapy and periodic tests of thyroid function, blood glucose levels, glucose tolerance tests, and tests for growth hormone antibodies (a risk that increases with the length of therapy). In addition, radiographs of the long bones will be taken to monitor for closure of the epiphyses, a sign that the drug must be stopped. Because the child who is taking growth hormone may experience sudden growth, he or she will need to be monitored for nutritional needs as well as psychological trauma that may occur with the sudden change in body image. Insulin therapy and replacement thyroid therapy may be needed, depending on the child's response to the drug.

The child's family or caregivers will need instructions on the following points:

- Storage of the drug (refrigeration is required)
- Preparation of the drug (the reconstitution procedure varies depending on the brand name product used)
- Administration of the drug (sterile technique, need to rotate injection sites, and need to monitor injection sites for atrophy or extravasation)

They also must be advised to report any lack of growth as well as signs of glucose intolerance (thirst, hunger, voiding pattern changes) or thyroid dysfunction (fatigue, thinning hair, slow pulse, puffy skin, intolerance to the cold).

The use of growth hormone involves an interrelationship among many subspecialists and expensive and regular medical evaluation and care. The key to the success of this therapy may be the attitude and cooperation of the young patient.

BOX 35.3 New Treatment for Growth Failure in Children

In late 2005, the U.S. Food and Drug Administration approved two drugs that contain human insulinlike growth factor-1 (IGF-1) and human insulinlike growth factor–binding protein-3. These factors promote linear growth in children and also have anabolic effects, sensitize cells to insulin, and have insulinlike effects on metabolism. They do not directly alter growth hormone levels. As more is learned about the intricate interrelationship of the various hormones, more specific drugs may be developed to target very specific disorders. The drugs, mecasermin (*Increlex*) and mecasermin rinfabate (*Iplex*), are approved for the long-term treatment of growth failure in children with severe primary IGF-1 deficiency or with growth hormone gene depletion who have developed neutralizing antibodies to growth hormone. *Increlex* is given by subcutaneous injection, initially 0.04–0.08 mg/kg (40–80 mcg/kg) b.i.d., and then increased by 0.04 mg/kg/dose to a maximum dose of 0.12 mg/kg b.i.d. *Iplex* only has to be injected once a day, which might be important to many parents administering the drug to their children. Dosage should be based on individual response and glucose levels. It is given by subcutaneous injection, initially 0.5 mg/kg/day, and then titrated to a maximum 2 mg/kg/day by subcutaneous injection, based on glucose and IGF-1 levels. The injection should be given at approximately the same time each day, either in the morning or evening. This drug must be kept frozen until ready to be used. With both of these drugs, hypoglycemia is common, and patients must be monitored to ensure that they eat after administration. Tonsillar hypertrophy is also common and the child should be monitored appropriately.

perfused tissues, particularly the liver and kidney. Excretion occurs through the urine and feces. Patients with liver or renal dysfunction may experience reduced clearance and increased concentrations of the drug. This drug should be avoided in pregnancy and lactation because of the potential for adverse effects on the fetus or neonate.

Contraindications and Cautions

Somatropin is contraindicated with any known allergy to the drug or ingredients in the drug. It is also contraindicated in the presence of closed epiphyses or with underlying cranial lesions.

Adverse Effects

The adverse effects that most often occur when using GH include the development of antibodies to GH and subsequent signs of inflammation and autoimmune-type reactions (much more common with somatrem); swelling and joint pain; and the endocrine reactions of hypothyroidism and insulin resistance.

BOX 35.4 New Delivery System for Growth Hormone

Saizen (somatropin) is a preparation of recombinant DNA–produced human growth hormone that is used to treat children with growth failure due to lack of growth hormone. The drug must be given by injection six or seven times a week. A new delivery form is now available to ease the discomfort and trauma of the frequent injections. The *cool.click* delivery system is a neon-colored, needle-free system that delivers the drug through the skin using a fine mist. Tests have shown a bioequivalency of this method with standard injection techniques, and the young patients who must use this drug are much less resistant to the dosing. Various drug companies anticipate similar delivery systems, which will provide a therapeutic dose of drugs without the associated discomfort of intramuscular or subcutaneous injection.

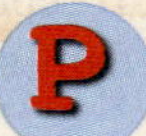

Prototype Summary: Somatropin

Indications: Long-term treatment of children with growth failure associated with various deficiencies, girls with Turner's syndrome, AIDS wasting and cachexia, growth hormone deficiency in adults; treatment of growth failure in children of small gestational age who do not achieve catch-up growth by 2 years of age

Actions: Replaces human growth hormone; stimulates skeletal growth, growth of internal organs, and protein synthesis

Pharmacokinetics:

Route	Onset	Peak
IM, Sub-Q	Varies	5–7.5 h

$T_{1/2}$: 15–50 min; metabolized in the liver and excreted in the urine and feces

Adverse effects: Development of antibodies to growth hormone, insulin resistance, swelling, joint pain, headache, injection site pain

Nursing Considerations for Patients Receiving Growth Hormone

Assessment: History and Examination

Screen for the following conditions, *which are contraindications to the use of the drug:* history of allergy to any GH or binder, and closed epiphyses or underlying cranial lesions.

Include screening *for baseline status before beginning therapy and for any potential adverse effects:* height, weight, thyroid function tests, glucose tolerance tests, and GH levels.

Nursing Diagnoses

The patient receiving any GH may have the following nursing diagnoses related to drug therapy:

- Imbalanced Nutrition: Less Than Body Requirements, related to metabolic changes
- Acute Pain related to need for injections
- Deficient Knowledge regarding drug therapy

Implementation With Rationale

- Reconstitute the drug following manufacturer's directions *because individual products vary;* administer intramuscularly or subcutaneously *for appropriate delivery of drug.*
- Monitor response carefully when beginning therapy *to allow appropriate dosage adjustments as needed.*
- Monitor thyroid function, glucose tolerance, and GH levels periodically *to monitor endocrine changes and to institute treatment as needed.*
- Provide thorough patient teaching, including measures to avoid adverse effects, warning signs of problems, and the need for regular evaluation (including blood tests) *to enhance patient knowledge about drug therapy and promote compliance.* Instruct a family member or caregiver in proper preparation and administration techniques *to ensure proper administration of the drug.*

Evaluation

- Monitor patient response to the drug (return of GH levels to normal; growth and development).
- Monitor for adverse effects (hypothyroidism, glucose intolerance, nutritional imbalance).
- Evaluate the effectiveness of the teaching plan (patient can name drug, dosage, adverse effects to watch for, and specific measures to avoid adverse effects; family member can demonstrate proper technique for preparation and administration of drug).
- Monitor the effectiveness of comfort measures and compliance with the regimen.

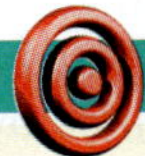

FOCUS POINTS

- Used mostly for diagnostic testing and for treating some cancers, hypothalamic releasing factors stimulate the anterior pituitary to release hormones, which in turn stimulate endocrine glands or cell metabolisms.
- In children, deficiency of growth hormone (GH) may be responsible for dwarfism; in adults it is associated with somatropin deficiency syndrome.
- GH may be replaced by a substance produced by recombinant DNA processes, which is safer than replacement drugs of the past.

Growth Hormone Antagonists

GH hypersecretion can occur at any time of life. This is often referred to as hyperpituitarism. If it occurs before the epiphyseal plates of the long bones fuse, it causes an acceleration in linear skeletal growth, producing **gigantism** of 7 to 8 feet in height with fairly normal body proportions. In adults after epiphyseal closure, linear growth is impossible. Instead, hypersecretion of GH causes enlargement in the peripheral parts of the body, such as the hands and feet, and the internal organs, especially the heart. **Acromegaly** is the term used to describe the onset of excessive GH secretion that occurs after puberty and epiphyseal plate closure.

Most conditions of GH hypersecretion are caused by pituitary tumors and are treated by radiation therapy or surgery. Drug therapy for GH excess can be used for those patients who are not candidates for surgery or radiation therapy. The drugs used to treat GH excess include a somatostatin analog (octreotide acetate [*Sandostatin*]), a GH analog (pegvisomant [*Somavert*]), and a dopamine agonist (bromocriptine [*Parlodel*]) (see Figure 35.1 and Table 35.3).

Therapeutic Actions and Indications

Somatostatin is an inhibitory factor released from the hypothalamus. It is not used to decrease GH levels, although it does do that very effectively. Because it has multiple effects on many secretory systems (for example, it inhibits release of gastrin, glucagon, and insulin) and a short duration of action, it is not desirable as a therapeutic agent. An analog of somatostatin, octreotide acetate, is considerably more potent in inhibiting GH release with less of an inhibitory effect on insulin release. Consequently, it is used instead of somatostatin.

Bromocriptine, a semisynthetic ergot alkaloid, is a dopamine agonist frequently used to treat acromegaly. It may be used alone or as an adjunct to irradiation. Dopamine agonists inhibit GH secretion in some patients with acromegaly; the opposite effect occurs in normal individuals. Bromocriptine's GH-inhibiting effect may be explained by the fact that dopamine increases somatostatin release from the hypothalamus. Both of these drugs are indicated for the treatment of acromegaly in patients who are not candidates for or cannot tolerate other therapy.

Pegvisomant (*Somavert*) is a GH analog that was approved in late 2003 for the treatment of acromegaly in patients who do not respond to other therapies. It binds to GH receptors on cells, inhibiting GH effects. It must be given by daily subcutaneous injections.

Pharmacokinetics

Octreotide is rapidly absorbed and widely distributed throughout the body. It is metabolized in the tissues, and about 30% is excreted unchanged in the urine. Patients with renal dysfunction may accumulate higher levels of the drug. There are no adequate studies of effects in pregnancy and during lactation, and use should be reserved for situations in which the benefits to the mother clearly outweigh any potential risks to the fetus or neonate.

Bromocriptine is effectively absorbed from the gastrointestinal (GI) tract and undergoes extensive first-pass metabolism in the liver. It is primarily excreted in the bile. The drug should not be used during pregnancy or lactation because of effects on the fetus and because it blocks lactation.

Pegvisomant is slowly absorbed from the subcutaneous tissue, reaching peak effects in 33 to 77 hours. It is cleared from the body slowly, with a half-life of 6 days. The drug is excreted in the urine. There are no well-controlled studies in pregnancy, and pegvisomant should be used during pregnancy only if the benefit clearly outweighs the potential risk to the fetus. It is not known if pegvisomant crosses into breast milk.

Contraindications and Cautions

These drugs are contraindicated in the presence of any known allergy to the drug. They should be used cautiously in the presence of any other endocrine disorder (e.g., diabetes, thyroid dysfunction) and in pregnancy or lactation.

Adverse Effects

Octreotide is associated with many GI complaints because of its effects on the GI tract. Constipation or diarrhea, flatulence, and nausea are not uncommon. Octreotide has also been associated with the development of acute cholecysti-

Table 35.3 DRUGS IN FOCUS

Growth Hormone Antagonists

Drug Name	Dosage/Route	Usual Indications
P bromocriptine mesylate (*Parlodel*)	1.25–2.5 mg/day PO	Treatment of acromegaly in patients who are not candidates for or cannot tolerate other therapy; not recommended for children <15 yr
octreotide (*Sandostatin*)	100–500 mcg Sub-Q t.i.d.; adjust dose in elderly patients	Treatment of acromegaly in adults who are not candidates for or cannot tolerate other therapy
pegvisomant (*Somavert*)	40 mg Sub-Q as a loading dose, then 10 mg/day Sub-Q	Treatment of acromegaly in adults who are not candidates for or who cannot tolerate other therapy

tis, cholestatic jaundice, biliary tract obstruction, and pancreatitis. Patients must be assessed for the possible development of any of these problems. Other, less common adverse effects include headache, sinus bradycardia or other cardiac arrhythmias, and decreased glucose tolerance. Octreotide must be administered subcutaneously, and it can be associated with discomfort and/or inflammation at injection sites.

Bromocriptine is given orally and is also associated with GI disturbances. Because of its dopamine-blocking effects, it may cause drowsiness and postural hypotension. It blocks lactation and should not be used by nursing mothers.

Pegvisomant is given by subcutaneous injection. Pain and inflammation at the injection site are common effects. Increased incidence of infection, nausea, and diarrhea, and changes in liver function may also occur.

Clinically Important Drug–Drug Interactions

Increased serum bromocriptine levels and increased toxicity occur if this drug is combined with erythromycin. This combination should be avoided.

The effectiveness of bromocriptine may decrease if it is combined with phenothiazines. If this combination is used, the patient should be monitored carefully.

Patients receiving pegvisomant may require higher dosages to receive adequate GH suppression if they are also taking opioids. The mechanism of action of this interaction is not understood.

Prototype Summary: *Bromocriptine Mesylate*

Indications: Treatment of Parkinson's disease, hyperprolactinemia associated with pituitary adenomas, female infertility associated with hyperprolactinemia, and acromegaly; short-term treatment of amenorrhea or galactorrhea

Actions: Acts directly on postsynaptic dopamine receptors in the brain

Pharmacokinetics:

Route	Onset	Peak	Duration
PO	Varies	1–3 h	14 h

$T_{1/2}$: 3 hours, then 45–50 hours; metabolized in the liver and excreted in the bile

Adverse effects: Dizziness, fatigue, light-headedness, nasal congestion, drowsiness, nausea, vomiting, abdominal cramps, constipation, diarrhea, headache

Nursing Considerations for Patients Receiving Growth Hormone Antagonists

Assessment: History and Examination

Screen for the following conditions, *which are contraindications to use of the drug:* history of allergy to any GH antagonist or binder; other endocrine disturbances; and pregnancy and lactation.

Include screening *for baseline status before beginning therapy and for any potential adverse effects:* orientation, affect, and reflexes; blood pressure, pulse, and orthostatic blood pressure; abdominal examination; glucose tolerance tests and GH levels.

Nursing Diagnoses

The patient receiving any GH antagonist may have the following nursing diagnoses related to drug therapy:

- Imbalanced Nutrition: More Than Body Requirements, related to metabolic changes
- Acute Pain related to need for injections (octreotide, pegvisomant)
- Deficient Knowledge regarding drug therapy

Implementation With Rationale

- Reconstitute octreotide and pegvisomant following manufacturer's directions; administer these drugs subcutaneously and rotate injection sites regularly *to prevent skin breakdown and to ensure proper delivery of the drug.*
- Monitor thyroid function, glucose tolerance, and GH levels periodically *to detect problems and to institute treatment as needed.*
- Arrange for baseline and periodic ultrasound evaluation of the gallbladder if using octreotide *to detect any gallstone development and to arrange for appropriate treatment.*
- Provide thorough patient teaching, including measures to avoid adverse effects, warning signs of problems, and need for regular evaluation (including blood tests), *to enhance patient knowledge about drug therapy and promote compliance.* Instruct a family member in proper preparation and administration techniques to ensure that there is another responsible person to administer the drug if needed.

Evaluation

- Monitor patient response to the drug (return of GH levels to normal, growth and development).

- Monitor for adverse effects (hypothyroidism, glucose intolerance, nutritional imbalance, GI disturbances, headache, dizziness, cholecystitis).
- Evaluate the effectiveness of the teaching plan (patient can name drug, dosage, adverse effects to watch for, and specific measures to avoid adverse effects; family member can demonstrate proper technique for preparation and administration of drug).
- Monitor the effectiveness of comfort measures and compliance with the regimen.

Posterior Pituitary Hormones

The posterior pituitary stores two hormones produced in the hypothalamus: antidiuretic hormone (ADH, also known as vasopressin) and oxytocin. Oxytocin stimulates milk ejection or "let down" in lactating women. In pharmacological doses, it can be used to initiate or improve uterine contractions in labor. This drug is discussed in Chapter 40.

ADH possesses antidiuretic, hemostatic, and vasopressor properties. Posterior pituitary disorders can occur secondary to metastatic cancer, lymphoma, disseminated intravascular coagulation (discussed in Chapter 48), or septicemia. Posterior pituitary disorders that are seen clinically involve ADH release and include **diabetes insipidus**, which results from insufficient secretion, and syndrome of inappropriate antidiuretic hormone (SIADH), which occurs with excessive secretion of ADH. Diabetes insipidus can be treated pharmacologically (see Critical Thinking Scenario 35-1).

Diabetes insipidus is characterized by the production of a large amount of dilute urine containing no glucose. Blood glucose levels are higher than normal, and the body responds with polyuria (lots of urine), polydipsia (lots of thirst), and dehydration. With this rare metabolic disorder, patients produce large quantities of dilute urine and are constantly thirsty. Diabetes insipidus is caused by a deficiency in the amount of posterior pituitary ADH and may result from pituitary disease or injury (e.g., head trauma, surgery, tumor). The condition can be acute and short in duration, or it can be a chronic, lifelong problem.

ADH itself is never used as therapy for diabetes insipidus. Instead, synthetic preparations of ADH, which are purer and have fewer adverse effects, are used. The ADH preparations that are available include vasopressin (*Pitressin Synthetic*), which is available in parenteral and nasal spray forms (Box 35.5), and desmopressin (*DDAVP*) (see Figure 35.1 and Table 35.4). The drug of choice depends on the individual response to the drug and the patient's ability or willingness to use a particular dosage form.

Therapeutic Actions and Indications

ADH is released in response to increases in plasma osmolarity or decreases in blood volume. It produces its antidiuretic activity in the kidneys, causing the cortical and medullary parts of the collecting duct to become permeable to water, thereby increasing water reabsorption and decreasing urine formation. These activities reduce plasma osmolarity and increase blood volume.

The ADH preparations that are available are indicated for the treatment of neurogenic diabetes insipidus. Desmopressin is also indicated for the treatment of hemophilia A and von Willebrand's disease, and it is used as a nasal spray for the treatment of nocturnal enuresis (bed wetting). Because of vasopressin's actions to increase GI motility, it is also indicated for the prevention and treatment of postoperative abdominal distention and to dispel gas formation before abdominal tests.

Pharmacokinetics

These drugs are rapidly absorbed and metabolized; they are excreted in the liver and kidneys. They should not be used during pregnancy because of the risk of uterine contractions that would harm the fetus. The effects of these drugs during lactation are not clear, so caution should be used with nursing mothers.

Contraindications and Cautions

ADH preparations are contraindicated with any known allergy to the drug or its components or with severe renal dysfunction. Caution should be used with any known vascular disease *because of its effects on vascular smooth muscle;* epilepsy; asthma; and pregnancy or lactation.

Adverse Effects

The adverse effects associated with the use of ADH preparations include water intoxication (drowsiness, lightheadedness, headache, coma, convulsions) related to the shift to water retention; tremor, sweating, vertigo, and headache related to water retention (a "hangover" effect); abdominal cramps, flatulence, nausea, and vomiting related to stimula-

BOX 35.5 FOCUS ON CLINICAL SKILLS

Administering a Nasal Spray

Instruct the patient to sit upright and press a finger over one nostril to close it. Then, with the spray bottle held upright, have the patient place the tip of the bottle about 1.5 cm (½") into the open nostril. A firm squeeze should deliver the drug to the desired mucosal area for absorption. Caution the patient not to use excessive force and not to tip the head back because these actions could result in ineffective administration.

CRITICAL THINKING SCENARIO 35-1

Diabetes Insipidus and Posterior Pituitary Hormones (Vasopressin)

The Situation

B.T. is a 56-year-old teacher with diabetes insipidus. Her condition was eventually regulated on vasopressin nasal spray, one or two sprays per nostril four times a day. B.T. seemed highly interested in her disease and therapy and learned to control her own dosage by symptom control. For several years, her symptoms were well controlled. Then at her last clinical visit, it was noted that she had postnasal ulcerations and nasal rhinitis. She also complained of several gastrointestinal symptoms, including upset stomach, abdominal cramps, and diarrhea.

Critical Thinking

Think about the pathophysiology of diabetes insipidus. What are the effects of vasopressin on the body, and what adverse effects might occur if the drug were being absorbed inappropriately?

Because B.T. has used the drug for so many years, she may have forgotten some of the teaching points about her disease and drug administration. Outline a care plan for B.T. that includes necessary teaching points and takes into consideration her long experience with her disease and her drug therapy. Think about specific warning signs that should be highlighted for B.T. and ways to involve her in the teaching program that might make it more pertinent to her and her needs.

Discussion

An essential aspect of the ongoing nursing process is continual evaluation of the effectiveness of the drug therapy. An evaluation of this situation shows that B.T.'s postnasal mucosa was ulcerated, possibly as a result of overexposure to the vasoconstrictive properties of the drug. B.T.'s gastrointestinal tract also seemed to show evidence of increased antidiuretic hormone effects. These factors suggest that perhaps the drug was being administered incorrectly, resulting in excessive exposure of the nasal mucosa to the drug, increased absorption, and increased levels of the drug reaching the systemic circulation.

The nurse should watch B.T. administer a dose of the drug to herself, then discuss the signs and symptoms of problems that B.T. should watch for. In this case, B.T. remembered most of the details of her drug teaching. But when administering the drug, she tilted her head back, tipped the bottle upside down, and then squirted the drug into each nostril. When the nurse questioned B.T. about her technique, she explained that she had seen an advertisement on TV about nasal sprays and realized that she had been doing it wrong all these years. The nurse explained the difference in the types of nasal sprays and reviewed the entire teaching plan with B.T. The drug was discontinued and B.T. was placed on subcutaneous antidiuretic hormone until the nasal ulcerations healed. As a patient becomes more familiar with drug therapy, the details about the drug may be forgotten.

It is important to remember that patient teaching needs regular updating and evaluation. This point is often forgotten when dealing with patients who have been taking a drug for years. However, remembering to assess the patient's knowledge about the drug can prevent problems such as B.T.'s from developing. Because B.T. is a teacher, she might be interested in developing a teaching protocol that will meet her needs and serve as an appropriate reminder about the disease and drug therapy. If B.T. is actively involved in preparing such a plan, it will be more effective and might be remembered much longer.

Nursing Care Guide for B.T.: Diabetes Insipidus and Posterior Pituitary Hormones

Assessment: history and examination

Assess for allergies to any anticholinergic agent and other drugs. Also assess for a history of COPD, narrow-angle glaucoma, myasthenia gravis, bowel or urinary obstruction, pregnancy or lactation, tachycardia, recent GI or urinary tract surgery.

Focus the physical assessment on the following:

CV: Blood pressure, pulse rate, peripheral perfusion, ECG

CNS: orientation, affect, reflexes, vision

Skin: color, lesions, texture, sweating

GU: urinary output, bladder tone

GI: abdominal examination

Respiratory: respiratory rate, adventitious sounds

Nursing diagnoses

Decreased Cardiac Output related to CV effects

Acute Pain related to GI, GU, CNS, CV effects

(continued)

Diabetes Insipidus and Posterior Pituitary Hormones (Vasopressin) *(continued)*

Constipation related to GI effects

Deficient Knowledge regarding drug therapy

Noncompliance related to adverse effects

Implementation

Ensure safe and appropriate administration of drug.

Provide comfort and safety measures, such as physical assistance or raised siderails if B.T. is hospitalized; temperature control; dark eyeglasses; small, frequent meals; artificial saliva, fluids; sugarless lozenges, mouth care; and bowel program.

Provide support and reassurance to deal with drug effects, discomfort, and GI effects.

Teach patient about drug therapy, including drug name, dosage, adverse effects, precautions, and warning signs of serious adverse effects to report.

Monitor blood pressure and pulse rate and adjust dosage as needed.

Evaluation

Evaluate drug effects, including decrease in signs and symptoms being treated.

Monitor for adverse effects: CV effects—tachycardia, heart failure; CNS—confusion, dreams; urinary retention; GI effects—constipation; visual blurring, photophobia.

Monitor for drug–drug interactions as indicated for each drug.

Evaluate effectiveness of patient teaching program and comfort and safety measures.

Patient Teaching for B.T.

☐ The anterior pituitary hormone vasopressin or antidiuretic hormone acts to promote the resorption of water in your kidneys, replacing the antidiuretic hormone that you are missing in your body. This lack of antidiuretic hormone is the cause of your diabetes insipidus. This drug will replace the missing hormone. This drug also causes your blood vessels to contract and may increase the activity of your GI tract. Some of the following adverse effects may occur:

- *Tremor, dizziness, vision changes:* If these occur, you should avoid driving a car or operating dangerous machinery, or performing any other tasks that require alertness.
- *GI cramping, passing of gas:* Eating small, frequent meals may help.
- *Nasal irritation, development of lesions:* Proper administration of the drug will decrease this effect.

☐ Use caution to administer the nasal solution correctly. Sit upright and press a finger over one nostril to close it. Hold the spray bottle upright and place the tip of the bottle about a ½" into the open nostril. A firm squeeze on the bottle will deliver the drug. Do not use excessive force when squeezing the bottle. Do not tip your head back during administration.

☐ Tell any doctor, nurse, or other health care provider involved in your care that you are taking this drug.

☐ Watch for any signs of water intoxication (drowsiness, light-headedness, headache, seizures, coma) and report this to your health care provider immediately.

☐ Report any nasal pain or runny nose, which might indicate that you are not administering the drug correctly.

☐ Keep this drug, and all medications, out of the reach of children. Do not share this drug with other people.

tion of GI motility; and local nasal irritation related to nasal administration. Hypersensitivity reactions have also been reported, ranging from rash to bronchial constriction.

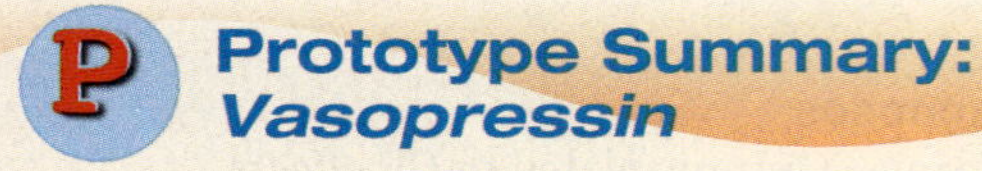

Prototype Summary: Vasopressin

Indications: Treatment of diabetes insipidus, prevention and treatment of postoperative abdominal distention, to dispel gas interfering with abdominal roentgenography

Actions: Has pressor and antidiuretic effects; increases GI motility

Pharmacokinetics:

Route	Onset	Peak	Duration
IM, Sub-Q	Varies	Unknown	2–8 h

$T_{1/2}$: 10–20 min; metabolized in the liver and excreted in the urine

Table 35.4 DRUGS IN FOCUS

Posterior Pituitary Hormones

Drug Name	Dosage/Route	Usual Indications
desmopressin (*DDAVP Stimate*)	Adult: 0.1–0.4 mL/day PO, IV, Sub-Q, intranasal for diabetes insipidus; 0.3 mcg/kg IV over 15–30 min for von Willebrand's disease; 20 mcg intranasal at bedtime for nocturnal enuresis Pediatric: 0.05–0.3 mL/day intranasal for diabetes insipidus; 0.3 mcg/kg IV over 15–30 min for von Willebrand's disease; 20 mcg intranasal at bedtime for nocturnal enuresis	Diabetes insipidus, von Willebrand's disease, hemophilia A, treatment of nocturnal enuresis
P vasopressin (*Pitressin Synthetic*)	5–10 International Units IM or Sub-Q b.i.d. to t.i.d. or administer on cotton pledgets by nasal spray or dropper	Diabetes insipidus, prevention of postoperative abdominal distention, to dispel gas for abdominal examination

Adverse effects: Tremor, sweating, vertigo, abdominal cramps, hypersensitivity reactions, water intoxication (drowsiness, light-headedness, headache, coma, convulsions)

Nursing Considerations for Patients Receiving Posterior Pituitary Hormones

Assessment: History and Examination

Screen for the following conditions, *which could be cautions or contraindications to use of the drug:* history of allergy to any ADH preparation or components; vascular diseases; epilepsy; renal dysfunction; pregnancy; and lactation.

Include screening *for baseline status before beginning therapy and for any potential adverse effects:* skin and lesions; orientation, affect, and reflexes; blood pressure and pulse; respiration and adventitious sounds; abdominal examination; renal function tests; and serum electrolytes.

Nursing Diagnoses

The patient receiving any posterior pituitary hormone may have the following nursing diagnoses related to drug therapy:

- Impaired Urinary Elimination
- Excess Fluid Volume related to water retention
- Deficient Knowledge regarding drug therapy

Implementation With Rationale

- Monitor patient fluid volume *to watch for signs of water intoxication and fluid excess;* arrange to decrease dosage as needed.
- Monitor patients with vascular disease for any sign of exacerbation *to provide for immediate treatment.*
- Monitor condition of nasal passages if given intranasally *to observe for nasal ulceration, which can occur and could affect absorption of the drug.*
- Provide thorough patient teaching, including measures to avoid adverse effects, warning signs of problems, and the need for regular evaluation, including blood tests, *to enhance patient knowledge about drug therapy and promote compliance.*

Evaluation

- Monitor patient response to the drug (maintenance of fluid balance).
- Monitor for adverse effects (GI problems, water intoxication, headache, skin rash).
- Evaluate the effectiveness of the teaching plan (patient can name drug, dosage, adverse effects to watch for, and specific measures to avoid adverse effects; patient can demonstrate proper administration of nasal preparations).
- Monitor the effectiveness of comfort measures and compliance with the regimen.

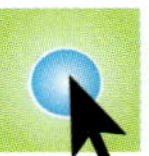

WEB LINKS

Patients and health care providers may want to consult the following Internet sources:

http://www.pens.org Information on GH therapy, pediatric challenges, and research—the Pediatric Endocrinology Nursing Society.

http://www.nih.gov Information on disease research and development, the latest drug therapy, and links to other resources—National Institutes of Health.

Points to Remember

- Hypothalamic releasing factors stimulate the anterior pituitary to release hormones.
- The hypothalamic releasing factors are used mostly for diagnostic testing and for treating some forms of cancer.
- Anterior pituitary hormones stimulate endocrine glands or cell metabolisms.
- Growth hormone (GH) deficiency can cause dwarfism in children and somatropin deficiency syndrome in adults.
- GH replacement is done with drugs produced by recombinant DNA processes; these agents are more reliable and cause fewer problems than drugs used in the past.
- GH excess causes gigantism in patients whose epiphyseal plates have not closed and acromegaly in patients with closed epiphyseal plates.
- GH antagonists include octreotide and bromocriptine. Blockage of other endocrine activity may occur when these drugs are used.
- Posterior pituitary hormones are produced in the hypothalamus and stored in the posterior pituitary. They include oxytocin and antidiuretic hormone (ADH).
- Lack of antidiuretic hormone produces diabetes insipidus, which is characterized by large amounts of dilute urine and excessive thirst.
- ADH replacement uses analogs of ADH and can be administered parenterally or intranasally.
- Fluid balance needs to be monitored when patients are taking ADH replacement drugs because water intoxication and dilution of essential electrolytes can occur.

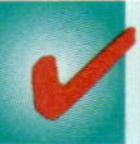

CHECK YOUR UNDERSTANDING

Answers to the questions in this chapter may be found in the Answer Key in the back of the book.

Multiple Choice

Select the best answer to the following.

1. Hypothalamic hormones are normally present in very small amounts. When used therapeutically, their main indication is
   a. diagnosis of endocrine disorders and treatment of specific cancers.
   b. treatment of multiple endocrine disorders.
   c. treatment of CNS-related abnormalities.
   d. treatment of autoimmune-related problems.

2. Somatropin (*Nutropin* and others) is a genetically engineered growth hormone that is used
   a. to diagnose hypothalamic failure.
   b. to treat precocious puberty.
   c. in the treatment of children with growth failure.
   d. to stimulate pituitary response.

3. Growth hormone deficiencies
   a. occur only in children.
   b. always result in dwarfism.
   c. are treated only in children because GH is usually produced only until puberty.
   d. can occur in adults as well as children.

4. Patients who are receiving growth hormone replacement therapy must be monitored very closely. Routine follow-up examinations would include
   a. a bowel program to deal with constipation.
   b. tests of thyroid function and glucose tolerance.
   c. a calorie check to control weight gain.
   d. tests of adrenal hormone levels.

5. Acromegaly and gigantism are both conditions related to excessive secretion of
   a. thyroid hormone.
   b. melanin-stimulating hormone.
   c. growth hormone.
   d. oxytocin.

6. Diabetes insipidus is a relatively rare disease characterized by
   a. excessive secretion of ADH.
   b. renal damage.
   c. the production of large amounts of dilute urine containing no glucose.
   d. insufficient pancreatic activity.

7. Treatment with ADH preparations is associated with adverse effects including
   a. constipation and paralytic ileus.
   b. cholecystitis and bile obstruction.
   c. nocturia and bed wetting.
   d. "hangover" symptoms, including headache, sweating, and tremors.

8. A patient who is receiving an ADH preparation for diabetes insipidus may need instruction in administering the drug
   a. orally or intramuscularly.
   b. orally or intranasally.

c. rectally or orally.
d. intranasally or by dermal patch.

Multiple Response

Select all that apply.

1. Octreotide (*Sandostatin*) would be the drug of choice in the treatment of acromegaly in a client with which of the following conditions?
   a. Diabetes
   b. Gallbladder disease
   c. Adrenal insufficiency
   d. Hypothalamic lesions
   e. Intolerance to other therapies
   f. Acromegaly in a client over the age of 18 years

2. A father brought his 15-year-old son to the endocrine clinic because the boy was only 5 feet tall. He wanted his son to receive growth hormone therapy because short stature would be a real detriment to his success as an adult. The boy would be considered for this therapy if under which of the following circumstances?
   a. If he were against the use of cadaver parts
   b. If his epiphyses were closed
   c. If his GH levels were very low
   d. If he were also diabetic
   e. If he had chronic renal failure
   f. If he had hypothyroidism

Web Exercise

You have been asked to give an inservice presentation to the staff of the pediatric endocrine unit where you are doing your current rotation. The topic is the use of growth hormone for treatment of Turner's syndrome and small stature. You want to ensure that your information is current because this presentation represents 25% of your grade. Go to the Internet to research current information.

Matching

Match the drug with its usual indication.

1. ______________________ CRF
2. ______________________ nafarelin
3. ______________________ cosyntropin
4. ______________________ pegvisomant
5. ______________________ goserelin
6. ______________________ histrelin
7. ______________________ leuprolide
8. ______________________ menotropins

A. Treatment of acromegaly
B. Treatment of specific cancers, endometriosis
C. Diagnosis of Cushing's disease
D. Treatment of prostatic cancers
E. Treatment of precocious puberty, endometriosis
F. Stimulation of ovulation and spermatogenesis
G. Diagnosis of adrenal failure
H. Treatment of precocious puberty

Bibliography and References

Andrews, M., & Boyle, J. (2002). *Transcultural concepts in nursing care.* Philadelphia: Lippincott Williams & Wilkins.

Drug facts and comparisons. (2006). St. Louis: Facts and Comparisons.

Gilman, A., Hardman, J. G., & Limbird, L. E. (Eds.). (2006). *Goodman and Gilman's the pharmacological basis of therapeutics* (11th ed.). New York: McGraw-Hill.

Girard, J. (1991). *Endocrinology of puberty.* Farmington, CT: Karger.

Guyton, A., & Hall, J. (2000). *Textbook of medical physiology.* Philadelphia: W. B. Saunders.

Karch, A. M. (2006). *2007 Lippincott's nursing drug guide.* Philadelphia: Lippincott Williams & Wilkins.

The medical letter on drugs and therapeutics. (2006). New Rochelle, NY: Medical Letter.

North, W. G., Moses, A. M., & Shafe, L. (Eds.). (1993). The neurohypophysis: A window on brain function. Proceedings of the 5th International Conference on Neurohypophysis, Hanover, New Hampshire, July 16–20, 1992. *Annals of the New York Academy of Sciences, 689,* 1–706.

Porth, C. (2005). *Pathophysiology: Concepts of altered health states* (7th ed.). Philadelphia: Lippincott Williams & Wilkins.

CHAPTER 36

Adrenocortical Agents

KEY TERMS

adrenal cortex
adrenal medulla
corticosteroids
diurnal rhythm
glucocorticoids
mineralocorticoids

LEARNING OBJECTIVES

Upon completion of this chapter, you will be able to:

1. Explain the control of the synthesis and secretion of the adrenocortical hormones and the physiological effects of these hormones.
2. Describe the therapeutic actions, indications, pharmacokinetics, contraindications, most common adverse reactions, and important drug–drug interactions associated with the adrenocortical agents.
3. Discuss the use of adrenocortical agents across the lifespan.
4. Compare and contrast the prototype drugs prednisone and fludrocortisone with other adrenocortical agents.
5. Outline the nursing considerations, including important teaching points, for patients receiving an adrenocortical agent.

GLUCOCORTICOIDS

beclomethasone
betamethasone
budesonide
cortisone
dexamethasone
flunisolide
hydrocortisone
methylprednisolone
prednisolone
P prednisone
triamcinolone

MINERALOCORTICOIDS

cortisone
P fludrocortisone
hydrocortisone

Adrenocortical agents are widely used to suppress the immune system and actually help people to feel better. These drugs do not, however, cure any inflammatory disorders. Once widely used to treat a number of chronic problems, adrenocortical agents are now reserved for short-term use to relieve inflammation during acute stages of illness.

The Adrenal Glands

The two adrenal glands are flattened bodies that sit on top of each kidney. Each gland is made up of an inner core called the **adrenal medulla** and an outer shell called the **adrenal cortex**.

The adrenal medulla is actually part of the sympathetic nervous system (SNS). It is a ganglion of neurons that releases the neurotransmitters norepinephrine and epinephrine into circulation when the SNS is stimulated. The secretion of these neurotransmitters directly into the bloodstream allows them to act as hormones, traveling from the adrenal medulla to react with specific receptor sites throughout the body. This is thought to be a backup system for the sympathetic system, adding an extra stimulus to the fight-or-flight response.

The adrenal cortex surrounds the medulla and consists of three layers of cells, each of which synthesizes chemically different types of steroid hormones that exert physiological effects throughout the body. The adrenal cortex produces hormones called **corticosteroids**. There are three types of corticosteroids: androgens, glucocorticoids, and mineralocorticoids. Box 36.1 discusses their use in different age groups.

Androgens (male and female sex hormones) actually have little effect compared with the sex hormones produced by the testes and ovaries. They are able to maintain a certain level of cellular stimulation and can contribute to cell-sensitive growth in some forms of cancers, particularly prostate, breast, and ovarian cancers. These drugs are addressed in Part VII: Drugs Acting on the Reproductive System.

Glucocorticoids are so named because they stimulate an increase in glucose levels for energy. They also increase the rate of protein breakdown and decrease the rate of protein formation from amino acids, another way of preserving energy. Glucocorticoids also cause lipogenesis, or the formation and storage of fat in the body. This stored fat will then be available to be broken down for energy when needed.

Mineralocorticoids affect electrolyte levels and homeostasis. These steroid hormones, such as aldosterone, directly affect the levels of electrolytes in the system. Potassium is lost

BOX 36.1 **Drug Therapy Across the Lifespan**

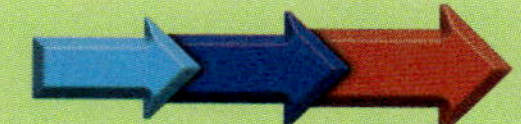

Corticosteroids

CHILDREN

Corticosteroids are used in children for the same indications as in adults. The dosage for children is determined by the severity of the condition being treated and the response to the drug, not on a weight or age formula.

Children need to be monitored closely for any effects on growth and development, and dosage adjustments should be made or drug discontinued if growth is severely retarded.

Topical use of corticosteroids should be limited in children; because their body surface area is comparatively large, the amount of the drug absorbed in relation to weight is greater than in an adult. Apply sparingly and do not use in the presence of open lesions. Do not occlude treated areas with dressings or diapers, which may increase the risk of systemic absorption.

Children need to be supervised when using nasal sprays or respiratory inhalants to ensure that proper technique is being used.

Children receiving long-term therapy should be protected from exposure to infection, and special precautions should be instituted to avoid injury. If injuries or infections do occur, the child should be seen by a primary care provider as soon as possible.

ADULTS

Adults should be reminded of the importance of taking these drugs in the morning, to approximate diurnal rhythm.

They should also be cautioned about the importance of tapering the drug, rather than stopping abruptly.

Several over-the-counter topical preparations contain corticosteroids, and adults should be cautioned to avoid combining these preparations with prescription topical corticosteroids. They also should be cautioned to apply any of these sparingly and to avoid applying them to open lesions or excoriated areas.

With long-term therapy, the importance of avoiding exposure to infection—crowded areas, people with colds or the flu, activities associated with injury—should be stressed. If an injury or infection should occur, the patient should be encouraged to seek medical care. Monitoring blood glucose levels should be done regularly.

These drugs should not be used during pregnancy because they cross the placenta and could cause adverse effects on the fetus. If the benefit to the mother clearly outweighs the potential risk to the fetus, they should be used with caution. Nursing mothers should find another method of feeding the baby if corticosteroids are needed, because of the potential for serious adverse effects on the baby.

OLDER ADULTS

Older adults are more likely to experience the adverse effects associated with these drugs, and the dosage should be reduced and the patient monitored very closely. Older adults are more likely to have hepatic and/or renal impairment, which could lead to accumulation of drug and resultant toxic effects. They are also more likely to have medical conditions that could be imbalanced by changes in fluid and electrolytes, metabolism changes, and other drug effects. Such conditions include diabetes, congestive heart failure, osteoporosis, coronary artery disease, and immune suppression. Careful monitoring of drug dosage and response to the drug should be done on a regular basis.

and sodium and water are retained in response to aldosterone. Hydrocortisone and cortisone also have the same effects when present in high levels.

Figure 36.1 displays the sites of action of the glucocorticoids and the mineralocorticoids.

Controls

The adrenal cortex responds to adrenocorticotropic hormone (ACTH) released from the anterior pituitary. ACTH, in turn, responds to corticotropin-releasing hormone (CRH) released from the hypothalamus. This happens regularly during a normal day in what is called **diurnal rhythm** (Box 36.2). A person who has a regular cycle of sleep and wakefulness will produce high levels of CRH during sleep, usually around midnight. A resulting peak response of increased ACTH and adrenocortical hormones occurs sometime early in the morning, around 6 to 9 AM. This high level of hormones then suppresses any further CRH or ACTH release. The corticosteroids are metabolized and excreted slowly throughout the day and fall to low levels by evening. At this point, the hypothalamus and pituitary sense low levels of the hormones and begin the production and release of CRH and ACTH again. This peaks around midnight, and the cycle starts again.

Activation of the stress reaction through the SNS bypasses the usual diurnal rhythm and causes release of ACTH and secretion of the adrenocortical hormones—an important aspect of the stress ("fight-or-flight") response. The stress response is activated with cellular injury or when a person perceives fear or feels anxious. These hormones have many actions, including the following:

- Increasing the blood volume (aldosterone effect)
- Causing the release of glucose for energy
- Slowing the rate of protein production (which reserves energy)
- Blocking the activities of the inflammatory and immune systems (which reserves a great deal of energy)

These actions are important during an acute stress situation, but they can cause adverse reactions in periods of extreme or prolonged stress. For instance, a postoperative patient who is very fearful and stressed may not heal well because protein building is blocked; infections may be hard to treat in such a patient because the inflammatory and immune systems are not functioning adequately.

Aldosterone is also released without ACTH stimulation when the blood surrounding the adrenal gland is high in potassium because high potassium is a direct stimulus for aldosterone release. Aldosterone causes the kidneys to excrete potassium in order to restore homeostasis.

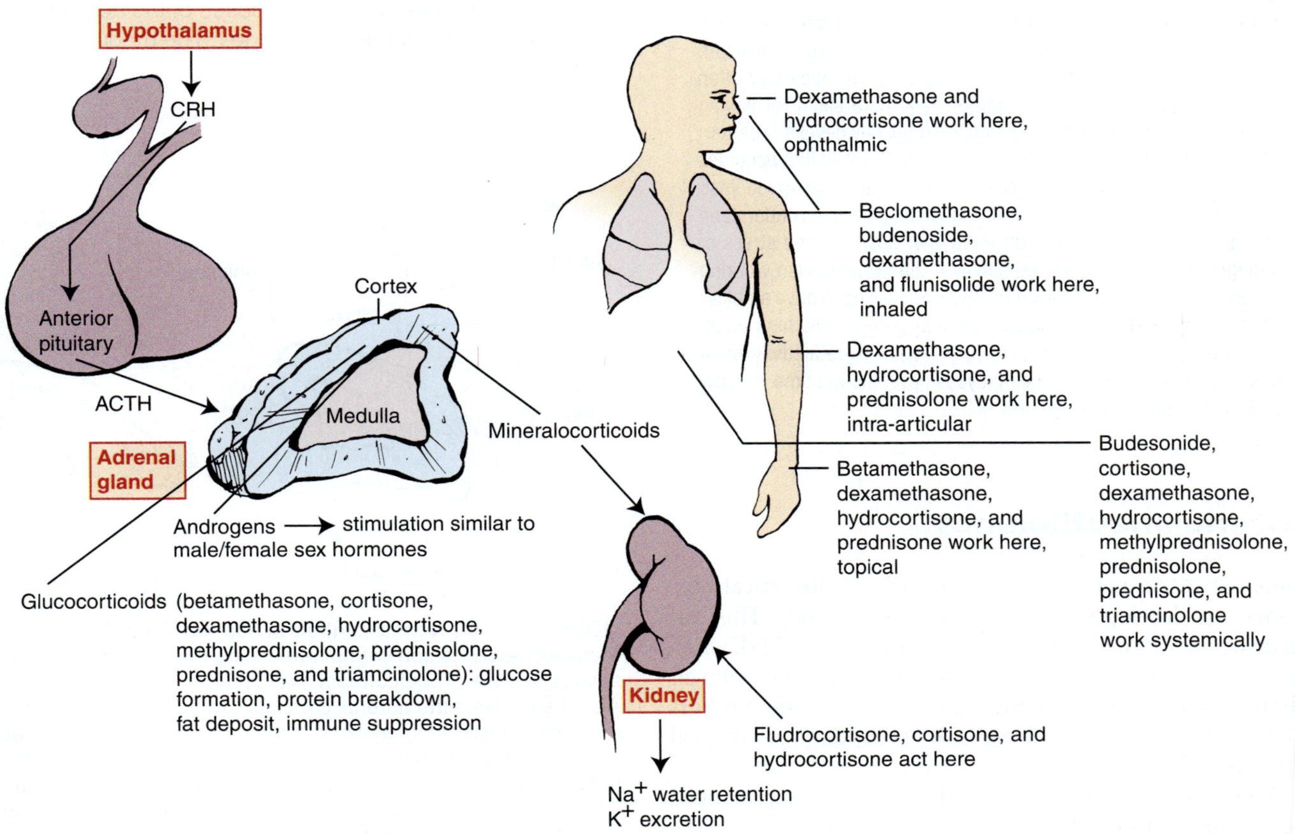

FIGURE 36.1 Sites of action of the adrenocortical agents.

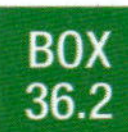

BOX 36.2 FOCUS ON THE **EVIDENCE**

Diurnal Rhythm

Research over the years shows that the adrenocortical hormones are released in a pattern called the diurnal rhythm. The secretion of corticotropin-releasing hormone (CRH), adrenocorticotropic hormone (ACTH), and cortisol are high in the morning in day-oriented people (those who have a regular cycle of wakefulness during the day and sleep during the night). In such individuals, the peak levels of cortisol usually come between 6 and 8 am. The levels then fall off slowly (with periodic spurts) and reach a low in the late evening, with lowest levels around midnight. It is thought that this cycle is related to the effects of sleeping on the hypothalamus, and that the hypothalamus is regulating its stimulation of the anterior pituitary in relation to sleep and activity. The cycle may also be connected to the hypothalamic response to light. This is important to keep in mind when treating patients with corticosteroids. In order to mimic the normal diurnal pattern, corticosteroids should be taken immediately on awakening in the morning.

Complications to this pattern arise, however, when patients work shifts or change their sleeping patterns (e.g., college students). In response, the hypothalamus shifts its release of CRH to correspond to the new cycle. For instance, if a person works all night and goes to bed at 8 AM, arising at 3 PM to carry on the day's activities before going to work at 11 PM, the hypothalamus will release CRH at about 3 PM in accordance with the new sleep–wake cycle. It usually takes 2 or 3 days for the hypothalamus to readjust. A patient on this schedule who is taking replacement corticosteroids would then need to take them at 3 PM, or on arising. Patients who work several different shifts in a single week may not have time to reregulate their hypothalamus, and the corticosteroid cycle may be thrown off. Patients who have to change their sleep patterns repeatedly often complain about feeling weak, getting sick more easily, or having trouble concentrating. College students frequently develop a pattern of sleeping all day, then staying up all night—a cycle that becomes hard to break as their bodies and endocrine systems try to readjust.

In nursing practice, it is a challenge to help patients understand how the body works and to offer ways to decrease the stress of changing sleep patterns—especially if the nurse is also working several different shifts. Many employers are willing to have employees work several days of the same shift before switching back, mainly because they have noticed an increase in productivity and a decrease in absences when employees have enough time to allow their bodies to adjust to the new shift.

Adrenal Insufficiency

Some patients experience a shortage of adrenocortical hormones and develop signs of adrenal insufficiency. This can occur when a patient does not produce enough ACTH, when the adrenal glands are not able to respond to ACTH, when an adrenal gland is damaged and cannot produce enough hormones (as in Addison's disease), or secondary to surgical removal of the glands.

A more common cause of adrenal insufficiency is prolonged use of corticosteroid hormones. When exogenous corticosteroids are used, they act to negate the regular feedback systems (Figure 36.2). The adrenal glands begin to atrophy because ACTH release is suppressed by the exogenous hormones, so the glands are no longer stimulated to produce or secrete hormones. It takes several weeks to recover from the atrophy caused by this lack of stimulation. To prevent this from happening, patients should receive only short-term steroid therapy and should be weaned slowly from the hormones so that the adrenals have time to recover and start producing hormones again.

Adrenal Crisis

Patients who have an adrenal insufficiency may do quite well until they experience a period of extreme stress, such as a motor vehicle accident, a surgical procedure, or a massive infection. Because they are not able to supplement the energy-consuming effects of the sympathetic reaction, they enter an adrenal crisis, which can include physiological exhaustion, hypotension, fluid shift, shock, and even death. Patients in adrenal crisis are treated with massive infusion of replacement steroids, constant monitoring, and life support procedures.

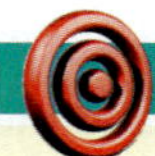

FOCUS POINTS

- There are two adrenal glands, one on top of each kidney.
- Each adrenal gland is composed of the adrenal medulla and the adrenal cortex. The medulla

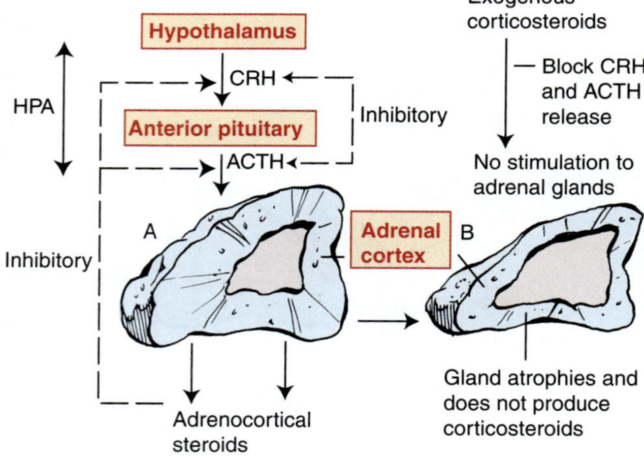

FIGURE 36.2 **(A)** Normal controls of adrenal gland. The hypothalamus releases corticotropin-releasing hormone (CRH), which causes release of corticotropin (ACTH) from the anterior pituitary. ACTH stimulates the adrenal cortex to produce and release corticosteroids. Increasing levels of corticosteroids inhibit the release of CRH and ACTH. **(B)** Exogenous corticosteroids act to inhibit CRH and ACTH release; the adrenal cortex is no longer stimulated and atrophies. Sudden stopping of steroids results in a crisis of adrenal hypofunction until hypothalamic–pituitary axis (HPA) controls stimulate the adrenal gland again.

releases norepinephrine and epinephrine into the bloodstream, and the cortex produces three types of hormones: androgens (male and female sex hormones), glucocorticoids, and mineralocorticoids.

- Corticosteroids help the body conserve energy for the fight-or-flight response.
- Prolonged use of corticosteroids suppresses the normal hypothalamic–pituitary axis and leads to adrenal atrophy from lack of stimulation.

Glucocorticoids

Several glucocorticoids are available for pharmacological use (Table 36.1). They differ mainly by route of administration and duration of action.

Beclomethasone (*Beclovent*) is available as a respiratory inhalant and nasal spray to block inflammation locally in the respiratory tract.

Betamethasone (*Celestone* and others) is a long-acting steroid. It is available for systemic, parenteral use in acute situations. It also is available orally for short-term relief of inflammation and as a topical application for local inflammatory conditions.

Budesonide (*Rhinocort, Entocort EC*) is a relatively new steroid for intranasal use. It relieves the signs and symptoms of allergic or seasonal rhinitis with few side effects. It was approved in 2001 as an oral agent for the treatment of mild-to-moderate active Crohn's disease.

Cortisone (*Cortone Acetate*) was one of the first corticosteroids made available. It is used orally and parenterally for replacement therapy in adrenal insufficiency, as well as acute inflammatory situations.

Dexamethasone (*Decadron* and others) is widely used and available in multiple forms for dermatological, ophthalmological, intra-articular, parenteral, and inhalational uses. It peaks quickly, and effects can last for 2 to 3 days.

Flunisolide (*AeroBid, Nasalide*) is another drug that has proved to be very successful as a respiratory inhalant or intranasal drug.

Hydrocortisone (*Cortef* and others) is a powerful corticosteroid that has both glucocorticoid and mineralocorticoid activity. For that reason, it is used as replacement therapy in patients with adrenal insufficiency. It has largely been replaced for other uses (e.g., intra-articular, intravenous) by other steroid hormones with less mineralocorticoid effect. It may be preferred for use as a topical or ophthalmic agent.

Methylprednisolone (*Medrol*) has little mineralocorticoid activity at therapeutic doses. Because it has significant anti-inflammatory and immunosuppressive effects, it is a drug of choice for inflammatory and immune disorders and is available in multiple forms, including oral, parenteral, intra-articular, and retention enema preparations. (See Box 36.3.)

Prednisolone (*Delta-Cortef* and others) is an intermediate-acting corticosteroid with effects lasting only a day or so. It is used for intralesional and intra-articular injection and is also available in oral and topical forms.

Prednisone (*Deltasone* and others) is available only as an oral agent and can be used as replacement therapy in cases of adrenal insufficiency. It is also used for short-term and acute therapy to decrease inflammation.

Triamcinolone (*Aristocort, Kenaject,* and others) is available in many forms for use in acute inflammatory conditions. It has been used to treat adrenal insufficiency when combined with a mineralocorticoid.

Therapeutic Actions and Indications

Glucocorticoids enter target cells and bind to cytoplasmic receptors, initiating many complex reactions that are responsible for anti-inflammatory and immunosuppressive effects. Hydrocortisone, cortisone, and prednisone also have some mineralocorticoid activity and affect potassium, sodium, and water levels in the body (Table 36.2).

Glucocorticoids are indicated for the short-term treatment of many inflammatory disorders, to relieve discomfort, and to give the body a chance to heal from the effects of inflammation. They block the actions of arachidonic acid, which leads to a decrease in the formation of prostaglandins and leukotrienes. Without these chemicals, the normal inflammatory reaction is blocked. They also impair the ability of phagocytes to leave the bloodstream and move to injured tissues, and they inhibit the ability of lymphocytes to act within the immune system, including a blocking of the production of antibodies. They can be used to treat local inflammation as topical agents, intranasal or inhaled agents, intra-articular injections, and ophthalmic agents. Systemic use is indicated for the treatment of some cancers, hypercalcemia associated with cancer, hematological disorders, and some neurological infections. When combined with mineralocorticoids, some of these drugs can be used in replacement therapy for adrenal insufficiency.

Pharmacokinetics

These drugs are absorbed well from many sites. They are metabolized by natural systems, mostly within the liver, and are excreted in the urine. The glucocorticoids are known to cross the placenta and to enter breast milk; they should be used during pregnancy and lactation only if the benefits to the mother clearly outweigh the potential risks to the fetus or neonate.

Contraindications and Cautions

These drugs are contraindicated in the presence of any known allergy to any steroid preparation; in the presence

Table 36.1 DRUGS IN FOCUS

Glucocorticoids

Drug Name	Dosage/Route	Usual Indications
beclomethasone (*Beclovent*)	Nasal spray, respiratory inhalant Adult: two inhalations (84–168 mcg) t.i.d. to q.i.d. for respiratory inhalant; one inhalation (42–84 mcg) in each nostril b.i.d. to q.i.d. for nasal spray Pediatric (6–12 yr): one or two inhalations t.i.d. to q.i.d. for respiratory inhalant Pediatric (>12 yr): one inhalation in each nostril b.i.d. to q.i.d. for nasal spray	Blocking inflammation in the respiratory tract
betamethasone (*Celestone*)	Oral, IM, IV intra-articular, topical Adult: 0.6–7.2 mg/day PO; up to 9 mg/day IV; 0.5–9.0 mg/day IM; apply topical preparation sparingly Pediatric: individualize dose based on severity and response, and monitor closely	Management of allergic intra-articular, topical, and inflammatory disorders
budesonide (*Rhinocort, Entocort EC*)	Intranasal—Adult and children >6 yr: 256 mcg/day given as two sprays in each nostril AM and PM	Relief of symptoms of seasonal and allergic rhinitis
cortisone (*Cortisone Acetate*)	Oral, IM Adult: 25–300 mg/day PO; 20–330 mg IM Pediatric: base dosage on response, monitor patient closely	Replacement therapy in adrenal insufficiency; treatment of allergic and inflammatory disorders
dexamethasone (*Decadron*)	Oral, IV, IM, inhalation, intranasal, ophthalmic, topical Adult and pediatric: individualize dosage based on response and severity—0.75–9 mg/day PO; 8–16 mg/day IM; 0.5–9 mg/day IV; two to three inhalations per day for inhalation; one to two sprays in each nostril b.i.d. for nasal spray; 1 gtt t.i.d. to q.i.d. for ophthalmic solutions; apply topical preparation sparingly	Management of allergic and topical inflammatory disorders, adrenal hypofunction
flunisolide (*Nasalide, AeroBid*)	Inhalant, intranasal Adult: 88–440 mcg intranasal b.i.d Pediatric: 500–600 mcg b.i.d. via diskhaler	Control of bronchial asthma; relief of symptoms of seasonal and allergic rhinitis
hydrocortisone (*Cortef*)	Oral, IV, IM, topical, ophthalmic, rectal, intra-articular Adult: 100–500 mg IM or IV q2–6h; 100 mg half strength by retention enema for 21 days; one applicatorful daily to b.i.d. intrarectal; apply topical sparingly; 5–20 mg/day PO based on response Pediatric: 20–240 mg/day PO, IM or Sub-Q; 100 mg half strength by retention enema for 21 days; one applicatorful daily to b.i.d. intrarectal; apply topical sparingly; 5–20 mg/day PO based on response	Replacement therapy, treatment of allergic and inflammatory disorders
methylprednisolone (*Medrol*)	Oral, IV, IM, intra-articular Adult: 40–120 mg/day PO or IM; 10–40 mg IV slowly Pediatric: base dosage on severity and response	Treatment of allergic and inflammatory disorders
prednisolone (*Delta-Cortef*)	Oral, IV, IM, ophthalmic, intra-articular Adult: 5–60 mg/day PO; 4–60 mg IM or IV; 1–2 gtt in affected eye t.i.d. to q.i.d. Pediatric: base dosage on severity and response	Treatment of allergic and inflammatory disorders
P prednisone (*Deltasone*)	Oral Adult: 0.1–0.15 mg/kg/day PO Pediatric: base dosage on severity and response	Replacement therapy for adrenal insufficiency; treatment of allergic and inflammatory disorders
triamcinolone (*Aristocort*)	Oral, IM, inhalant, intra-articular, topical Adult: 4–60 mg/day PO; 2.5–60 mg/day IM; two inhalations t.i.d. to q.i.d. Pediatric: individualize dosage based on severity and response; 6–12 yr, one to two inhalations t.i.d. to q.i.d.	Treatment of allergic and inflammatory disorders, management of asthma

of an acute infection *which could become serious or even fatal if the immune and inflammatory responses are blocked;* and with lactation *because the anti-inflammatory and immunosuppressive actions could be passed to the baby.*

Caution should be used in patients with diabetes *because the glucose-elevating effects disrupt glucose control;* acute peptic ulcers *because steroid use is associated with the development of ulcers;* other endocrine disorders *which could be sent into imbalance; or pregnancy.*

BOX 36.3 CULTURAL CONSIDERATIONS FOR DRUG THERAPY

Steroid Toxicity in African Americans

African Americans develop increased toxicity to the corticosteroid methylprednisolone—particularly when it is used for immunosuppression after renal transplantation. This toxicity can include severe steroid-induced diabetes mellitus. African Americans are almost four times as likely as whites to develop end-stage renal disease, so this complication is not an unusual problem. If an African American patient is being treated with methylprednisolone, extreme care should be taken to adjust dosages appropriately and to treat adverse effects as they arise.

Adverse Effects

The adverse effects associated with the glucocorticoids are related to the route of administration that is used. Systemic use is associated with endocrine disorders; fluid retention and potential congestive heart failure (CHF); increased appetite and weight gain; fragile skin and loss of hair; weakness and muscle atrophy as protein breakdown occurs and protein is not built; and increased susceptibility to infections and the development of cancers (with long-term use). Children are at risk for growth retardation associated with suppression of the hypothalamic–pituitary system. Local use is associated with local inflammations and infections, as well as burning and stinging sensations (Box 36.4).

Clinically Important Drug–Drug Interactions

Therapeutic and toxic effects increase if corticosteroids are given with erythromycin, ketoconazole, or troleandomycin. Serum levels and effectiveness may decrease if corticosteroids are combined with salicylates, barbiturates, phenytoin, or rifampin.

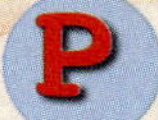

Prototype Summary: Prednisone

Indications: Replacement therapy in adrenal cortical insufficiency, short-term management of various inflammatory and allergic disorders, hypercalcemia associated with cancer, hematological disorders, ulcerative colitis, acute exacerbations of multiple sclerosis, palliation in some leukemias, trichinosis with systemic involvement

Actions: Enters target cells and binds to intracellular corticosteroid receptors, initiating many complex reactions responsible for its anti-inflammatory and immunosuppressive effects

Pharmacokinetics:

Route	Onset	Peak	Duration
PO	Varies	1–2 h	1–1.5 days

$T_{1/2}$: 3.5 hours; metabolized in the liver and excreted in the urine

Adverse effects: Vertigo, headache, hypotension, shock, sodium and fluid retention, amenorrhea, increased appetite, weight gain, immunosuppression, aggravation or masking of infections, impaired wound healing

Table 36.2 Selected Corticosteroids: Equivalent Strength, Glucocorticoid and Mineralocorticoid Effects, and Duration of Effects

Drug	Equivalent Dose (mg)	Glucocorticoid Effects	Mineralocorticoid Effects	Duration of Effects
Short-Acting Corticosteroids				
cortisone	25	+	++++	8–12 h
hydrocortisone	20	+	++++	8–12 h
Intermediate-Acting Corticosteroids				
prednisone	5	++++	++	18–36 h
prednisolone	5	++++	++	18–36 h
triamcinolone	4	+++++	—	18–36 h
methylprednisolone	4	+++++	—	18–36 h
Long-Acting Corticosteroids				
dexamethasone	0.75	+++++++++	—	36–54 h
betamethasone	0.75	+++++++++	—	35–54 h

BOX 36.4 Adverse Effects of Corticosteroid Use Associated With Varying Routes of Administration

Systemic: Systemic effects are most likely to occur when the corticosteroid is given by the oral, intravenous, intramuscular, or subcutaneous route. Systemic absorption is possible, however, if other routes of administration are not used correctly or if tissue breakdown or injury allows direct absorption.

Central nervous system: vertigo, headache, paresthesias, insomnia, convulsions, psychosis

Gastrointestinal: peptic or esophageal ulcers, pancreatitis, abdominal distention, nausea, vomiting, increased appetite, weight gain

Cardiovascular: hypotension, shock, congestive heart failure secondary to fluid retention, thromboembolism, thrombophlebitis, fat embolism, arrhythmias secondary to electrolyte disturbances

Hematological: sodium and fluid retention, hypokalemia, hypocalcemia, increased blood sugar, increased serum cholesterol, decreased thyroid hormone levels

Musculoskeletal: muscle weakness, steroid myopathy, loss of muscle mass, osteoporosis, spontaneous fractures

Eyes, ears, nose, and throat: cataracts, glaucoma

Dermatological: frail skin, petechiae, ecchymoses, purpura, striae, subcutaneous fat atrophy

Endocrine: amenorrhea, irregular menses, growth retardation, decreased carbohydrate tolerance, diabetes

Other: immunosuppression, aggravation or masking of infections, impaired wound healing, suppression of hypothalamic–pituitary axis

Intramuscular repository injections: atrophy at the injection site
Retention enema: local pain, burning; rectal bleeding
Intra-articular injection: osteonecrosis, tendon rupture, infection
Intraspinal: meningitis, adhesive arachnoiditis, conus medullaris syndrome
Intrathecal administration: arachnoiditis
Topical: local burning, irritation, acneiform lesions, striae, skin atrophy
Respiratory inhalant: oral, laryngeal, and pharyngeal irritation; fungal infections
Intranasal: headache, nausea, nasal irritation, fungal infections, epistaxis, rebound congestion, perforation of the nasal septum, anosmia, urticaria
Ophthalmic: infections, glaucoma, cataracts
Intralesional: blindness when used on the face and head (rare)

Nursing Considerations for Patients Receiving Glucocorticoids

Assessment: History and Examination

Screen for the following conditions, *which could be cautions or contraindications to use of the drug:* history of allergy to any steroid preparations, acute infections, peptic ulcer disease, pregnancy, lactation, endocrine disturbances, and renal dysfunction.

Include screening *for baseline status before beginning therapy and for any potential adverse effects:* weight; temperature; orientation and affect; grip strength; eye examination; blood pressure, pulse, peripheral perfusion, and vessel evaluation; respiration and adventitious breath sounds; glucose tolerance, renal function, serum electrolytes, and endocrine function tests as appropriate.

Nursing Diagnoses

The patient receiving any glucocorticoid may have the following nursing diagnoses related to drug therapy:

- Decreased Cardiac Output related to fluid retention
- Excess Fluid Volume related to water retention
- Disturbed Sensory Perception (Visual, Kinesthetic)
- Risk for Infection related to immunosuppression
- Ineffective Coping related to body changes caused by the drug
- Deficient Knowledge regarding drug therapy

Implementation With Rationale

- Administer drug daily at 8 to 9 AM *to mimic normal peak diurnal concentration levels and thereby minimize suppression of the hypothalamic–pituitary axis.*
- Space multiple doses evenly throughout the day *to try to achieve homeostasis.*
- Use minimal dose for minimal amount of time *to minimize adverse effects.*
- Taper doses when discontinuing from high doses or from long-term therapy *to give the adrenal glands a chance to recover and produce adrenocorticoids.*
- Arrange for increased dosage when the patient is under stress *to supply increased demand for corticosteroids associated with the stress reaction.*
- Use alternate-day maintenance therapy with short-acting drugs whenever possible *to decrease the risk of adrenal suppression.*
- Do not give live virus vaccines when the patient is immunosuppressed *because there is an increased risk of infection.*

- Protect the patient from unnecessary exposure to infection and invasive procedures *because the steroids suppress the immune system and the patient is at increased risk for infection.*
- Assess the patient carefully for any potential drug–drug interactions *to avoid adverse effects.*
- Provide thorough patient teaching, including measures to avoid adverse effects; warning signs of problems; and the need for regular evaluation, including blood tests, *to enhance patient knowledge of drug therapy and promote compliance.* Explain the need to protect the patient from exposure to infections *to prevent serious adverse effects.*

Evaluation

- Monitor patient response to the drug (relief of signs and symptoms of inflammation, return of adrenal function to within normal limits).
- Monitor for adverse effects (increased susceptibility to infections, skin changes, endocrine dysfunctions, fatigue, fluid retention, peptic ulcer, psychological changes).
- Evaluate the effectiveness of the teaching plan (patient can name drug, dosage, adverse effects to watch for, specific measures to avoid adverse effects).
- Monitor the effectiveness of comfort measures and compliance with the regimen (see Critical Thinking Scenario 36-1).

Mineralocorticoids

The classic mineralocorticoid is aldosterone. Aldosterone holds sodium—and with it, water—in the body and causes the excretion of potassium by acting on the renal tubule. Aldosterone is no longer available for pharmacological use. When used in high doses, the glucocorticoids cortisone and hydrocortisone have a mineralocorticoid effect. However, this effect usually is not enough to maintain electrolyte balance in adrenal insufficiency.

Fludrocortisone (*Florinef*) is a more powerful mineralocorticoid and is preferred for replacement therapy, in combination with a glucocorticoid. Hydrocortisone and cortisone also exert mineralocorticoid effects at certain doses (Table 36.3).

Therapeutic Actions and Indications

The mineralocorticoids increase sodium reabsorption in renal tubules and increase potassium and hydrogen excretion, leading to water and sodium retention (see Figure 36.1). These drugs are indicated, in combination with a glucocorticoid, for replacement therapy in primary and secondary adrenal insufficiency. They are also indicated for the treatment of salt-wasting adrenogenital syndrome when taken with appropriate glucocorticoids. Fludrocortisone is being tried for the treatment of severe orthostatic hypotension because its sodium and water retention effects can lead to increased blood pressure.

Pharmacokinetics

These drugs are absorbed slowly and distributed throughout the body. They undergo hepatic metabolism to inactive forms. They are known to cross the placenta and to enter breast milk. They should be avoided during pregnancy and lactation because of the potential for adverse effects in the fetus or baby.

Contraindications and Cautions

These drugs are contraindicated in the presence of any known allergy to the drug; with severe hypertension, CHF, or cardiac disease *because of the resultant increased blood pressure;* and with lactation. Caution should be used in pregnancy, in the presence of any infection, and with high sodium intake (*severe hypernatremia could occur*).

Adverse Effects

Adverse effects commonly associated with the use of mineralocorticoids are related to the increased fluid volume seen with sodium and water retention (e.g., headache, edema, hypertension, CHF, arrhythmias, weakness, hypokalemia). Allergic reactions, ranging from skin rash to anaphylaxis, have also been reported.

Clinically Important Drug–Drug Interactions

Decreased effectiveness of salicylates, barbiturates, hydantoins, rifampin, and anticholinesterases has been reported when these drugs are combined with mineralocorticoids. Such combinations should be avoided if possible, but if they are necessary, the patient should be monitored closely and the dosage increased as needed.

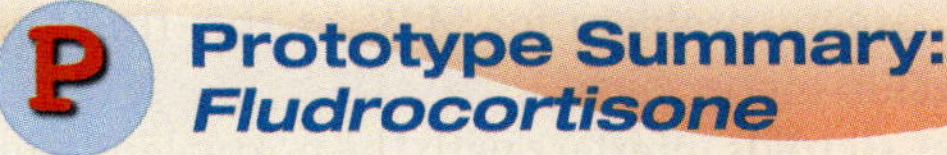

Indications: Partial replacement therapy in cortical insufficiency conditions, treatment of salt-losing adrenogenital syndrome; unlabeled use: treatment of hypotension

(text continues on page 572)

CRITICAL THINKING SCENARIO 36-1

Adrenocorticosteroids

THE SITUATION

M.W., a 48-year-old woman, was diagnosed with severe rheumatoid arthritis 7 years ago. She has been retired, on disability, from her job as an art teacher in the local high school. Her pain is no longer controlled by aspirin, and her physician ordered 5 mg prednisone t.i.d. Over the next 4 weeks, M.W.'s symptoms were markedly relieved; she was able to start painting again, and she became much more mobile. She also noted that for the first time in years she felt "really good." Her appetite increased, she was no longer fatigued, and her outlook on life was markedly improved. At her follow-up visit, M.W. had gained 9 pounds; she had slight edema in both ankles, and her blood pressure was 150/92. An inflamed, oozing lesion was found on her right hand, which she stated became infected a few weeks ago after she cut her hand while peeling potatoes. Her range of motion and joints were markedly improved. The physician decided that M.W. was past her crisis, and the prednisone should be tapered to 5 mg/day over a 4-week period.

CRITICAL THINKING

Think about the pathophysiology of rheumatoid arthritis. What effects did the prednisone have on the process at work in M.W.'s joints?

What effects does the adrenocorticoid steroid have on the rest of M.W.'s body?

What can be expected to occur when a patient is on prednisone for a month?

What precautions should be taken?

What nursing interventions are appropriate for M.W. at this visit?

DISCUSSION

The most urgent problem for M.W. at this time is the infected lesion on her hand.

Because steroids interfere with the normal inflammatory and immune response to infection, the lesion could progress to a very serious problem. The lesion should be cultured, cleansed, and dressed. M.W. should be instructed in how to care for her hand and how to protect it from water or further injury. An antibiotic might be prescribed and then evaluated for its appropriateness when the culture report comes back.

The real nursing challenge with M.W. will be helping her to cope with and understand the need to taper her prednisone. The drug teaching information for prednisone should be thoroughly reviewed with M.W., pointing out the side effects of drug therapy that she is already experiencing and explaining, again, the effect that prednisone has on her body. A calendar should be prepared for M.W. to help her schedule the tapering of the drug. It usually progresses from 5 mg b.i.d. for 2 weeks to 5 mg/day. M.W. will need a great deal of encouragement and support to cope with the decrease in therapeutic benefit caused by the need to reduce the prednisone dosage. She has felt so good and done so much better while receiving the drug that she may have a real dread of losing those benefits. She should be encouraged to discuss her feelings and to call in for support if she needs it. M.W. should be given an appointment for a return visit in 2 weeks to evaluate the lesion on her hand and to check her progress in the tapering of the drug. She should be urged to call if the lesion looks worse to her or if she has any difficulties with her drug therapy.

M.W.'s case is a common example of the clinical problems that are encountered when a patient with a chronic inflammatory condition begins steroid therapy. These patients require strong nursing support and continual teaching.

NURSING CARE GUIDE FOR M.W.: ADRENOCORTICOSTEROIDS

Assessment: History And Examination

Assess for allergies to any steroids and for heart failure, pregnancy, hypertension, acute infection, peptic ulcer, vaccination with a live virus, or endocrine disorders.

Also assess for concurrent use of ketoconazole, troleandomycin, estrogens, barbiturates, phenytoin, rifampin, or salicylates.

Focus the physical examination on the following:

Neurological: orientation, reflexes, affect

General: temperature, weight, site of hand infection

CV: pulse, cardiac auscultation, blood pressure, edema

Respiratory: respiratory rate, adventitious sounds

Adrenocorticosteroids *(continued)*

Laboratory tests: urinalysis, blood glucose level, stool guaiac test, renal function tests, culture and sensitivity of wound specimen

Nursing Diagnoses

Decreased Cardiac Output related to fluid retention

Disturbed Sensory Perception related to CNS effects

Risk for Infection related to immunosuppression

Ineffective Coping related to body changes caused by drug

Excess Fluid Volume related to water retention

Deficient Knowledge regarding drug therapy

Implementation

Administer around 9 AM to mimic normal diurnal rhythm.

Use minimal dose for minimal period of time dosage is needed.

Arrange for increased doses during times of stress.

Taper gradually to allow adrenal glands to recover and produce own steroids.

Protect patient from unnecessary exposure to infection.

Provide support and reassurance to deal with drug therapy.

Provide patient teaching regarding drug name, dosage, adverse effects, precautions, and warning signs to report.

Evaluation

Evaluate drug effects: relief of signs and symptoms of inflammation.

Monitor for adverse effects: infection, peptic ulcer, fluid retention, hypertension, electrolyte imbalance, or endocrine changes.

Monitor for drug–drug interactions as listed.

Evaluate effectiveness of patient teaching program.

Evaluate effectiveness of comfort and safety measures and support offered.

Patient Teaching For M.W.

☐ The drug that has been prescribed for you is called prednisone. Prednisone is from a class of drugs called corticosteroids, which are similar to steroids produced naturally in your body. They affect a number of bodily functions, including your body's glucose levels, blocking your body's inflammatory and immune responses, and slowing the healing process.

☐ You should never stop taking your drug suddenly. If your prescription is low or you are unable to take the medication for any reason, notify your health care provider.

☐ Some of the following adverse effects may occur:

- *Increased appetite:* This may be a welcome change, but if you notice a continual weight gain, you may want to watch your calories.
- *Restlessness, trouble sleeping:* Some people experience elation and a feeling of new energy; frequent rest periods should be taken.
- *Increased susceptibility to infection:* Because your body's normal defenses will be decreased, you should avoid crowded places and people with known infections. If you notice any signs of illness or infection, notify your health care provider at once.
- Report any of the following to your health care provider: *sudden weight gain; fever or sore throat; black, tarry stools; swelling of the hands or feet; any signs of infection; or easy bruising.*

☐ If you are taking this drug for a prolonged period, limit your intake of salt and salted products and add proteins to your diet.

☐ Avoid the use of any over-the-counter medication without first checking with your health care provider. Several of these medications can interfere with the effectiveness of this drug.

☐ Tell any doctor, nurse, or other health care provider involved in your care that you are taking this drug.

☐ Because this drug affects your body's natural defenses, you will need special care during any stressful situations. You may want to wear or carry medical identification showing that you are taking this medication. This identification alerts any medical personnel taking care of you in an emergency to the fact that you are taking this drug.

☐ It is important to have regular medical follow-up. If your drug dosage is being tapered, notify your health care provider if any of the following occur: fatigue, nausea, vomiting, diarrhea, weight loss, weakness, or dizziness.

☐ Keep this drug out of the reach of children. Do not give this medication to anyone else or take any similar medication that has not been prescribed for you.

Table 36.3 DRUGS IN FOCUS

Mineralocorticoids

Drug Name	Dosage/Route	Usual Indications
cortisone (*Cortisone Acetate*)	Oral, IM Adult: 25–300 mg/day PO or 20–330 mg/day IM Pediatric: base dosage on severity and response	Replacement therapy in adrenal insufficiency, treatment of allergic and inflammatory disorders
P fludrocortisone (*Florinef*)	Adult: 0.1–0.2 mg/day PO	Replacement therapy and treatment of salt-losing adrenogenital syndrome with a glucocorticoid; not recommended for children
hydrocortisone (*Cortef*)	Oral, IV, IM, topical, ophthalmic, rectal, intra-articular Adult: 20–240 mg/day PO; 100–500 mg IM or IV q2–6h; 100 mg half-strength by retention enema; one applicatorful rectal foam q.i.d. to b.i.d.; apply topical preparation sparingly Pediatric: base dosage on response and severity; 20–240 mg/day PO; 20–240 mg/day IM or Sub-Q 100 mg half-strength by retention enema; one applicatorful rectal foam q.i.d. to b.i.d.; apply topical preparation sparingly	Replacement therapy, treatment of allergic and inflammatory disorders

Actions: Increases sodium reabsorption in the renal tubules and increases potassium and hydrogen excretion, leading to water and sodium retention

Pharmacokinetics:

Route	Onset	Peak	Duration
PO	Gradual	1.7 h	18–36 h

$T_{1/2}$: 3.5 hours; metabolized in the liver and excreted in the urine

Adverse effects: Frontal and occipital headaches, arthralgia, weakness, increased blood volume, edema, hypertension, CHF, rash, anaphylaxis

Nursing Considerations for Patients Receiving Mineralocorticoids

Assessment: History and Examination

Screen for the following conditions, *which could be cautions or contraindications to use of the drug:* allergy to these drugs; history of CHF, hypertension, or infections; high sodium intake; lactation; and pregnancy.

Include screening *for baseline status before beginning therapy and for any potential adverse effects:* blood pressure, pulse, and adventitious breath sounds; weight and temperature; tissue turgor; reflexes and bilateral grip strength; and serum electrolyte levels.

Nursing Diagnoses

The patient receiving any mineralocorticoid may have the following nursing diagnoses related to drug therapy:

- Imbalanced Nutrition: More Than Body Requirements, related to metabolic changes
- Excess Fluid Volume related to sodium retention
- Impaired Urinary Elimination related to sodium retention
- Deficient Knowledge regarding drug therapy

Implementation With Rationale

- Use only in conjunction with appropriate glucocorticoids *to maintain control of electrolyte balance.*
- Increase dosage in times of stress *to prevent adrenal insufficiency and to meet increased demands for corticosteroids under stress.*
- Monitor for hypokalemia (weakness, serum electrolytes) *to detect the loss early and treat appropriately.*
- Discontinue if signs of overdosage (excessive weight gain, edema, hypertension, cardiomegaly) occur *to prevent the development of more severe toxicity.*
- Provide thorough patient teaching, including measures to avoid adverse effects; warning signs of problems; and the need for regular evaluation, including blood tests, *to enhance patient knowledge about drug therapy and promote compliance.*

Evaluation

- Monitor patient response to the drug (maintenance of electrolyte balance).

- Monitor for adverse effects (fluid retention, edema, hypokalemia, headache).
- Evaluate the effectiveness of the teaching plan (patient can name drug, dosage, adverse effects to watch for, specific measures to avoid adverse effects).
- Monitor the effectiveness of comfort measures and compliance with the regimen.

WEB LINKS

Patients and health care providers may want to consult the following Internet sources:

http://www.healthfinder.gov Information on where to go to learn about diseases, drugs, and other therapies.

http://www.nih.gov Information on disease research and development, latest drug therapy, and links to other resources—National Institutes of Health.

http://www.medicinenet.com Information on where to go to find support groups, information on specific diseases, and treatments.

http://www.arthritis.org Information on rheumatoid and inflammatory diseases.

http://www.arthritis.about.com

Points to Remember

- There are two adrenal glands, one on top of each kidney.
- Each adrenal gland is composed of the adrenal medulla and the adrenal cortex. The adrenal medulla is basically a sympathetic nerve ganglion that releases norepinephrine and epinephrine into the bloodstream in response to sympathetic stimulation.
- The adrenal cortex produces three types of corticosteroids: androgens (male and female sex hormones), glucocorticoids, and mineralocorticoids.
- The corticosteroids are released normally in a diurnal rhythm, with the hypothalamus producing peak levels of corticotropin-releasing hormone (CRH) around midnight; peak adrenal response occurs around 9 AM. The steroid levels drop slowly during the day to reach low levels in the evening, when the hypothalamus begins CRH secretion, with peak levels again occurring around midnight. Corticosteroids are also released as part of the sympathetic stress reaction to help the body conserve energy for the fight-or-flight response.
- Prolonged use of corticosteroids suppresses the normal hypothalamic–pituitary axis and leads to adrenal atrophy from lack of stimulation. Corticosteroids need to be tapered slowly after prolonged use to allow the adrenals to resume steroid production.
- The glucocorticoids increase glucose production, stimulate fat deposition and protein breakdown, and inhibit protein formation. They are used clinically to block inflammation and the immune response and in conjunction with mineralocorticoids to treat adrenal insufficiency.
- The mineralocorticoids stimulate retention of sodium and water and excretion of potassium. They are used therapeutically in conjunction with glucocorticoids to treat adrenal insufficiency.
- Adverse effects of corticosteroids are related to exaggeration of the physiological effects; they include immunosuppression, peptic ulcer formation, fluid retention, and edema.
- Corticosteroids are used topically and locally to achieve the desired anti-inflammatory effects at a particular site without the systemic adverse effects that limit the usefulness of the drugs.

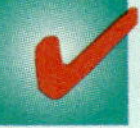

CHECK YOUR UNDERSTANDING

Answers to the questions in this chapter may be found in the Answer Key in the back of the book.

Multiple Choice

Select the best answer to the following.

1. Adrenocortical agents are widely used
   a. to cure chronic inflammatory disorders.
   b. for short-term treatment to relieve inflammation.
   c. for long-term treatment of chronic disorders.
   d. to relieve minor aches and pains and to make people feel better.

2. The adrenal medulla
   a. is the outer core of the adrenal gland.
   b. is the site of production of aldosterone and corticosteroids.
   c. is actually a neural ganglion of the sympathetic nervous system.
   d. consists of three layers of cells that produce different hormones.

3. Glucocorticoids are hormones that
   a. are released in response to high glucose levels.
   b. help to regulate electrolyte levels.
   c. help to regulate water balance in the body.

  d. promote the preservation of energy through increased glucose levels, protein breakdown, and fat formation.

4. Diurnal rhythm in a person with a regular sleep cycle would show
   a. high levels of ACTH during the night while sleeping.
   b. rising levels of corticosteroids throughout the day.
   c. peak levels of ACTH and corticosteroids early in the morning.
   d. hypothalamic stimulation to release CRH around noon.

5. Patients who have been receiving corticosteroid therapy for a prolonged period and suddenly stop the drug will experience an adrenal crisis because their own adrenal glands will not be producing any adrenal hormones. Your assessment of a patient for the possibility of adrenal crisis may include
   a. physiological exhaustion, shock, and fluid shift.
   b. acne development and hypertension.
   c. water retention and increased speed of healing.
   d. hyperglycemia and water retention.

6. A patient is started on a regimen of prednisone because of a crisis in her ulcerative colitis. Nursing care of this patient would need to include
   a. immunizations to prevent infections.
   b. increased calories to deal with metabolic changes.
   c. fluid restriction to decrease water retention.
   d. administration of the drug around 8 or 9 AM to mimic normal diurnal rhythm.

7. A patient who is taking corticosteroids is at increased risk for infection and should
   a. be protected from exposure to infections and invasive procedures.
   b. take anti-inflammatory agents regularly throughout the day.
   c. receive live virus vaccine to protect him/her from infection.
   d. be at no risk if elective surgery is needed.

8. Mineralocorticoids are used to maintain electrolyte balance in situations of adrenal insufficiency. Mineralocorticoids
   a. are usually given alone.
   b. can be given only intravenously.
   c. are always given in conjunction with appropriate glucocorticoids.
   d. are separate in their function from the glucocorticoids.

Multiple Response

Select all that apply.

1. Patients who are taking corticosteroids would be expected to report which of the following?
   a. Weight gain
   b. Round or "moon face" appearance
   c. Feeling of well-being
   d. Weight loss
   e. Excessive hair growth
   f. Fragile skin

2. Corticosteroid hormones are released during a sympathetic stress reaction. They would act to do which of the following?
   a. Increase blood volume
   b. Cause the release of glucose for energy
   c. Increase the rate of protein production
   d. Block the effects of the inflammatory and immune systems
   e. Store glucose to preserve energy
   f. Block protein production to save energy

Word Scramble

Unscramble the following letters to form the names of adrenocortical agents.

1. sonnderpie ____________________
2. toolninemacir ____________________
3. sathatobeemen ____________________
4. coorsdyrthinoe ____________________
5. soddubenie ____________________
6. solidfunlie ____________________
7. sorticone ____________________
8. mexdateshaoen ____________________

True or False

Indicate whether the following statements are true (T) or false (F).

_____ 1. There are two adrenal glands, one on either side of the kidney.

_____ 2. The adrenal cortex is basically a sympathetic nerve ganglia that releases norepinephrine and epinephrine into the bloodstream in response to sympathetic stimulation.

_____ 3. The adrenal medulla produces three corticosteroids: androgens (male and female sex hormones), glucocorticoids, and mineralocorticoids.

_____ 4. The corticosteroids are released normally in a diurnal rhythm.

_____ 5. Prolonged use of corticosteroids will suppress the normal hypothalamic–pituitary axis and lead to adrenal atrophy from lack of stimulation.

_____ 6. The glucocorticoids decrease glucose production, stimulate fat deposition and protein breakdown, and increase protein formation.

_____ 7. The mineralocorticoids stimulate sodium and water excretion and potassium retention.

_____ 8. Adverse effects of corticosteroids are related to exaggeration of their physiological effects, including immunosuppression, peptic ulcer formation, fluid retention, and edema.

_____ 9. Corticosteroids are used topically and locally to achieve the desired anti-inflammatory effects.

_____ 10. Glucocorticoids are used in conjunction with mineralocorticoids to treat adrenal insufficiency

Bibliography and References

Andrews, M., & Boyle, J. (2002). *Transcultural concepts in nursing care.* Philadelphia: Lippincott Williams & Wilkins.

Drug facts and comparisons. (2006). St. Louis: Facts and Comparisons.

Gilman, A., Hardman, J. G., & Limbird, L. E. (Eds.). (2006). *Goodman and Gilman's the pharmacological basis of therapeutics* (11th ed.). New York: McGraw-Hill.

Guyton, A., & Hall, J. (2000). *Textbook of medical physiology.* Philadelphia: W. B. Saunders.

Karch, A. M. (2006). *2007 Lippincott's nursing drug guide.* Philadelphia: Lippincott Williams & Wilkins.

The medical letter on drugs and therapeutics. (2006). New Rochelle, NY: Medical Letter.

North, W. G., Moses, A. M., & Shafe, L. (Eds.). (1993). The neurohypophysis: A window on brain function. Proceedings of the 5th International Conference on Neurohypophysis, Hanover, New Hampshire, July 16–20, 1992. *Annals of the New York Academy of Sciences, 689,* 1–706.

Porth, C. (2005). *Pathophysiology: Concepts of altered health states* (7th ed.). Philadelphia: Lippincott Williams & Wilkins.

CHAPTER 37

Thyroid and Parathyroid Agents

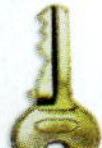

KEY TERMS

bisphosphonates
calcitonin
cretinism
follicles
hypercalcemia
hyperparathyroidism
hyperthyroidism
hypocalcemia
hypoparathyroidism
hypothyroidism
iodine
levothyroxine
liothyronine
metabolism
myxedema
Paget's disease
parathormone
postmenopausal osteoporosis
thioamides
thyroxine

LEARNING OBJECTIVES

Upon completion of this chapter, you will be able to:

1. Explain the control of the synthesis and secretion of thyroid hormones and parathyroid hormones, applying this to alterations in the control process (e.g., using thyroid hormones to treat obesity, Paget's disease, etc.).
2. Describe the therapeutic actions, indications, pharmacokinetics, contraindications, most common adverse reactions, and important drug–drug interactions associated with thyroid, antithyroid, antihypocalcemic, and antihypercalcemic agents.
3. Discuss the use of thyroid, antithyroid, and calcium regulating drugs across the lifespan.
4. Compare and contrast the prototype drugs levothyroxine, propylthiouracil, strong iodine products, calcitriol, alendronate, and calcitonin with thyroid or parathyroid agents in their class.
5. Outline the nursing considerations, including important teaching points, for patients receiving drugs used to affect thyroid or parathyroid function.

THYROID HORMONES

P levothyroxine
liothyronine
liotrix
thyroid desiccated

ANTITHYROID AGENTS

Thioamides

methimazole
P propylthiouracil

Iodines

radioactive iodide I^{131}
P strong iodine products, potassium iodide

ANTIHYPOCALCEMIC AGENTS

P calcitriol
dihydrotachysterol

ANTIHYPERCALCEMIC AGENTS

Bisphosphonates

P alendronate
etidronate
ibandronate
pamidronate
risedronate
tiludronate
zoledronic acid

Calcitonins

calcitonin, human
P calcitonin, salmon

This chapter reviews drugs that are used to affect the function of the thyroid and parathyroid glands. These two glands are closely situated in the middle of the neck and share a common goal of calcium homeostasis. In most respects, however, these glands are very different in structure and function.

The Thyroid Gland

Structure

The thyroid gland is located in the middle of the neck, where it surrounds the trachea like a shield (Figure 37.1). Its name comes from the Greek words *thyros* (shield) and *eidos* (gland). The thyroid is a vascular gland with two lobes, one on each side of the trachea, and a small isthmus connecting the lobes. The gland is made up of cells arranged in circular **follicles**. The center of each follicle is composed of colloid tissue, in which the thyroid hormones produced by the gland are stored.

The thyroid gland produces two slightly different thyroid hormones, using iodine that is found in the diet: tetraiodothyronine or **levothyroxine** (T_4), so named because it contains four iodine atoms, and triiodothyronine or **liothyronine** (T_3), so named because it contains three iodine atoms. The thyroid cells remove **iodine** from the blood, concentrate it, and prepare it for attachment to tyrosine, an amino acid. A person must obtain sufficient amounts of dietary iodine to produce thyroid hormones.

When thyroid hormone is needed in the body, the stored thyroid hormone molecule is absorbed into the thyroid cells, where the T_3 and T_4 are broken off and released into circulation. These hormones are carried on plasma proteins, which can be measured as protein-bound iodine (PBI) levels. The thyroid gland produces more T_4 than T_3. More T_4 is released into circulation, but T_3 is approximately four times more active than T_4. Most T_4 (with a half-life of about 12 hours) is converted to T_3 (with a half-life of about 1 week) at the tissue level.

Control

Thyroid hormone production and release are regulated by the anterior pituitary hormone called thyroid-stimulating hormone (TSH). The secretion of TSH is regulated by

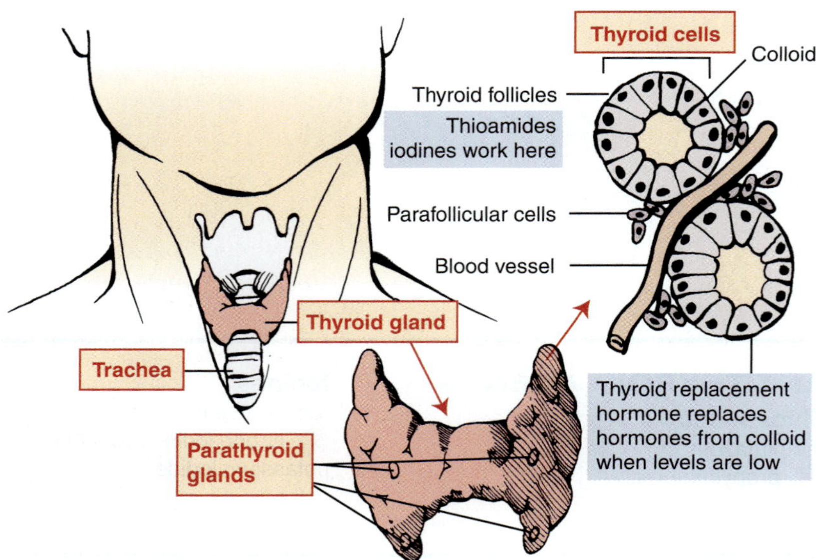

FIGURE 37.1 The thyroid and parathyroid glands. The basic unit of the thyroid gland is the follicle.

thyrotropin-releasing hormone (TRH), a hypothalamic regulating factor. A delicate balance exists among the thyroid, the pituitary, and the hypothalamus in regulating the levels of thyroid hormone. The thyroid gland produces increased thyroid hormones in response to increased levels of TSH. The increased levels of thyroid hormones send a negative feedback message to the pituitary to decrease TSH release, and at the same time, to the hypothalamus, to decrease TRH release. A drop in TRH levels subsequently results in a drop in TSH levels, which in turn leads to a drop in thyroid hormone levels. In response to low blood serum levels of thyroid hormone, the hypothalamus sends TRH to the anterior pituitary, which responds by releasing TSH, which in turn stimulates the thyroid gland to again produce and release thyroid hormone. The rising levels of thyroid hormone are sensed by the hypothalamus, and the cycle begins again. This intricate series of negative feedback mechanisms keeps the level of thyroid hormone within a narrow range of normal (Figure 37.2).

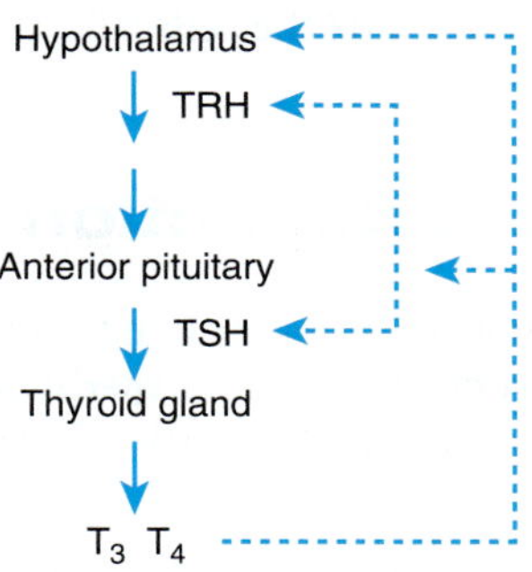

FIGURE 37.2 In response to low blood serum levels of thyroid hormone, the hypothalamus sends the thyrotropin-releasing hormone (TRH) to the anterior pituitary, which responds by releasing the thyroid-stimulating hormone (TSH) to the thyroid gland; it, in turn, responds by releasing the thyroid hormone (T_3 and T_4) into the bloodstream. The anterior pituitary is also sensitive to the increase in blood serum levels of the thyroid hormone and responds by decreasing production and release of TSH. As thyroid hormone production and release subside, the hypothalamus senses the lower serum levels and the process is repeated by the release of TRH again. This intricate series of negative feedback mechanisms keeps the level of thyroid hormone within normal limits.

Function

The thyroid hormone regulates the rate of **metabolism**—that is, the rate at which energy is burned—in almost all the cells of the body. The thyroid hormones affect heat production and body temperature; oxygen consumption and cardiac output; blood volume; enzyme system activity; and metabolism of carbohydrates, fats, and proteins. Thyroid hormone is also an important regulator of growth and development, especially within the reproductive and nervous systems. Because the thyroid has such widespread effects throughout the body, any dysfunction of the thyroid gland will have numerous systemic effects.

Cells found around the follicle of the thyroid gland, called parafollicular cells, produce another hormone, **calcitonin**. This hormone affects calcium levels and acts to balance the effects of the parathyroid hormone, **parathormone**. The release of calcitonin is not controlled by the hypothalamic–pituitary axis but is regulated locally at the cellular level. The cells release calcitonin when the concentration of calcium around them rises. The calcitonin released into the bloodstream works to reduce calcium levels by blocking bone resorption and enhancing bone formation, pulling calcium out of the serum for deposit into bone (Figure 37.3). If the

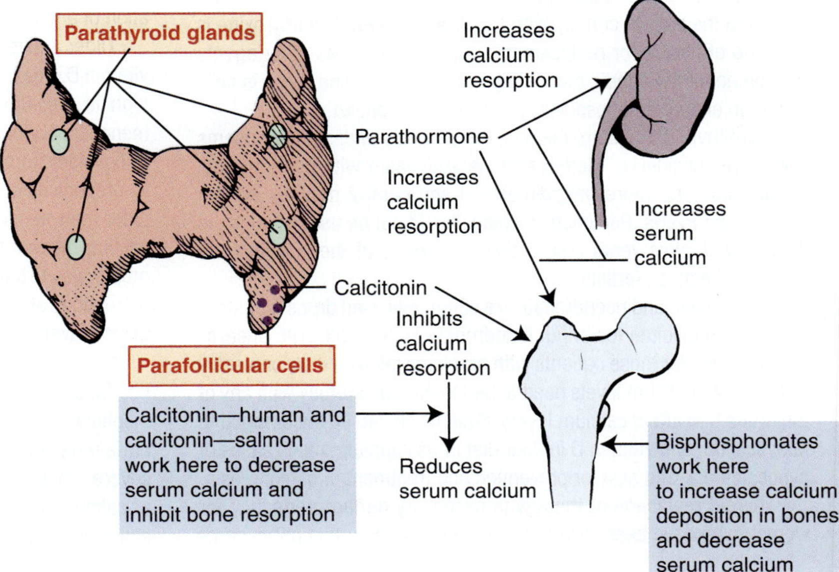

FIGURE 37.3 Calcium control. Parathormone and calcitonin work to maintain calcium homeostasis in the body.

calcium level surrounding the cells falls, they will no longer produce calcitonin.

Thyroid Dysfunction

Thyroid dysfunction involves either underactivity, called **hypothyroidism**, or overactivity, called **hyperthyroidism.** This dysfunction can affect any age group (Box 37.1).

Hypothyroidism

Hypothyroidism is a lack of sufficient levels of thyroid hormones to maintain a normal metabolism. This condition occurs in a number of pathophysiological states:

- Absence of the thyroid gland
- Lack of sufficient iodine in the diet to produce the needed level of thyroid hormone

BOX 37.1 DRUG THERAPY ACROSS THE LIFESPAN

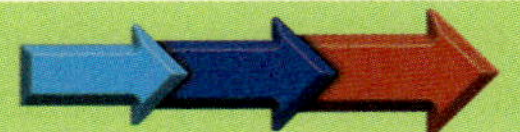

Thyroid and Parathyroid Agents

CHILDREN

Thyroid replacement therapy is required when a child is hypothyroid. Levothyroxine is the drug of choice in children. Dosage is determined based on serum thyroid hormone levels and the response of the child, including growth and development. Dosage in children tends to be higher than in adults because of the higher metabolic rate of the growing child. Usually, the starting dose to consider is 10 to 15 mcg/kg per day.

Regular monitoring, including growth records, is necessary to determine the accurate dosage as the child grows. Maintenance levels at the adult dosage usually occurs after puberty and when active growing stops.

If an antithyroid agent is needed, propylthiouracil (*PTU*) is the drug of choice because it is less toxic. Radioactive agents are not used in children, unless other agents are ineffective, because of the effects of radiation on chromosomes and developing cells.

Hypercalcemia is relatively rare in children, although it may be seen with certain malignancies. If a child develops a malignancy-related hypercalcemia, the bisphosphonates may be used, with dosage adjustments based on age and weight. Serum calcium levels should be monitored very closely in the child and dosage adjustments made as necessary.

ADULTS

Adults who require thyroid replacement therapy need to understand that this will be a lifelong replacement need. An established routine of taking the tablet first thing in the morning, with a full glass of water, may help the patient comply with the drug regimen. Levothyroxine is the drug of choice for replacement, but in some cases other agents may be needed. Periodic monitoring of thyroid hormone levels is necessary to ensure that dosage needs have not changed.

If antithyroid drugs are needed, the patient's underlying problems should be considered. Methimazole is associated with bone marrow suppression and more gastrointestinal and central nervous system effects than *PTU* is. Radioactive iodine should not be used in adults in their reproductive years unless they are aware of the possibility of adverse effects on fertility.

Alendronate and risendronate are commonly used drugs for osteoporosis and calcium lowering. Ibandronate is available with once-a-month dosing for those patients with problems taking a daily or weekly drug. Serum calcium levels need to be monitored carefully with any of the drugs that affect calcium levels. Patients should be encouraged to take calcium and vitamin D in their diet or as supplements in cases of hypocalcemia, and also for prevention and treatment of osteoporosis.

Thyroid replacement therapy is necessary during pregnancy for women who have been maintained on this regimen. It is not uncommon for hypothyroidism to develop during pregnancy. Levothyroxine is again the drug of choice.

If an antithyroid drug is essential during pregnancy, *PTU* is the drug of choice because it is less likely to cross the placenta and cause problems for the fetus. Radioactive agents should not be used. Bisphosphonates should be used during pregnancy only if the benefit to the mother clearly outweighs the potential risk to the fetus. Nursing mothers who need thyroid replacement therapy should continue with their prescribed regimen and report any adverse reactions in the baby. Bisphosphonates and antithyroid drugs should not be used during lactation because of the potential for adverse reactions in the baby—another method of feeding the baby should be used.

OLDER ADULTS

Because the signs and symptoms of thyroid disease mimic many other problems that are common to older adults—hair loss, slurred speech, fluid retention, congestive heart failure, and so on—it is important to screen older adults for thyroid disease carefully before beginning any therapy. The dosage should be started at a very low level and increased based on the patient response. Levothyroxine is the drug of choice for hypothyroidism. Periodic monitoring of thyroid hormone levels as well as cardiac and other responses is essential with this age group.

If antithyroid agents are needed, radioactive iodine may be the drug of choice because it has fewer adverse effects than the other agents and surgery. The patient should be monitored closely for the development of hypothyroidism, which usually occurs within a year after initiation of antithyroid therapy.

Older adults may have dietary deficiencies related to calcium and vitamin D. They should be encouraged to eat dairy products and foods high in calcium and to supplement their diet if necessary. Postmenopausal women, who are prone to develop osteoporosis, may want to consider hormone replacement therapy and calcium supplements to prevent osteoporosis. Many postmenopausal women, and some older men, respond well to the effect of bisphosphonates in moving calcium back into the bone. They need specific instructions on the proper way to take these drugs and may not be able to comply with the restrictions about staying upright and swallowing the tablet with a full glass of water.

Older adults have a greater incidence of renal impairment, and kidney function should be evaluated before starting any of these drugs. Bisphosphonates should be used in lower doses in patients with moderate renal impairment and are not recommended for those who have severe renal impairment. With any of these drugs, regular monitoring of calcium levels is important to ensure that therapeutic effects are achieved with a minimum of adverse effects.

- Lack of sufficient functioning thyroid tissue due to tumor or autoimmune disorders
- Lack of TSH due to pituitary disease
- Lack of TRH related to a tumor or disorder of the hypothalamus

Hypothyroidism is the most common type of thyroid dysfunction. It is estimated that approximately 5% to 10% of women older than 50 years of age are hypothyroid. Hypothyroidism is also a common finding in the elderly. The symptoms of hypothyroidism can be varied and vague and are frequently overlooked. The signs and symptoms of hypothyroidism, including obesity, are often mistaken for signs of normal aging (Box 37.2). Goiter, or enlargement of the thyroid gland, occurs when the thyroid is overactive. This effect frequently occurs when the thyroid is overstimulated by TSH, which can happen if the thyroid gland does not make sufficient thyroid hormones to turn off the hypothalamus and anterior pituitary. In the body's attempt to produce the needed amount of thyroid hormone, the thyroid is continually stimulated by increasing levels of TSH.

Children who are born without a thyroid gland or who have a nonfunctioning gland develop a condition called **cretinism.** If untreated, these children will have poor growth and development and mental retardation because of the lack of thyroid hormone stimulation. Severe adult hypothyroidism is called **myxedema**. Myxedema usually develops gradually as the thyroid slowly stops functioning. It can develop as a result of autoimmune thyroid disease (Hashimoto's disease), viral infection, or overtreatment with antithyroid drugs or because of surgical removal or irradiation of the thyroid gland. Patients with myxedema exhibit many signs and symptoms of decreased metabolism, including lethargy, hypoactive reflexes, hypotension, bradycardia, pale and coarse skin, loss of hair, intolerance to the cold, decreased appetite, decreased body temperature, thickening of the tongue and vocal cords, decreased sexual function, and even sterility. Patients with hypothyroidism are treated with replacement thyroid hormone therapy.

BOX 37.2 FOCUS ON THE EVIDENCE

Thyroid Hormones for Obesity

Treatment trends for obesity have changed over the years. Not long ago, one of the suggested treatments was the use of thyroid hormone. The thinking was that obese people had slower metabolisms and therefore would benefit from a boost in metabolism from extra thyroid hormone.

If an obese patient is truly hypothyroid, this might be a good idea. Unfortunately, many of the patients who received thyroid hormone for weight loss were not tested for thyroid activity and ended up with excessive thyroid hormone in their systems. This situation triggered a cascade of events. The exogenous thyroid hormone disrupted the hypothalamic–pituitary–thyroid control system, resulting in decreased production of thyrotropin-releasing hormone (TRH) and thyroid-stimulating hormone (TSH) as the hypothalamus and pituitary sensed the rising levels of thyroid hormone. Because the thyroid was no longer stimulated to produce and secrete thyroid hormone, thyroid levels would actually fall. Lacking stimulation by TSH, the thyroid gland would start to atrophy. If exogenous thyroid hormone were stopped, the atrophied thyroid would not be able to immediately respond to the TSH stimulation and produce thyroid hormone. Ultimately, these patients experienced an endocrine imbalance. What's more, they also did not lose weight—and in the long run may actually have gained weight as the body's compensatory mechanisms tried to deal with the imbalances.

Today, thyroid hormone is no longer considered a good choice for treating obesity. Other drugs have come and gone, and new drugs are released each year to attack other aspects of the problem. Many patients, especially middle-aged people who may recall that thyroid was once used for weight loss, ask for thyroid hormone as an answer to their weight problem. Patients have even been known to "borrow" thyroid replacement hormones from others for a quick weight loss solution or to order the drug over the Internet without supervision or monitoring.

Obese patients need reassurance, understanding, and education about the risks of borrowed thyroid hormone. Insistent patients should undergo thyroid function tests. If the results are normal, patients should receive teaching about the controls and actions of thyroid hormone in the body and an explanation of why taking these hormones can cause problems. Obesity is a chronic and frustrating problem that poses continual challenges for health care providers.

Hyperthyroidism

Hyperthyroidism occurs when excessive amounts of thyroid hormones are produced and released into the circulation. Graves' disease, a poorly understood condition that is thought to be an autoimmune problem, is the most common cause of hyperthyroidism. Patients with hyperthyroidism may exhibit many signs and symptoms of overactive cellular metabolism, including increased body temperature, tachycardia, palpitations, hypertension, flushing, thin skin, an intolerance to heat, amenorrhea, weight loss, and goiter. Treatment of hyperthyroidism may involve surgical removal of the gland or portions of the gland; treatment with radiation to destroy parts or all of the gland; or drug treatment to block the production of **thyroxine** in the thyroid gland or to destroy parts or all of the gland. The metabolism of these patients then must be regulated with replacement thyroid hormone therapy.

Table 37.1 outlines the signs and symptoms of thyroid dysfunction.

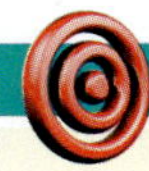

FOCUS POINTS

- The thyroid gland uses iodine to produce the thyroid hormones that regulate body metabolism.
- Control of the thyroid gland involves an intricate balance among TRH, TSH, and circulating levels of thyroid hormone.
- Hypothyroidism is treated with replacement thyroid hormone; hyperthyroidism is treated with thioamides or iodines.

Table 37.1 Signs and Symptoms of Thyroid Dysfunction

System	Hypothyroidism	Hyperthyroidism
Central nervous system	Depressed—hypoactive reflexes, lethargy, sleepiness, slow speech, emotional dullness	Stimulated—hyperactive reflexes, anxiety, nervousness, insomnia, tremors, restlessness
Cardiovascular	Depressed—bradycardia, hypotension, anemia, oliguria, decreased sensitivity to catecholamines	Stimulated—tachycardia, palpitations, increased pulse pressure, systolic hypertension, increased sensitivity to catecholamines
Skin, hair, nails	Pale, coarse, dry, thickened; puffy eyes and eyelids; hair coarse and thin; nails thick and hard	Flushed, warm, thin, moist, sweating; hair fine and soft; nails soft and thin
Metabolic rate	Decreased—lower body temperature; intolerance to cold; decreased appetite, higher levels of fat and cholesterol, weight gain, and hypercholesterolemia	Increased—low-grade fever; intolerance to heat; increased appetite with weight loss; muscle wasting and weakness, thyroid myopathy
Generalized myxedema	Accumulation of mucopolysaccharides in the heart, tongue, vocal cords; periorbital edema, cardiomyopathy, hoarseness, and thickened speech	Localized with accumulation of mucopolysaccharides in eyeballs, ocular muscles; periorbital edema, lid lag, exophthalmos; pretibial edema
Ovaries	Decreased function—menorrhagia, habitual abortion, sterility	Altered; tendency toward oligomenorrhea, amenorrhea
Goiter	Rare; simple nontoxic type may occur	Diffuse, highly vascular; very frequent

Thyroid Hormone

Several replacement hormone products are available for treating hypothyroidism. These products contain both natural and synthetic thyroid hormone. Replacement hormones act to replace low or absent levels of the thyroid hormones and to suppress overproduction of TSH by the pituitary (see Figure 37.1 and Table 37.2). Levothyroxine (*Synthroid, Levoxyl, Levothroid*), a synthetic salt of T_4, is the most frequently used replacement hormone because of its predictable bioavailability and reliability.

Thyroid desiccated (*Armour Thyroid* and others) is prepared from dried animal thyroid glands and contains both T_3 and T_4. Although the ratio of the hormones is unpredictable and the required dosage and effects vary widely, this drug is inexpensive, making it attractive to some.

Liothyronine (*Cytomel, Triostat*) is a synthetic salt of T_3. Because it contains only T_3, liothyronine has a rapid onset and a long duration of action. It also has a greater incidence of cardiac side effects and is not recommended for use in patients with potential cardiac problems.

Liotrix (*Thyrolar*) is a synthetic preparation of T_4 and T_3 in a standard 4:1 ratio. Because it is associated with several cardiac and central nervous system (CNS) effects, it may not be the drug of choice for patients who have cardiac problems or are prone to anxiety reactions.

Therapeutic Actions and Indications

The thyroid replacement hormones increase the metabolic rate of body tissues, increasing oxygen consumption, respi-

Table 37.2 DRUGS IN FOCUS

Thyroid Hormones

Drug Name	Dosage/Route	Usual Indications
P levothyroxine (*Synthroid, Levoxyl, others*)	Adult: 0.05–0.2 mg/day PO Pediatric: 0.025–0.4 mg/day PO	Replacement therapy in hypothyroidism; suppression of thyroid-stimulating hormone (TSH) release; treatment of myxedema coma and thyrotoxicosis
liothyronine (*Cytomel, Triostat*)	Adult: 25–100 mcg/day PO Pediatric: 20–50 mcg/day PO	Replacement therapy in hypothyroidism; suppression of TSH release; treatment of thyrotoxicosis; synthetic hormone used in patients allergic to dessicated thyroid **Special considerations:** not for use with cardiac or anxiety problems
iotrix (*Thyrolar*)	Adult: 60–120 mg/day PO Pediatric: 25–150 mcg/day PO based on age and weight	Replacement therapy in hypothyroidism; suppression of TSH release; treatment of thyrotoxicosis **Special considerations:** not for use with cardiac dysfunction
thyroid desiccated (*Armour Thyroid*)	Adult: 60–120 mg/day PO Pediatric: 15–90 mg/day PO	Replacement therapy in hypothyroidism; suppression of TSH release; treatment of thyrotoxicosis

ration, heart rate, growth and maturation, and the metabolism of fats, carbohydrates, and proteins. They are indicated for replacement therapy in hypothyroid states, treatment of myxedema coma, suppression of TSH in the treatment and prevention of goiters, and management of thyroid cancer. In conjunction with antithyroid drugs, they also are indicated to treat thyroid toxicity, prevent goiter formation during thyroid overstimulation, and treat thyroid overstimulation during pregnancy.

Pharmacokinetics

These drugs are well absorbed from the gastrointestinal (GI) tract and bound to serum proteins. Deiodination of the drugs occurs at several sites, including the liver, kidney, and other body tissues. Elimination is primarily in the bile. Thyroid hormone does not cross the placenta and seems to have no effect on the fetus. Thyroid replacement therapy should not be discontinued during pregnancy, and the need for thyroid replacement often becomes apparent during pregnancy. Thyroid hormone does enter breast milk in small amounts. Caution should be used during lactation.

Contraindications and Cautions

These drugs should not be used with any known allergy to the drugs or their binders, during acute thyrotoxicosis (unless used in conjunction with antithyroid drugs), or during acute myocardial infarction (unless complicated by hypothyroidism), *because the thyroid hormones could exacerbate these conditions.* Caution should be used during lactation, *because the drug enters breast milk and could suppress the infant's own thyroid production,* and with hypoadrenal conditions such as Addison's disease.

Adverse Effects

When the correct dosage of the replacement therapy is being used, few if any adverse effects are associated with these drugs. Skin reactions and loss of hair are sometimes seen, especially during the first few months of treatment in children. Symptoms of hyperthyroidism may occur as the drug dose is regulated. Some of the less predictable effects are associated with cardiac stimulation (arrhythmias, hypertension), CNS effects (anxiety, sleeplessness, headache), and difficulty swallowing (taking the drug with a full glass of water may help).

Clinically Important Drug–Drug Interactions

Decreased absorption of the thyroid hormones occurs if they are taken concurrently with cholestyramine. If this combination is needed, the drugs should be taken 2 hours apart.

The effectiveness of oral anticoagulants is increased if they are combined with thyroid hormone. Because this may lead to increased bleeding, the dosage of the oral anticoagulant should be reduced and the bleeding time checked periodically.

Decreased effectiveness of digitalis glycosides can occur when these drugs are combined. Consequently, digitalis levels should be monitored and increased dosage may be required.

Theophylline clearance is decreased in hypothyroid states. As the patient approaches normal thyroid function, theophylline dosage may need to be adjusted frequently.

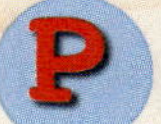

Prototype Summary: *Levothyroxine*

Indications: Replacement therapy in hypothyroidism; pituitary TSH suppression in the treatment of euthyroid goiters and in the management of thyroid cancer; thyrotoxicosis in conjunction with other therapy; myxedema coma

Actions: Increases the metabolic rate of body tissues, increasing oxygen consumption, respiration, and heart rate; the rate of fat, protein, and carbohydrate metabolism; and growth and maturation

Pharmacokinetics:

Route	Onset	Peak	Duration
PO	Slow	1–3 wk	1–3 wk
IV	6–8 h	24–48 h	unknown

$T_{1/2}$: 6–7 days; metabolized in the liver and excreted in the bile

Adverse effects: Tremors, headache, nervousness, palpitations, tachycardia, allergic skin reactions, loss of hair in the first few months of therapy in children, diarrhea, nausea, vomiting

Nursing Considerations for Patients Receiving Thyroid Hormones

Assessment: History and Examination

Screen for the following conditions, *which could be contraindications or cautions to use of the drug:* history of allergy to any thyroid hormone or binder, lactation, Addison's disease, acute myocardial infarction not complicated by hypothyroidism, and thyrotoxicosis.

Include screening *for baseline status before beginning therapy and for any potential adverse effects:* presence of any skin lesions; orientation and affect; baseline pulse, blood pressure, and electrocardiogram (ECG); respiration and adventitious sounds; and thyroid function tests.

Nursing Diagnoses

The patient receiving any thyroid hormone may have the following nursing diagnoses related to drug therapy:

- Decreased Cardiac Output related to cardiac effects
- Imbalanced Nutrition: Less Than Body Requirements related to changes in metabolism
- Ineffective Tissue Perfusion related to thyroid activity
- Deficient Knowledge regarding drug therapy

Implementation With Rationale

- Administer a single daily dose before breakfast each day, *to ensure consistent therapeutic levels.*
- Administer with a full glass of water *to help prevent difficulty swallowing.*
- Monitor response carefully when beginning therapy, *to adjust dosage according to patient response.*
- Monitor cardiac response, *to detect cardiac adverse effects.*
- Assess the patient carefully, *to detect any potential drug–drug interactions if giving thyroid hormone in combination with other drugs.*
- Arrange for periodic blood tests of thyroid function, *to monitor the effectiveness of the therapy.*
- Provide thorough patient teaching, including measures to avoid adverse effects, warning signs of problems, and the need for regular evaluation if used for longer than recommended, *to enhance patient knowledge of drug therapy and promote compliance.*

Evaluation

- Monitor patient response to the drug (return of metabolism to normal, prevention of goiter).
- Monitor for adverse effects (tachycardia, hypertension, anxiety, skin rash).
- Evaluate the effectiveness of the teaching plan (patient can name drug, dosage, adverse effects to watch for, and specific measures to avoid adverse effects).
- Monitor the effectiveness of comfort measures and compliance to the regimen (see Critical Thinking Scenario 37-1).

Antithyroid Agents

Drugs used to block production of thyroid hormone and to treat hyperthyroidism include the **thioamides** and iodide solutions (Table 37.3). Although these groups of drugs are not chemically related, they both block the formation of thyroid hormones within the thyroid gland (see Figure 37.1).

The Thioamides

Propylthiouracil (*PTU*) is the most frequently used thioamide; it is associated with several GI effects. The other available thioamide is methimazole (*Tapazole*). Hematological adverse effects are more common with methimazole, so the patient needs to have a complete blood count and differential monitored regularly. GI effects are somewhat less pronounced with methimazole, so it may be the drug of choice for patients who are unable to tolerate *PTU.*

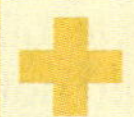

FOCUS ON PATIENT SAFETY

Name confusion has been reported between propylthiouracil (*PTU*) and *Purinethol* (mercaptopurine), an antineoplastic agent. Serious adverse effects could occur. Use extreme caution when using these drugs.

Therapeutic Actions and Indications

The thioamides prevent the formation of thyroid hormone within the thyroid cells, lowering the serum levels of thyroid hormone. They also partially inhibit the conversion of T_4 to T_3 at the cellular level. Thioamides are indicated for the treatment of hyperthyroidism.

Pharmacokinetics

These drugs are well absorbed from the GI tract and are then concentrated in the thyroid gland. Some excretion can be detected in the urine. Methimazole crosses the placenta and is found in a high ratio in breast milk. *PTU* has a low potential for crossing the placenta and for entering breast milk. If an antithyroid drug is needed during pregnancy, *PTU* is the drug of choice, but caution should still be used. Another method of feeding the baby should be chosen if an antithyroid drug is needed during lactation because of the potential for adverse effects on the baby, including the development of neonatal goiter.

Contraindications and Cautions

Thioamides are contraindicated in the presence of any known allergy to antithyroid drugs and during pregnancy. (If an antithyroid drug is absolutely essential and the mother has been informed about the risk of cretinism in the infant, propylthiouracil is the drug of choice.) These drugs should be used cautiously during lactation *because of the risk of antithyroid activity in the infant.* (Again, if an antithyroid drug is needed, propylthiouracil is the drug of choice.)

CRITICAL THINKING SCENARIO 37-1

Hypothyroidism

The Situation

H.R., a 38-year-old white woman, complains of "exhaustion, lethargy, and sleepiness." Her past history is sketchy, her speech seems slurred, and her attention span is limited. Mr. R., her husband, reports feeling frustrated with H.R., stating that she has become increasingly lethargic, disorganized, and uninvolved at home. He also notes that she has gained weight and lost interest in her appearance. Physical examination reveals the following remarkable findings: pulse rate, 52; blood pressure, 90/62; temperature, 96.8°F (oral); pale, dry, and thick skin; periorbital edema; thick and asymmetric tongue; height, 5 ft 5 in; weight, 165 lb. The immediate impression is that of hypothyroidism. Laboratory tests confirm this, revealing elevated TSH and very low levels of triiodothyronine (T_3) and thyroxine (T_4). *Synthroid,* 0.2 mg qd PO, is prescribed.

Critical Thinking

What teaching plans should be developed for this patient?

What interventions would be appropriate in helping Mr. and Mrs. R. accept the diagnosis and the pathophysiological basis for Mrs. R's complaints and problems?

What body image changes will H.R. experience as her body adjusts to the thyroid therapy?

How can H.R. be helped to adjust to these changes and re-establish her body image and self-concept?

Discussion

Hypothyroidism develops slowly. With it comes fatigue, lethargy, and lack of emotional affect—conditions that result in the patient's losing interest in appearance, activities, and responsibilities. In this case, the patient's husband, not knowing that there was a physical reason for the problem, became increasingly frustrated and even angry. Mr. R. should be involved in the teaching program so that his feelings can be taken into consideration. Any teaching content should be written down for later reference. (When H.R. starts to return to normal, her attention span and interest should return; anything that was missed or forgotten can be referred to in the written teaching program.)

H.R. may be encouraged to bring a picture of herself from a year or so ago to help her to understand and appreciate the changes that have occurred. Many patients are totally unaware of changes in their appearance and activity level because the disease progresses so slowly and brings on lethargy and lack of emotional affect.

The teaching plan should include information about the function of the thyroid gland and the anticipated changes that will be occurring to H.R. over the next week and beyond. The importance of taking the medication daily should be emphasized. The need to return for follow-up to evaluate the effectiveness of the medication and the effects on her body should also be stressed. Both H.R. and her husband will need support and encouragement to deal with past frustrations and the return to normal. Lifelong therapy will probably be needed, so further teaching will be important once things have stabilized.

Nursing Care Guide For H.R.: Thyroid Hormone

Assessment: History And Examination

Review the patient's history for allergies to any of these drugs, Addison's disease, acute myocardial infarction not complicated by hypothyroidism, lactation, and thyrotoxicosis.

Focus the physical examination on the following:

Neurological: orientation and affect

Skin: color and lesions

CV: pulse, cardiac auscultation, blood pressure and ECG findings

Respiratory: respirations, adventitious sounds

Hematological: thyroid function tests

Nursing Diagnoses

Decreased Cardiac Output related to cardiac effects

Imbalanced Nutrition: Less Than Body Requirements related to effects on metabolism

Ineffective Tissue Perfusion related to thyroid effects.

Deficient Knowledge regarding drug therapy

Implementation

Administer once a day before breakfast with a full glass of water.

Provide comfort, safety measures (e.g., temperature control, rest as needed, safety precautions).

(continued)

Hypothyroidism *(continued)*

Provide support and reassurance to deal with drug effects and lifetime need.

Provide patient teaching regarding drug name, dosage, adverse effects, precautions, and warning signs to report.

Evaluation

Evaluate drug effects: return of metabolism to normal; prevention of goiter.

Monitor for adverse effects: anxiety, tachycardia, hypertension, skin reaction.

Monitor for drug–drug interactions as indicated for each drug.

Evaluate effectiveness of patient teaching program and comfort and safety measures.

Patient Teaching For H.R.

- ☐ This hormone is designed to replace the thyroid hormone that your body is not able to produce. The thyroid hormone is responsible for regulating your body's metabolism, or the speed with which your body's cells burn energy. Thyroid hormone actions affect many body systems; so it is very important that you take this medication only as prescribed.
- ☐ Never stop taking this drug without consulting with your health care provider. The drug is used to replace a very important hormone and will probably have to be taken for life. Stopping the medication can lead to serious problems.
- ☐ Take this drug before breakfast each day with a full glass of water.
- ☐ Thyroid hormone usually causes no adverse effects. You may notice a slight skin rash or hair loss in the first few months of therapy. You should notice the signs and symptoms of your thyroid deficiency subsiding, and you will feel "back to normal."
- ☐ Report any of the following to your health care provider: chest pain, difficulty breathing, sore throat, fever, chills, weight gain, sleeplessness, nervousness, unusual sweating or intolerance to heat.
- ☐ Avoid taking any over-the-counter medication without first checking with your health care provider because several of these medications can interfere with the effectiveness of this drug.
- ☐ Tell any doctor, nurse, or other health care provider involved in your care that you are taking this drug. You may also want to wear or carry medical identification showing that you are taking this medication. This would alert any health care personnel taking care of you in an emergency to the fact that you are taking this drug.
- ☐ While you are taking this drug, you will need regular medical follow-up, including blood tests to check the activity of your thyroid gland, to evaluate your response to the drug and any possible underlying problems.
- ☐ Keep this drug, and all medications, out of the reach of children. Do not give this medication to anyone else or take any similar medication that has not been prescribed for you.

Adverse Effects

The adverse effects most commonly seen with these drugs are the effects of thyroid suppression: drowsiness, lethargy, bradycardia, nausea, skin rash, and so on. Propylthiouracil is associated with nausea, vomiting, and GI complaints. Methimazole is also associated with bone marrow suppression, so the patient using this drug must have frequent blood tests to monitor for this effect.

Clinically Important Drug–Drug Interactions

An increased risk for bleeding exists when *PTU* is administered with oral anticoagulants. Changes in serum levels of theophylline, metoprolol, propranolol, and digitalis may lead to changes in the effects of *PTU* as the patient moves from hyperthyroid to euthyroid state.

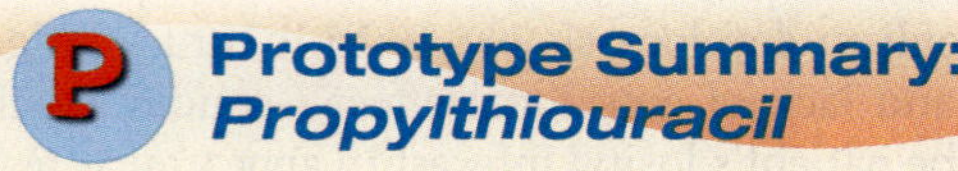

Prototype Summary: *Propylthiouracil*

Indications: Treatment of hyperthyroidism

Actions: Inhibits the synthesis of thyroid hormones, partially inhibits the peripheral conversion of T_4 to T_3

Pharmacokinetics:

Route	Onset
PO	Varies

$T_{1/2}$: 1–2 hours; metabolized in the liver and excreted in the urine

Table 37.3 DRUGS IN FOCUS

Antithyroid Agents

Drug Name	Dosage/Route	Usual Indications
Thioamides		
methimazole (*Tapazole*)	Adult: 15 mg/day PO initially, up to 30–60 mg/day may be needed; maintenance, 5–15 mg/day PO Pediatric: 0.4 mg/kg/day PO initially; maintenance, 15–20 mg/m²/day PO in three divided doses	Treatment of hyperthyroidism
P propylthiouracil (*PTU*)	Adult: 300–900 mg/day PO initially; maintenance, 100–150 mg/day PO Pediatric: 50–300 mg/day PO based on age and response	Treatment of hyperthyroidism
Iodines		
sodium iodide I^{131} (generic)	Adult (>30 yr): 4–10 millicuries PO as needed	Treatment of hyperthyroidism, destruction of thyroid tissue in patients who are not candidates for surgery if thyroid destruction is needed
P strong iodine solution, potassium iodide (*Thyro-Block*)	Adult: one tablet, or 2–6 gtt PO daily to t.i.d. Pediatric (>1 yr): adult dose Pediatric (<1 yr): ½ tablet or 3 gtt PO daily to t.i.d.	Treatment of hyperthyroidism, thyroid blocking in radiation emergencies

Adverse effects: Paresthesias, neuritis, vertigo, drowsiness, skin rash, urticaria, skin pigmentation, nausea, vomiting, epigastric distress, nephritis, bone marrow suppression, arthralgia, myalgia, edema

Iodine Solutions

Low doses of iodine are needed in the body for the formation of thyroid hormone. High doses, however, block thyroid function. Therefore, iodine preparations are sometimes used to treat hyperthyroidism. Radioactive iodine (I^{131}) is sometimes used as a diagnostic agent or to destroy thyroid tissue in cases of severe Graves' disease. It is usually reserved for use in patients who are older than 30 years of age because of the adverse effects associated with the radioactivity. Strong iodine products, potassium iodide (*Thyro-Block*), and sodium iodide are taken orally and have a rapid onset of action, with effects seen within 24 hours and peak effects seen in 10 to 15 days. The effects are short-lived and may even precipitate further thyroid enlargement and dysfunction. For this reason, and because of the availability of the more predictable thioamides, iodides are not used as often as they once were in the clinical setting.

Therapeutic Actions and Indications

These drugs cause the thyroid cells to become oversaturated with iodine and stop producing thyroid hormone. In some cases, the thyroid cells are actually destroyed. The strong iodine products are reserved for presurgical suppression of the thyroid gland, for treatment of acute thyrotoxicosis until thioamide levels can take effect, or for thyroid blocking during radiation therapy.

The strong iodine products are also used to block thyroid function in radiation emergencies. Radioactive iodine is taken up into the thyroid cells, which are then destroyed by the beta-radiation given off by the radioactive iodine. Except during radiation emergencies, the use of radioactive iodine is reserved for those patients who are not candidates for surgery, women who cannot become pregnant, and elderly patients with such severe, complicating conditions that immediate thyroid destruction is needed.

Pharmacokinetics

These drugs are rapidly absorbed from the GI tract and widely distributed throughout the body fluids. Excretion occurs through the urine. Radioactive iodine can cause serious fetal harm and is rated pregnancy category X. It enters breast milk, and another method of feeding the baby should be used if radioactive iodine is needed. The strong iodine products cross the placenta and can cause hypothyroidism and goiter in the fetus or newborn. They should not be used during pregnancy unless the benefit to the mother clearly outweighs the potential risk to the fetus. They are known to enter breast milk, but the effects on the neonate are not known. Caution should be used.

Contraindications and Cautions

The use of strong iodine products is contraindicated in the presence of pregnancy, *because of the effect on the thyroid glands of the mother and the fetus,* and with pulmonary edema or pulmonary tuberculosis.

Adverse Effects

The most common adverse effect of these drugs is hypothyroidism; the patient will need to be started on replacement thyroid hormone to maintain homeostasis. Other adverse effects include iodism (metallic taste and burning in the mouth, sore teeth and gums, diarrhea, cold symptoms, and stomach upset), staining of teeth, skin rash, and the development of goiter.

Clinically Important Drug–Drug Interactions

Because the use of drugs to destroy thyroid function reverts the patient from hyperthyroidism to hypothyroidism, patients who are taking drugs that are metabolized differently in hypothyroid and hyperthyroid states or drugs that have a small margin of safety that could be altered by the change in thyroid function should be monitored closely. These drugs include anticoagulants, theophylline, digoxin, metoprolol, and propranolol.

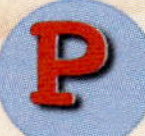

Prototype Summary: Strong Iodine Products

Indications: Adjunct therapy for hyperthyroidism; thyroid blocking in a radiation emergency

Actions: Inhibits the synthesis of thyroid hormones and inhibits the release of these hormones into the circulation

Pharmacokinetics:

Route	Onset	Peak	Duration
PO	24 h	10–15 days	6 wk

$T_{1/2}$: Unknown; metabolized in the liver and excreted in the urine

Adverse effects: Rash, hypothyroidism, goiter, swelling of the salivary glands, iodism (metallic taste, burning mouth and throat, sore teeth and gums, head cold symptoms, stomach upset, diarrhea), allergic reactions

Nursing Considerations for Patients Receiving Antithyroid Agents

Assessment: History and Examination

Screen for the following conditions, *which could be cautions or contraindications to use of the drug:* history of allergy to any antithyroid drug, pregnancy, and lactation.

Include screening *for baseline status before beginning therapy and for any potential adverse effects:* skin lesions; orientation and affect; baseline pulse, blood pressure, and ECG; respiration and adventitious sounds; and thyroid function tests.

Nursing Diagnoses

The patient receiving any antithyroid drug may have the following nursing diagnoses related to drug therapy:

- Decreased Cardiac Output related to cardiac effects
- Imbalanced Nutrition: More Than Body Requirements related to changes in metabolism
- Risk for Injury related to bone marrow suppression
- Deficient Knowledge regarding drug therapy

Implementation With Rationale

- Administer propylthiouracil three times a day, around the clock, *to ensure consistent therapeutic levels.*
- Give iodine solution through a straw, *to decrease staining of teeth;* tablets can be crushed.
- Monitor response carefully and arrange for periodic blood tests, *to assess patient response and to monitor for adverse effects.*
- Monitor patients receiving iodine solution for any sign of iodism, *so the drug can be stopped immediately if such signs appear.*
- Provide thorough patient teaching, including measures to avoid adverse effects, warning signs of problems, and the need for regular evaluation if used for longer than recommended, *to enhance patient knowledge of drug therapy and promote compliance.*

Evaluation

- Monitor patient response to the drug (lowering of thyroid hormone levels).
- Monitor for adverse effects (bradycardia, anxiety, blood dyscrasias, skin rash).
- Evaluate the effectiveness of the teaching plan (patient can name drug, dosage, adverse effects to watch for, specific measures to avoid adverse effects).
- Monitor the effectiveness of comfort measures and compliance to the regimen.

The Parathyroid Glands

Structure and Function

The parathyroid glands are actually four very small groups of glandular tissue located on the back of the thyroid gland. These cells produce parathyroid hormone (PTH), or parathormone.

PTH is the most important regulator of serum calcium levels in the body. PTH has many actions, including the following:

- Stimulation of osteoclasts or bone cells to release calcium from the bone
- Increased intestinal absorption of calcium
- Increased calcium resorption from the kidneys
- Stimulation of cells in the kidney to produce calcitriol, the active form of vitamin D, which stimulates intestinal transport of calcium into the blood

Control

Calcium is an electrolyte that is used in many of the body's metabolic processes. These processes include membrane transport systems, conduction of nerve impulses, muscle contraction, and blood clotting. To achieve all of these effects, serum levels of calcium must be maintained between 9 and 11 mg/dL. This is achieved through regulation of serum calcium by two hormones, PTH and calcitonin (Figure 37.4).

Calcitonin is released when serum calcium levels rise. Calcitonin, produced in the thyroid gland, works to reduce calcium levels by blocking bone resorption and enhancing bone formation. This action pulls calcium out of the serum for deposit into the bone. PTH secretion is also directly regulated by serum calcium levels. When serum calcium levels are low, PTH release is stimulated. When serum calcium levels are high, PTH release is blocked.

Another electrolyte, magnesium, also affects PTH secretion by mobilizing calcium and inhibiting the release of PTH when concentrations rise above or fall below normal. An increased serum phosphate level indirectly stimulates parathyroid activity. Renal tubular phosphate reabsorption is balanced by calcium secretion into the urine, which causes a drop in serum calcium, stimulating PTH secretion. The hormones PTH and calcitonin work together to maintain the delicate balance of serum calcium levels in the body and to keep serum calcium levels within the normal range.

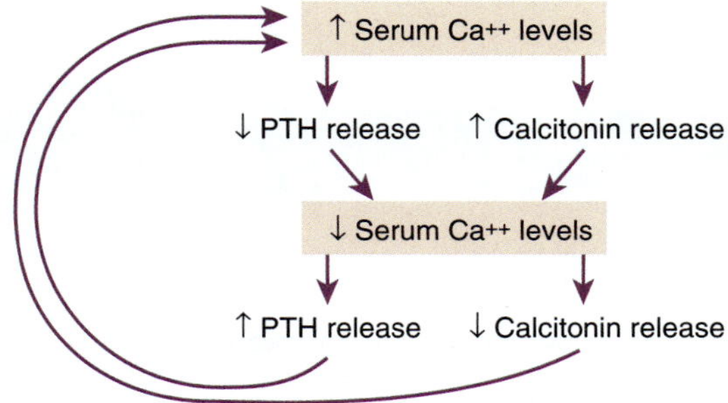

FIGURE 37.4 Control of serum Ca^{++} levels by parathormone (PTH) and calcitonin, showing the negative feedback cycle in effect.

Parathyroid Dysfunction and Related Disorders

The absence of PTH, a condition called **hypoparathyroidism**, is relatively rare. It is most likely to occur with the accidental removal of the parathyroid glands during thyroid surgery. The treatment of hypoparathyroidism consists of calcium and vitamin D therapy to increase serum calcium levels. There is currently no replacement PTH available.

The excessive production of PTH, called **hyperparathyroidism**, can occur as a result of parathyroid tumor or certain genetic disorders. Patients with hyperparathyroidism may present with decalcification of bone and deposits of calcium in body tissues including the kidney, resulting in kidney stones. Primary hyperparathyroidism occurs more often in women in their 60s and 70s. Secondary hyperparathyroidism occurs most frequently in patients with chronic renal failure (see Box 37.3 for more information). When

BOX 37.3 Treatments for Secondary Hyperparathyroidism

In 2004, a new drug in a new class of calcimimetic agents, cinacalcet hydrochloride (*Sensipar*) was approved for treatment of secondary hyperparathyroidism in patients undergoing dialysis for chronic kidney disease and for treatment of hypercalcemia in patients with parathyroid carcinoma. Cinacalcet is a calcimimetic drug that increases the sensitivity of the calcium-sensing receptor to activation by extracellular calcium. In increasing the receptors' sensitivity, cinacalcet lowers parathyroid hormone (PTH) levels, causing a concomitant decrease in serum calcium levels.

The usual initial adult doses for secondary hyperparathyroidism are 30 mg/day PO, after which PTH, serum calcium, and serum phosphorus levels are monitored to achieve the desired therapeutic effect. The usual dosage range is 60–180 mg/day. The drug must be used in combination with vitamin D and/or phosphate binders.

For parathyroid carcinoma, the initial dosage is 30 mg PO b.i.d., titrated every 2–4 weeks to maintain serum calcium levels within a normal range; 30–90 mg b.i.d. up to 90 mg three to four times daily may be needed. Side effects that the patient may experience include nausea, vomiting, diarrhea, and dizziness.

Another treatment available for secondary hyperparathyroidism related to renal failure is paricalcitol (*Zemplar*). Paricalcitol is an analog of vitamin D. Vitamin D levels are decreased in renal disease, leading to an increase in PTH levels and signs and symptoms of hyperparathyroidism. *Zemplar* is taken orally or can be injected during hemodialysis. The body recognizes the vitamin D and subsequently decreases the synthesis and storage of PTH, allowing a control over calcium levels.

The usual dose is 1–4 mcg PO from once a day to three times a week, based on the patient's calcium levels, or 0.04–0.1 mcg/kg injected during hemodialysis. The drug is rapidly absorbed with peak levels within 3 hours. The drug has a half-life of 12–20 hours. Patients will need regular serum calcium checks and dosage will be adjusted based on individual response. Adverse effects are usually mild, as long as the calcium levels are monitored. Diarrhea, headache, and mild hypertension have been reported.

plasma concentrations of calcium are elevated secondary to high PTH levels, inorganic phosphate levels are usually decreased. Pseudorickets (renal fibrocystic osteosis or renal rickets) may occur as a result of this phosphorus retention (hyperphosphatemia), which results from increased stimulation of the parathyroid glands and increased PTH secretion.

The genetically linked disorder **Paget's disease** is a condition of overactive osteoclasts that are eventually replaced by enlarged and softened bony structures. Patients with this disease complain of deep bone pain, headaches, and hearing loss and usually have cardiac failure and bone malformation.

Postmenopausal osteoporosis can occur when dropping levels of estrogen allow calcium to be pulled out of the bone, resulting in weakened and honeycombed bone structure. Estrogen normally causes calcium deposits in the bone; osteoporosis is one of the many complications that accompany the loss of estrogen at menopause (Box 37.4).

BOX 37.4 Gender Considerations: Osteoporosis

Osteoporosis is the most common bone disease found in adults. It results from a lack of bone-building cell (osteoclast) activity and a decrease in bone matrix and mass, with less calcium and phosphorus being deposited in the bone. This can occur with advancing age, when the endocrine system is slowing down and the stimulation to build bone is absent; with menopause, when the calcium-depositing effects of estrogen are lost; with malnutrition states, when vitamin C and proteins essential for bone production are absent from the diet; and with a lack of physical stress on the bones from lack of activity, which promotes calcium removal and does not stimulate osteoclast activity. The inactive, elderly, postmenopausal woman with a poor diet is a prime candidate for osteoporosis. Fractured hips and wrists, shrinking size, and curvature of the spine are all evidence of osteoporosis in this age group. Besides the use of bisphosphonates to encourage calcium deposition in the bone, several other interventions can help prevent severe osteoporosis in this group or in any other people with similar risk factors.

- *Aerobic exercise*—Walking, even 10 minutes a day, has been shown to help increase osteoclast activity. Encourage people to walk around the block or to park their car far from the door and walk. Exercise does not have to involve vigorous gym activity to be beneficial.
- *Proper diet*—Calcium and proteins are essential for bone growth. The person who eats only pasta and avoids milk products could benefit from calcium supplements and encouragement to eat protein at least 2 to 3 times a week. Weight loss can also help to improve activity and decrease pressure on bones at rest.
- *Hormone replacement therapy (HRT)*—For women, HRT has been very successful in decreasing the progression of osteoporosis. Results of the Women's Health Study showed an increase in cardiovascular events with long-term HRT, making it a less desirable treatment. Women who are at high risk for breast cancer or who do not elect to take HRT may be good candidates for bisphosphonates.

The risk of osteoporosis should be taken into consideration as part of the health care regimen for all people as they age. Prevention can save a great deal of pain and debilitation in the long run.

Antihypocalcemic Agents

Deficient levels of PTH result in **hypocalcemia**, or calcium deficiency. Vitamin D stimulates calcium absorption from the intestine and restores the serum calcium to a normal level. Hypoparathyroidism is treated primarily with vitamin D and, if necessary, dietary supplements of calcium. Calcitriol (*Rocaltrol*) is the most commonly used form of vitamin D. Dihydrotachysterol (*Hytakerol*) is also used (Table 37.4.)

Therapeutic Actions and Indications

Vitamin D compounds regulate the absorption of calcium and phosphate from the small intestine, mineral resorption in bone, and reabsorption of phosphate from the renal tubules. Working along with PTH and calcitonin to regulate calcium homeostasis, vitamin D actually functions as a hormone. Use of these agents is indicated for the management of hypocalcemia in patients undergoing chronic renal dialysis and for the treatment of hypoparathyroidism.

Table 37.4 DRUGS IN FOCUS

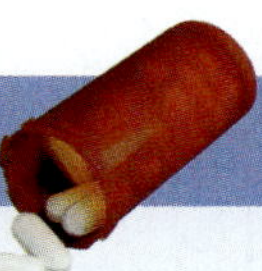

Antihypocalcemic Agents

Drug Name	Usual Dosage	Usual Indications
P calcitriol (*Rocaltrol*)	0.5–2 mcg/day PO in the morning	Management of hypocalcemia and reduction of parathormone levels
dihydrotachysterol (*Hytakerol*)	0.8–2.4 mg/day PO initially, maintenance 0.2–1 mg/day PO based on serum calcium levels	Management of hypocalcemia

Pharmacokinetics

These drugs are well absorbed from the GI tract and widely distributed throughout the body. They are stored in the liver, fat, muscle, skin, and bones. After being metabolized in the liver, they are primarily excreted in the urine. Patients with liver or renal dysfunction may experience increased levels of the drugs and/or toxic effects. At therapeutic levels, these drugs should be used during pregnancy only if the benefit to the mother clearly outweighs the potential for adverse effects on the fetus. Calcitriol has been associated with hypercalcemia in the baby when used by nursing mothers. Another method of feeding the baby should be used if these drugs are needed during lactation.

Contraindications and Cautions

These drugs should not be used in the presence of any known allergy to vitamin D, hypercalcemia, vitamin D toxicity, or pregnancy. Caution should be used with a history of renal stones or during lactation, *when high calcium levels could cause problems.*

Adverse Effects

The adverse effects most commonly seen with these drugs are related to GI effects: metallic taste, nausea, vomiting, dry mouth, constipation, and anorexia. CNS effects such as weakness, headache, somnolence, and irritability may also occur. These are possibly related to the changes in electrolytes that occur with these drugs.

Clinically Important Drug–Drug Interactions

The risk of hypermagnesemia increases if these drugs are taken with magnesium-containing antacids. This combination should be avoided.

Reduced absorption of these compounds may occur if they are taken with cholestyramine or mineral oil, because they are fat-soluble vitamins. If this combination is used, the drugs should be separated by at least 2 hours.

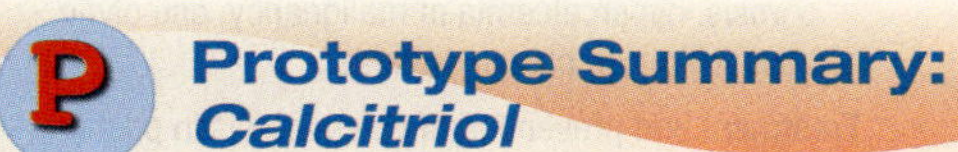

Prototype Summary: Calcitriol

Indications: Management of hypocalcemia in patients on chronic renal dialysis, management of hypocalcemia associated with hypoparathyroidism

Actions: A Vitamin D compound that regulates the absorption of calcium and phosphate from the small intestine, mineral resorption in bone, and reabsorption of phosphate from the renal tubules, increasing the serum calcium level

Pharmacokinetics:

Route	Onset	Peak	Duration
PO	Slow	4 h	3–5 days

$T_{1/2}$: 5–8 hours; metabolized in the liver and excreted in the bile

Adverse effects: Weakness, headache, nausea, vomiting, dry mouth, constipation, muscle pain, bone pain, metallic taste

Nursing Considerations for Patients Receiving Antihypocalcemic Agents

Assessment: History and Examination

Screen for the following conditions, *which could be cautions or contraindications to use of the drug:* history of allergy to vitamin D, hypercalcemia, vitamin toxicity, renal stone, and pregnancy or lactation.

Include screening *for baseline status before beginning therapy and for any potential adverse effects:* the presence of any skin lesions; orientation and affect; liver evaluation; serum calcium, magnesium, and alkaline phosphate levels; and radiographs of bones as appropriate.

Nursing Diagnoses

The patient receiving any antihypocalcemic drug may have the following nursing diagnoses related to drug therapy:

- Acute Pain related to GI or CNS effects
- Imbalanced Nutrition: Less Than Body Requirements related to GI effects
- Deficient Knowledge regarding drug therapy

Implementation With Rationale

- Monitor serum calcium concentration before and periodically during treatment, *to allow for adjustment of dosage to maintain calcium levels within normal limits.*
- Provide supportive measures *to help the patient deal with GI and CNS effects of the drug* (analgesics, small and frequent meals, help with activities of daily living).

- Arrange for a nutritional consultation if GI effects are severe, *to ensure nutritional balance.*
- Provide thorough patient teaching, including measures to avoid adverse effects, warning signs of problems, and the need for regular evaluation, *to enhance the patient's knowledge about drug therapy and promote compliance.*

Evaluation

- Monitor patient response to the drug (return of serum calcium levels to normal).
- Monitor for adverse effects (weakness, headache, GI effects).
- Evaluate the effectiveness of the teaching plan (patient can name drug, dosage, adverse effects to watch for, and specific measures to avoid adverse effects).
- Monitor the effectiveness of comfort measures and compliance to the regimen.

Antihypercalcemic Agents

Drugs used to treat PTH excess or high levels of serum calcium (**hypercalcemia**) include the **bisphosphonates** and calcitonin (human and salmon). These drugs act on the serum levels of calcium and not directly on the parathyroid gland or PTH.

Bisphosphonates

The bisphosphonates include etidronate (*Didronel*), ibandronate (*Boniva*), pamidronate (*Aredia*), risedronate (*Actonel*), tiludronate (*Skelid*), alendronate (*Fosamax*), and zoledronic acid (*Zometa*), as shown in Table 37.5. These drugs act to slow or block bone resorption; by doing this, they help to lower serum calcium levels.

Therapeutic Actions and Indications

The bisphosphonates slow normal and abnormal bone resorption but do not inhibit normal bone formation and mineralization. These drugs are used in the treatment of Paget's disease and of postmenopausal osteoporosis in women, and alendronate is used to treat osteoporosis in men. Pamidronate, etidronate, and zoledronic acid are also used for the treatment of hypercalcemia of malignancy and of osteolytic bone lesions in certain cancer patients, Ibandronate is approved only for the prevention and treatment of postmenopausal osteoporosis and is available in a once-a-month dose form. Tiludronate is reserved for use in the treatment of Paget's disease if there is no response to other therapy. Risedronate is used daily for 2 months to treat Paget's disease in symptomatic people who are at risk for complications.

Pharmacokinetics

These drugs are well absorbed from the small intestine and do not undergo metabolism. They are excreted relatively unchanged in the urine. Patients with renal dysfunction may experience toxic levels of the drug and should be evaluated for a dosage reduction. Fetal abnormalities have been associated with these drugs in animal trials, and they should not

Table 37.5 DRUGS IN FOCUS

Bisphosphonates

Drug Name	Dosage/Route	Usual Indications
P alendronate (*Fosamax*)	10 mg/day PO; for males and for postmenopausal osteoporosis, 70 mg PO every week or 10 mg/day PO for treatment, 35 mg PO every week or 5 mg/day PO for prevention	Treatment of Paget's disease, postmenopausal osteoporosis treatment and prevention, treatment of glucocorticoid-induced osteoporosis, osteoporosis in men
etidronate (*Didronel*)	5–10 mg/kg/day PO; 7.5 mg/kg/day IV for 3 days for hypercalcemia of malignancy	Treatment of Paget's disease, postmenopausal osteoporosis, hypercalcemia of malignancy, osteolytic bone lesions in cancer patients
ibandronate (*Boniva*)	2.5 mg/day PO or 150 mg PO once per month on the same day each month	Treatment and prevention of osteoporosis in postmenopausal women
pamidronate (*Aredia*)	60–90 mg IV	Treatment of hypercalcemia of malignancy, osteolytic bone lesions in cancer patients
risedronate (*Actonel*)	30 mg/day PO for 2 mo; reduce dosage in renal dysfunction; 5 mg/day PO for osteoporosis	Treatment of symptomatic Paget's disease; osteoporosis
tiludronate (*Skelid*)	400 mg/day PO for 3 mo; reduce dosage with renal impairment	Treatment of Paget's disease that is not responsive to other treatment
zoledronic acid (*Zometa*)	4 mg IV as a single infusion over not less than 15 min	Treatment of hypercalcemia of malignancy

be used during pregnancy unless the benefit to the mother clearly outweighs the potential risk to the fetus. Extreme caution should be used when nursing because of the potential for adverse effects on the baby. Alendronate should not be used by nursing mothers.

Contraindications and Cautions

These drugs should not be used in the presence of hypocalcemia, *which could be made worse by lowering calcium levels;* during pregnancy or lactation, *because of the potential for adverse effects on the fetus or neonate;* or with a history of any allergy to bisphosphonates.

Caution should be used in patients with renal dysfunction, *which could interfere with excretion of the drug,* or with upper GI disease, *which could be aggravated by the drug.* Alendronate and risedronate should not be given to anyone who is unable to remain upright for 30 minutes after taking the drug, *because serious esophageal erosion can occur.* Taking the drug with a full glass of water and remaining upright for at least 30 minutes facilitates delivery of the drug to the stomach. These drugs need to be taken on arising in the morning, with a full glass of water, fully 30 minutes before any other food or beverage. The patient must then remain upright for at least 30 minutes. Zoledronic acid should be used cautiously in aspirin-sensitive asthmatic patients. Alendronate and risedronate are now available in a once-a-week formulation to decrease the number of times the patient must take the drug, which should increase compliance with the drug regimen.

Adverse Effects

The most common adverse effects seen with bisphosphonates are headache, nausea, and diarrhea. There is also an increase in bone pain in patients with Paget's disease, but this effect usually passes after a few days to a few weeks. Esophageal erosion has been associated with alendronate, ibandronate and risedronate if the patient has not remained upright for at least 30 minutes after taking the tablets.

Clinically Important Drug–Drug Interactions

Oral absorption of bisphosphonates is decreased if they are taken concurrently with antacids, calcium products, iron, or multiple vitamins. If these drugs need to be taken, they should be separated by at least 30 minutes.

GI distress may increase if bisphosphonates are combined with aspirin; this combination should be avoided if possible.

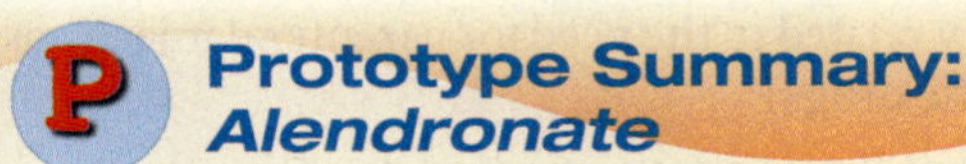

Prototype Summary: Alendronate

Indications: Treatment and prevention of osteoporosis in postmenopausal women and in men; treatment of glucocorticoid-induced osteoporosis; treatment of Paget's disease in certain patients

Actions: Slows normal and abnormal bone resorption without inhibiting bone formation and mineralization

Pharmacokinetics:

Route	Onset	Duration
PO	Slow	Days

$T_{1/2}$: >10 days; not metabolized, but excreted in the urine

Adverse effects: Headache, nausea, diarrhea, increased or recurrent bone pain, esophageal erosion

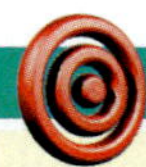

FOCUS POINTS

- Parathyroid glands produce PTH, which, together with calcitonin, maintains the body's calcium balance.
- A low calcium level (hypocalcemia) is treated with vitamin D and calcium replacement therapy.
- Hypercalcemia and hypercalcemic states are associated with postmenopausal osteoporosis, Paget's disease, and malignancies.

Calcitonins

The calcitonins are hormones secreted by the thyroid gland to balance the effects of PTH. They are available as synthetic human calcitonin (*Cibacalcin*) or salmon calcitonin (*Calcimar* and others), as shown in Table 37.6.

Therapeutic Actions and Indications

These hormones inhibit bone resorption; lower serum calcium levels in children and in patients with Paget's disease; and increase the excretion of phosphate, calcium, and sodium from the kidney. Human calcitonin is now approved only for orphan drug use in treating Paget's disease. Salmon calcitonin, which has a longer duration of action, has more approved uses. For example, it is recommended for the treatment of Paget's disease, for the treatment of postmenopausal osteoporosis in conjunction with vitamin D and calcium supplements, and for the emergency treatment of hypercalcemia. Human calcitonin can be given only by injection. Salmon calcitonin can be given by injection and most recently as a nasal spray.

Pharmacokinetics

These drugs are metabolized in the body tissues to inactive fragments, which are excreted by the kidney. They cross the placenta and have been associated with adverse effects on the fetus in animal studies. They should be used in pregnancy only if the benefit to the mother clearly outweighs

Table 37.6 DRUGS IN FOCUS

Calcitonins

Drug Name	Dosage/Route	Usual Indications
calcitonin, human (*Cibacalcin*)	0.5 mg/day Sub-Q	Treatment of Paget's disease
P calcitonin, salmon (*Calcimar* and others)	Paget's disease: 50–100 International Units/day Sub-Q or IM Postmenopausal osteoporosis: 100 International Units/day Sub-Q or IM with calcium and vitamin D Hypercalcemia: 4–8 International Units/kg Sub-Q or IM q12h	Treatment of Paget's disease, postmenopausal osteoarthritis, emergency treatment of hypercalcemia
calcitonin, salmon (*Fortical*)	Postmenopausal osteoporosis: one spray (200 International Units)/day intranasally; alternate nostrils daily	

the potential risk to the fetus. These drugs inhibit lactation in animals; it is not known whether they are excreted in breast milk.

Contraindications and Cautions

These drugs should not be used during lactation, *because the calcium-lowering effects could cause problems for the baby.* Salmon calcitonin should not be used with a known allergy to salmon or fish products. Caution should be used in patients with renal dysfunction or pernicious anemia, *which could be exacerbated by these drugs.*

Adverse Effects

The most common adverse effects seen with these drugs are flushing of the face and hands, skin rash, nausea and vomiting, urinary frequency, and local inflammation at the site of injection. Many of these side effects lessen with time, the time varying with each individual patient.

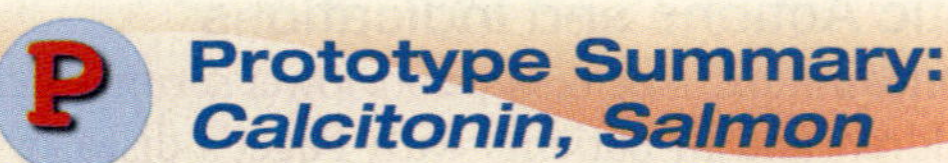

Prototype Summary: Calcitonin, Salmon

Indications: Paget's disease, postmenopausal osteoporosis, emergency treatment of hypercalcemia

Actions: Inhibits bone resorption; lowers elevated serum calcium in children and patients with Paget's disease; increases the excretion of filtered phosphate, calcium, and sodium by the kidney

Pharmacokinetics:

Route	Onset	Peak	Duration
IM, Sub-Q	15 min	3–4 h	8–24 h
Nasal	Rapid	31–39 min	8–24 h

$T_{1/2}$: 1.43 hours; metabolized in the kidneys and excreted in urine

Adverse effects: Flushing of face and hands, nausea, vomiting, local inflammatory reactions at injection site, nasal irritation if nasal form is used

Nursing Considerations for Patients Receiving Antihypercalcemic Agents

Assessment: History and Examination

Screen for the following conditions, *which could be cautions or contraindications to use of the drug:* history of allergy to any of these products, or to fish products with salmon calcitonin; pregnancy or lactation; hypocalcemia; and renal dysfunction.

Include screening *for baseline status before beginning therapy and for any potential adverse effects:* presence of any skin lesions; orientation and affect; abdominal examination; serum electrolytes; and renal function tests.

Nursing Diagnoses

The patient receiving any antihypercalcemic agent may have the following nursing diagnoses related to drug therapy:

- Acute Pain related to GI or skin effects
- Imbalanced Nutrition: Less Than Body Requirements related to GI effects
- Anxiety related to the need for parenteral injections (specific drugs)
- Deficient Knowledge regarding drug therapy

Implementation With Rationale

- Ensure adequate hydration with any of these agents, *to reduce risk of renal complications.*

- Arrange for concomitant vitamin D, calcium supplements, and hormone replacement therapy *if used to treat postmenopausal osteoporosis.*
- Rotate injection sites and monitor for inflammation if using calcitonins, *to prevent tissue breakdown and irritation.*
- Monitor serum calcium regularly, *to allow for dosage adjustment as needed.*
- Assess the patient carefully for any potential drug–drug interactions if giving in combination with other drugs, *to prevent serious effects.*
- Arrange for periodic blood tests of renal function if using gallium, *to monitor for renal dysfunction.*
- Provide comfort measures and analgesics, *to relieve bone pain if it returns as treatment begins.*
- Provide thorough patient teaching, including measures to avoid adverse effects, warning signs of problems, the need for regular evaluation if used for longer than recommended, and proper administration of nasal spray *to enhance patient knowledge about drug therapy and promote compliance.*

Evaluation

- Monitor patient response to the drug (return of calcium levels to normal; prevention of complications of osteoporosis; control of Paget's disease).
- Monitor for adverse effects (skin rash; nausea and vomiting; hypocalcemia; renal dysfunction).
- Evaluate the effectiveness of the teaching plan (patient can name drug, dosage, adverse effects to watch for, specific measures to avoid adverse effects).
- Monitor the effectiveness of comfort measures and compliance to the regimen.

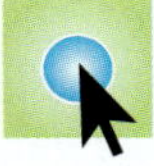

WEB LINKS

Patients and health care providers may want to consult the following Internet sources:

http://www.the-thyroid-society.org Information on thyroid diseases, support groups, treatments, research.

http://www.endo-society.org Information on endocrine diseases, screening, and treatment.

http://www.nof.org Information on osteoporosis—support groups, screening, treatment, and research.

http://www.osteorec.com Information on national and international research on osteoporosis and related bone diseases.

Points to Remember

- The thyroid gland uses iodine to produce thyroid hormones. Thyroid hormones control the rate at which most body cells use energy (metabolism).
- Control of the thyroid gland is an intricate balance between TRH, released by the hypothalamus; TSH, released by the anterior pituitary; and circulating levels of thyroid hormone.
- Hypothyroidism, or lower-than-normal levels of thyroid hormone, is treated with replacement thyroid hormone.
- Hyperthyroidism, or higher-than-normal levels of thyroid hormone, is treated with thioamides, which block the thyroid from producing thyroid hormone, or with iodines, which prevent thyroid hormone production or destroy parts of the gland.
- The parathyroid glands are located behind the thyroid gland and produce PTH, which works with calcitonin, produced by thyroid cells, to maintain the calcium balance in the body.
- Hypocalcemia, or low levels of calcium, is treated with vitamin D products and calcium replacement therapy.
- Hypercalcemia and hypercalcemic states include postmenopausal osteoporosis and Paget's disease, as well as hypercalcemia related to malignancy.
- Hypercalcemia is treated with bisphosphonates or calcitonin. Bisphosphonates slow or block bone resorption, which lowers serum calcium levels. Calcitonin inhibits bone resorption; lowers serum calcium levels in children and patients with Paget's disease; and increases the excretion of phosphate, calcium, and sodium from the kidney.

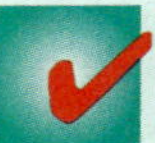

CHECK YOUR UNDERSTANDING

Answers to the questions in this chapter may be found in the Answer Key in the back of the book.

Multiple Choice

Select the best answer to the following.

1. The thyroid gland produces the thyroid hormones T_3 and T_4, which are dependent on the availability of
   a. iodine produced in the liver.
   b. iodine found in the diet.
   c. iron absorbed from the gastrointestinal tract.
   d. parathyroid hormone to promote iodine binding.

2. The thyroid gland is dependent on the hypothalamic–pituitary axis for regulation. Increasing the levels of thyroid hormone (by taking replacement thyroid hormone) would
   a. increase hypothalamic release of TRH.
   b. increase pituitary release of TSH.
   c. suppress hypothalamic release of TRH.
   d. stimulate the thyroid gland to produce more T_3 and T_4.

3. Goiter, or enlargement of the thyroid gland, is usually associated with
   a. hypothyroidism.
   b. iodine deficiency.
   c. hyperthyroidism.
   d. underactive thyroid tissue.

4. Thyroid replacement therapy is indicated for the treatment of
   a. obesity.
   b. myxedema.
   c. Graves' disease.
   d. acute thyrotoxicosis.

5. Assessing a patient's knowledge of his or her thyroid replacement therapy would show good understanding if the patient stated:
   a. "My wife may use some of my drug, since she wants to lose weight."
   b. "I should only need this drug for about 3 months."
   c. "I can stop taking this drug as soon as I feel like my old self."
   d. "I should call if I experience unusual sweating, weight gain, or chills and fever."

6. Administration of propylthiouracil would include giving the drug
   a. once a day in the morning.
   b. around the clock to assure therapeutic levels.
   c. once a day at bedtime to decrease adverse effects.
   d. if the patient is experiencing slow heart rate, skin rash, or excessive bleeding.

7. The parathyroid glands produce PTH, which is important in the body as
   a. a modulator of thyroid hormone.
   b. a regulator of potassium.
   c. a regulator of calcium.
   d. an activator of vitamin D.

8. A drug of choice for the treatment of postmenopausal osteoporosis would be
   a. risedronate.
   b. alendronate.
   c. tiludronate.
   d. calcitriol.

Multiple Response

Select all that apply.

1. A patient who is receiving a bisphosphonate for the treatment of postmenopausal osteoporosis should be taught
   a. to also take vitamin D, calcium, and hormone replacement.
   b. to restrict fluids as much as possible.
   c. to take the drug before any food for the day, with a full glass of water.
   d. to stay upright for at least one-half hour after taking the drug.
   e. to take the drug with meals to avoid GI upset.
   f. to avoid exercise to prevent bone fractures.

2. Hypothyroidism is a very common and often missed disorder. Signs and symptoms of hypothyroidism include
   a. increased body temperature.
   b. thickening of the tongue.
   c. bradycardia.
   d. loss of hair.
   e. excessive weight loss.
   f. oily skin.

Matching

Match the following words with the appropriate choice.

1. ____________________ iodine
2. ____________________ thyroxine
3. ____________________ liothyronine
4. ____________________ calcitonin

5. ________________________ hypothyroidism
6. ________________________ cretinism
7. ________________________ myxedema
8. ________________________ hyperthyroidism
9. ________________________ thioamides
10. ________________________ Paget's disease

A. T_4
B. Hormone produced by the thyroid
C. Lack of thyroid hormone in the infant
D. Excess levels of thyroid hormone
E. Dietary element used to produce thyroid hormone
F. T_3
G. Drugs used to prevent the formation of thyroid hormone
H. Severe lack of thyroid hormone in adults
I. Disorder of overactive osteoclasts
J. Lack of sufficient thyroid hormone to maintain metabolism

Word Scramble

Unscramble the following letters to form words related to thyroid and parathyroid glands.

1. ccnniiloat ________________________
2. oxtnihery ________________________
3. mertiiscn ________________________
4. sseothapnsoihbp ________________________
5. thromonearap ________________________
6. inodei ________________________
7. oooossstepir ________________________
8. mhstirdeipoyrhy ________________________
9. madeyemx ________________________
10. irloontihnye ________________________

Bibliography and References

AMA drug evaluations. (2004). Chicago: American Medical Association.

Drug facts and comparisons. (2006). St. Louis: Fact and Comparisons.

Gilman, A., Hardman, J. G., & Limbird, L. E. (Eds.). (2006). *Goodman and Gilman's the pharmacological basis of therapeutics* (11th ed.). New York: McGraw-Hill.

Karch, A. M. (2006). *2007 Lippincott's nursing drug guide.* Philadelphia: Lippincott Williams & Wilkins.

The medical letter on drugs and therapeutics. (2006). New Rochelle, NY: Medical Letter.

CHAPTER 38

Antidiabetic Agents

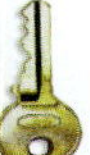

KEY TERMS

diabetes mellitus
glycogen
glycosuria
glycosylated hemoglobin
hyperglycemia
hypoglycemia
insulin
ketosis
polydipsia
polyphagia
sulfonylureas

LEARNING OBJECTIVES

Upon completion of this chapter, you will be able to:

1. Describe the pathophysiology of diabetes mellitus, including alterations in metabolic pathways and changes to basement membranes.
2. Describe the therapeutic actions, indications, pharmacokinetics, contraindications, most common adverse reactions, and important drug–drug interactions associated with insulin and other antidiabetic and glucose-elevating agents.
3. Discuss the use of antidiabetic and glucose-elevating agents across the lifespan.
4. Compare and contrast the prototype drugs insulin, chlorpropamide, glyburide, and metformin with other antidiabetic agents in their class.
5. Outline the nursing considerations, including important teaching points, for patients receiving an antidiabetic or glucose-elevating agent.

PARENTERAL ANTIDIABETIC AGENT

P insulin

OTHER ANTIDIABETIC AGENTS

Sulfonylureas: First Generation

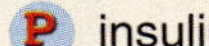

P chlorpropamide
tolazamide
tolbutamide

Sulfonylureas: Second Generation

glimepiride
glipizide
P glyburide

Nonsulfonylureas

acarbose
exenatide
P metformin
miglitol
nateglinide
pioglitazone
pramlintide
repaglinide
rosiglitazone

GLUCOSE-ELEVATING AGENTS

diazoxide
glucagon

Diabetes mellitus is the most common of all metabolic disorders. It is estimated that 8 million people in the United States have been diagnosed with diabetes mellitus, and there are many others not yet diagnosed. Diabetes is a complicated disorder that affects many end organs and causes numerous clinical complications. Currently, treatment of diabetes is aimed at tightly regulating the blood sugar level through the use of insulin or insulin-stimulating drugs.

Glucose Regulation

Glucose is the leading energy source for the human body. Glucose is stored in the body for rapid release in times of stress and so that the serum concentration of glucose can be maintained at a level that provides a constant supply of glucose to the neurons. The minute-to-minute control of glucose levels is the function of the endocrine pancreas gland.

The Pancreas and Insulin

The pancreas is both an endocrine gland, producing hormones, and an exocrine gland, releasing sodium bicarbonate and pancreatic enzymes directly into the common bile duct to be released into the small intestine, where they neutralize the acid chyme from the stomach and aid digestion. The endocrine part of the pancreas produces hormones in collections of tissue called the islets of Langerhans. These islets contain endocrine cells that produce specific hormones. The alpha cells release glucagon in response to low glucose levels. The beta cells release insulin in response to high glucose levels. Delta cells produce somatostatin, which blocks the secretion of insulin and glucagon. These hormones work together to maintain the serum glucose level within normal limits.

Insulin is the hormone produced by the beta cells of the islets of Langerhans. The hormone is released into circulation when the levels of glucose around these cells rise. Insulin circulates through the body and reacts with specific insulin receptor sites to stimulate the transport of glucose into the cells to be used for energy, a process called facilitated diffusion. Insulin also stimulates the synthesis of **glycogen** (glucose stored for immediate release during times of stress or low glucose), the conversion of lipids into fat stored in the form of adipose tissue, and the synthesis of needed proteins from amino acids.

Insulin is released after a meal, when the blood glucose levels rise. It circulates and affects metabolism, allowing the body to either store or use the nutrients from the meal effectively. As a result of the insulin release, blood glucose levels fall and insulin release drops off. Sometimes, an insufficient amount of insulin is released. This may occur because the pancreas cannot produce enough insulin, the insulin receptor sites have lost their sensitivity to insulin, or the person does not have enough receptor sites to support his or her body size, as in obesity.

When an insufficient amount of insulin is released, several metabolic changes occur, beginning with **hyperglycemia** or increased blood sugar. Hyperglycemia results in **glycosuria**: sugar is spilled into the urine because the concentration of glucose in the blood is too high for complete reabsorption. Because this sugar-rich urine is an ideal environment for bacteria, cystitis is a common finding. The patient experiences fatigue because the body's cells cannot use the glucose that is there; they need insulin to facilitate transport of the glucose into the cells. **Polyphagia** (increased hunger) occurs because the hypothalamic centers cannot take in glucose and sense that they are starving. **Polydipsia** (increased thirst) occurs because the tonicity of the blood is increased owing to the increased glucose and waste products in the blood and the loss of fluid with glucose in the urine. (The hypothalamic cells that are sensitive to fluid levels sense a need to increase fluid in the system, and the patient feels thirsty.)

Lipolysis, or fat breakdown, occurs as the body breaks down stored fat for energy because glucose is not usable. The patient experiences **ketosis** as metabolism shifts to the use of fat and the ketone wastes cannot be removed effectively. Acidosis also occurs because the liver cannot remove all of the waste products (acid being a primary waste product) that result from the breakdown of glucose, fat, and proteins. Muscles break down because proteins are no longer being built and because the body breaks down proteins for their essential amino acids. The breakdown of proteins results in an increase in nitrogen wastes, which is manifested in an elevated blood urea nitrogen (BUN) concentration and sometimes in protein in the urine. Patients with hyperglycemia do not heal quickly because of this breakdown of proteins and the lack of a stimulus to build proteins. All of these actions eventually contribute to development of the complications associated with chronic hyperglycemia or diabetes.

Diabetes Mellitus

Diabetes mellitus (literally, "honey urine") is characterized by complex disturbances in metabolism. Diabetes affects carbohydrate, protein, and fat metabolism. The most frequently recognized clinical signs of diabetes are hyperglycemia (fasting blood sugar level greater than 126 mg/dL) and glycosuria (the presence of sugar in the urine). The alterations in the body's ability to effectively deal with carbohydrate, fat, and protein metabolism over the long term results in a thickening of the basement membrane (a thin layer of collagen filament that lies just below the endothelial lining of blood vessels) in large and small blood vessels. This thickening leads to changes in oxygenation of the lining of the vessel; damage to the vessel lining, which leads to narrowing and decreased blood flow through the vessel; and an inability of oxygen to rapidly diffuse across the membrane to the tissues. These changes result in an increased incidence of a number of disorders, including the following:

- *Atherosclerosis:* Heart attacks and strokes related to the development of atherosclerotic plaques in the vessel lining
- *Retinopathy:* With resultant loss of vision as tiny vessels in the eye are narrowed and closed
- *Neuropathies:* With motor and sensory changes in the feet and legs and progressive changes in other nerves as the oxygen supply to these nerves is slowly cut off
- *Nephropathy:* With renal dysfunction related to changes in the basement membrane of the glomerulus

The overall metabolic disturbances associated with diabetes are thought to be caused by a lack of the hormone insulin. There is debate over whether lack of insulin leads to the basement membrane changes and complications of diabetes, or whether the basement membrane thickening is the initial problem that leads to lack of insulin. Whichever comes first, replacement or stimulation of insulin release is the mainstay for treatment of diabetes mellitus. The diagnosis of diabetes mellitus has involved monitoring of fasting blood glucose levels and sometimes challenging the system with glucose for a glucose tolerance test.

Recent research indicates that the body's response to food may be a more important indicator of impending diabetes, and it is now believed that a fasting blood glucose level may not be as important as a postprandial blood glucose level, which reveals the body's ability to respond to a glucose challenge. The importance of looking at a variety of different glucose markers is being stressed today. **Glycosylated hemoglobin** levels, or an HbA1c test, provide a 3-month average of glucose levels. Red blood cells are freely permeable to glucose, and this test gives an average range of glucose exposure over the life of the red blood cell, about 120 days. This test does not require fasting before blood is drawn or the oral intake of glucose before testing. Elevations above 6% may be an early indicator of a prediabetic state, before changes are noted in the fasting blood sugar level. Once a baseline is established, the goal of therapy for a diabetic patient is an HbA1c level less than 7%. Researchers believe that very early intervention—diet, exercise, and lifestyle changes—may delay the onset of diabetes and the complications, including coronary artery disease, that come with it (Abraira & Duckworth, 2003).

Diabetes mellitus is classified as either type 1, insulin-dependent diabetes mellitus (IDDM), or type 2, non–insulin-dependent diabetes mellitus (NIDDM). Type 1 diabetes is usually associated with rapid onset, mostly in younger people, and is connected in many cases to viral destruction of the beta cells of the pancreas. Type 1 diabetes always requires insulin replacement. (See Critical Thinking Scenario 38-1, pps. 608–609, for an example of handling this type of diabetes.)

Type 2 diabetes usually occurs in mature adults and has a slow and progressive onset. However, studies released in 2001 reported that the incidence of type 2 diabetes in teenagers and young adults is increasing markedly (Levetan, 2001). Questions are being raised about the impact of early diet and lack of exercise in contributing to this new increase in type 2 diabetes in young people. The treatment of type 2 diabetes usually begins with changes in diet and exercise. Dieting controls the amount and timing of glucose introduction into the body, and weight loss decreases the number of insulin receptor sites that need to be stimulated. Exercise increases the movement of glucose into the cells by activation of the sympathetic nervous system (SNS) and by the increase of potassium in the blood that occurs directly after exercising. Potassium acts as part of a polarizing system during exercise that pushes glucose into the cells. Clinical studies have shown that controlling serum glucose levels can decrease the risk of complications by up to 40% (ADA, 2002). Box 38.1 describes the treatment of diabetes for all age groups. Cultural variations among diabetics are described in Box 38.2.

When diet and exercise no longer work, oral agents (discussed later) are tried, to stimulate the production of insulin in the pancreas, increase the sensitivity of the insulin receptor sites, or control the entry of glucose into the system. Injection of insulin may eventually be needed to replace the missing insulin. This concept is often confusing to patients who are learning about diabetes. NIDDM (type 2) often evolves until insulin is needed. Timing of the injections of insulin is correlated with food intake and anticipated increases in blood glucose levels as well as exercise levels and anticipated stress (ADA, 2002). See Box 38.3 for more information about managing glucose levels during stress.

Hyperglycemia

Hyperglycemia, or high blood sugar, results when there is insufficient insulin to deal with the glucose in the system. Clinical signs and symptoms of hyperglycemia include fatigue, lethargy, irritation, glycosuria, polyphagia, polydipsia, and itchy skin (from accumulation of wastes that the liver cannot clear). If the hyperglycemia goes unchecked, the patient will experience ketoacidosis and central nervous system (CNS) changes that can progress to coma. Signs of impending dangerous complications of hyperglycemia include the following:

- Fruity breath as the ketones build up in the system and are excreted through the lungs
- Dehydration as fluid and important electrolytes are lost through the kidneys
- Slow, deep respirations (Kussmaul's respirations) as the body tries to rid itself of high acid levels
- Loss of orientation and coma

This level of hyperglycemia needs to be treated immediately with insulin.

Hypoglycemia

Hypoglycemia, or a blood sugar concentration lower than 40 mg/dL, occurs in a number of clinical situations, including starvation, and if treatment of hyperglycemia with insu-

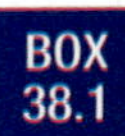

BOX 38.1 DRUG THERAPY ACROSS THE LIFESPAN

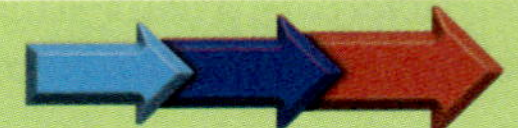

Antidiabetic Agents

CHILDREN

Oral antidiabetic agents have not been proven to be safe or effective for use in children. With the increasing number of children being diagnosed with type 2 diabetes, the use of these agents in children may be tested.

Treatment of diabetes in children is a difficult challenge of balancing diet, activity, growth and stress needs, and insulin requirements. Children need to be carefully monitored for any sign of hypoglycemia or hyperglycemia and treated quickly, because their fast metabolism and lack of body reserves can push them into a severe state quickly.

Insulin dosage, especially in infants, may be so small that the dose is difficult to calibrate. Insulin often needs to be diluted to a volume that can be detected on the syringe. A second person should always check the calculations and dosage of insulin being given to small children.

Teenage children often present a real challenge for diabetes management. The desire to be "normal" often leads to a resistance to dietary restrictions and insulin injections. The metabolism of the teenager is also in flux, leading to complications in regulating insulin dosage. A team approach, including the child, family members, teachers, coaches, and even friends, may be the best way to help the child deal with the disease and the required therapy. New delivery methods for insulin may help this age group cope with the drug therapy in the future.

ADULTS

Adults need extensive education about the disease as well as the drug therapy. Warning signs and symptoms should be stressed repeatedly as the adult learns to juggle insulin needs with exercise, stressors, other drug effects, and diet. Adults maintained on oral agents need to be monitored for changes in response to the drugs. Often additional drugs are added or dosages are changed as the disease progresses over time.

Exercise and diet should always be emphasized as the mainstay of dealing with diabetes. Adults need to be cautioned about the use of over-the-counter and herbal or alternative therapies. Many of these products contain agents that alter blood glucose levels and will change insulin or oral agent requirements. Adults should always be asked specifically whether they use any of these agents and adjustments made accordingly.

Insulin therapy is the best choice for diabetics during pregnancy and lactation, times of high stress and metabolic demands. Needs may change on a daily basis, and the mother should have ready support and extensive teaching about what to do if hypoglycemia or hyperglycemia occurs. Labor and delivery is often a critical time in diabetes management because of the stress and sudden changes in body fluid volume and hormone levels. The obstetrician and the endocrinologist or primary care provider should consult frequently about the best way to support the patient through this period.

OLDER ADULTS

Older adults can have many underlying problems that complicate diabetic therapy. Poor vision and/or coordination may make it difficult to prepare a syringe. A week's supply of syringes can be prepared and refrigerated for the usual dose of insulin.

Dietary deficiencies related to changes in taste, absorption, or attitude may lead to wide fluctuations in blood sugar levels, making it difficult to control diabetes. Many areas offer nutritional assistance programs for older adults (e.g., Meals on Wheels) or can refer patients to appropriate agencies that might be able to offer assistance.

Older adults have a greater incidence of renal or hepatic impairment, and kidney and liver function should be evaluated before starting any of these drugs. Combinations of oral agents may not be feasible with severe dysfunction, and the patient may need to use insulin to control blood glucose levels.

Older adults should still receive periodic educational reminders about diet, the need for exercise, skin and foot care, and warning signs to report to the health care provider.

The older patient is also more likely to experience end organ damage related to the diabetes—loss of vision, kidney problems, coronary artery disease, infections—and the drug regimen of these patients can become quite complex. Careful screening for drug interactions is an important aspect of the assessment of these patients.

lin or oral agents lowers the blood sugar too far. The body immediately reacts to lowered blood sugar because the cells require glucose to survive, the neurons being among the cells most sensitive to the lack of glucose. The initial reaction to falling blood sugar is parasympathetic stimulation—increased gastrointestinal (GI) activity to increase digestion and absorption. Rather rapidly, the SNS responds with a "fight or flight" reaction that increases blood glucose levels by initiating the breakdown of fat and glycogen to release glucose for rapid energy. The pancreas releases glucagon, a hormone that counters the effects of insulin and works to increase glucose levels. In many cases, the response to the hypoglycemic state causes a hyperglycemic state. Balancing the body's responses to glucose is sometimes difficult when one is trying to treat and control diabetes. Table 38.1 offers a comparison of the signs and symptoms of hyperglycemia and hypoglycemia.

Replacement Insulin

Replacement insulin (Table 38.2) is used to treat type 2 diabetes mellitus in adults who have no response to diet, exercise, and oral agents, and for type 1 diabetics who require replacement insulin. Originally, insulin was prepared from pork and beef pancreas. Today, virtually all insulin is prepared by recombinant DNA technology and is human insulin produced by genetically altered bacteria. This more pure form of insulin is not associated with the sensitivity problems that many patients developed with the animal products. Animal insulins may still be obtained for patients who are most responsive to them, but they are not generally used. Box 38.4 describes the various forms of insulin delivery that are currently available or under study for future use.

BOX 38.2 CULTURAL CONSIDERATIONS FOR DRUG THERAPY

Diabetes and Blood Glucose Variations

Certain cultures tend to have a genetically predetermined variation in blood glucose levels, possibly caused by a variation in metabolism. For example, Native Americans, Hispanic Americans, and Japanese Americans have higher blood glucose levels than white Americans do. The clinical importance of this fact relates to proper screening of patients for hypoglycemia and diabetes mellitus. Patients in these cultural groups who have fasting glucose tolerance tests need to have the standard readjusted before a diagnosis is made. Such patients also require an understanding of potential differences in normal levels on home glucose monitoring units when they are regulating insulin at home.

Cultural groups that are more likely to develop diabetes mellitus include African Americans, Native Americans, and Hispanic Americans. People in these groups should be screened regularly for diabetes. They also can benefit from teaching about warning signs of diabetes.

Therapeutic Actions and Indications

Insulin is a hormone that promotes the storage of the body's fuels; facilitates the transport of various metabolites and ions across cell membranes; and stimulates the synthesis of glycogen from glucose, of fats from lipids, and of proteins from amino acids. Insulin does these things by reacting with specific receptor sites on the cell. Figure 38.1 shows the sites of action of replacement insulin and other drugs used to treat diabetic conditions.

Replacement insulin is used to treat type 1 diabetes mellitus; type 2 diabetes mellitus in patients whose diabetes cannot be controlled by diet or other agents; severe ketoacidosis or diabetic coma; and hyperkalemia with infusion of glucose to produce a shift of potassium into the cells (polarizing solution). It also is used for short courses of therapy during periods of stress (e.g., surgery, disease) in type 2 diabetics, for newly diagnosed patients getting stabilized, for patients with poor control of glucose levels, and for patients with gestational diabetes. Various preparations of insulin are available to provide short- and long-term coverage (Table 38.3). Frequently, patients use more than one preparation to provide insulin coverage at different times during the day.

Pharmacokinetics

The various insulins available are processed within the body like endogenous insulin. The peak, onset, and duration of the different preparations vary with each type of insulin because of the placement or addition of glycine and/or arginine chains. Insulin does not cross the placenta, and it is the drug of choice for managing diabetes during pregnancy. Insulin does enter breast milk, but it is destroyed in the GI tract and does not

BOX 38.3 FOCUS ON THE EVIDENCE

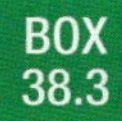

Managing Glucose Levels During Stress

The body has many compensatory mechanisms for ensuring that blood glucose levels stay within a safe range. The sympathetic stress reaction elevates blood glucose levels to provide ready energy for fight or flight (see Chapter 29). The stress reaction causes the breakdown of glycogen to release glucose, and the breakdown of fat and proteins to release other energy.

Stress Reactions

The stress reaction elevates the blood glucose concentration above the normal range. In severe stress situations—such as an acute myocardial infarction or an automobile accident—the blood glucose level can be very high (300–400 mg/dL). The body uses that energy to fight the insult or flee from the stressor.

Nurses in acute care situations need to be aware of this reflex elevation in glucose when caring for patients in acute stress, especially patients in emergency situations whose medical history is unknown. The usual medical response to a blood glucose concentration of 400 mg/dL would be the administration of insulin. In many situations, that is exactly what is done, especially if the patient's history is not known and the effects of such a high glucose level could cause severe systemic reactions. Insulin administration causes a drop in the blood glucose level as glucose enters cells to be either used for energy or converted to glycogen for storage.

However, a problem may arise in the acute care setting, particularly in a nondiabetic patient. Relieving the stress reaction can also drop glucose levels as the stimulus to increase these levels is lost and the glucose that was there is used for energy. A patient in this situation, who has been treated with insulin, is at risk for development of potentially severe hypoglycemia. The body's response to low glucose levels is a sympathetic stress reaction, which again elevates the blood glucose concentration. If treated, the patient potentially can enter a cycle of high and low glucose levels.

Best Nursing Practice

Nurses are often the ones in closest contact with the highly stressed patient—in the emergency room, the intensive care unit, the postanesthesia room—and should be constantly aware of the normal and reflex changes in blood glucose that accompany stress. Careful monitoring, with awareness of stress and the relief of stress, can prevent a prolonged treatment program to maintain blood glucose levels within the range of normal, a situation that is not "normal" during a stress reaction.

Diabetic patients who are in severe stress situations require changes in their insulin dosages. They should be allowed some elevation of blood glucose, even though their inability to produce sufficient insulin will make it difficult for their cells to make effective use of the increased glucose levels. It is a clinical challenge to balance glucose levels with the needs of the patient because so many factors can affect the glucose level.

Source: American Diabetes Association. Standards of Medical Care for Patients with Diabetes Mellitus. (2002). *Clinical Diabetes,* 20, 24–33.

Table 38.1 Signs and Symptoms of Hypoglycemia and Hyperglycemia

System	Hypoglycemia	Hyperglycemia
Central nervous system	Headache, blurred vision, diplopia; drowsiness progressing to coma; ataxia; hyperactive reflexes	Decreased level of consciousness, sluggishness progressing to coma; hypoactive reflexes
Neuromuscular	Paresthesias; weakness; muscle spasms; twitching progressing to seizures	Weakness, lethargy
Cardiovascular	Tachycardia; palpitations; normal to high blood pressure	Tachycardia; hypotension
Respiratory	Rapid, shallow respirations	Rapid, deep respirations (Kussmaul's); acetone-like or fruity breath
Gastrointestinal	Hunger, nausea	Nausea; vomiting; thirst
Other	Diaphoresis; cool and clammy skin; normal eyeballs	Dry, warm, flushed skin; soft eyeballs
Laboratory tests	Urine glucose—negative; blood glucose low	Urine glucose—strongly positive; urine ketone levels—positive; blood glucose levels—high
Onset	Sudden; patient appears anxious, drunk; associated with overdose of insulin, missing a meal, increased stress	Gradual; patient is slow and sluggish; associated with lack of insulin, increased stress

affect the nursing baby. Insulin-dependent mothers may have inhibited milk production, however, and the effectiveness of nursing should be evaluated periodically.

Contraindications and Cautions

Because insulin is used as a replacement hormone, there are no contraindications. Care should be taken during pregnancy and lactation to monitor glucose levels closely and adjust the insulin dosage accordingly. Patients with allergies to beef or pork products should use only human insulins.

Adverse Effects

The most common adverse effects to insulin use are hypoglycemia and ketoacidosis, which can be controlled with proper dosage adjustments, and local reactions at injection sites.

Clinically Important Drug–Drug Interactions

Caution should be used when giving a patient stabilized on insulin any drug that decreases glucose levels (e.g., monoamine oxidase inhibitors, beta-blockers, salicylates, alcohol). Dosage adjustments are needed when any of these drugs is added or removed. Care should also be taken when combining insulin with any beta-blocker. The blocking of the SNS also blocks many of the signs and symptoms of hypoglycemia, hindering the patient's ability to recognize problems. Patients taking beta-blockers need to learn other ways to recognize hypoglycemia. Patients should also be warned about possible interactions with various herbal therapies (Box 38.5).

Nursing Considerations for Patients Taking Insulin

Assessment: History and Examination

Screen for history of allergy to any insulin and for pregnancy or lactation *so that appropriate monitoring and dosage adjustments can be completed.* Include screening for baseline status before beginning therapy and for any potential adverse effects: presence of any skin lesions; orientation and reflexes; baseline pulse and

Table 38.2 DRUGS IN FOCUS

Parenteral Antihyperglycemic Agent

Drug Name	Dosage/Route	Usual Indications
P Insulin (various types)	Varies based on patient response, diet, and activity level	Treatment of diabetes; treatment of diabetes type 2 that cannot be controlled by other means; treatment of severe ketoacidosis; treatment of newly diagnosed diabetes; treatment of hyperkalemia as part of a polarizing solution; treatment of gestational diabetes

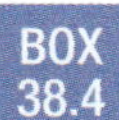

Insulin Delivery—Past, Present, and Future

Past

Subcutaneous Injection—The delivery of insulin by subcutaneous injection was first introduced in the 1920s and changed the way that diabetic patients were managed clinically, giving them a chance for a normal lifestyle. Research is ongoing to find more efficient and acceptable ways to deliver insulin to diabetic patients.

Present

Subcutaneous Insulin Injection—This remains the primary delivery system.

Insulin Jet Injector—This cylindrical device shoots a fine spray of insulin through the skin under very high pressure. Although it is appealing for people who don't like needles or have problems disposing of needles properly, it can be very expensive.

Insulin Pen—This syringe-like device actually looks like a pen. It has a small needle at the tip and a barrel that holds insulin. The patient "dials" the amount of insulin to be given and injects the insulin subcutaneously by pressing on the top of the pen. This is advantageous for people who need insulin two or three times during the day but cannot easily transport syringes and needles. It is a subtle way to give insulin, and is popular with students and business people on the go. It is important to rotate the syringe 15 to 20 times before injecting the insulin, to disperse it. Patients often forget this point after using the pens for awhile, and as a result, may inject far too much or too little insulin when it is needed. Periodic reinforcement of the administration instructions is important.

External Insulin Pump—This pump device can be worn on a belt or hidden in a pocket and is attached to a small tube inserted into the subcutaneous tissue of the abdomen. The device slowly leaks a base rate of insulin into the abdomen all day; the patient can pump or inject booster doses throughout the day to correspond with meals and activity. The device does have several disadvantages. For example, it is awkward, the tubing poses an increased risk of infection and requires frequent changing, and the patient has to frequently check blood glucose levels throughout the day to monitor response.

Long-Acting Insulin—The year 2001 brought the release of a subcutaneous insulin that lasts two to three times longer than NPH insulin. This should decrease the need for multiple injections and may increase glucose control, especially for patients with erratic glucose levels during the night. Long-term effects of this type of insulin therapy are not yet known.

Future

Implantable Insulin Pump—This pump is surgically implanted into the abdomen and delivers base insulin as well as insulin boluses as needed directly into the abdomen to be absorbed by the liver, just as pancreatic insulin is. The disadvantages are risk of infection, mechanical problems with the pump, and lack of long-term data on its effectiveness. This method is not yet available for general use.

Insulin Patch—The patch is placed on the skin and delivers a constant low dose of insulin. When the patient eats a meal, tabs are pulled on the patch to release more insulin. The problem with this delivery method is that insulin does not readily pass through the skin, so there is tremendous variability in its effects. This route is not yet commercially available.

Inhaled Insulin—The lung tissue is one of the best sites for insulin absorption. An aerosol delivery system has been developed that delivers a powdered insulin formulation directly into the lung tissue. Research has been very promising, suggesting that this may be a more reliable method of delivering insulin in the future. However, Phase III studies showed an increase in insulin antibody formation in patients using inhaled insulin in clinical trials, sending the drug back for further refinement and research. Inhaled insulin (*Exubera*) was approved for marketing in early 2006 (see Box 38.6).

For the most up-to-date information on insulin delivery research, visit the following web site: http://www.niddk.nih.gov.

blood pressure; respiration, adventitious breath sounds; urinalysis and blood glucose level.

Nursing Diagnoses

The patient receiving insulin may have the following nursing diagnoses related to drug therapy:

- Imbalanced Nutrition: Less Than Body Requirements, related to metabolic effects
- Disturbed Sensory Perception (Kinesthetic, Visual, Auditory, Tactile) related to glucose levels
- Risk for Infection related to injections and disease process
- Ineffective Coping related to diagnosis and injection therapy
- Deficient Knowledge regarding drug therapy

Implementation With Rationale

- Gently rotate vial and avoid vigorous shaking *to ensure uniform suspension of insulin.*
- Give maintenance doses by the subcutaneous route only (Box 38.7), and rotate injection sites regularly *to avoid damage to muscles and to prevent subcutaneous atrophy.* Give regular insulin intramuscularly or intravenously in emergency situations.

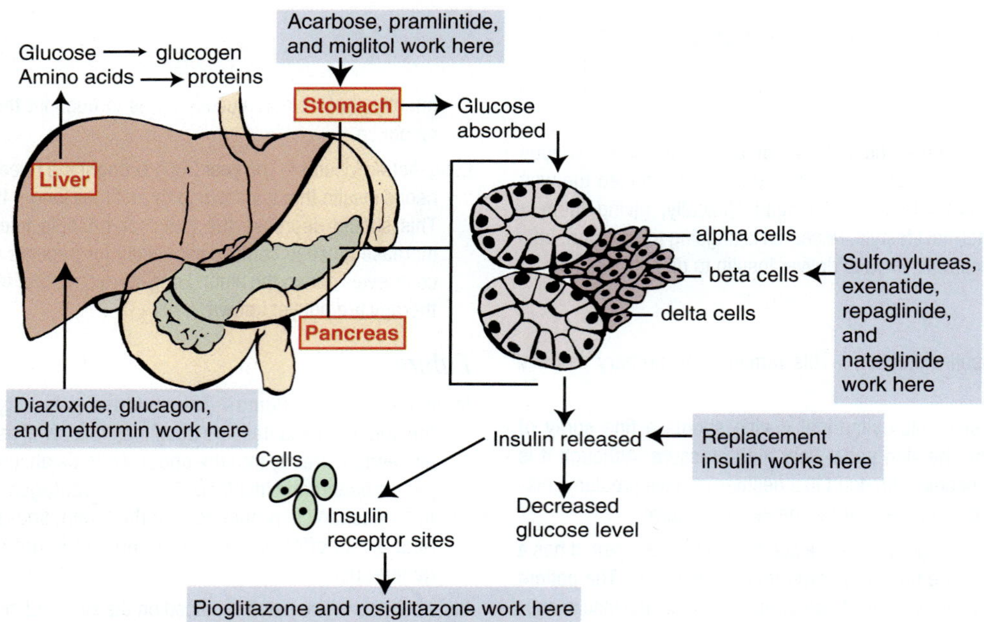

FIGURE 38.1 Sites of action of drugs used to treat diabetic conditions.

Table 38.3 Comparison of Insulin Types

Type	Onset	Peak	Duration
Regular (*Humulin R*)	30–60 min	2–4 h	8–12 h
Semilente NPH (*Humulin N*)	1–1.5 h 60–90 min	5–10 h 4–12 h	12–16 h 24 h
Lente (*Humulin L*)	1–2.5 h	7–15 h	24 h
PZI (*Humulin U*)	4–8 h	14–24 h	36 h
Ultralente (*Humulin U Ultralente*)	4–8 h	10–30 h	20–36 h
Lispro (*Humalog*)	<15 min	30–90 min	2–5 h
Aspart (*NovoLog*)	15 min	1–3 h	3–5 h
Glargine (*Lantus*)	60–70 min	—	24 h
Glulisine (*Apidra*)	2–5 min	30–90 min	1–2.5 h
Detemir (*Levemir*)	1–2 h	6–8 h	24 h
Combination insulins			
NPH and regular (*Humulin 70/30, Novolin 70/30, Humulin 50/50, Humalog 75/25*)	30–60 min, then 1–2 h	2–4 h, then 6–12 h	6–8 h, then 18–24 h
Inhalational (*Exubera*)	10–20 min	2 h	6 h

Insulin is available in various preparations with a wide range of peaks and durations of action. A patient may receive a combination of regular and NPH insulin in the morning to cover the glucose peak from breakfast (regular onset, 30–60 min) and the lunch and dinner glucose peaks. The patient may then require another injection before bed. The types of insulin used are determined by the anticipated eating and exercise activities of any particular patient. It is very important to make sure one is using the correct insulin preparation when administering the drug. Insulin glargine (*Lantus*) and insulin detemir (*Levemir*) cannot be mixed in solution with any other drug, including other insulins.

BOX 38.5 HERBAL AND ALTERNATIVE THERAPIES

Patients being treated with antidiabetic therapies are at an increased risk of developing hypoglycemia if they use juniper berries, ginseng, garlic, fenugreek, coriander, dandelion root, or celery. If a patient uses these therapies, blood glucose levels should be monitored closely and appropriate dosage adjustment made in their prescribed drug.

BOX 38.6 New Delivery Form of Insulin Approved

In early 2006, the Food and Drug Administration (FDA) approved the first new delivery form for insulin since insulin was introduced. Up until this time, injection was the only available delivery form for insulin. Now insulin can be delivered through inhalation, using an insulin inhaler delivery system. *Exubera* is approved for the treatment of adult patients with diabetes mellitus for the control of hyperglycemia. In patients with type 1 diabetes, it is designed to be used in combination with longer-acting insulins; patients with type 2 diabetes can use it as monotherapy or in combination with other antidiabetic agents. *Exubera* has a shorter onset of action than regular insulin and should be taken within 10 minutes of eating a meal. All patients should have pulmonary function tests done before and periodically during therapy, and patients who smoke or who have chronic obstructive pulmonary disorder, asthma, or other lung disease are not candidates for use of this drug, because the membranes in their lungs will not predictably absorb the drug. Hypoglycemia is the most common adverse effect of this form of insulin. Pulmonary function has been shown to decline while using this form of insulin; periodic testing to evaluate pulmonary function should detect this effect. If a decline of 20% occurs, the drug should be stopped and traditional delivery methods used. Patients require teaching in the correct use and care of the inhaler used with *Exubera*. No long-term studies are available, and the FDA will carefully monitor the drug.

- Monitor response carefully, *to avoid adverse effects;* blood glucose monitoring is the most effective way to evaluate insulin dosage.
- Use caution when mixing types of insulin; administer mixtures of regular and NPH or regular and lente insulins within 15 minutes after combining them; do not mix *Lantus* or *Levemir* insulin with any other insulin *to prevent precipitation and ineffective dosing.*
- Store insulin in a cool place away from direct sunlight. Predrawn syringes are stable for 1 week if refrigerated; *they offer a good way to ensure the proper dosage for patients who have limited vision.*
- Monitor patients during times of trauma or severe stress *for potential dosage adjustment needs.*

BOX 38.7 FOCUS ON **CLINICAL SKILLS**

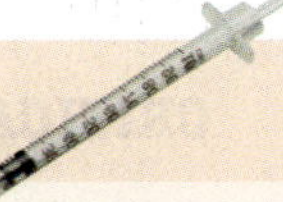

Insulin is usually given by subcutaneous injection. Using an insulin syringe with a 25-gauge, ½-inch needle, inject the insulin into the loose connective tissue underneath the skin. The areas of the body that are best able to be pinched up to access this tissue are the abdomen, the upper thigh, and the upper arm. Insert the needle at a 45-degree angle, and pull the plunger back to ensure that there is no blood and that the needle is not in a vein. Inject the insulin if no blood is returned. Rotate sites regularly to prevent tissue damage.

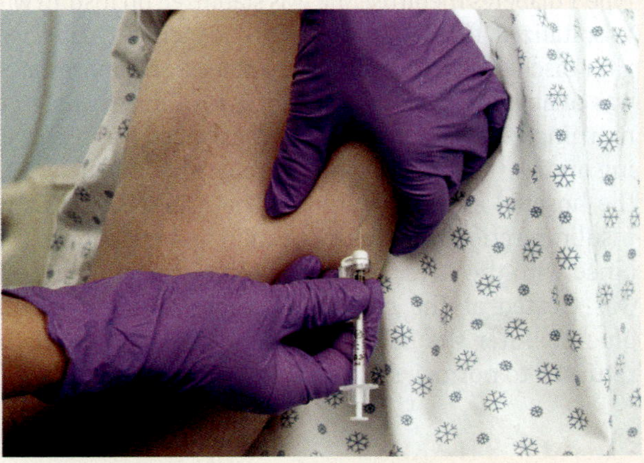

Insert the needle at a 45-degree angle. (Photo by Rick Brady, with permission from Taylor, C., Lillis, C., and LeMone, P. (2005). *Fundamentals of nursing: The art and science of nursing care* (5th ed.). Philadelphia: Lippincott Williams & Wilkins.

Evaluation

- Monitor patient response to the drug (stabilization of blood glucose levels).
- Monitor for adverse effects (hypoglycemia, ketoacidosis, injection site irritation).
- Evaluate the effectiveness of the teaching plan (patient can name drug, dosage, adverse effects to watch for, specific measures to avoid adverse effects, proper administration technique).
- Monitor the effectiveness of comfort measures and compliance to the regimen.
- Instruct patients who are also receiving beta-blockers about ways to monitor glucose levels and signs and symptoms of glucose abnormalities, *to prevent hypoglycemic and hyperglycemic episodes when SNS and warning signs are blocked.*
- Provide thorough patient teaching, including measures to avoid adverse effects, warning signs of problems, proper administration techniques, and the need to monitor disease status, *to enhance patient knowledge about drug therapy and promote compliance.*

CRITICAL THINKING SCENARIO 38-1

Type 1 Diabetes Mellitus

The Situation

M.J. is a 22-year-old woman who has newly diagnosed type 1 diabetes mellitus. She was stabilized on insulin while hospitalized for diagnosis and management. One week after discharge, M.J. experienced nausea and anorexia. She was unable to eat, but she took her insulin as usual in the morning. That afternoon, she experienced profuse sweating and was tremulous and apprehensive, so she went to the hospital emergency room. The initial diagnosis was insulin reaction from taking insulin and not eating, combined with the stress of her gastrointestinal distress. M.J. was treated at the emergency room with intravenous glucose. After she had rested and her glucose levels had returned to normal, she was discharged to home.

Critical Thinking

What instructions should M.J. receive before she leaves? Think about the ways that stress can alter the blood glucose levels. Then consider the stress that a newly diagnosed type 1 diabetic patient undergoes while trying to cope with the diagnosis, learn self-injection, and think about complications of the disease that may arise in the future.

What teaching approaches could help M.J. to decrease her stress and to effectively plan her medical regimen? What sort of support would be useful for M.J. as she adjusts to her new life?

Discussion

The diagnosis of type 1 diabetes is a life-changing event. M.J. had to learn about the disease and how to test her own blood and give herself injections; manage a new diet and exercise program; and cope with the knowledge that the long-term complications of diabetes can be devastating. Many patients who are regulated on insulin in the hospital experience a change in insulin demand after discharge. The sympathetic nervous system (SNS) is active in the hospital, and one of the effects of SNS activity is increased glucose levels—preparing the body for fight or flight. For some patients, returning home eases the stress that activated the SNS, and glucose levels fall. If the patient continues to use the same insulin dose, hypoglycemia can occur. Other patients may feel protected in the hospital and experience stress when they are sent home. They may feel anxious about taking care of themselves while coping with everyday problems and tensions. These patients need an increased insulin dose because their stress reaction intensifies when they get home, driving their blood glucose level up.

Patients are taught how to measure their own blood glucose levels before they leave the hospital. After they get used to doing this and regulating their own insulin based on glucose concentrations, they usually manage well. The first few days to weeks are often the hardest. The nurse should review with M.J. how to test her glucose, draw up her insulin, and regulate the dose. The nurse also should give M.J. written information that she can refer to later.

In addition, the nurse should give M.J. a chance to talk and to vent her feelings about her diagnosis and her future. To help decrease M.J.'s stress and to avoid problems during this adjustment period, the nurse can give M.J. a telephone number to call if she has problems or questions. M.J. should return in a few days to review her progress and have any questions answered. In the meantime, the nurse should encourage M.J. to write down any questions or problems that arise so that they can be addressed during the follow-up visit. Support and encouragement will be crucial to helping M.J. adjust to her disease and her drug therapy. She can also be referred to the American Diabetic Association, which in many communities offers support services to help diabetics.

Nursing Care Guide For M.J.: Type 1 Diabetes Mellitus

Assessment: History And Examination

Review the patient's history for allergies to drug products, pregnancy, breast-feeding, and other drugs in current use. M.J. denies allergies, pregnancy, and lactation. She is taking no other medications.

Focus the physical examination on the following:

Neuro: orientation, reflexes; M.J. appears shaky and pupils are dilated

Skin: coloration and/or lesions; M.J.'s appearance (pale, sweaty) is consistent with diaphoresis

CV: pulse, 110; blood pressure, 155/92

Resp: respiratory rate, 24; lungs clear on auscultation

Lab tests: urinalysis—negative for glucose, positive for ketones; blood glucose level, 72

Type 1 Diabetes Mellitus *(continued)*

Nursing Diagnoses

Imbalanced Nutrition: Less Than Body Requirements, related to metabolic effects

Disturbed Sensory Perception (Kinesthetic, Visual, Auditory, Tactile) related to effects on glucose levels

Risk for Infection related to injections and disease process

Ineffective Coping related to diagnosis and injections

Deficient Knowledge regarding drug therapy

Implementation

Provide patient teaching regarding drug name, dosage, adverse effects, precautions, warning signs to report, and proper administration technique.

Assist M.J. to restore blood glucose to normal levels by using insulin and constant monitoring of blood glucose levels during normal times and during times of stress and trauma so that insulin dosage can be adjusted to needed amount.

Review proper subcutaneous injection technique and site rotation.

Provide support and reassurance to help M.J. deal with drug injections, this hypoglycemic episode, and her lifetime need for insulin.

Teach M.J. how to store insulin in cool place away from light and to use caution when mixing insulin types.

Review with M.J. the name and type of insulin, dosage, adverse effects, precautions, warning signs of adverse effects to report, and proper administration technique.

Evaluation

Evaluate drug effects: return of glucose levels to normal.

Monitor for adverse effects: hypoglycemia and/or injection site reaction.

Monitor for drug–drug interactions as indicated for insulin.

Evaluate effectiveness of patient teaching program and comfort and safety measures.

Patient Teaching For M.J.

- ☐ Insulin is a hormone that is normally produced by your pancreas. It helps to regulate your energy balance by affecting the way the body uses sugar and fats. The lack of insulin produces a disease called diabetes mellitus. By injecting insulin each day, you can help your body use the sugars and fats in your food effectively.
- ☐ Check the expiration date on your insulin. Store the insulin at room temperature and avoid extremes of heat and light. Gently rotate the vial between your palms before use to dispense any crystals that may have formed. Do not shake the vial, because vigorous shaking can inactivate the drug. Rotate your injection sites on a regular basis.
- ☐ A prescription is required to get the syringes that you will need to administer your insulin. Keep the syringes sealed until ready to use, and dispose of them appropriately. Rotate your injection sites regularly to prevent tissue damage and to ensure that the proper amount of insulin is absorbed.
- ☐ You should be aware of the signs and symptoms of hypoglycemia (too much insulin). If any of these occur, eat or drink something high in sugar, such as candy, orange juice, honey, or sugar. The signs and symptoms to watch for include the following: nervousness, anxiety, sweating, pale and cool skin, headache, nausea, hunger, shakiness. These may happen if you skip a meal, exercise too much, or experience extreme stress. If these symptoms happen very often, notify your health care provider. If you cannot eat because of illness or other problems, do not take your usual insulin dose. Contact your health care provider for assistance.
- ☐ Avoid the use of any over-the-counter medications or herbal therapies without first checking with your health care provider. Several of these medications and many commonly used herbs can interfere with the effectiveness of insulin. Avoid the use of alcohol, because it increases the chances of having hypoglycemic attacks.
- ☐ Tell any doctor, nurse, or other health care provider involved in your care that you are taking this drug. You may want to wear or carry a MedicAlert tag showing that you are on this medication. This would alert any medical personnel taking care of you in an emergency to the fact that you are taking this drug.
- ☐ Report any of the following to your health care provider: *loss of appetite, blurred vision, fruity odor to your breath, increased urination, increased thirst, nausea, vomiting.*
- ☐ While you are taking this drug, it is important to have regular medical follow-up, including blood tests to monitor your blood glucose levels, to evaluate you for any adverse effects of your diabetes.
- ☐ Keep this drug and your syringes out of the reach of children. Use proper disposal techniques for your needles and syringes. Do not give this medication to anyone else or take any similar medication that has not been prescribed for you.

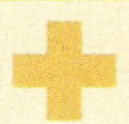

FOCUS ON **PATIENT SAFETY**

Name confusion has occurred between *Lantus* insulin and lente insulin. The pharmacokinetics and dosage vary greatly. Use caution to make sure you know which insulin was intended for your patient. *Lantus* insulin cannot be mixed in a syringe with any other insulin or any other drug. Use caution when working with *Lantus* insulin.

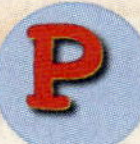

Prototype Summary: *Insulin*

Indications: Treatment of type 1 diabetes; treatment of type 2 diabetes when other agents have failed; short-term treatment of type 2 diabetes during periods of stress; management of diabetic ketoacidosis, hyperkalemia, marked insulin resistance

Actions: Replacement of endogenous insulin

Pharmacokinetics:

Route	Onset	Peak	Duration
Regular	30–60 min	2–3 h	8–12 h
Semilente	1–1.5 h	5–10 h	12–16 h
NPH	1–1.5 h	4–12 h	24 h
Lente	1–2.5 h	7–15 h	24 h
PZI	4–8 h	14–24 h	36 h
Ultralente	4–8 h	10–30 h	20–36 h
Lispro	<15 min	30–90 min	2–5 h
Aspart	15 min	1–3 h	3–5 h
Glargine	60–70 min	None	24 h
Glulisine	2–5 min	30–90 min	1–2.5 h
Detemir	1–2 h	6–8 h	24 h
Inhalation	10–20 min	2 h	6 h

$T_{1/2}$: Varies with each preparation; metabolized at the cellular level

Adverse effects: Hypersensitivity reaction, local reactions at injection site, hypoglycemia, ketoacidosis

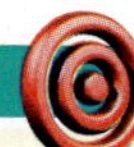

FOCUS POINTS

- Insulin replaces the endogenous hormone when the body does not produce enough insulin or when there are not enough insulin receptor sites to provide adequate glucose control.
- Dosage of insulin will vary with food intake, exercise, and stress levels.
- Patients need to learn to recognize the signs of hypoglycemia and hyperglycemia to effectively manage their drug therapy.

Oral Antidiabetic Agents

Oral drugs are successful in controlling type 2 diabetes in patients who still have a functioning pancreas. The **sulfonylureas** were the first oral agents introduced. They stimulate the pancreas to release insulin. Other oral agents, called nonsulfonylureas, have been introduced more recently. The nonsulfonylureas act to decrease insulin resistance or alter glucose absorption and uptake. They often are combined with a sulfonylurea for effectiveness.

Sulfonylureas

The sulfonylureas (Table 38.4) bind to potassium channels on pancreatic beta cells to increase insulin secretion. They may improve insulin binding to insulin receptors and increase the number of insulin receptors. They are also known to increase the effect of antidiuretic hormone on renal cells. They are effective only in patients who have functioning beta cells. They are not effective for all diabetics and may lose their effectiveness over time with others. All of the sulfonylureas can cause hypoglycemia.

First-Generation Sulfonylureas

The first-generation sulfonylureas include chlorpropamide (*Diabinese*), tolbutamide (*Orinase*), and tolazamide (*Tolinase*). Chlorpropamide is the most frequently used of the group because it has the most predictable effects and has proved to be very reliable. Tolbutamide is preferred for patients with renal dysfunction, who may not be able to excrete chlorpropamide, because it is more easily cleared from the body. Tolazamide, which is used less frequently, is usually tried after the first two drugs have been shown to be ineffective. It is not as predictably effective in many patients, but it can be very effective in some patients who do not respond to chlorpropamide. Tolbutamide and tolazamide are sometimes used in combination with insulin to reduce the insulin dosage and decrease the risk of hypoglycemia in certain type 2 diabetics who have begun to use insulin to control their blood glucose level.

The first-generation sulfonylureas were associated with an increased risk of cardiovascular disease and death in a somewhat controversial study (Chalmers, 1975). They are now thought to possibly cause an increase in cardiovascular deaths.

Table 38.4 DRUGS IN FOCUS

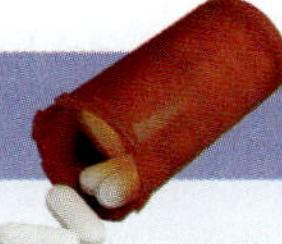

Sulfonylureas

Drug Name	Dosage/Route	Usual Indications
First Generation		
P chlorpropamide (*Diabinese*)	100–250 mg/day PO; use lower doses with geriatric patients	Adjunct to diet for the management of type 2 diabetes
tolazamide (*Tolinase*)	100–250 mg/day PO; use lower doses with geriatric patients	Adjunct to diet for the management of type 2 diabetes; adjunct to insulin for management in certain type 2 diabetics, reducing the insulin dose and decreasing the risks of hypoglycemia
tolbutamide (*Orinase*)	0.25–3 g/day PO; use lower doses with geriatric patients	Adjunct to diet for the management of type 2 diabetes; adjunct to insulin for management in certain type 2 diabetics, reducing the insulin dose and decreasing the risks of hypoglycemia
Second Generation		
glimepiride (*Amaryl*)	1–4 mg/day PO ; use lower doses with geriatric patients	Adjunct to diet for the management of type 2 diabetes; adjunct to insulin for management in certain type 2 diabetics, reducing the insulin dose and decreasing the risks of hypoglycemia
glipizide (*Glucotrol*)	5 mg PO daily, titrate based on response; do not exceed 15 mg/day; use lower doses with geriatric and hepatic-impaired patients; ER: 5 mg/day, adjust to a maximum of 20 mg/day	Adjunct to diet for the management of type 2 diabetes; adjunct to insulin for management in certain type 2 diabetics, reducing the insulin dose and decreasing the risks of hypoglycemia
P glyburide (*DiaBeta, Micronase, Glynase PresTab*)	1.25–20 mg/day PO (*DiaBeta, Micronase*), 0.75–12 mg/day PO (*Glynase*); use lower doses with geriatric patients	Adjunct to diet for the management of type 2 diabetes; adjunct to insulin for management in certain type 2 diabetics, reducing the insulin dose and decreasing the risks of hypoglycemia

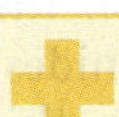

FOCUS ON **PATIENT SAFETY**

Name confusion has been reported between chlorpropamide (the antidiabetic agent *Diabinese*) and chlorpromazine (the antipsychotic agent *Thorazine*). A mix-up can be deadly. Use caution to make sure you know which drug was ordered for your patient.

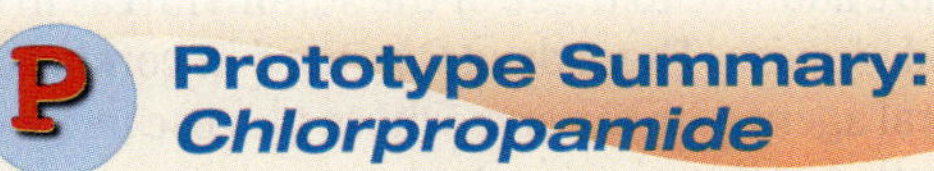

Prototype Summary: Chlorpropamide

Indications: Adjunct to diet and exercise to lower blood glucose level in type 2 diabetics

Actions: Stimulates the release of insulin from functioning cells in the pancreas; may improve binding of insulin to insulin receptor sites or increase the number of insulin receptor sites

Pharmacokinetics:

Route	Onset	Peak	Duration
Oral	1 hr	3–4 h	60 h

$T_{1/2}$: 36 hours; metabolized in the liver and excreted in the urine and bile

Adverse effects: GI discomfort, anorexia, heartburn, vomiting, nausea, hypoglycemia

Second-Generation Sulfonylureas

These drugs have several advantages over the first-generation drugs, including the following:

- Second-generation sulfonylureas are excreted in urine and bile, making them safer for patients with renal dysfunction.
- They do not interact with as many protein-bound drugs as the first-generation drugs do.
- They have a longer duration of action, making it possible to take them only once or twice a day, thus increasing compliance.

The second-generation drugs include glimepiride (*Amaryl*), glipizide (*Glucotrol*), and glyburide (*DiaBeta* and others). Glimepiride is a much less expensive drug than most of the other sulfonylureas, which has advantages for some people. Prescribers may try different agents (first- or second-generation drugs) before finding the one that is most effective for a given patient.

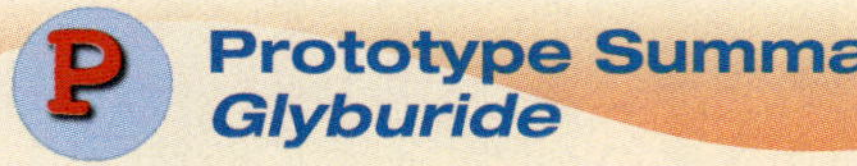

Prototype Summary: Glyburide

Indications: Adjunct to diet and exercise in the management of type 2 diabetes; with metformin or insulin for stabilization of diabetic patients

Actions: Stimulates insulin release from functioning beta cells in the pancreas; may improve insulin binding to insulin receptor sites or increase the number of insulin receptor sites

Pharmacokinetics:

Route	Onset	Duration
Oral	1 h	24 h

$T_{1/2}$: 4 hours; metabolized in the liver and excreted in bile and urine

Adverse effects: GI discomfort, anorexia, nausea, vomiting, heartburn, diarrhea, allergic skin reactions, hypoglycemia

Therapeutic Actions and Indications

The sulfonylureas stimulate insulin release from the beta cells in the pancreas (see Figure 38.1). They improve insulin binding to insulin receptors and may actually increase the number of insulin receptors. They are indicated as an adjunct to diet and exercise to lower blood glucose levels in type 2 diabetes mellitus. They have the unlabeled use of being an adjunct to insulin to improve glucose control in type 2 diabetics.

Pharmacokinetics

These drugs are rapidly absorbed from the GI tract and undergo hepatic metabolism. They are excreted in the urine. The peak effects and duration of effects differ because of the activity of various metabolites of the different drugs. These drugs are not for use during pregnancy. Insulin should be used if an antidiabetic agent is needed during pregnancy. Some of these drugs cross into breast milk, and adequate studies are not available on others. Because of the risk of hypoglycemic effects in the baby, these drugs should not be used during lactation. Another method of feeding the baby should be used.

Contraindications and Cautions

Sulfonylureas are contraindicated in the presence of known allergy to any sulfonylureas and in diabetes complicated by fever, severe infection, severe trauma, major surgery, ketoacidosis, severe renal or hepatic disease, pregnancy, or lactation. These drugs are also contraindicated for use in type 1 diabetics.

Adverse Effects

The most common adverse effects related to the sulfonylureas are hypoglycemia (caused by an imbalance in levels of glucose and insulin) and GI distress, including nausea, vomiting, epigastric discomfort, heartburn, and anorexia. (Anorexia should be monitored, because affected patients may not eat after taking the sulfonylurea, which could lead to hypoglycemia.) Allergic skin reactions have been reported with some of these drugs and, as mentioned earlier, there may be an increased risk of cardiovascular mortality, particularly with the first-generation agents.

Clinically Important Drug–Drug Interactions

Care should be taken with any drug that acidifies the urine, because excretion of the sulfonylurea may be decreased. Caution should also be used with beta-blockers, which may mask the signs of hypoglycemia, and with alcohol, which can lead to altered glucose levels when combined with sulfonylureas. The safety and efficacy of these drugs for use in children have not been established.

Nonsulfonylureas

The nonsulfonylureas (Table 38.5) are oral agents that are structurally unrelated to the sulfonylureas. They frequently are effective when used in combination with sulfonylureas or insulin. These drugs include the alpha-glucosidase inhibitors acarbose (*Precose*) and miglitol (*Glyset*); the biguanide, metformin (*Glucophage*); the meglitinides, repaglinide (*Prandin*) and nateglinide (*Starlix*); and the thiazolidinediones, pioglitazone (*Actos*) and rosiglitazone (*Avandia*).

Acarbose and miglitol are inhibitors of alpha-glucosidase (an enzyme that breaks down glucose for absorption); they delay the absorption of glucose. They have only a mild effect on glucose levels and have been associated with severe hepatic toxicity. They do not enhance insulin secretion, so their effects are additive to those of the sulfonylureas in controlling blood glucose. These drugs are used in combination with other oral agents for patients whose glucose levels cannot be controlled with a single agent.

Metformin decreases the production and increases the uptake of glucose. It is effective in lowering blood glucose levels and does not cause hypoglycemia as the sulfonylureas do. It has been associated with the development of lactic acidosis. Both acarbose and metformin can cause GI distress. Box 38.8 describes some of the new fixed-combination oral agents, which provide two different agents in one tablet to make it easier for the patient to be compliant.

Newer oral agents include repaglinide and nateglinide, which act like the sulfonylureas to increase insulin release. These are rapid-acting drugs with a very short half-life. They are used just before meals to lower postprandial glucose lev-

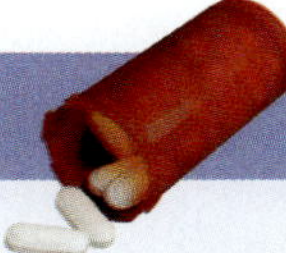

Table 38.5 DRUGS IN FOCUS

Nonsulfonylureas

Drug Name	Dosage/Route	Usual Indications
acarbose (*Precose*)	100 mg PO t.i.d. at the start of each meal	Adjunct to diet to lower blood glucose in type 2 diabetics; in combination with sulfonylureas to control blood sugar in patients whose diabetes cannot be controlled with either drug alone
exenatide (*Baraclude*)	5 mcg by Sub-Q injection within 60 min before morning and evening meals; may be increased to 10 mcg b.i.d. after 1 mo	Adjunct to diet and oral agents to improve glycemic control in patients with type 2 diabetes
P metformin (*Glucophage*)	500–850 mg/day PO in divided doses; reduce dosage in geriatric and renal-impaired patients; maximum dose: 2550 mg/day Children 10–16 yr: 500 mg/day PO with a maximum dose of 2000 mg/day; do not use ER form	Adjunct to diet to lower blood glucose in type 2 diabetics
miglitol (*Glyset*)	50–100 mg PO t.i.d. with the first bite of each meal	Adjunct to diet to lower blood glucose in type 2 diabetics; in combination with sulfonylureas to control blood sugar in patients whose diabetes cannot be controlled with either drug alone
nateglinide (*Starlix*)	120 mg PO t.i.d. with each meal	Adjunct to diet to lower blood glucose in type 2 diabetics; in combination with metformin to control blood sugar in patients whose diabetes cannot be controlled with either drug alone
pioglitazone (*Actos*)	15–30 mg/day PO as a single dose; use caution with hepatic impairment	Adjunct to diet to lower blood glucose in type 2 diabetics; in combination with insulin or sulfonylureas to control blood sugar in patients whose diabetes cannot be controlled with either drug alone
pramlintide acetate (*Symlin*)	*Type 2 diabetes:* 60 mcg by Sub-Q injection immediately before major meals; may be increased to 120 mcg *Type 1 diabetes:* Initially 15 mcg by Sub-Q injection; maintenance 30–60 mcg/dose	Adjunct to type 2 or type 1 diabetics using mealtime insulin but without glycemic control
repaglinide (*Prandin*)	0.5–4 mg PO before meals, do not exceed 16 mg/day	Adjunct to diet to lower blood glucose in type 2 diabetics; in combination with metformin to control blood sugar in patients whose diabetes cannot be controlled with either drug alone
rosiglitazone (*Avandia*)	4–8 mg/day PO as a single dose; use caution with hepatic impairment	Adjunct to diet to lower blood glucose in type 2 diabetics; in combination with insulin or sulfonylureas to control blood sugar in patients whose diabetes cannot be controlled with either drug alone

els. These drugs can be used in combination with metformin. Because they are new, long-term effects are not known.

The thiazolidinediones are drugs that decrease insulin resistance; they are used in combination with sulfonylureas or metformin to treat patients with insulin resistance. The first drug of this class, troglitazone, was withdrawn from the market after reports of serious hepatotoxicity. The two drugs that are available now—pioglitazone and rosiglitazone—are not associated with the same severe liver toxicity. Patients should still be monitored for any change in liver function while they are taking these drugs.

Therapeutic actions and indications, pharmacokinetics, contraindications and cautions, adverse effects, and clinically important drug–drug interactions for nonsulfonylureas are basically the same as for the sulfonylureas. The safety and efficacy of these drugs for use in children have not been established.

The newest of the antidiabetic agents, both released in 2005, include pramlintide (*Symlin*) and exenatide (*Baraclude*).

Symlin works to modulate gastric emptying after a meal, causes a feeling of fullness or satiety, and prevents the post-meal rise in glucagons that usually elevates glucose levels. It is a synthetic form of human amylin, a hormone produced by the beta cells in the pancreas, important in regulating post-meal glucose levels. It is injected subcutaneously immediately before a major meal and can be used in combination with insulins and oral agents. It has a rapid onset of action and peaks in 21 minutes. It should be injected before each major meal of the day, at least 2" away from any insulin injection site. It cannot be combined in the syringe with insulin. This drug should not be used if the patient is unable to eat.

Baraclude is an incretin that mimics the enhancement of glucose-dependent insulin secretion by the beta cells in the pancreas, depresses elevated glucagon secretion, and slows gastric emptying to help moderate and lower blood glucose levels. It is given by subcutaneous injection twice a day, within 60 minutes before the morning and evening meals. It has a rapid onset of action and peaks within 2 hours; its effects last 8 to 10 hours. It is given in combination with oral agents to improve glycemic control in type 2 diabetes patients who cannot achieve glycemic control on oral agents alone. It should not be given if the patient is unable to eat.

BOX 38.8 Fixed-Combination Oral Agents Available

Several fixed-combination oral antidiabetic agents have become available in the last 5 years. These combination products are intended to decrease the number of tablets the patient needs to take each day and thereby increase compliance with the drug regimen. The patient should be stabilized on the individual product first and then switched to the combination product after the correct dosage combination for that patient has been established. The patient should be reminded that diet and exercise are still the key parts of the antidiabetic treatment regimen.

- *Glucovance* is a combination of glyburide and metformin and is available in three sizes: 1.25 mg glyburide with 250 mg metformin, 2.5 mg glyburide with 500 mg metformin, and 5 mg glyburide with 500 mg metformin.
- *Metaglip* is a combination of glipizide and metformin and is available in three sizes: 2.5 mg glipizide with 250 or 500 mg metformin and 5 mg glipizide with 500 mg metformin.
- *Avandamet* is a combination of rosiglitazone and metformin and is available in three sizes: 1, 2, or 4 mg rosiglitazone with 500 mg metformin.
- *Avandaryl* is a combination of rosiglitazone and glimepiride and is available in three sizes: 1, 2, or 4 mg glimepiride with 4 mg rosiglitazone.
- *Actoplus Met* is a combination of pioglitazone and metformin and is available in two sizes: 500 or 850 mg metformin with 15 mg pioglitazone.

Prototype Summary: Metformin

Indications: Adjunct to diet and exercise for the treatment of type 2 diabetics over 10 years of age; extended release form for patients over 17 years of age

Actions: May increase the peripheral use of glucose, increase production of insulin, decrease hepatic glucose production, and alter intestinal absorption of glucose

Pharmacokinetics:

Route	Onset	Peak	Duration
Oral	Slow	2–2.5 h	10–16 h

$T_{1/2}$: 6.2 and then 17 hours; metabolized in the liver and excreted in the urine

Adverse effects: Hypoglycemia, lactic acidosis, GI upset, nausea, anorexia, diarrhea, heartburn, allergic skin reaction

Nursing Considerations for Patients Taking Oral Antidiabetic Agents

Assessment: History and Examination

Screen for the following conditions, *which could be cautions or contraindications to use of the drug:* history of allergy to any of the oral agents; severe renal or hepatic dysfunction; and pregnancy or lactation.

Include screening for baseline status before beginning therapy and for any potential adverse effects: presence of any skin lesions; orientation and reflexes; baseline pulse and blood pressure; adventitious breath sounds; abdominal sounds and function; urinalysis and blood glucose concentration; and renal and liver function tests.

Nursing Diagnoses

The patient receiving oral antidiabetic agents may have the following nursing diagnoses related to drug therapy:

- Imbalanced Nutrition: Less Than Body Requirements, related to metabolic effects
- Disturbed Sensory Perception (Kinesthetic, Visual, Auditory, Tactile) related to glucose levels
- Ineffective Coping related to diagnosis and therapy
- Deficient Knowledge regarding drug therapy

Implementation With Rationale

- Administer the drug as prescribed in the appropriate relationship to meals, *to ensure therapeutic effectiveness.*
- Monitor nutritional status, *to provide nutritional consultation as needed.*
- Monitor response carefully; blood glucose monitoring is the most effective way *to evaluate dosage.*
- Monitor liver enzymes of patients receiving pioglitazone or rosiglitazone very carefully *to avoid liver toxicity;* arrange to discontinue the drug *to avert serious liver damage if liver toxicity develops.*
- Monitor patients during times of trauma, pregnancy, or severe stress, *and arrange to switch to insulin coverage as needed.*
- Provide thorough patient teaching, including measures to avoid adverse effects, warning signs of problems, proper administration technique, and the need to monitor disease status, *to enhance patient knowledge of drug therapy and promote compliance.*

Evaluation

- Monitor patient response to the drug (stabilization of blood glucose levels).
- Monitor for adverse effects (hypoglycemia, GI distress).
- Evaluate the effectiveness of the teaching plan (patient can name drug, dosage, adverse effects to watch for, specific measures to avoid adverse effects).
- Monitor the effectiveness of comfort measures and compliance to the regimen.

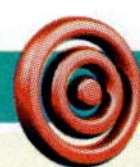

FOCUS POINTS

- Sulfonylureas work only if the pancreas has functioning beta cells.
- In times of severe stress, patients regulated on oral agents usually need to be switched to insulin to control blood glucose levels.
- Proper diet and exercise are the backbone of antidiabetic therapy; oral drugs are adjuncts to help control blood glucose levels.

Glucose-Elevating Agents

Some adverse conditions are associated with hypoglycemia, or abnormally low blood sugar level (less than 40 mg/dL), including pancreatic disorders, kidney disease, certain cancers, disorders of the anterior pituitary, and unbalanced treatment of diabetes mellitus (which can occur if the patient takes the wrong dose of insulin or oral agents or if something interferes with food intake or changes stress or exercise levels). Two agents are used to elevate glucose in these conditions: diazoxide (*Proglycem*), which can be taken orally, and glucagon (*GlucaGen*), the hormone produced by the alpha cells of the pancreas to elevate glucose levels (Table 38.6). Glucagon can be given only parenterally and is preferred for emergency situations. Pure glucose can also be given orally or intravenously to increase glucose levels. Oral glucose tablets or gels (*Glutose, Insta-Glucose, B-D Glucose*) are available over the counter for patients to keep on hand for management of moderate hypoglycemic episodes.

Therapeutic Actions and Indications

These agents increase the blood glucose level by decreasing insulin release and accelerating the breakdown of glycogen in the liver to release glucose. They are indicated for the treatment of hypoglycemic reactions related to insulin or oral antidiabetic agents; treatment of hypoglycemia related to pancreatic or other cancers; and short-term treatment of acute hypoglycemia related to anterior pituitary dysfunction.

Pharmacokinetics

Glucagon and diazoxide are rapidly absorbed and widely distributed throughout the body. They are excreted in the urine. Diazoxide has been associated with adverse effects on the fetus and should not be used during pregnancy. There are no adequate studies on glucagon and pregnancy, so use should be reserved for those situations in which the benefits to the mother outweigh any potential risks to the fetus. Caution should be used during lactation, because the drugs may cause hyperglycemic effects in the baby.

Contraindications and Cautions

Diazoxide is contraindicated with known allergies to sulfonamides or thiazides. Both drugs are contraindicated for use during pregnancy and lactation. Caution should be used in patients with renal or hepatic dysfunction or cardiovascular disease.

Adverse Effects

Glucagon is associated with GI upset, nausea, and vomiting. Diazoxide has been associated with vascular effects including hypotension, headache, cerebral ischemia, weakness, congestive heart failure, and arrhythmias; these reactions are

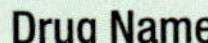

Table 38.6 DRUGS IN FOCUS

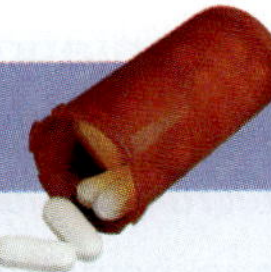

Glucose-Elevating Agents

Drug Name	Dosage/Route	Usual Indications
diazoxide (*Proglycem, Hyperstat*)	Adults and children: 3–8 mg/kg/day PO in two to three divided doses q8–12h	Oral management of hypoglycemia; intravenous use for management of severe hypertension
glucagon (*GlucaGen*)	Adults and children >20 kg: 0.5–1 mg Sub-Q, IM, or IV Children <20 kg: 0.5 mg Sub-Q, IM, or IV	To counteract severe hypoglycemic reactions

associated with diazoxide's ability to relax arteriolar smooth muscle.

Clinically Important Drug–Drug Interactions

Taking diazoxide in combination with thiazide diuretics causes an increased risk of toxicity, because diazoxide is structurally similar to these diuretics.

Increased anticoagulation effects have been noted when glucagon is combined with oral anticoagulants. If this combination is needed, the dosage should be adjusted.

Nursing Considerations for Patients Taking Glucose-Elevating Agents

Assessment: History and Examination

Screen for the following conditions, *which could be cautions or contraindications to use of the drug:* history of allergy to thiazides if using diazoxide; severe renal or hepatic dysfunction, cardiovascular disease; and pregnancy or lactation.

Physical assessment should include screening *for baseline status before beginning therapy and for any potential adverse effects:* orientation and reflexes; baseline pulse, blood pressure, and adventitious sounds; abdominal sounds and function; urinalysis and blood glucose level; renal and liver function tests.

Nursing Diagnoses

The patient receiving glucose-elevating agents may have the following nursing diagnoses related to drug therapy:

- Imbalanced Nutrition: More Than Body Requirements, related to metabolic effects, and Less Than Body Requirements, related to GI upset
- Disturbed Sensory Perception (Kinesthetic, Visual, Auditory, Tactile) related to glucose levels
- Deficient Knowledge regarding drug therapy

Implementation With Rationale

- Monitor blood glucose levels daily, *to evaluate the effectiveness of the drug.*
- Have insulin on standby during emergency use *to treat severe hyperglycemia if it occurs.*
- Monitor nutritional status, *to provide nutritional consultation as needed.*
- Monitor patients receiving diazoxide for potential cardiovascular effects, including blood pressure, heart rhythm and output, and weight changes, *to avert serious adverse reactions.*
- Provide thorough patient teaching, including measures to avoid adverse effects, warning signs of problems, proper administration technique, and the need to monitor glucose levels daily, *to enhance patient knowledge of drug therapy and promote compliance.*

Evaluation

- Monitor patient response to the drug (stabilization of blood glucose levels).
- Monitor for adverse effects (hyperglycemia, GI distress).
- Evaluate the effectiveness of the teaching plan (patient can name drug, dosage, adverse effects to watch for, specific measures to avoid adverse effects).
- Monitor the effectiveness of comfort measures and compliance to the regimen.

WEB LINKS

Patients and health care providers may want to consult the following Internet sources:

http://www.diabetes.org Information on diabetes, drugs, research, diet, recipes, support groups, activities.

http://www.niddk.nih.gov Information on diabetes research and information.

http://www.castleweb.com/diabetes Information on research, treatment, and care of children with diabetes.

Points to Remember

- Diabetes mellitus is the most common metabolic disorder. It is characterized by high blood glucose levels and alterations in the metabolism of fats, proteins, and glucose.
- Diabetes mellitus is complicated by many end-organ problems. These are related to thickening of basement membranes and the resultant decrease in blood flow to these areas.
- Treatment of diabetes involves tight control of blood glucose levels using diet and exercise, a combination of oral agents to stimulate insulin release or alter glucose absorption, or the injection of replacement insulin.
- Replacement insulin was once obtained from beef and pork pancreas. Today, most replacement insulin is human, derived from genetically altered bacteria.
- The amount and type of insulin given must be regulated daily. Patients taking insulin must learn to inject the

drug, to test their own blood, and to recognize the signs of hypoglycemia and hyperglycemia.

- Insulin is used for type 1 diabetes and for type 2 diabetes in times of stress or when other therapies have failed.
- Other antidiabetic agents include first- and second-generation sulfonylureas, which stimulate the pancreas to release insulin, and other agents that alter glucose absorption, decrease insulin resistance, or decrease the formation of glucose. These agents are often used in combination to achieve effectiveness.
- Glucose-elevating agents are used to increase glucose when levels become dangerously low. Imbalance in glucose levels while taking insulin or oral agents is a common cause of hypoglycemia.

CHECK YOUR UNDERSTANDING

Answers to the questions in this chapter may be found in the Answer Key in the back of the book.

Multiple Choice

Select the best answer to the following.

1. Currently, the medical management of diabetes mellitus is aimed at
   a. controlling caloric intake.
   b. increasing exercise levels.
   c. tightly regulating blood sugar levels.
   d. decreasing fluid loss.

2. The HbA1c blood test is a good measure of overall glucose control because
   a. it reflects the level of glucose after a meal.
   b. the patient needs to fast for 8 hours before having the test done, ensuring an accurate level.
   c. it reflects a 3-month average glucose level in the body.
   d. the test can be affected by the glucose challenge.

3. A patient with hyperglycemia will present with
   a. polyuria, polydipsia, and polyphagia.
   b. polycythemia, polyuria, and polyphagia.
   c. polyadenitis, polyuria, and polydipsia.
   d. polydipsia, polycythemia, and polyarteritis.

4. The long-term alterations in fat, carbohydrate, and protein metabolism associated with diabetes mellitus result in
   a. obesity.
   b. thickening of the capillary basement membrane and end-organ damage.
   c. chronic obstructive pulmonary disease.
   d. lactose intolerance.

5. Insulin is available in several forms or suspensions, which differ in their
   a. effect on the pancreas.
   b. onset of action and duration of action.
   c. means of administration.
   d. tendency to cause adverse effects.

6. A patient on a fixed income would benefit from a second-generation sulfonylurea to control blood glucose levels. The drug of choice for this patient would be
   a. glipizide.
   b. glyburide.
   c. tolbutamide.
   d. glimepiride.

7. Miglitol differs from the sulfonylureas in that it
   a. greatly stimulates pancreatic insulin release.
   b. greatly increases the sensitivity of insulin receptor sites.
   c. delays the absorption of glucose, leading to lower glucose levels.
   d. cannot be used in combination with other antidiabetic agents.

8. Teaching subjects for the patient with diabetes should include
   a. diet, exercise, hygiene, and lifestyle changes that are needed.
   b. the importance of avoiding exercise, which could alter blood glucose.
   c. the need for protection from exposure to any infection.
   d. the importance of avoiding pregnancy.

Multiple Response

Select all that apply.

1. Treatment of diabetes may include which of the following?
   a. Replacement therapy with insulin
   b. Control of glucose absorption through the GI tract
   c. Drugs that stimulate insulin release or increase sensitivity of insulin receptor sites
   d. Surgical clearing of the capillary basement membranes
   e. Slowing of gastric emptying
   f. Diet and exercise programs

2. A client is recently diagnosed with diabetes. In reviewing his past history, which of the following would be early indicators of the problem?
   a. Lethargy
   b. Fruity smelling breath
   c. Boundless energy
   d. Weight loss
   e. Increased sweating
   f. Getting up often at night to go to the bathroom

Web Exercise

J.L. is a 53-year-old traveling salesman recently diagnosed with type 2 diabetes. He and his family are referred to the nurse for education about his disease, diet, drugs, and medical regimen. Go to the Internet to find the latest information for J.L. and to prepare the best teaching resources for him and his family.

Fill in the Blanks

1. The most common metabolic disorder in this country is ____________________.

2. The pancreas produces three different hormones, all related to glucose control. These three hormones are ____________________, ____________________, and ____________________.

3. Insulin stimulates the synthesis of ____________________ (stored glucose for immediate release during times of stress or low glucose), the conversion of ____________________ into fat stored in the form of adipose tissue, and the synthesis of needed ____________________ from amino acids.

4. Hyperglycemia results in ____________________ as sugar is spilled into the urine.

5. Hyperglycemia will also cause ____________________ (increased eating) because the hypothalamic centers cannot take in glucose and sense that they are starving.

6. ____________________ (increased thirst) occurs with hyperglycemia because the tonicity of the blood is increased due to the increased glucose and waste products in the blood and to the loss of fluid with glucose in the urine.

7. When a person with diabetes needs to break down fats for energy, he or she will experience ____________________ as the metabolism shifts from using sugar to the use of fat and the ketone wastes that result cannot be removed effectively.

8. The first steps for controlling diabetes should always be ____________________ and ____________________.

9. The ____________________ were the first oral antidiabetic agents. They stimulate the pancreas to produce more insulin.

10. ____________________ is an oral antidiabetic agent that decreases the production of glucose and increases its uptake into cells.

Bibliography and References

Abraira, C., & Duckworth, W. (2003). The need for glycemic trials in type 2 diabetes. *Clinical Diabetes, 21,* 107–111.

American Diabetes Association. (2002). Standards of medical care for patients with diabetes mellitus. *Diabetes Care, 25,* 213–229.

American Diabetes Association. (2003). Tests of glycemia in diabetes. *Diabetes Care, 26,* S106–S108.

Andrews, M., & Boyle, J. (2004). *Transcultural concepts in nursing care.* Philadelphia: Lippincott Williams & Wilkins.

Chalmers, T. C. (1975). Settling the University Group Diabetes Program controversy. *Journal of the American Medical Association, 231,* 624.

Drug facts and comparisons. (2006). St. Louis: Facts and Comparisons.

Gilman, A., Hardman, J. G., & Limbird, L. E. (Eds.). (2006). *Goodman and Gilman's the pharmacological basis of therapeutics* (11th ed.). New York: McGraw-Hill.

Henderson, D. (1998). Microvascular complications of diabetes. *American Journal of Nursing, 98*(6).

Karch, A. M. (2006). *2007 Lippincott's nursing drug guide.* Philadelphia: Lippincott Williams & Wilkins.

Levetan, C. (2001). Into the mouths of babes: The diabetes epidemic in children. *Clinical Diabetes, 19,* 102–104.

Marks, J. (1998). Diabetes management in the future: A whiff and a long shot? *Clinical Diabetes, 16*(3).

Pickup, J., & Keen, H. (2002). Continuous subcutaneous insulin infusion at 25 years: Evidence base for expanding use of insulin pump therapy for type 1 diabetes. *Diabetes Care, 25,* 593–598.

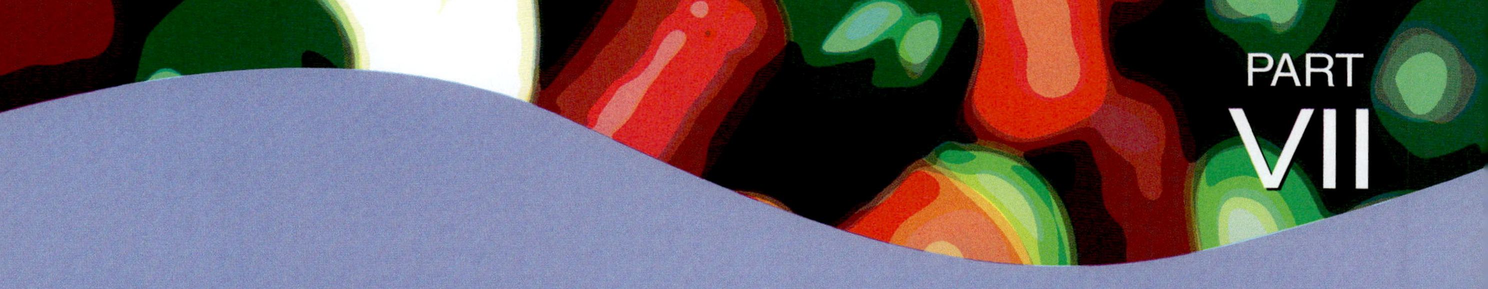

PART VII

Drugs Acting on the Reproductive System

CHAPTER 39

Introduction to the Reproductive System

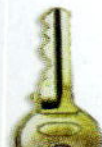

KEY TERMS

corpus luteum
estrogen
follicle
inhibin
interstitial or Leydig cells
menopause
menstrual cycle
ova
ovaries
progesterone
puberty
seminiferous tubules
sperm
testes
testosterone
uterus

LEARNING OBJECTIVES

Upon completion of this chapter, you will be able to:

1. Label a diagram of the parts of the female and male reproductive systems and explain the function of each part.
2. Outline the controls of the male and female reproductive systems, using this outline to explain the cyclical nature of the female reproductive system.
3. List five effects of each of the sex hormones: estrogen, progesterone, and testosterone.
4. Describe the changes that occur to the female body during pregnancy.
5. Describe the phases of the human sexual response and briefly describe the clinical presentation of each stage.

The glands that produce sexual hormones originate from the same fetal cells in both males and females. In the female, those cells stay in the abdomen and develop into the **ovaries**. In the male, the cells migrate out of the abdomen to form the **testes**, which are suspended from the body in the scrotum. Both male and female glands respond to follicle-stimulating hormone (FSH) and luteinizing hormone (LH), which are released from the anterior pituitary in response to stimulation from gonadotropin-releasing hormone (GnRH) released from the hypothalamus.

Female Reproductive System

The female reproductive system is composed of two ovaries, which store the **ova**, or eggs, and which act as endocrine glands that produce **estrogen** and **progesterone**; the **uterus**, which is the womb for the developing embryo and fetus; and the fallopian tubes, which provide a pathway for released ova from the ovaries to the uterus. Accessory parts include the vagina, clitoris, labia, and breast tissue (Figure 39.1).

Ovaries

The ovaries contain all of the ova that a woman will have at birth. The ova slowly degenerate over time or are released for possible fertilization throughout a woman's life. Each ovum is contained in a storage site called a **follicle**, which produces the female sex hormones, estrogen and progesterone. The primary goal of these hormones is to prepare the body for pregnancy and to maintain the pregnancy until delivery.

In a nonpregnant woman, the levels of these hormones fluctuate in a cyclical fashion until all of the ova are gone and **menopause**, the cessation of menses, occurs. In a pregnant woman, the placenta takes over production of estrogen and progesterone, and high levels of both hormones help to maintain the pregnancy. The adrenal glands also produce small amounts of androgens, which include testosterone and some estrogens.

Controls

The developing hypothalamus is sensitive to the androgens released by the adrenal glands and does not release GnRH during childhood. As the hypothalamus matures, it loses its sensitivity to the androgens and starts to release GnRH. This occurs at **puberty**, or sexual development. The onset of puberty leads to a number of hormonal changes.

To begin with, GnRH stimulates the anterior pituitary to release FSH and LH. FSH and LH stimulate the follicles on the outer surface of the uterus to grow and develop. These follicles are called graafian follicles; they produce progesterone, which is retained in the follicle, and estrogen, which is released into circulation. When the circulating estrogen

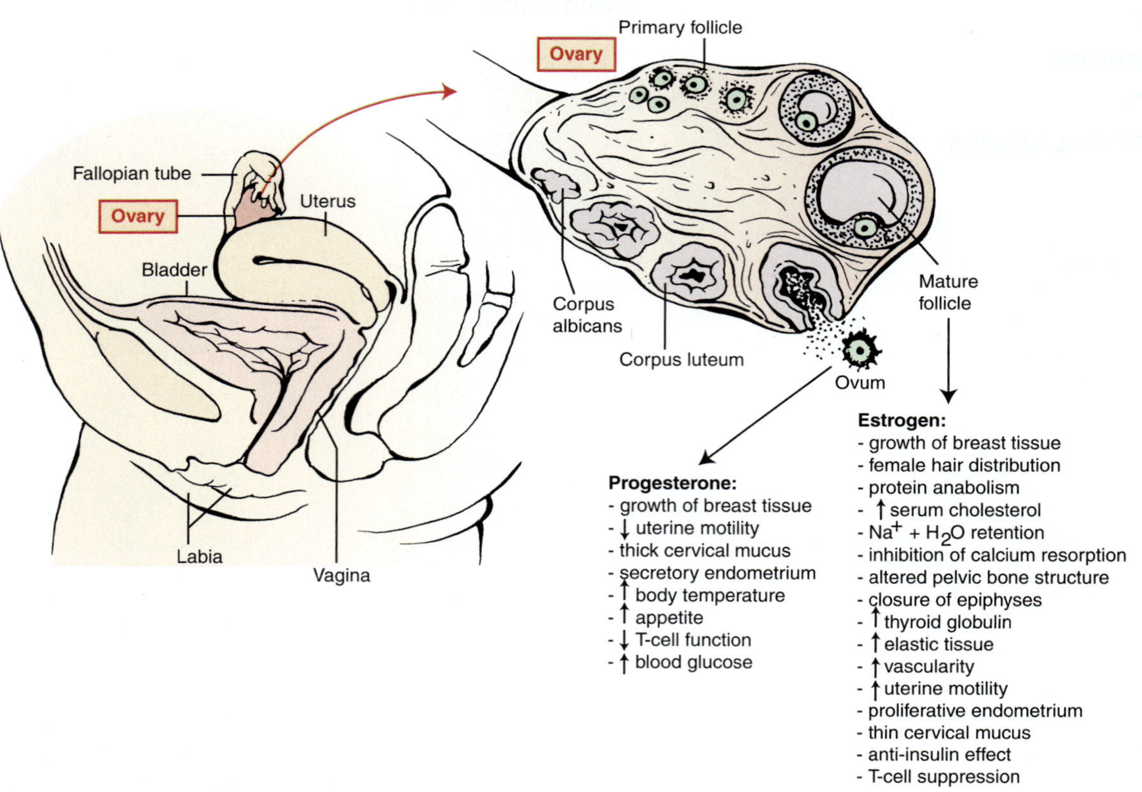

FIGURE 39.1 The female reproductive system.

level rises high enough, it stimulates a massive release of LH from the anterior pituitary. This is called the "LH surge." This burst of LH causes one of the developing follicles to burst and release the ovum and all the hormones that are inside the follicle into the system. LH also causes the rest of the developing follicles to shrink in on themselves, or involute, and eventually disappear. The release of an ovum from the follicle is called ovulation.

The ovum is released into the abdomen near the end of one of the fallopian tubes, and the constant movement of cilia within the tube helps to propel the ovum into the fallopian tube and then into the uterus. The ruptured follicle becomes a functioning endocrine gland called the **corpus luteum**. It will continue to produce estrogen and progesterone for 10 to 14 days unless pregnancy occurs. If the ovum is fertilized and implants in the uterine wall, one of the first hormones that is produced by the junction of the fertilized embryo with the uterine wall is human chorionic gonadotropin. This hormone stimulates the corpus luteum to continue to produce estrogen and progesterone until placental levels of these hormones are high enough to sustain the pregnancy.

If pregnancy does not occur, the corpus luteum involutes and becomes a white scar on the ovary. This scar is called the corpus albicans. Initially, the rising levels of estrogen and progesterone produced by the corpus luteum act as a negative feedback system to the hypothalamus and the pituitary, stopping the production and secretion of GnRH, FSH, and LH. Later in the cycle, the corpus luteum atrophies, the falling levels of estrogen and progesterone stimulate the hypothalamus to release GnRH, and the cycle begins again.

After all of the follicles are used up, the ovaries no longer produce estrogen and progesterone, and menopause occurs. The hypothalamus and pituitary produce increased levels of GnRH, FSH, and LH for a while in an attempt to stimulate the ovaries to produce estrogen and progesterone. If that does not happen, the levels of these hormones fall back within a normal range in response to their own negative feedback systems. Menopause is associated with loss of many of the effects of these two hormones on the body, including retention of calcium in the bones, lowered serum lipid levels, and maintenance of secondary sex characteristics.

Because of its position in the brain, the hypothalamus is influenced by many internal and external factors. For example, high levels of stress can stop the reproductive cycle: Tremendous amounts of energy are expended in reproduction, and if the body needs energy for fight or flight, the hypothalamus shuts down the reproductive activities. In addition to stress, starvation, extreme exercise, and emotional problems are all associated with a decrease in reproductivity, related to the controls of the hypothalamus.

Interestingly, light has been found to have an influence on the functioning of the hypothalamus. Increased light levels boost the release of FSH and LH and increase the release of estrogen and progesterone. This is thought to contribute to the early sexual maturation of girls near the equator. Longer and earlier exposure to light leads to earlier GnRH release by the hypothalamus and earlier sexual development.

Hormones

The hormones produced in the ovaries are estrogen and progesterone. These two hormones influence many other body systems while preparing the body for pregnancy or maintenance of pregnancy.

Estrogen

The estrogens produced by the ovaries include estradiol, estrone, and estriol. The estrogens enter cells and bind to receptors within the cytoplasm to promote messenger RNA (mRNA) activity, which results in specific proteins for cell activity or structure. The effects of estrogen on the body are summarized in Box 39.1. Many of these effects are first noticed at menarche (the onset of the menstrual cycle), when the hormones begin cycling for the first time. Female characteristics are associated with the effects of estrogen on many of the body's systems—wider hips, soft skin, breast growth, and so on.

Progesterone

Progesterone is released into circulation after ovulation. Its effects are summarized in Box 39.2. Progesterone's effects on body temperature are monitored in the "rhythm method" of birth control to indicate that ovulation has just occurred.

The Menstrual Cycle

The cyclic effects of the female sex hormones on the body produce the **menstrual cycle**. The onset of the menstrual cycle at puberty is called the menarche. Each cycle starts with release of FSH and LH and stimulation of the follicles on the ovary. For about the next 14 days, the developing follicles release estrogen into the body. The many effects of estrogen may be noticed by the woman (e.g., breast tenderness, water retention, thin cervical mucosa, increased susceptibility to infections, development of a secretory endometrium).

By about day 14, the estrogen levels have caused the LH surge, and ovulation occurs. The woman experiences increased body temperature, increased appetite, breast tenderness, bloating and abdominal fullness, constipation, and so on—the effects associated with progesterone. The uterus becomes thicker and more vascular as the cycle progresses and develops a proliferative endometrium. After ovulation, the lining of the uterus begins to produce glucose and other nutrients that would nurture a growing embryo; this is called a secretory endometrium. If pregnancy does not occur, after about 14 days the corpus luteum involutes and the levels of estrogen and progesterone drop off (Figure 39.2).

The dropping levels of estrogen and progesterone trigger the release of FSH and LH again, along with the start of another menstrual cycle. Lowered hormone levels also cause the inner lining of the uterus to slough off because it is no longer stimulated by the hormones. High levels of

BOX 39.1 Clinical Assessment of the Effects of Estrogen

- Growth of genitalia (in preparation for childbirth)
- Growth of breast tissue (in preparation for pregnancy and lactation)
- Characteristic female pubic hair distribution (a triangle)
- Stimulation of protein building (important for the developing fetus)
- Increased total blood cholesterol (for energy for the mother as well as the developing fetus) with an increase in high-density lipoprotein levels ("good" cholesterol, which serves to protect the female blood vessels against atherosclerosis)
- Retention of sodium and water (to provide cooling for the heat generated by the developing fetus and to increase diffusion of sodium and water to the fetus through the placenta)
- Inhibition of calcium resorption from the bones (helps to deposit calcium in the fetal bone structure; when this property is lost at menopause, osteoporosis or loss of calcium from the bone is common)
- Alteration of pelvic bone structure to a wider and flaring pelvis (to promote easier delivery)
- Closure of the epiphyses (to conserve energy for the fetus by halting growth of the mother)
- Increased thyroid hormone globulin (metabolism needs to be increased greatly during pregnancy, and the increase in thyroid hormone facilitates this)
- Increased elastic tissue of the skin (to allow for the tremendous stretch of the abdominal skin during pregnancy)
- Increased vascularity of the skin (to allow for radiation loss of heat generated by the developing fetus)
- Increased uterine motility (estrogen is high when the ovum first leaves the ovary, and increased uterine motility helps to move the ovum toward the uterus and to propel the sperm toward the ovum)
- Thin, clear cervical mucus (allows easy penetration of the sperm into the uterus as ovulation occurs; used in fertility programs as an indication that ovulation will soon occur)
- Proliferative endometrium (to prepare the lining of the uterus for implantation with the fertilized egg)
- Anti-insulin effect with increased glucose levels (to allow increased diffusion of glucose to the developing fetus)
- T-cell inhibition (to protect the nonself-cells of the embryo from the immune surveillance of the mother)

plasminogen in the uterus prevent clotting of the lining as the vessels shear off. Prostaglandins in the uterus stimulate uterine contraction to clamp off vessels as the lining sheds away. This causes menstrual cramps, which can be very uncomfortable for some women. This loss of the uterine lining, called menstruation, repeats approximately every 28 days. Figure 39.3 displays the various phases of the menstrual cycle.

Pregnancy

When the ovum is fertilized by a sperm, a new cell is produced that rapidly divides to produce the embryo. The embryo implants in the wall of the uterus, and the interface between the fetal cells and the uterus produces the placenta, a large, vascular organ that serves as a massive endocrine gland and a transfer point for nutrients from the mother to the fetus. The placenta maintains high levels of estrogens and proges-

BOX 39.2 Clinical Assessment of the Effects of Progesterone

- Decreased uterine motility (to provide increased chance that implantation can occur)
- Development of a secretory endometrium (to provide glucose and a rich blood supply for the developing placenta and embryo)
- Thickened cervical mucus (to protect the developing embryo and keep out bacteria and other pathogens; this is lost at the beginning of labor as the mucous plug)
- Breast growth (to prepare for lactation)
- Increased body temperature (a direct hypothalamic response to progesterone, which stimulates metabolism and promotes activities for the developing embryo; this increase in temperature is monitored in the "rhythm method" of birth control to indicate that ovulation has occurred)
- Increased appetite (this is a direct effect on the satiety centers of the hypothalamus and results in increased nutrients for the developing embryo)
- Depressed T-cell function (again, this protects the nonself-cells of the developing embryo from the immune system)
- Anti-insulin effect (to generate a higher blood glucose concentration to allow rapid diffusion of glucose to the developing embryo)

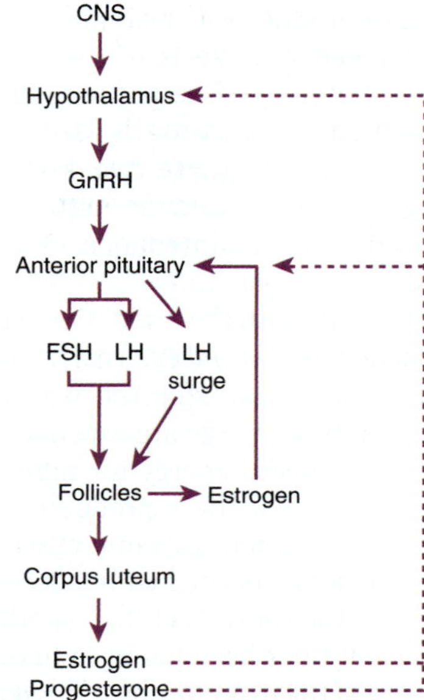

FIGURE 39.2 Interaction of the hypothalamic, pituitary, and ovarian hormones that underlies the menstrual cycle of the female. Dotted lines indicate negative feedback surge. CNS, central nervous system; FSH, follicle-stimulating hormone; GnRH, gonadotropin-releasing hormone; LH, luteinizing hormone.

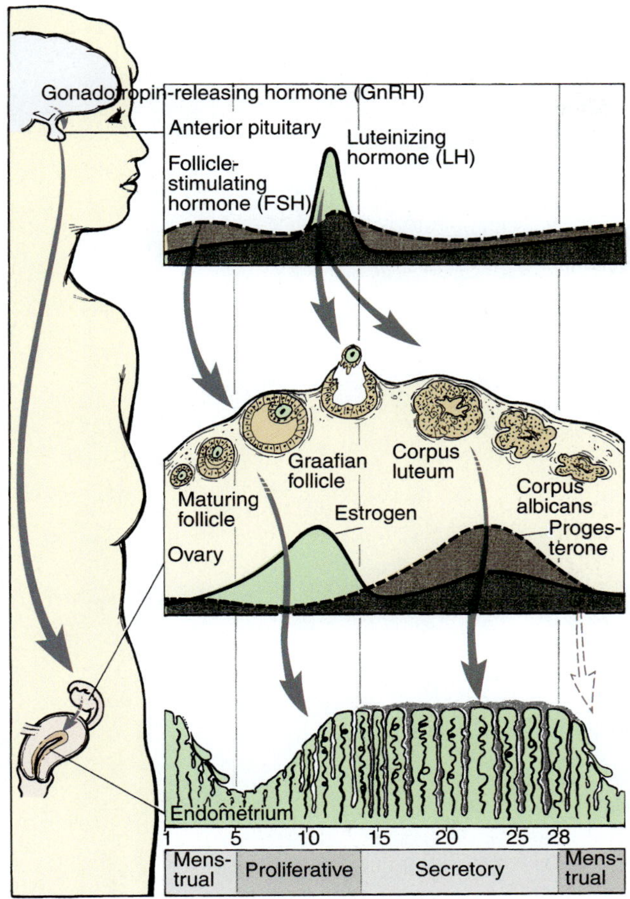

FIGURE 39.3 Relation of pituitary and ovarian hormone levels to the menstrual cycle and to ovarian and endometrial function.

terone to support the uterus and the developing fetus. When the placenta ages, the levels of progesterone and estrogens fall off.

Eventually, the tendency to block uterine activity (an effect of progesterone) is overcome by the stimulation to increase uterine activity caused by oxytocin (a hypothalamic hormone stored in the posterior pituitary). At this point, local prostaglandins stimulate uterine contraction and the onset of labor. Once the fetus and the placenta have been expelled from the uterus, the hormone levels plummet toward the nonpregnant state. This is a time of tremendous adjustment for the body as it tries to reachieve homeostasis.

FOCUS POINTS

- The female ovary stores ova and produces the sex hormones estrogen and progesterone.
- The hypothalamus releases GnRH at puberty to stimulate the anterior pituitary release of FSH and LH, thus stimulating the production and release of the sex hormones. Levels are controlled by a series of negative feedback systems.
- Female sex hormones prepare the body for pregnancy and the maintenance of the pregnancy. If pregnancy does not occur, the prepared inner lining of the uterus sloughs off as menstruation in the menstrual cycle.
- Menopause occurs when the supply of ova is exhausted and the woman's body no longer produces the hormones estrogen and progesterone.

Male Reproductive System

The male reproductive system originates from the same fetal cells as in the female. The two endocrine glands that develop in the male are called the testes. The testes continually produce **sperm** as well as the hormone **testosterone**. The other parts of the male reproductive system include the vas deferens, which stores produced sperm and carries sperm from the testes to be ejaculated from the body; the prostate gland, which produces enzymes to stimulate sperm maturation as well as lubricating fluid; the penis, which includes two corpora cavernosa and a corpus spongiosum, structures that allow massively increased blood flow and erection; the urethra, through which urine as well as the sperm and seminal fluid are delivered; and other glands and ducts that promote sperm and seminal fluid development (Figure 39.4).

Testes

During fetal development, the two testes migrate down the abdomen and descend into the scrotum outside the body. There they are protected from the heat of the body to prevent injury to the sperm-producing cells. The testes are made up of two distinct parts: the **seminiferous tubules**, which produce the sperm, and the **interstitial or Leydig cells**, which produce the hormone testosterone.

Controls

The activity of the male sex glands is not thought to be cyclical like that of the female. The hypothalamus in the male child is also sensitive to circulating levels of adrenal androgens and suppresses GnRH release. After the hypothalamus matures, this sensitivity is lost and the hypothalamus releases GnRH. This in turn stimulates the anterior pituitary to release FSH and LH, or what is sometimes called interstitial cell-stimulating hormone (ICSH) in males. FSH directly stimulates the seminiferous tubules to produce sperm, a process called spermatogenesis. FSH also stimulates the Sertoli cells in the seminiferous tubules to produce estrogens, which provide negative feedback to the pituitary and hypothalamus to cause a decrease in the release of GnRH, FSH, and LH.

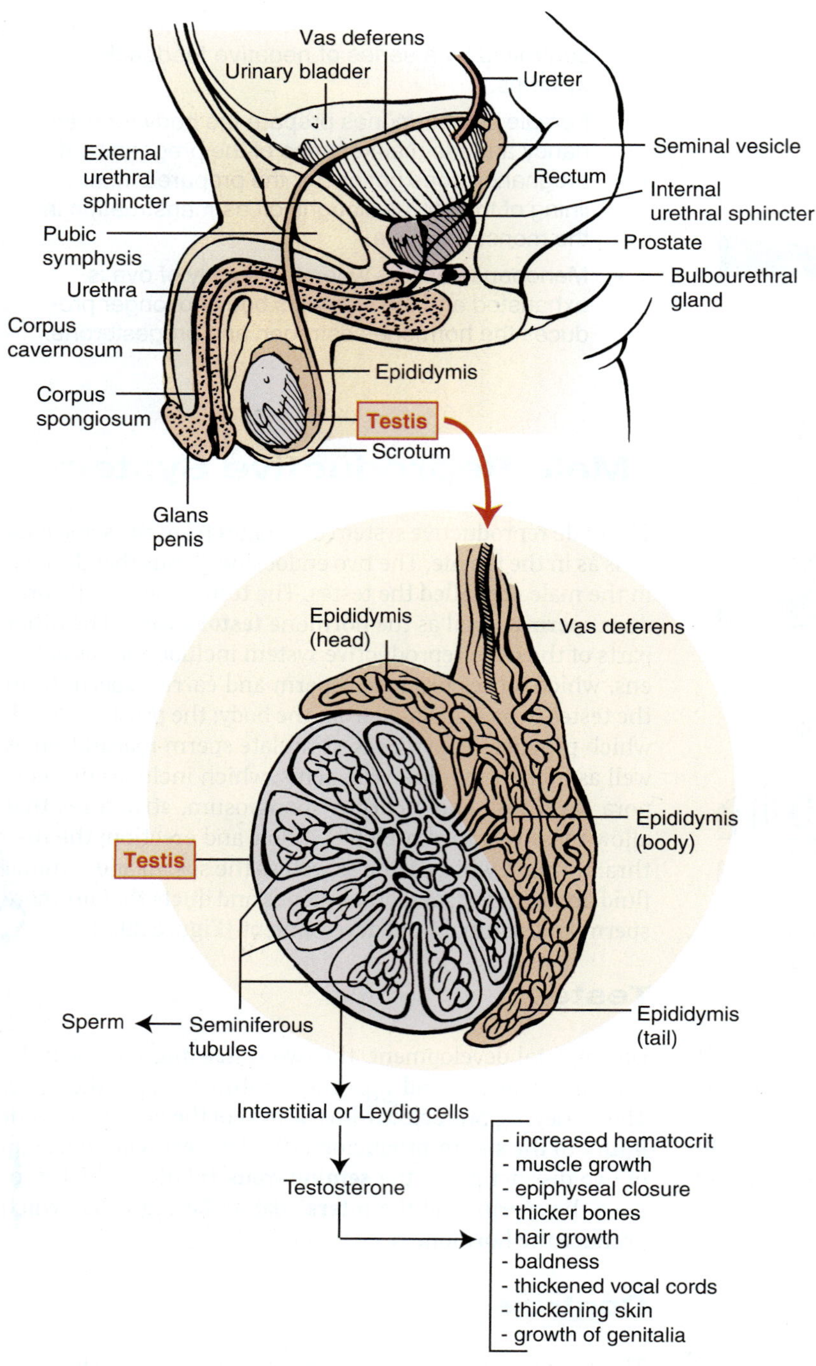

FIGURE 39.4 The male reproductive system.

The Sertoli cells also produce a substance called **inhibin** (an estrogen-like molecule). The inhibin is sensed by the hypothalamus and anterior pituitary, and a negative feedback response occurs, decreasing the circulating level of FSH. When the FSH level falls low enough, the hypothalamus is stimulated to again release GnRH to stimulate FSH release. This feedback system prevents overproduction of sperm in the testes (Figure 39.5). Inhibin has been investigated for many years as a possible male birth control drug, because it is thought to affect only sperm production.

The LH or ICSH stimulates the interstitial (Leydig) cells to produce testosterone. The concentration of testosterone acts in a similar negative feedback system with the hypothalamus. When the concentration is high enough, the hypothalamus decreases GnRH release, leading to a subsequent decrease in FSH and LH release. The levels of testosterone are thought to remain within a fairly well-defined

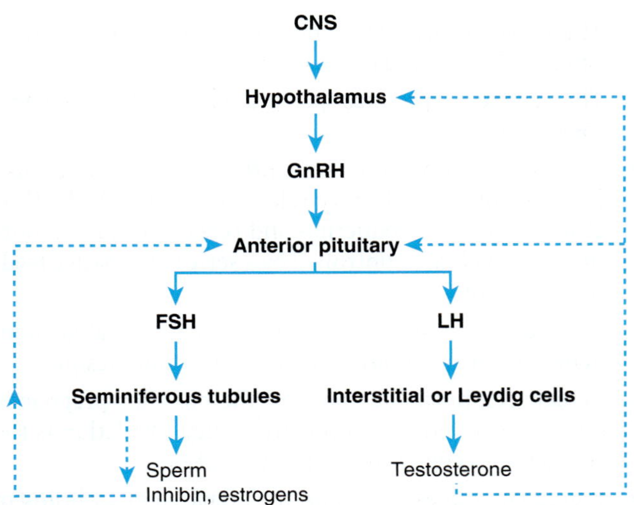

FIGURE 39.5 Interaction of the hypothalamic, pituitary, and testicular hormones that underlies the male sexual hormone system. CNS, central nervous system; FSH, follicle-stimulating hormone; GnRH, gonadotropin-releasing hormone; LH, luteinizing hormone.

range of normal. It has been documented, however, that light affects the male sexual hormones in a similar fashion to its effect on female hormones. "Spring fever," with increased exposure time to sunlight, does increase testosterone levels in men. Other factors that may also have an influence on male hormone levels are likely to be identified in the future.

With age, the seminiferous tubules and interstitial cells atrophy and the male climacteric, a period of lessened sexual activity, occurs. This is similar to female menopause, and the hypothalamus and anterior pituitary put out larger amounts of GnRH, FSH, and LH in an attempt to stimulate the gland. If no increase in testosterone or inhibin occurs, the levels of GnRH, FSH, and LH eventually return to normal levels.

Hormones

Testosterone is responsible for many sexual and metabolic effects in the male. Like estrogen, testosterone enters the cell and reacts with a cytoplasmic receptor site to influence mRNA activity, resulting in the production of proteins for cell structure or function. The effects of testosterone on the body are summarized in Box 39.3.

Castration, or removal of the testes, before puberty results in lack of development of the normal male characteristics as well as sterility. However, once puberty and the physical changes brought about by testosterone have occurred, the androgens released by the adrenal glands are sufficient to sustain the male characteristics. This is important information for adult patients undergoing testicular surgery or chemical castration.

BOX 39.3 Clinical Assessment of the Effects of Testosterone

Growth of male and sexual accessory organs (penis, prostate gland, seminal vesicles, vas deferens)

Growth of testes and scrotal sac

Thickening of vocal cords, producing the deep, male voice

Hair growth on the face, body, arms, legs, and trunk

Male-pattern baldness

Increased protein anabolism and decreased protein catabolism (this causes larger and more powerful muscle development)

Increased bone growth in length and width, which ends when the testosterone stimulates closure of the epiphyses

Thickening of the cartilage and skin, leading to the male gait

Vascular thickening

Increased hematocrit

The Human Sexual Response

Humans and ferrets are the only animals known to be sexually stimulated and responsive at will. Many animals require particular endocrine stimuli, called an estrous cycle, for sexual response to occur. Humans can be sexually stimulated by thoughts, sights, touch, or a variety of combined stimuli. The human sexual response consists of four phases:

- A period of stimulation with mild increases in sensitivity and beginning stimulation of the sympathetic nervous system
- A plateau stage when stimulation levels off
- A climax, which results from massive sympathetic stimulation of the body
- A period of recovery or resolution, when the effects of the sympathetic stimulation are resolved (Figure 39.6)

It was once believed that male and female responses were very different, but it is now thought that the physiology of the responses is quite similar. Sexual stimulation and activity are a normal response and, in healthy individuals, are probably necessary for complete health of the body's systems. The sympathetic stimulation causes increased heart rate, increased blood pressure, sweating, pupil dilation, glycogenolysis (breakdown of stored glycogen to glucose for energy), and other sympathetic responses. This stimulation could be dangerous in some cardiovascular conditions that could be exacerbated by the sympathetic effects. In the male, the increased blood flow to the penis causes erection, which is necessary for penetration of the female and deposition of the sperm. Any drug therapy or disease process that interferes with the sympathetic response or the innervation of the sexual organs will change the person's ability to experience

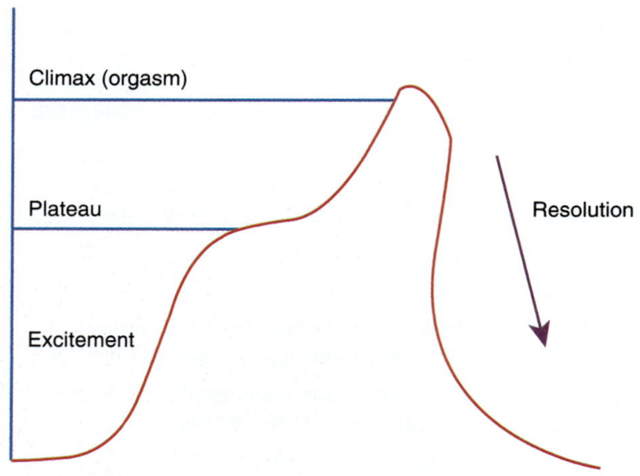

FIGURE 39.6 Human sexual response.

the human sexual response. This is important to keep in mind when doing patient teaching and when evaluating the effects of a drug.

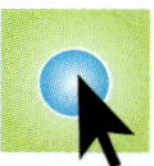

WEB LINK

Patients and health care providers may want to explore the following Internet source:

http://www.InnerBody.com Explore the virtual reproductive system.

Points to Remember

- Male and female reproductive systems arise from the same fetal cells.
- The female ovaries store ova and produce the sex hormones estrogen and progesterone.
- The male testes produce sperm and the sex hormone testosterone.
- The hypothalamus releases GnRH at puberty to stimulate the anterior pituitary release of FSH and LH, thus stimulating the production and release of the sex hormones. Levels are controlled by a series of negative feedback systems.
- Female sex hormones are released in a cyclical fashion. Male sex hormones are released in a steadier fashion.
- Female sex hormones prepare the body for pregnancy and the maintenance of the pregnancy. Ovulation is the release of an egg for possible fertilization.
- If pregnancy does not occur, the prepared inner lining of the uterus is sloughed off as menstruation in the menstrual cycle, so that the lining can be prepared again when ovulation reoccurs.
- Menopause in women and the male climacteric in men occur when the body can no longer produce sex hormones; the hypothalamus and anterior pituitary respond by releasing increasing levels of GnRH, FSH, and LH in an attempt to achieve higher levels of sex hormones.
- The testes produce sperm in the seminiferous tubules, in response to FSH stimulation, and testosterone in the interstitial cells, in response to LH stimulation.
- Testosterone is responsible for the development of male sex characteristics. These characteristics can be maintained by the androgens from the adrenal gland once the body has undergone the changes of puberty.
- The human sexual response involves activation of the sympathetic nervous system to allow a four-phase response: stimulation, plateau, climax, and resolution.

CHECK YOUR UNDERSTANDING

Answers to the questions in this chapter may be found in the Answer Key in the back of the book.

Multiple Choice

Select the best answer to the following.

1. In a nonpregnant woman, the levels of the sex hormones fluctuate in a cyclical fashion until
   a. all of the ova are gone and menopause occurs.
   b. the FSH and LH are depleted.
   c. the hypothalamus no longer senses FSH and LH.
   d. the menarche, when the hypothalamus becomes more sensitive.
2. A woman develops ova, or eggs
   a. continually until menopause.
   b. during fetal life.
   c. until menopause.
   d. starting with puberty
3. Control of the female sex hormones starts with the release of GnRH from the hypothalamus. Because of this, the cycling of these hormones may be influenced by
   a. body temperature.
   b. stress or emotional problems.
   c. age.
   d. androgen release.

4. The rhythm method of birth control depends on the effects of progesterone
   a. to increase uterine motility.
   b. to decrease and thicken cervical secretions.
   c. to elevate body temperature.
   d. to depress appetite.

5. The menstrual cycle
   a. always repeats itself every 28 days.
   b. is associated with the cyclical effects of the changing hormone levels.
   c. is necessary for a human sexual response.
   d. cannot occur if ovulation does not occur.

6. In the male reproductive system
   a. the seminiferous tubules produce sperm and testosterone.
   b. the interstitial cells produce sperm.
   c. the seminiferous tubules produce sperm and the interstitial cells produce testosterone.
   d. the interstitial cells produce sperm and testosterone.

7. Spring fever occurs as a result of increased light. In males, this increase in light causes an increase in the production of
   a. inhibin.
   b. adrenal androgens.
   c. estrogen.
   d. testosterone.

8. The human sexual response depends on stimulation of
   a. the sympathetic nervous system.
   b. the parasympathetic nervous system.
   c. the hypothalamic sex drive center.
   d. adrenal androgens.

Multiple Response

Select all that apply.

1. Estrogen has many effects on the body. Estrogenic effects would include
   a. increased levels of high-density lipoproteins.
   b. increased calcium density in the bone.
   c. closing of the epiphyses.
   d. development of a thick cervical plug.
   e. increased body temperature.
   f. triangle-shaped body hair distribution.

2. Testosterone has many effects on the body. Testosterone effects would include
   a. thickening of skin and vocal cords.
   b. development of a wide and flat pelvis.
   c. development of facial hair.
   d. closure of the epiphyses.
   e. increased hematocrit.
   f. increased aggression.

Web Exercise

You have been asked to speak about sexual development to the fifth grade class at your local middle school. Go to the Internet and find appropriate information to be used for this presentation. Remember that visual learning is important at this age (9 to 11 years). Prepare a handout that you can use to help explain the normal sexual development of males and females. http://www.InnerBody.com would be a good place to start.

True or False

Indicate whether the following statements are true (T) or false (F).

_____ 1. Male and female reproductive systems arise from different fetal cells.

_____ 2. The male testes store sperm and produce the sex hormone testosterone.

_____ 3. The hypothalamus releases GnRH at puberty to stimulate the anterior pituitary release of FSH and LH, thus stimulating the production and release of the sex hormones.

_____ 4. Levels of sex hormones are controlled by local response to specific hormone stimulation.

_____ 5. Ovulation is the release of an egg into the abdomen.

_____ 6. Menopause in women and the male climacteric in men occur when the body no longer responds to the circulating sex hormones.

_____ 7. The testes produce sperm in the seminiferous tubules, in response to LH stimulation, and testosterone in the interstitial cells, in response to FSH stimulation.

_____ 8. Testosterone is responsible for the development of male sex characteristics, which can be maintained by the androgens from the adrenal gland once the body has undergone the changes of puberty.

Bibliography and References

Girard, J. (1991). *Endocrinology of puberty.* Farmington, CT: Karger.

Guyton, A., & Hall, J. (2004). *Textbook of medical physiology.* Philadelphia: WB Saunders.

Karch, A. M. (2006). *2007 Lippincott's nursing drug guide.* Philadelphia: Lippincott Williams & Wilkins.

Muske, L. E. (1993). *The neurobiology of reproductive behavior.* Farmington, CT: Karger.

CHAPTER

40

Drugs Affecting the Female Reproductive System

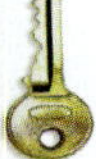

KEY TERMS

abortifacients

fertility drugs

oxytocics

progestins

tocolytics

LEARNING OBJECTIVES

Upon completion of this chapter, you will be able to:

1. Discuss the effects of estrogen and progesterone on the female body and use this information to explain the therapeutic and adverse effects of these agents when used clinically.
2. Describe the therapeutic actions, indications, pharmacokinetics, contraindications, most common adverse reactions, and important drug–drug interactions associated with the estrogens, estrogen receptor modulators, progestins, fertility drugs, oxytocics, and abortifacients.
3. Discuss the use of drugs that affect the female reproductive system across the lifespan.
4. Compare and contrast the prototype drugs estradiol, raloxifene, norethindrone, clomiphene, oxytocin, and dinoprostone with other agents in their class.
5. Outline the nursing considerations, including important teaching points to stress, for patients receiving drugs used to affect the female reproductive system.

ESTROGENS

P estradiol
estrogens, conjugated
estrogens, esterified
estropipate

ESTROGEN RECEPTOR MODULATORS

P raloxifene
toremifene

PROGESTINS

levonorgestrel
medroxyprogesterone
P norethindrone acetate
norgestrel
progesterone

FERTILITY DRUGS

cetrorelix
chorionic gonadotropin
chorionic gonadotropin alpha
P clomiphene
follitropin alfa
follitropin beta
ganirelix
menotropins
urofollitropin
urofollitropin, purified

OXYTOCICS

ergonovine
methylergonovine
P oxytocin

ABORTIFACIENTS

carboprost
P dinoprostone
mifepristone

The female reproductive system uses a cycling balance to maintain homeostasis. Changing any factor in the system can have a wide variety of effects on the entire body. Drugs that are used to affect the female reproductive system include the female steroid hormones estrogen and the **progestins** (the endogenous female hormone progesterone and its various derivatives); estrogen receptor modulators, which are not hormones but affect specific estrogen receptor sites; **fertility drugs**, which stimulate the female reproductive system; **oxytocics**, which stimulate uterine contractions and assist labor; **abortifacients**, which are used to induce abortion; and **tocolytics**, which are used to relax the gravid uterus to prolong pregnancy (Figure 40.1). Box 40.1 discusses the effects of these drugs across the lifespan.

Estrogens

Estrogens are used in many clinical situations; for example, in small doses, they are used for hormone replacement therapy (HRT) when ovarian activity is blocked or absent. They are also used less often for palliative and preventive therapy during menopause, when many of the beneficial effects of estrogen are lost. (Box 40.2 lists combination products used as HRT.) Estrogens produce a wide variety of systemic effects, including protecting the heart from atherosclerosis, retaining calcium in the bones, and maintaining the secondary female sex characteristics (see Box 39.1 in Chapter 39 for a complete list of estrogen effects). However, the results of a study by the Women's Health Initiative showed some serious negative reactions to HRT (Box 40.3 and Box 40.4).

Estrogens that are available for use include estradiol (*Estrace, Climara,* and others), which is widely used and is found in combination form as an oral contraceptive; conjugated estrogens (*Premarin*), once one of the most popular drugs for postmenopausal treatment; esterified estrogen (*Menest*); and estropipate (*Ortho-Est, Ogen*), a slow-acting oral agent associated with severe hepatic effects. Figure 40.2 and Table 40.1 summarize the various available forms of estrogens.

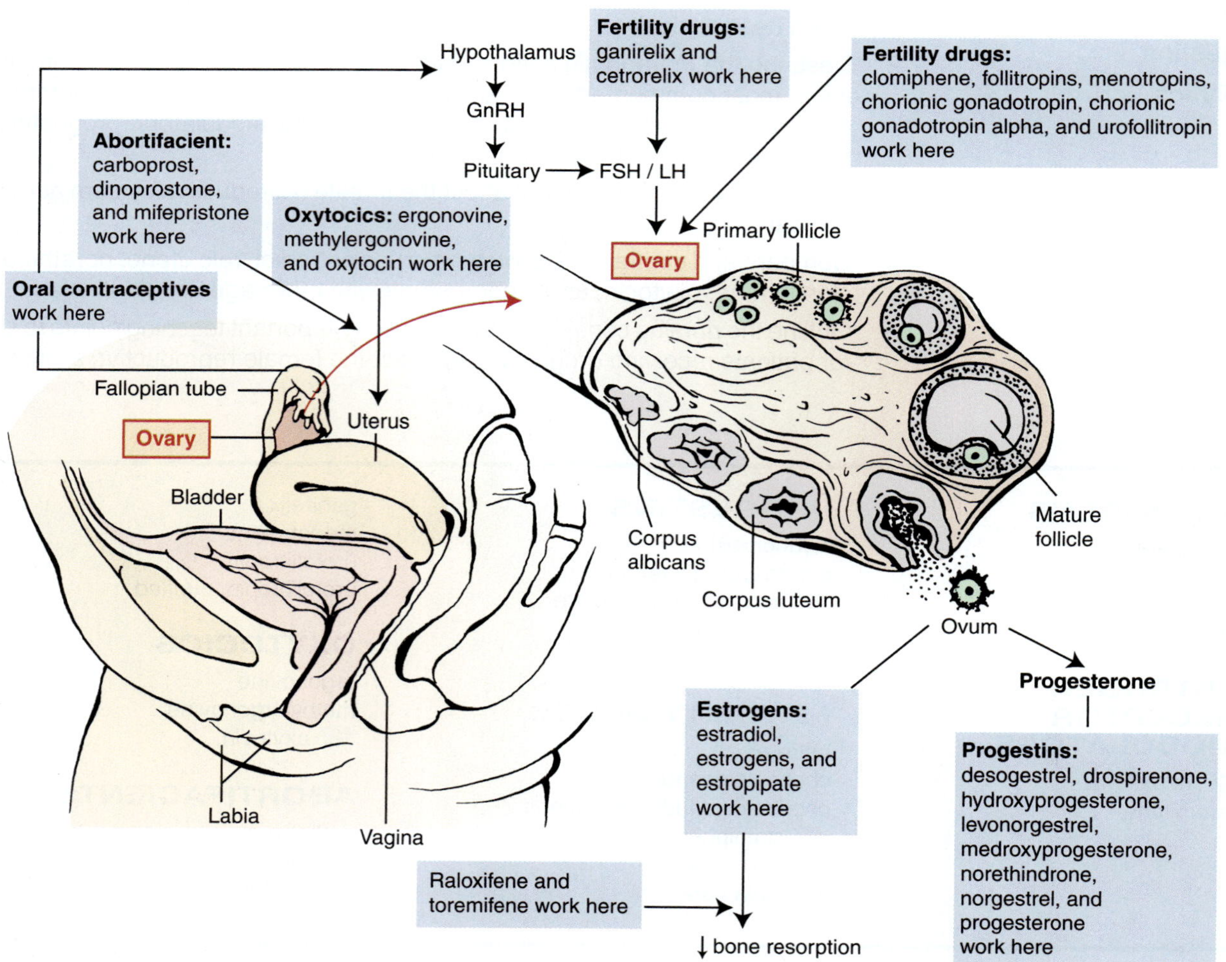

FIGURE 40.1 Sites of action of drugs affecting the female reproductive system.

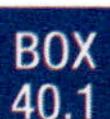

BOX 40.1 DRUG THERAPY ACROSS THE LIFESPAN

Drugs Affecting the Female Reproductive System

CHILDREN

The estrogens and progestins have undergone little testing in children. Because of their effects on closure of the epiphyses, they should be used only with great caution in growing children.

If oral contraceptives are prescribed for teenage girls, the smallest dose possible should be used and the child should be monitored carefully for metabolic and other effects.

ADULTS

If any of these drugs are used in males for the treatment of specific cancers, the patient should be advised about the possibility of estrogenic effects and appropriate support should be offered.

Women who are receiving any of these drugs should receive an annual medical examination, including breast examination and Pap smear, to monitor for adverse effects and underlying medical conditions. The potential for adverse effects should be discussed and comfort measures provided. Women taking estrogen should be advised not to smoke because of the increased risk of thrombotic events.

When combinations of these hormones are used as part of fertility programs, women need a great deal of psychological support and comfort measures to cope with the many adverse effects associated with these drugs. The risk of multiple births should be explained, as should the need for frequent monitoring.

When abortifacients are used, patients need a great deal of psychological support. Written lists of signs and symptoms to report and what to expect are more effective than just verbal lists in this time of potential stress.

These agents are not for use during pregnancy or lactation because of the potential for adverse effects on the fetus or neonate.

OLDER ADULTS

Hormone replacement therapy (HRT) is no longer commonly used by postmenopausal women. Reports of benefits and risks are frequent and conflicting, and patients need support and reliable information to make informed decisions about the use of these drugs.

If patients are also using alternative therapies, their effects on the HRT and other possible prescription drugs need to be carefully evaluated.

Therapeutic Actions and Indications

As explained previously, estrogens are important for the development of the female reproductive system and secondary sex characteristics. They affect the release of pituitary follicle-stimulating hormone (FSH) and luteinizing hormone (LH); cause capillary dilatation, fluid retention, and protein anabolism and thin the cervical mucus; conserve calcium and phosphorus and encourage bone formation; inhibit ovulation; and prevent postpartum breast discomfort. Estrogens also are responsible for the proliferation of the endometrial lining. An absence or decrease in estrogen produces the signs and symptoms of menopause in the uterus, vagina, breasts, and cervix. Estrogens are known to compete with androgens for receptor sites; this trait makes them beneficial in certain androgen-dependent prostate cancers.

Estrogens are indicated for the following conditions (Figure 40.3):

- Palliation of moderate to severe vasomotor symptoms, atrophic vaginitis, and kraurosis vulvae (atrophy of the female genitalia) associated with menopause
- Treatment of female hypogonadism, female castration, and primary ovarian failure
- Prevention of postpartum breast engorgement; in combination with progestins as oral contraceptives
- Contraception after coitus when taken in a particular sequence
- Retardation of osteoporosis in postmenopausal women
- Palliation in certain types of prostatic and mammary cancers

BOX 40.2 Combination Drugs Used for Menopause

Many fixed-combination drugs containing estrogen and a progestin are available specifically for relieving the signs and symptoms associated with menopause in women who have an intact uterus. The benefits include reduction in the risk of osteoporosis and coronary artery disease with short-term use. These drugs are taken as one tablet, once a day. Patients should receive regular medical follow-up and monitoring while taking these drugs.

Estradiol/norethindrone (*Activella*)

Estradiol/norgestimate (*Ortho-Prefest*)

Ethinyl estradiol/norethindrone acetate (*Femhrt 1/5*)

Estrogen/medroxyprogesterone (*Premphase*)

Estrogen/medroxyprogesterone/conjugated estrogens (*Prempro*)

Estradiol/drospirenone (*Angeliq*)

Also available is a combination patch (which should be changed twice each week).

Estrogen/norethindrone (*Combipatch*)

Pharmacokinetics

Oral estrogens are well absorbed through the gastrointestinal (GI) tract and undergo extensive hepatic metabolism.

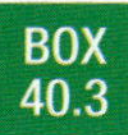

BOX 40.3 FOCUS ON THE **EVIDENCE**

Menopause and HRT—The Women's Health Initiative

Women experience the menarche (onset of the menstrual cycle) in adolescence and menopause (cessation of the menstrual cycle) in midlife. The exact age at which a woman experiences menopause or "the change" of life varies. The family history of onset of menopause is a good guide for when the effects can be expected. Just as the physical changes associated with puberty can take a few years to be accomplished, so too can the changes associated with menopause. The signs and symptoms of menopause (vaginal dryness, hot flashes, moodiness, loss of bone density, increased risk of cardiovascular disease, somnolence) are related to the loss of estrogen and progesterone effects on the body.

Hormone Replacement Therapy or Not?

For centuries, women have proceeded through this time in their lives without pharmacological intervention, although many herbal and alternative therapies may be helpful to ease the transition through menopause (see Box 40.4). Women who rely on these therapies need to be cautioned about potential drug–drug interactions and advised to always report the use of these agents to their health care providers. Today, with more research and safer drugs available to counteract some of the effects of menopause, many women choose to use hormone replacement therapy (HRT) if the adverse effects of menopause become too uncomfortable or difficult to tolerate. The use of HRT can decrease the discomforts associated with menopause, although various forms of HRT have been associated with increased risks of breast and cervical cancer. Many women are reluctant to consider HRT because of these effects. The newer drugs used in HRT have been shown to be associated with only a possible increase in risk of breast and cervical cancer, but with long-term use, are associated with an increased risk of cardiovascular events. Patients with many risk factors for developing these cancers are at greater risk than patients with no risk factors. Other drugs, the estrogen receptor modulators, have antiestrogen effects on the breast and may remove the cancer risk. But these drugs may be less reliable in their management of the signs and symptoms of menopause and have not been correlated with a reduction in the risk of coronary artery disease.

Early Research

The Women's Health Initiative was a long-term, multisite study of the effects of hormones on menopausal women. When the initial reports were published, after the third and fourth years of the study, it seemed that the use of HRT was protective in many ways. It seemed that women using HRT had decreased coronary artery disease and cardiovascular events, decreased osteoporosis and bone fractures, decreased breast and colon cancer, and improved memory. HRT was then being prescribed to prevent a number of these chronic conditions.

Later Research

In 2002, however, the study was stopped when it was found that women using HRT for 5 or more years had an increased incidence cardiovascular disease and stroke, as well as blood clots, gallstones, and ovarian cancer. The news headlines were confusing at best; many women simply stopped HRT, and women new to menopause would not even consider it.

Applying the Evidence

The woman who is entering menopause should have all of the information available before deciding whether HRT is for her. This can be a very difficult decision for many women, because the risks involved may outweigh the benefits or vice-versa. The nurse is often in the best position to provide information, listen to concerns, and help the patient decide what is best for her.

A complete family and personal history of cancer and coronary artery disease risk factors should be completed to help the patient balance the benefits versus the risks of this therapy. If the decision is made to use HRT, the patient may need support in dealing with the effects of the drugs and may have to try several different preparations before the one best suited to her is found. This can be a very frustrating time, so the patient will need a consistent, reliable person to turn to with questions and for support. As researchers continue to study women's health issues, better therapies may be developed to help women through this transition in life. Keeping up with the research as it is reported can be a difficult task, but if you work with women in clinical practice it is a necessity.

The current recommendation of the U.S. Preventative Services Task Force is that women should feel comfortable taking HRT to reduce the symptoms of menopause for short-term therapy (fewer than 5 years). The task force summarized all of the studies and noted that long-term use of HRT provides a decreased risk of osteoporosis and related fractures, possibly a reduced risk of dementia, and a reduction in risk of colon cancer. The negative aspects of this therapy include a definite but small increased risk for heart disease, stroke, and breast cancer. The harms of long-term use outweigh the benefits for most women. The benefits of short-term use, however, must be considered if a woman is having a difficult time getting through menopause (U.S. Preventative Services Task Force, 2002).

Critics of the study also point out that the women in the study were much older than most early postmenopausal groups who could benefit from HRT; they concluded that more research is needed on this issue (Neves-e-Castro, 2003).

They are excreted in the urine. Estrogens cross the placenta and enter breast milk. They should not be used during pregnancy or breast-feeding because of associated adverse effects on the fetus and neonate.

Contraindications and Cautions

Estrogens are contraindicated in the presence of any known allergies to estrogens and in patients with pregnancy (*serious fetal defects have occurred*); idiopathic vaginal bleeding; breast cancer; any estrogen-dependent cancer; history of thromboembolic disorders, *because of the increased risk of thrombus and embolus development;* or hepatic dysfunction, *because of the effects of estrogen on liver function.*

Estrogens should be used with caution during breast-feeding, *because of possible effects on the neonate;* with metabolic bone disease, *because of the bone-conserving effect of*

BOX 40.4 HERBAL AND ALTERNATIVE THERAPIES

black cohosh—40 mg/day active ingredient, should not be used for longer than 60 days; monitor for dizziness, nausea, vomiting, visual disturbances; contains alcohol—do not combine with disulfiram, metronidazole

borage—90–500 mg/day PO in softgel capsules, not for long-term use; use caution with seizure disorders or liver impairment

chaste tree—150–325 mg PO once or twice daily; may cause increased blood pressure—avoid use with antihypertensives or beta-blockers; may cause rash and itching

clary—8 gtt in 1 oz of water daily as an atomizer or dissolved in bath water; may cause sedation—avoid use with alcohol; not for internal use

devil's claw—1.5–6 g/day PO depending on preparation; increases stomach acid and may interfere with many prescription drugs; use with caution

dong quai—500 mg/day PO; causes photosensitivity—avoid exposure to the sun; do not use with warfarin—increased bleeding can occur

false unicorn root—1–2 mL PO t.i.d.; do not use with estrogen or progestins—may alter uterine effects

red clover—4 g PO t.i.d. as tea; 30–60 gtt PO t.i.d. of liquid extract; do not use with heparin or warfarin because of increased bleeding effects; do not combine with hormone replacement therapy because of risk of increased estrogenic effects

soy—25 g/day PO; do not use with calcium, iron, or zinc products; may decrease effects of estrogen, raloxifene, tamoxifen—alert health care provider if combining these drugs

wild yam—1–6 g/day PO; contains progesterone—do not use with hormone replacement therapy; may cause increased blood glucose and other toxic effects; do not combine with disulfiram or metronidazole—severe reaction may occur

estrogen; with renal insufficiency, *because of the effect on fluid and electrolytes and because estrogens are excreted in the urine;* and with hepatic impairment, *because of the many effects on the liver and GI tract and because estrogens are metabolized in the liver.*

Adverse Effects

Many of the most common adverse effects associated with estrogens involve the genitourinary (GU) tract. They include breakthrough bleeding, menstrual irregularities, dysmenorrhea, amenorrhea, and changes in libido. Other effects can result from the systemic effects of estrogens, including fluid retention, electrolyte disturbances, headache, dizziness, mental changes, weight changes, and edema. GI effects also are fairly common and include nausea, vomiting, abdominal cramps and bloating, and colitis. Potentially serious GI effects, including acute pancreatitis, cholestatic jaundice, and hepatic adenoma, have been reported with the use of estrogens.

Clinically Important Drug–Drug Interactions

If estrogens are given in combination with drugs that enhance hepatic metabolism of the estrogens (e.g., barbiturates, rifampin, tetracyclines, phenytoin), serum estrogen levels may decrease. Whenever a drug is added to or removed from a drug regimen that contains estrogens, the nurse should evaluate that drug for possible interactions and consult with the prescriber for appropriate dosage adjustments.

Estrogens have been associated with increased therapeutic and toxic effects of corticosteroids, so patients taking both drugs should be monitored very closely.

Smoking while taking estrogens should be strongly discouraged, because the combination with nicotine increases the risk for development of thrombi and emboli.

Grapefruit juice can inhibit the metabolism of estradiols, leading to increased serum levels. Patients should be discouraged from drinking large quantities of grapefruit juice.

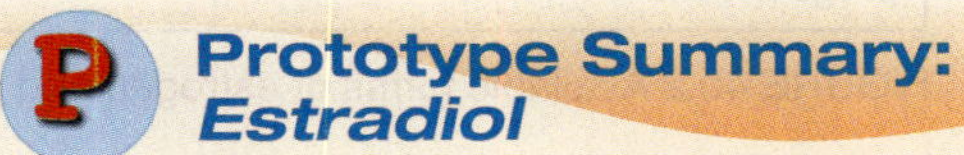

Prototype Summary: *Estradiol*

Indications: Palliation of moderate to severe vasomotor symptoms associated with menopause; prevention of postmenopausal osteoporosis; treatment of female hypogonadism, female castration; female ovarian failure; palliation of inoperable and progressing breast cancer and inoperable prostatic cancer

Actions: Most potent endogenous female sex hormone, responsible for estrogen effects on the body

Pharmacokinetics:

Route	Onset	Peak	Duration
PO	Slow	Days	Unknown

Topical preparations are not generally absorbed systemically.

$T_{1/2}$: Not known; with hepatic metabolism and excretion in the urine

Adverse effects: Corneal changes, photosensitivity, peripheral edema, chloasma, hepatic adenoma, nausea, vomiting, abdominal cramps, bloating, breakthrough bleeding, change in menstrual flow, dysmenorrhea, premenstrual-like syndrome

Estrogen Receptor Modulators

Estrogen receptor modulators were developed to produce some of the positive effects of estrogen replacement, yet limit the adverse effects. The two estrogen receptor modula-

	Oral	Injection	Vaginal cream or gel	Transdermal patch	Vaginal ring	Implanted uterine device
Estrogens						
estradiol	x	x	x	x	x	–
estrogens, conjugated	x	x	x	–	–	–
estrogens, esterified	x	–	–	–	–	–
estrone	–	x	–	–	–	–
estropipate	x	–	x	–	–	–
Progestins						
etonogestrel	–	–	–	–	x	–
hydroxyprogesterone	–	x	–	–	–	–
levonorgestrel	x	–	–	–	–	x
medroxyprogesterone	x	x	–	–	–	–
norelgestromin	–	–	–	x	–	–
norethindrone	x	–	–	–	–	–
norgestrel	x	–	–	–	–	–
progesterone	–	x	x	–	–	x

FIGURE 40.2 Available forms of estrogen and progestin.

tors that are currently available are raloxifene (*Evista*), which is used to prevent and treat osteoporosis (Table 40.2), and toremifene (*Fareston*), which is used as an antineoplastic agent because of its effects on estrogen receptor sites (see Chapter 14 for information on toremifene). The long-term effects of these two drugs are not yet known.

Therapeutic Actions and Indications

Raloxifene has modulating effects on estrogen receptor sites, stimulating some and blocking others. It is used therapeutically to stimulate specific estrogen receptor sites so as to increase bone mineral density without stimulating the endometrium in women. It is indicated for the treatment of postmenopausal osteoporosis.

Pharmacokinetics

Raloxifene is well absorbed from the GI tract and is metabolized in the liver. Excretion occurs through the feces. It is known to cross the placenta and enter into breast milk, so it should not be used during pregnancy or lactation.

Table 40.1 DRUGS IN FOCUS

Estrogens

Name	Usual Dosage	Usual Indications
P estradiol (*Estrace*)	1–2 mg/day PO; 1–5 mg IM every 3–4 wk; 10–20 mg valerate in oil IM q4wk or 1–5 mg cypionate in oil IM every 3–4 wk; 2–4 g intravaginal cream daily; apply vaginal ring once every 90 days	Palliation of signs and symptoms of menopause, prostate cancer, inoperable breast cancer; treatment of female hypogonadism, postpartum breast engorgement
estrogens, conjugated (*C.E.S., Premarin*)	0.3–1.25 mg/day PO	Palliation of signs and symptoms of menopause, prostate cancer, inoperable breast cancer; treatment of female hypogonadism, postpartum breast engorgement; to retard the progress of osteoporosis
estrogens, esterified (*Menest*)	0.3–1.25 mg/day PO	Palliation of signs and symptoms of menopause, prostate cancer, inoperable breast cancer; treatment of female hypogonadism
estropipate (*Ortho-Est, Ogen*)	0.625–5 mg/day PO	Palliation of signs and symptoms of menopause; treatment of female hypogonadism

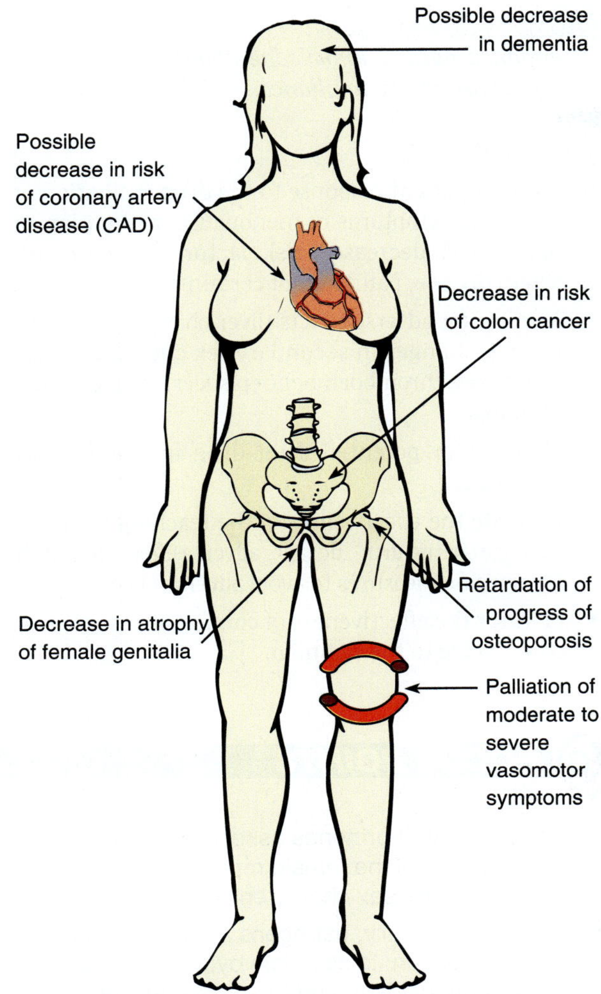

FIGURE 40.3 Sites of action of the estrogens.

Contraindications and Cautions

Raloxifene is contraindicated in the presence of any known allergy to raloxifene, and in pregnancy and lactation, *because of potential effects on the fetus or neonate.* Caution should be used in patients with a history of venous thrombosis or smoking, *because of an increased risk of blood clot formation if smoking and estrogen are combined.*

Adverse Effects

Raloxifene has been associated with GI upset, nausea, and vomiting. Changes in fluid balance may also cause headache, dizziness, visual changes, and mental changes. Hot flashes, skin rash, edema, and vaginal bleeding may occur, secondary to specific estrogen receptor stimulation. Venous thromboembolism is a potentially dangerous side effect that has been reported.

Clinically Important Drug–Drug Interactions

Cholestyramine reduces the absorption of raloxifene. Highly protein-bound drugs, such as diazepam (*Valium*), ibuprofen (*Motrin*), indomethacin (*Indocin*), and naproxen (*Naprosyn*) may interfere with binding sites. Warfarin taken with raloxifene may decrease the prothrombin time (PT); patients using this combination must be monitored closely.

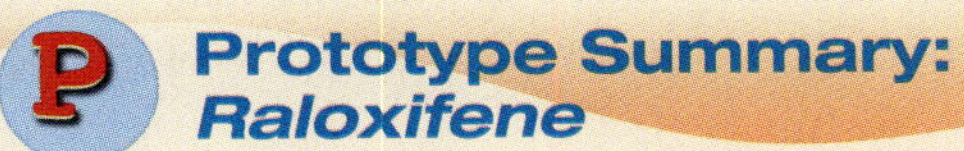

Indications: Prevention and treatment of osteoporosis in postmenopausal women

Actions: Increases bone mineral density without stimulating the endometrium; modulates effects of endogenous estrogen at specific receptor sites

Pharmacokinetics:

Route	Onset	Peak	Duration
PO	Varies	4–7 h	24 h

$T_{1/2}$: 27.7 hours, with hepatic metabolism and excretion in the feces

Adverse effects: Venous thromboembolism, hot flashes, skin rash, nausea, vomiting, vaginal bleeding, depression, light-headedness

Table 40.2 DRUGS IN FOCUS

Estrogen Receptor Modulators

Drug Name	Dosage/Route	Usual Indications
P raloxifene (*Evista*)	60 mg/day PO	Treatment of postmenopausal osteoporosis
toremifene (*Fareston*)	60 mg/day PO until disease progression occurs	Treatment of advanced breast cancer in postmenopausal women with estrogen receptor–positive and estrogen receptor–unknown tumors

Nursing Considerations for Patients Receiving Estrogens or Estrogen Receptor Modulators

Assessment: History and Examination

Screen for the following conditions, *which could be cautions or contraindications to use of the drug:* history of allergy to any estrogen or estrogen product, pregnancy, breast-feeding, hepatic dysfunction, cardiovascular disease, breast or genital cancer, renal disease, metabolic bone disease, history of thromboembolism, smoking, and idiopathic vaginal bleeding.

Include screening *for baseline status before beginning therapy and for any potential adverse effects:* skin color, lesions, texture; affect, orientation, mental status, reflexes; blood pressure, pulse, cardiac auscultation, edema, perfusion; abdominal examination, liver examination, pelvic examination, Pap smear, urinalysis, breast examination, and ophthalmic examination (particularly if the patient wears contact lenses).

Nursing Diagnoses

The patient receiving estrogens or estrogen receptor modulators may have the following nursing diagnoses related to drug therapy:

- Excess Fluid Volume related to fluid retention
- Acute Pain related to systemic side effects
- Ineffective Tissue Perfusion (Cerebral, Cardiopulmonary, Peripheral)
- Deficient Knowledge regarding drug therapy

Implementation With Rationale

- Administer drug as prescribed, *to prevent adverse effects;* administer with food if GI upset is severe, *to relieve GI distress.*
- Provide analgesics *for relief of headache as appropriate.*
- Arrange for at least an annual physical examination, including pelvic examination, Pap smear, and breast examination, *to avert adverse effects and monitor drug effects.*
- Monitor liver function periodically for the patient on long-term therapy, *to ensure that the drug is discontinued at any sign of hepatic dysfunction.*
- Provide support and reassurance *to deal with the drug and drug effects.*
- Provide thorough patient education, including measures to avoid adverse effects, warning signs of problems, and the need for regular evaluation, *to enhance patient knowledge about drug therapy and to promote compliance.*

Evaluation

- Monitor patient response to the drug (palliation of signs and symptoms of menopause, prevention of pregnancy, decreased risk factors for coronary artery disease, palliation of certain cancers).
- Monitor for adverse effects (liver changes, GI upset, edema, changes in secondary sex characteristics, headaches, thromboembolic episodes, breakthrough bleeding).
- Monitor for potential drug–drug interactions as indicated.
- Evaluate the effectiveness of the teaching plan: patient can name drug, dosage, adverse effects to watch for, specific measures to avoid adverse effects.
- Monitor the effectiveness of comfort measures and compliance to the regimen.

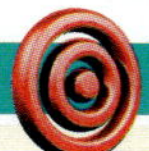

FOCUS POINTS

- Estrogens are hormones associated with the development of the female reproductive system and secondary sex characteristics.
- Pharmacologically, estrogens are used to prevent conception, to stimulate ovulation in women with hypogonadism, and to a lesser extent to replace hormones after menopause.

Progestins

Progestins are used as contraceptives, most effectively in combination with estrogens (Box 40.5 lists the currently available contraceptives); to treat amenorrhea and functional uterine bleeding; and as part of fertility programs. Like the estrogens, some progestins are useful in treating specific cancers with specific receptor site sensitivity (see Chapter 14). A number of progestins are available for use. Levonorgestrel was once available as an implant system to prevent pregnancy (*Norplant System*) but now is available only in combination-form oral contraceptives or as a uterine insert (*Mirena*). It is also used as the "morning after" pill (*Preven, Plan B*) (Box 40.6). Medroxyprogesterone (*Provera*) is available orally for treatment of amenorrhea and by injection for cancer palliation therapy. Norethindrone (*Aygestin*) is used in combination oral contraceptives and alone for the treatment of amenorrhea. Norgestrel (*Ovrette*) is an oral contraceptive that is most effective when used in combination

BOX 40.5

Contraceptives: Forms and Dosing

Oral contraceptives are available as monophasic, biphasic, and triphasic preparations. One tablet is taken orally for 21 days, beginning on the fifth day of the cycle (day 1 of the cycle is the first day of menstrual bleeding). Inert tablets or no tablets are taken for the next 7 days, and then a new course of 21 days is started.

Missed doses—If one tablet is missed, take it as soon as possible or take two tablets the next day. If two consecutive tablets are missed, take two tablets daily for the next 2 days; then resume the regular schedule. If three consecutive tablets are missed, begin a new cycle of tablets 7 days after the last tablet was taken, and use an additional method of birth control until the start of the next menstrual period.

Postcoital or emergency contraception ("morning after" regimen)—The dosing regimen must be started within 72 hours after unprotected intercourse, and a follow-up dose of the same number of pills must be taken 12 hours after the first dose. The dosages are as follows:

Ovral	Two white tablets
Nordette	Four light orange tablets
Lo/Ovral	Four white tablets
Triphasil	Four yellow tablets
Levlen	Four light orange tablets
Tri-Levlen	Four yellow tablets
Preven	Postcoital contraception kit includes a pregnancy test, used first to ensure that there is no pregnancy; four tablets containing levonorgestrel and ethinyl estradiol are then taken—two within 72 h after intercourse and two 12 h later
Plan B (levonorgestrel)	Take one tablet 72 h after intercourse and a second tablet 12 h later.

Monophasic Oral Contraceptives

Alesse, Avian 28, Lessina	20 mcg estradiol, 0.10 mg levonorgestrel
Apri, Desogen, Ortho-Cept	30 mcg ethinyl estradiol, 0.15 mg desogestrel
Brevicon, Modicon	35 mcg estradiol, 0.5 mg norethindrone
Cryselle, Lo/Ovral, Low-Ogestrel	30 mcg ethinyl estradiol, 0.3 mg norgestrel
Demulen 1/35, Zovia 1/35E	35 mcg ethinyl estradiol, 1 mg ethynodiol diacetate
Demulen 1/50, Zovia 1/50E	50 mcg estradiol, 1 mg ethynodiol diacetate
Kariva	20 mcg ethinyl estradiol, 0.15 mg desogestrel
Levlen, Levora 0.15/30, Nordette, Portia	30 mcg ethinyl estradiol, 0.15 mg levonorgestrel
Levlite	0.10 mg levonorgestrel, 0.02 mg ethinyl estradiol
Loestrin 21 1/20, Microgestin Fe 1/20	20 mcg estradiol, 1 mg norethindrone
Loestrin 21 1.5/30, Microgestin Fe 1.5/30	30 mcg ethinyl estradiol, 1.5 mg norethindrone
Necon 1/35, Norinyl 1+35, Ortho-Novum 1/35	35 mcg ethinyl estradiol, 1 mg norethindrone
Necon 1/50, Norinyl 1+50	50 mcg mestranol, 1 mg norethindrone
Ortho-Novum 1/50, Ovcon 50	50 mcg ethinyl estradiol, 1 mg norethindrone
Ovral-28, Ogestrel	50 mcg ethinyl estradiol, 0.5 mg norgestrel
Seasonale	0.15 mg levonorgestrel, 0.03 mg ethinyl estradiol for 84 days, 7 days inactive
Yasmin	30 mcg ethinyl estradiol, 3 mg drospirenone

Biphasic Oral Contraceptives

Necon 10/11, Ortho-Novum 10/11	phase 1, 10 tablets: 0.5 mg norethindrone, 35 mcg ethinyl estradiol; phase 2, 11 tablets: 1 mg norethindrone, 35 mcg ethinyl estradiol
Mircette	phase 1, 21 tablets: 0.15 mg desogestrel, 20 mcg ethinyl estradiol; phase 2, five tablets: 10 mcg ethinyl estradiol

Triphasic Oral Contraceptives

Cyclessa	phase 1, seven tablets: 0.1 mg desogestrel, 25 mcg ethinyl estradiol; phase 2, seven tablets: 0.125 mg desogestrel, 25 mcg ethinyl estradiol; phase 3, seven tablets: 0.15 mg desogestrel, 25 mcg ethinyl estradiol
Empress, Tri-Levlen, Triphasil, Trivora-28	phase 1, six tablets: 0.05 mg levonorgestrel, 30 mcg ethinyl estradiol; phase 2, five tablets: 0.075 mg evonorgestrel, 40 mcg ethinyl estradiol; phase 3, 10 tablets: 0.125 mg levonorgestrel, 30 mcg ethinyl estradiol

(continued)

BOX 40.5 Contraceptives: Forms and Dosing *(Continued)*

Estrostep 21, Estrostep Fe	phase 1, five tablets: 1 mg norethindrone, 20 mcg ethinyl estradiol; phase 2, seven tablets: 1 mg norethindrone, 30 mcg ethinyl estradiol; phase 3, nine tablets: 1 mg norethindrone, 35 mcg ethinyl estradiol
Ortho-Novum 7/7/7, Necon 7/7/7	phase 1, seven tablets: 0.5 mg norethindrone, 35 mcg ethinyl estradiol; phase 2, seven tablets: 0.75 mg norethindrone, 35 mcg ethinyl estradiol; phase 3, seven tablets: 1 mg norethindrone, 35 mcg ethinyl estradiol
Ortho Tri-Cyclen	phase 1, seven tablets: 0.18 mg norgestimate, 35 mcg ethinyl estradiol; phase 2, seven tablets: 0.215 mg norgestimate, 35 mcg ethinyl estradiol; phase 3, seven tablets: 0.25 mg norgestimate, 35 mcg ethinyl estradiol
Ortho Tri-Cyclen LO	phase 1, seven tablets: 0.18 mg norgestimate, 25 mcg ethinyl estradiol; phase 2, seven tablets: 0.215 mg norgestimate, 25 mcg ethinyl estradiol; phase 3, seven tablets: 0.25 mg norgestimate, 25 mcg ethinyl estradiol
Tri-Norinyl	phase 1, seven tablets: 0.5 mg norethindrone, 35 mcg ethinyl estradiol; phase 2, nine tablets: 1 mg norethindrone, 35 mcg ethinyl estradiol; phase 3, five tablets: 0.5 mg norethindrone, 35 mcg ethinyl estradiol

Injectables

Depo-Provera	150 mg medroxyprogesterone, given 1 mL by deep IM injection q3mo

Intrauterine System

Mirena	52 mg levonorgestrel: inserted into the uterus, releases low-dose levonorgestrel over a 5-yr period
Progestaset	38 mg progesterone inserted into the uterus each year

Transdermal System

Ortho Evra	6 mg norelgestromin, 0.75 mg ethinyl estradiol; three patches per cycle, each worn for 1 wk; releases estrogen and progestin to prevent ovulation; found to be as safe and effective as oral contraceptives and easier to remember to use for some patients

Vaginal Ring

NuvaRing	0.12 mg etonogestrol, 0.015 mg ethinyl estradiol ring inserted vaginally once a month and kept in place for 3 wk; after 1 wk's rest, a new ring is inserted

form. Progesterone (*Progestasert* and others) is available in several forms for the treatment of amenorrhea, for contraception, and in fertility programs. Desogestrel and drospirenone are only available in combination-form oral contraceptives. See Figure 40.2 for a summary of the various forms in which progestins are available. See Table 40.3 for more information about each type of progestin.

Therapeutic Actions and Indications

The progestins transform the proliferative endometrium into a secretory endometrium, inhibit the secretion of FSH and LH, prevent follicle maturation and ovulation, inhibit uterine contractions, and may have some anabolic and estrogenic effects. When they are used as contraceptives, the exact mechanism of action is not known, but it is thought that circulating progestins and estrogens "trick" the hypothalamus and pituitary and prevent the release of gonadotropin-releasing hormone (GnRH), FSH, and LH, thus preventing follicle development and ovulation. The low levels of these hormones do not produce a lush endometrium that is receptive to implantation, and if ovulation and fertilization were to occur, the chances of implantation would be remote.

Progestins are indicated for contraception; as treatment of primary and secondary amenorrhea; as treatment for functional uterine bleeding; and in some fertility protocols. Some

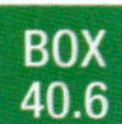

BOX 40.6 FOCUS ON THE **EVIDENCE**

OTC Availability of the "Morning After" Pill

In late 2003 and again in 2005, the Food and Drug Administration (FDA) was advised to approve the over-the-counter (OTC) use of the morning-after birth control products *Plan B* (levonorgestrel) and *Preven* (levonorgestrel and ethinyl estradiol). These drugs are used within 72 hours after intercourse and are 89% effective in preventing pregnancy.

Available OTC in two states, the drugs' history of use prompted the Reproductive Health Drugs Advisory Committee to recommend national approval. Critics, however, are concerned that women will not receive appropriate education and follow-up after the use of these products and will not receive appropriate screening. Supporters believe that these drugs will decrease the number of unwanted pregnancies and abortions in the population of women who would take advantage of the availability of these drugs. For the full report and continuing discussion of the controversy, visit the FDA web site, *www.fda.gov*.

progestins are also effective as palliative treatment in specific cancers (see Chapter 14).

Pharmacokinetics

The progestins are well absorbed, undergo hepatic metabolism, and are excreted in the urine. They are known to cross the placenta and to enter breast milk. They are not to be used during pregnancy or breast-feeding, because of the potential for adverse effects on the fetus or neonate.

Contraindications and Cautions

Progestins are contraindicated in the presence of any known allergies to progestins; pregnancy (*serious fetal defects have occurred*); idiopathic vaginal bleeding; breast cancer or genital cancer; history of thromboembolic disorders, including cerebrovascular accident, *because of the increased risk of thrombus and embolus development;* hepatic dysfunction, *because of the effects of progestins on the liver function;* pelvic inflammatory disease (PID), sexually transmitted diseases, endometriosis, or pelvic surgery, *because of the effects of progestins on the uterus;* and breast-feeding, *because of potential effects on the neonate.*

Progestins should be used with caution in patients with epilepsy, migraine headaches, asthma, or cardiac or renal dysfunction, *because of the potential exacerbation of these conditions.*

Adverse Effects

Adverse effects associated with progestins vary with the administration route used. Oral contraceptives are associated with thromboembolic disorders (particularly when combined with nicotine), increased blood pressure, weight gain, and headache. Dermal patch contraceptives are associated with the same systemic effects as well as local skin irritation. Vaginal gel use is associated with headache, nervousness, constipation, breast enlargement, and perineal pain. Intrauterine systems are associated with abdominal pain, endometriosis, abortion, PID, and expulsion of the intrauterine device. Vaginal use is associated with local irritation and swelling. Parenteral routes are associated with breakthrough bleeding, spotting, changes in the menstrual cycle, breast tenderness, thrombophlebitis, vision changes, weight gain, and fluid retention and pain at the injection site.

Clinically Important Drug–Drug Interactions

Interaction with barbiturates, carbamazepine, phenytoin, or rifampin may reduce the effect of progestins.

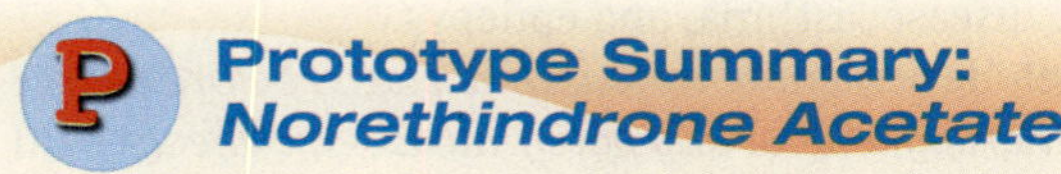

Prototype Summary: *Norethindrone Acetate*

Indications: Treatment of amenorrhea, abnormal uterine bleeding due to hormonal imbalance; treatment

Table 40.3 DRUGS IN FOCUS

Progestins

Drug Name	Dosage/Route	Usual Indications
medroxyprogesterone (*Provera*)	5–10 mg/day PO for 5–10 days; 400–1000 mg/wk IM for cancer therapy	Treatment of amenorrhea; palliation of certain cancers
P norethindrone (*Aygestin*)	2.5–10 mg/day PO	Contraception, treatment of amenorrhea
norgestrel (*Ovrette*)	0.075–0.35 mg/day PO	Contraception
progesterone (*generic*)	5–10 mg/day IM for 6–8 days; 90 mg/day intravaginally	Contraception, treatment of amenorrhea, fertility programs

of endometriosis; component of some hormonal contraceptives

Actions: Progesterone derivative that transforms the proliferative endometrium into a secretory endometrium; inhibits the secretion of pituitary FSH and LH, which prevents ovulation; inhibits uterine contractions

Pharmacokinetics:

Route	Onset	Peak	Duration
PO	Varies	Unknown	Unknown

$T_{1/2}$: Unknown, with hepatic metabolism and excretion in the feces and urine

Adverse effects: Venous thromboembolism, loss of vision, diplopia, migraine headache, rash, acne, chloasma, alopecia, breakthrough bleeding, spotting, amenorrhea, fluid retention, edema, increase in weight

Nursing Considerations for Patients Receiving Progestins

Assessment: History and Examination

Screen for the following conditions, *which could be cautions or contraindications to use of the drug:* history of allergy to any progestin product, pregnancy, breastfeeding, hepatic dysfunction, cardiovascular disease, breast or genital cancer, renal disease, history of thromboembolism, smoking, idiopathic vaginal bleeding, pelvic disease, asthma, and epilepsy.

Include screening *for baseline status before beginning therapy and for any potential adverse effects:* skin color, lesions, texture; affect, orientation, mental status, reflexes; blood pressure, pulse, cardiac auscultation, edema, perfusion; abdominal examination, liver examination, pelvic examination, Pap test, urinalysis, breast examination, and ophthalmic examination (particularly if the patient wears contact lenses). For more information, see Critical Thinking Scenario 40-1.

Nursing Diagnoses

Nursing diagnoses are the same as for estrogens.

Implementation With Rationale

Follow the same implementation guidelines as for estrogens.

Evaluation

Evaluation guidelines are the same as for estrogens.

Fertility Drugs

Women without primary ovarian failure who cannot get pregnant after 1 year of trying may be candidates for the use of fertility drugs. These drugs act to stimulate follicle development and ovulation in functioning ovaries and are combined with human chorionic gonadotropin (HCG) to maintain the follicles once ovulation has occurred. The following fertility drugs are in use today.

Cetrorelix (*Cetrotide*) is an injected drug that inhibits premature LH surges in women undergoing controlled ovarian stimulation by acting as a GnRH antagonist. Chorionic gonadotropin (*Chorex, Profasi, Pregnyl*) is an injected drug that is used to stimulate ovulation by acting like GnRH and affecting FSH and LH release. Chorionic gonadotropin alpha (*Ovidrel*) is an injected drug that stimulates final follicular development and ovulation in infertile women. Clomiphene (*Clomid* and others) is a commonly used oral agent that is also used for the treatment of male infertility. Follitropin alfa (*Gonal-F*) and follitropin beta (*Follistim*) are FSH molecules produced by recombinant DNA technology; they are injected to stimulate follicular development in infertility and for harvesting of ova for in vitro fertilization. Ganirelix (*Antagon*) is an injected drug that inhibits premature LH surges in women undergoing controlled ovarian hyperstimulation as part of a fertility program. Menotropins (*Pergonal, Humegon*) is a purified gonadotropin (similar to FSH and LH) that is also used to stimulate spermatogenesis. Urofollitropin (*Fertinex*) is an injected preparation derived from the urine of postmenopausal women; it has been associated with immune-type reactions. With the development of newer, purer drugs, urofollitropin is used less often. Urofollitropin, purified (*Bravelle*) is a less toxic form of urofollitropin that is used to induce ovulation in women with pituitary suppression and to stimulate multiple follicle development in ovulatory patients. See Table 40.4 for more information on all of these drugs.

Therapeutic Actions and Indications

Fertility drugs work either directly or by stimulating the hypothalamus to increase FSH and LH levels, leading to ovarian follicular development and maturation of ova. Given in sequence with HCG to maintain the follicle and hormone production, these drugs are used to treat infertility in women with functioning ovaries whose partners are fertile. Fertility drugs also may be used to stimulate multiple follicle development for the harvesting of ova for in vitro fertilization. Menotropins also stimulate spermatogenesis in men with low sperm counts and otherwise normally functioning testes.

Pharmacokinetics

These drugs are well absorbed and are treated like endogenous hormones within the body, undergoing hepatic metabolism

CRITICAL THINKING SCENARIO 40-1

Birth Control

THE SITUATION

J.M. is a 25-year-old woman who is being seen in her gynecologist's office for a routine annual physical examination and Pap test. J.M. reports that she has just become sexually active and would like to start using contraceptives. She has some concerns about stories she has heard about "the pill" and would like to know the safest and most effective birth control to use.

CRITICAL THINKING

What teaching and counseling issues will be important for J.M. at this time?

What important issues should be discussed when explaining the benefits and drawbacks of various contraceptive measures?

What teaching information needs to be stressed with J.M. if she elects to use oral contraceptives?

DISCUSSION

This appointment presents a good opportunity for the health care provider to allow J.M. to discuss this new aspect of her life. She may have questions about the experience and about things she should be doing or should be questioning. The risk of sexually transmitted diseases as well as pregnancy can be discussed. J.M. needs full information about the various forms of birth control that are available for use. Nonpharmacological measures, such as condoms, and the rhythm method, and their reliability can be discussed.

The use of hormones for birth control should then be explained, including the 96% to 98% reliability of these methods when used correctly. The numerous delivery methods for these hormones should be outlined. A variety of possibilities exist, from the transdermal patch to injection to the vaginal ring to the traditional tablet. J.M. elected to go with an oral contraceptive (OC). J.M. will need teaching about drug and herbal interactions with the OC and will need to have written instructions on what to do if a dose is missed. The action that should be taken if a dose is missed can be very complicated and involves knowing on which day in the cycle the dose was missed.

It is also important to stress that the OC will not protect J.M. from sexually transmitted diseases and that precautions will need to be taken to avoid exposure to these diseases. She should also be advised not to smoke, because smoking combined with OC use increases the risk for emboli. The adverse effects that she might experience should be reviewed, and the importance of an annual pelvic examination and Pap test should be stressed. A trusting nurse–patient relationship is important at this time so that J.M. can feel free to call with questions or problems in the future.

NURSING CARE GUIDE FOR J.M.: ORAL CONTRACEPTIVES

Assessment: History And Examination

Assess the patient's health history for allergies to any estrogens; pregnancy, lactation; breast or genital cancer; hepatic dysfunction; coronary artery disease; thromboembolic disease; renal disease; idiopathic vaginal bleeding; metabolic bone disease; diabetes

Focus the physical examination on the following:

Neuro: orientation, reflexes, affect, mental status

Skin: color, lesions

CV: pulse, cardiac auscultation, blood pressure, edema, perfusion

GI: abdominal examination, liver examination

GU: pelvic examination, Pap smear, urinalysis

Eye: ophthalmologic examination

Nursing Diagnoses

Excess Fluid Volume related to fluid retention

Acute Pain related to systemic side effects

Ineffective Tissue Perfusion

Deficient Knowledge regarding drug therapy

Implementation

Administer medication as prescribed.

Administer with meals.

Provide analgesics for headache if appropriate.

Provide at least annual physical examination, including Pap smear and breast examination.

Provide support and reassurance to deal with drug therapy.

Provide patient teaching regarding drug name, dosage, adverse effects, precautions, warnings to report, safe administration.

(continued)

Birth Control *(continued)*

Evaluation

Evaluate drug effects: prevention of pregnancy; relief of signs and symptoms of menopause; decreased risk of coronary artery disease.

Monitor for adverse effects: signs of liver dysfunction; gastrointestinal upset; edema; changes in secondary sex characteristics; headaches; thromboembolic episodes; breakthrough bleeding.

Monitor for drug–drug interactions as indicated for each drug.

Evaluate effectiveness of patient teaching program and comfort and safety measures.

Patient Teaching For J.M.

- ☐ An oral contraceptive (OC), or birth control pill, contains specific amounts of female sex hormones that work to make the body unreceptive to pregnancy and to prevent ovulation (the release of the egg from the ovary). Because these hormones affect many systems in your body, it is important to have regular physical checkups while you are taking this drug.
- ☐ Many drugs affect the way that OCs work. To be safe, avoid the use of over-the-counter drugs and other drugs, unless you first check with your health care provider.
- ☐ Some of the following adverse effects may occur:
    - *Headache, nervousness*—Check with your health care provider about the use of an analgesic; this effect usually passes after a few months on the drug.
    - *Nausea, loss of appetite*—This usually passes with time; consult your health care provider if it is a problem.
    - *Swelling, weight gain*—Water retention is a normal effect of these hormones. Limiting salt intake may help. You may have trouble with contact lenses if you wear them, because the body often retains fluid, which may change the shape of your eye. This usually adjusts over time.
    - *Blood clots in women who smoke cigarettes*—Cigarette smoking can aggravate serious side effects of OCs, such as the formation of blood clots. When taking OCs, it is advisable to cut down, or preferably to stop, cigarette smoking.
- ☐ Tell any doctor, nurse, or other health care provider that you are taking this drug.
- ☐ Report any of the following to your health care provider: pain in the calves or groin; chest pain or difficulty breathing; lump in the breast; severe headache, dizziness, visual changes; severe abdominal pain; yellowing of the skin; pregnancy.
- ☐ Bleeding (a false menstrual period) should occur during the time that the drug is withdrawn. Report bleeding at *any* other time to your health care provider.
- ☐ It is important to have regular medical checkups, including Pap tests, while you are taking this drug. If you decide to stop the drug to become pregnant, consult with your health care provider.
- ☐ A patient package insert is included with the drug. Read this information and feel free to ask any questions that you might have.
- ☐ Keep this drug and all medications out of the reach of children.

and renal excretion. They should not be used during pregnancy or lactation because of the potential for adverse hormonal effects on the fetus or neonate.

Contraindications and Cautions

These drugs are contraindicated in the presence of primary ovarian failure (*they only work to stimulate functioning ovaries*); thyroid or adrenal dysfunction, *because of the effects on the hypothalamic–pituitary axis;* ovarian cysts; pregnancy (*serious fetal defects have occurred*); idiopathic uterine bleeding; and known allergy to any fertility drug.

Caution should be used in women who are breast-feeding and in those with thromboembolic diseases, *because of the risk of increased thrombus formation;* and in women with respiratory diseases, *because of alterations in fluid volume and blood flow.*

Adverse Effects

Adverse effects associated with fertility drugs include a greatly increased risk of multiple births and birth defects; ovarian overstimulation (abdominal pain, distention, ascites, pleural effusion); and headache, fluid retention, nausea, bloating, uterine bleeding, ovarian enlargement, gynecomastia, and

Table 40.4 DRUGS IN FOCUS

Fertility Drugs

Drug Name	Dosage/Route	Usual Indications
cetrorelix (*Cetrotide*)	3 mg Sub-Q during early follicular phase *or* 0.25 mg Sub-Q on day 5 or 6 of stimulation and then every day until HCG is administered	Inhibition of premature luteinizing hormone (LH) surge in women undergoing controlled ovarian stimulation
chorionic gonadotropin (*Chorex, Profasi, Pregnyl*)	500–10,000 International Units Sub-Q depending on timing and indication	Ovulation induction, hypogonadism, prepubertal cryptorchidism
chorionic gonadotropin alpha (*Ovidrel*)	250 mcg Sub-Q, timing depending on indication	Induction of final follicular maturation and ovulation induction
P clomiphene (*Clomid* and others)	50–100 mg/day PO with length of therapy and timing dependent on the particular situation	Treatment of infertility
follitropin alfa (*Gonal-F*)	75–150 International Units/day Sub-Q, dosage increases based on response; do not exceed 300 International Units/day	Stimulation of follicular development for harvesting of ova
follitropin beta (*Follistim*)	75–225 International Units/day Sub-Q, dosage increases based on response; do not exceed 300 International Units/day	Stimulation of follicular development for harvesting of ova
ganirelix (*Antagon*)	250 mcg/day Sub-Q during early follicular phase	Inhibition of premature LH surges in women undergoing controlled ovarian hyperstimulation
menotropins (*Pergonal, Repronex*)	Treatment scheduled with HCG; 150 International Units FSH/150 International Units LH IM for 9–12 days is often used	Stimulation of ovulation in women and spermatogenesis in men
urofollitropin (*Fertinex*)	75–150 International Units/day IM for 7–12 days cycled with HCG, dosage dependent on response	Stimulation of ovulation for the treatment of infertility and to stimulate follicular development for harvesting of ova
urofollitropin, purified (*Bravelle*)	150 International Units/day Sub-Q or IM, maximum daily dose of 450 International Units	Induction of ovulation in patients who have previously received pituitary suppression, stimulation of multiple follicles in ovulatory patients

febrile reactions (possibly due to stimulation of progesterone release).

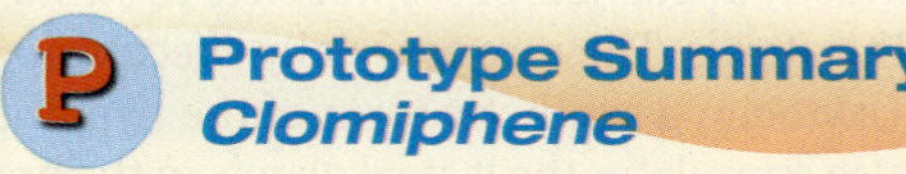

Prototype Summary: Clomiphene

Indications: Treatment of ovarian failure in patients with normal liver function and normal endogenous estrogens; unlabeled use: treatment of male sterility

Actions: Binds to estrogen receptors, decreasing the number of available estrogen receptors, which gives the hypothalamus the false signal to increase FSH and LH secretion, leading to ovarian stimulation

Pharmacokinetics:

Route	Onset	Peak	Duration
PO	5–8 days	Unknown	6 wk

$T_{1/2}$: 5 days, with hepatic metabolism and excretion in the feces

Adverse effects: Vasomotor flushing, visual changes, abdominal discomfort, distention and bloating, nausea, vomiting, ovarian enlargement, breast tenderness, ovarian overstimulation, multiple pregnancies

Nursing Considerations for Patients Receiving Fertility Drugs

Assessment: History and Examination

Screen for the following conditions, *which could be cautions or contraindications to use of the drug:* history of allergy to any fertility drug, pregnancy, lactation, ovarian failure, thyroid or adrenal dysfunction, ovarian cysts, idiopathic uterine bleeding, thromboembolic diseases, and respiratory diseases.

Include screening *for baseline status before beginning therapy and for any potential adverse effects:* skin, lesions; orientation, affect, reflexes; blood pressure, pulse; respiration, adventitious sounds; hormone levels, Pap smear, breast examination.

Nursing Diagnoses

The patient receiving fertility drugs may have the following nursing diagnoses related to drug therapy:

- Disturbed Body Image related to drug treatment and diagnosis
- Acute Pain related to headache, fluid retention, GI upset
- Sexual Dysfunction
- Deficient Knowledge regarding drug therapy

Implementation With Rationale

- Assess the cause of dysfunction before beginning therapy, *to ensure appropriate use of the drug.*
- Complete a pelvic examination before each cycle of drug therapy, *to rule out ovarian enlargement, pregnancy, or uterine problems.*
- Check urine estrogen and estradiol levels before beginning therapy, *to verify ovarian function.*
- Administer with an appropriate dosage of HCG as indicated, *to ensure beneficial effects.*
- Discontinue the drug at any sign of ovarian overstimulation, and arrange for hospitalization *to monitor and support patient* if this occurs.
- Provide women with a calendar of treatment days, explanations of adverse effects to anticipate, and instructions on when intercourse should occur, *to increase the therapeutic effectiveness of the drug.*
- Provide warnings about the risk and hazards of multiple births, *so the patient can make informed decisions about drug therapy.*
- Provide thorough patient education, including measures to avoid adverse effects, warning signs of problems, and the need for regular evaluation *to enhance patient knowledge about drug therapy and to promote compliance.*

Evaluation

- Monitor patient response to the drug (ovulation).
- Monitor for adverse effects (abdominal bloating, weight gain, ovarian overstimulation, multiple births).
- Evaluate the effectiveness of the teaching plan (patient can name drug, dosage, adverse effects to watch for, specific measures to avoid adverse effects).
- Monitor the effectiveness of comfort measures and compliance with the regimen.

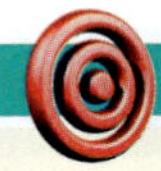

FOCUS POINTS

- Progestins maintain pregnancy and are also involved with development of secondary sex characteristics.
- Combined with estrogens, progestins are used to prevent conception, to treat uterine bleeding, and to improve comfort in some patients with cancers.
- In women with functioning ovaries, fertility drugs increase follicle development by stimulating FSH and LH to increase the chances for pregnancy.

Oxytocics

Oxytocic drugs are used to stimulate contraction of the uterus, much like the action of the hypothalamic hormone oxytocin, which is stored in the posterior pituitary. These drugs include ergonovine (*Ergotrate*), which is given intramuscularly or intravenously and is used to prevent and treat postpartum and postabortion uterine atony; methylergonovine (*Methergine*), which can be given intramuscularly or intravenously directly after delivery, then continued in the oral form to promote uterine involution; and oxytocin (*Pitocin, Syntocinon*), which is used to induce labor and to promote uterine contractions after labor. Oxytocin is also available in a nasal form to stimulate milk "let down" in lactating women. See Table 40.5 for more information.

Therapeutic Actions and Indications

The oxytocics directly affect neuroreceptor sites to stimulate contraction of the uterus. They are especially effective in the gravid uterus. Oxytocin, a synthetic form of the hypothalamic hormone, also stimulates the lacteal glands in the breast to contract, promoting milk ejection in lactating women.

Oxytocics are indicated for the prevention and treatment of uterine atony after delivery. This is important to prevent postpartum hemorrhage. Ergonovine is being investigated for use in diagnostic tests for angina during arteriography studies because it has been shown to induce coronary artery contraction. Methylergonovine has been successfully used to stimulate the last stage of labor. Oxytocin is used in a nasal form to stimulate milk "let down" in lactating women. It is also being evaluated as a diagnostic agent to test abnormal fetal heart rates (oxytocin challenge) and to treat breast engorgement.

Pharmacokinetics

The oxytocics are rapidly absorbed, metabolized in the liver, and excreted in urine and feces. They cross the placenta and enter breast milk. Because of their effects on the uterus, they

Table 40.5 DRUGS IN FOCUS

Oxytocics

Drug Name	Dosage/Route	Usual Indications
ergonovine (*Ergotrate*)	0.2 mg IM, may repeat doses q2–4h as needed	Prevention and treatment of postpartum and post-abortion uterine atony
methylergonovine (*Methergine*)	0.2 mg IM or IV, may repeat q2–4h; 0.2 mg PO t.i.d. during the puerperium for up to 1 wk	Promotion of postpartum uterine involution
P oxytocin (*Pitocin, Syntocinon*)	1–2 milliunits/min IV through an infusion pump, increase as needed, do not exceed 20 milliunits/min; 10 units IM after delivery of the placenta One spray in each nostril 2–3 min before breast-feeding	Induction of labor; promotion of uterine contractions postpartum; nasally to stimulate milk "let down" in lactating women

are not used during pregnancy. Oxytocin is used during lactation because of its effects on milk ejection, but the baby should be evaluated for any adverse effects associated with the hormone.

Contraindications and Cautions

Oxytocics are contraindicated in the presence of any known allergy to oxytocics and with cephalopelvic disproportion, unfavorable fetal position, complete uterine atony, or early pregnancy. Caution should be used in patients with coronary disease, hypertension, lactation, or previous cesarean section *because of the effects on artery contraction and uterine contraction.*

Adverse Effects

The adverse effects most often associated with the oxytocics are related to excessive effects (e.g., uterine hypertonicity and spasm, uterine rupture, postpartum hemorrhage, decreased fetal heart rate). GI upset, nausea, headache, and dizziness are not uncommon. Ergonovine and methylergonovine can produce ergotism (e.g., nausea, blood pressure changes, weak pulse, dyspnea, chest pain, numbness and coldness in extremities, confusion, excitement, delirium, convulsions, and even coma). Oxytocin has caused severe water intoxication with coma and even maternal death when used for a prolonged period. This is thought to occur because of related effects of antidiuretic hormone (ADH), which is also stored in the posterior pituitary and may be released in response to oxytocin activity, causing water retention in the kidney.

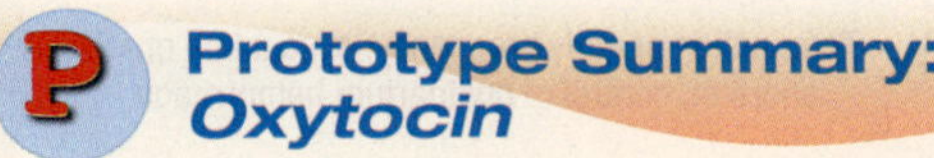

Prototype Summary: *Oxytocin*

Indications: To initiate or improve uterine contractions for early vaginal delivery; to stimulate or reinforce labor in selected cases of uterine inertia; to manage inevitable or incomplete abortion; second-trimester abortion; to control postpartum bleeding or hemorrhage; to treat lactation deficiency

Actions: Synthetic form stimulates the uterus, especially the gravid uterus; causes myoepithelium of the lacteal glands to contract, resulting in milk ejection in lactating women

Pharmacokinetics:

Route	Onset	Peak	Duration
IV	Immediate	Unknown	60 min
IM	3–5 min	Unknown	2–3 h

$T_{1/2}$: 1–6 min, with tissue metabolism and excretion in the urine

Adverse effects: Cardiac arrhythmias, hypertension, fetal bradycardia, nausea, vomiting, uterine rupture, pelvic hematoma, uterine hypertonicity, severe water intoxication, anaphylactic reaction

Nursing Considerations for Patients Receiving Oxytocics

Assessment: History and Examination

Screen for the following conditions, *which could be cautions or contraindications to use of the drug:* history of allergy to oxytocics, early pregnancy, lactation, uterine atony, hypertension, history of cesarean section, undesirable fetal position, and cephalopelvic disproportion.

Include screening *for baseline status before beginning therapy and for any potential adverse effects:* skin, lesions; orientation, affect, reflexes; blood pressure, pulse; respiration, adventitious sounds; fetal position, fetal heartbeat, uterine tone, and timing of contractions; and bleeding studies and complete blood count.

Nursing Diagnoses

The patient receiving oxytocics may have the following nursing diagnoses related to drug therapy:

- Acute Pain related to uterine contractions, headache, fluid retention, GI upset
- Excess Fluid Volume related to ergotism or water intoxication
- Deficient Knowledge regarding drug therapy

Implementation With Rationale

- Ensure fetal position (if appropriate) and cephalopelvic proportions, *to prevent serious complications of delivery.*
- Regulate oxytocin delivery between contractions if being given to stimulate labor *to regulate dosage appropriately.*
- Monitor blood pressure periodically during and after administration, *to monitor for adverse effects.* Discontinue the drug if blood pressure rises dramatically.
- Monitor uterine tone and involution and amount of bleeding, *to ensure safe and therapeutic drug use.*
- Discontinue the drug at any sign of uterine hypertonicity, *to avoid potentially life-threatening effects;* provide life support as needed.
- Monitor fetal heartbeat if given during labor, *to ensure safety of the fetus.*
- Provide nasal oxytocin at bedside with the bottle sitting upright. The patient should be instructed to invert the squeeze bottle and exert gentle pressure to deliver the drug just before nursing *to achieve greatest therapeutic effect.*
- Provide thorough patient education, including measures to avoid adverse effects and warning signs of problems to report, *to enhance patient knowledge about drug therapy and to promote compliance.*

Evaluation

- Monitor patient response to the drug (uterine contraction, prevention of hemorrhage, milk "let down").
- Monitor for adverse effects (blood pressure changes, uterine hypertonicity, water intoxication, ergotism).
- Evaluate the effectiveness of the teaching plan (patient can name drug, dosage, adverse effects to watch for, specific measures to avoid adverse effects).
- Monitor the effectiveness of comfort measures and compliance with the regimen.

Abortifacients

Abortifacients are drugs used to evacuate the uterus by stimulating intense uterine contractions (Table 40.6). These drugs include carboprost (*Hemabate*), dinoprostone (*Cervidil, Prepidil Gel, Prostin E2*), and mifepristone (RU-486, *Mifeprex*). Carboprost is an intramuscular drug used to terminate early pregnancy, evacuate a missed abortion, or control postpartum hemorrhage. Dinoprostone is a prostaglandin that stimulates uterine contractions; it is given by intravaginal suppository. Besides evacuating the uterus, it is also used to stimulate cervical ripening before labor. Mifepristone is a newer, controversial drug that acts as an antagonist of progesterone sites in the endometrium, allowing local prostaglandins to stimulate uterine contractions and dislodge or prevent the implantation of any fertilized egg. This drug is given orally and takes 5 to 7 days to produce the desired effect.

Therapeutic Actions and Indications

The abortifacients stimulate uterine activity, dislodging any implanted trophoblast and preventing implantation of any fer-

Table 40.6 DRUGS IN FOCUS

Abortifacients

Drug Name	Dosage/Route	Usual Indications
carboprost (*Hemabate*)	250 mcg IM at intervals of 1.5–3.5 h, not to exceed 12 mg total dose; 250 mcg IM to control postpartum bleeding, not to exceed 2 mg total dose	Termination of early pregnancy, evacuation of missed abortion, control of postpartum hemorrhage
P dinoprostone (*Cervidil, Propedil Gel, Prostin E2*)	20 mg vaginal suppository, may repeat q3–5h as needed for termination of pregnancy; 0.5 mg gel via cervical catheter, repeated in 6 h if needed for cervical ripening, then wait 6–12 h before using oxytocin	Evacuation of the uterus, cervical ripening before labor
mifepristone (*Mifeprex, RU-486*)	600 mg PO as a single dose; if pregnancy not terminated by day 3, 400 mcg misoprostol PO; if not terminated by day 14, surgical intervention is suggested	Termination of early pregnancy

tilized egg. These drugs are approved for use to terminate pregnancy 12 to 20 weeks from the date of the last menstrual period. Mifepristone is approved for use during the first 49 days of the pregnancy. Carboprost and dinoprostone are also approved for use to evacuate the uterus after a missed abortion or fetal death. Carboprost also is used to treat postpartum hemorrhage that is not responsive to the usual therapy. Because of its local prostaglandin effects, dinoprostone can also be used to stimulate cervical ripening before induction of labor.

Pharmacokinetics

These drugs are well absorbed, metabolized in the liver, and excreted in the urine. Because of their effects on the uterus, they are used during pregnancy only to end the pregnancy. They are not recommended for use during lactation because of the potential for serious effects on the neonate. If these drugs are to be used by a lactating mother, another method of feeding the baby should be used.

Contraindications and Cautions

Abortifacients should not be used with any known allergy to abortifacients or prostaglandins; after 20 weeks from the last menstrual period; or with active PID or acute cardiovascular, hepatic, renal, or pulmonary disease.

Caution should be used with any history of asthma, hypertension, or adrenal disease and with acute vaginitis (inflammation of the vagina) or scarred uterus.

Adverse Effects

Adverse effects associated with abortifacients include abdominal cramping, heavy uterine bleeding, perforated uterus, and uterine rupture, all of which are related to exaggeration of the desired effects of the drug. Other side effects include headache, nausea and vomiting, diarrhea, diaphoresis (sweating), backache, and rash.

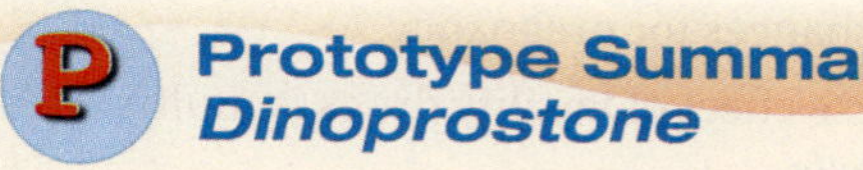

Prototype Summary: Dinoprostone

Indications: Termination of pregnancy 12 to 20 weeks from the first day of the last menstrual period; evacuation of the uterus in the management of missed abortion or intrauterine fetal death; management of nonmetastatic gestational trophoblastic disease; initiation of cervical ripening

Actions: Stimulates the myometrium of the pregnant uterus to contract, evacuating the contents of the uterus

Pharmacokinetics:

Route	Onset	Peak	Duration
Intravaginal	10 min	15 min	2–3 h

$T_{1/2}$: 5–10 hours, with tissue metabolism and excretion in the urine

Adverse effects: Headache, paresthesias, hypotension, vomiting, diarrhea, nausea, uterine rupture, uterine or vaginal pain, chills, diaphoresis, backache, fever

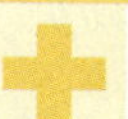

FOCUS ON **PATIENT SAFETY**

Name confusion has been reported among *Prostin VR Pediatric* (alprostadil), *Prostin FZ* (dinoprostone), and *Prostin 15* (carboprost, available in Europe). Confusion has also been reported between *Prepidil* (dinoprostone) and bepridil, a calcium channel blocker. Use extreme caution to make sure that your patient is receiving the correct drug.

Nursing Considerations for Patients Receiving Abortifacients

Assessment: History and Examination

Screen for the following conditions, *which could be cautions or contraindications to use of the drug:* history of allergy to any abortifacient or prostaglandin preparation; active PID; cardiac, hepatic, pulmonary, or renal disease; history of asthma; and hypotension, hypertension, epilepsy, scarred uterus, or acute vaginitis.

Include screening *for baseline status before beginning therapy and for any potential adverse effects:* skin, lesions; orientation, affect; blood pressure, pulse; respiration, adventitious sounds; vaginal discharge, pelvic examination, uterine tone; and liver and renal function tests, leukocyte count, and urinalysis.

Nursing Diagnoses

The patient receiving abortifacients may have the following nursing diagnoses related to drug therapy:

- Acute Pain related to uterine contractions, headache, fluid retention, GI upset
- Ineffective Coping related to abortion or fetal death
- Deficient Knowledge regarding drug therapy

Implementation With Rationale

- Administer via route indicated, following the manufacturer's directions for storage and preparation, *to ensure safe and therapeutic use of the drug.*
- Confirm the age of the pregnancy before administering the drug, *to ensure appropriate use of the drug.*

- Confirm that abortion or uterine evacuation is complete, *to avoid potential bleeding problems;* prepare for dilation and curettage if necessary.
- Monitor blood pressure periodically during and after administration, *to assess for adverse effects;* discontinue the drug if blood pressure rises dramatically.
- Monitor uterine tone and involution and the amount of bleeding during and for several days after use of the drug, *to ensure appropriate response and recovery from the drug.*
- Provide support and appropriate referrals, *to help the patient deal with abortion or fetal death.*
- Provide thorough patient teaching, including measures to avoid adverse effects and warning signs of problems to report, *to enhance patient knowledge about drug therapy and to promote compliance.*

Evaluation

- Monitor patient response to the drug (evacuation of uterus).
- Monitor for adverse effects (GI upset, nausea, blood pressure changes, hemorrhage, uterine rupture).
- Evaluate the effectiveness of the teaching plan (patient can name drug, dosage, adverse effects to watch for, specific measures to avoid adverse effects).
- Monitor the effectiveness of comfort measures and compliance to the regimen.

Tocolytics

Uterine contractions that become strong before term can lead to premature labor and delivery, which can have detrimental effects on the neonate, including death. Drugs used to relax the uterine smooth muscle and prevent contractions leading to premature labor and delivery are called tocolytics. They are usually reserved for use after 20 weeks of gestation, when the neonate has a chance of survival outside the uterus. Only one tocolytic agent was available in the United States—ritodrine (*Yutopar*). Because of serious adverse effects associated with the drug, it was withdrawn from the market in 2003. If premature contractions occur, terbutaline, a beta$_2$-selective adrenergic agonist, is often used. Stimulation of these receptors calms uterine contractions, but the patient will need to be monitored for sympathetic stimulation.

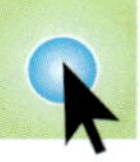

WEB LINKS

Health care providers and patients may want to explore the following Internet sources:

http://www.babycenter.com/refcap/4091.html Information on fertility drugs—research, explanations, related information.

http://fbhc.org/Patients/BetterHealth/Menopause/home.html Information on menopause, specifically for patients, and teaching aids with explanations, drugs, choices, and support groups.

http://www.menopause-online.com Information on HRT, updated regularly with studies, controversies, and treatment choices, cross-referenced to research studies.

http://www.menopause.org Information on women's health in midlife and beyond from the North American Menopause Society.

http://www.reproline.jhu.edu Information on contraceptives—good teaching guidelines, explanations, and choices.

http://www.asrm.com Information on estrogens—research, uses, and controversies, for professionals.

Points to Remember

- Estrogens are female sex hormones that are important in the development of the female reproductive system and secondary sex characteristics.
- Estrogens are used pharmacologically mainly to replace hormones lost at menopause so as to prevent many of the signs and symptoms associated with menopause, including the development of coronary artery disease; to stimulate ovulation in woman with hypogonadism; and in combination with progestins for oral contraceptives.
- Progestins are female sex hormones that are responsible for maintenance of a pregnancy and for the development of some secondary sex characteristics.
- Progestins are used in combination with estrogens for contraception, to treat uterine bleeding, and for palliation in certain cancers with sensitive receptor sites.
- Fertility drugs stimulate FSH and LH in women with functioning ovaries to increase follicle development and improve the chances for pregnancy.
- A major adverse effect of fertility drugs is multiple births and birth defects.
- Oxytocic drugs act like the hypothalamic hormone oxytocin to stimulate uterine contractions and induce or speed up labor. They are most frequently used to control bleeding and promote postpartum involution of the uterus.
- Abortifacients are drugs that stimulate uterine activity to cause uterine evacuation. These drugs can be used to induce abortion in early pregnancy or to promote uterine evacuation after intrauterine fetal death.
- Tocolytics are drugs that relax the uterine smooth muscle; they are used to stop premature labor in patients after 20 weeks' gestation.

CHECK YOUR UNDERSTANDING

Answers to the questions in this chapter may be found in the Answer Key in the back of the book.

Multiple Choice

Select the best answer to the following.

1. A postmenopausal woman is started on estrogens to control her unpleasant menopausal symptoms. She should be instructed that, as a result of the drug therapy, she may experience
   a. constipation.
   b. breakthrough bleeding.
   c. weight loss.
   d. persistently elevated body temperature.

2. An estrogen receptor modulator might be the drug of choice in the treatment of postmenopausal osteoporosis in a patient with a family history of breast or uterine cancer. The postmenopausal patient taking an estrogen receptor modulator should be taught that she might experience.
   a. constipation and dry, itchy skin.
   b. flushing and dry vaginal mucosa.
   c. hot flashes and vaginal bleeding.
   d. no associated adverse effects.

3. Combination estrogens and progestins are commonly used as oral contraceptives. It is thought that this combination has its effect by
   a. acting like circulating estrogen and progesterone to block the hypothalamic release of FSH and LH, preventing follicle development and ovulation.
   b. directly suppressing the ovaries and preventing ovulation.
   c. keeping the endometrium constantly lush and blood filled.
   d. preventing menstruation, which prevents pregnancy.

4. Any patient who is taking estrogens, progestins, or combination products should be cautioned to avoid smoking because
   a. nicotine increases the metabolism of the hormones and they may not be effective.
   b. the combination leads to an increased risk of potentially dangerous thromboembolic episodes.
   c. nicotine amplifies the adverse effects of the hormones.
   d. nicotine blocks hormone receptor sites and they may no longer be effective.

5. Oxytocin, a synthetic form of the hypothalamic hormone, is used to
   a. induce abortion.
   b. stimulate milk "let down" in the lactating woman.
   c. increase fertility and the chance of conception.
   d. relax the gravid uterus and prevent preterm labor.

6. The use of an abortifacient drug would be contraindicated in a woman
   a. who is 15 weeks pregnant.
   b. who is older than 50 years of age.
   c. who has had four cesarean sections in the past.
   d. who is 10 weeks pregnant.

7. A young woman decides to start on oral contraceptives because she feels that it is not the right time for her to get pregnant. You would evaluate her teaching about the drug to be effective if she tells you:
   a. "I shouldn't smoke for the first month to make sure I don't react severely to the pills."
   b. "If I forget to take a pill, I will need to just start over the next day with a new series of pills."
   c. "I may experience difficulty with my contact lenses. I may not be able to wear my lenses while taking these pills, or I might have to be fitted for a new pair."
   d. "If I have to take an antibiotic while I am using these pills, I should take double pills on those days that I am using the antibiotic."

Multiple Response

Select all that apply.

1. Estrogens produce a wide variety of systemic effects. Effects attributed to estrogen include
   a. protecting the heart from atherosclerosis.
   b. retaining calcium in the bones.
   c. maintaining the secondary female sex characteristics.
   d. relaxing the gravid uterus to prolong pregnancy.
   e. stimulating the uterus to increase the chances of conception.
   f. relaxing blood vessels.

2. A client is taking *Clomid* (clomiphene) after 6 years of inability to conceive a child. The client will need to be informed about which of the following?
   a. The need for a complete physical and pelvic examination before each course of drug therapy
   b. The risks and hazards of multiple births
   c. The importance of scheduling treatments and intercourse to increase the chance of conception
   d. The need to avoid intercourse during drug therapy
   e. The need to report blurred vision
   f. That light-headedness, dizziness, and drowsiness are common side effects

3. A client is receiving an oxytocic drug to stimulate labor. The nursing care of this client would include which of the following?
   a. Monitoring of fetal heart beat during labor
   b. Regulation of drug delivery between contractions
   c. Administration of blood pressure–lowering drugs to balance hypertensive effects
   d. Monitoring of maternal blood pressure periodically during and after administration
   e. Close monitoring of maternal blood loss following delivery
   f. Isolation of mother and newborn to prevent infection

Word Scramble

Unscramble the following letters to form the names of commonly used estrogens and estrogen receptor modulators.

1. morefinete ______________________
2. dotrailse ______________________
3. noreest ______________________
4. foxnarliee ______________________
5. notsiederl ______________________
6. potrestapei ______________________
7. stillbesthiedyrotl ______________________
8. cehnleosriontari ______________________

Fill in the Blanks

1. Drugs that stimulate uterine contractions are called ______________________.
2. Drugs that are used to relax the gravid uterus to prolong pregnancy are referred to as ______________________.
3. Loss of estrogen is associated with many problems at menopause, including ______________ or a loss of calcium from the bones, ______________ associated with vascular spasms, and an increased risk of ______________ ______________, the leading cause of death among women.
4. Women are strongly discouraged from smoking when taking estrogen replacement therapy because of an increased risk of ______________ and ______________ development.
5. ______________ is an estrogen receptor modulator, stimulating some receptors and blocking others.
6. Medroxyprogesterone is available as *Depo-Provera,* a form of birth control that is delivered every 3 months by ______________.
7. Women without primary ovarian failure who cannot become pregnant after a year of trying may be candidates for the use of ______________.
8. Drugs that can be used to induce abortion in early pregnancy or to promote uterine evacuation after intrauterine fetal death are called ______________.

Bibliography and References

Abernathy, K. (1997). Hormone replacement therapy. *Professional Nurse, 21,* 717–719.

Anderson, G., et al. (2003). Effects of estrogen plus progestin on gynecological cancers and associated diagnostic procedures. *Journal of the American Medical Association, 290,* 1739–1748.

Cauley, J. A., Robbins, J., Chen, Z., et al. (2003). Effects of estrogen plus progestin on risk of fractures and bone mineral density. *Journal of the American Medical Association, 290,* 1729–1738.

Drug facts and comparisons. (2006). St. Louis: Facts and Comparisons.

Gilman, A., Hardman, J. G., & Limbird, L. E. (Eds.). (2006). *Goodman and Gilman's the pharmacological basis of therapeutics* (11th ed.). New York: McGraw-Hill.

Greendale, G. A., & Sowers, M. (1997). The menopause transition. *Endocrinology and Metabolism Clinics of North America, 26,* 262–277.

Karch, A. M. (2006). *2007 Lippincott's nursing drug guide.* Philadelphia: Lippincott Williams & Wilkins.

Manson, J. E., Hsia, J., Johnson, K. C., et al. (2003). Estrogen plus progestin and the risk of coronary heart disease. *New England Journal of Medicine, 349,* 523–534.

Neves-e-Castro, M. (2003). Menopause in crisis post-Women's Health Initiative? *Human Reproduction, 18,* 2512–2518.

U.S. Preventative Services Task Force. (2002). Post-menopausal hormone replacement therapy to prevent chronic conditions: Recommendations. *Annals of Internal Medicine, 127,* 1–48.

CHAPTER

41

Drugs Affecting the Male Reproductive System

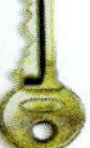

KEY TERMS

anabolic steroids

androgenic effects

androgens

hirsutism

hypogonadism

penile erectile dysfunction

LEARNING OBJECTIVES

Upon completion of this chapter, you will be able to:

1. Discuss the effects of testosterone and androgens on the male body and use this information to explain the therapeutic and adverse effects of these agents when used clinically.
2. Describe the therapeutic actions, indications, pharmacokinetics, contraindications, most common adverse reactions, and important drug–drug interactions associated with androgens, anabolic steroids, and drugs used to treat erectile dysfunction.
3. Discuss the use of drugs that affect the male reproductive system across the lifespan.
4. Compare and contrast the prototype drugs testosterone, oxandrolone, and sildenafil with other agents in their class.
5. Outline the nursing considerations, including important teaching points, for patients receiving drugs used to affect the male reproductive system.

ANDROGENS

danazol

testolactone

(P) testosterone

ANABOLIC STEROIDS

nandrolone

(P) oxandrolone

oxymetholone

DRUGS FOR TREATING PENILE ERECTILE DYSFUNCTION

alprostadil

(P) sildenafil

tadalafil

vardenafil

Drugs that are used to affect the male reproductive system include male steroid hormones or **androgens**, which act like the male sex hormone, testosterone; **anabolic steroids**, which are synthetic testosterone preparations that have more anabolic (tissue-building) effects than **androgenic effects** (effects associated with development of male sexual characteristics); and drugs that act to improve penile dysfunction. This last group includes alprostadil, which is a prostaglandin, and sildenafil, tadalafil and vardenafil, which are selective inhibitors of cyclic guanosine monophosphate (cGMP), a reactive tissue enzyme inhibitor) that increase nitric oxide in the corpus cavernosum to improve erection (Figure 41.1). Box 41.1 describes the effect of these drugs across the lifespan.

Androgens

The primary natural androgen, testosterone (*Duratest, Testoderm,* and others), is the classic androgen in use today. It is used for replacement therapy in cases of **hypogonadism** (underdeveloped testes) and to treat certain breast cancers. These drugs are all class III controlled substances. Other androgens include danazol (*Danocrine*), a synthetic andro-

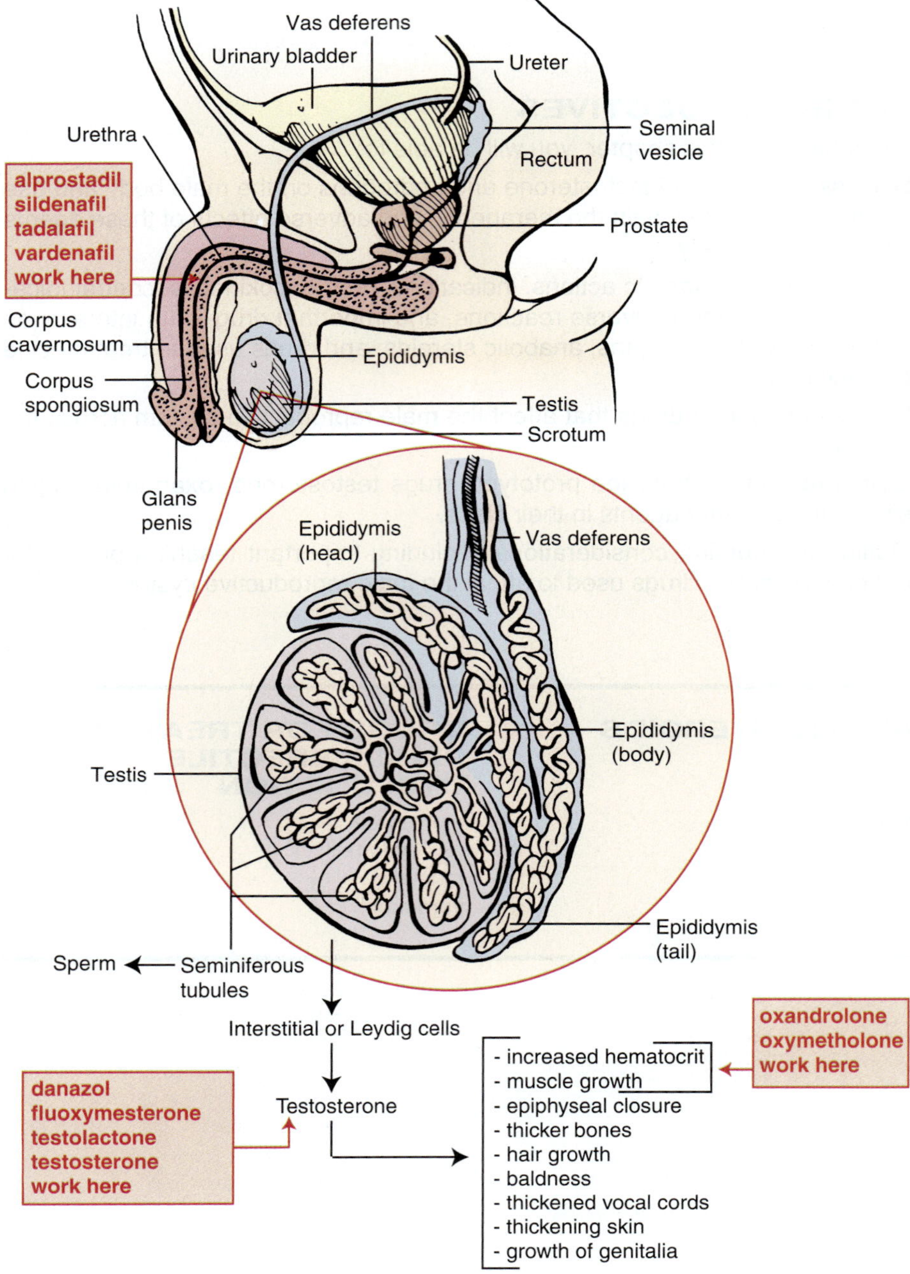

FIGURE 41.1 Sites of action of drugs affecting the male reproductive system.

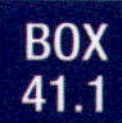
BOX 41.1 DRUG THERAPY ACROSS THE LIFESPAN
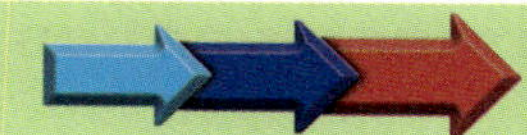

Drugs Affecting the Male Reproductive System

CHILDREN

These drugs are used in children as replacement therapy and to increase red blood cell production in renal failure. Because of the effects of these hormones on epiphyseal closure, children should be closely monitored with hand and wrist radiographs pretreatment and every 6 months. If precocious puberty occurs, the drug should be stopped.

Adolescents who are prescribed androgens should be alerted to the potential for increased acne and other effects.

Adolescent athletes need constant education about the risks associated with the use of anabolic steroids to improve athletic prowess and the lack of scientific evidence of beneficial effects.

ADULTS

Adults also need reinforcement of the information about anabolic steroid use and athletics.

Women who are prescribed these drugs may experience masculinizing effects and may need support in coping with these body changes. Men who are receiving these drugs for replacement therapy may need to learn self-injection techniques and may benefit from information on depot forms or dermal systems. Periodic liver function tests are important in monitoring the effects of these drugs on the liver.

These drugs are not indicated for use in pregnancy or lactation because of the potential for serious effects on the fetus or neonate.

OLDER ADULTS

Older adults may have problems with androgen therapy because of underlying conditions that are aggravated by the drug effects. Hypertension, congestive heart failure, and coronary artery disease may be aggravated by the fluid retention associated with these drugs. Benign prostatic hypertrophy, a common problem in older men, may be aggravated by androgenic effects that may enlarge the prostate further, leading to urinary difficulties and increased risk of prostate cancer.

Many older adults have hepatic dysfunction, and these drugs can be hepatotoxic. Older patients should be monitored very carefully and dosage should be reduced. If signs of liver failure or hepatitis occur, the drug should be stopped immediately.

gen that is used primarily to block the release of follicle-stimulating hormone and luteinizing hormone in women, and testolactone (*Teslac*), a synthetic androgen used for the treatment of specific breast cancers. See Table 41.1 for more information about these androgens.

Therapeutic Actions and Indications

The androgens are forms of testosterone. They are responsible for the growth and development of male sex organs and the maintenance of secondary sex characteristics (see Figure 41.1). They act to increase the retention of nitrogen, sodium, potassium, and phosphorus and to decrease the urinary excretion of calcium. Testosterones increase protein anabolism and decrease protein catabolism (breakdown). They also increase the production of red blood cells.

Androgens (testosterone and testolactone) can be indicated for the treatment of hypogonadism and delayed puberty in male patients. They are also indicated for the treatment of certain breast cancers in postmenopausal women; for the prevention of ovulation to treat endometriosis (danazol); for the prevention of postpartum breast engorgement (testosterone); and for the treatment of hereditary angioedema (danazol). Testosterone is long-acting and is available in several forms, including depot (deep, slow-release) injections and a dermal patch. Testolactone is short-acting and is available only in oral form. Danazol is long-acting and also is available only in oral form.

Table 41.1 DRUGS IN FOCUS

Androgens

Drug Name	Usual Dosage	Usual Indications
danazol (*Danocrine*)	100–600 mg/day PO, depending on use and response	Blockade of follicle-stimulating hormone and luteinizing hormone release in women, treatment of endometriosis, prevention of angioedema
fluoxymesterone (*Halotestin*)	5–20 mg/day PO for replacement therapy; 10–40 mg/day PO for certain breast cancers	Replacement therapy in hypogonadism, certain breast cancers
testolactone (*Teslac*)	250 mg PO q.i.d.	Treatment of specific breast cancers
P testosterone (*Duratest, Testoderm*)	50–400 mg IM every 2–4 wk, dose varies with preparation; some long-acting depository forms are available; dermatological patch 4–6 mg/day, replace patch daily	Replacement therapy in hypogonadism, certain breast cancers

Pharmacokinetics

The androgens are well absorbed and widely distributed throughout the body. They are metabolized in the liver and excreted in the urine. Androgens are contraindicated for use in pregnancy because of adverse effects on the fetus. It is not known whether androgens enter breast milk, but because of the potential for adverse effects, another method of feeding the baby should be used if these drugs are needed during lactation.

Contraindications and Cautions

These drugs are contraindicated with any known allergy to the drug or ingredients in the drug; during pregnancy and lactation, *because of potential effects on the neonate;* and in the presence of prostate or breast cancer in men. They should be used cautiously in the presence of any liver dysfunction or cardiovascular disease, *because these disorders could be exacerbated by the effects of the hormones.*

Adverse Effects

Androgenic effects include acne, edema, **hirsutism** (increased hair distribution), deepening of the voice, oily skin and hair, weight gain, decrease in breast size, and testicular atrophy. Antiestrogen effects—flushing, sweating, vaginitis, nervousness, and emotional lability—can be anticipated when these drugs are used with women. Other common effects include headache (possibly related to fluid and electrolyte changes), dizziness, sleep disorders and fatigue, rash, and altered serum electrolytes. A potentially life-threatening effect that has been documented is hepatocellular cancer. This may occur because of the effect of testosterone on hepatic cells. Patients on long-term therapy should have hepatic function tests monitored regularly—before beginning therapy and every 6 months during therapy.

Clinically Significant Drug–Laboratory Test Interferences

While a patient is taking androgens, there may be a decrease in thyroid function as well as increased creatinine and creatinine clearance, results that are not associated with disease states. These effects can last up to 2 weeks after the discontinuation of therapy.

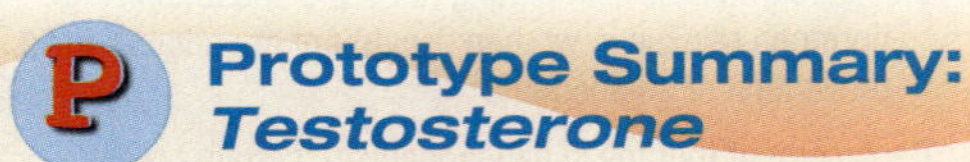

Prototype Summary: *Testosterone*

Indications: Replacement therapy in hypogonadism, inoperable breast cancer

Actions: Primary natural androgen, responsible for growth and development of male sex organs and maintenance of secondary sex characteristics; increases the retention of nitrogen, sodium, potassium, and phosphorus; decreases urinary excretion of calcium; increases protein anabolism; stimulates RBC production

Pharmacokinetics:

Route	Onset	Peak
IM	Slow	1–3 days
IM cypionate	Slow	2–4 wk
IM enanthate	Slow	2–4 wk
Dermal	Rapid	24 h

$T_{1/2}$: 10–100 min, with hepatic metabolism and excretion in the urine and feces

Adverse effects: Dizziness, headache, sleep disorders, fatigue, rash, androgenic effects (acne, deepening voice, oily skin), hypoestrogenic effects (flushing, sweating, vaginitis), polycythemia, nausea, hepatocellular carcinoma

Nursing Considerations for Patients Receiving Androgens

Assessment: History and Examination

Screen for the following conditions, *which could be cautions or contraindications to use of the drug:* history of allergy to any testosterone or androgen, pregnancy, lactation, hepatic dysfunction, cardiovascular disease, and breast or prostate cancer in men.

Include screening *for baseline status before beginning therapy and for any potential adverse effects:* skin color, lesions, texture, hair distribution; affect, orientation, peripheral sensation; abdominal examination; serum electrolytes, serum cholesterol, and liver function tests; and radiographs of the long bones in children.

Nursing Diagnoses

The patient receiving any androgen may also have the following nursing diagnoses related to drug therapy:

- Disturbed Body Image related to androgenic effects
- Acute Pain related to need for injections
- Sexual Dysfunction related to androgenic effects
- Deficient Knowledge regarding drug therapy

Implementation With Rationale

- Reconstitute the drug according to the manufacturer's directions, *to ensure proper reconstitution and to administer as prescribed.*

- Remove old dermal system before applying new system to clean, dry, intact skin *to ensure accurate administration and decrease risk of toxic levels.*
- Monitor response carefully when beginning therapy, *so that the dosage can be adjusted accordingly.*
- Monitor liver function periodically with long-term therapy, and *arrange to discontinue the drug at any sign of hepatic dysfunction.*
- Provide thorough patient teaching, including measures to avoid adverse effects, warning signs of problems, and the need for regular evaluation, including blood tests. Instruct a family member or caregiver in proper preparation and administration techniques as appropriate, *to enhance patient knowledge about drug therapy and to promote compliance with the drug regimen.*

Evaluation

- Monitor patient response to the drug (onset of puberty, maintenance of male sexual characteristics, palliation of breast cancer, blockage of ovulation, prevention of postpartum breast engorgement, relief of angioedema).
- Monitor for adverse effects (androgenic effects, hypoestrogen effects, serum electrolyte imbalance, headache, sleep disturbances, rash, hepatocellular carcinoma).
- Evaluate the effectiveness of the teaching plan (patient can name drug, dosage, adverse effects to watch for, specific measures to avoid adverse effects; family member or caregiver can demonstrate proper technique for preparation and administration of drug as appropriate).
- Monitor the effectiveness of comfort measures and compliance to the regimen.

Anabolic Steroids

The anabolic steroids are analogs of testosterone that have been developed to produce the tissue-building effects of testosterone with less androgenic effect. These are controlled substances that are known to be used illegally for the enhancement of athletic performance through increased muscle mass, increased hematocrit, and, theoretically, an increase in strength and endurance. The adverse effects of these drugs can be deadly when they are used in the amounts needed for enhanced athletic performance. Cardiomyopathy, hepatic carcinoma, personality changes, and sexual dysfunction are all associated with the excessive and nonindicated use of anabolic steroids. There is an increased effort to encourage the use of herbal products to improve athletic performance. These products are advertised as "safe" alternatives (Box 41.2).

Nandrolone is an anabolic steroid indicated for the treatment of anemia associated with chronic renal failure; however, it is infamous as an agent used illegally by athletes to improve performance. Oxandrolone (*Oxandrin*) is an anabolic steroid that has several uses: to promote weight gain in debilitated patients, to increase protein anabolism in patients receiving prolonged corticosteroid therapy, and to treat certain cancers. Oxymetholone (*Anadrol-50*) is used to treat various anemias. See Table 41.2 for more information about these anabolic steroids.

BOX 41.2 HERBAL AND ALTERNATIVE THERAPIES

With an increasing awareness of the risks associated with anabolic steroid use and increasing pressures to make it difficult to get these drugs, even illegally, there is an increased push in advertising of alternative or "natural" products that are reported to enhance athletic performance.

Bee pollen—Reported to contain amino acids and other minerals and enzymes. There are no scientific studies regarding its effectiveness. Serious allergic reactions have been reported with the use of this product. Random studies have found a wide variety of ingredients in each product, depending on the season, growing conditions, and geographical area.

Creatine—Contains a substance that is found in muscle and naturally occurs in red meats and other dietary sources. No scientific data are available on its actual effects on energy or athletic performance. It interacts with many other drugs, including nonsteroidal anti-inflammatory drugs, cimetidine, probenecid, and trimethoprim, and can cause serious effects on kidney functioning. Users should be advised to drink plenty of fluids while taking this drug and to monitor for swelling, muscle cramps, and dizziness. Suggested only for short-term use.

Damiana—Used to increase muscle strength, as an aphrodisiac, and to boost mental health. It can cause liver toxicity. It interferes with antidiabetic agents and causes elevated blood sugar concentrations. Users should report muscle spasms or hallucinations.

Spirulina—Used to increase energy and boost metabolism. It may contain toxic metals and can cause serious reactions in children and pets. It interferes with vitamin B_{12} absorption. No scientific studies validate the claims of its effectiveness.

Wild yam—Found to have many estrogen-like effects, this herb is used to increase athletic performance because it may contain a constituent of dehydroepiandrosterone (DHEA) used to slow the aging process and to improve energy and stamina. Preparations interact with disulfiram and metronidazole because they contain alcohol. It is known to be toxic to the liver. Users may experience estrogen-like effects including breast pain. Users should be monitored closely and urged to report any adverse effects.

Patients who are taking a prescribed androgen or anabolic steroid for a medical condition should be advised to avoid taking any of these herbal remedies because of a risk of adverse effects.

Table 41.2 DRUGS IN FOCUS

Anabolic Steroids

Drug Name	Usual Dosage	Usual Indication
nandrolone (*generic*)	Males: 100–200 mg/wk IM Females: 50–100 mg/wk IM Pediatric: 25–50 mg IM every 3–4 wk	Anemia associated with renal dysfunction, treatment of some breast cancers; HIV wasting syndrome
oxandrolone (*Oxandrin*)	Adult: 2.5 mg PO two to four times daily Pediatric: <0.1 mg/kg/day PO, monitor closely, may be repeated intermittently	Promotion of weight gain in debilitated patients; treatment of certain cancers; relief of bone pain of osteoporosis; promotion of catabolism with prolonged corticosteroid use
oxymetholone (*Anadrol-50*)	1–5 mg/kg/day PO	Treatment of anemias in adults

Therapeutic Actions and Indications

Anabolic steroids promote body tissue-building processes, reverse catabolic or tissue-destroying processes, and increase hemoglobin and red blood cell mass.

Indications for particular anabolic steroids vary with the drug. They can be used to treat anemias, certain cancers, and angioedema, and to promote weight gain and tissue repair in debilitated patients and protein anabolism in patients who are receiving long-term corticosteroid therapy.

Pharmacokinetics

Like the androgens, the anabolic steroids are well absorbed and widely distributed throughout the body. They are metabolized in the liver and excreted in the urine. Anabolic steroids are contraindicated for use in pregnancy because of adverse effects to the fetus. It is not known whether anabolic steroids enter breast milk, but because of the potential for adverse effects, another method of feeding the baby should be used if these drugs are needed during lactation.

Contraindications and Cautions

These drugs are contraindicated in the presence of any known allergy to anabolic steroids; during pregnancy and lactation, *because of potential masculinization in the neonate;* and in the presence of liver dysfunction (*because these drugs are metabolized in the liver and are known to cause liver toxicity*), coronary disease (*because of cholesterol-raising effects through effects on the liver*), or prostate or breast cancer in males.

Adverse Effects

In prepubertal males, adverse effects include virilization (e.g., phallic enlargement, hirsutism, increased skin pigmentation). Postpubertal males may experience inhibition of testicular function, gynecomastia, testicular atrophy, priapism (a painful and continual erection of the penis), baldness, and change in libido (increased or decreased). Women may experience hirsutism, hoarseness, deepening of the voice, clitoral enlargement, baldness, and menstrual irregularities. As with the androgens, serum electrolyte changes, liver dysfunction (including life-threatening hepatitis), insomnia, and weight gain may occur. There is an increased risk of prostate problems, especially in geriatric patients.

Clinically Important Drug–Drug Interactions

Because the anabolic steroids affect the liver, there is a potential for interaction with oral anticoagulants and a potentially decreased need for antidiabetic agents, which may not be metabolized normally. Patients should be monitored closely and appropriate dosage adjustments made.

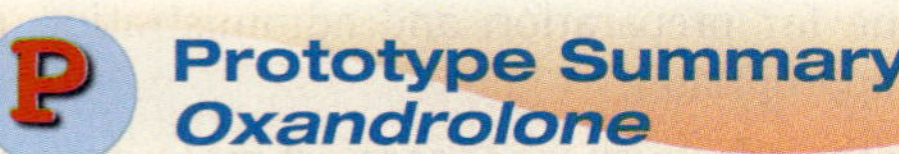

Prototype Summary: *Oxandrolone*

Indications: Adjunctive therapy to promote weight gain after weight loss associated with extensive surgery, chronic infections, or trauma; to offset protein catabolism associated with prolonged corticosteroid use; orphan drug uses: short stature syndrome, human immunodeficiency virus (HIV) cachexia and wasting

Actions: Testosterone analog with androgenic and anabolic activity, promotes tissue building, reverses catabolic processes, increases red blood cell mass

Pharmacokinetics:

Route	Onset
PO	Slow

$T_{1/2}$: 9 hours, with hepatic metabolism and excretion in the urine

Adverse effects: Excitation; insomnia; virilization; hepatitis; liver cell tumors; blood lipid changes; retention of sodium, water, and chloride; acne; masculinization of females; inhibition of testicular function; priapism; baldness; loss of libido in postpubertal males

Nursing Considerations for Patients Receiving Anabolic Steroids

Assessment: History and Examination

Screen for the following conditions, *which could be cautions or contraindications to use of the drug:* history of allergy to any androgens or anabolic steroids; pregnancy or lactation, *because of masculinization of the neonate;* prostrate or breast cancer; coronary disease; and hepatic dysfunction.

Include screening *for baseline status before beginning therapy and for any potential adverse effects:* skin color, texture, hair distribution; affect, orientation; abdominal examination; liver evaluation; serum electrolytes, cholesterol levels; and radiographs of the long bones in children.

Nursing Diagnoses

The patient receiving an anabolic steroid may have the following nursing diagnoses related to drug therapy:

- Disturbed Body Image related to systemic effects
- Acute Pain related to gastrointestinal (GI), central nervous system effects
- Deficient Knowledge regarding drug therapy

Implementation With Rationale

- Administer with food if GI effects are severe, *to relieve GI distress.*
- Monitor endocrine function, hepatic function, and serum electrolytes before and periodically during therapy, *so that dosage can be adjusted appropriately and severe adverse effects can be avoided.*
- Arrange for radiographs of the long bones of children every 3 to 6 months, *so that the drug can be discontinued if bone growth reaches the norm for the child's age.*
- Provide thorough patient teaching, including measures to avoid adverse effects and warning signs of problems, as well as the need for regular evaluation including blood tests, *to enhance patient knowledge about drug therapy and to promote compliance with drug regimen.* (See the patient teaching information in Critical Thinking Scenario 41-1.)

Evaluation

- Monitor patient response to the drug (increase in hematocrit, protein anabolism).
- Monitor for adverse effects (androgenic effects, serum electrolyte disturbances, epiphyseal closure, hepatic dysfunction, personality changes, cardiac effects).
- Evaluate the effectiveness of the teaching plan (patient can name drug, dosage, adverse effects to watch for, specific measures to avoid adverse effects).
- Monitor the effectiveness of comfort measures and compliance to the regimen.

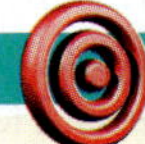

FOCUS POINTS

- Androgens are the male sex hormones that are responsible for the development and maintenance of male sex characteristics and secondary sex characteristics or androgenic effects.
- Androgens are used for replacement therapy or to block other hormonal effects.
- Anabolic steroids are testosterone analogs with more anabolic or protein-building effects than androgenic effects.
- Deadly effects may result from abuse of anabolic steroids by athletes trying to build muscle mass and improve performance.

Drugs for Treating Penile Erectile Dysfunction

Two very different drugs are approved for the treatment of **penile erectile dysfunction**, a condition in which the corpus cavernosum does not fill with blood to allow for penile erection. Penile erection can be compromised by the aging process and by vascular and neurological conditions. Alprostadil (*Caverject, MUSE*) is a prostaglandin that relaxes vascular smooth muscle and allows filling of the corpus cavernosum when it is injected directly into the cavernosum. Sildenafil (*Viagra*), tadalafil (*Cialis*), and vardenafil (*Levitra*) selectively inhibit receptors, called the phosphodiesterase type 5 receptors (PDE5), and increase nitrous oxide levels, allowing blood flow into the corpus cavernosum. These drugs have the advantage of being oral drugs that can be timed in coordination with sexual activity, based on the drug's onset. See Table 41.3 for more information about all four of these drugs. Box 41.3 contains more information about *Viagra.*

CRITICAL THINKING SCENARIO 41-1

Adverse Effects of Anabolic Steroids

The Situation

Senior nursing student K.S. recently became engaged. Her fiancé is a college senior who is training as a javelin thrower in hopes of competing in the Olympics. K.S. noticed that her fiancé had been suffering from GI upset for the last 3 weeks and more recently had developed tremors and muscle cramps. K.S. first suspected that he was suffering from a viral infection, but when the symptoms did not resolve, she became concerned. K.S. tried to get her fiancé to see a doctor, but he refused. Eventually, he admitted that he had begun using anabolic steroids to develop his muscles and improve his athletic prowess. He said that the friend who gave him the drugs told him that stomach upset was normal. He refuses to see a physician because he knows that the use of these drugs is illegal. He believes that using the anabolic steroids for a while will put him closer to his goal. K.S. accepts his explanation but is upset about the use of anabolic steroids. She consults with her clinical instructor about the effects of these drugs.

Critical Thinking

What does K.S. need to know? *Think about the systemic effects of anabolic steroids and the possible long-term effects from their abuse.*

What implications do these effects have for the athlete? *Consider the concern that K.S. must be experiencing. Suggest ways for K.S. to share the information about the actual effects of anabolic steroids with her fiancé and still cope with her own feelings and concerns.*

What are the ethical and legal issues involved when a heath care provider knows about illegal drug use and abuse? *Outline a plan for helping K.S. and her fiancé cope with this issue and its implications for their futures.*

Discussion

Use of anabolic steroids is illegal in almost all organized athletic contests. Random drug testing is done to rule out use of these and other drugs. Not surprisingly, K.S. feels insecure about her fiancé's decision. She needs to know that her discussion will be confidential and that she will receive support for her concerns and her fears. K.S. needs to review the effects of anabolic steroids. Although they do promote muscle development, there has never been any evidence that they actually improve athletic performance. The potential adverse effects of these drugs can be deadly, especially if K.S.'s fiancé is receiving the drugs from a friend and has no medical evaluation or dosage guidance to reduce the risk. Personality changes, cardiomyopathy, liver cancer, and impotence are just a few of the possible adverse effects.

K.S. is in a precarious position. She does not want to interfere with her fiancé's dreams or cause problems in their relationship. She should be encouraged to explain the adverse effects of the drugs to her fiancé, pointing out that he is already experiencing some of them. Adverse effects associated with the drugs can ultimately interfere with, not enhance, his athletic performance. She might be encouraged to practice what she will tell her fiancé and to seek other support as needed.

The sale or distribution of anabolic steroids without a prescription is illegal, and this fact further complicates the situation for K.S. Because she is planning to become a health care provider, she may be obligated by state law to report this information to the authorities. K.S. should research these issues and discuss them further with her clinical instructor and other resource people.

Nursing Care Guide for K.S.: Androgens, Anabolic Steroids

A patient receiving an anabolic steroid for a medical condition, would have the following care plan

Assessment: History And Examination

Assess the patient's health history for allergies to any steroids, breast or prostate cancer in men; hepatic dysfunction; coronary artery disease; pregnancy or breastfeeding in women; concurrent use of insulin or oral anticoagulants

Focus the physical examination on the following:

Neuro: orientation, reflexes, affect

Skin: color, lesions, hair

CV: pulse, cardiac auscultation, blood pressure, edema

GI: abdominal examination, liver examination

Laboratory tests: serum electrolytes, hepatic function tests, long bone x-ray studies

Adverse Effects of Anabolic Steroids *(continued)*

Nursing Diagnoses

Disturbed Body Image related to drug effects

Sexual Dysfunction

Acute Pain related to injections

Deficient Knowledge regarding drug therapy

Implementation

Administer as prescribed.

Monitor liver function before and periodically during therapy.

Monitor patient response and adjust dose as appropriate.

Provide support and reassurance to deal with drug therapy.

Provide patient teaching regarding drug name, dosage, adverse effects, precautions, warnings to report, and safe administration.

Evaluation

Evaluate drug effects: maintenance of male sex characteristics, suppression of lactation in women.

Monitor for adverse effects: androgenic effects, hypoestrogenic effects, hepatic dysfunction, electrolyte imbalance, endocrine changes.

Monitor for drug–drug interactions: decreased need for insulin, increased bleeding with oral anticoagulants.

Evaluate effectiveness of patient teaching program and comfort and safety measures.

Patient Teaching For K.S.

If the patient is taking these drugs to increase body mass following severe weight loss due to trauma, you would teach about the following. Sharing this information with those considering the unprescribed use of the drugs might be helpful.

- ☐ Androgens or anabolic steroids have properties similar to those of the male sex hormones. Because the formulation has widespread effects, there are often many adverse effects associated with its use.
- ☐ These drugs are controlled substances because the tendency for people, and athletes in particular, to abuse these drugs can cause serious medical problems. When the drug is used as prescribed, it is safe, but you will need to be monitored.
- ☐ Some of the following adverse effects may occur:
  - *GI upset, nausea, vomiting:* Taking the drug with food usually helps relieve these effects.
  - *Acne:* This is a hormonal effect; washing your face regularly and avoiding oily foods may help.
  - *Increased facial hair, decreased head hair:* These are hormonal effects; if they become bothersome, consult with your health care provider.
  - *Menstrual irregularities (women):* This is a normal effect of the androgens; if you suspect that you might be pregnant, consult with your health care provider immediately.
  - *Weight gain, increased muscle development:* These are common hormonal effects.
  - *Change in sex drive:* This can be distressing and difficult to deal with; consult with your health care provider if this is a serious concern.
  - Report any of the following to your health care provider: *swelling in fingers or legs; continual erection; uncontrollable sex drive; yellowing skin; fever, chills, or rash; chest pain or difficulty breathing; hoarseness, loss of hair or growth of facial hair (women).*
- ☐ Tell any doctor, nurse, or other health care provider involved in your care that you are taking this drug.
- ☐ Take this medicine only as directed. Also, schedule regular medical follow-up, including blood tests, to monitor your response to this drug.
- ☐ Keep this drug and all medications out of the reach of children. Do not give this medication to anyone else or take any similar medication that has not been prescribed for you.

Therapeutic Actions and Indications

The prostaglandin alprostadil is injected and acts locally to relax vascular smooth muscle and promote blood flow into the corpus cavernosum, causing penile erection. Alprostadil is metabolized to inactive compounds in the lungs and excreted in the urine. The drug is not indicated for use in women and is not classified for use in pregnancy or lactation. Because the effects on pregnancy are not known, if alprostadil is being used, condoms should be used during intercourse with a pregnant woman.

The PDE5 inhibitors are taken orally and act to increase nitrous oxide levels in the corpus cavernosum. Nitrous oxide activates the enzyme cGMP, which causes smooth muscle relaxation, allowing the flow of blood into

Table 41.3 DRUGS IN FOCUS

Drugs Used to Treat Penile Erectile Dysfunction

Drug Name	Usual Dosage	Usual Indications
alprostadil (*Caverject, MUSE*)	2.5 mcg injected intracavernously, titrate the dose to one that will allow a satisfactory erection that is maintained no longer than 1 hr; mean dose after 6 mo is reported to be 20.7 mcg	Penile erectile dysfunction
sildenafil (*Viagra*)	25–100 mg PO taken 1 h before sexual stimulation	Penile erectile dysfunction
sildenafil (*Revaton*)	20 mg PO t.i.d, at least 4–6 h apart	Treatment of pulmonary arterial hypertension
tadalafil (*Cialis*)	10 mg PO taken before sexual activity; range 5–20 mg PO; limit use to once a day	Penile erectile dysfunction
vardenafil (*Levitra*)	5–10 mg PO taken 1 h before sexual stimulation; range 5–20 mg; limit use to once a day	Penile erectile dysfunction

the corpus cavernosum. They prevent the breakdown of cGMP by phosphodiesterase, leading to increased cGMP levels and prolonged smooth muscle relaxation, thus promoting the flow of blood into the corpus cavernosum, resulting in penile erection. Sildenafil (*Revaton*) is also approved for the treatment of pulmonary arterial hypertension. By relaxing smooth muscle, the pulmonary artery relaxes and there is less resistance and pressure in the pulmonary bed. All three drugs are well absorbed from the GI tract, undergo metabolism in the liver, and are excreted in the feces. The differences among the three drugs lie in their onset and duration of action. Sildenafil has a median onset of 27 minutes and a duration of 4 hours. Patients are encouraged to take the drug 1 hour before anticipated sexual stimulation. Vardenafil has a mean onset of action of 26 minutes and a duration of 4 hours; it is also intended to be taken 1 hour before sexual stimulation. Tadalafil has an onset of action of 45 minutes and a duration of 36 hours. A patient might select this drug if the timing of sexual stimulation is not known and may be several hours away. None of these drugs is indicated for use in women, so no adequate studies have been done during pregnancy and lactation.

The prostaglandin alprostadil and the PDE5 inhibitors are indicated for the treatment of penile erectile dysfunction.

Contraindications and Cautions

These drugs are contraindicated in the presence of any anatomical obstruction or condition that might predispose to priapism. They cannot be used with penile implants, and they are not indicated for use in women (although sildenafil has been studied for the treatment of sexual dysfunction in women, without positive results). However, sildenafil is used in women for the treatment of pulmonary arterial hypertension.

Caution should be used in patients with bleeding disorders. The PDE5 inhibitors should also be used cautiously in those patients with coronary artery disease, active peptic ulcer, retinitis pigmentosa, optic neuropathy, hypotension or severe hypertension, congenital prolonged QT interval, or severe hepatic or renal disorders, *because of the risk of exacerbating these diseases.*

Adverse Effects

Adverse effects associated with alprostadil are local effects such as pain at the injection site, infection, priapism, fibrosis, and rash. The PDE5 inhibitors are associated with more systemic effects, including headache, flushing (related to relaxation of vascular smooth muscle), dyspepsia, urinary tract infection, diarrhea, dizziness, possible optic neuropathy, and rash.

Clinically Important Drug–Drug Interactions

The PDE5 inhibitors cannot be taken in combination with any organic nitrates or alpha-adrenergic blockers; serious cardiovascular effects, including death, have occurred. There is also a possibility of increased vardenafil or tadalafil levels and effects if PDE5 inhibitors are taken with ketoconazole, itraconazole, or erythromycin; monitor the patient and reduce dosage as needed.

Vardenafil and tadalafil serum levels can increase if combined with indinavir or ritonavir. If these drugs are being used, limit dosage of the PDE5 inhibitor.

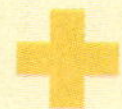

FOCUS ON PATIENT SAFETY

Patients who are using PDE5 inhibitors need to be advised to avoid drinking grapefruit juice while using the drug. Grapefruit juice can cause a decrease in the metabolism of the PDE5 inhibitor, leading to increased serum levels and a risk of toxicity. They should also be advised to avoid taking the drug with or just after a high-fat meal. The presence of fat in the GI tract will delay the absorption and onset of action of the drug, which could cause problems for patients who are timing onset of action with their sexual activity.

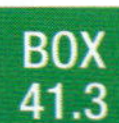

BOX 41.3 FOCUS ON THE **EVIDENCE**

Viagra—Wonder Drug?

The release of the drug *Viagra* to treat penile erectile dysfunction caused a tremendous stir in American society. This was the first oral drug developed to treat a disorder that was common in aging men but was seldom mentioned or discussed. *Viagra,* which facilitates penile erection approximately 1 hour after it is taken, returned sexual function to many of these men.

For many months after its release, the drug was the center of controversy, news coverage, and debate. Stand-up comedians, television situation comedies, and Internet joke networks were buzzing with the latest *Viagra* jokes. Insurance companies debated covering the cost of this drug. Was it like cosmetic surgery, and not a necessary treatment, or was it a necessary part of human physiology? Most insurance companies ended up covering the cost of *Viagra.*

Women's rights groups voiced concern that no drug was approved and covered to help facilitate a woman's sexual response. *Viagra* is in trial stages for the treatment of sexual dysfunction in women; early reports seem to indicate that it is not effective. However, *Viagra* has proved to be very effective at increasing sexual functioning for many men. Its success has led to the development of two new drugs in the same class of PDE5 inhibitors, tadalafil (*Cialis*) and vardenafil (*Levitra*).

The use of these drugs is not without risks. Deaths have occurred when these drugs were combined with nitrates (e.g., nitroglycerin) or alpha-adrenergic blockers. Headache, flushing, stomach upset, and urinary tract infections often occur. These drugs can be used only once daily, and they do not work without sexual stimulation. Absorption is delayed if they are taken with a high-fat meal, and patients need to plan accordingly. Patients also should be reminded that they need to use protection against sexually transmitted diseases.

When *Viagra* was the hot, new drug, there was tremendous demand for it from the public. This demand put health care providers in the position of ensuring that the drug was right for the patient's actual needs. The cause of penile erectile dysfunction should be determined, if at all possible. If this is a problem that the patient has never before discussed with the health care provider, there could be an underlying medical condition that should be addressed. The adverse effects, timing of administration, and drug combinations to avoid should be discussed with the patient before the drug is prescribed.

With pharmaceutical companies now advertising in magazines, on television, and over the Internet, health care providers are often asked for specific prescription drugs based on media advertising. This relatively new phenomenon in health care presents new challenges to the health care provider to ensure quality patient teaching to help the patient understand the actual uses, effects, and rationales for a specific drug therapy.

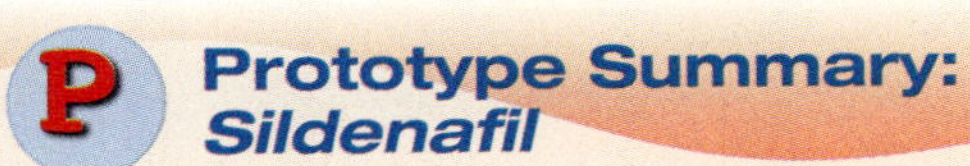

Prototype Summary: *Sildenafil*

Indications: Treatment of erectile dysfunction in the presence of sexual stimulation; treatment of pulmonary arterial hypertension

Actions: Inhibits PDE5 receptors, leading to a release of nitrous oxide, which activates cGMP to cause a prolonged smooth muscle relaxation, allowing the flow of blood into the corpus cavernosum and facilitating erection

Pharmacokinetics:

Route	Onset	Peak	Duration
PO	15–30 min	30–120 min	4 h

$T_{1/2}$: 4 hours, with hepatic metabolism and excretion in the feces and urine

Adverse effects: Headache, abnormal vision, flushing, dyspepsia, urinary tract infection, rash

Nursing Considerations for Patients Receiving Drugs to Treat Penile Erectile Dysfunction

Assessment: History and Examination

Screen for the following conditions, *which could be cautions or contraindications to the use of the drug:* history of allergy to any of the preparations, penile structural abnormalities, penile implants, bleeding disorders, active peptic ulcer, coronary artery disease, hypotension or severe hypertension, congenital prolonged QT interval, or severe hepatic or renal disorders.

Include screening *for baseline status before beginning therapy and for any potential adverse effects:* skin, lesions; orientation, affect, reflexes; blood pressure, pulse; respiration, adventitious sounds; local inspection of penis; and bleeding time and liver function tests.

Nursing Diagnoses

The patient receiving drugs for treating penile dysfunction may have the following nursing diagnoses related to drug therapy:

- Disturbed Body Image related to drug effects and indication
- Acute Pain related to injection of alprostadil
- Sexual Dysfunction
- Deficient Knowledge regarding drug therapy

Implementation With Rationale

- Assess the cause of dysfunction before beginning therapy, *to ensure appropriate use of these drugs.*

- Monitor patients with vascular disease for any sign of exacerbation, *so that the drug can be discontinued before severe adverse effects occur.*
- Instruct the patient in the injection of alprostadil, storage of the drug, filling of the syringe, sterile technique, site rotation, and proper disposal of needles, *to ensure safe and proper administration of the drug.*
- Monitor patients who are taking PDE5 inhibitors for use of nitrates or alpha-blockers, *to avert potentially serious cardiovascular drug–drug interactions.*
- Provide thorough patient teaching, including measures to avoid adverse effects and warning signs of problems, as well as the need for regular evaluation, *to enhance patient knowledge about drug therapy and to promote compliance with the drug regimen.*

Evaluation

- Monitor patient response to the drug (improvement in penile erection).
- Monitor for adverse effects (dizziness, flushing, local inflammation or infection, fibrosis, diarrhea, dyspepsia).
- Evaluate the effectiveness of the teaching plan (patient can name drug, dosage, adverse effects to watch for, specific measures to avoid adverse effects; patient can demonstrate proper administration of injected drug).
- Monitor the effectiveness of comfort measures and compliance to the regimen.

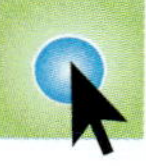

WEB LINKS

Health care providers and patients may want to consult the following Internet sources:

http://www.maleinfertilitymds.com Information on male fertility—research, explanations, related information, endocrinology research.

http://www.aace.com Information on testosterone and testosterone replacement.

http://www.urologychannel.com Information on erectile dysfunction—overview, teaching aids, patient information, support groups.

http://www.ama-assn.org Information for professionals, research, new drugs.

http://www.uro.com Information on current research, professional issues.

Points to Remember

- Androgens are male sex hormones, specifically testosterone or testosterone-like compounds.
- Androgens are responsible for the development and maintenance of male sex characteristics and secondary sex characteristics or androgenic effects.
- Side effects related to androgen use involve excess of the desired effects as well as potentially deadly hepatocellular carcinoma.
- Androgens can be used for replacement therapy or to block other hormone effects, as is seen with their use in the treatment of specific breast cancers.
- Anabolic steroids are analogs of testosterone that have been developed to have more anabolic or protein-building effects than androgenic effects.
- Anabolic steroids have been abused to enhance muscle development and athletic performance, often with deadly effects.
- Anabolic steroids are used to increase hematocrit and improve protein anabolism in certain depleted states.
- Penile erectile dysfunction can inhibit erection and male sexual function.
- Alprostadil, a prostaglandin, can be injected into the penis to stimulate erection.
- The PDE5 inhibitors are oral agents that act quickly to promote vascular filling of the corpus cavernosum and promote penile erection. They differ in duration and time of onset. They are effective only in the presence of sexual stimulation.
- Dangerous cardiovascular effects, including death, have occurred when the PDE5 inhibitors are combined with organic nitrates or alpha-blockers. Careful patient teaching is very important to avoid this drug–drug interaction.

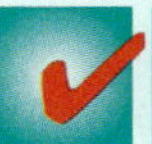

CHECK YOUR UNDERSTANDING

Answers to the questions in this chapter may be found in the Answer Key in the back of the book.

Multiple Choice

Select the best answer to the following.

1. Testosterone is approved for use in
   a. treatment of breast cancers.
   b. increasing muscle strength in athletes.
   c. oral contraceptives.
   d. increasing hair distribution in male pattern baldness.

2. Illegal use of large quantities of unprescribed anabolic steroids to enhance athletic performance has been associated with
   a. increased sexual prowess.
   b. muscle rupture from overexpansion.
   c. development of COPD.
   d. cardiomyopathy and liver cancers.

3. Anabolic steroids would be indicated for the treatment of
   a. anemia.
   b. angioedema.
   c. debilitation and severe weight loss.
   d. breast cancers in males.

4. Erectile penile dysfunction is a condition in which
   a. problems with childhood authority figures prevent a male erection.
   b. the corpus cavernosum does not fill with blood to allow for penile erection.
   c. the sympathetic nervous system fails to function.
   d. past exposure to sexually transmitted disease causes physical damage within the penis.

5. A potentially deadly drug–drug interaction can occur if a PDE5 inhibitor (sildenafil, tadalafil, or vardenafil) is combined with
   a. corticosteroids.
   b. oral contraceptives.
   c. organic nitrates.
   d. halothane anesthetics.

6. To achieve erection, a patient taking sildenafil (*Viagra*) would require
   a. sexual stimulation of the penis.
   b. no additional stimulation.
   c. privacy.
   d. 10 to 15 minutes after taking the oral drug.

7. Men taking alprostadil for treatment of erectile dysfunction must
   a. take the drug orally about 1 hour before anticipated intercourse.
   b. arrange for sexual stimulation to promote erection.
   c. learn to inject the drug directly into the penis.
   d. avoid the use of nitrates for cardiovascular disorders.

8. *Viagra* is known to
   a. cause unexpected and enlarged erections.
   b. make a person young and agile.
   c. promote interpersonal relationships between partners.
   d. increase nitrous oxide levels in the corpus cavernosum, causing vascular relaxation and promoting blood flow into the corpus cavernosum.

Multiple Response

Select all that apply.

1. In assessing a client for androgenic effects, you would expect to find which of the following?
   a. Hirsutism
   b. Deepening of the voice
   c. Testicular enlargement
   d. Acne
   e. Elevated body temperature
   f. Sudden growth

2. A child treated with anabolic steroids because of anemia associated with renal disease will need
   a. early sex education classes because of the effects of the drug.
   b. x-rays of the long bones every 3 to 6 months so the drug can be stopped when the bone size is appropriate to the child's age.
   c. to learn to shave.
   d. to learn to cope with an altered body image.
   e. regular monitoring of liver function tests.
   f. monitoring for the development of edema.

True or False

Indicate whether the following statements are true (T) or false (F).

_____ 1. Androgens are male sex hormones, specifically testosterone or testosterone-like compounds.

_____ 2. Androgens are responsible for the development and maintenance of male sex characteristics and secondary sex characteristics or estrogenic effects.

_____ 3. Adverse effects related to androgen use involve potentially deadly hepatocellular carcinoma.

_____ 4. Androgens can be used for replacement therapy or to block other hormone effects.

_____ 5. Anabolic steroids are analogs of estrogen that have been developed to have protein building effects.

_____ 6. Anabolic steroids are used pharmacologically to enhance muscle development and athletic performance, often with deadly effects.

_____ 7. Anabolic steroids are used to increase hematocrit and improve protein anabolism in certain depleted states.

_____ 8. Erectile penile dysfunction can inhibit erection and male sexual function.

_____ 9. Alprostadil, a prostaglandin, is an oral agent used to stimulate penile erection.

_____ 10. Sildenafil is an injected agent that acts quickly to promote vascular filling of the corpus cavernosum and promote penile erection.

Fill in the Blanks

1. ____________________ effects are associated with development of male sexual characteristics.

2. ____________________ effects are tissue-building effects associated with androgen use.

3. ____________________ is the primary natural androgen.

4. Because they cause an increase in red blood cell production, androgens may be indicated to treat various ____________________.

5. ____________________ is a condition in which the corpus cavernosum does not fill with blood to allow for penile erection.

6. Alprostadil is a ____________________ that relaxes vascular smooth muscle and allows filling of the corpus cavernosum when ____________________ directly into the cavernosum.

7. ____________________ is taken orally and acts to increase nitrous oxide levels in the corpus cavernosum.

8. The penile erection that accompanies oral use of *Viagra* occurs only with ____________________.

Bibliography and References

Abramowicz, M. (Ed.). (2003). Tadalafil for erectile dysfunction. *The Medical Letter on Drugs and Therapeutics, 45,* 101–102.

Davis, S. R., & Burger, H. G. (1996). Androgens and postmenopausal women. *Journal of Endocrinology and Metabolism, 81,* 2759–2763.

Drug facts and comparisons. (2006). St. Louis: Facts and Comparisons.

Gilman, A., Hardman, J. G., & Limbird, L. E. (Eds.). (2006). *Goodman and Gilman's the pharmacological basis of therapeutics* (11th ed.). New York: McGraw-Hill.

Karch, A. M. (2006). *2007 Lippincott's nursing drug guide.* Philadelphia: Lippincott Williams & Wilkins.

The medical letter on drugs and therapeutics. (2006). New Rochelle, NY: Medical Letter.

Miller, K. L. (1996). Hormone replacement therapy in the elderly. *Annals of Pharmacotherapy, 31,* 915–917.

Walsh, P. C., et al. (Eds.). (2002). *Campbell's urology* (8th ed.). Philadelphia: W. B. Saunders.

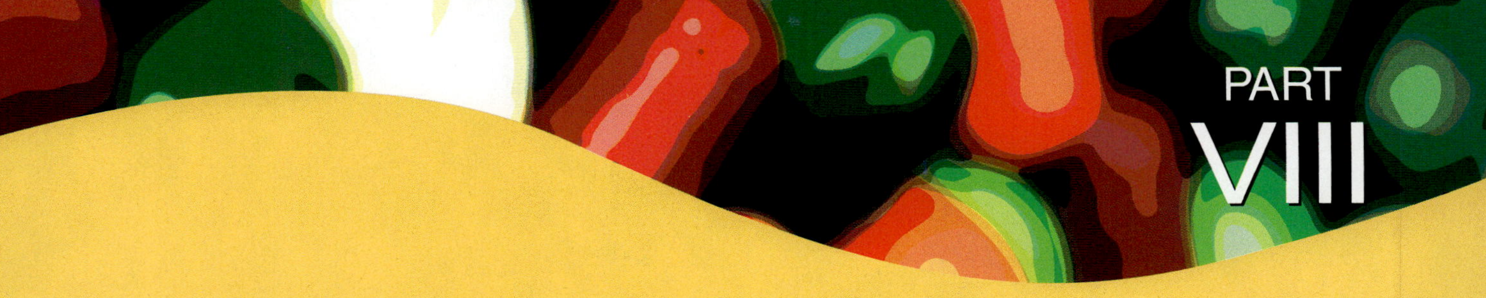

PART VIII

Drugs Acting on the Cardiovascular System

CHAPTER 42

Introduction to the Cardiovascular System

KEY TERMS

actin
arrhythmia
arteries
atrium
auricle
automaticity
capillary
capacitance system
cardiac cycle
conductivity
diastole
dysrhythmia
electrocardiogram (ECG)
fibrillation
myocardium
myosin
oncotic pressure
pulse pressure
resistance system
sarcomere
sinoatrial (SA) node
Starling's law of the heart
syncytia
systole
troponin
veins
ventricle

LEARNING OBJECTIVES

Upon completion of this chapter, you will be able to:

1. Label a diagram of the heart, including all chambers, valves, great vessels, coronary vessels, and the conduction system.
2. Describe the flow of blood during the cardiac cycle, including flow to the cardiac muscle.
3. Outline the conduction system of the heart and correlate the normal ECG pattern with the underlying electrical activity in the heart.
4. Discuss four normal controls of blood pressure.
5. Describe the capillary fluid shift, including factors that influence the movement of fluid in clinical situations.

The cardiovascular system is responsible for delivering oxygen and nutrients to all of the cells of the body and for removing waste products for excretion. The cardiovascular system consists of a pump—the heart—and an interconnected series of tubes that continually move blood throughout the body.

The Heart

The heart is a hollow, muscular organ that is divided into four chambers. The heart may actually be viewed as two joined hearts: a right heart and a left heart, each of which is divided into two parts, an upper part called the **atrium** (literally "porch" or entryway) and a lower part called the **ventricle**.

Attached to each atrium is an appendage called the **auricle**, which collects blood that is then pumped into the ventricles by atrial contraction. The right auricle is quite large; the left is very small. The ventricles pump blood out of the heart to the lungs or the body. Between the atria and ventricles are two cardiac valves—thin tissues that are anchored to an annulus, or fibrous ring, which also gives the hollow organ some structure and helps to keep the organ open and divided into distinct chambers.

A partition called a septum separates the right half of the heart from the left. The right half receives deoxygenated blood from everywhere in the body through the **veins** (vessels that carry blood toward the heart) and directs that blood into the lungs. The left half receives the now oxygenated blood from the lungs and directs it into the aorta. The aorta delivers blood into the systemic circulation by way of **arteries** (vessels that carry blood away from the heart) (Figure 42.1). The heart is the pump that keeps blood flowing through 60,000 miles of tubes, constituting the cardiovascular system, to deliver oxygen and nutrients to all the cells of the body and to remove metabolic waste products from the tissues.

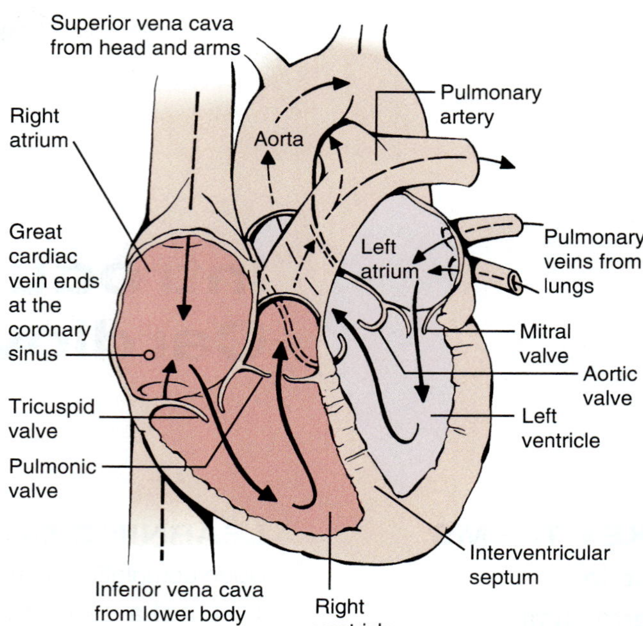

FIGURE 42.1 Blood flow into and out of the heart. Deoxygenated blood enters the right atrium from the great cardiac vein and the superior and inferior venae cavae and falls through the tricuspid valve into the right ventricle, which contracts and sends the blood through the pulmonic valve into the pulmonary artery and to the lungs. Oxygenated blood from the lungs enters the left atrium through the pulmonary veins and passes through the mitral valve into the left ventricle, which contracts and ejects the blood through the aortic valve into the aorta and out to the systemic circulation.

The Cardiac Cycle

The heart, which contracts thousands of millions of times in a lifetime, possesses structural and functional properties that are different from those of other muscles. The fibers of the cardiac muscle, or **myocardium**, form two intertwining networks called the atrial and ventricular **syncytia**. These interlacing structures enable first the atria and then the ventricles to contract synchronously when excited by the same stimulus.

Simultaneous contraction is a necessary property for a muscle that acts as a pump. A hollow pumping mechanism must also pause long enough in the pumping cycle to allow the chambers to fill with fluid. Heart muscle relaxes long enough to ensure adequate filling; the more completely it fills, the stronger the subsequent contraction. This occurs because the muscle fibers of the heart, stretched by the increased volume of blood that has returned to them, spring back to normal size. This is similar to stretching a rubber band, which returns to its normal size after it is stretched—the further it is stretched, the stronger the spring back to normal. This property is defined in **Starling's law of the heart** (see page 673).

During **diastole**, the period of cardiac muscle relaxation, blood returns to the heart from the systemic and pulmonary veins, which flow into the right and left atria, respectively. When the pressure generated by the blood volume in the atria is greater than the pressure in the ventricles, blood flows through the atrioventricular (AV) valves into the ventricles. The valve on the right side of the heart is called the tricuspid valve because it is composed of three leaflets or cusps (see Figure 42.1). The valve on the left side of the heart, called the mitral or bicuspid valve, is composed of two leaflets or cusps (see Figure 42.1). Just before the ventricles are stimulated to contract, the atria contract, pushing about 1 more tablespoon of blood into each ventricle. The much more powerful ventricles then contract, pumping blood out to the lungs through the pulmonary valve or out to the aorta through the aortic valve and into the systemic circulation. The contraction of the ventricles is referred to as **systole**. Each period of systole followed by a period of diastole is called a **cardiac cycle**. The heart's series of one-way valves keeps the blood flowing in the correct direction, as follows (see Figure 42.1):

- *Deoxygenated blood:* Right atrium, through tricuspid valve to right ventricle, through pulmonary valve to the lungs
- *Oxygenated blood:* Through the pulmonary veins to the left atrium, through the mitral valve to the left ventricle, through the aortic valve to the aorta

The AV valves close very tightly when the ventricles contract, preventing blood from flowing backward into the atria and keeping it moving forward through the system. The pulmonary and aortic valves open with the pressure of ventricular contraction and close tightly during diastole, keeping blood from flowing backward into the ventricles. These valves operate much like one-way automatic doors: you can go through in the intended direction, but if you try to go the wrong way, the doors close and stop your movement. The proper functioning of the cardiac valves is important in maintaining the functioning of the cardiovascular system.

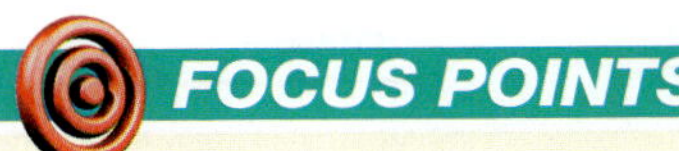

FOCUS POINTS

- The heart, a hollow muscle with four chambers comprising two upper atria and two lower ventricles, pumps oxygenated blood to the body's cells and also collects waste products from the tissues.
- The two-step process known as the cardiac cycle includes diastole (resting period when the veins carry blood back to the heart) and systole (contraction period when the heart pumps blood out to the arteries for distribution to the body).
- Deoxygenated blood is carried by the veins to the right side of the heart, which directs the blood to the lungs where it takes on oxygen.
- Oxygenated blood from the lungs circulates to the left side of the heart to be pumped out to every cell in the body through the arteries.

Conduction System of the Heart

Each cycle of cardiac contraction and relaxation is controlled by impulses that arise spontaneously in certain pacemaker cells of the **sinoatrial (SA) node** of the heart. These impulses are conducted from the pacemaker cells by a specialized conducting system that activates all of the parts of the heart muscle almost simultaneously. These continuous, rhythmic contractions are controlled by the heart itself; the brain does not stimulate the heart to beat. This safety feature allows the heart to beat as long as it has enough nutrients and oxygen to survive, regardless of the status of the rest of the body. This property protects the vital cardiovascular function in many disease states; it is the same property that allows the heart to continue functioning in a patient who is "brain dead."

The conduction system of the heart consists of the SA node, atrial bundles, AV node, bundle of His, bundle branches, and Purkinje fibers (Figure 42.2). The SA node, located in the top of the right atrium, acts as the pacemaker of the heart. Atrial bundles conduct the impulse through the atrial muscle. The AV node slows the impulse, allowing for the delay needed for ventricular filling, and sends it from the atria into the ventricles by way of the bundle of His, which enters the septum and then divides into three bundle branches. These bundle branches, which conduct the impulses through the ventricles, break into a fine network of conducting fibers called the Purkinje fibers, which deliver the impulse to the ventricular cells.

Automaticity

The cells of the impulse-forming and conducting system are rather primitive, uncomplicated cells called pale or P cells. Because of their simple cell membrane, these cells possess a special property that differentiates them from other cells: They can generate action potentials or electrical impulses without being excited to do so by external stimuli. This property is called **automaticity**.

All cardiac cells possess some degree of automaticity. During diastole or rest, these cells undergo a spontaneous depolarization because they decrease the flow of potassium ions out of the cell and probably leak sodium into the cell, causing an action potential. This action potential is basically the same as the action potential of the neuron (see

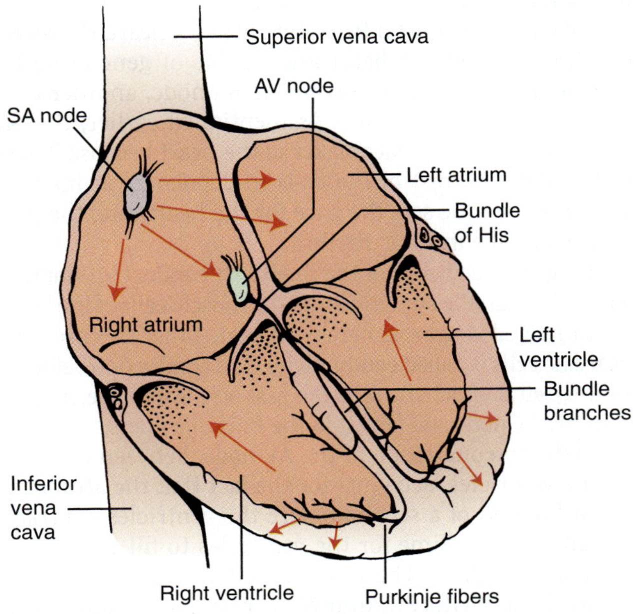

FIGURE 42.2 The conducting system of the heart. Impulses originating in the sinoatrial (SA) node are transmitted through the atrial bundles to the atrioventricular (AV) node and down the bundle of His and the bundle branches by way of the Purkinje fibers through the ventricles.

Chapter 19). The action potential of the cardiac muscle cell consists of five phases:

- Phase 0 occurs when the cell reaches a point of stimulation. The sodium gates open along the cell membrane, and sodium rushes into the cell, resulting in a positive flow of electrons into the cell—an electrical potential. This is called depolarization.
- Phase 1 is the very short period when the sodium ion concentrations are equal inside and outside the cell.
- Phase 2, or the plateau stage, occurs as the cell membrane becomes less permeable to sodium. Calcium slowly enters the cell, and potassium begins to leave the cell. The cell membrane is trying to return to its resting state, a process called repolarization.
- Phase 3 is a period of rapid repolarization as the gates are closed and potassium rapidly moves out of the cell.
- Phase 4 occurs when the cell comes to rest as the sodium–potassium pump returns the membrane to its previous state, with sodium outside and potassium inside the cell, and spontaneous depolarization begins again.

Each area of the heart has an action potential that appears slightly different from the other action potentials, reflecting the complexity of the cells in that particular area. Because of these differences in the action potential, each area of the heart has a slightly different rate of rhythmicity. The SA node generates an impulse about 90 to 100 times a minute, the AV node about 40 to 50 times a minute, and the complex ventricular muscle cells only about 10 to 20 times a minute (Figure 42.3).

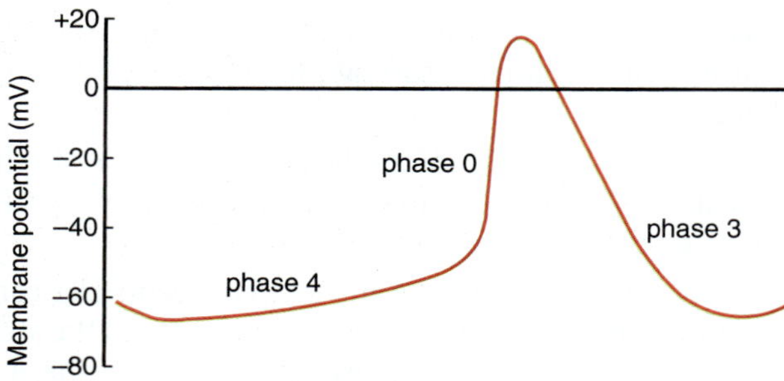

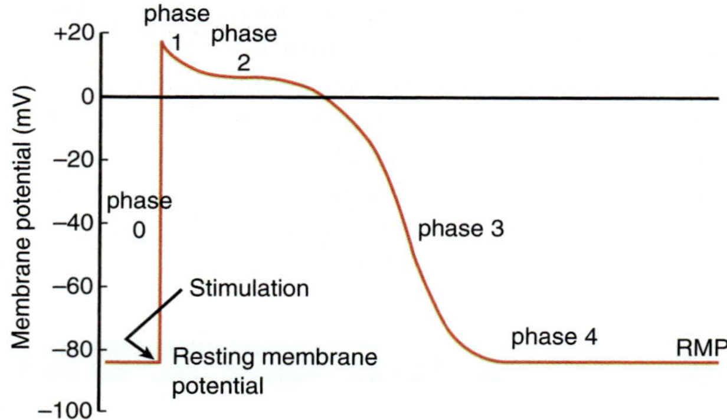

FIGURE 42.3 Action potentials recorded from a cell in the sinoatrial (SA) node **(A)** showing diastolic depolarization in phase 4, and recorded from a ventricular muscle cell **(B)**. In *phase 0,* the cell is stimulated, sodium rushes into the cell, and the cell is depolarized. In *phase 1,* sodium levels equalize. In *phase 2,* the plateau phase, calcium enters the cell (the slow current), and potassium and sodium leave. In *phase 3,* the slow current stops, and sodium and potassium leave the cell. In *phase 4,* the resting membrane potential (RMP) returns and the pacemaker potential begins in the SA node cell.

Conductivity

Normally, the SA node sets the pace for the heart rate because it depolarizes faster than any cell in the heart. However, the other cells in the heart are capable of generating an impulse if anything happens to the SA node, another protective feature of the heart. As mentioned earlier, the SA node is said to be the pacemaker of the heart because it acts to stimulate the rest of the cells to depolarize at its rate. When the SA node sets the pace for the heart rate, the person is said to be in sinus rhythm.

The specialized cells of the heart can conduct an impulse rapidly through the system so that the muscle cells of the heart are stimulated at approximately the same time. This property of cardiac cells is called **conductivity**. The conduction velocity, or the speed at which the cells can pass on the impulse, is slowest in the AV node and fastest in the Purkinje fibers.

A delay in conduction at the AV node, between the atria and the ventricles, accounts for the fact that the atria contract a fraction of a second before the ventricles contract. This allows extra time for the ventricles to fill completely before they contract. The almost simultaneous spread of the impulse through the Purkinje fibers permits a simultaneous and powerful contraction of the ventricle muscles, making them an effective pump.

After a cell membrane has conducted an action potential, there is a span of time, called the absolute refractory period, in which it is impossible to stimulate that area of membrane. The absolute refractory period is the minimal amount of time that must elapse between two stimuli applied at one site in the heart for each of these stimuli to cause an action potential. This time reflects the responsiveness of the heart cells to stimuli. Cardiac drugs may affect the refractory period of the cells to make the heart more or less responsive.

Autonomic Influences

The heart can generate action potentials on its own and could function without connection to the rest of the body. The autonomic nervous system (see Chapter 29) can influence the heart rate and rhythm and the strength of contraction. The parasympathetic nerves, primarily the vagus or tenth cranial nerve, can slow the heart rate and decrease the speed of conduction through the AV node. This allows the heart to rest and conserve its strength. The parasympathetic influence on the SA node is the dominant influence most of the time, keeping the resting heart rate at 70 to 80 beats per minute (bpm).

The sympathetic nervous system stimulates the heart to beat faster, speeds conduction through the AV node, and causes the heart muscle to contract harder. This action is important during exercise or stress, when the body's cells need to have more oxygen delivered. These two branches of the autonomic nervous system work together to help the heart meet the body's demands. Drugs that influence either of these branches of the autonomic nervous system have autonomic effects on the heart.

Mechanical Activity

The end result of the electrical stimulation of the heart cells is the unified contraction of the atria and ventricles, which moves the blood throughout the vascular system. The basic unit of the cardiac muscle is the **sarcomere**. A sarcomere is made up of two contractile proteins: **actin**, a thin filament, and **myosin**, a thick filament with small projections on it. These proteins readily react with each other, but at rest they are kept apart by the protein **troponin** (Figure 42.4).

When a cardiac muscle cell is stimulated, calcium enters the cell though channels in the cell membrane and also from storage sites within the cell. This occurs during phase 3 of the action potential, when the cell is starting to repolarize. The calcium reacts with the troponin and inactivates it. This action allows the actin and myosin proteins to react with each other, forming actomyosin bridges. These bridges then break quickly, and the myosin slides along to form new bridges.

As long as calcium is present, the actomyosin bridges continue to form. This action slides the proteins together, shortening or contracting the sarcomere. Cardiac muscle cells are linked together: when one cell is stimulated to contract, they are all stimulated to contract.

The shortening of numerous sarcomeres causes the contraction and pumping action of the heart muscle. As the cell reaches its repolarized state, calcium is removed from the cell by a sodium–calcium pump, and calcium released from storage sites within the cell returns to the storage sites. The contraction process requires energy and oxygen for the chemical reaction that allows the formation of the actomyosin bridges, and calcium to allow the bridge formation to occur.

The degree of shortening (the strength of contraction) is determined by the amount of calcium present—the more calcium is present, the more bridges will be formed—and by the stretch of the sarcomere before contraction begins. The further apart the actin and myosin proteins are before the cell is stimulated, the more bridges will be formed and the stronger the contraction will be. This correlates with Starling's law of the heart. The more the cardiac muscle is stretched, the greater the contraction will be. The more blood you put into the heart, the greater the contraction will be to empty the heart, up to a point. However, if the bridges are stretched too far apart, they will not be able to reach each other to form the actomyosin bridges, and no contraction will occur (see Figure 42.4).

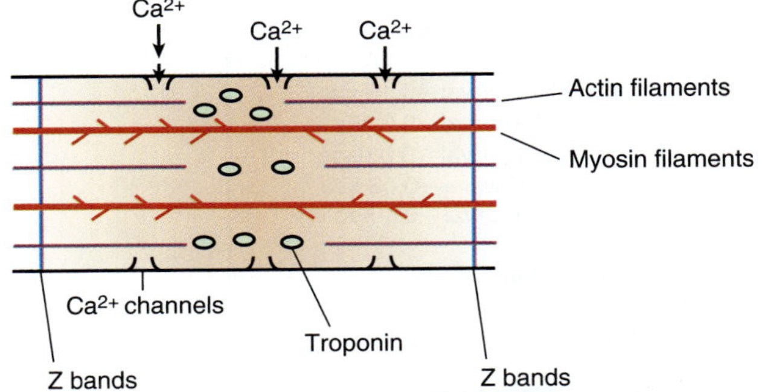

FIGURE 42.4 A sarcomere, the functioning unit of cardiac muscle.

Cardiac Arrhythmias

Various factors, such as drugs, acidosis, decreased oxygen levels, changes in the electrolytes in the area, and buildup of waste products, can change the cardiac rate and rhythm. A disruption in cardiac rate or rhythm is called an **arrhythmia** or a **dysrhythmia**. Arrhythmias interfere with the work of the heart and can disrupt cardiac output, which affects every cell in the body. Arrhythmias can arise because of changes in the automaticity or conductivity of the heart cells. Some arrhythmias occur when there is a shift in the pacemaker of the heart from the SA node to some other site, called an ectopic focus. This occurs most frequently with damage to the heart muscle and can be seen in the form of premature contractions or extrasystoles. These premature beats may be unimportant and sporadic, but in some cases they can be the prelude to more serious or even fatal arrhythmias if the coordinated pumping action of the muscle is lost.

A lack of, or decrease in, conductivity through the AV node produces a condition called heart block. In first-degree heart block, all of the impulses from the SA node arrive in the ventricles, but after a longer time than normal. In second-degree heart block, some of the impulses are lost and do not get through, resulting in a slow rate of ventricular contraction. In third-degree or complete heart block, no impulses from the SA node get through to the ventricles, and the much slower ventricular automaticity takes over. Very serious arrhythmias arise when the combination of ectopic foci and altered conduction set off an irregular, uncoordinated twitching of the atrial or ventricular muscle, called **fibrillation**. In this situation, the pumping action of the heart is lost, and the cardiac output falls. Individuals can live quite normally with atrial fibrillation, but if the ventricles fibrillate, there is total loss of cardiac output, and death can occur if treatment is not initiated quickly.

The Electrocardiogram

Electrocardiography is a process of recording the patterns of electrical impulses as they move through the heart. It is an important diagnostic tool in the care of the cardiac patient. The electrocardiography machine detects the patterns of electrical impulse generation and conduction through the heart and translates that information to a recorded pattern, which is displayed on a cardiac monitor or printed out on calibrated paper as a wave form. It must be remembered that an **electrocardiogram (ECG)** is a measure of electrical activity; it provides no information about the mechanical activity of the heart. The important aspect of cardiac output—the degree to which the heart is doing its job of pumping blood out to all of the tissues—needs to be carefully assessed by looking at and evaluating the patient.

Normal Sinus Rhythm

The normal ECG pattern is made up of five main waves: the P wave, which is formed as impulses originating in the SA node or pacemaker pass through the atrial tissues; the QRS complex, which represents depolarization of the bundle of His (Q) and the ventricles (RS); and the T wave, which represents repolarization of the ventricles (Figure 42.5).

The P wave immediately precedes the contraction of the atria. The QRS complex immediately precedes the contraction of the ventricles and then relaxation of the ventricles during the T wave. The repolarization of the atria (the Ta wave) occurs during the QRS complex and usually is not seen on an ECG. In certain conditions of atrial hypertrophy, the Ta wave may appear around the QRS complex.

The critical points of the ECG are as follows:

P–R interval: Reflects the normal delay of conduction at the AV node

Q–T interval: Reflects the critical timing of repolarization of the ventricles

S–T segment: Reflects important information about the repolarization of the ventricles

Abnormalities in the shape or timing of each part of an ECG tracing reveal the presence of particular cardiac disorders. A person with a normal ECG pattern and a heart rate within

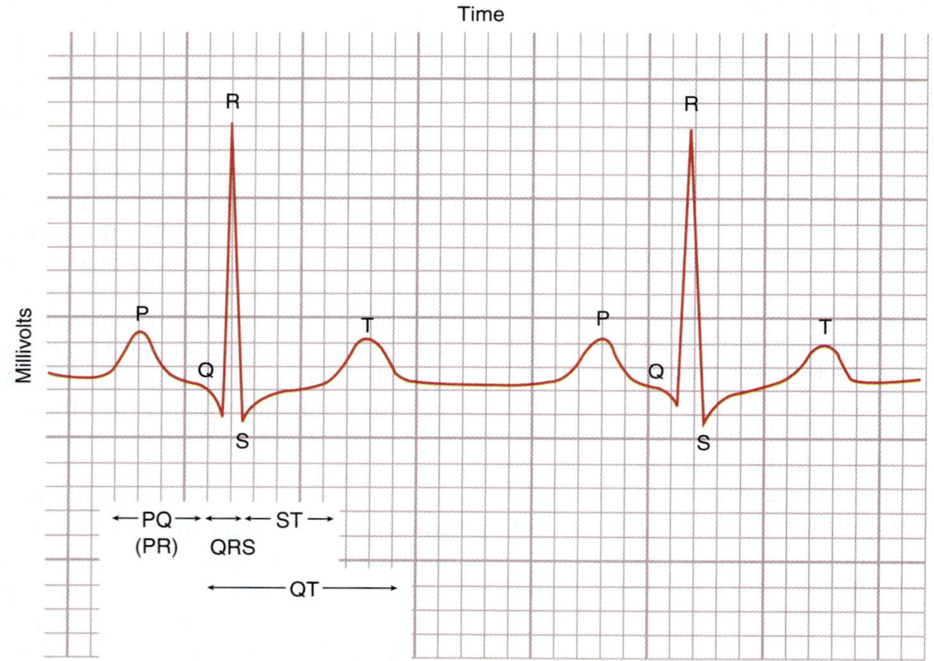

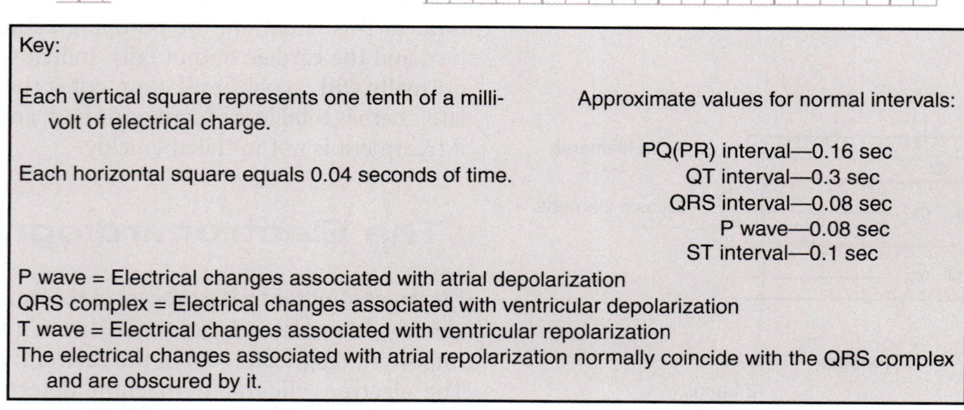

Key:

Each vertical square represents one tenth of a millivolt of electrical charge.

Each horizontal square equals 0.04 seconds of time.

Approximate values for normal intervals:

PQ(PR) interval—0.16 sec
QT interval—0.3 sec
QRS interval—0.08 sec
P wave—0.08 sec
ST interval—0.1 sec

P wave = Electrical changes associated with atrial depolarization
QRS complex = Electrical changes associated with ventricular depolarization
T wave = Electrical changes associated with ventricular repolarization
The electrical changes associated with atrial repolarization normally coincide with the QRS complex and are obscured by it.

FIGURE 42.5 The normal electrocardiogram pattern.

the normal range for that person's age group is said to be in normal sinus rhythm.

Types of Arrhythmias

A disruption in cardiac rate or rhythm is called an arrhythmia (or dysrhythmia). Arrhythmias are significant because they interfere with the work of the heart and can disrupt the cardiac output, which eventually will affect every cell in the body.

Sinus Arrhythmias

The SA node is influenced by the autonomic nervous system to change the rate of firing in order to meet the body's demands for oxygen. A faster-than-normal heart rate, usually anything faster than 100 beats/min in an adult, with a normal-appearing ECG pattern is called sinus tachycardia. Sinus bradycardia is a slower-than-normal heart rate (usually less than 60 beats/min) with a normal-appearing ECG pattern.

Supraventricular Arrhythmias

Arrhythmias that originate above the ventricles but not in the SA node are called supraventricular arrhythmias. These arrhythmias feature an abnormally shaped P wave, because the site of origin is not the sinus node; however, they show normal QRS complexes, because the ventricles are still conducting impulses normally. Supraventricular arrhythmias include the following:

- *Premature atrial contractions (PACs),* which reflect an ectopic focus in the atria that is generating an impulse out of the normal rhythm
- *Paroxysmal atrial tachycardia (PAT),* sporadically occurring runs of rapid heart rate originating in the atria
- *Atrial flutter,* characterized by sawtooth-shaped P waves reflecting a single ectopic focus that is generating a regular, fast atrial depolarization
- *Atrial fibrillation,* with irregular P waves representing many ectopic foci firing in an uncoordinated manner through the atria

With atrial flutter, often one of every two or one of every three impulses is transmitted to the ventricles. The person may have a 2:1 or 3:1 ratio of P waves to QRS complexes. The ventricles beat faster than normal, losing some efficiency. With atrial fibrillation, so many impulses are bombarding the AV node that an unpredictable number of impulses are transmitted to the ventricles. The ventricles are stimulated to beat in a fast, irregular, and often inefficient manner.

Atrioventricular Block

AV block, also called heart block, reflects a slowing or lack of conduction at the AV node. This can occur because of structural damage, hypoxia, or injury to the heart muscle. First-degree heart block is characterized by a lengthening of the P–R interval beyond the normal 0.16 to 0.20 seconds. Each P wave is followed by a QRS complex. In second-degree heart block, a QRS complex may follow one, two, three, or four P waves. Third-degree heart block, or complete heart block, shows a total dissociation of P waves from QRS complexes and T waves. Because the P waves can come at any time, the P–R interval is not constant. The QRS complexes appear at a very slow rate and may not be sufficient to meet the body's needs.

Ventricular Arrhythmias

Impulses that originate below the AV node originate from ectopic foci that do not use the normal conduction pathways. The QRS complexes appear wide and prolonged, and the T waves are inverted, reflecting the slower conduction across cardiac tissue that is not part of the rapid conduction system. Premature ventricular contractions (PVCs) can arise from a single ectopic focus in the ventricles, with all of them having the same shape, or from many ectopic foci, which produces PVCs with different shapes. Runs or bursts of PVCs from many different foci are more ominous because they can reflect extensive damage or hypoxia in the myocardium. Runs of several PVCs at a rapid rate are called ventricular tachycardia. Ventricular fibrillation is seen as a bizarre, irregular, distorted wave. It is potentially fatal because it reflects a lack of any coordinated stimulation of the ventricles; this leads to inability to contract in a coordinated fashion, with the result that no blood is pumped to the body or the brain.

The Cardiovascular System

The purpose of the heart's continual pumping action is to keep blood flowing to and from all of the body's tissues. Blood delivers oxygen and much-needed nutrients to the cells for producing energy, and it carries away carbon dioxide and other waste products of metabolism. The steady circulation of blood is essential for the proper functioning of all of the body's organs, including the heart itself.

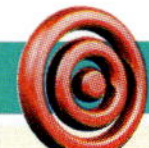

FOCUS POINTS

- Impulses generated in the heart—not the brain—stimulate contraction of the heart muscle.
- The heart's conduction (or stimulatory) system, the cardiac cycle, consists of the sinoatrial (SA) node, the atrial bundles, the atrioventricular (AV) node, the bundle of His, the bundle branches, and the Purkinje fibers.
- In normal sinus rhythm, the SA node generates an impulse that is transmitted through the atrial bundles, delayed slightly at the AV node, then sent over the bundle of His into the ventricles.
- When the generation of impulses is altered, the result is known as an arrhythmia (or dysrhythmia) that can upset the normal balance in the cardiovascular system. A decrease in cardiac output, which affects all of the cells of the body, follows.

Circulation

The circulation of the blood follows two courses:

- *Heart–lung or pulmonary circulation:* The right side of the heart sends blood to the lungs, where carbon dioxide and some waste products are removed from the blood and oxygen is picked up by the red blood cells.
- *Systemic circulation:* The left side of the heart sends oxygenated blood out to all of the cells in the body.

The blood moves through the circulatory system from areas of high pressure to areas of lower pressure. The system is a "closed" system; that is, it has no openings or holes that would allow blood to leak out. The closed nature of the system is what keeps the pressure differences in the proper relationship so that blood always flows in the direction in which it is intended to flow (Figure 42.6).

CONCEPTS in action ANIMATION

Pulmonary and Systemic Circulation

The right atrium is a very-low-pressure area in the cardiovascular system. All of the deoxygenated blood from the body flows into the right atrium from the inferior and superior venae cavae (see Figure 42.1) and from the great cardiac vein, which returns deoxygenated blood from the heart muscle. As the blood flows into the atrium, the pressure increases. When the pressure becomes greater than the pressure in the right ventricle, most of the blood flows into the right ventricle; this is called the rapid-filling phase. At this point in the cardiac cycle, the atrium is stimulated to contract and pushes the remaining blood into the right ventricle. The ventricle is then stimulated to contract; it generates pressure that pushes open the pulmonic valve (see Figure 42.1) and sends blood into the pulmonary artery, which takes the blood into the lungs, a very-low-pressure area. The blood then circulates around the alveoli of the lungs, picking up oxygen and getting rid of carbon dioxide; flows through pulmonary capillaries (the tiny blood vessels that connect arteries and veins) into the pulmonary veins; and then flows into the left atrium. When the pressure of blood volume in the left atrium is greater than the pressure in the large left ventricle, this oxygenated blood flows into the left ventricle. The left atrium contracts and pushes any remaining blood into the left ventricle, which is stimulated to contract and generates tremendous pressure to push the blood out the aorta, carrying it throughout the body. In a normal heart, the right and left atria contract at the same time and the right and left ventricles contract at the same time.

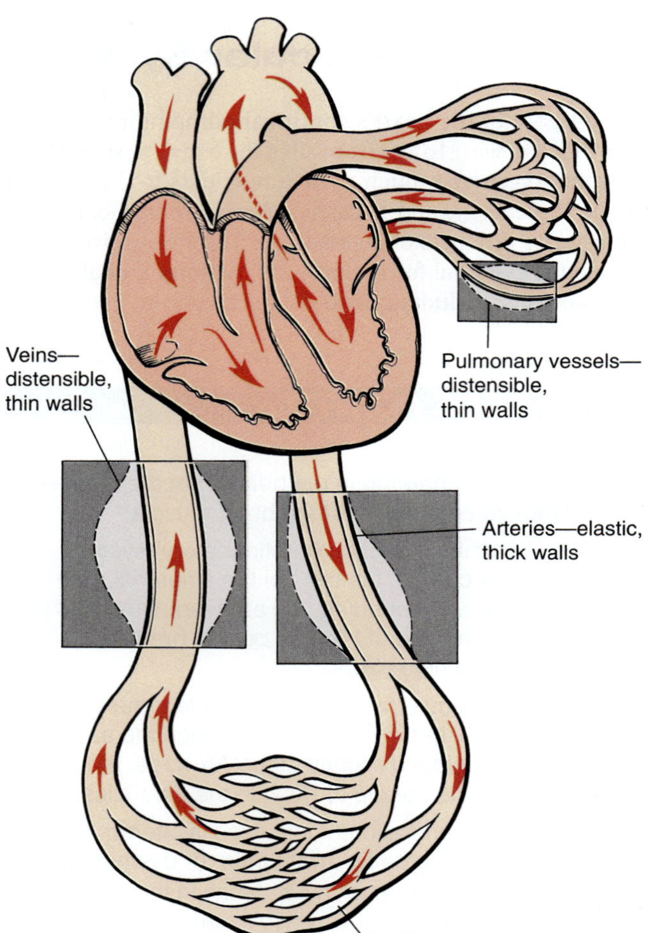

FIGURE 42.6 Blood flow through the systemic and pulmonary vasculature circuits.

Arteries, Capillaries, and Veins

The aorta and other large arteries have thick, muscular walls. The entire arterial system contains muscles in the walls of the vessels all the way to the terminal branches or arterioles, which consist of fragments of muscle and endothelial cells. These muscles offer resistance to the blood that is sent pumping into the arterial system by the left ventricle, generating pressure. The arterial system is referred to as a **resistance system**. The vessels can either constrict or dilate, increasing or decreasing resistance, based on the needs of the body. The arterioles are able to completely shut off blood flow to some areas of the body; that is, they can shunt blood to another area where it is needed more. The arterioles, because of their ability to increase or decrease resistance in the system, are one of the main regulators of blood pressure.

Blood from the tiny arterioles flows into the **capillary** system, which connects the arterial and venous systems. These microscopic vessels are composed of loosely connected endothelial cells. Oxygen, fluid, and nutrients are able to pass through the arterial end of the capillaries and enter the interstitial area between tissue cells. Fluid at the venous end of the capillary is drawn back into the vessel and contains carbon dioxide and other waste products. This shifting of fluid in the capillaries, called the capillary fluid shift, is carefully regulated by a balance between hydrostatic (fluid pressure) forces on the arterial end of the capillary and **oncotic pressure** (the pulling pressure of the large, vascular proteins) on the venous end of the capillary. In a normal situation, the higher pressure at the arterial end of a capillary forces fluid out of the vessel and into the tissue, and the now-concentrated proteins (which are too large to leave the capillary) exert a pull on the fluid at the venous end of the capillary to pull it back in. A disruption in the hydrostatic pressure or in the concentration of proteins in the capillary can lead to fluid's being left in the tissue, a condition referred to as edema. The capillaries merge into venules, which merge into veins, which are responsible for returning the blood to the heart (Figure 42.7).

The veins are thin-walled, very elastic, low-pressure vessels that can hold large quantities of blood if necessary. The venous system is referred to as a **capacitance system** because the veins have the capacity to hold large quantities of fluid as they distend with fluid volume. These capacitance vessels have a great deal of influence on the venous return to the heart, the amount of blood that is delivered to the right atrium.

Coronary Circulation

The heart muscle itself requires a constant supply of oxygenated blood to keep contracting. The myocardium receives its blood through two main coronary arteries that branch off the base of the aorta from an area called the sinuses of Valsalva. These arteries encircle the heart in a pattern resembling a crown, which is why they are called coronary arteries.

The artery arising from the left side of the aorta bifurcates, or divides, into two large vessels called the left circumflex artery (which travels down the left side of the heart and feeds most of the left ventricle) and the left anterior descending coronary artery (which travels down the front of the heart and feeds the septum and anterior areas, including much of the conduction system). The artery arising from the right side of the aorta feeds most of the right side of the heart, including the SA node.

The coronary arteries receive blood during diastole, when the muscle is at rest and relaxed so that blood can flow freely down into the muscle. When the ventricle contracts, it forces the aortic valve open, and the leaflets of the valve cover the openings of the coronary arteries. When the ventricles relax, the blood is no longer pumped forward and starts to flow back toward the ventricle. The blood flowing down the sides of the aorta closes the aortic valve and fills up the coronary arteries. The pressure that fills the coronary arteries is the difference between the systolic ejection pressure and the diastolic resting pressure. This is called the **pulse pressure** (systolic minus diastolic blood pressure readings). The pulse pressure is monitored clinically to evaluate the filling pressure of the coronary arteries. The oxygenated blood that is fed into the heart by the coronary circulation reaches every cardiac muscle fiber as the vessels divide and subdivide throughout the myocardium (Figure 42.8).

The heart has a pattern of circulation called end-artery circulation. The arteries go into the muscle and end without a great deal of backup or collateral circulation. Normally this is an efficient system and is able to meet the needs of the heart muscle. The heart's supply of and demand for oxygen is met by changes in the delivery of oxygen through the coronary system. Problems can arise, however, when an imbalance

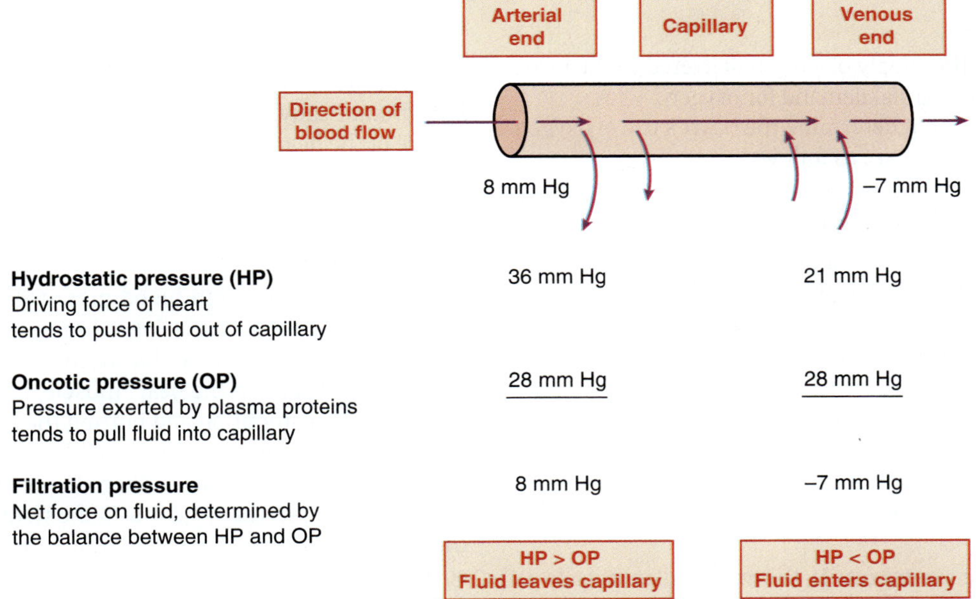

FIGURE 42.7 The net shift of fluid out of and into the capillary is determined by the balance between the hydrostatic pressure (HP) and the oncotic pressure (OP). HP tends to push fluid out of the capillary, and the OP tends to pull it back into the capillary. At the arterial end of the capillary bed, the blood pressure is higher than at the venous end. At the arterial end, HP exceeds OP, and fluid filters out. At the venous end, HP has fallen and HP is less than OP; fluid is pulled back into the capillary from the surrounding tissue. The lymphatic system also returns fluids and substances from the tissues to the circulation.

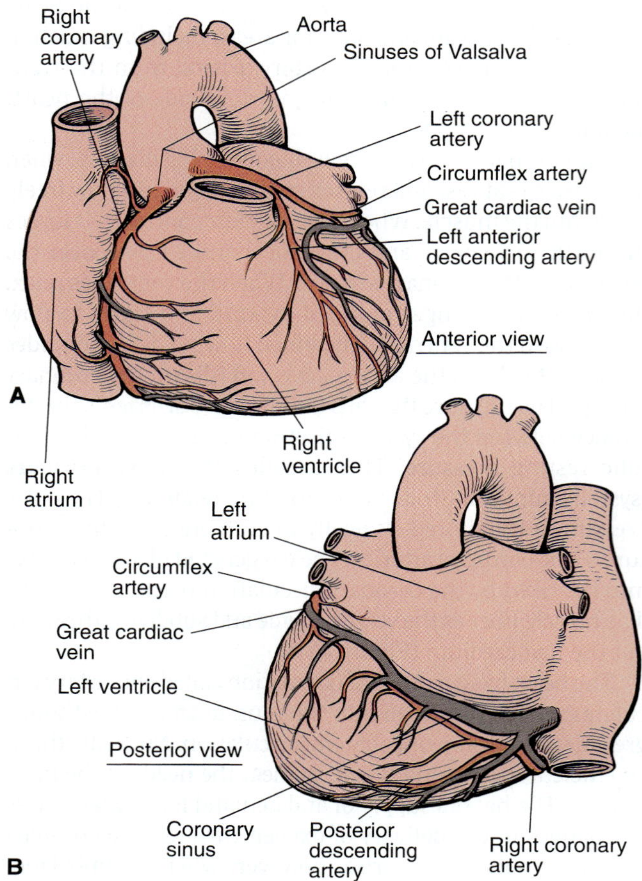

FIGURE 42.8 Coronary arteries and veins. **(A)** Anterior view; **(B)** posterior view.

develops between the supply of oxygen delivered to the heart muscle and the myocardial demand for oxygen.

The main forces that determine the heart's use of oxygen or oxygen consumption are as follows:

- *Heart rate:* The more the heart has to pump, the more oxygen it will require to do that.
- *Preload (amount of blood that is brought back to the heart to be pumped around):* The more blood that is returned to the heart, the harder it will have to work to pump the blood around. The volume of blood in the system is a determinant of preload.
- *Afterload (resistance against which the heart has to beat):* The higher the resistance in the system, the harder the heart will have to contract to force open the valves and pump the blood along. Blood pressure is a measure of afterload.
- *Stretch on the ventricles:* If the ventricular muscle is stretched before it is stimulated to contract, more actomyosin bridges will be formed (which will take more energy); or, if the muscle is stimulated to contract harder than usual (which happens with sympathetic stimulation), more bridges will be formed, which will require more energy.

The muscle can be stretched, as in ventricular hypertrophy related to chronic hypertension or cardiac muscle damage, or in heart failure when the ventricle does not empty completely and blood backs up in the system.

The supply of blood to the myocardium can be altered if the heart fails to pump effectively and cannot deliver blood to the coronary arteries. This happens in congestive heart failure and cases of hypotension. The supply is most frequently altered, however, when the coronary vessels become narrowed and unresponsive to stimuli to dilate and deliver more blood. This happens in atherosclerosis or coronary artery disease. The end result of this narrowing can be total blockage of a coronary artery, leading to hypoxia and eventual death of the cells that depend on that vessel for oxygen. This is called a myocardial infarction (MI), and it is the leading cause of death in the United States.

Systemic Arterial Pressure

The contraction of the left ventricle, which sends blood surging out into the aorta, creates a pressure that continues to force blood into all of the branches of the aorta. This pressure against arterial walls is greatest during systole (cardiac contraction) and falls to its lowest level during diastole. Measurement of both the systolic and the diastolic pressure indicates both the pumping pressure of the ventricle and the generalized pressure in the system, or the pressure the ventricle has to overcome to pump blood out of the heart.

Hypotension

The pressure in the arteries needs to remain relatively high to ensure that blood is delivered to every cell in the body and to keep the blood flowing from high-pressure to low-pressure areas. Hypotension can occur if the blood pressure falls dramatically, either from loss of blood volume or from failure of the heart muscle to pump effectively. Severe hypotension can progress to shock and even death as cells are cut off from their oxygen supply.

Hypertension

Constant, excessive high blood pressure, called hypertension, can damage the fragile inner lining of blood vessels and cause a disruption of blood flow to the tissues. It also puts a tremendous strain on the heart muscle, increasing myocardial oxygen consumption and putting the heart muscle itself at risk. Hypertension can be caused by neurostimulation of the blood vessels that causes them to constrict and to raise pressure, or by increased volume in the system. In most cases, the cause of hypertension is not known, and drug therapy to correct it is aimed at changing one or more of the normal reflexes that control vascular resistance or the force of cardiac muscle contraction.

Vasomotor Tone

The smooth muscles in the walls of the arteries receive constant input from nerve fibers of the sympathetic nervous system. These impulses work to dilate the vessels if more blood flow is needed in an area; to constrict vessels if increased pressure is needed in the system; and to maintain muscle tone so that the vessel remains patent and responsive.

The coordination of these impulses is regulated through the medulla in an area called the cardiovascular center. If increased pressure is needed, this center increases sympathetic flow to the vessels. If pressure rises too high, this is sensed by baroreceptors or pressure receptors and the sympathetic flow is decreased. Chapter 43 discusses the drugs that are used to influence the stimulation of vessels to alter blood pressure.

Renin–Angiotensin System

Another determinant of blood pressure is the renin–angiotensin system. This system is activated when blood flow to the kidneys is decreased. Cells in the kidney release an enzyme called renin. Renin is transported to the liver, where it converts angiotensinogen (produced in the liver) to angiotensin I. Angiotensin I travels to the lungs, where it is converted by angiotensin-converting enzyme (ACE) to angiotensin II. Angiotensin II travels through the body and reacts with angiotensin II receptor sites on blood vessels to cause a severe vasoconstriction. This increases blood pressure and should increase blood flow to the kidneys to decrease the release of renin. Angiotensin II also causes the release of aldosterone from the adrenal cortex, which causes retention of sodium and water, leading to the release of antidiuretic hormone (ADH) to retain water and increase blood volume. Increasing blood volume increases blood flow to the kidney. This system works constantly, whenever a position change alters flow to the kidney or blood volume or pressure changes, to help maintain the blood pressure within a range that ensures perfusion (delivery of blood to all of the tissues) (Figure 42.9).

Venous Pressure

Pressure in the veins may also sometimes rise above normal. This can happen if the heart is not pumping effectively and cannot pump out all of the blood that is trying to return to it. This results in a backup or congestion of blood waiting to enter the heart. Pressure rises in the right atrium and then in the veins that are trying to return blood to the heart as they encounter resistance. The venous system begins to back up, or become congested with blood.

Congestive Heart Failure and Edema

If the heart muscle fails to do its job of effectively pumping blood through the system, blood backs up and the system becomes congested. This is called congestive heart failure (CHF). The rise in venous pressure that results from this backup of blood increases the hydrostatic pressure on the venous end of the capillaries. The hydrostatic pressure pushing fluid out of the capillary is soon higher than the oncotic pressure that is trying to pull the fluid back into the vessel, causing fluid to be lost into the tissues. This shift of fluid accounts for the edema seen with CHF. Pulmonary edema

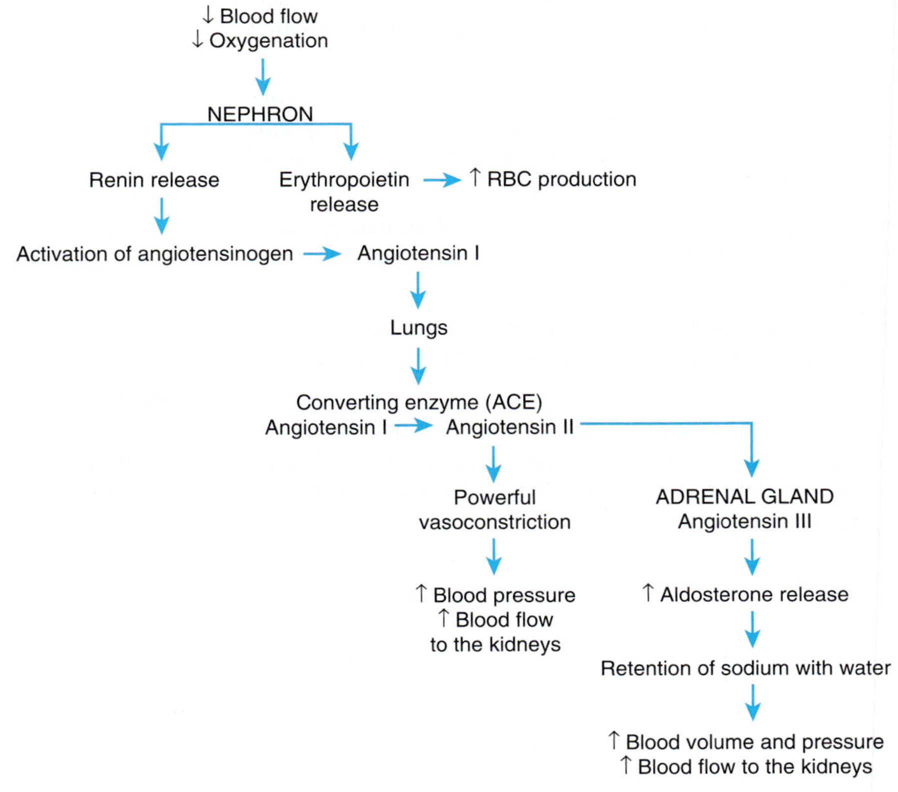

FIGURE 42.9 The renin–angiotensin system for reflex maintenance of blood pressure control.

results when the left side of the heart is failing; peripheral, abdominal, and liver edema occur when the right side of the heart is failing.

Other factors that can contribute to this loss of fluid in the tissues include protein loss and fluid retention. Protein loss can lead to a fall in oncotic pressure and an inability to pull fluid back into the vascular system. Protein levels fall in renal failure, when protein is lost in the urine, and in liver failure, when the liver is no longer able to produce plasma proteins. Fluid retention, which often is stimulated by aldosterone and ADH as described earlier, can increase the hydrostatic pressure so much that fluid is pushed out under higher pressure and the balancing pressure to pull it back into the vessel is not sufficient. Drugs that are used to treat CHF may affect the vascular system at any of these areas in an attempt to return a balance to the pressures in the system.

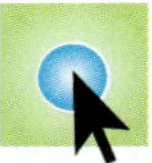

WEB LINK

To explore the virtual cardiovascular system, consult the following Internet source:
http://www.InnerBody.com

Points to Remember

- The heart is a hollow muscle that is divided into a right and a left side by a thick septum, and into four chambers—the two upper atria and the two lower ventricles.
- The heart is responsible for pumping oxygenated blood to every cell in the body and for picking up waste products from the tissues.
- The cardiac cycle consists of a period of rest, or diastole, when blood is returned to the heart by veins, and a period of contraction, or systole, when the blood is pumped out of the heart.
- The right side of the heart receives all of the deoxygenated blood from the body through the veins and directs it into the lungs.
- The left side of the heart receives oxygenated blood from the lungs and pumps it out to every cell in the body through the arteries.
- The heart muscle possesses the properties of automaticity (the ability to generate an action potential in the absence of stimulation) and conductivity (the ability to rapidly transmit an action potential).
- The heart muscle is stimulated to contract by impulses generated in the heart, not by stimuli from the brain. The autonomic nervous system can affect the heart to increase (sympathetic) or decrease (parasympathetic) activity.
- The normal conduction or stimulatory system of the heart consists of the SA node, the atrial bundles, the AV node, the bundle of His, the bundle branches, and the Purkinje fibers.
- In normal sinus rhythm, cells in the SA node generate an impulse that is transmitted through the atrial bundles and delayed slightly at the AV node before being sent down the bundle of His into the ventricles. When cardiac muscle cells are stimulated, they contract.
- Alterations in the generation of conduction of impulses in the heart cause arrhythmias (dysrhythmias), which can upset the normal balance in the cardiovascular system and lead to a decrease in cardiac output, affecting all of the cells of the body.
- Heart muscle contracts by the sliding of actin and myosin filaments in a functioning unit called a sarcomere. Contraction requires energy and calcium to allow the filaments to react with each other and slide together.
- The heart muscle needs a constant supply of blood, which is furnished by the coronary arteries. Increase in demand for oxygen can occur with changes in heart rate, preload, afterload, or stretch on the muscle.
- The cardiovascular system is a closed pressure system that uses arteries (muscular, pressure or resistance tubes) to carry blood from the heart, veins (flexible, distensible capacitance vessels) to return blood to the heart, and capillaries (which connect arteries to veins) to keep blood flowing from areas of high pressure to areas of low pressure.
- Blood pressure is maintained by stimulus from the sympathetic system and reflex control of blood volume and pressure by the renin–angiotensin system and the aldosterone–ADH system. Alterations in blood pressure (hypotension or hypertension) can upset the balance of the cardiovascular system and lead to problems in blood delivery.
- Fluid shifts out of the blood at the arterial ends of capillaries to deliver oxygen and nutrients to the tissues. It is pushed out of the vessel by the hydrostatic or fluid pressure in the arterial side of the system. Fluid returns to the system at the venous end of the capillaries because of the oncotic pull of proteins in the vessels. Disruptions in these pressures can lead to edema or loss of fluid in the tissues.

CHECK YOUR UNDERSTANDING

Answers to the questions in this chapter may be found in the Answer Key in the back of the book.

Multiple Choice

Select the best answer to the following.

1. When referring to the heart valves,
   a. the closing of the AV valves is what is responsible for heart sounds.
   b. small muscles attached to the AV valves are responsible for opening and closing the valves with each cycle's contraction.
   c. the aortic valve opens when the pressure in the left ventricle becomes slightly greater than the pressure in the aorta.
   d. the valves leading to the great vessels are called cuspid valves.

2. In the heart,
   a. the ventricles will not contract unless they are stimulated by action potentials arising from the SA node in the right atrium.
   b. fibrillation of the atria will cause blood pressure to fall to zero.
   c. spontaneous depolarization of the muscle membrane can occur in the absence of nerve stimulation.
   d. the muscle can continue to contract for a long period of time in the absence of oxygen through the use of anaerobic glycolysis to synthesize ATP.

3. The activity of the heart depends on both the inherent properties of the cardiac muscle cells and the activity of the autonomic nerves to the heart. Therefore,
   a. cutting all of the autonomic nerves to the heart will produce a decrease in heart rate.
   b. blocking the parasympathetic nerves to the heart decreases the heart rate.
   c. stimulating the sympathetic nerves to the heart increases the time available to fill the ventricles during diastole.
   d. dehydration leads to an increase in heart rate.

4. A heart transplantation patient has no nerve connections to the transplanted heart. In such an individual, one would expect to find
   a. a slower than normal resting heart rate.
   b. atria that contract at a different rate than ventricles.
   c. an increase in heart rate during emotional stress.
   d. inability to exercise because there is no way to increase heart rate or force of contraction to increase cardiac output.

5. The baroreceptors in the carotid sinus and aortic arch
   a. are in appropriate position to protect the brain from sudden changes in blood pressure and thus blood flow.
   b. decrease the frequency of impulses sent to the cardiovascular center when arterial blood pressure is increased.
   c. monitor the magnitude of concentration of oxygen in the vessels.
   d. react to high levels of carbon dioxide.

6. Cardiac cells differ from skeletal muscle cells in that
   a. they contain actin and myosin.
   b. they possess automaticity and conductivity.
   c. calcium must be present for muscle contraction to occur.
   d. they do not require oxygen to survive.

7. Clinically, dysrhythmias or arrhythmias cause
   a. alterations in cardiac output that could affect all cells.
   b. changes in capillary filling pressures.
   c. alterations in osmotic pressure.
   d. valvular dysfunction.

8. A client is brought to the emergency room with a suspected MI. The client is very upset because he had just had an ECG in his doctor's office and it was fine. The explanation of this common phenomenon would include the fact that
   a. the ECG only reflects changes in cardiac output.
   b. the ECG is not a very accurate test.
   c. the ECG only measures the flow of electrical current through the heart and does not indicate mechanical activity or blood flow to the muscle.
   d. the ECG is not related to the heart problems.

9. Blood flow to the myocardium differs from blood flow to the rest of the cells of the body in that
   a. blood perfuses the myocardium during systole.
   b. blood flow is determined by many local factors including buildup of acid.
   c. blood perfuses the myocardium during diastole.
   d. oxygenated blood flows to the myocardium via veins.

Multiple Response

Select all that apply.

1. During diastole, which of the following would occur?
   a. Opening of the atrioventricular valves
   b. Relaxation of the myocardial muscle

c. Flow of blood from the atria to the ventricles
d. Contraction of the ventricles
e. Closing of the semilunar valves
f. Filling of the coronary arteries

2. The sympathetic nervous system would be expected to have which of the following effects?
a. Stimulate the heart to beat faster
b. Speed conduction through the AV node
c. Cause the heart muscle to contract harder
d. Slow conduction through the AV node
e. Decrease overall vascular volume
f. Increase total peripheral resistance

Definitions

Define the following terms.

1. troponin ______________________________

____

2. actin ______________________________

____

3. myosin ______________________________

____

4. arrhythmia ______________________________

____

5. Starling's law of the heart ______________________________

____

6. fibrillation ______________________________

____

7. capillary ______________________________

____

8. resistance system ______________________________

____

Matching

Match the word with the appropriate definition.

1. ____________________ atrium
2. ____________________ ventricle
3. ____________________ auricle
4. ____________________ vein
5. ____________________ artery
6. ____________________ myocardium
7. ____________________ syncytia
8. ____________________ diastole
9. ____________________ systole
10. ____________________ automaticity
11. ____________________ conductivity
12. ____________________ pulse pressure

A. Resting phase of the heart
B. Reflects the filling pressure of the coronary arteries
C. Bottom chamber of the heart
D. Vessel that takes blood away from the heart
E. Vessel that returns blood to the heart
F. Appendage on the atria of the heart
G. Property of heart cells to generate an action potential
H. Top chamber of the heart
I. Property of heart cells to rapidly conduct an action potential of electrical impulse
J. Intertwining network of muscle fibers
K. Contracting phase of the heart
L. Muscle of the heart

Bibliography and References

Ganong, W. (2003). *Review of medical physiology* (20th ed.). Norwalk, CT: Appleton & Lange.

Gilman, A., Hardman, J. G., & Limbird, L. E. (Eds.). (2006). *Goodman and Gilman's the pharmacological basis of therapeutics* (11th ed.). New York: McGraw-Hill.

Guyton, A., & Hall, J. (2004). *Textbook of medical physiology.* Philadelphia: W. B. Saunders.

Karch, A. M. (2006). *2007 Lippincott's nursing drug guide.* Philadelphia: Lippincott Williams & Wilkins.

Porth, C. M. (2005). *Pathophysiology: Concepts of altered health states* (7th ed.). Philadelphia: Lippincott Williams & Wilkins.

CHAPTER 43

Drugs Affecting Blood Pressure

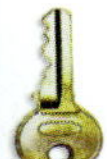

KEY TERMS

ACE inhibitor
angiotensin II receptors
baroreceptor
cardiovascular center
essential hypertension
hypotension
peripheral resistance
renin–angiotensin system
shock
stroke volume

LEARNING OBJECTIVES

Upon completion of this chapter, you will be able to:

1. Outline the normal controls of blood pressure and explain how the various drugs used to treat hypertension or hypotension affect these controls.
2. Describe the therapeutic actions, indications, pharmacokinetics, contraindications, most common adverse reactions, and important drug–drug interactions associated with the angiotensin-converting inhibitors, angiotensin II receptor blockers, calcium channel blockers, vasodilators, ganglionic blockers, and the antihypotensive agent.
3. Discuss the use of drugs that affect blood pressure across the lifespan.
4. Compare and contrast the prototype drugs captopril, losartan, diltiazem, nitroprusside, mecamylamine, and midodrine with other agents in their class and with other agents used to affect blood pressure.
5. Outline the nursing considerations, including important teaching points, for patients receiving drugs used to affect blood pressure.

ANTIHYPERTENSIVE AGENTS

Angiotensin-Converting Enzyme Inhibitors

benazepril
P captopril
enalapril
fosinopril
lisinopril
moexipril
perindopril
quinapril
ramipril
trandolapril

Angiotensin II Receptor Blockers

candesartan
eprosartan
irbesartan
P losartan
olmesartan
telmisartan
valsartan

Calcium Channel Blockers

amlodipine
P diltiazem
felodipine
isradipine
nicardipine
nifedipine
nisoldipine
verapamil

Vasodilators

diazoxide
hydralazine
minoxidil
P nitroprusside

Ganglionic Blocker

mecamylamine

ANTIHYPOTENSIVE AGENT

midodrine

The cardiovascular system is a closed system of blood vessels that is responsible for delivering oxygenated blood to the tissues and removing waste products from the tissues. The blood in this system flows from areas of higher pressure to areas of lower pressure. The area of highest pressure in the system is always the left ventricle during systole. The pressure in this area propels the blood out of the aorta and into the system. The lowest pressure is in the right atrium, which collects all of the deoxygenated blood from the body. The maintenance of this pressure system is controlled by specific areas of the brain and various hormones. If the pressure becomes too high, the person is said to be hypertensive. If the pressure becomes too low and blood cannot be delivered effectively, the person is said to be hypotensive. Helping the patient to maintain the blood pressure within normal limits is the goal when drug therapy is instituted.

Blood Pressure Control

The pressure in the cardiovascular system is determined by three elements:

- Heart rate
- **Stroke volume**, or the amount of blood that is pumped out of the ventricle with each heartbeat (primarily determined by the volume of blood in the system)
- Total **peripheral resistance**, or the resistance of the muscular arteries to the blood being pumped through.

The small arterioles are thought to be the most important factors in determining peripheral resistance. Because they have the smallest diameter, they are able to almost stop blood flow into capillary beds when they constrict, building up tremendous pressure in the arteries behind them as they prevent the blood from flowing through. The arterioles are very responsive to stimulation from the sympathetic nervous system; they constrict when the sympathetic system is stimulated, increasing total peripheral resistance and blood pressure. The body uses this responsiveness to regulate blood pressure on a minute-to-minute basis, to ensure that there is enough pressure in the system to deliver sufficient blood to the brain.

Baroreceptors

As the blood leaves the left ventricle through the aorta, it influences specialized cells in the arch of the aorta called **baroreceptors** (pressure receptors). Similar cells are located in the carotid arteries, which deliver blood to the brain. If there is sufficient pressure in these vessels, the baroreceptors are stimulated, sending that information to the brain. If the pressure falls, the stimulation of the baroreceptors falls off. That information is also sent to the brain.

The sensory input from the baroreceptors is received in the medulla, in an area called the **cardiovascular center** or vasomotor center. If the pressure is high, the medulla stimulates vasodilation and a decrease in cardiac rate and output, causing the pressure in the system to drop. If the pressure is low, the medulla directly stimulates an increase in cardiac rate and output and vasoconstriction; this increases total peripheral resistance and raises the blood pressure. The medulla mediates these effects through the autonomic nervous system (see Chapter 29).

The baroreceptor reflex functions continually to maintain blood pressure within a predetermined range of normal. For example, if you have been lying down flat and suddenly stand up, the blood will rush to your feet (an effect of gravity). You may even feel light-headed or dizzy for a short time. When you stand and the blood flow drops, the baroreceptors are not stretched. The medulla senses this drop in stimulation of the baroreceptors and stimulates a rise in heart rate and cardiac output and a generalized vasoconstriction, which increases total peripheral resistance and blood pressure. These increases should raise pressure in the system, which restores blood flow to the brain and stimulates the baroreceptors. The stimulation of the baroreceptors leads to a decrease in stimulatory impulses from the medulla, and the blood pressure falls back within normal limits (Figure 43.1).

Renin–Angiotensin System

Another compensatory system is activated when the blood pressure within the kidneys falls. Because the kidneys require a constant perfusion to function properly, they have a compensatory mechanism to help ensure that blood flow is maintained. This mechanism is called the **renin–angiotensin system**. (It is also sometimes referred to as the renin–angiotensin–aldosterone system.)

Low blood pressure or poor oxygenation of a nephron causes the release of renin from the juxtaglomerular cells, a group of cells that monitor blood pressure and flow into the glomerulus. Renin is released into the bloodstream and arrives in the liver to convert the compound angiotensinogen (produced in the liver) to angiotensin I. Angiotensin I travels in the bloodstream to the lungs, where the metabolic cells of the alveoli use angiotensin-converting enzyme (ACE) to convert angiotensin I to angiotensin II. Angiotensin II reacts with specific angiotensin II receptor sites on blood vessels to cause intense vasoconstriction. This effect raises the total peripheral resistance and raises the blood pressure, restoring blood flow to the kidneys and decreasing the release of renin.

Angiotensin II, probably after conversion to angiotensin III, also stimulates the adrenal cortex to release aldosterone. Aldosterone acts on the nephrons to cause the retention of sodium and water. This effect increases blood volume, which should also contribute to increasing blood pressure. The sodium-rich blood stimulates the osmoreceptors in the hypothalamus to cause the release of antidiuretic hormone (ADH), which in turn causes retention of water in the nephrons, further increasing the blood volume. This increase in blood volume increases the blood pressure, which should increase blood flow to the kidneys. This should lead to a decrease in

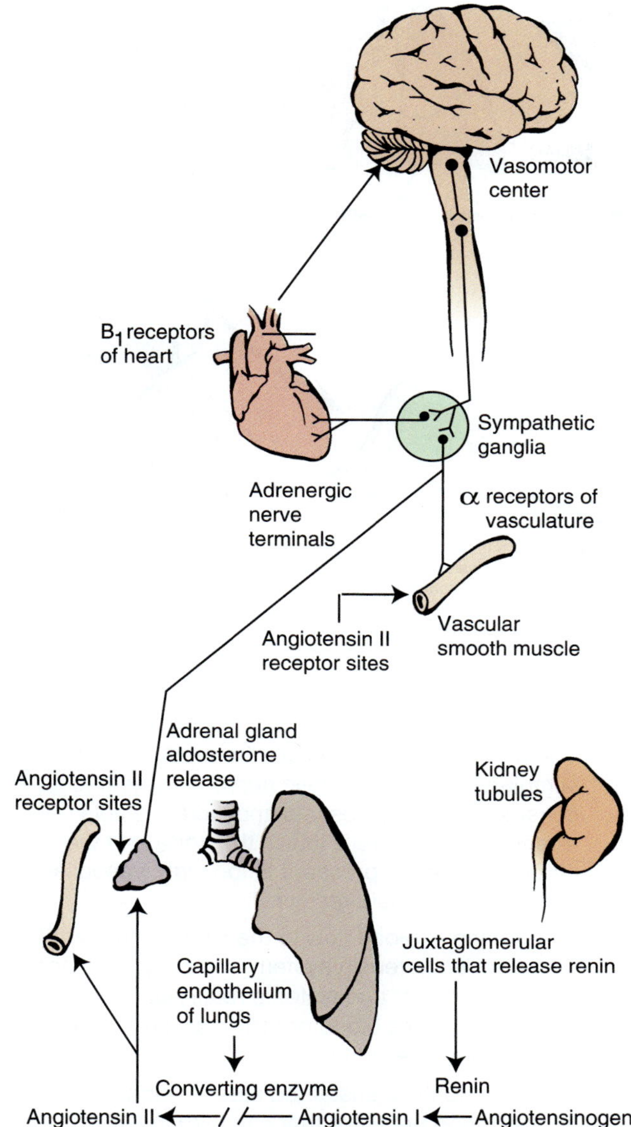

FIGURE 43.1 Control of blood pressure. The vasomotor center in the medulla responds to stimuli from aortic and carotid baroreceptors to cause sympathetic stimulation. The kidneys release renin to activate the renin–angiotensin system, causing vasoconstriction and increased blood volume.

the release of renin, thus causing the compensatory mechanisms to stop (Figure 43.2).

Hypertension

When a person's blood pressure is above normal limits for a sustained period, a diagnosis of hypertension is made (Table 43.1). It is estimated that at least 20% of the people in the United States have hypertension, and many are unaware of it.

Ninety percent of the people with hypertension have what is called **essential hypertension**, or hypertension with no known cause. People with essential hypertension usually have elevated total peripheral resistance. Their organs are being perfused effectively, and they usually display no symptoms. A few people develop secondary hypertension, or high blood pressure resulting from a known cause. For instance, a tumor in the adrenal medulla, called a pheochromocytoma, can cause hypertension that resolves after the tumor is removed.

The underlying danger of hypertension of any type is the prolonged force on the vessels of the vascular system. The muscles in the arterial system eventually thicken, leading to a loss of responsiveness in the system. The left ventricle thickens because the muscle must constantly work hard to expel blood at a greater force. The thickening of the heart muscle and the increased pressure that the muscle has to generate every time it contracts increase the workload of the heart and the risk of coronary artery disease (CAD) as well. The force of the blood being propelled against them damages the inner linings of the arteries, making these vessels susceptible to atherosclerosis and to narrowing of the lumen of the vessels (see Chapter 46). Tiny vessels can be damaged and destroyed, leading to losses of vision (if the vessels are in the retina), kidney function (if the vessels include the glomeruli in the nephrons), or cerebral function (if the vessels are small and fragile vessels in the brain).

Untreated hypertension increases a person's risk for the following conditions: CAD and cardiac death, stroke, renal failure, and loss of vision. Because hypertension has no symptoms, it is difficult to diagnose and treat, and it is often called the "silent killer." All of the drugs used to treat hypertension have adverse effects, many of which are seen as unacceptable by otherwise healthy people. Nurses face a difficult challenge trying to convince patients to comply with their drug regimens when they experience adverse effects and do not see any positive effects on their bodies. Research into the cause of hypertension is ongoing. Many theories have been proposed for the cause of the disorder, and it may well be a mosaic of factors. Factors that are known to increase blood pressure in some people include high levels of psychological stress, exposure to high-frequency noise, a high-salt diet, lack of rest, and genetic predisposition. (See Boxes 43.1 and 43.2.)

CONCEPTS in action ANIMATION

Hypotension

If blood pressure becomes too low, the vital centers in the brain as well as the rest of the tissues of the body may not receive enough oxygenated blood to continue functioning. **Hypotension** can progress to **shock**, when the body is in serious jeopardy as waste products accumulate and cells die from lack of oxygen. Hypotensive states can occur in the following situations:

- When the heart muscle is damaged and unable to pump effectively

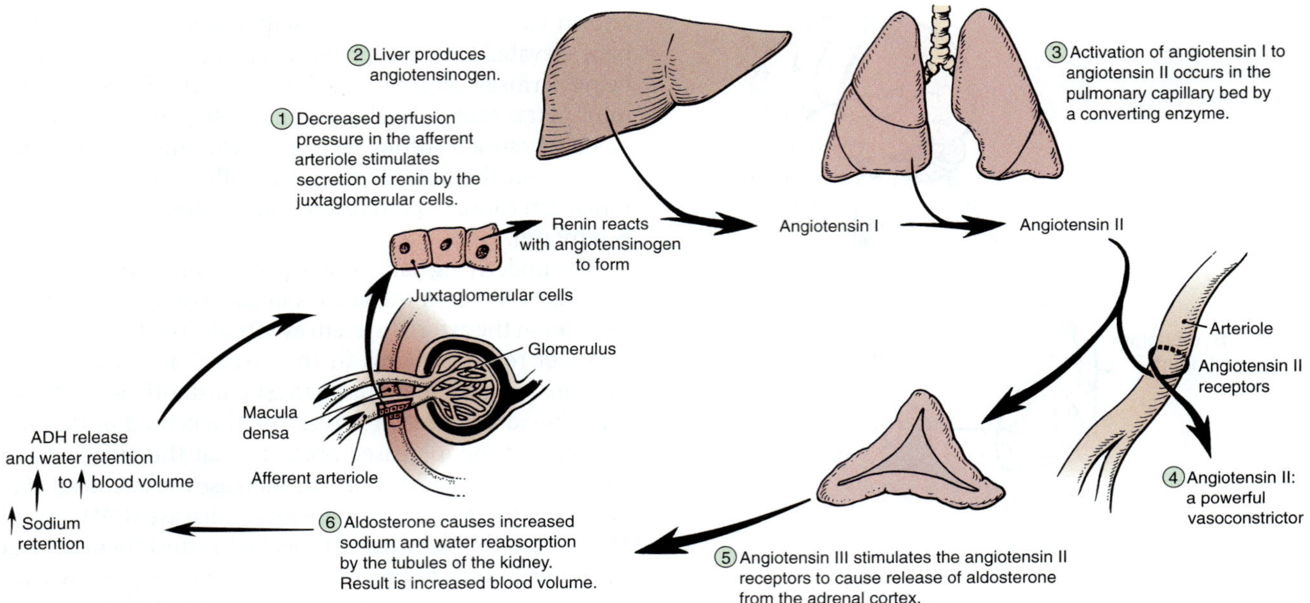

② Liver produces angiotensinogen.
① Decreased perfusion pressure in the afferent arteriole stimulates secretion of renin by the juxtaglomerular cells.
③ Activation of angiotensin I to angiotensin II occurs in the pulmonary capillary bed by a converting enzyme.
Renin reacts with angiotensinogen to form
Angiotensin I
Angiotensin II
Juxtaglomerular cells
Glomerulus
Arteriole
Angiotensin II receptors
Macula densa
ADH release and water retention
↑ to ↑ blood volume
Afferent arteriole
↑ Sodium retention
④ Angiotensin II: a powerful vasoconstrictor
⑥ Aldosterone causes increased sodium and water reabsorption by the tubules of the kidney. Result is increased blood volume.
⑤ Angiotensin III stimulates the angiotensin II receptors to cause release of aldosterone from the adrenal cortex.

FIGURE 43.2 The renin–angiotensin system.

- With severe blood loss, when volume drops dramatically
- When there is extreme stress and the body's levels of norepinephrine are depleted, leaving the body unable to respond to stimuli to raise blood pressure

FOCUS POINTS

- The cardiovascular system depends on pressure changes to circulate blood to the tissues and back to the heart.
- Heart rate, stroke volume, and peripheral vascular resistance are factors that determine blood pressure.
- Constriction and relaxation of the arterioles result in peripheral resistance.
- The baroreceptors stimulate the medulla, which stimulates the sympathetic nervous system to constrict the blood vessels and increase fluid retention if pressure is low in the aorta and the carotid arteries. If pressure is too high, vasodilation and loss of fluid results.
- A decrease in blood flow to the kidneys triggers the renin–angiotensin system, whereby the blood vessels constrict and water is retained. This activity increases blood pressure and restores blood flow to the kidney.
- Hypertension is a sustained state of higher-than-normal blood pressure that can lead to blood vessel damage, atherosclerosis, and damage to small vessels in end organs.
- The cause of essential hypertension is unknown; treatment varies among individuals.

Table 43.1 Categories Rating the Severity of Hypertension

Blood Pressure Classification	Systolic Blood Pressure (mm Hg)	Diastolic Blood Pressure (mm Hg)
Normal	<120	and <80
Prehypertension	120–139	or 80–89
Stage 1 hypertension	140–159	or 90–99
Stage 2 hypertension	≥160	or ≥100

Source: National Heart, Lung, and Blood Institute. (May 2003). *7th Report of the Joint National Commission on Prevention, Detection, Evaluation, and Treatment of High Blood Pressure.* Washington, DC: U.S. Department of Health and Human Services, National Institutes of Health.

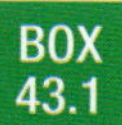

BOX 43.1 FOCUS ON THE **EVIDENCE**

"White Coat" Hypertension

The diagnosis of hypertension is accompanied by the impact of serious ramifications, such as increased risk for numerous diseases and cardiovascular death, the potential need for significant lifestyle changes, and the potential need for drug therapy, which may include many unpleasant adverse effects. Consequently, it is important that a patient be correctly diagnosed before being labeled hypertensive.

Researchers in the 1990s discovered that some patients were hypertensive only when they were in their doctor's office having their blood pressure measured. This was correlated to a sympathetic stress reaction (which elevates systolic blood pressure) and a tendency to tighten the muscles (isometric exercise, which elevates diastolic blood pressure) while waiting to be seen and during the blood pressure measurement. The researchers labeled this phenomenon "white coat" hypertension.

The American Heart Association has put forth new guidelines for the diagnosis of hypertension. A patient should have three consecutive blood pressure readings above normal, when taken by a nurse, over a period of 2 to 3 weeks. (It was assumed that nurses were not as threatening or stress provoking as doctors.) These guidelines point out the importance of using the correct technique when taking a patient's blood pressure, especially because the results can have such a tremendous impact on a patient. It is good practice to periodically review the process for performing this routine task. For example, the nurse should

- Select a cuff that is the correct size for the patient's arm (a cuff that is too small may give a high reading; a cuff that is too large may give a lower reading).
- Try to put the patient at ease; remember that waiting alone in a cold room can be stressful to the body and mind and can increase the blood pressure.
- Ensure that the arm that will be used for the cuff is supported.
- Make sure the rest of the patient's muscles are not tensed while the blood pressure is being taken.
- Place both the cuff and the stethoscope directly on the patient instead of on clothing.
- Listen carefully and record the first sound heard, the muffling of sounds, and the absence of sound (the actual diastolic pressure is thought to be between these two sounds).

Blood pressure machines found in grocery stores and pharmacies often give higher readings than the actual blood pressure, so patients should not be encouraged to use these machines for follow-up readings. The American Heart Association offers many good guidelines for accurate blood pressure measurement. Nurses are often the health care providers most likely to be taking and recording patient blood pressure, so it is important to always use proper technique and to make accurate records.

BOX 43.2 CULTURAL CONSIDERATIONS FOR DRUG THERAPY

Antihypertensive Therapy

In the United States, African Americans are at highest risk for developing hypertension, with men more likely than women to develop the disease. African Americans have documented differences in response to antihypertensive therapy. For example, African Americans are

- Most responsive to single-drug therapy (as opposed to combination drug regimens)
- More responsive to diuretics, calcium channel blockers, and alpha-adrenergic blockers
- Less responsive to angiotensin-converting enzyme inhibitors and beta-blockers

Increased adverse effects (depression, fatigue, drowsiness) often occur when using thiazide and thiazide-like diuretics, potentially requiring the use of different diuretics or lower doses of the thiazide diuretics.

Screening for hypertension among African Americans is very important to detect hypertension early and to prevent the organ damage that occurs with prolonged hypertension. Because African Americans are more responsive to diuretics, the treatment approach should include the first-line use of a diuretic in combination with diet and other lifestyle changes. The use of calcium channel blockers or alpha-adrenergic blockers should follow.

Antihypertensive Agents

Because an underlying cause of hypertension is usually unknown, altering the body's regulatory mechanisms is the best treatment currently available. Drugs used to treat hypertension work to alter the normal reflexes that control blood pressure. Treatment for essential hypertension does not cure the disease but is aimed at maintaining the blood pressure within normal limits to prevent the damage that hypertension can cause. Not all patients respond the same way to antihypertensive drugs, because different factors may contribute to each person's hypertension. Patients may have complicating conditions, such as diabetes or acute myocardial infarction (AMI), that make it unwise to use certain drugs.

Several different types of drugs, which affect different areas of blood pressure control, may need to be used in combination to actually maintain a patient's blood pressure within normal limits. Trials of drugs and combinations of drugs are often needed to develop an individual regimen that is effective without producing adverse effects that are unacceptable to the patient (Box 43.3). Research is ongoing into the treatment of more specific hypertensions (e.g., pulmonary hypertension). The development of drugs that target specific blood vessel sites and chemicals could lead to a new approach to the treatment of essential hypertension in the future (Box 43.4).

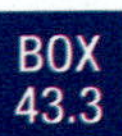

BOX 43.3 DRUG THERAPY ACROSS THE LIFESPAN

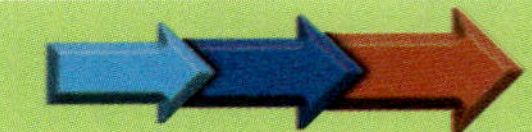

Drugs Affecting Blood Pressure

CHILDREN

National standards for determining normal levels of blood pressure in children are quite new. It has been determined that hypertension may start as a childhood disease, and more screening studies are being done to establish normal values for each age group.

Children are thought to be more likely to have secondary hypertension, caused by renal disease or congenital problems such as coarctation of the aorta.

Treatment of childhood hypertension should be done very cautiously, because the long-term effects of the antihypertensive agents are not known. Lifestyle changes should be instituted before drug therapy if at all possible. Weight loss and increased activity may bring an elevated blood pressure back to normal in many children.

If drug therapy is used, a mild diuretic may be tried first, with monitoring of blood glucose and electrolyte levels on a regular basis. Beta-blockers have been used with success in some children; adverse effects may limit their usefulness in others. The safety and efficacy of the angiotensin-converting enzyme (ACE) inhibitors and the angiotensin receptor blockers (ARBs) have not been established in children. Calcium channel blockers have been used to treat hypertension in children and may be a first consideration if drug therapy is needed. Careful follow-up of the growing child is essential to monitor for changes in blood pressure as well as adverse effects.

ADULTS

Adults receiving any of these drugs need to be instructed about adverse reactions that should be reported immediately. They need to be reminded of safety precautions that may be needed in hot weather or with conditions that cause fluid depletion (e.g., diarrhea, vomiting). If they are taking any other drugs, the interacting effects of the various drugs should be evaluated. The importance of other measures to help lower blood pressure—weight loss, smoking cessation, increased activity—should be stressed.

The safety for the use of these drugs during pregnancy has not been established. ACE inhibitors and ARBs should not be used during pregnancy, and women of child-bearing age should be advised to use barrier contraceptives to prevent pregnancy while taking these drugs. Calcium channel blockers and vasodilators should not be used in pregnancy unless the benefit to the mother clearly outweighs the potential risk to the fetus. The drugs do enter breast milk and can cause serious adverse effects in the baby. Caution should be used or another method of feeding the baby should be used if one of these drugs is needed during lactation.

OLDER ADULTS

Older adults frequently are prescribed one of these drugs. They are more susceptible to the toxic effects of the drugs and are more likely to have underlying conditions that could interfere with drug metabolism and excretion. Renal or hepatic impairment can lead to accumulation of the drugs in the body. If renal or hepatic dysfunction is present, the dosage should be reduced and the patient monitored very closely.

The total drug regimen of the older patient should be coordinated, with careful attention to interactions among drugs and alternative therapies.

Older adults need to use special caution in any situation that could lead to a fall in blood pressure, such as loss of fluids from diarrhea or vomiting, lack of fluid intake, or excessive heat with decreased sweating that comes with age. Dizziness, falls, or syncope can occur if the blood pressure falls too far in these situations. The blood pressure should always be taken immediately before an antihypertensive is administered to an older adult in an institutional setting, to avoid excessive lowering of blood pressure.

Older patients should be especially cautioned about sustained-release antihypertensives that cannot be cut, crushed, or chewed, to avoid the potential for excessive dosing if these drugs are inappropriately cut.

Stepped-Care Approach to Treating Hypertension

The importance of treating hypertension has been proven in numerous research studies. If hypertension is controlled, the patient's risk of cardiovascular death and disease is reduced. The risk of developing cardiovascular complications is directly related to the patient's degree of hypertension (see Table 43.1). Lowering the degree of hypertension lowers the risk.

The Seventh Joint National Committee on Prevention, Detection, Evaluation and Treatment of Hypertension, from the National Institutes of Health, has established a stepped-care approach to treating hypertension that has proved effective in national studies (Box 43.5).

Four steps are involved.

Step 1: Lifestyle modifications are instituted. These include weight reduction, smoking cessation, reduction in the use of alcohol and salt in the diet (all of these conditions have been shown to increase blood pressure), and an increase in physical exercise (which has been shown to decrease blood pressure and improve cardiovascular tone and reserve).

Step 2: If the measures in step 1 are not sufficient to lower the blood pressure to an acceptable level, drug therapy is added. The drug of choice may be a diuretic, which decreases serum sodium levels and blood volume; a beta-blocker, which leads to a decrease in heart rate and strength of contraction as well as vasodilation; an ACE inhibitor, which blocks the conversion of angiotensin I to angiotensin II; an angiotensin II receptor blocker (ARB), which blocks the effects of angiotensin on the blood vessel; a calcium channel blocker, which relaxes muscle contraction; or other autonomic blockers.

Step 3: If the patient's response to step 2 is inadequate, the drug dose or class may be changed or another drug may be added for a combined effect. Many antihypertensive agents are available in fixed combinations to help

BOX 43.4 Treatment of Pulmonary Arterial Hypertension

In late 2001, bosentan (*Tracleer*) became the first endothelin receptor antagonist to be approved for use in the treatment of pulmonary arterial hypertension. This drug specifically blocks receptor sites for endothelin (ET_A and ET_B) in the endothelium and vascular smooth muscles; these endothelins are chemicals that are elevated in the plasma and lung tissues of patients with pulmonary arterial hypertension. Blockade of these receptor sites allows the vessels to relax and dilate, relieving the pressure in the arteries. *Tracleer* is an oral drug that is given to adults, initially as 62.5 mg PO b.i.d. for 4 wk, and then increased to 125 mg PO b.i.d. if the patient's exercise tolerance improves on the drug. Patients need to be monitored closely for any change in their respiratory function, signs of liver toxicity, or signs of peripheral vasodilation, including flushing, headache, hypotension, and palpitations. The drug is pregnancy category X and is known to interact with other drugs, including ketoconazole, the statins, glyburide, and oral contraceptives.

Treprostinil (*Remodulin*) was introduced shortly after bosentan. It has a similar mechanism of action. It is a drug that can be given only by continuous subcutaneous infusion. The patient needs to learn how to care for the infusion port and use the pump. Dosage adjustments are made based on the patient's response and exercise tolerance. Headache and injection site pain are common and may be relieved by the use of analgesics. The drug cannot be discontinued abruptly, but it needs to be tapered to prevent a rebound worsening of the condition.

In 2005, sildenafil, a drug known for the treatment of erectile dysfunction, was approved for the treatment of pulmonary arterial hypertension. *Revatio* is an oral drug, with 20 mg given three times a day. The doses should be at least 4–6 h apart. *Revatio* inhibits cGMP; this allows nitrous oxide in the blood vessel to cause smooth muscle relaxation and decreases vessel pressure (see Chapter 41).

BOX 43.5 Stepped-Care Management of Hypertension

Step 1: Lifestyle modifications

- Weight reduction
- Reduction of sodium intake
- Moderation of alcohol intake
- Smoking cessation
- Physical activity increase

Step 2: Inadequate response

- Continue lifestyle modifications
- Initial drug selection:
  1. Diuretic or beta-blocker
  2. ACE inhibitor, calcium channel blocker, alpha-blocker, alpha- and beta-blocker

Step 3: Inadequate response

1. Increase drug dose, *or*
2. Substitute another drug, *or*
3. Add a second drug from another class

Step 4: Inadequate response

Add a second or third agent or diuretic if not already prescribed

decrease the number of pills a patient needs to take each day. Fixed-combination drugs should only be used when the patient has been stabilized on each drug separately (Box 43.6).

Step 4: This step includes all of the above measures with the addition of more antihypertensive agents until the desired level of blood pressure control is achieved.

Hypertensive treatment is further complicated by the presence of other chronic conditions. The Joint National Committee published an algorithm for the treatment of hypertension to help prescribers select an antihypertensive agent in light of complicating conditions (Figure 43.3). A patient's response to a given antihypertensive agent is very individual, so the drug of choice for one patient may have little to no effect on another patient.

Diuretics

Diuretics are drugs that increase the excretion of sodium and water from the kidney (see Chapter 51) (Figure 43.4). These drugs are often the first agents tried in mild hypertension; they affect blood sodium levels and blood volume. A somewhat controversial study, the ALLHAT study, reported in 2002 that patients taking the less expensive, less toxic diuretics did better and had better blood pressure control than patients using other antihypertensive agents. Although these drugs increase urination and can disturb electrolyte and acid–base balances, they are usually tolerated well by most patients (Box 43.7).

Sympathetic Nervous System Blockers

Drugs that block the effects of the sympathetic nervous system (see Chapter 31) are useful in blocking many of the compensatory effects of the sympathetic nervous system (see Figure 43.4).

- Beta-blockers block vasoconstriction, decrease heart rate, decrease cardiac muscle contraction, and tend to increase blood flow to the kidneys, leading to a decrease in the release of renin. These drugs have many adverse effects and are not recommended for all people. They are often used as monotherapy in step 2 treatment, and in some patients they control blood pressure adequately.
- Alpha- and beta-blockers are useful in conjunction with other agents and tend to be somewhat more powerful, blocking all of the receptors in the sympathetic system. Patients often complain of fatigue, loss of libido, inability to sleep, and gastrointestinal (GI) and genitourinary

BOX 43.6 Fixed-Combination Drugs for the Treatment of Hypertension

Many patients require more than one type of antihypertensive to achieve good control of their blood pressure. There are now many fixed-combination drugs available for treating hypertension. This allows for fewer tablets or capsules each day, making it easier for the patient to be compliant with drug therapy. The patient should be stabilized on each drug first and then an appropriate combination product can be used.

The drugs available in combination include:

atenolol with chlorthalidone (*Tenoretic*)
amlodipine with benazepril (*Lotrel*)
bisoprolol with hydrochlorothiazide (*Ziac*)
candesartan with hydrochlorothiazide (*Atacand HCT*)
chlorthalidone with clonidine (*Combipres*)
enalapril with diltiazem (*Teczem ER Tablets*)
enalapril with felodipine (*Lexxel ER Tablets*)
enalapril with hydrochlorothiazide (*Vaseretic*)
eprosartan with hydrochlorothiazide (*Teveten HCT*)
fosinopril with hydrochlorothiazide (*Monopril-HCT*)
hydrochlorothiazide with benazepril (*Lotensin HCT*)
hydrochlorothiazide with captopril (*Capozide*)
hydrochlorothiazide with propranolol (*Inderide*)
irbesartan with hydrochlorothiazide (*Avalide*)
lisinopril with hydrochlorothiazide (*Prinzide, Zestoretic*)
losartan with hydrochlorothiazide (*Hyzaar*)
methyldopa with chlorothiazide (*Aldoclor*)
methyldopa with hydrochlorothiazide (*Aldoril D*)
metoprolol with hydrochlorothiazide (*Lopressor HCT*)
moexipril with hydrochlorothiazide (*Uniretic*)
nadolol with bendroflumethiazide (*Corzide*)
olmesartan with hydrochlorothiazide (*Benicar HCT*)
prazosin with polythiazide (*Minizide*)
quinapril with hydrochlorothiazide (*Accuretic*)
telmisartan with hydrochlorothiazide (*Micardis HCT*)
trandolapril with verapamil (*Tarka*)
valsartan with hydrochlorothiazide (*Diovan HCT*)

disturbances, and they may be unwilling to continue taking these drugs.

- Alpha-adrenergic blockers inhibit the postsynaptic alpha$_1$-adrenergic receptors, decreasing sympathetic tone in the vasculature and causing vasodilation, which leads to a lowering of blood pressure. However, these drugs also block presynaptic alpha$_2$-receptors, preventing the feedback control of norepinephrine release. The result is an increase in the reflex tachycardia that occurs when blood pressure decreases. These drugs are used to diagnose and manage episodes of pheochromocytoma, but they have limited usefulness in essential hypertension because of the associated adverse effects.
- Alpha$_1$-blockers are used to treat hypertension because of their ability to block the postsynaptic alpha$_1$-receptor sites. This decreases vascular tone and promotes vasodilation, leading to a fall in blood pressure. These drugs do not block the presynaptic alpha$_2$-receptor sites, and therefore the reflex tachycardia that accompanies a fall in blood pressure does not occur.
- Alpha$_2$-agonists stimulate the alpha$_2$-receptors in the central nervous system (CNS) and inhibit the cardiovascular centers, leading to a decrease in sympathetic outflow from the CNS and a resultant drop in blood pressure. These drugs are associated with many adverse CNS and GI effects as well as cardiac dysrhythmias.

Angiotensin-Converting Enzyme Inhibitors

The **ACE inhibitors** block the conversion of angiotensin I to angiotensin II in the lungs (see Figure 43.4). This stops that phase of the renin–angiotensin system before vasoconstriction can occur or aldosterone can be released. The ACE inhibitors may be used as monotherapy in step 2 of hypertension management, or they may be combined with diuretics. ACE inhibitors that are used include the following agents (Table 43.2):

- Benazepril (*Lotensin*), a frequently used oral drug, is approved only for use in treating hypertension; it is usually well tolerated but has been associated with an unrelenting cough.
- Captopril (*Capoten*) is indicated for use in hypertension and in treating congestive heart failure (CHF), diabetic nephropathy, and left ventricular dysfunction after MI; it has been associated with a sometimes fatal pancytopenia, cough, and unpleasant GI distress.
- Enalapril (*Vasotec*), an oral drug, is used for the treatment of hypertension, CHF, and left ventricular dysfunction; it has the advantage of parenteral use (enalaprilat [*Vasotec IV*]) if oral use is not feasible or rapid onset is desirable.
- Fosinopril (*Monopril*) is a well-tolerated oral drug used for the treatment of hypertension and for adjunctive therapy in CHF; it is also associated with a cough.
- Lisinopril (*Prinivil, Zestril*) is an oral drug used in treating hypertension and CHF, and it is used in stable patients within 24 hours after acute MI to improve the likelihood of survival.
- Moexipril (*Univasc*) is a less well-tolerated oral drug used in the treatment of hypertension; it is associated with many unpleasant GI and skin effects, cough, and cardiac arrhythmias; fatal MI and pancytopenia have sometimes been associated with this drug.
- Perindopril (*Aceon*) is an oral drug that is used alone or in combination with other antihypertensive agents to

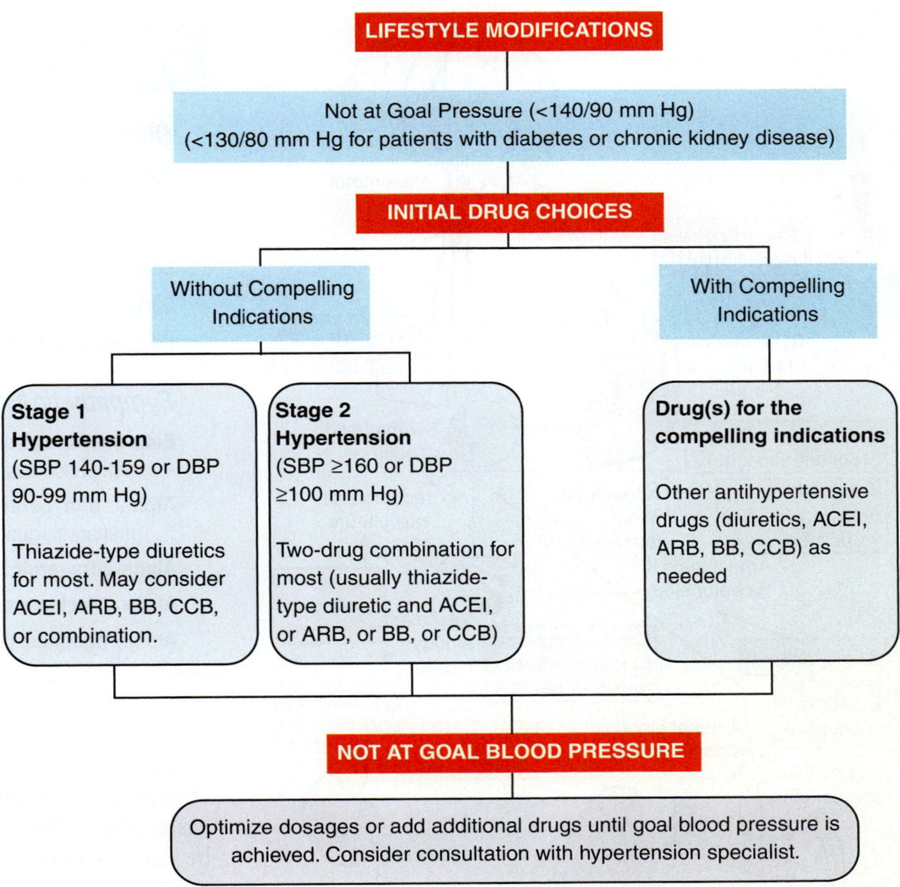

FIGURE 43.3 Algorithm for the treatment of hypertension. (From the *Report of the Seventh Joint National Committee on Prevention, Detection, Evaluation, and Treatment of High Blood Pressure.* [May 2003]. Bethesda, MD: National Heart, Lung & Blood Institute, National Institutes of Health).

control blood pressure. It is associated with a sometimes fatal pancytopenia as well as a serious to fatal airway obstruction (found to occur more frequently in African American patients).

- Quinapril (*Accupril*) is used orally for the treatment of hypertension and as an adjunct treatment of CHF; it is not associated with as many adverse effects as some of the other agents are.
- Ramipril (*Altace*) is used orally for the treatment of hypertension and as an adjunct treatment of CHF; it is not associated with as many adverse effects as some of the other agents are.
- Trandolapril (*Mavik*) is used orally for the treatment of hypertension and for CHF after an acute MI and is fairly well-tolerated.

Therapeutic Actions and Indications

ACE inhibitors prevent ACE from converting angiotensin I to angiotensin II, a powerful vasoconstrictor and stimulator of aldosterone release. This action leads to a decrease in blood pressure and in aldosterone secretion, with a resultant slight increase in serum potassium and a loss of serum sodium and fluid.

These drugs are indicated for the treatment of hypertension, alone or in combination with other drugs. They are also used in conjunction with digoxin and diuretics for the treatment of CHF and left ventricular dysfunction. Their therapeutic effect in these cases is thought to be related to a decrease in cardiac workload associated with the decrease in peripheral resistance and blood volume.

Pharmacokinetics

These drugs are well absorbed, widely distributed, metabolized in the liver, and excreted in the urine and feces. They are known to cross the placenta and have been associated with serious fetal abnormalities. These drugs should not be used during pregnancy. Women of child-bearing age who choose to use one of these drugs should be encouraged to use barrier contraceptives to avoid pregnancy while taking the drug. Several of these

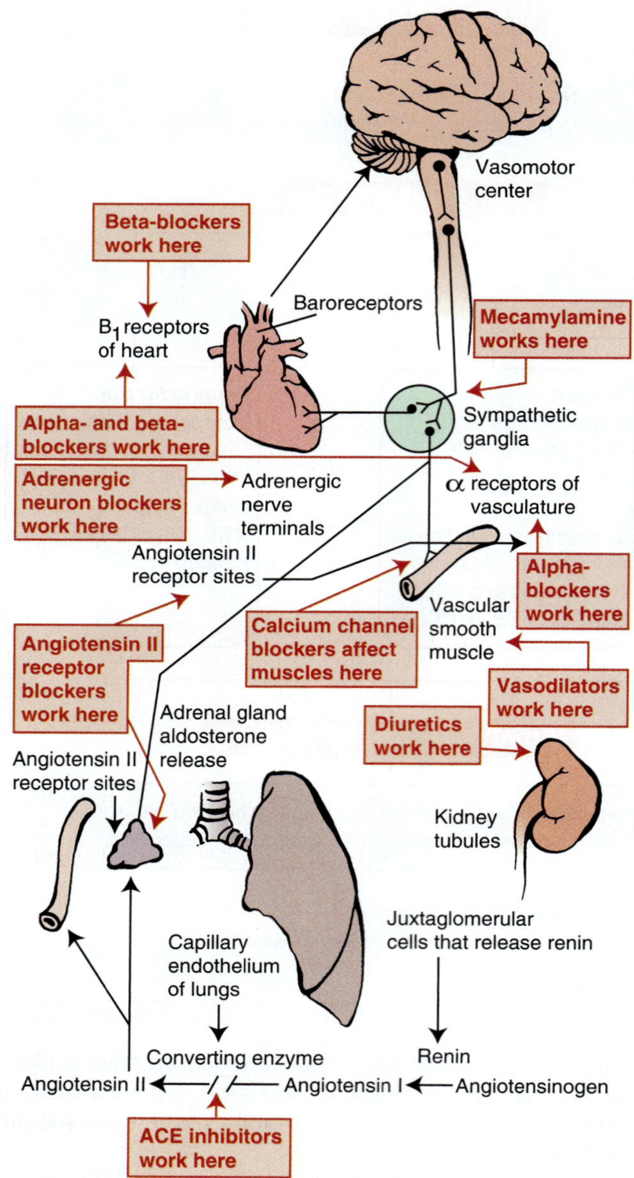

FIGURE 43.4 Sites of action of antihypertensive drugs.

drugs have been detected in breast milk. Because of the potential for serious adverse effects in the neonate, another method of feeding the baby should be used during lactation, or another antihypertensive should be chosen.

Contraindications and Cautions

ACE inhibitors are contraindicated in the presence of allergy to any of the ACE inhibitors; with impaired renal function, which could be exacerbated by the effects of this drug in decreasing renal blood flow; with pregnancy, because of the potential for adverse effects on the fetus; and during lactation, because of potential decrease in milk production and effects on the neonate.

BOX 43.7 Other Drug Classes Used to Treat Hypertension

Diuretics (see Chapter 51)

Thiazide and thiazide-like diuretics: bendroflumethiazide, chlorothiazide, hydrochlorothiazide, hydroflumethiazide, methyclothiazide, trichlormethiazide, chlorthalidone, indapamide, metolazone

Loop diuretics: bumetanide, ethacrynic acid, furosemide torsemide

Carbonic anhydrase inhibitors: acetazolamide, methazolamide

Potassium-sparing diuretics: amiloride, spironolactone, triamterene

Sympathetic Nervous System Drugs (see Chapter 31)

Beta-blockers: acebutolol, atenolol, betaxolol, bisoprolol, carteolol, metoprolol, nadolol, penbutolol, pindolol, propranolol, timolol

Alpha- and beta-blockers: carvedilol, labetalol, guanabenz, guanadrel, guanethidine

Alpha-adrenergic blockers: phenoxybenzamine, phentolamine

Alpha$_1$-blockers: doxazosin, prazosin, terazosin

Alpha$_2$-agonists: clonidine, guanfacine, methyldopa

Caution should be used in patients with CHF, because the change in hemodynamics could be detrimental in some cases; and in those with salt/volume depletion, which could be exacerbated by the drug effects.

Adverse Effects

The adverse effects most commonly associated with the ACE inhibitors are related to the effects of vasodilation and alterations in blood flow. Such effects include reflex tachycardia, chest pain, angina, CHF, and cardiac arrhythmias; GI irritation, ulcers, constipation, and liver injury; renal insufficiency, renal failure, and proteinuria; and rash, alopecia, dermatitis, and photosensitivity. Many of these drugs cause an unrelenting cough, possibly related to effects in the lungs, where the ACE is inhibited, that may lead patients to discontinue the drug. Some of these drugs have been associated with fatal pancytopenia and MI.

Clinically Important Drug–Drug Interactions

The risk of hypersensitivity reactions increases if these drugs are taken with allopurinol.

Clinically Important Drug–Food Interactions

Absorption of oral ACE inhibitors decreases if they are taken with food. They should be taken on an empty stomach, 1 hour before or 2 hours after meals.

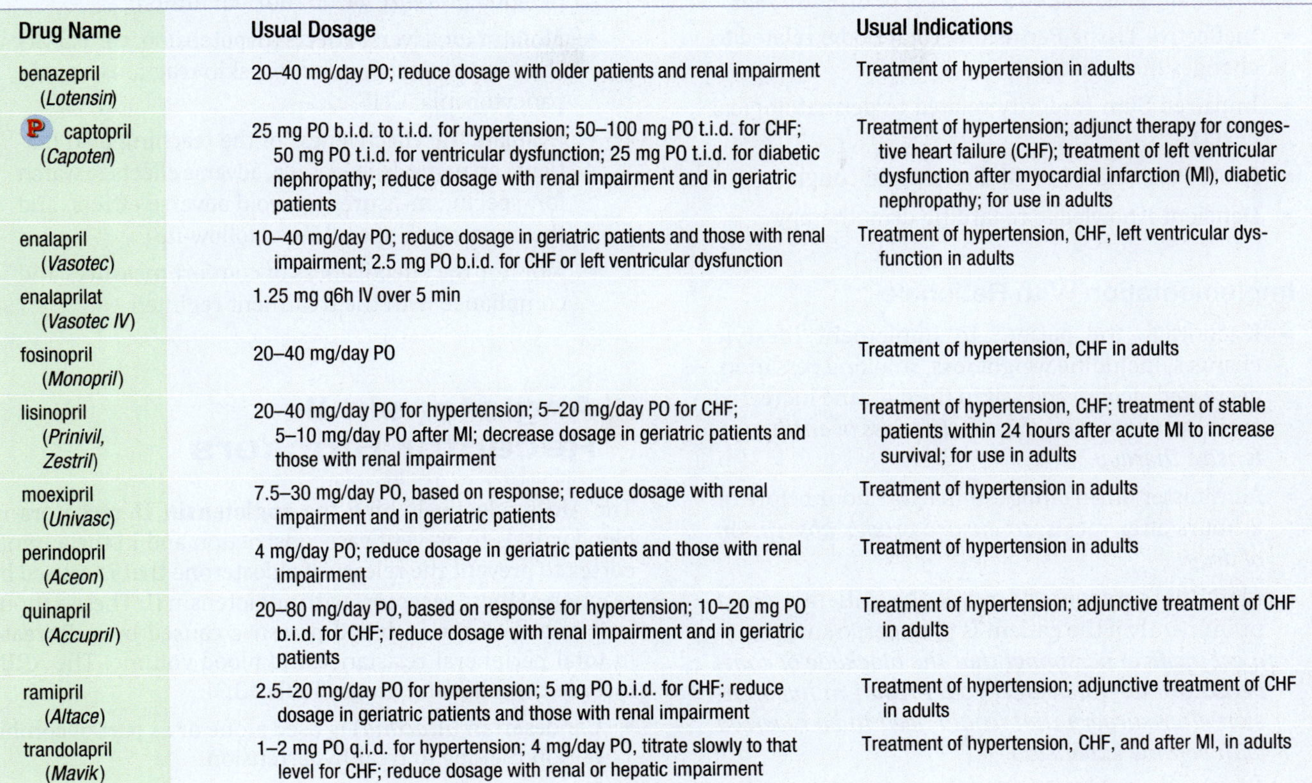

Table 43.2 DRUGS IN FOCUS

Angiotensin-Converting Enzyme Inhibitors

Drug Name	Usual Dosage	Usual Indications
benazepril (*Lotensin*)	20–40 mg/day PO; reduce dosage with older patients and renal impairment	Treatment of hypertension in adults
P captopril (*Capoten*)	25 mg PO b.i.d. to t.i.d. for hypertension; 50–100 mg PO t.i.d. for CHF; 50 mg PO t.i.d. for ventricular dysfunction; 25 mg PO t.i.d. for diabetic nephropathy; reduce dosage with renal impairment and in geriatric patients	Treatment of hypertension; adjunct therapy for congestive heart failure (CHF); treatment of left ventricular dysfunction after myocardial infarction (MI), diabetic nephropathy; for use in adults
enalapril (*Vasotec*)	10–40 mg/day PO; reduce dosage in geriatric patients and those with renal impairment; 2.5 mg PO b.i.d. for CHF or left ventricular dysfunction	Treatment of hypertension, CHF, left ventricular dysfunction in adults
enalaprilat (*Vasotec IV*)	1.25 mg q6h IV over 5 min	
fosinopril (*Monopril*)	20–40 mg/day PO	Treatment of hypertension, CHF in adults
lisinopril (*Prinivil, Zestril*)	20–40 mg/day PO for hypertension; 5–20 mg/day PO for CHF; 5–10 mg/day PO after MI; decrease dosage in geriatric patients and those with renal impairment	Treatment of hypertension, CHF; treatment of stable patients within 24 hours after acute MI to increase survival; for use in adults
moexipril (*Univasc*)	7.5–30 mg/day PO, based on response; reduce dosage with renal impairment and in geriatric patients	Treatment of hypertension in adults
perindopril (*Aceon*)	4 mg/day PO; reduce dosage in geriatric patients and those with renal impairment	Treatment of hypertension in adults
quinapril (*Accupril*)	20–80 mg/day PO, based on response for hypertension; 10–20 mg PO b.i.d. for CHF; reduce dosage with renal impairment and in geriatric patients	Treatment of hypertension; adjunctive treatment of CHF in adults
ramipril (*Altace*)	2.5–20 mg/day PO for hypertension; 5 mg PO b.i.d. for CHF; reduce dosage in geriatric patients and those with renal impairment	Treatment of hypertension; adjunctive treatment of CHF in adults
trandolapril (*Mavik*)	1–2 mg PO q.i.d. for hypertension; 4 mg/day PO, titrate slowly to that level for CHF; reduce dosage with renal or hepatic impairment	Treatment of hypertension, CHF, and after MI, in adults

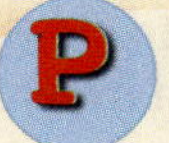

Prototype Summary: Captopril

Indications: Treatment of hypertension, CHF, diabetic nephropathy, left ventricular dysfunction after an MI

Actions: Blocks ACE from converting angiotensin I to angiotensin II, leading to a decrease in blood pressure, a decrease in aldosterone production, and a small increase in serum potassium levels along with sodium and fluid loss

Pharmacokinetics:

Route	Onset	Peak
Oral	15 min	30–90 min

$T_{1/2}$: 2 hours; excreted in urine

Adverse effects: Tachycardia, MI, rash, pruritus, gastric irritation, aphthous ulcers, peptic ulcers, dysgeusia, proteinuria, bone marrow suppression, cough

Nursing Considerations for Patients Receiving ACE Inhibitors

Assessment: History and Examination

Screen for the following conditions, *which could be cautions or contraindications to use of the drug:* any known allergies to these drugs; impaired kidney function, *which could be exacerbated by these drugs;* pregnancy or lactation, *because of the potential adverse effects on the fetus or neonate;* salt/volume depletion, *which could be exacerbated by these drugs;* and CHF.

Include screening *for baseline status before beginning therapy and for any potential adverse effects.* Assess the following: body temperature and weight; skin color, lesions, and temperature; pulse, blood pressure, baseline electrocardiogram (ECG), and perfusion; respirations and adventitious breath sounds; bowel sounds and abdominal examination; and renal function tests, complete blood count with differential, and serum electrolytes.

Nursing Diagnoses

The patient receiving an ACE inhibitor may have the following nursing diagnoses related to drug therapy:

- Ineffective Tissue Perfusion (Total Body) related to changes in cardiac output
- Impaired Skin Integrity related to dermatological effects
- Acute Pain related to GI distress and cough
- Deficient Knowledge regarding drug therapy

Implementation With Rationale

- Encourage the patient to implement lifestyle changes, including weight loss, smoking cessation, decreased alcohol and salt in the diet, and increased exercise, *to increase the effectiveness of antihypertensive therapy.*
- Administer on an empty stomach, 1 hour before or 2 hours after meals, *to ensure proper absorption of drug.*
- Alert the surgeon and mark the patient's chart prominently if the patient is to undergo surgery, *to alert medical personnel that the blockage of compensatory angiotensin II could result in hypotension after surgery that would need to be reversed with volume expansion.*
- Give parenteral forms only if an oral form is not feasible; transfer to an oral form as soon as possible, *to avert an increased risk of adverse effects.*
- Consult with the prescriber to reduce dosage in patients with renal failure, *to account for their decreased production of renin and lower-than-normal levels of angiotensin II.*
- Monitor the patient carefully in any situation that might lead to a drop in fluid volume (e.g., excessive sweating, vomiting, diarrhea, dehydration), *to detect and treat excessive hypotension that may occur.*
- Provide comfort measures *to help the patient tolerate drug effects.* These include small, frequent meals; access to bathroom facilities; bowel program as needed; environmental controls; safety precautions; and appropriate skin care as needed.
- Provide thorough patient teaching, including the name of the drug, dosage prescribed, measures to avoid adverse effects, warning signs of problems, and the need for periodic monitoring and evaluation *to enhance patient knowledge about drug therapy and to promote compliance.*
- Offer support and encouragement *to help the patient deal with the diagnosis and the drug regimen.*

Evaluation

- Monitor patient response to the drug (maintenance of blood pressure within normal limits).
- Monitor for adverse effects (hypotension, cardiac arrhythmias, renal dysfunction, skin reactions, cough, pancytopenia, CHF).
- Evaluate the effectiveness of the teaching plan (patient can name drug, dosage, adverse effects to watch for, specific measures to avoid adverse effects, and the importance of continued follow-up).
- Monitor the effectiveness of comfort measures and compliance with the treatment regimen

Angiotensin II Receptor Blockers

The ARBs selectively bind the **angiotensin II receptors** in blood vessels to prevent vasoconstriction and in the adrenal cortex to prevent the release of aldosterone that is caused by reaction of these receptors with angiotensin II. These actions lead to a decrease in blood pressure caused by a decrease in total peripheral resistance and blood volume. The ARBs include the following drugs (Table 43.3):

- Candesartan (*Atacand*) is used alone or as part of combination therapy to treat hypertension.
- Eprosartan (*Teveten*) is used alone or as part of combination therapy to treat hypertension in adults.
- Irbesartan (*Avapro*) is used as monotherapy in the treatment of hypertension but can be combined with other antihypertensives if needed. It is also used to slow the progression of kidney disease in patients with hypertension and type 2 diabetes.
- Losartan (*Cozaar*) can be used alone or as part of combination therapy for hypertension, as well as for treatment of diabetic neuropathy with an elevated serum creatinine and proteinuria in patients with hypertension and type 2 diabetes.
- Olmesartan (*Benicar*) is used alone or as part of combination therapy to treat hypertension. This is the newest angiotensin II receptor blocker.
- Telmisartan (*Micardis*) is used alone or as part of combination therapy to treat hypertension.
- Valsartan (*Diovan*) can be used alone or as part of combination therapy for hypertension and for the treatment of heart failure in patients who are intolerant to ACE inhibitors

Therapeutic Actions and Indications

The ARBs selectively bind with angiotensin II receptor sites in vascular smooth muscle and in the adrenal gland to block

Table 43.3 DRUGS IN FOCUS

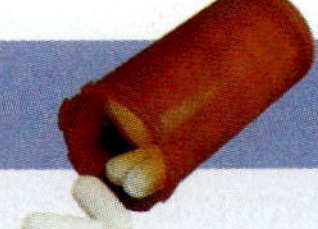

Angiotensin II Receptor Blockers

Drug Name	Usual Dosage	Usual Indications
candesartan (*Atacand*)	16–32 mg/day PO	Alone or as part of combination therapy to treat hypertension in adults
eprosartan (*Teveten*)	400–800 mg/day PO	Alone or as part of combination therapy to treat hypertension in adults
irbesartan (*Avapro*)	150–300 mg/day PO	Monotherapy in the treatment of hypertension in adults; slowing progression of diabetic nephropathy
P losartan (*Cozaar*)	25–100 mg/day PO	Alone or as part of combination therapy to treat hypertension in adults; slowing progression of diabetic nephropathy
olmesartan (*Benicar*)	20–40 mg/day PO	Alone or as part of combination therapy to treat hypertension in adults
telmisartan (*Micardis*)	40–80 mg/day PO	Alone or as part of combination therapy to treat hypertension in adults
valsartan (*Diovan*)	80–320 mg/day PO based on response	Alone or as part of combination therapy to treat hypertension in adults

vasoconstriction and the release of aldosterone. These actions block the blood pressure–raising effects of the renin–angiotensin system and lower blood pressure. They are indicated to be used alone or in combination therapy for the treatment of hypertension and for the treatment of CHF in patients who are intolerant to ACE inhibitors. Recently, they also were found to slow the progression of renal disease in patients with hypertension and type 2 diabetes. This action is thought to be related to the effects of blocking angiotensin receptors in the vascular endothelium.

Pharmacokinetics

These agents are well absorbed and undergo metabolism in the liver by the cytochrome P450 system. They are excreted in feces and in urine. Known to cross the placenta, the ARBs have been associated with serious fetal abnormalities and even death when given in the second or third trimester. Women of child-bearing age should be advised to use barrier contraceptives to avoid pregnancy; if a pregnancy does occur, the ARB should be discontinued immediately. Candesartan, eprosartan, irbesartan, olmesartan, and telmisartan should not be used during the second or third trimester of pregnancy because of associated fetal abnormalities and death. Losartan and valsartan should not be used at any time during pregnancy. It is not known whether the ARBs enter breast milk during lactation; however, because of the potential for serious adverse effects in the neonate, these drugs should not be used in lactating women.

Contraindications and Cautions

The ARBs are contraindicated in the presence of allergy to any of these drugs; during pregnancy, *because of associated fetal death and severe abnormalities;* and during lactation, *because of potential adverse effects on the neonate.* Caution should be used in the presence of hepatic or renal dysfunction, *which could alter the metabolism and excretion of these drugs,* and with hypovolemia, *because of the blocking of potentially life-saving compensatory mechanisms.*

Adverse Effects

The adverse effects most commonly associated with ARBs include the following: headache, dizziness, syncope, and weakness, which could be associated with drops in blood pressure; hypotension; GI complaints including diarrhea, abdominal pain, nausea, dry mouth, and tooth pain; symptoms of upper respiratory tract infections and cough; and rash, dry skin, and alopecia. In preclinical trials, these drugs have been associated with the development of cancers.

Clinically Important Drug–Drug Interactions

The risk of decreased serum levels and loss of effectiveness increases if the ARB is taken in combination with phenobarbital. If this combination is used, the patient should be monitored closely and dosage adjustments made.

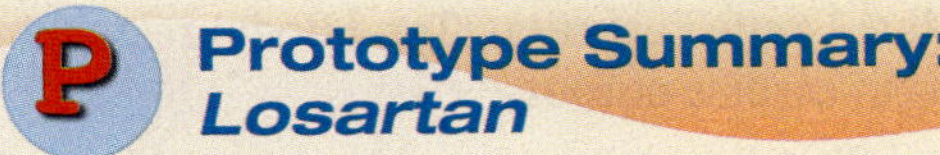

Prototype Summary: Losartan

Indications: Alone or as part of combination therapy for the treatment of hypertension; treatment of diabetic nephropathy with an elevated serum creatinine and proteinuria in patients with type 2 diabetes and hypertension

Actions: Selectively blocks the binding of angiotensin II to specific tissue receptors found in the vascular smooth muscle and adrenal glands; blocks the vasoconstriction and release of aldosterone associated with the renin–angiotensin system

Pharmacokinetics:

Route	Onset	Peak	Duration
Oral	Varies	1–3 h	24 h

$T_{1/2}$: 2 hours, then 6–9 hours; metabolized in the liver and excreted in urine and feces

Adverse effects: Dizziness, headache, diarrhea, abdominal pain, symptoms of upper respiratory tract infection, cough, back pain, fever, muscle weakness, hypotension

Nursing Considerations for Patients Receiving Angiotensin II Receptor Blockers

Assessment: History and Examination

Screen for the following conditions, *which could be cautions or contraindications to use of the drug:* any known allergies to these drugs; impaired kidney or liver function, *which could be exacerbated by these drugs;* pregnancy and lactation, *because of the potential adverse effects on the fetus and neonate;* and hypovolemia, *which could potentiate the blood pressure–lowering effects.*

Include screening *for baseline status before beginning therapy and for any potential adverse effects.* Assess the following: body temperature and weight; skin color, lesions, and temperature; pulse, blood pressure, baseline ECG, and perfusion; respirations and adventitious breath sounds; bowel sounds and abdominal examination; and renal and liver function tests.

Nursing Diagnoses

The patient receiving an ARB may have the following nursing diagnoses related to drug therapy:

- Ineffective Tissue Perfusion (Total Body) related to changes in cardiac output
- Impaired Skin Integrity related to dermatological effects
- Acute Pain related to GI distress, cough, skin effects, and headache
- Deficient Knowledge regarding drug therapy

Implementation With Rationale

- Encourage the patient to implement lifestyle changes, including weight loss, smoking cessation, decreased alcohol and salt in the diet, and increased exercise, *to increase the effectiveness of antihypertensive therapy.*
- Administer without regard to meals; give with food, *to decrease GI distress if needed.*
- Alert the surgeon and mark the patient's chart prominently if the patient is to undergo surgery, *to notify medical personnel that the blockage of compensatory angiotensin II could result in hypotension after surgery that would need to be reversed with volume expansion.*
- Ensure that the female patient is not pregnant before beginning therapy, and suggest the use of barrier contraceptives while she is taking this drug, *to avert potential fetal abnormalities and fetal death, which have been associated with these drugs.*
- Find an alternative method of feeding the baby if the patient is nursing, *to prevent the potentially dangerous blockade of the renin–angiotensin system in the neonate.*
- Monitor the patient carefully in any situation that might lead to a drop in fluid volume (e.g., excessive sweating, vomiting, diarrhea, dehydration), *to detect and treat excessive hypotension that may occur.*
- Provide comfort measures, *to help the patient tolerate drug effects,* including small, frequent meals; access to bathroom facilities; safety precautions if CNS effects occur; environmental controls; appropriate skin care as needed; and analgesics as needed.
- Provide thorough patient teaching, including the name of the drug, dosage prescribed, measures to avoid adverse effects, warning signs of problems, and the need for periodic monitoring and evaluation, *to enhance patient knowledge about drug therapy and to promote compliance.*
- Offer support and encouragement *to help the patient deal with the diagnosis and the drug regimen.*

Evaluation

- Monitor patient response to the drug (maintenance of blood pressure within normal limits).
- Monitor for adverse effects (hypotension, GI distress, skin reactions, cough, headache, dizziness).
- Evaluate effectiveness of the teaching plan (patient can name drug, dosage, adverse effects to watch for, measures to avoid adverse effects, and the importance of continued follow-up).
- Monitor the effectiveness of comfort measures and compliance to the regimen.

Calcium Channel Blockers

The calcium channel blockers prevent the movement of calcium into the cardiac and smooth muscle cells when the cells are stimulated. This blocking of calcium interferes with the muscle cell's ability to contract, leading to a loss of smooth muscle tone, vasodilation, and a decrease in peripheral resistance. These effects decrease blood pressure, cardiac workload, and myocardial oxygen consumption. Calcium channel blockers are very effective in the treatment of angina (see Chapter 46) because they decrease the cardiac workload (see Critical Thinking Scenario 43-1).

Not all calcium channel blockers are used to treat hypertension. Some are considered safe and effective in treating hypertension only if they are given as sustained-release or extended-release preparations. The calcium channel blockers used in treating hypertension include the following (Table 43.4):

- Amlodipine (*Norvasc*), an oral drug that may be used alone or in combination with other agents to treat hypertension, also is used for angina.
- Diltiazem (*Cardizem, Tiamate*) is a sustained-release preparation recommended for the treatment of hypertension.
- Felodipine (*Plendil*) is not used for angina but is indicated alone or in combination with other agents for the treatment of hypertension.
- Isradipine (*DynaCirc*) is not used for angina but is indicated alone or in combination with thiazide diuretics for the treatment of hypertension.
- Nicardipine (*Cardene*) is used alone or in combination with other agents to treat hypertension and angina; it is also available in intravenous form for short-term use when oral administration is not feasible.
- Nifedipine (*Procardia XL*) is a sustained-release preparation indicated for the treatment of hypertension.
- Nisoldipine (*Sular*) comes in extended-release tablets and is indicated for the treatment of hypertension as monotherapy or as part of combination therapy.
- Verapamil (*Calan SR*) comes in extended-release tablets and is indicated for the treatment of essential hypertension; other preparations are used for angina and treating various arrhythmias.

Therapeutic Actions and Indications

Calcium channel blockers inhibit the movement of calcium ions across the membranes of myocardial and arterial muscle cells, altering the action potential and blocking muscle cell contraction. This effect depresses myocardial contractility, slows cardiac impulse formation in the conductive tissues, and relaxes and dilates arteries, causing a fall in blood pressure and a decrease in venous return.

Pharmacokinetics

These drugs are generally well absorbed, metabolized in the liver, and excreted in the urine. These drugs cross the placenta and enter breast milk. Fetal toxicity has been reported in animal studies, and, although there are no well defined studies about effects during pregnancy, they should not be used during pregnancy unless the benefit to the mother clearly outweighs any potential risk to the fetus. Because of the potential for serious adverse effects on the baby, another method of feeding the infant should be used if these drugs are required during lactation.

Contraindications and Cautions

These drugs are contraindicated in the presence of allergy to any of these drugs; with heart block or sick sinus syndrome, *which could be exacerbated by the conduction-slowing effects of these drugs;* with renal or hepatic dysfunction, *which could alter the metabolism and excretion of these drugs;* and with pregnancy or lactation, *because of the potential for adverse effects on the fetus or neonate.*

Adverse Effects

The adverse effects associated with these drugs relate to their effects on cardiac output and on smooth muscle. CNS effects include dizziness, light-headedness, headache, and fatigue. GI problems include nausea and hepatic injury related to direct toxic effects on hepatic cells. Cardiovascular effects include hypotension, bradycardia, peripheral edema, and heart block. Skin flushing and rash may also occur.

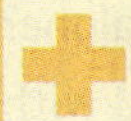

FOCUS ON PATIENT SAFETY

Several drugs that are used to treat hypertension cannot be cut, crushed, or chewed. This is very important information to share with patients. Sometimes patients cut tablets in half to facilitate swallowing, or to get twice the number of days for any given prescription. Most drugs formulated for extended release or sustained release are delivered in a matrix system that slowly dispenses the drug into the system. If the coating of the matrix is cut, all of the drug is released at once, leading to the release of too much drug at one time and, consequently, toxic levels of the drug when first taking it. Then the patient receives no drug as the day goes on. Some antihypertensives to be aware of are diltiazem, nifedipine, nisoldipine, and verapamil.

Clinically Important Drug–Drug Interactions

Drug–drug interactions vary with each of the calcium channel blockers used to treat hypertension. A potentially serious

(text continues on page 700)

CRITICAL THINKING SCENARIO 43-1

Initiating Antihypertensive Therapy

The Situation

B.R., a 46-year-old African American male business executive, was seen for a routine insurance physical. His examination was normal except for a blood pressure reading of 164/102 mm Hg. He also was approximately 20 lb overweight. Urinalysis and blood work results were all within normal limits. He was given a 1200-calorie-per-day diet to follow and was encouraged to reduce his salt and alcohol intake, start exercising, and stop smoking. He was asked to return in 3 weeks for a follow-up appointment (step 1). Three weeks later, B.R. returned with a 7-pound weight loss and an average blood pressure reading (of three readings) of 145/92 mm Hg. Discussion was held about starting B.R. on a diuretic (step 2) in addition to the lifestyle changes that B.R. was undertaking. B.R. was reluctant to take a diuretic and, after much discussion, was prescribed a calcium channel blocker. B.R. asked for a couple more weeks to try to bring his blood pressure down with lifestyle changes before starting the drug.

Critical Thinking

What nursing interventions should be done at this point? *Consider the risk factors that B.R. has for hypertension and the damage that hypertension can cause.*

What are the chances that B.R. can bring his blood pressure within a normal range with lifestyle changes alone?

What additional teaching points should be covered with B.R. before a treatment decision is made?

What implication does the diagnosis of hypertension have for B.R.'s insurance and job security?

What effects could diuretic therapy have on B.R.'s busy business day?

Discussion

B.R. was asked to change many things in his life over the last 3 weeks. These changes themselves can be stressful and can increase a person's blood pressure. B.R.'s reluctance to take a diuretic is understandable for a business executive who might not want his day interrupted by many bathroom stops. African Americans often respond well to diuretic therapy, with a return to normal blood pressure, but they also tend to have more adverse central nervous system effects with the most commonly used diuretics, the thiazides. This may have an impact on B.R.'s business and home life. The decision to use a calcium channel blocker may decrease some of the stress B.R. was feeling about the diuretic.

African Americans tend to respond well to monotherapy with calcium channel blockers, alpha-blockers, or diuretics. B.R. should receive a complete teaching program outlining what is known about hypertension and all of the risk factors involved with the disease. The good effects of weight loss, exercise, and other lifestyle changes should be stressed, and B.R. should be praised for his success over the last 3 weeks.

B.R. may benefit from trying for a couple more weeks to make lifestyle changes that will help bring his blood pressure into normal range. He will then feel that he has some control and input into the situation, and if drug therapy is needed, he may be more willing to comply with the prescribed treatment. The diagnosis of hypertension may be delayed for these 2 weeks while B.R. changes his lifestyle. Such a diagnosis should be made only after three consecutive blood pressure readings in the high range are recorded. B.R. may be able to have his blood pressure checked at work in a comfortable environment, which will improve the accuracy of the reading.

In the past, many insurance companies, and some employers, viewed hypertension as a hiring and insurability risk. As a business executive, B.R. may be well aware of this increased risk category—another reason to give him a little more time. He may wish to look into biofeedback for relaxation, a fitness program, smoking cessation programs (if appropriate), and stress reduction. As long as B.R. receives regular follow-up and frequent blood pressure checks, it may be a good idea to allow him to take some control and continue lifestyle changes. If at the end of the 2 weeks no further progress has been made or B.R.'s blood pressure has risen, drug therapy should be considered. Teaching should be aimed at helping B.R. to incorporate the drug effects into his lifestyle, to improve his compliance and tolerance of the therapy.

Nursing Care Guide For B.R.: Calcium Channel Blockers

Assessment: History And Examination

Concentrate the health history on allergies to any calcium channel blocker, renal dysfunction, salt/volume depletion, or heart failure and concurrent use of barbiturates, hydantoins, erythromycin, cimetidine, ranitidine, antifungal agents, and/or grapefruit juice.

Initiating Antihypertensive Therapy *(continued)*

Focus the physical examination on the following:

CV: blood pressure, pulse, perfusion, baseline ECG

CNS: orientation, affect

Skin: color, lesions, texture, temperature

Resp: respiration, adventitious sounds

GI: abdominal examination, bowel sounds

Laboratory tests: renal function tests, CBC, electrolyte levels

Nursing Diagnoses

Ineffective Tissue Perfusion related to changes in cardiac output

Impaired Skin Integrity related to skin effects

Acute Pain related to GI effects of drug

Deficient Knowledge regarding drug therapy

Implementation

Encourage lifestyle changes to increase drug effectiveness.

Do not cut, crush, or chew this tablet. Give with food if GI upset occurs.

Provide comfort and safety measures.

Reduce dosage if patient has renal failure.

Monitor for any situation that might lead to a drop in blood pressure.

Provide support and reassurance to deal with drug effects.

Provide patient teaching regarding drug, dosage, adverse effects, signs and symptoms of problems to report, and safety precautions.

Evaluation

Evaluate drug effects: maintenance of blood pressure within normal limits.

Monitor for adverse effects: nausea, dizziness; hypotension, congestive heart failure, skin reactions.

Monitor for drug–drug interactions as listed.

Evaluate effectiveness of patient teaching program and comfort and safety measures.

Patient Teaching For B.R.

- ☐ The drug that has been prescribed to treat your hypertension is called a calcium channel blocker. When used to treat high blood pressure, this drug is called an antihypertensive. High blood pressure is a disorder that may have no symptoms but that can cause serious problems, such as heart attack, stroke, or kidney problems, if left untreated.
- ☐ It is very important to take your medication every day, as prescribed, even if you feel perfectly well without the medication. It is possible that you may feel worse because of the adverse effects associated with the medication when you take it. Even if this happens, it is crucial that you take your medication.
- ☐ If you find that the adverse effects of this drug are too uncomfortable, discuss the possibility of taking a different antihypertensive medication with your health care provider.
- ☐ This drug should be taken on an empty stomach, 1 hour before or 2 hours after meals.
- ☐ Common effects of these drugs include:
  - *Dizziness, drowsiness, light-headedness:* These effects often pass after the first few days. Until they do, avoid driving or performing hazardous or delicate tasks that require concentration. If these effects occur, change positions slowly to decrease the light-headedness.
  - *Nausea, vomiting, change in taste perception:* Small, frequent meals may help ease these effects, which may pass with time. If they persist and become too uncomfortable, consult with your health care provider.
  - *Skin rash, mouth sores:* Frequent mouth care may help. Keep the skin dry and use prescribed skin care (lotions, coverings, medication) if needed.
  - Report any of the following to your health care provider: *difficulty breathing; mouth sores; swelling of the feet, hands, or face; chest pain; palpitations; sore throat; fever or chills.*
- ☐ Do not stop taking this drug for any reason. Consult with your health care provider if you have problems taking this medication.
- ☐ You should avoid the use of grapefruit juice while you are taking this drug, because the combination grapefruit juice and a calcium channel blocker may case toxic effects.
- ☐ Tell any doctor, nurse, or others involved in your health care that you are taking this drug.
- ☐ Avoid taking over-the-counter medications while you are taking this drug. If you feel that you need one of these, consult with your health care provider for the best choice. Many of these drugs may interfere with the antihypertensive effect that usually occurs with this drug.
- ☐ Be extremely careful in any situation that might lead to a drop in blood pressure (e.g., excessive sweating, vomiting, diarrhea, dehydration). If you experience light-headedness or dizziness in any of these situations, consult your health care provider immediately.
- ☐ Keep this drug, and all medications, out of the reach of children.

Table 43.4 DRUGS IN FOCUS

Calcium Channel Blockers Used in Hypertension

Drug Name	Usual Dosage	Usual Indications
amlodipine (*Norvasc*)	5–10 mg/day PO, reduce dosage with hepatic impairment and in geriatric patients	Alone or in combination with other agents for the treatment of hypertension in adults
P diltiazem (*Cardizem, Dilacor CR*)	60–120 mg PO b.i.d.	Extended release preparation used to treat hypertension in adults
felodipine (*Plendil*)	10–15 mg/day PO; do not exceed 10 mg/day in geriatric patients or in those with hepatic impairment	Alone or in combination with other agents for the treatment of hypertension in adults
isradipine (*DynaCirc*)	2.5–10 mg PO b.i.d.; 5–10 mg/day PO—controlled release	Alone or in combination with other agents for the treatment of hypertension in adults
nicardipine (*Cardene*)	20–40 mg PO t.i.d.; 0.5–2.2 mg/h IV based on response, switch to oral form as soon as feasible; reduce dosage in geriatric patients and in those with hepatic or renal impairment; 30–60 mg PO b.i.d.—sustained release	Alone or in combination with other agents to treat hypertension and angina; IV form for short-term use when oral route is not feasible; for use in adults
nifedipine (*Procardia XL*)	30–60 mg/day PO	Sustained-release (SR) preparation only; indicated for the treatment of hypertension in adults
nisoldipine (*Sular*)	20–40 mg/day PO; reduce dosage in geriatric patients and in those with hepatic impairment	Extended-release (ER) tablets for the treatment of hypertension as monotherapy or as part of combination therapy in adults
verapamil (*Calan SR*)	120–240 mg/day PO, reduce dosage in the morning; ER capsules: 100–300 mg/day PO at bedtime	ER formulations for the treatment of essential hypertension

effect to note is an increase in serum levels and toxicity of cyclosporine if taken with diltiazem.

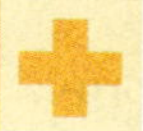

FOCUS ON PATIENT SAFETY

The calcium channel blockers are a class of drugs that interact with grapefruit juice. When grapefruit juice is present in the body, the concentrations of calcium channel blockers increase, sometimes to toxic levels. Advise patients to avoid the use of grapefruit juice if they are taking a calcium channel blocker. If a patient on a calcium channel blocker reports toxic effects, ask whether he or she is drinking grapefruit juice.

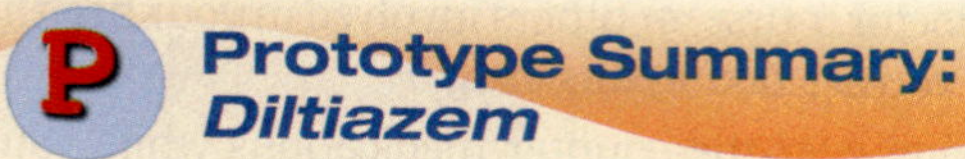

Prototype Summary: *Diltiazem*

Indications: Treatment of essential hypertension in the extended-release form

Actions: Inhibits the movement of calcium ions across the membranes of cardiac and arterial muscle cells, depressing the impulse and leading to slowed conduction, decreased myocardial contractility, and dilation of arterioles, which lowers blood pressure and decreases myocardial oxygen consumption

Pharmacokinetics:

Route	Onset	Peak	Duration
Oral, ER	30–60 min	6–11 h	12 h

$T_{1/2}$: 5–7 hours; metabolized in the liver and excreted in urine

Adverse effects: Dizziness, light-headedness, headache, peripheral edema, bradycardia, atrioventricular block, flushing, nausea

Nursing Considerations for Patients Receiving Calcium Channel Blockers

The main use of calcium channel blockers is for the treatment of angina. See Chapter 46 for the nursing considerations of calcium channel blockers.

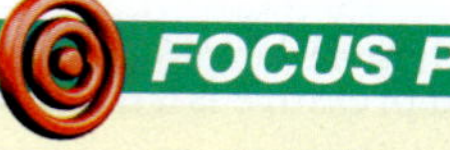

FOCUS POINTS

- Drug treatment of hypertension aims to change one or more of the normal reflexes that control blood pressure.

- Sodium levels and fluid volume are decreased by diuretic agents.
- ACE inhibitors prevent the conversion of angiotensin I to angiotensin II, leading to a fall in blood pressure.
- ARBs prevent the body from responding to angiotensin II, causing a loss of effectiveness of the renin–angiotensin system.
- Calcium channel blockers interfere with the ability of muscles to contract, which leads to vasodilation, which in turn reduces blood pressure.

Vasodilators

If other drug therapies do not achieve the desired reduction in blood pressure, it is sometimes necessary to use a direct vasodilator. Vasodilators produce relaxation of the vascular smooth muscle, decreasing peripheral resistance and reducing blood pressure. They do not block the reflex tachycardia that occurs when blood pressure drops. Most of the vasodilators are reserved for use in severe hypertension or hypertensive emergencies. The vasodilators that might be used to treat severe hypertension include the following (Table 43.5):

- Diazoxide (*Hyperstat*) is used as an intravenous drug in hospitalized patients with severe hypertension. This drug also increases blood glucose levels by blocking insulin release, so it must be used with extreme caution with functional hypoglycemia.
- Hydralazine (*Apresoline*) is available for oral, intravenous, and intramuscular use for the treatment of severe hypertension. It is thought to maintain or increase renal blood flow while relaxing smooth muscle.
- Minoxidil (*Loniten*) is an oral agent used only for the treatment of severe and unresponsive hypertension. It is associated with reflex tachycardia and increased renin release leading to volume increase. (The oral drug is associated with changes in body hair growth and distribution, which led to a topical preparation [*Rogaine*] for the treatment of baldness.)
- Nitroprusside (*Nitropress*) is used intravenously for the treatment of hypertensive crisis and to maintain controlled hypotension during surgery; toxic levels cause cyanide toxicity.

Therapeutic Actions and Indications

The vasodilators act directly on vascular smooth muscle to cause muscle relaxation, leading to vasodilation and drop in blood pressure. They are indicated for the treatment of severe hypertension that has not responded to other therapy.

Pharmacokinetics

These drugs are rapidly absorbed and widely distributed. They are metabolized in the liver and primarily excreted in urine. They cross the placenta and enter breast milk. They should not be used during pregnancy unless the benefit to the mother clearly outweighs the potential risk to the fetus. If they are needed by a nursing mother, another method of feeding the baby should be selected. Do not use these drugs during lactation.

Contraindications and Cautions

The vasodilators are contraindicated in the presence of known allergy to the drug; with pregnancy and lactation, *because of the potential for adverse effects on the fetus or neonate;* and with any condition that could be exacerbated by a sudden fall in blood pressure, such as cerebral insufficiency. Caution should be used in patients with peripheral vascular disease, CAD, CHF, or tachycardia, *all of which could be exacerbated by the fall in blood pressure.*

Table 43.5 DRUGS IN FOCUS

Vasodilators

Drug Name	Usual Dosage	Usual Indications
diazoxide (*Hyperstat*)	1–3 mg/kg IV, by rapid bolus over 30 sec; may be repeated q5–15min as needed	IV use for the treatment of severe hypertension in hospitalized adults
hydralazine (*Apresoline*)	Adult: 20–40 mg IM or IV repeated as necessary Pediatric: 1.7–3.5 mg/kg per 24 h IV or IM in four to six divided doses	Treatment of severe hypertension
minoxidil (*Loniten*)	Adult: 10–40 mg/day PO in divided doses Pediatric (<12 yr): 0.25–1 mg/kg/day PO as a single dose	Treatment of severe hypertension unresponsive to other therapy
P nitroprusside (*Nitropress*)	All patients: 3 mcg/kg/min, do not exceed 10 mcg/kg/min	IV use for the treatment of hypertensive crisis; to maintain controlled hypotension during surgery

Adverse Effects

The adverse effects most frequently seen with these drugs are related to the changes in blood pressure. These include dizziness, anxiety, and headache; reflex tachycardia, CHF, chest pain, edema; skin rash and lesions (abnormal hair growth with minoxidil); and GI upset, nausea, and vomiting. Cyanide toxicity (dyspnea, headache, vomiting, dizziness, ataxia, loss of consciousness, imperceptible pulse, absent reflexes, dilated pupils, pink color, distant heart sounds, and shallow breathing) may occur with nitroprusside, which is metabolized to cyanide and which also suppresses iodine uptake and can cause hypothyroidism.

Clinically Important Drug–Drug Interactions

Each of these drugs works differently in the body, so each drug should be checked for potential drug–drug interactions before use.

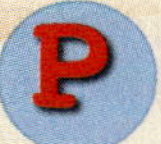

Prototype Summary: *Nitroprusside*

Indications: Hypertensive crisis, maintenance of controlled hypotension during anesthesia, acute CHF

Actions: Acts directly on vascular smooth muscle to cause vasodilation and drop of blood pressure; does not inhibit cardiovascular reflexes and tachycardia; renin release will occur

Pharmacokinetics:

Route	Onset	Peak	Duration
IV	1–2 min	rapid	1–10 min

$T_{1/2}$: 2 min; metabolized in the liver and excretion in urine

Adverse effects: Apprehension, headache, retrosternal pressure, palpitations, cyanide toxicity, diaphoresis, nausea, vomiting, abdominal pain, irritation at the injection site

Nursing Considerations for Patients Receiving Vasodilators

Assessment: History and Examination

Screen for the following conditions, *which could be cautions or contraindications to use of the drug:* any known allergies to these drugs; impaired kidney or liver function; pregnancy or lactation, *because of the potential adverse effects on the fetus or neonate;* and cardiovascular dysfunction, *which could be exacerbated by a fall in blood pressure.*

Include screening *for baseline status before beginning therapy and for any potential adverse effects.* Assess the following: body temperature and weight; skin color, lesions, and temperature; pulse, blood pressure, baseline ECG, and perfusion; respirations and adventitious breath sounds; bowel sounds and abdominal examination; renal and liver function tests; and blood glucose.

Nursing Diagnoses

The patient receiving a vasodilator may have the following nursing diagnoses related to drug therapy:

- Ineffective Tissue Perfusion (Total Body) related to changes in cardiac output
- Impaired Skin Integrity related to dermatological effects
- Acute Pain related to GI distress, skin effects, or headache
- Deficient Knowledge regarding drug therapy

Implementation With Rationale

- Encourage the patient to implement lifestyle changes, including weight loss, smoking cessation, decreased alcohol and salt in the diet, and increased exercise, *to increase the effectiveness of antihypertensive therapy.*
- Monitor blood pressure closely during administration, *to evaluate for effectiveness and to ensure quick response if blood pressure falls rapidly or too much.*
- Monitor blood glucose and serum electrolytes, *to avoid potentially serious adverse effects.*
- Monitor the patient carefully in any situation that might lead to a drop in fluid volume (e.g., excessive sweating, vomiting, diarrhea, dehydration), *to detect and treat excessive hypotension that may occur.*
- Provide comfort measures *to help the patient tolerate drug effects,* including small, frequent meals; access to bathroom facilities; safety precautions if CNS effects occur; environmental controls; appropriate skin care as needed; and analgesics as needed.
- Provide thorough patient teaching, including the name of the drug, dosage prescribed, measures to avoid adverse effects, warning signs of problems, and the need for periodic monitoring and evaluation, *to enhance patient knowledge about drug therapy and to promote compliance.*

- Offer support and encouragement, *to help the patient deal with the diagnosis and the drug regimen.*

Evaluation

- Monitor patient response to the drug (maintenance of blood pressure within normal limits).
- Monitor for adverse effects (hypotension, GI distress, skin reactions, tachycardia, headache, dizziness).
- Evaluate the effectiveness of the teaching plan (patient can name drug, dosage, adverse effects to watch for, specific measures to avoid adverse effects, and the importance of continued follow-up).
- Monitor the effectiveness of comfort measures and compliance with the regimen.

Other Antihypertensive Agents

One other drug that has proved useful in the treatment of severe hypertension is mecamylamine (*Inversine*). Mecamylamine is a ganglionic blocker that occupies cholinergic receptor sites of autonomic neurons, blocking the effects of acetylcholine at both sympathetic and parasympathetic ganglia. It decreases the effectiveness of both of these branches of the autonomic system. Blocking the sympathetic system leads to vasodilation, decreased blood pressure, and a blocking of reflex tachycardia as well as the release of catecholamines from the adrenal gland. It can cause severe hypotension, CHF, and CNS symptoms of dizziness, syncope, weakness, and vision changes; parasympathetic blocking symptoms of dry mouth, glossitis, nausea, vomiting, constipation, and urinary retention; and impotence. It is reserved for use in severe or malignant hypertension when other drugs have not proved successful. The patient receiving this drug must be monitored very closely because of the loss of autonomic reflexes.

Antihypotensive Agents

As mentioned earlier, if blood pressure becomes too low (hypotension), the vital centers in the brain and the rest of the tissues of the body may not receive sufficient oxygenated blood to continue functioning. Severe hypotension or shock puts the body in serious jeopardy; it is often an acute emergency situation, with treatment required to save the patient's life. The first-choice drug for treating shock is usually a sympathomimetic drug.

Sympathetic Adrenergic Agonists

Sympathomimetic drugs react with sympathetic adrenergic receptors to cause the effects of a sympathetic stress response: increased blood pressure, increased blood volume, and increased strength of cardiac muscle contraction. These actions increase blood pressure and may restore balance to the cardiovascular system while the underlying cause of the shock (e.g., volume depletion, blood loss) is treated. The sympathomimetic drugs are discussed in Chapter 30. Box 43.8 lists the sympathomimetics used in the treatment of severe hypotension and shock.

Midodrine

Midodrine (*ProAmatine*) is a drug that is used to treat orthostatic hypotension—hypotension that occurs with position change—that interferes with a person's ability to function and has not responded to any other therapy (Table 43.6).

Therapeutic Actions and Indications

Midodrine activates alpha-receptors in arteries and veins to produce an increase in vascular tone and an increase in blood pressure. It is indicated for the symptomatic treatment of orthostatic hypotension in patients whose lives are impaired by the disorder and who have not had a response to any other therapy.

Pharmacokinetics

Midodrine is rapidly absorbed from the GI tract, reaching peak levels within 1 to 2 hours. It is metabolized in the liver and excreted in the urine with a half-life of 3 to 4 hours. It should be reserved in pregnancy for cases in which the benefit to the mother clearly outweighs the potential risk to the fetus. It is not known whether midodrine enters breast milk, so caution should be used during lactation.

Contraindications and Cautions

Midodrine is contraindicated in the presence of supine hypertension, CAD, or pheochromocytoma, *because of the risk of precipitating a hypertensive emergency;* with acute renal disease, *which might interfere with excretion of the drug;* with urinary retention, *because the stimulation of alpha-receptors can exacerbate this problem;* and with thy-

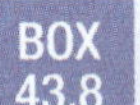

Sympathomimetic Drugs Used to Treat Severe Hypotension and Shock

Sympathomimetic Drugs (see Chapter 30)

- dobutamine
- dopamine
- ephedrine
- epinephrine
- isoproterenol
- metaraminol

Table 43.6 DRUGS IN FOCUS

Antihypotensive–Midodrine

Drug Name	Usual Dosage	Usual Indications
midodrine (*ProAmatine*)	10 mg PO t.i.d.	Treatment of orthostatic hypotension in adults

rotoxicosis, *which could further increase blood pressure.* Caution should be used with pregnancy and lactation, *because of the potential for adverse effects on the fetus or neonate;* with visual problems, *which could be exacerbated by vasoconstriction;* and with renal or hepatic impairment, *which could alter the metabolism and excretion of the drug.*

Adverse Effects

The most common adverse effects associated with this drug are related to the stimulation of alpha-receptors and include piloerection, chills, and rash; hypertension and bradycardia; dizziness, vision changes, vertigo, and headache; and problems with urination.

Clinically Important Drug–Drug Interactions

There is a risk of increased effects and toxicity of cardiac glycosides, beta-blockers, alpha-adrenergic agents, and corticosteroids if they are taken with midodrine. Patients who are receiving any of these combinations should be monitored carefully for the need for a dosage adjustment.

Nursing Considerations for Patients Receiving Midodrine

Assessment: History and Examination

Screen for the following conditions, *which could be contraindications or cautions to use of the drug:* any known allergy to midodrine; impaired kidney or liver function; pregnancy or lactation *because of the potential adverse effects on the fetus or neonate;* cardiovascular dysfunction; visual problems; urinary retention; and pheochromocytoma.

Include screening *for baseline status before beginning therapy and for any potential adverse effects.* Assess the following: body temperature and weight; skin color, lesions, and temperature; pulse, blood pressure, orthostatic blood pressure, and perfusion; respiration and adventitious sounds; bowel sounds and abdominal examination; and renal and liver function tests.

Nursing Diagnoses

The patient receiving midodrine may have the following nursing diagnoses related to drug therapy:

- Ineffective Tissue Perfusion (Total Body) related to changes in cardiac output
- Disturbed Sensory Perception (Visual, Kinesthetic, Tactile) related to CNS effects
- Acute Pain related to GI distress, piloerection, chills, or headache
- Deficient Knowledge regarding drug therapy

Implementation With Rationale

- Monitor blood pressure carefully, *to monitor effectiveness and blood pressure changes.*
- Do not administer the drug to patients who are bedridden, but only to patients who are up and mobile, *to ensure therapeutic effects and decrease the risk of severe hypertension.*
- Monitor heart rate regularly when beginning therapy, *to monitor for bradycardia, which commonly occurs at the beginning of therapy; if bradycardia persists, it may indicate a need to discontinue the drug.*
- Monitor patients with known visual problems carefully, *to ensure that the drug is discontinued if visual fields change.*
- Encourage patients to void before taking a dose of the drug, *to decrease the risk of urinary retention problems.*
- Provide comfort measures *to help the patient tolerate drug effects,* including small, frequent meals; access to bathroom facilities; safety precautions if CNS effects occur; environmental controls; appropriate skin care as needed; and analgesics as needed.
- Provide thorough patient teaching, including the name of the drug, dosage prescribed, measures to avoid adverse effects, warning signs of problems, and the need for periodic monitoring and evaluation, *to enhance patient knowledge about drug therapy and to promote compliance.*
- Offer support and encouragement, *to help the patient deal with the diagnosis and the drug regimen.*

Evaluation

- Monitor patient response to the drug (maintenance of blood pressure within normal limits).
- Monitor for adverse effects (hypertension, dizziness, visual changes, piloerection, chills, urinary problems).
- Evaluate the effectiveness of the teaching plan (patient can name drug, dosage, adverse effects to watch for, specific measures to avoid adverse effects, and the importance of continued follow-up).
- Monitor the effectiveness of comfort measures and compliance with the regimen.

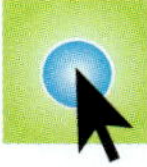

WEB LINKS

Health care providers and patients may want to consult the following Internet sources:

http://www.heartinfo.org Information on research, alternative methods of therapy, and pharmacology.

http://www.fda.gov/hearthealth/ Information and instructions related to products, such as medications and devices, to prevent, diagnose, and treat cardiovascular disease.

http://www.ash-us.org Patient information on hypertension, treatments, and lifestyle adjustments.

http://www.americanheart.org Patient information, support groups, diet, exercise, and research information on hypertension and other cardiovascular diseases.

http://www.medscape.com Specific information on the care of the pediatric hypertensive patient; enter "pediatric hypertension" in the search box.

http://www.nhlbi.nih.gov/guidelines/hypertension Data released in 2003 by the Seventh Joint National Committee on the Prevention, Detection, Evaluation and Treatment of High Blood Pressure.

Points to Remember

- The cardiovascular system is a closed system that depends on pressure differences to ensure the delivery of blood to the tissues and the return of that blood to the heart.
- Blood pressure is related to heart rate, stroke volume, and the total peripheral resistance against which the heart has to push the blood.
- Peripheral resistance is primarily controlled by constriction or relaxation of the arterioles. Constricted arterioles raise pressure; dilated arterioles lower pressure.
- Control of blood pressure involves baroreceptor (pressure receptor) stimulation of the medulla to activate the sympathetic nervous system, which causes vasoconstriction and increased fluid retention when pressure is low in the aorta and carotid arteries, and vasodilation and loss of fluid when pressure is too high.
- The kidneys activate the renin–angiotensin system when blood flow to the kidneys is decreased.
- Renin activates conversion of angiotensinogen to angiotensin I in the liver; angiotensin I is converted by angiotensin-converting enzyme (ACE) to angiotensin II in the lungs; angiotensin II then reacts with specific receptor sites on blood vessels to cause vasoconstriction to raise blood pressure and in the adrenal gland to cause release of aldosterone, which leads to retention of fluid and increased blood volume.
- Hypertension is a sustained state of higher-than-normal blood pressure that can lead to damage to blood vessels, increased risk of atherosclerosis, and damage to small vessels in end organs. Because hypertension often has no signs or symptoms, it is called the silent killer.
- Essential hypertension has no underlying cause, and treatment can vary widely from individual to individual. Treatment approaches include lifestyle changes first, followed by careful addition and adjustment of various antihypertensive drugs.
- Drug treatment of hypertension is aimed at altering one or more of the normal reflexes that control blood pressure: diuretics decrease sodium levels and volume; sympathetic nervous system drugs alter the sympathetic response and lead to vascular dilation and decreased pumping power of the heart; ACE inhibitors prevent the conversion of angiotensin I to angiotensin II; ARBs prevent the body from responding to angiotensin II; calcium channel blockers interfere with the ability of muscles to contract and lead to vasodilation; and vasodilators directly cause the relaxation of vascular smooth muscle.
- Hypotension is a state of lower-than-normal blood pressure that can result in decreased oxygenation of the tissues, cell death, tissue damage, and even death. Hypotension is most often treated with sympathomimetic drugs, which stimulate the sympathetic receptor sites to cause vasoconstriction, fluid retention, and return of normal pressure.

CHECK YOUR UNDERSTANDING

Answers to the questions in this chapter may be found in the Answer Key in the back of the book.

Multiple Choice

Select the best answer to the following.

1. The baroreceptors are the most important factor in minute-to-minute control of blood pressure. The baroreceptors
   a. are evenly distributed throughout the body to maintain pressure in the system.
   b. sense pressure and immediately send that information to the medulla in the brain.
   c. are directly connected to the sympathetic nervous system.
   d. are as sensitive to oxygen levels as to pressure changes.

2. Essential hypertension is the most commonly diagnosed form of high blood pressure. Essential hypertension is
   a. caused by a tumor in the adrenal gland.
   b. associated with no known cause.
   c. related to renal disease.
   d. caused by liver dysfunction.

3. Hypertension is associated with
   a. loss of vision.
   b. strokes.
   c. atherosclerosis.
   d. all of the above.

4. The stepped-care approach to the treatment of hypertension would include
   a. lifestyle modification, including exercise, diet, and decreased smoking and alcohol intake.
   b. use of a diuretic, beta-blocker, or ACE inhibitor to supplement lifestyle changes.
   c. a combination of antihypertensive drug classes to achieve desired control.
   d. all of the above.

5. ACE inhibitors work on the renin–angiotensin system to prevent the conversion of angiotensin I to angiotensin II. Because this blocking occurs in the cells in the lung, which is usually the site of this conversion, use of ACE inhibitors often results in
   a. spontaneous pneumothorax.
   b. pneumonia.
   c. unrelenting cough.
   d. respiratory depression.

6. A client taking an ACE inhibitor is scheduled for surgery. The nurse should
   a. stop the drug.
   b. alert the surgeon and mark the client's chart prominently, because the blockage of compensatory angiotensin II could result in hypotension after surgery that would need to be reversed with volume expansion.
   c. cancel the surgery and consult with the prescriber.
   d. monitor fluid levels and make the sure the fluids are restricted before surgery.

7. A patient who is hypertensive becomes pregnant. The drug of choice for this patient would be
   a. an angiotensin II receptor blocker.
   b. an ACE inhibitor.
   c. a diuretic.
   d. a calcium channel blocker.

8. Midodrine, an antihypotensive drug, should be used
   a. only with patients who are confined to bed.
   b. in the treatment of acute shock.
   c. in patients with known pheochromocytoma.
   d. to treat orthostatic hypotension in patients whose lives are impaired by the disorder.

Multiple Response

Select all that apply.

1. Pressure within the vascular system is determined by which of the following?
   a. Peripheral resistance
   b. Stroke volume
   c. Sodium load
   d. Heart rate
   e. Total intravascular volume
   f. Rate of erythropoietin release

2. The renin–angiotensin system is associated with which of the following?
   a. Intense vasoconstriction and blood pressure elevation
   b. Blood flow through the kidneys
   c. Production of surfactant in the lungs
   d. Release of aldosterone from the adrenal cortex
   e. Retention of sodium and water in the kidneys
   f. Liver production of fibrinogen

Matching

Match the following drugs with their appropriate class of antihypertensive agents. (Some classes may be used more than once.)

1. ______________________ candesartan
2. ______________________ quinapril
3. ______________________ mecamylamine
4. ______________________ losartan
5. ______________________ nitroprusside
6. ______________________ tolazoline
7. ______________________ lisinopril
8. ______________________ valsartan
9. ______________________ nicardipine
10. ______________________ minoxidil
11. ______________________ fosinopril
12. ______________________ amlodipine

A. Angiotensin-converting enzyme inhibitor
B. Angiotensin II receptor blocker
C. Calcium channel blocker
D. Vasodilator
E. Ganglionic blocker

True or False

Indicate whether the following statements are true (T) or false (F).

_____ 1. The cardiovascular system is an open system that depends on pressure differences to ensure the delivery of blood.

_____ 2. Blood pressure is related to heart rate, stroke volume, and the total peripheral resistance.

_____ 3. Constricted arterioles lower pressure; dilated arterioles raise pressure.

_____ 4. Control of blood pressure involves baroreceptor (pressure receptor) stimulation of the medulla to activate the parasympathetic nervous system.

_____ 5. The kidneys activate the renin–angiotensin system when blood flow to the kidneys is decreased.

_____ 6. Renin activates angiotensinogen to angiotensin I in the lung using angiotensin-converting enzyme.

_____ 7. Hypertension is a sustained state of higher-than-normal blood pressure.

_____ 8. Essential hypertension has no underlying cause, and treatment can vary widely.

_____ 9. Angiotensin II receptor blockers prevent the body from responding to angiotensin II and blocking calcium channels.

_____ 10. Hypotension can result in decreased oxygenation of the tissues, cell death, tissue damage, and even death.

Bibliography and References

ALLHAT Officers and ALLHAT Collaborative Research Group. (2002). Major outcomes in high-risk hypertensive patients randomized to angiotensin-converting enzyme inhibitor or calcium channel blocker vs diuretic: the Antihypertensive and Lipid-Lowering Treatment to Prevent Heart Attack Trial (ALLHAT). *Journal of the American Medical Association 288:*2981–2997.

Andrews, M., & Boyle, J. (2004). *Transcultural concepts in nursingcare.* Philadelphia: Lippincott Williams & Wilkins.

Drug facts and comparisons. (2006). St. Louis: Facts and Comparisons.

Gilman, A., Hardman, J. G., & Limbird, L. E. (Eds.). (2006). *Goodman and Gilman's the pharmacological basis of therapeutics* (11th ed.). New York: McGraw-Hill.

Karch, A. M. (2006). *2007 Lippincott's nursing drug guide.* Philadelphia: Lippincott Williams & Wilkins.

The medical letter on drugs and therapeutics. (2006). New Rochelle, NY: Medical Letter.

Porth, C. M. (2005). *Pathophysiology: Concepts of altered health states* (7th ed.). Philadelphia: Lippincott Williams & Wilkins.

CHAPTER 44

Cardiotonic Agents

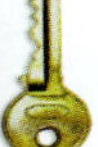

KEY TERMS

cardiomegaly

cardiomyopathy

congestive heart failure (CHF)

dyspnea

hemoptysis

nocturia

orthopnea

positive inotropic

pulmonary edema

tachypnea

LEARNING OBJECTIVES

Upon completion of this chapter, you will be able to:

1. Describe the pathophysiological process of heart failure and the resultant clinical signs, and explain the body's compensatory mechanisms when this occurs.
2. Describe the therapeutic actions, indications, pharmacokinetics, contraindications, most common adverse reactions, and important drug–drug interactions associated with the cardiac glycoside, the phosphodiesterase inhibitors, and the digoxin antidote.
3. Discuss the use of cardiotonic agents across the lifespan.
4. Compare and contrast the prototype drugs digoxin and inamrinone, and digoxin immune Fab.
5. Outline the nursing considerations, including important teaching points, for patients receiving cardiotonic agents.

CARDIAC GLYCOSIDE

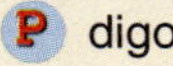 digoxin

PHOSPHODIESTERASE INHIBITORS

P inamrinone

milrinone

DIGOXIN ANTIDOTE

digoxin immune Fab

Congestive heart failure (CHF) is a condition in which the heart fails to effectively pump blood around the body. Because the cardiac cycle normally involves a tight balance between the pumping of the right and left sides of the heart, any failure of the muscle to pump blood out of either side of the heart can result in a backup of blood cells. If this happens, the blood vessels become congested; eventually, the body's cells are deprived of oxygen and nutrients, and waste products build up in the tissues. The primary treatment for CHF involves helping the heart muscle to contract more efficiently to bring the system back into balance.

Review of Cardiac Muscle Function

The underlying problem in CHF usually involves muscle function: (1) the muscle could be damaged by atherosclerosis or **cardiomyopathy** (a disease of the heart muscle that leads to an enlarged heart and eventually to complete muscle failure and death); (2) the muscle could be forced to work too hard to maintain an efficient output, as with hypertension or valvular disease; or (3) the structure of the heart could be abnormal, as with congenital cardiac defects.

The basic unit of the heart muscle, the sarcomere, contains two contractile proteins, actin and myosin, which are highly reactive with each other but at rest are kept apart by troponin. When a cardiac muscle cell is stimulated, calcium enters the cell and inactivates the troponin, allowing the actin and myosin to form actomyosin bridges. The formation of these bridges allows the muscle fibers to slide together or contract (Figure 44.1). (See Chapter 42 for a review of heart muscle contraction processes.)

The contraction process requires energy, oxygen, and calcium to allow the formation of the actomyosin bridges. The degree of shortening, or the strength of contraction, is determined by the amount of calcium present (the more calcium that is present, the more bridges will be formed) and by the stretch of the sarcomere before contraction begins (the farther apart the actin and myosin proteins are before the cell is stimulated, the more bridges will be formed and the stronger the contraction will be). This correlates with Starling's law of the heart: The more the cardiac muscle is stretched, the greater the contraction will be. The more blood you put into the heart, the greater the contraction will be to empty the heart, up to a point. If the bridges are stretched too far apart, they will not be able to reach each other to form the actomyosin bridges, and no contraction

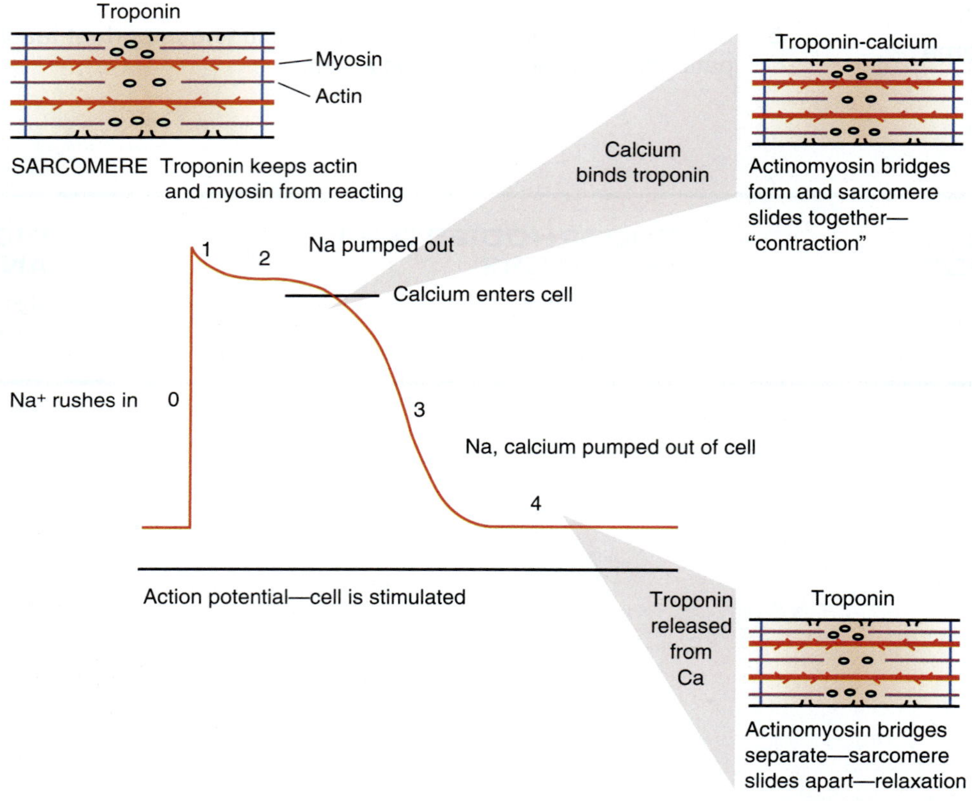

FIGURE 44.1 The sliding filaments of myocardial muscles. Calcium entering the cell deactivates troponin and allows actin and myosin to react, causing contraction. Calcium pumped out of the cell frees troponin to separate actin and myosin; the sarcomere filament slides apart and the cell relaxes.

will occur. This extreme response can be seen with severe cardiomyopathy: The muscle cells are stretched and distorted and eventually stop contracting because they can no longer respond.

Congestive Heart Failure

CHF, a condition that was once called "dropsy" or decompensation, is a syndrome that can occur with any of the disorders that damage or overwork the heart muscle.

- Coronary artery disease (CAD) is the leading cause of CHF, accounting for approximately 95% of the cases diagnosed (see Chapter 47 for a discussion of CAD). CAD results in an insufficient supply of blood to meet the oxygen demands of the myocardium. Consequently, the muscles become hypoxic and can no longer function efficiently. When CAD evolves into a myocardial infarction (MI), muscle cells die or are damaged, leading to an inefficient pumping effort.
- Cardiomyopathy can occur as a result of a viral infection, alcoholism, anabolic steroid abuse, or a collagen disorder. It causes muscle alterations and ineffective contraction and pumping.
- Hypertension eventually leads to an enlarged cardiac muscle because the heart has to work harder than normal to pump against the high pressure in the arteries. Hypertension puts constant, increased demands for oxygen on the system because the heart is pumping so hard all of the time.
- Valvular heart disease leads to an overload of the ventricles because the valves do not close tightly, which allows blood to leak backward into the ventricles. This overloading causes muscle stretching and increased demand for oxygen and energy as the heart muscle has to constantly contract harder. (Valvular heart disease is rarely seen today owing to the success of cardiac surgery and effective treatment for rheumatic fever.)

The end result of all of these conditions is that the heart muscle cannot pump blood effectively throughout the vascular system. If the left ventricle pumps inefficiently, blood backs up into the lungs, causing pulmonary vessel congestion and fluid leakage into the alveoli and lung tissue. In severe cases, **pulmonary edema** (rales, wheezes, blood-tinged sputum, low oxygenation, development of a third heart sound [S_3]) can occur. If the right side of the heart is the primary problem, blood backs up in the venous system leading to the right side of the heart. Liver congestion and edema of the legs and feet reflect right-sided failure. Because the cardiovascular system works as a closed system, one-sided failure, if left untreated, eventually leads to failure of both sides, and the signs and symptoms of total CHF occur.

CONCEPTS in action **ANIMATION**

Compensatory Mechanisms in Congestive Heart Failure

Because effective pumping of blood to the cells is essential for life, the body has several compensatory mechanisms that function if the heart muscle starts to fail (Figure 44.2). Decreased cardiac output stimulates the baroreceptors in the aortic arch and the carotid arteries, causing a sympathetic stimulation (see Chapter 29). This sympathetic stimulation causes an increase in heart rate, blood pressure, and rate and depth of respirations, as well as a **positive inotropic** effect (increased force of contraction) on the heart and an increase in blood volume (through the release of aldosterone). The decrease in cardiac output also stimulates the release of renin from the kidneys and activates the renin–angiotensin system, which further increases blood pressure and blood volume.

If these compensatory mechanisms are working effectively, the patient may have no signs or symptoms of CHF and is said to be compensated. Over time, however, all of these effects increase the workload of the heart, contributing to further development of CHF. Eventually, the heart muscle stretches out from overwork, and the chambers of the heart dilate secondary to the increased blood volume that they have had to handle. This hypertrophy (enlargement) of the heart muscle, called **cardiomegaly**, leads to inefficient pumping and eventually to increased CHF.

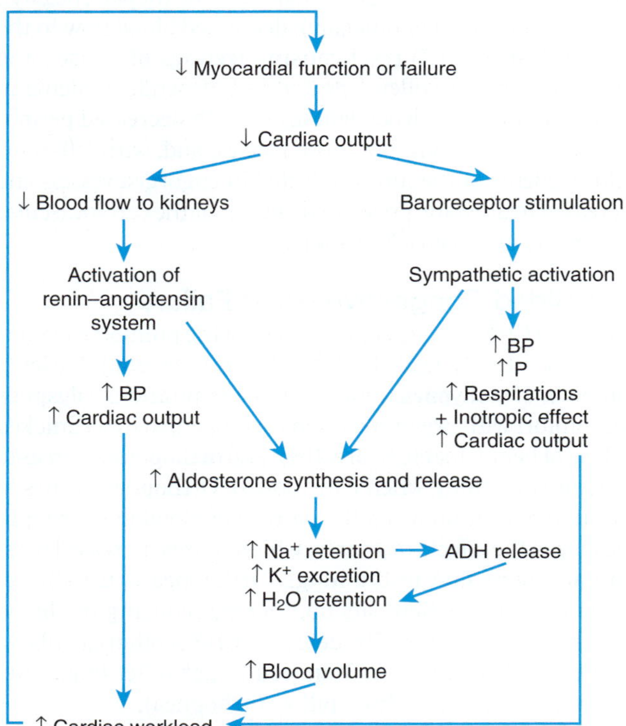

FIGURE 44.2 Compensatory mechanisms in congestive heart failure (CHF), which lead to increased cardiac workload and further CHF. ADH, antidiuretic hormone; BP, blood pressure; P, pulse.

Cellular Changes in Congestive Heart Failure

The myocardial cells are changed with prolonged CHF. Unlike healthy heart cells, the cells of the failing heart seem to lack the ability to produce energy and use it for effective contractions. They are no longer able to effectively move calcium ions into and out of the cell. This defect in the calcium movement process may lead to further deterioration, because the muscle contracts ineffectively and is unable to deliver blood to the cardiac muscle itself.

Signs and Symptoms of Congestive Heart Failure

The patient with CHF presents a predictable clinical picture that reflects not only the problems with heart pumping but also the compensatory mechanisms that are working to balance the problem. Cardiomegaly can be detected using radiography, electrocardiography (ECG), or direct percussion and palpation. The heart rate will be rapid secondary to sympathetic stimulation, and the patient may develop atrial flutter or fibrillation as atrial cells are stretched and damaged. Anxiety often occurs as the body stimulates the sympathetic stress reaction. Heart murmurs may develop when the muscle is no longer able to support the papillary muscles or the annuli supporting the cardiac valves. Peripheral congestion and edema occur as the blood starts to engorge vessels as it waits to be pumped through the heart. Enlarged liver (hepatomegaly); enlarged spleen (splenomegaly); decreased blood flow to the gastrointestinal (GI) tract causing feelings of nausea and abdominal pain; swollen legs and feet; dependent edema in the coccyx or other dependent areas, with decreased peripheral pulses and hypoxia of those tissues; and, with left-sided failure, edema of the lungs reflected in engorged vessels and increased hydrostatic pressure throughout the cardiovascular system, are also seen (Figure 44.3).

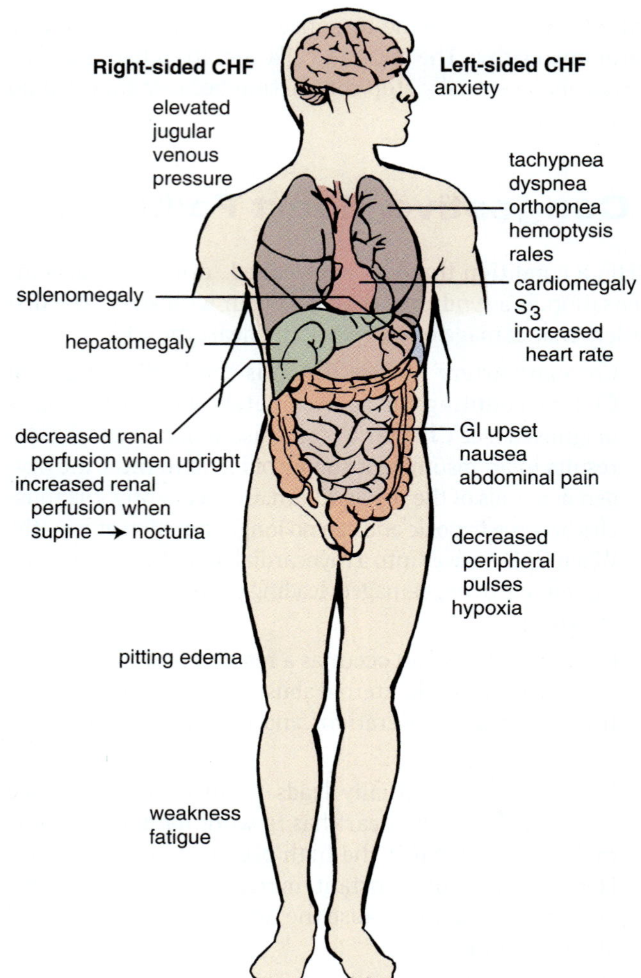

FIGURE 44.3 Signs and symptoms of congestive heart failure (CHF).

Left-Sided Congestive Heart Failure

Left-sided CHF reflects engorgement of the pulmonary veins, which eventually leads to difficulty in breathing. Patients complain of **tachypnea** (rapid, shallow respirations); **dyspnea** (discomfort with breathing often accompanied by a panicked feeling of being unable to breathe); and **orthopnea** (increased difficulty breathing when lying down). Orthopnea occurs in the supine position when the pattern of blood flow changes because of the effects of gravity, which causes increased pressure and perfusion in the lungs. Orthopnea is usually relieved when the patient sits up, thereby reducing the blood flow through the lungs. The degree of CHF is often calculated by the number of pillows required to get relief (e.g., one-pillow, two-pillow, or three-pillow orthopnea).

The patient with left-sided CHF may also experience coughing and **hemoptysis** (coughing up of blood). Rales may be present, signaling the presence of fluid in the lung tissue. In severe cases, the patient may develop pulmonary edema; this can be life-threatening because, as the spaces in the lungs fill up with fluid, there is no place for gas exchange to occur (Figure 44.4).

Right-Sided Congestive Heart Failure

Right-sided CHF usually occurs as a result of chronic obstructive pulmonary disease (COPD) or other lung diseases that elevate the pulmonary pressure. It often results when the right side of the heart, normally a very low-pressure system, must generate more and more force to move the blood into the lungs (Figure 44.5).

In right-sided CHF, venous return to the heart is decreased because of the increased pressure in the right side of the heart. This causes a congestion and backup of blood in the systemic system. Jugular venous pressure (JVP) rises and can be seen in distended neck veins, reflecting increased central venous pressure (CVP). The liver enlarges and becomes congested with blood, which leads initially to pain and tenderness and eventually to liver dysfunction and jaundice.

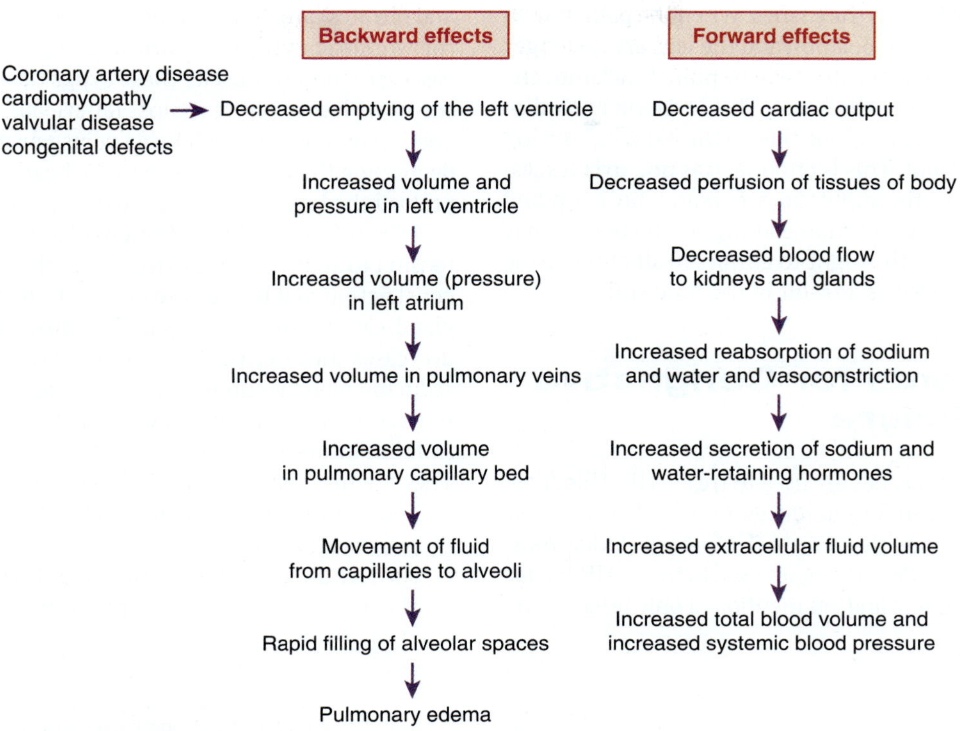

FIGURE 44.4 Highly schematic representation of the pathophysiology of left-sided heart failure.

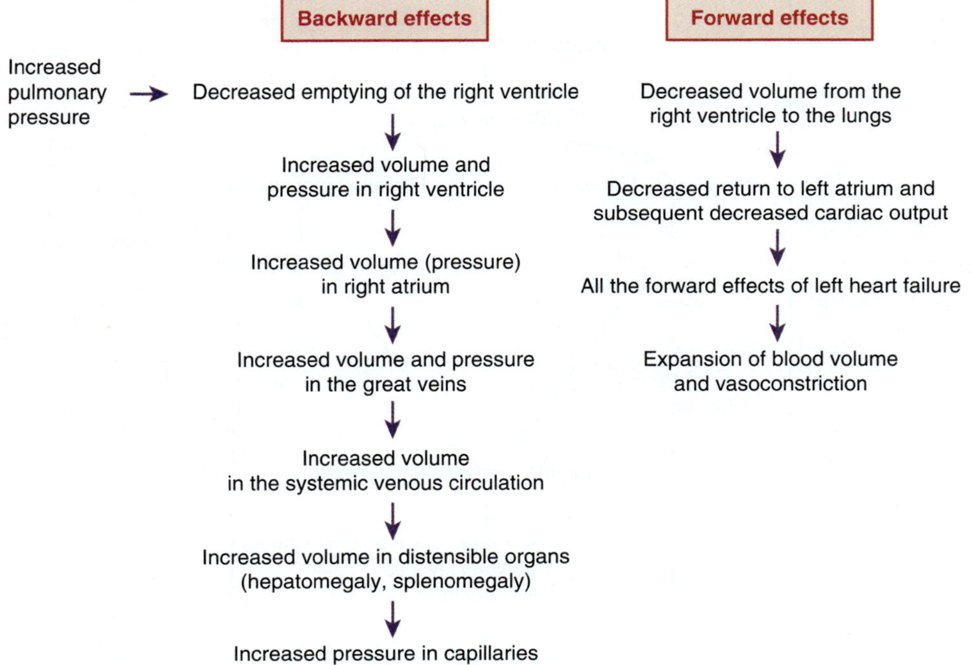

FIGURE 44.5 Highly schematic representation of the pathophysiology of right-sided heart failure.

Dependent areas develop edema or swelling of the tissues as fluid leaves the congested blood vessels and pools in the tissues. Pitting edema in the legs is a common finding, reflecting a pool of fluid in the tissues. When the patient with right-sided CHF changes position and the legs are no longer dependent, for example, the fluid will be pulled back into circulation and returned to the heart. This increase in cardiovascular volume increases blood flow to the kidneys, causing increased urine output. This is often seen as **nocturia** (excessive voiding during the night) in a person who is up and around during the day and supine at night. The person may need to get up during the night to eliminate all of the urine that has been produced as a result of the fluid shift.

Treatments for Congestive Heart Failure

Several different approaches are used to treat CHF. This chapter focuses on the cardiotonic drugs (also called inotropic drugs) that work to directly increase the force of cardiac muscle contraction. Other drug therapies used to treat CHF are discussed in other chapters and are mentioned only briefly here.

Vasodilators

Vasodilators (angiotensin-converting enzyme [ACE] inhibitors and nitrates) are used to treat CHF because they can decrease the workload of the overworked cardiac muscle. By relaxing vascular smooth muscle, these drugs decrease the pressure the heart has to pump against (afterload). They also cause a pooling of blood in stretchable veins when the vessels relax, decreasing the venous return to the heart and decreasing the preload the heart muscle has to deal with.

ACE inhibitors block the enzyme that converts angiotensin I to angiotensin II in the lungs, thus blocking the vasoconstriction and the release of aldosterone from the adrenal gland caused by angiotensin II (Figure 44.6). This in turn decreases the afterload by relieving vasoconstriction and by reducing blood volume through its effects on decreasing the release of aldosterone, which also decreases the afterload. ACE inhibitors are the vasodilators of choice in treating CHF. They are most effective in mild CHF and in patients who are at high risk for development of CHF or who have only beginning signs and symptoms.

Nitrates directly relax vascular muscle and cause a decrease in blood pressure and a pooling of blood in the veins (see

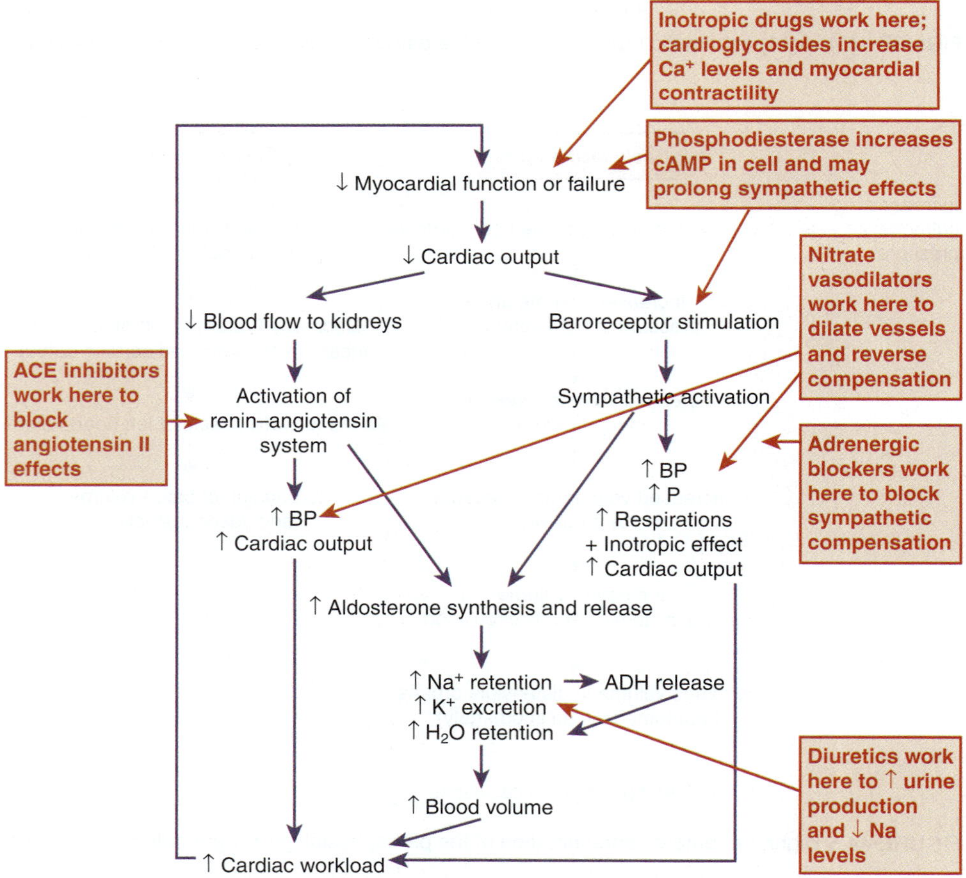

FIGURE 44.6 Sites of action of drugs used to treat congestive heart failure (CHF).

Figure 44.6). These two actions also decrease preload and afterload. Nitrates are often used to treat more severe CHF. (See Chapters 43 and 46 for additional information.) In 2005, a combination drug containing a nitrate and vasodilator was approved specifically for treating CHF in African American patients (see Box 44.1).

Diuretics

Diuretics are used to decrease blood volume, which decreases venous return and blood pressure (see Figure 44.6). The end result is a decrease in afterload and preload and a decrease in the heart's workload. Diuretics are available in mild to potent compounds and are frequently used as adjunctive therapy in the treatment of all degrees of CHF. (See Chapter 51 for additional information.)

Beta-Adrenergic Agonists

Beta-adrenergic agonists stimulate the beta receptors in the sympathetic nervous system, increasing calcium flow into the myocardial cells and causing increased contraction, a positive inotropic effect (see Figure 44.6). Other sympathetic stimulation effects can cause increased CHF, because the heart's workload is increased by most sympathetic activity. Dobutamine is the beta-agonist most frequently used to treat CHF. Because it must be given by intravenous infusion in an acute care setting, it is usually reserved for treatment of acute CHF. (See Chapter 30 for additional information.)

BOX 44.1 CULTURAL CONSIDERATIONS FOR DRUG THERAPY

Drugs for Congestive Heart Failure

In 2005, for the first time, the Food and Drug Administration approved a drug for use in a specific cultural group. The approval caused a great deal of debate and controversy because of the implications of having a drug approved only for use in African American patients. As a result of much debate, the drug was approved for use in self-identified African American patients with severe to moderate congestive heart failure (CHF). The drug, *BiDil*, is a fixed-combination drug containing isosorbide dinitrate and hydralazine. This combination of vasodilators was studied in 1999 in the Vasodilator–Heart Failure Study and was found to be only moderately effective in general, but was very effective in the subset of African American patients. Further studies were done, and the African American Heart Failure Study (A-HeFT) found that this combination of drugs had a significant impact in decreasing deaths and hospitalizations related to CHF in African American patients. African American patients have been found to be less responsive to angiotensin-converting inhibitors, a standard therapy for hypertension and CHF; this new combination showed real promise for treating this population. It is thought that there are race-related differences in endothelial functioning and responsiveness that could explain these findings. *BiDil* contains 20 mg isosorbide dinitrate and 37.5 mg hydralazine. In this combination, the drugs are rapidly absorbed and reach peak levels within 1 hour. They are both metabolized in the liver and have half-lives of 4 hours (hydralazine) and 3 to 6 hours (isosorbide). *BiDil* should not be taken with any of the phosphodiesterase inhibitors (sildenafil, vardenafil, tadalafil) because of the risk of serious hypotension. Adverse effects that occurred commonly with the use of this drug were headache, dizziness, and orthostatic hypotension.

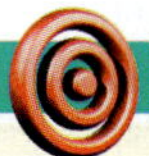

FOCUS POINTS

- In CHF, the heart pumps blood so ineffectively that blood builds up, causing congestion in the cardiovascular system.
- CHF can result from damage to the heart muscle combined with an increased workload related to CAD, hypertension, cardiomyopathy, valvular disease, or congenital heart abnormalities. As the heart pump fails, the muscle cells can no longer work to move calcium into the cell, and cardiac contractions become weak and ineffective.
- Signs and symptoms of CHF result from the backup of blood in the vascular system and the loss of fluid in the tissues. Right-sided CHF is characterized by edema, liver congestion, elevated jugular venous pressure, and nocturia, whereas left-sided failure is marked by tachypnea, dyspnea, orthopnea, hemoptysis, anxiety, and poor oxygenation of the blood.
- Treatment agents include vasodilators (to lighten the heart's workload); diuretics (to reduce blood volume and workload); beta-blockers (to decrease the heart's workload by activating sympathetic reaction); and cardiotonic (inotropic) agents (to stimulate more effective muscle contractions).

Cardiotonic Drugs

Cardiotonic (inotropic) drugs affect the intracellular calcium levels in the heart muscle, leading to increased contractility. This increase in contraction strength leads to increased cardiac output, which causes increased renal blood flow and increased urine production. Increased renal blood flow decreases renin release, breaking the effects of the renin–angiotensin system, and increases urine output, leading to decreased blood volume. Together, these effects decrease the heart's workload and help to relieve CHF. Two types of cardiotonic drugs are used: the classic cardiac glycosides, which have been used for hundreds of years, and the newer phosphodiesterase inhibitors. See Box 44.2 for the use of cardiotonic drugs in different age groups.

Cardiac Glycosides

The cardiac glycosides were originally derived from the foxglove or digitalis plant. These plants were once ground up to

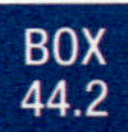

BOX 44.2 **DRUG THERAPY ACROSS THE LIFESPAN**

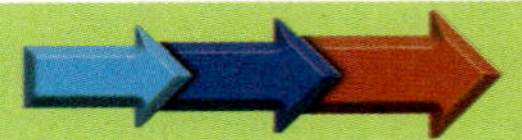

Cardiotonic Agents

CHILDREN

Digoxin is used widely in children with heart defects and related cardiac problems. The margin of safety for the dosage of the drug is very small with children. The dosage needs to be very carefully calculated and should be double-checked by another nurse before administration.

Children should be monitored closely for any sign of impending digitalis toxicity and should have serum digoxin levels monitored

The phosphodiesterase inhibitors are not recommended for use in children.

ADULTS

Adults receiving any of these drugs need to be instructed as to what adverse reactions to report immediately. They should learn to take their own pulse and should be encouraged to keep track of rate and regularity on a calendar. They may be asked to weigh themselves in the same clothing and at the same time of the day to monitor for fluid retention. Any changes in diet, gastrointestinal activity, or medications should be reported to the health care provider because of the potential for altering serum levels and causing toxic reactions or ineffective dosing.

Patients should also be advised against switching between brands of digoxin, because there have been reports of different bioavailabilities, leading to toxic reactions.

The safety for the use of these drugs during pregnancy has not been established. They should not be used in pregnancy unless the benefit to the mother clearly outweighs the potential risk to the fetus. The drugs do enter breast milk, but they have not been associated with any adverse effects in the neonate. Caution should be used, however, if one of these drugs is needed during lactation.

OLDER ADULTS

Older adults frequently are prescribed one of these drugs. They, like children at the other end of the life spectrum, are more susceptible to the toxic effects of the drugs and are more likely to have underlying conditions that could interfere with their metabolism and excretion.

Renal impairment can lead to accumulation of digoxin in the body. If renal dysfunction is present, the dosage needs to be reduced and the patient monitored very closely for signs of digoxin toxicity.

Inamrinone is metabolized in the liver, and patients with liver dysfunction may be at increased risk for toxicity. The dosage needs to be reduced and the patient monitored continually.

The total drug regimen of the older patient should be coordinated, with careful attention to interacting drugs or alternative therapies.

For backup in situations of stress or illness, a significant other should be instructed in how to take the patient's pulse and the adverse effects to watch for while the patient is taking this drug.

make digitalis leaf. Today, digoxin (*Lanoxin, Lanoxicaps*) is the drug most often used to treat CHF; it has a very rapid onset of action and is available for parenteral and oral use (Table 44.1). (Note that *Lanoxin* and *Lanoxicaps* have very different bioavailabilities; see Box 44.3.) It is excreted unchanged in the urine, making it a safe drug for patients with liver dysfunction. Digoxin has a very narrow margin of safety (meaning that the therapeutic dose is very close to the toxic dose), so extreme care must be taken when using this drug. Digoxin toxicity is a real possibility in clinical practice because of the narrow margin of safety. A digoxin antidote, digoxin immune Fab, has been developed to rapidly treat digoxin toxicity (see Box 44.4).

Therapeutic Actions and Indications

The cardiac glycosides increase intracellular calcium and allow more calcium to enter myocardial cells during depolarization (see Figure 44.6), causing the following effects:

- Increased force of myocardial contraction (a positive inotropic effect)
- Increased cardiac output and renal perfusion (which has a diuretic effect, increasing urine output and decreasing blood volume while decreasing renin release and activation of the renin–angiotensin system)
- Slowed heart rate, owing to slowing of the rate of cellular repolarization (a negative chronotropic effect)

Table 44.1 DRUGS IN FOCUS

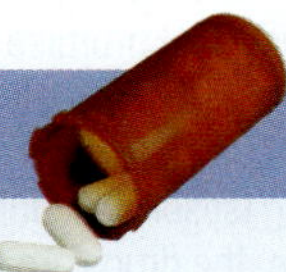

Cardiac Glycosides

Drug Name	Usual Dosage	Usual Indications
P digoxin (*Lanoxin, Lanoxicaps*)	Adult: loading dose 0.75–1.25 mg PO or 0.125–0.25 mg IV, then maintenance dose of 0.125–0.25 mg/day PO; decrease dosage with renal impairment Pediatric (dosage based on age): 10–60 mcg/kg PO or 8–50 mcg/kg IV loading dose, maintenance is 25%–30% of loading dose	Treatment of acute congestive heart failure, atrial arrhythmias

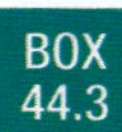

BOX 44.3

FOCUS ON THE **EVIDENCE**

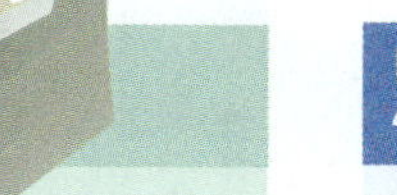

Lanoxin Versus Lanoxicaps

Digoxin comes in two similar-sounding, brand-name preparations: *Lanoxin* and *Lanoxicaps.* These drugs both provide digoxin, but the bioavailability of these two drugs is dramatically different.

Differences

Lanoxicaps are absorbed much more effectively—a 0.2-mg dose of *Lanoxicaps* is the equivalent of a 0.25-mg dose of *Lanoxin*, and the 0.1-mg capsule of *Lanoxicaps* is equivalent to the 0.125-mg tablet of *Lanoxin.* Digoxin has a very small margin of safety to begin with, and the room for error is much smaller with *Lanoxicaps.*

Safe Administration

Extreme care must be taken when administering either of these drugs to ensure that the right dose goes with the right brand name. Patient education should clearly identify the drug and dose being ordered. Patients should be warned not to trade or share medication because of the potential for serious problems. Here is an example of what can happen: A patient on vacation ran out of his *Lanoxin* tablets, which were ordered at 0.25 mg/day, and borrowed 0.1 mg *Lanoxicaps* from a friend. He took two and a half *Lanoxicaps* each day because he knew he should have 0.25 mg. As a result, the patient experienced digoxin toxicity and required hospitalization.

The names of these two drugs are so similar that it is easy to make a mistake in a patient care setting. By being alert to the possibility of a problem, the nurse may avert adverse consequences for the patient.

BOX 44.4

Digoxin Antidote: Digoxin Immune Fab

Digoxin immune Fab (*Digibind, Digifab*) is an antigen-binding fragment (Fab) derived from specific anti-digoxin antibodies. These antibodies bind molecules of digoxin, making them unavailable at their site of action. The digoxin antibody–antigen complexes accumulate in the blood and are excreted through the kidney. Digoxin immune Fab is used for the treatment of life-threatening digoxin intoxication (serum levels >10 ng/mL with serum potassium >5 mEq/L in a setting of digoxin intoxication) and potential life-threatening digoxin overdose.

The amount of digoxin immune Fab that is infused intravenously is determined by the amount of digoxin ingested or by the serum digoxin level if the ingested amount is unknown. The patient's cardiac status should be monitored continually while the drug is given and for several hours after the infusion is finished. Because there is a risk of hypersensitivity reaction to the infused protein, life-support equipment should be on standby.

Serum digoxin levels will be very high and unreliable for about 3 days after the digoxin immune Fab infusion because of the high levels of digoxin in the blood. The patient should not be redigitalized for several days to 1 week after digoxin immune Fab has been used, because of the potential of remaining fragments in the blood. The drug comes in two preparations: *Digibind* and *Digifab.* The dosing of the two preparations is subtly different, and care must be taken to check the brand name before administering the drug.

- Decreased conduction velocity through the atrioventricular node

The overall effect is a decrease in the myocardial workload and relief of CHF (Table 44.2). The cardiac glycosides are indicated for the treatment of CHF, atrial flutter, atrial fibrillation, and paroxysmal atrial tachycardia.

Pharmacokinetics

Digoxin is rapidly absorbed and widely distributed throughout the body. Digoxin is primarily excreted unchanged in the urine. Because of this, caution should be used in the presence

Table 44.2 Congestive Heart Failure and Response to Cardiac Glycosides

	Response	
Signs and Symptoms*	***During Congestive Heart Failure***	***After Full Digitalization†***
Heart rate, rhythm, and size	Heart hypertrophied, dilated; rate rapid, irregular; "palpitations"; auscultation—S_3	Dilatation decreased, hypertrophy remains; rate, 70–80 beats/min, may be regular; auscultation—no S_3
Lungs	Dyspnea on exertion; orthopnea; tachypnea; paroxysmal nocturnal dyspnea; wheezing, rales, cough, hemoptysis (pulmonary edema)	↓ Rate of respiration; wheezes, rales gone
Peripheral congestion	Pitting edema of dependent parts; hepatomegaly; ↑ jugular venous pressure; cyanosis; oliguria; nocturia	↑ Cardiac output and renal blood flow leads to ↑ urine flow, ↓ edema, ↓ signs and symptoms of poor perfusion
Other	Weakness, fatigue, anorexia, insomnia, nausea, vomiting, abdominal pain	↑ Appetite: ↑ strength, energy

*Because the clinical picture in heart failure varies with the stage and degree of severity, the signs and symptoms may vary considerably in different patients.

†Digitalization will not overcome similar symptoms when they are caused by conditions other than heart failure. Overdosage may actually cause symptoms similar to those of heart failure (e.g., anorexia, nausea, vomiting, cardiac arrhythmias, peripheral congestion).

of renal impairment, because the drug may not be excreted and could accumulate, causing toxicity. It is not known whether digoxin causes fetal toxicity; it should be given during pregnancy only if the benefit to the mother clearly outweighs the risk to the fetus. Digoxin does enter breast milk, but it has not been shown to cause problems for the neonate. Caution should be used, however, during lactation.

Contraindications and Cautions

Cardiac glycosides are contraindicated in the presence of allergy to any digitalis preparation. These drugs also are contraindicated in the following conditions: ventricular tachycardia or fibrillation, *which are potentially fatal arrhythmias and should be treated with other drugs;* heart block or sick sinus syndrome, *which could be made worse by slowing of conduction through the atrioventricular node;* idiopathic hypertrophic subaortic stenosis (IHSS), *because the increase in force of contraction could obstruct the outflow tract to the aorta and cause severe problems;* acute MI, *because the increase in force of contraction could cause more muscle damage and infarct;* renal insufficiency, *because the drug is excreted through the kidneys and toxic levels could develop;* and electrolyte abnormalities (e.g., increased calcium, decreased potassium, decreased magnesium), *which could alter the action potential and change the effects of the drug.*

Cardiac glycosides should be used cautiously in patients who are pregnant or lactating *because of the potential for adverse effects on the fetus or neonate.* Pediatric and geriatric patients also are at higher risk (see Box 44.5).

Adverse Effects

The adverse effects most frequently seen with the cardiac glycosides include headache, weakness, drowsiness, and vision changes (a yellow halo around objects is often reported with digoxin toxicity). GI upset and anorexia also commonly occur. A risk of arrhythmia development exists because the glycosides affect the action potential and conduction system of the heart.

Clinically Important Drug–Drug Interactions

There is a risk of increased therapeutic effects and toxic effects of digoxin if it is taken with verapamil, amiodarone, quinidine, quinine, erythromycin, tetracycline, or cyclosporine. If digoxin is combined with any of these drugs, it may be necessary to decrease the digoxin dose to prevent toxicity. If one of these drugs has been part of a medical regimen with digoxin and is discontinued, the digoxin dose may need to be increased. The risk of cardiac arrhythmias could increase if these drugs are taken with potassium-losing diuretics. If this combination is used, the patient's potassium levels should be checked regularly and appropriate replacement done. Digoxin may be less effective if it is combined with thyroid hormones, metoclopramide, or penicillamine, and increased digoxin dosage may be needed.

Absorption of oral digoxin may be decreased if it is taken with cholestyramine, charcoal, colestipol, bleomycin, cyclophosphamide, or methotrexate. If it is used in combination with any of these agents, the drugs should not be taken at the same time, but should be administered 2 to 4 hours apart. See Box 44.6 for information about the interactions between digoxin and common herbal remedies.

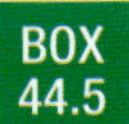

BOX 44.5 FOCUS ON THE EVIDENCE

Preventing Digoxin Toxicity in Children and the Elderly

Pediatric and geriatric patients are at increased risk for digoxin toxicity. Individuals in both of these groups have body masses that are smaller than the average adult body mass, and they may have immature or aging kidneys. Digoxin is excreted unchanged in the kidneys, so any change in kidney function can result in increased serum digoxin levels and subsequent digoxin toxicity. Extreme care should be taken when administering digoxin to patients in either of these age groups.

Pediatric Findings

Many institutions require that pediatric digoxin doses be checked by a second nurse before administration. This practice provides an extra check to help prevent the toxicity of this potentially dangerous drug. The patient should then be assessed before the drug is given, including careful cardiac auscultation and apical pulse measurement to monitor heart rate and rhythm to detect any possible toxic effects.

Geriatric Findings

Geriatric patients may not receive the same kind of attention as a policy, but they should be monitored for any factor that might affect digoxin levels when the drug is administered. Such factors may include

- Renal function (Is the blood urea nitrogen concentration elevated?)
- Low body mass (Is the patient underweight, undernourished, taking laxatives?)
- Current pulse, including quality and rhythm
- Hydration (Is the skin loose? Are the mucous membranes dry? The presence of these conditions could signal potential electrolyte disturbances.)

Many geriatric patients eventually need a decrease in dose, from 0.25 mg once a day to 0.125 mg once a day or 0.25 mg every other day. The nurse administering the drug is often in the best position to detect any changes in the patient's condition that might indicate a need for further evaluation.

BOX 44.6 HERBAL AND ALTERNATIVE THERAPIES

St. John's wort and psyllium have been shown to decrease the effectiveness of digoxin; this combination should be avoided. Increased digoxin toxicity has been reported with ginseng, hawthorn, and licorice. Patients should be advised to avoid these combinations.

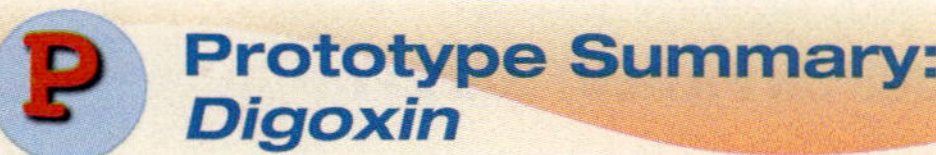

Indications: Treatment of CHF, atrial fibrillation

Actions: Increases intracellular calcium and allows more calcium to enter the myocardial cell during depolarization; this causes a positive inotropic effect (increased force of contraction), increased renal perfusion with a diuretic effect and decrease in renin release, a negative chronotropic effect (slower heart rate), and slowed conduction through the atrioventricular (AV) node

Pharmacokinetics:

Route	Onset	Peak	Duration
Oral	30–120 min	2–6 h	6–8 days
IV	5–30 min	1–5 h	4–5 days

$T_{1/2}$: 30–40 hours; largely excreted unchanged in the urine

Adverse effects: Headache, weakness, drowsiness, visual disturbances, arrhythmias, GI upset

Nursing Considerations for Patients Receiving Cardiac Glycosides

Assessment: History and Examination

Screen for the following conditions, *which could be cautions or contraindications to use of the drug:* known allergies to any digitalis product; impaired kidney function, *which could alter the excretion of the drug;* ventricular tachycardia or fibrillation; heart block or sick sinus syndrome; IHSS; acute MI; electrolyte abnormalities (increased calcium, decreased potassium, or decreased magnesium), *which could increase the toxicity of the drug;* and pregnancy or lactation, *because of the potential adverse effects on the fetus or neonate.*

Include screening *for baseline status before beginning therapy and for any potential adverse effects.* Assess the following: weight, skin color, and lesions; affect, orientation, and reflexes; pulse, blood pressure, perfusion, baseline electrocardiogram (ECG), and cardiac auscultation; respirations and adventitious sounds; abdominal examination and bowel sounds; renal function tests; and serum electrolyte levels.

Nursing Diagnoses

The patient receiving a cardiac glycoside may have the following nursing diagnoses related to drug therapy:

- Risk for Deficient Fluid Volume related to diuresis
- Ineffective Tissue Perfusion (Total Body) related to change in cardiac output
- Impaired Gas Exchange related to changes in cardiac output
- Deficient Knowledge regarding drug therapy

Implementation With Rationale

- Consult with the prescriber about the need for a loading dose when beginning therapy, *to achieve desired results as soon as possible.*
- Monitor apical pulse for 1 full minute before administering the drug, *to monitor for adverse effects.* Hold the dose if the pulse is less than 60 beats/min in an adult or less than 90 beats/min in an infant; retake pulse in 1 hour. If pulse remains low, document pulse, withhold the drug, and notify the prescriber, *because the pulse rate could indicate digoxin toxicity.*
- Monitor pulse for any change in quality or rhythm, *to detect arrhythmias or early signs of toxicity.*
- Check the dosage and preparation carefully, *because digoxin has a very small margin of safety, and inadvertent drug errors can cause serious problems.*
- Check pediatric dosage with extreme care, *because children are more apt to develop digoxin toxicity.* Have the dosage double-checked by another nurse before administration.
- Follow dilution instructions carefully for intravenous use; use promptly *to avoid drug degradation.*
- Administer intravenous doses very slowly over at least 5 minutes, *to avoid cardiac arrhythmias and adverse effects.*
- Avoid intramuscular administration, *which could be quite painful.*
- Arrange for the patient to be weighed at the same time each day, in the same clothes, *to monitor for fluid retention and CHF.*
- Avoid administering the oral drug with food or antacids, *to avoid delays in absorption.*
- Maintain emergency equipment on standby: potassium salts, lidocaine (*for treatment of arrhythmias*), phenytoin (*for treatment of seizures*), atropine (*to increase heart rate*), and a cardiac monitor, *in case severe toxicity should occur.*
- Monitor the patient for therapeutic digoxin level (0.5 to 2 ng/mL), *to evaluate therapeutic dosing and to monitor for the development of toxicity.*
- Provide comfort measures *to help the patient tolerate drug effects.* These include small, frequent meals;

access to bathroom facilities if GI upset is severe; environmental controls; safety precautions; adequate lighting if vision changes occur; positioning for comfort; and frequent rest periods to balance supply and demand of oxygen.

- Provide thorough patient teaching, including the name of the drug, dosage prescribed, proper administration, measures to avoid adverse effects, warning signs of problems, and the need for periodic monitoring and evaluation, *to enhance patient knowledge about drug therapy and to promote compliance* (see Critical Thinking Scenario 44-1).
- Offer support and encouragement, *to help the patient deal with the diagnosis and the drug regimen.*

Evaluation

- Monitor patient response to the drug (improvement in signs and symptoms of CHF, resolution of atrial arrhythmias, serum digoxin level of 0.5 to 2 ng/mL).
- Monitor for adverse effects (vision changes, arrhythmias, CHF, headache, dizziness, drowsiness, GI upset, nausea).
- Evaluate the effectiveness of the teaching plan (patient can name drug, dosage, proper administration, adverse effects to watch for, specific measures to avoid adverse effects, and the importance of continued follow-up).
- Monitor the effectiveness of comfort measures and compliance to the regimen.

Phosphodiesterase Inhibitors

The phosphodiesterase inhibitors belong to a second class of drugs that act as cardiotonic (inotropic) agents. Inamrinone (*Inocor*) is available only for intravenous use and is approved only for use in patients with CHF who have not responded to digoxin, diuretics, or vasodilators. Milrinone (*Primacor*) is available only for intravenous use for the short-term management of CHF in patients who are receiving digoxin and diuretics. Because these drugs have been associated with the development of potentially fatal ventricular arrhythmias, their use is limited to severe situations (Table 44.3).

Therapeutic Actions and Indications

The phosphodiesterase inhibitors block the enzyme phosphodiesterase. This blocking effect leads to an increase in myocardial cell cyclic adenosine monophosphate (cAMP), which increases calcium levels in the cell (see Figure 44.6). Increased cellular calcium causes a stronger contraction and prolongs the effects of sympathetic stimulation, which can lead to vasodilation, increased oxygen consumption, and arrhythmias. These drugs are indicated for the short-term treatment of CHF that has not responded to digoxin or diuretics alone or that has had a poor response to digoxin, diuretics, and vasodilators.

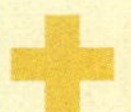

FOCUS ON PATIENT SAFETY

Inamrinone used to be called amrinone, but the U.S. Food and Drug Administration (FDA) required that the name be changed to help reduce errors. Name confusion occurred many times between amrinone and amiodarone, both drugs used in cardiac conditions. Be cautious when using amiodarone or inamrinone, because name confusion may still occur.

Pharmacokinetics

These drugs are widely distributed after injection. They are metabolized in the liver and excreted primarily in the urine. There are no adequate studies about the effects of these drugs during pregnancy, and their use should be reserved for situations in which the benefit to the mother clearly outweighs the potential risk to the fetus. It is not known whether these drugs enter breast milk, so caution should be used if patient is breast-feeding.

Contraindications and Cautions

Phosphodiesterase inhibitors are contraindicated in the presence of allergy to either of these drugs or to bisulfites. They also are contraindicated in the following conditions: severe aortic or pulmonic valvular disease, *which could be exacerbated by increased contraction;* acute MI, *which could be exacerbated by increased oxygen consumption and increased force of contraction;* fluid volume deficit, *which could be made worse by increased renal perfusion;* and ventricular arrhythmias, *which could be exacerbated by these drugs.*

Caution should be used in the elderly, *who are more likely to develop adverse effects,* and in pregnant or lactating women, *because of potential adverse effects on the fetus or neonate.*

Adverse Effects

The adverse effects most frequently seen with these drugs are ventricular arrhythmias (which can progress to fatal ventricular fibrillation), hypotension, and chest pain. GI effects include nausea, vomiting, anorexia, and abdominal pain. Thrombocytopenia occurs frequently with inamrinone, and it also can occur with milrinone. Hypersensitivity reactions associated with these drugs include vasculitis, pericarditis, pleuritis, and ascites. Burning at the injection site is also a frequent adverse effect.

Clinically Important Drug–Drug Interactions

Precipitates form when these drugs are given in solution with furosemide. Avoid this combination in solution. Use alternate lines if both of these drugs are being given intravenously.

CRITICAL THINKING SCENARIO 44-1

Inadequate Digoxin Absorption

The Situation

G.J. is an 82-year-old white woman with a 50-year history of rheumatic mitral valve disease. She has been stabilized on digoxin for 10 years in a compensated state of congestive heart failure (CHF). G.J. recently moved into an extended care facility because she was having difficulty caring for herself independently. She was examined by the admitting facility physician and was found to be stable. Note was made of an irregular pulse of 76 beats/min with electrocardiographic documentation of her chronic atrial fibrillation.

Three weeks after her arrival at the nursing home, G.J. began to develop progressive weakness, dyspnea on exertion, two-pillow orthopnea, and peripheral 2+ pitting edema. These signs and symptoms became progressively worse, and 5 days after the first indication that her CHF was returning, G.J. was admitted to the hospital with a diagnosis of CHF. Physical examination revealed a heart rate of 96 beats/min with atrial fibrillation, third heart sound, rales, wheezes, 2+ pitting edema bilaterally up to the knees, elevated jugular venous pressure, cardiomegaly, weak pulses, and poor peripheral perfusion. G.J.'s serum digoxin level was 0.12 ng/mL (therapeutic range, 0.5 to 2 ng/mL). G.J. was treated with diuretics and was redigitalized in the hospital with close cardiac monitoring.

After her condition stabilized, G.J. reported that she knew she had been taking her digoxin every day because she recognized the pill. The only difference she could identify was that she was given the pill in the afternoon with a dish of ice cream, while at home she always took it on an empty stomach first thing in the morning. The nursing home staff confirmed that G.J. had received the drug daily in the afternoon and that it was the same brand name she had used at home.

Critical Thinking

What nursing interventions should be done at this point? *Think about the signs and symptoms of CHF and how they show the progression of the heart failure.*

How could the change in the timing of drug administration be related to the decreased serum digoxin levels noted on G.J.'s admission?

Consider the factors that affect absorption of a drug. What alterations in dosing could be suggested that would prevent this from happening to G.J. again?

What potential problems with trust could develop for G.J. on her return to the nursing home? Suggest an explanation for what happened to G.J. and possible ways that this problem could have been averted.

Discussion

G.J.'s immediate needs involve trying to alleviate the alteration to her cardiac output that occurred when she lost the therapeutic effects of digoxin. Positioning, cool environment, small and frequent meals, and rest periods can help to decrease the workload on her heart. Digoxin has a small margin of safety and requires an adequate serum level to be therapeutic. G.J. was not absorbing enough digoxin to achieve a therapeutic serum level; consequently, her body began to go through the progression of CHF, first right-sided and then left-sided.

Nursing Care Guide For G.J.: Digoxin

Assessment: History And Examination

Assess the patient's health history for allergies to any digitalis product, renal dysfunction, IHSS, pregnancy, lactation, arrhythmias, heart block, and electrolyte abnormalities

Focus the physical examination on the following areas:

CV: blood pressure, pulse, perfusion, ECG

Neuro (CNS): orientation, affect, reflexes, vision

Skin: color, lesions, texture, perfusion

Resp: respiratory rate and character, adventitious sounds

GI: abdominal examination, bowel sounds

Laboratory tests: serum electrolytes, body weight

Nursing Diagnoses

Decreased Cardiac Output related to cardiac effect

Deficient Fluid Volume related to diuretic effects

Ineffective Tissue Perfusion related to changes in cardiac output

Impaired Gas Exchange related to changes in cardiac output

Deficient Knowledge regarding drug therapy

Implementation

Administer a loading dose to provide rapid therapeutic effects.

(continued)

Inadequate Digoxin Absorption *(continued)*

Monitor apical pulse for 1 full minute before administering to assess for adverse and therapeutic effects.

Check dosage very carefully.

Provide comfort and safety measures: give small, frequent meals; ensure access to bathroom facilities; avoid intramuscular injection; administer intravenously over 5 min; keep emergency equipment on standby.

Provide support and reassurance to deal with drug effects.

Provide patient teaching regarding drug, dosage, adverse effects, what to report, safety precautions.

Evaluation

Evaluate drug effects: relief of signs and symptoms of CHF, resolution of atrial arrhythmias, serum digoxin levels 0.5 to 2 ng/mL.

Monitor for adverse effects, including arrhythmias, vision changes (yellow halo), GI upset, headache, drowsiness

Monitor for drug–drug interactions as indicated for each drug.

Evaluate effectiveness of patient teaching program.

Evaluate effectiveness of comfort and safety measures.

Patient Teaching For G.J.

- ☐ Digoxin is a digitalis preparation. Digitalis has many helpful effects on the heart; for example, it helps the heart to beat more slowly and efficiently. These effects promote better circulation and should help to reduce the swelling in your ankles or legs. It also should increase the amount of urine that you produce every day.
- ☐ Digoxin is a very powerful drug and must be taken exactly as prescribed. It is important to have regular medical checkups to ensure that the dosage of the drug is correct for you and that it is having the desired effect on your heart.
- ☐ Do not stop taking this drug without consulting your health care provider. Never skip doses and never try to "catch up" any missed doses, because serious adverse effects could occur.
- ☐ Learn to take your own pulse. Take it each morning before engaging in any activity. Write your pulse rate on a calendar so you will be aware of any changes and can notify your health care provider if the rate or rhythm of your pulse shows a consistent change.

  Your normal pulse rate is __________.
- ☐ Try to monitor your weight fairly closely. Weigh yourself every other day, at the same time of the day and in the same amount of clothing. Record your weight on your calendar for easy reference. If you gain or lose 3 lb or more in 1 day, it may indicate a problem with your drug. Consult your health care provider.
- ☐ Some of the following adverse effects may occur:
  - *Dizziness, drowsiness, headache:* Avoid driving or performing hazardous tasks or delicate tasks that require concentration if these occur. Consult your health care provider for an appropriate analgesic if the headache is a problem.
  - *Nausea, gastrointestinal upset, loss of appetite:* Small, frequent meals may help; monitor your weight loss; if it becomes severe, consult your health care provider.
  - *Vision changes, "yellow" halos around objects:* These effects may pass with time. Take extra care in your activities for the first few days. If these reactions do not go away after 3 to 4 days, consult with your health care provider.
  - Report any of the following to your health care provider: *unusually slow or irregular pulse; rapid weight gain; "yellow vision"; unusual tiredness or weakness; skin rash or hives; swelling of the ankles, legs, or fingers; difficulty breathing.*
- ☐ Tell any doctor, nurse, dentist, or other health care provider that you are taking this drug.
- ☐ Keep this drug, and all medications, out of the reach of children.
- ☐ Avoid the use of over-the-counter medications while you are taking this drug. If you think that you need one of these, consult with your health care provider for the best choice. Many of these drugs contain ingredients that could interfere with your digoxin.
- ☐ Consider wearing or carrying a medical identification to alert any medical personnel who might take care of you in an emergency that you are taking this drug.
- ☐ Schedule regular medical check-ups to evaluate the actions of the drug and to adjust the dosage if necessary.

Table 44.3 DRUGS IN FOCUS

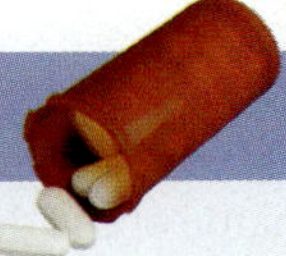

Phosphodiesterase Inhibitors

Drug Name	Usual Dosage	Usual Indications
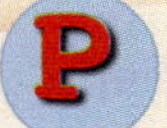 inamrinone (*Inocor*)	0.75 mg/kg IV bolus over 2–3 min; may be repeated in 30 min as needed; then 5–10 mcg/kg/min IV; do not exceed 10 mg/kg/day	Treatment of adults with congestive heart failure (CHF) not responsive to digoxin, diuretics, or vasodilators
milrinone (*Primacor*)	50 mcg/kg IV bolus over 10 min; then 0.375–0.75 mcg/kg/min IV infusion; do not exceed 1.13 mg/kg/day; reduce dosage in renal impairment	Short-term management of CHF in adults receiving digoxin and diuretics

P Prototype Summary: Inamrinone

Indications: Short-term treatment of CHF in patients who have not responded to digitalis, diuretics, or vasodilators

Actions: Blocks the enzyme phosphodiesterase, which leads to an increase in myocardial cell cAMP, which increases calcium levels in the cell, causing a stronger contraction and prolonged response to sympathetic stimulation; directly relaxes vascular smooth muscle

Pharmacokinetics:

Route	Onset	Peak	Duration
IV	Immediate	10 min	2 h

$T_{1/2}$: 3.6–5.8 hours; metabolized in the liver and excreted in urine and feces

Adverse effects: Arrhythmias, hypotension, nausea, vomiting, thrombocytopenia, pericarditis, pleuritis, fever, chest pain, burning at injection site

Nursing Considerations for Patients Receiving Phosphodiesterase Inhibitors

Assessment: History and Examination

Screen for the following conditions, *which could be cautions or contraindications to use of the drug:* any known allergies to these drugs or to bisulfites; acute aortic or pulmonic valvular disease, acute MI or fluid volume deficit, and ventricular arrhythmias, *which could be exacerbated by these drugs;* and pregnancy and lactation, *because of the potential adverse effects on the fetus or neonate.*

Include screening *for baseline status before beginning therapy and for any potential adverse effects.* Assess the following: skin color, lesions, and temperature; affect, orientation, and reflexes; pulse, blood pressure, perfusion, and baseline ECG; respirations and adventitious sounds; abdominal examination; and serum electrolytes and complete blood count.

Nursing Diagnoses

The patient receiving a phosphodiesterase inhibitor may have the following nursing diagnoses related to drug therapy:

- Decreased Cardiac Output related to arrhythmias or hypotension
- Risk for Injury related to CNS or cardiovascular effects
- Ineffective Tissue Perfusion (Total Body) related to hypotension, thrombocytopenia, or arrhythmias
- Deficient Knowledge regarding drug therapy

Implementation With Rationale

- Protect the drug from light, *to prevent drug degradation.*
- Monitor pulse and blood pressure periodically during administration, *to monitor for adverse effects so that dosage can be altered if needed to avoid toxicity.*
- Monitor input and output and record daily weights, *to evaluate resolution of CHF.*
- Monitor platelet counts before and regularly during therapy, *to ensure that the dose is appropriate;* consult with the prescriber about the need to decrease the dose at the first sign of thrombocytopenia.
- Monitor injection sites and provide comfort measures *if infusion is painful.*
- Provide life support equipment on standby *in case of severe reaction to the drug or development of ventricular arrhythmias.*
- Provide comfort measures *to help the patient tolerate drug effects.* These include small, frequent meals, access to bathroom facilities if GI upset is severe and if diuresis occurs, environmental controls, safety precautions, and orientation to surroundings.

- Provide thorough patient teaching, including the name of the drug, dosage prescribed, proper administration, measures to avoid adverse effects, warning signs of problems, and the need for periodic monitoring and evaluation, *to enhance patient knowledge about drug therapy and to promote compliance.*
- Offer support and encouragement, *to help the patient deal with the diagnosis and the drug regimen.*

Evaluation

- Monitor patient response to the drug (alleviation of signs and symptoms of CHF).
- Monitor for adverse effects (hypotension, cardiac arrhythmias, GI upset, thrombocytopenia).
- Evaluate the effectiveness of the teaching plan (patient can name drug, dosage, adverse effects to watch for, specific measures to avoid adverse effects, and the importance of continued follow-up).
- Monitor the effectiveness of comfort measures and compliance to the regimen.

WEB LINKS

Health care providers and patients may want to consult the following Internet sources:

http://www.jhbmc.jhu.edu/cardiology Information on diet, exercise, drug therapy, and cardiac rehabilitation.

http://www.jhbmc.jhu.edu/cardiology/rehab/patientinfo.html Patient information on the latest resources, diets, and programs.

http://www.americanheart.org Patient information, support groups, diet, exercise, and research information on heart disease and CHF.

http://www.aacn.org Specific information on the acute care of CHF from the American Association of Critical Care Nurses:

Points to Remember

- CHF is a condition in which the heart muscle fails to effectively pump blood through the cardiovascular system, leading to a buildup of blood or congestion in the system.
- CHF can be the result of a damaged heart muscle and increased demand to work harder secondary to CAD, hypertension, cardiomyopathy, valvular disease, or congenital heart abnormalities.
- The sarcomere, the functioning unit of the heart muscle, is made up of protein fibers—thin actin fibers and thick myosin fibers.
- Actin and myosin fibers react with each other and slide together, contracting the sarcomere, when calcium is present to inactivate troponin, an inhibitory compound that prevents this reaction. This sliding action requires the use of energy.
- Calcium enters the cell during the action potential after the cell has been stimulated. It gains entrance to the cell through calcium channels in the cell membrane and from storage sites within the cell.
- Failing cardiac muscle cells lose the ability to effectively use energy to move calcium into the cell, and contractions become weak and ineffective.
- Treatment for CHF can include the use of vasodilators (to reduce the heart's workload); diuretics (to reduce blood volume and the heart's workload); beta-blockers (which decrease the heart's workload precipitated by the activation of the sympathetic reaction); and cardiotonic (inotropic) agents (which directly stimulate the muscle to contract more effectively).
- Signs and symptoms of CHF reflect the backup of blood in the vascular system and the loss of fluid in the tissues. Edema, liver congestion, elevated jugular venous pressure, and nocturia reflect right-sided CHF. Tachypnea, dyspnea, orthopnea, hemoptysis, anxiety, and low blood oxygenation reflect left-sided CHF.
- Cardiac glycosides increase the movement of calcium into the heart muscle. This results in increased force of contraction, which increases blood flow to the kidneys (causing a diuretic effect), slows the heart rate, and slows conduction through the atrioventricular node. All of these effects decrease the heart's workload, helping to bring the system back into balance or compensation.
- Phosphodiesterase inhibitors block the breakdown of cAMP in the cardiac muscle. This allows more calcium to enter the cell (leading to more intense contraction) and increases the effects of sympathetic stimulation (which can lead to vasodilation but also can increase pulse, blood pressure, and workload on the heart). Because these drugs are associated with severe effects, they are reserved for use in extreme situations.

CHECK YOUR UNDERSTANDING

Answers to the questions in this chapter may be found in the Answer Key in the back of the book.

Multiple Choice

Select the best answer to the following.

1. Patients with CHF present clinically with
   a. cardiac arrest.
   b. congestion of blood vessels with slowing in delivery of nutrients and removal of waste products.
   c. a myocardial infarction.
   d. a pulmonary embolism.

2. Calcium is needed in the cardiac muscle
   a. to break apart actin–myosin bridges.
   b. to activate troponin.
   c. to allow actin–myosin bridges to form, causing contraction.
   d. to maintain the electrical rhythm.

3. A patient with right-sided CHF might exhibit edema
   a. in any gravity-dependent areas.
   b. in the hands and fingers.
   c. around the eyes.
   d. when lying down.

4. ACE inhibitors and other vasodilators are used in the early treatment of CHF. They act to
   a. cause loss of volume.
   b. increase arterial pressure and perfusion.
   c. cause pooling of the blood and decreased venous return to the heart, decreasing the workload of the muscle.
   d. increase the release of aldosterone and improve fluid balance.

5. Cardiotonic drugs are drugs that
   a. block the sympathetic nervous system.
   b. block the renin–angiotensin system.
   c. block the parasympathetic influence on the heart muscle.
   d. affect intracellular calcium levels in the heart muscle, leading to increased contractility.

6. A patient taking *Lanoxin* (digoxin) for the treatment of CHF would be advised to
   a. make up any missed doses the next day.
   b. report changes in vision or in heart rate.
   c. avoid exposure to the sun.
   d. switch to generic tablets if they are less expensive.

7. A nurse is about to administer *Lanoxin* to a patient whose apical pulse is 48 beats/min. She should
   a. give the drug and notify the prescriber.
   b. retake the pulse in 15 minutes and give the drug if the pulse has not changed.
   c. retake the pulse in 1 hour and withhold the drug if the pulse is still less than 60 beats/min.
   d. withhold the drug and notify the prescriber.

8. Before giving digoxin to an infant, the nurse would
   a. notify the prescriber that the dose is about to be given.
   b. check the apical pulse and have another nurse double-check the dose.
   c. make sure the infant has eaten and has a full stomach.
   d. check the apical pulse and give the drug very slowly.

Multiple Response

Select all that apply.

1. CHF occurs when the heart fails to pump effectively. Which of the following could cause CHF?
   a. Coronary artery disease
   b. Chronic hypertension
   c. Cardiomyopathy
   d. Fluid overload
   e. Pneumonia
   f. Cirrhosis

2. A client develops left-sided CHF after an MI. Which of the following would the nurse expect during the client assessment?
   a. Orthopnea
   b. Polyuria
   c. Tachypnea
   d. Dyspnea
   e. Blood-tinged sputum
   f. Swollen ankles

Web Exercise

J.D. calls your clinic asking for information about CHF. Her mother has been diagnosed with CHF, and J.D. is moving her to town so that she can care for her. However, J.D. does not know anything about CHF and wants to find out what she can expect. Use the Internet to obtain information that might be useful to J.D.; www.fda.gov/hearthealth might be a good starting point.

Word Scramble

Unscramble the following letters to form words related to the cardiotonic agents.

1. pnseyad ______________________
2. oneiirnlm ______________________
3. catoniur ______________________
4. topranheo ______________________
5. haptaceny ______________________
6. voteginsec thrae firaleu ______________________
7. nixgodi ______________________
8. potymsehis ______________________
9. yohitdarpaocmy ______________________
10. unimem abf ______________________

Bibliography and References

Abramowicz, M. (1996). Drugs for chronic heart failure. *Medical Letter, 38,* 985.

Drug facts and comparisons. (2006). St. Louis: Facts and Comparisons.

Gilman, A., Hardman, J. G., & Limbird, L. E. (Eds.). (2006). *Goodman and Gilman's the pharmacological basis of therapeutics* (11th ed.). New York: McGraw-Hill.

Karch, A. M. (2006). *2007 Lippincott's nursing drug guide.* Philadelphia: Lippincott Williams & Wilkins.

The medical letter on drugs and therapeutics. (2006). New Rochelle, NY: Medical Letter.

Porth, C. M. (2005). *Pathophysiology: Concepts of altered health states* (7th ed.). Philadelphia: Lippincott Williams & Wilkins.

CHAPTER 45

Antiarrhythmic Agents

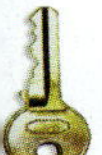

KEY TERMS

antiarrhythmics
bradycardia
cardiac output
Cardiac Arrhythmia Suppression Trial (CAST)
heart blocks
hemodynamics
premature ventricular contraction (PVC)
premature atrial contraction (PAC)
proarrhythmic
tachycardia

LEARNING OBJECTIVES

Upon completion of this chapter, you will be able to:

1. Describe the cardiac action potential and the processes occurring during each phase, and use this information to explain the changes made by each class of antiarrhythmic agents.
2. Describe the therapeutic actions, indications, pharmacokinetics, contraindications, most common adverse reactions, and important drug–drug interactions associated with antiarrhythmic agents.
3. Discuss the use of antiarrhythmic agents across the lifespan.
4. Compare and contrast the prototype drugs lidocaine, propranolol, sotalol, and diltiazem with other agents in their class and with other classes of antiarrhythmics.
5. Outline the nursing considerations, including important teaching points, for patients receiving antiarrhythmic agents.

CLASS IA ANTIARRHYTHMICS

disopyramide
moricizine
procainamide
quinidine

CLASS IB ANTIARRHYTHMICS

P lidocaine
mexiletine

CLASS IC ANTIARRHYTHMICS

flecainide
propafenone

CLASS II ANTIARRHYTHMICS

acebutolol
esmolol
P propranolol

CLASS III ANTIARRHYTHMICS

amiodarone
bretylium
dofetilide
ibutilide
P sotalol

CLASS IV ANTIARRHYTHMICS

P diltiazem
verapamil

OTHER

adenosine
digoxin

As discussed in earlier chapters, disruptions in impulse formation and in the conduction of impulses through the myocardium are called arrhythmias. (They also are called dysrhythmias by some health care providers.) Arrhythmias occur in the heart because all of the cells of the heart possess the property of automaticity (discussed later in this chapter) and therefore can generate an excitatory impulse. Disruptions in the normal rhythm of the heart can interfere with myocardial contractions and affect the **cardiac output**, the amount of blood pumped with each beat. Arrhythmias that seriously disrupt cardiac output can be fatal. Drugs used to treat arrhythmias suppress automaticity or alter the conductivity of the heart.

Review of Cardiac Conduction

As discussed in Chapter 42, each cycle of cardiac contraction and relaxation is controlled by impulses that arise spontaneously in the sinoatrial (SA) node of the heart. These impulses are conducted from the pacemaker cells by a specialized conducting system that activates all parts of the heart muscle almost simultaneously. These continuous, rhythmic contractions are controlled by the heart itself. This property allows the heart to beat as long as it has enough nutrients and oxygen to survive, regardless of the status of the rest of the body. The conduction system of the heart comprises the following:

- The SA node, located in the top of the right atrium, which acts as the pacemaker of the heart
- Atrial bundles that conduct the impulse through the atrial muscle
- The atrioventricular (AV) node, which slows the impulse and sends it from the atria into the ventricles by way of the bundle of His
- The bundle of His, which enters the septum and then divides into three bundle branches
- The bundle branches, which conduct the impulses through the ventricles; these branches break into a fine network of conducting fibers called the Purkinje fibers
- The Purkinje fibers, which deliver the impulse to the ventricular cells (Figure 45.1).

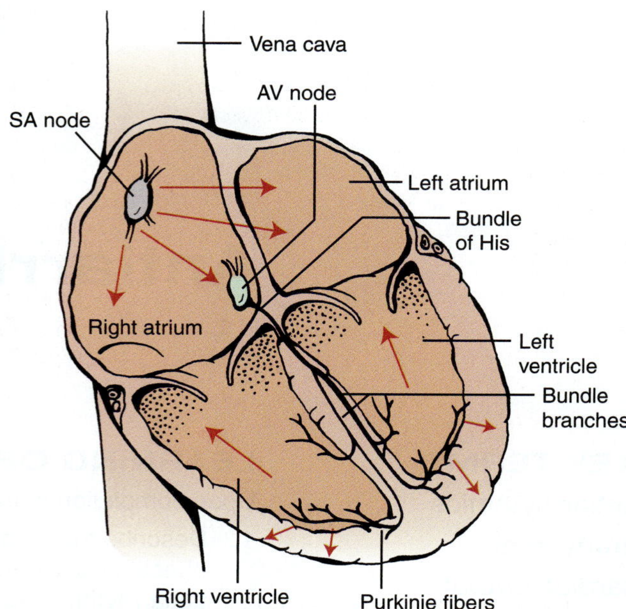

FIGURE 45.1 The conducting system of the heart. Impulses originating in the sinoatrial (SA) node are transmitted through the atrial bundles to the atrioventricular (AV) node and down the bundle of His and the bundle branches by way of the Purkinje fibers through the ventricles.

Automaticity of the Heart

All cardiac cells possess some degree of automaticity, as described in Chapter 42. These cells undergo a spontaneous depolarization during diastole or rest because they decrease the flow of potassium ions out of the cell and probably leak sodium into the cell, causing an action potential. This action potential is basically the same as the action potential of the neuron (described in Chapter 19).

The action potential of the cardiac muscle cell consists of five phases:

Phase 0 occurs when the cell reaches a point of stimulation. The sodium gates open along the cell membrane, and sodium rushes into the cell; this positive flow of electrons into the cell results in an electrical potential. This is called depolarization.

Phase 1 is a very short period during which the sodium ion concentration equalizes inside and outside of the cell.

Phase 2, or the plateau stage, occurs as the cell membrane becomes less permeable to sodium, calcium slowly enters the cell, and potassium begins to leave the cell. The cell membrane is trying to return to its resting state, a process called repolarization.

Phase 3 is a time of rapid repolarization as the sodium gates are closed and potassium flows out of the cell.

Phase 4 occurs when the cell comes to rest; the sodium–potassium pump returns the membrane to its resting membrane potential, and spontaneous depolarization begins again.

Each area of the heart has a slightly different-appearing action potential that reflects the complexity of the cells in that area. Because of these differences in the action potential, each area of the heart has a slightly different rate of rhythmicity. The SA node generates an impulse about 80 to 90 times a minute, the AV node about 40 to 50 times a minute, and the complex ventricular muscle cells about 10 to 20 times a minute.

Cardiac Arrhythmias

As noted earlier, various factors can change the cardiac rate and rhythm. Arrhythmias can be caused by changes in rate (**tachycardia**, which is a faster-than-normal heart rate, or **bradycardia**, which is a slower-than-normal heart rate); by stimulation from an ectopic focus, such as **premature atrial contractions (PACs)** or **premature ventricular contractions (PVCs)**, atrial flutter, atrial fibrillation (see Box 45.1), or ventricular fibrillation; or by alterations in conduction through the muscle, such as **heart blocks** and bundle branch blocks. Figure 45.2 displays an electrocardiogram (ECG) strip showing normal sinus rhythm; Figures 45.3, 45.4, 45.5, and 45.6 are ECG strips showing various arrhythmias.

Causes of Arrhythmias

The underlying causes of arrhythmias can arise from changes to the automaticity or conductivity of the heart cells. These changes can be caused by several factors, including

- Electrolyte disturbances that alter the action potential
- Decreases in oxygen delivered to the cells, which lead to hypoxia or anoxia and which change the cell's action potential and ability to maintain a membrane potential
- Structural damage that changes the conduction pathway through the heart
- Acidosis or accumulation of waste products that alters the action potential in that area

BOX 45.1 Understanding Atrial Fibrillation

Atrial fibrillation (AF) is a relatively common arrhythmia of the atria. It has been associated with coronary artery disease (CAD), myocardial inflammation, valvular disease, cardiomegaly, and rheumatic heart disease. The cells of the atria are connected side to side and top to bottom and are relatively simple cells. In contrast, the cells of the ventricles are connected only from top to bottom, with one cell connected only to one or two other cells. It is much easier, therefore, for an ectopic focus in the atria to spread that impulse throughout the entire atria, setting up a cycle of chaotic depolarization and repolarization. It is more difficult to stimulate fibrillation in the ventricles, because one ectopic site cannot rapidly spread impulses to many other cells, only to the cells connected in its two- or three-cell set.

Fibrillation results in lack of any coordinated pumping action, because the muscles are not stimulated to contract and pump out blood. In the ventricles, this is a life-threatening situation. If the ventricles do not pump blood, no blood is delivered to the brain, the tissues of the body, or the heart muscle itself. However, loss of pumping action in the atria per se does not usually cause much of a problem. The atrial contraction is like an extra kick of blood into the ventricles; it provides a nice backup to the system, but the blood will still flow normally without that kick.

Danger of Blood Clots

One of the problems with AF occurs when it exists for longer than 1 week. The auricles (those appendages hanging on the atria to collect blood; see Chapter 42) fill with blood that is not effectively pumped into the ventricles. Over time, this somewhat stagnant blood tends to clot. Because the auricles are sacks of striated muscle fibers, blood clots form around these fibers. In this situation, if the atria were to contract in a coordinated manner, there is a substantial risk that those clots or emboli would be pumped into the ventricles and then into the lungs (from the right auricle), which could lead to pulmonary emboli, or to the brain or periphery (from the left auricle), which could cause a stroke or occlusion of peripheral vessels.

Treatment Choices

Treatment of AF can be complicated if the length of time the patient has been in AF is not known. If a patient goes into AF acutely, drug therapy is available for rapid conversion. For example, ibutilide is often very effective when given intravenously for rapid conversion of the AF. Intramuscular quinidine also may convert AF effectively. In some situations, digoxin has been effective in converting AF. Electrocardioversion, a DC current shock to the chest, may break the cycle of fibrillation and convert a patient to sinus rhythm, after which the rhythm will need to be stabilized with drug therapy. Quinidine is often the drug of choice for long-term stabilization.

If the onset of AF is not known and it is suspected that the atria may have been fibrillating for longer than 1 week, the patient is better off staying in AF without drug therapy or electrocardioversion. Prophylactic oral anticoagulants are given to decrease the risk of clot formation and emboli being pumped into the system. Conversion in this case could result in potentially life-threatening embolization of the lungs, brain, or other tissues.

SVT: Another Danger

The other danger of AF is rapid ventricular response to the atrial stimuli, a condition called supraventricular tachycardia (SVT). With the atria firing impulses, possibly 200 to 300 a minute, the number of stimuli conducted into the ventricles is erratic and irregular. If the ventricle is responding too rapidly—more than 120 times a minute—the filling time of the ventricles is greatly reduced, causing cardiac output to fall dramatically. In these situations, and when AF is anticipated (such as with atrial flutter or paroxysmal atrial tachycardia), drugs may be given to slow conduction and protect the ventricles from rapid rates. Flecainide, propafenone, and propranolol are often used to convert rapid SVT. Esmolol, diltiazem, and verapamil are used intravenously to convert SVT with rapid ventricular response, which could progress to AF.

Implications for Nurses

Careful patient assessment is essential before beginning treatment for AF. If a history cannot be established from patient information and medical records are not available, it is usually recommended that AF be left untreated and anticoagulant therapy be started. This can pose a challenge for the nurse in trying to teach patients about why their rapid and irregular heart rate will not be treated and explaining all of the factors involved in the long-term use of oral anticoagulants.

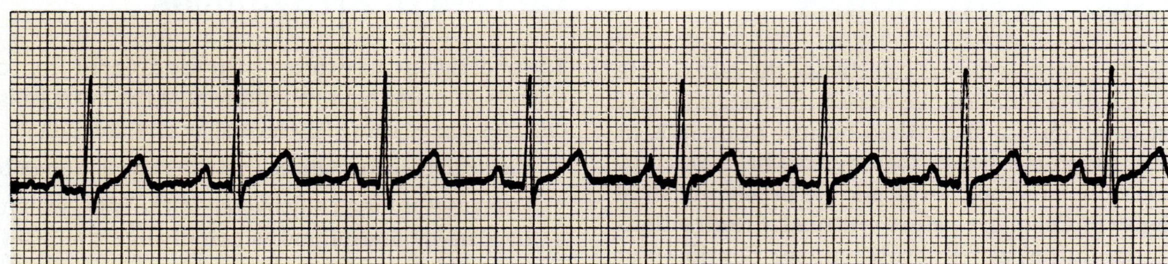

FIGURE 45.2 Normal sinus rhythm. Rhythm: regular. Rate: 60 to 100 beats/min. P-R interval: 0.12 to 0.20 seconds. QRS: 0.06 to 0.10 seconds.

In some cases, changes to the heart's automaticity or conductivity may result from drugs that alter the action potential or cardiac conduction.

Hemodynamics

The study of the forces that move blood throughout the cardiovascular system is called **hemodynamics**. The ability of the heart to effectively pump blood depends on the coordinated contraction of the atrial and ventricular muscles. The muscular walls of these chambers are activated to contract by impulses that arise at the SA node, travel through the atria, are delayed slightly at the AV node, and then stimulate the His–Purkinje system through the ventricles. The conduction system is designed so that atrial stimulation is followed by total atrial contraction and ventricular stimulation is followed by total ventricular contraction.

To be an effective pump, these muscles need to contract together. If this orderly initiation and conduction of impulses is altered, the result can be a poorly coordinated contraction of the ventricles that is unable to deliver an adequate supply of oxygenated blood to the brain and other organs, including the heart muscle itself. If these hemodynamic alterations are severe, serious complications can occur. For example, lack of sufficient blood flow to the brain can cause syncope or precipitate stroke; lack of sufficient blood flow to the myocardium can exacerbate atherosclerosis and cause angina or myocardial infarction (MI).

FOCUS POINTS

- Arrhythmias (also called dysrhythmias) are disruptions in the normal rate or rhythm of the heart.
- The cardiac conduction system determines the heart's rate and rhythm. Landmarks of the system include the SA node, which directs electrical impulses through the atria to the AV node, then through the bundle of His into the ventricles, and down bundle branches to the Purkinje fibers.
- The property by which the cardiac cells generate an action potential internally to stimulate the cardiac muscle without other stimulation is known as automaticity.
- Changes in the heart rate, uncoordinated heart muscle contractions, or blocks that alter the movement of impulses through the system can disrupt automaticity.
- Electrolyte disturbances, decreases in the oxygen delivered to the cells, structural damage in the conduction pathway, drug effects, acidosis, or the accumulation of waste products can trigger arrhythmias.
- Arrhythmias change the mechanics of blood circulation (hemodynamics), which can interrupt delivery of blood to the brain, other tissues, and the heart itself.

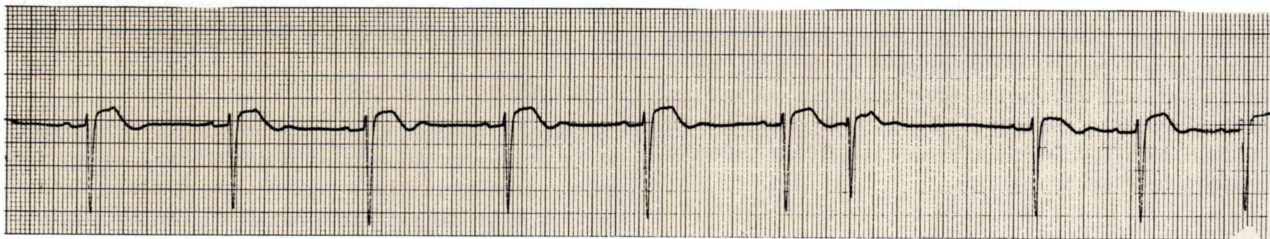

FIGURE 45.3 Premature atrial contractions (PACs). Rhythm: irregular due to the origination of a beat outside the normal conduction system (ectopic). Rate: normal sinus rate, except for PACs. P-R interval: P wave is abnormal and interval may be slightly shortened in ectopic beat. QRS: normal.

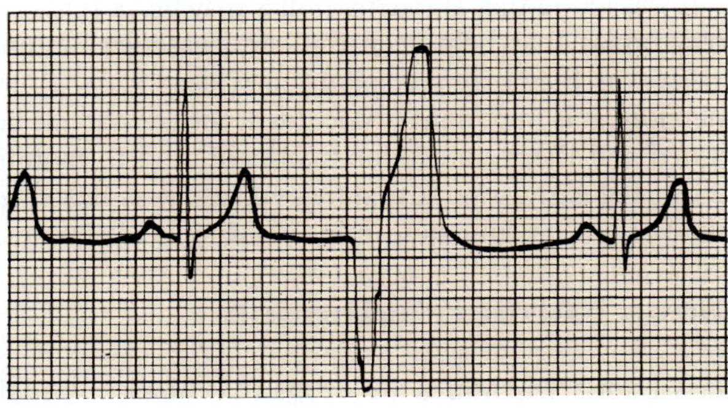

A

Premature ventricular contraction (PVC).

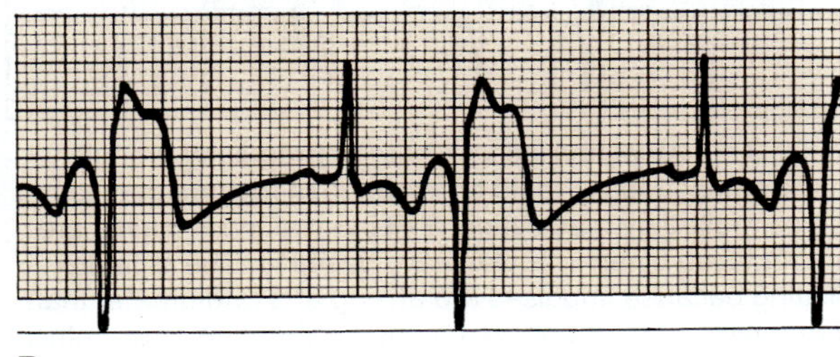

B

Ventricular bigeminy. (Every other beat is a PVC.)

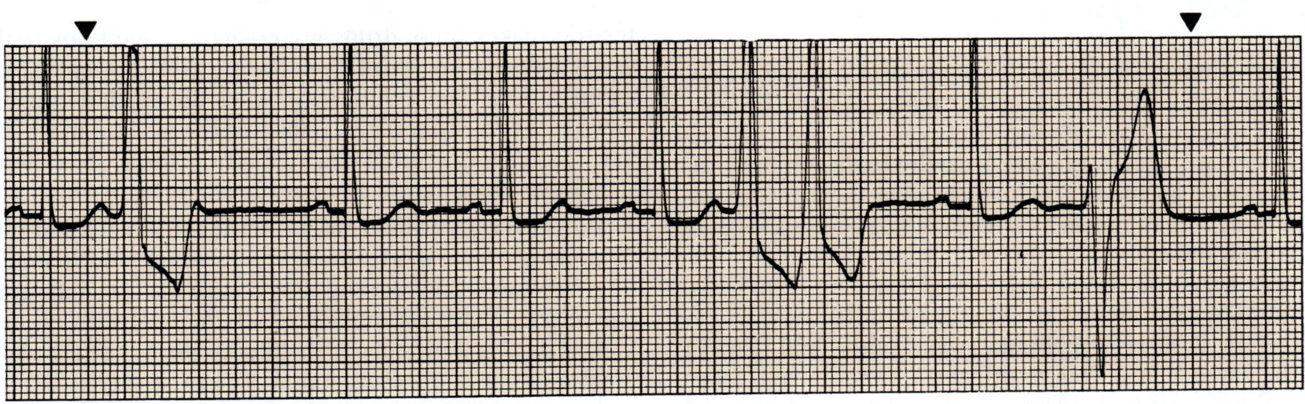

C

Multiformed PVCs.

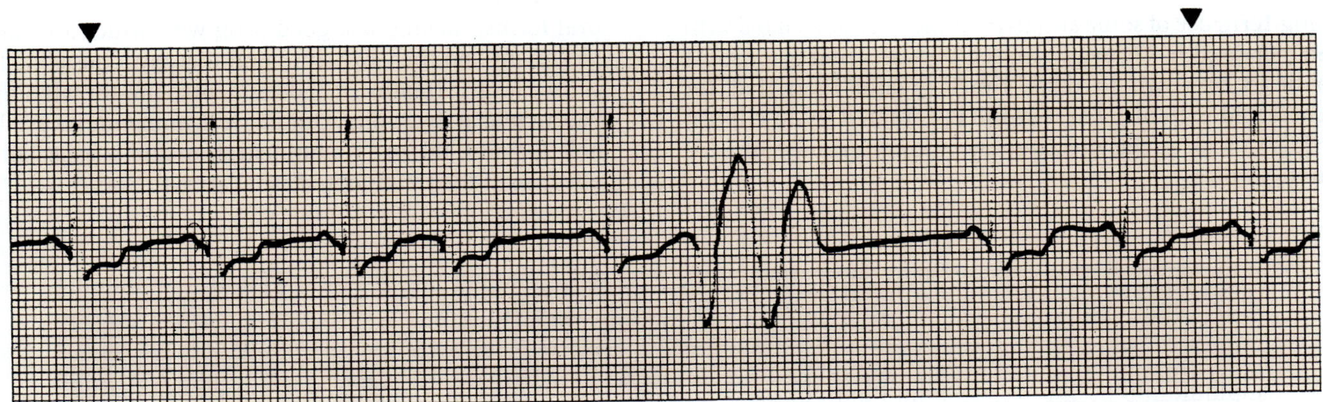

D

Heart block with PVCs.

FIGURE 45.4 Premature ventricular contractions (PVCs) or ventricular premature beats (VPBs). Rhythm: irregular. Rate: variable; only interrupts the cycle of the ectopic, ventricular contraction. P-R: normal in sinus beats, not measurable in PVCs. QRS: wide, bizarre, greater than 0.12 seconds.

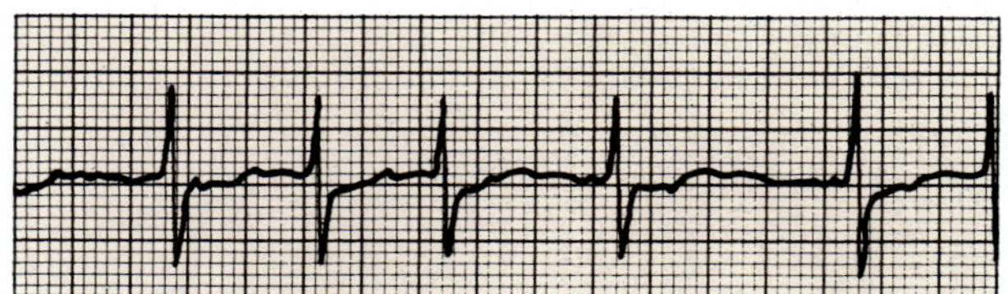

FIGURE 45.5 Atrial fibrillation. Rhythm: Irregularly irregular. Rate: variable; usually rapid on initiation of rhythm; decreases when controlled by medication. P-R interval: no P waves are seen, replaced by an irregular wavy baseline. The atria are fibrillating because impulses are arising at a rate greater than 350 per minute. The ventricles respond when the atrioventricular (AV) node is stimulated to threshold and can receive the impulse. QRS: normal.

Antiarrhythmic Drugs

Antiarrhythmics affect the action potential of the cardiac cells, altering their automaticity, conductivity, or both. Because of this effect, antiarrhythmic drugs can also produce new arrhythmias—that is, they are **proarrhythmic**. Antiarrhythmics are used in emergency situations when the hemodynamics arising from the patient's arrhythmia are severe and could potentially be fatal.

Antiarrhythmics were widely used on a long-term basis, to suppress any abnormal arrhythmia, until the publication of the **Cardiac Arrhythmia Suppression Trial (CAST)** in the early 1990s. This multicenter, randomized, long-term study, conducted by the National Heart, Lung and Blood Institute, looked at the mortality rate of patients with asymptomatic, non–life-threatening arrhythmias who were treated with antiarrhythmics. The results showed that long-term use of some antiarrhythmics was associated with an increased risk of death. In fact, the risk of death for some patients was two to three times greater than that for untreated patients. These results prompted more clinical trials to look at the effectiveness of long-term use of antiarrhythmics.

It was found that antiarrhythmics may block some reflex arrhythmias that help keep the cardiovascular system in balance, or they may precipitate new, deadly arrhythmias. Therefore, it is important to document the arrhythmia being treated and the rationale for treatment, and to monitor a patient regularly, when using these drugs. (See Box 45.2 for information on using these drugs in different age groups.)

Class I Antiarrhythmics

Class I antiarrhythmics are drugs that block the sodium channels in the cell membrane during an action potential (Figure 45.7). The class I drugs are local anesthetics or membrane-stabilizing agents. They bind more quickly to sodium channels that are open or inactive—ones that have been stimulated and are not yet repolarized. This characteristic makes these drugs preferable in conditions such as tachycardia, in which the sodium gates are open frequently. The class I antiarrhythmics are further broken down into three subclasses, reflecting the manner in which their blockage of sodium channels affects the action potential (Table 45.1).

- *Class Ia drugs* depress phase 0 of the action potential and prolong the duration of the action potential. Disopyramide (*Norpace*) is an oral drug that is available for adults and children and is recommended for the treatment of life-threatening ventricular arrhythmias. Moricizine (*Ethmozine*) is one of the drugs found to increase cardiac deaths because of its proarrhythmic effects. It is available in oral form, for adults only, and should be used only if the benefit clearly outweighs the risk. Procainamide (*Pronestyl*) is available in intramuscular (IM), intravenous (IV), and oral forms, making it a good drug with which to start treatment and then switch to oral therapy if possible. It is used for the treatment of documented life-threatening ventricular arrhythmias. Quinidine (*Quinaglute*) is available for oral, IM, or IV administration and is especially effective in the treatment of atrial arrhythmias.

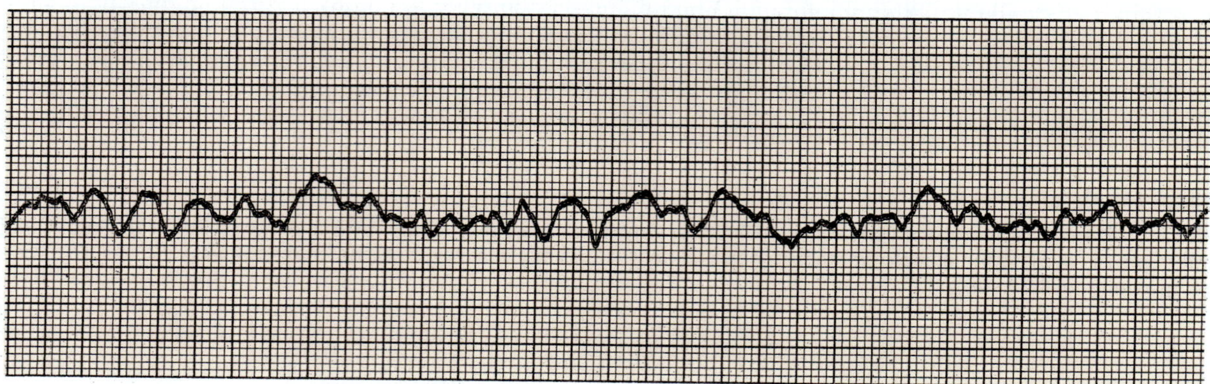

FIGURE 45.6 Ventricular fibrillation. Rhythm: irregular. Rate: not measurable. P-R interval: not measurable. QRS: not measurable, replaced by an irregular wavy baseline. No coordinated electrical or mechanical activity in the ventricle, no cardiac output.

BOX 45.2 DRUG THERAPY ACROSS THE LIFESPAN

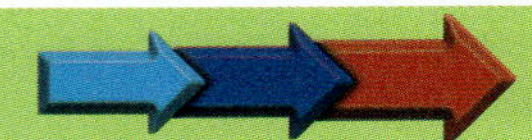

Antiarrhythmic Agents

CHILDREN

Antiarrhythmic agents are not used as often in children as they are in adults. Children who do require these drugs, after cardiac surgery or because of congenital heart problems, need to be monitored very closely to deal with the related adverse effects that can occur with these drugs.

Digoxin is approved for use in children to treat arrhythmias and has an established recommended dosage. If other antiarrhythmics are used, the dosage should be carefully calculated using weight and age and should be double-checked by another nurse before administration.

Adenosine, propranolol, procainamide, and digoxin have been successfully used to treat supraventricular arrhythmias, with propranolol and digoxin being the drugs of choice for long-term management. Verapamil should be avoided in children.

Many arrhythmias in children are now treated by ablation techniques to destroy the arrhythmia-producing cells. This has been very successful in treating Wolff–Parkinson–White and related syndromes in children. If lidocaine is used for ventricular arrhythmias related to cardiac surgery or digoxin toxicity, serum levels should be monitored regularly to determine the appropriate dosage and to avoid the potential for serious proarrhythmias and other adverse effects. The child should have continual cardiac monitoring.

ADULTS

Adults receive these drugs most often as emergency measures. Patient monitoring and careful evaluation of the total drug regimen should be a routine procedure to ensure the most effective treatment with the least chance of adverse effects. Frequent monitoring and medical follow-up is very important for these patients.

The safety for the use of these drugs during pregnancy has not been established. They should not be used in pregnancy unless the benefit to the mother clearly outweighs the potential risk to the fetus. The drugs do enter breast milk, and some have been associated with adverse effects on the neonate. Class I, III, and IV agents should not be used during lactation; if they are needed, another method of feeding the baby should be used.

OLDER ADULTS

Older adults frequently are prescribed one of these drugs. Older adults are more likely to develop adverse effects associated with the use of these drugs, including arrhythmias, hypotension, and congestive heart failure. They are also more likely to have renal and/or hepatic impairment related to underlying medical conditions, which could interfere with the metabolism and excretion of these drugs.

The dosage for older adults should be started at a lower level than that recommended for other adults. The patient should be monitored very closely and the dosage adjusted based on patient response. If other drugs are added or removed from the drug regimen, appropriate dosage adjustments may need to be made.

FOCUS ON **PATIENT SAFETY**

Confusion of the drug names *Procanbid* (procainamide) and *Procan SR* (a Canadian drug) has been reported, as well as confusion between the drug names *Procanbid* and probenecid. Use caution when administering any of these drugs, because dosages vary.

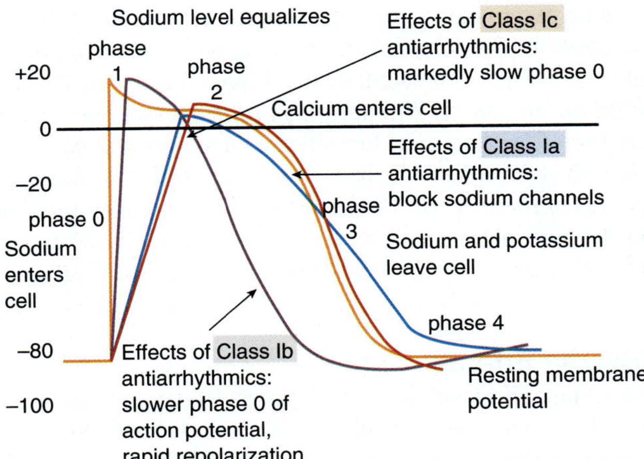

FIGURE 45.7 The cardiac action potentials, showing the effects of class Ia, Ib, and Ic antiarrhythmics.

- *Class Ib drugs* depress phase 0 somewhat and actually shorten the duration of the action potential. Lidocaine (*Xylocaine*), a frequently used antiarrhythmic, is administered by the IM or IV route to manage acute ventricular arrhythmias in patients with MI or during cardiac surgery. It also can be a bolus injection in emergencies when monitoring is not available to document the exact arrhythmia. Mexiletine (*Mexitil*) is an oral drug that is approved only for use in life-threatening arrhythmias. The CAST showed that its use may not affect mortality.
- *Class Ic drugs* markedly depress phase 0, with a resultant extreme slowing of conduction. They have little effect on the duration of the action potential. Flecainide (*Tambocor*) is a class Ic drug that was found to increase the risk of death in the CAST study. It is available as an oral drug for use in the treatment of life-threatening ventricular arrhythmias and for the prevention of paroxysmal atrial tachycardia (PAT) in symptomatic patients without structural heart disease. Propafenone (*Rythmol*) is another oral class Ic drug that can be used to treat potentially life-threatening ventricular arrhythmias and for prevention of PAT in symptomatic patients who are without structural heart defects.

Therapeutic Actions and Indications

The class I antiarrhythmics stabilize the cell membrane by binding to sodium channels, depressing phase 0 of the action

Table 45.1 DRUGS IN FOCUS

Class I Antiarrhythmics

Drug Name	Usual Dosage	Usual Indications
Class Ia		
disopyramide (*Norpace*)	Adult: 400–800 mg/day PO in divided doses q6–12h; use lower doses with older patients Pediatric: 6–30 mg/kg/day PO in divided doses q6h, base dosage on age	Treatment of life-threatening ventricular arrhythmias
moricizine (*Ethmozine*)	600–900 mg/day PO in divided doses q8h; start with <600 mg/day in older patients and those with hepatic impairment Pediatric: Do not use if <18 yr	Treatment of life-threatening ventricular arrhythmias
procainamide (*Pronestyl*)	Adult: 50 mg/kg/day PO in divided doses q3h; 0.5–1 g IM q4–8h; 500–600 mg IV over 25–30 min, then 2–6 mg/min IV Pediatric: 15–50 mg/kg/day PO in divided doses q3–6h; 20–30 mg/kg/day IM in divided doses q4–6h; 3–6 mg/kg IV over 5 min, then 20–80 mcg/kg/min IV	Treatment of life-threatening ventricular arrhythmias
quinidine (*generic*)	400–600 mg PO q2–3h; 600 mg IM, then 400 mg IM q2h as needed; 330 mg IV at a rate of 1 mL/min	Treatment of atrial arrhythmias in adults
Class Ib		
P lidocaine (*Xylocaine*)	Adult: 300 mg of 10% solution IM; 50–100 mg IV bolus at the rate of 20–50 mg/min; 1–4 mg/min IV infusion Pediatric: safety and efficacy not established; 1 mg/kg IV followed by 30 mcg/kg/min IV infusion has been recommended	Treatment of life-threatening ventricular arrhythmias during myocardial infarction or cardiac surgery; emergency treatment of ventricular arrhythmias when diagnostic tests are not available
mexiletine (*Mexitil*)	200 mg PO q8h up to 1200 mg/day PO may be needed	Treatment of life-threatening ventricular arrhythmias in adults
Class Ic		
flecainide (*Tambocor*)	50–100 mg PO q12h; reduce dosage as needed with older patients or renal impairment	Treatment of life-threatening ventricular arrhythmias in adults; prevention of paroxysmal atrial tachycardia (PAT) in symptomatic patients with no structural heart defect
propafenone (*Rythmol*)	150–300 mg PO based on patient response; start with lower dose and increase slowly with older patients	Treatment of life-threatening ventricular arrhythmias in adults; prevention of PAT in symptomatic patients with no structural heart defect

potential, and changing the duration of the action potential. They have a local anesthetic effect. These drugs are indicated for the treatment of potentially life-threatening ventricular arrhythmias and should not be used to treat other arrhythmias because of the risk of a proarrhythmic effect. Quinidine is especially effective in the treatment of atrial arrhythmias. Flecainide and propafenone are also used to prevent PAT in symptomatic patients who do not have structural heart defects.

Pharmacokinetics

These drugs are widely distributed after injection or after rapid absorption through the gastrointestinal (GI) tract. They undergo extensive hepatic metabolism and are excreted in urine. These drugs cross the placenta; although no specific adverse effects have been associated with their use, it is suggested that they be used in pregnancy only if the benefits to the mother clearly outweigh the potential risks to the fetus. These drugs enter breast milk and, because of the potential for adverse effects on the neonate, they should not be used during lactation. Another method of feeding the baby should be chosen.

Contraindications and Cautions

These drugs are contraindicated in the presence of allergy to any of these drugs; with bradycardia or heart block unless an artificial pacemaker is in place, *because changes in conduction could lead to complete heart block;* with congestive heart failure (CHF), hypotension, or shock, *which could be exacerbated by effects on the action potential;* with lactation, *because of the potential for adverse effects on the neonate;* and with electrolyte disturbances, *which could alter the effectiveness of these drugs.* Caution should be used with renal or hepatic dysfunction, *which could interfere with the biotransformation and excretion of these drugs,* and during pregnancy, *because of the potential for adverse effects on the fetus.*

Adverse Effects

The adverse effects of the class I antiarrhythmics are associated with their membrane-stabilizing effects and effects on action potentials. Central nervous system (CNS) effects can include dizziness, drowsiness, fatigue, twitching, mouth numbness, slurred speech, vision changes, and tremors that can progress to convulsions. GI symptoms include changes in taste, nausea, and vomiting. Cardiovascular effects include the development of arrhythmias (including heart blocks), hypotension, vasodilation, and the potential for cardiac arrest. Respiratory depression progressing to respiratory arrest can also occur. Other adverse effects include rash, hypersensitivity reactions, loss of hair, and potential bone marrow depression.

Clinically Important Drug–Drug Interactions

Several drug–drug interactions have been reported with these agents, so the possibility of an interaction should always be considered before any drug is added to a regimen containing an antiarrhythmic. The risk for arrhythmia increases if these agents are combined with other drugs that are known to cause arrhythmias, such as digoxin and the beta blockers.

Because quinidine competes for renal transport sites with digoxin, the combination of these two drugs can lead to increased digoxin levels and digoxin toxicity. If these drugs are used in combination, the patient's digoxin level should be monitored and appropriate dosage adjustment made. Serum levels and toxicity of the class I antiarrhythmics increase if they are combined with cimetidine; extreme caution should be used if patients are receiving this combination.

The risk of bleeding effects of these drugs increases if they are combined with oral anticoagulants; patients receiving this combination should be monitored closely and have their anticoagulant dose reduced as needed. Check individual drug monographs for specific interactions associated with each drug.

Clinically Important Drug–Food Interactions

Quinidine requires a slightly acidic urine (normal state) for excretion. Patients receiving quinidine should avoid foods that alkalinize the urine (e.g., citrus juices, vegetables, antacids, milk products), which could lead to increased quinidine levels and toxicity. Grapefruit juice has been shown to interfere with the metabolism of quinidine, leading to increased serum levels and toxic effects; this combination should be avoided.

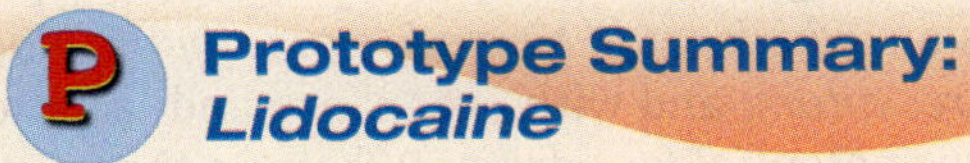

Prototype Summary: *Lidocaine*

Indications: Management of acute ventricular arrhythmias during cardiac surgery or MI

Actions: Decreases depolarization, decreasing automaticity of the ventricular cells; increases ventricular fibrillation threshold

Pharmacokinetics:

Route	Onset	Peak	Duration
IM	5–10 min	5–15 min	2 h
IV	Immediate	Immediate	10–20 min

$T_{1/2}$: 10 min, then 1.5–3 hours; metabolized in the liver and excreted in urine

Adverse effects: Dizziness, light-headedness, fatigue, arrhythmias, cardiac arrest, nausea, vomiting, anaphylactoid reactions, hypotension, vasodilation

Nursing Considerations for Patients Receiving Class I Antiarrhythmics

Assessment: History and Examination

Screen for the following conditions, *which could be cautions or contraindications to use of the drug:* any known allergies to these drugs; impaired liver or kidney function, *which could alter the metabolism and excretion of the drug;* any condition that could be exacerbated by the depressive effects of the drugs (e.g., heart block, CHF, hypotension, shock, respiratory dysfunction, electrolyte disturbances); and pregnancy and lactation, *because of the potential for adverse effects on the fetus or neonate.*

Include screening *for baseline status before beginning therapy and for any potential adverse effects.* Assess the following: body temperature and weight; skin color, lesions, and temperature; affect, orientation, reflexes, and speech; pulse, blood pressure, perfusion, and baseline ECG; respirations and adventitious sounds; bowel sounds and abdominal examination; and renal and liver function tests.

Nursing Diagnoses

The patient receiving an antiarrhythmic may have the following nursing diagnoses related to drug therapy:

- Disturbed Sensory Perception (Visual, Auditory, Kinesthetic, Gustatory, Tactile) related to CNS effects
- Risk for Injury related to CNS effects
- Decreased Cardiac Output related to cardiac effects
- Deficient Knowledge regarding drug therapy

Implementation With Rationale

- Continually monitor cardiac rhythm when initiating or changing dose, *to detect potentially serious adverse effects and to evaluate drug effectiveness.*
- Maintain life support equipment on standby, *to treat severe adverse reactions that might occur.*
- Give parenteral forms only if the oral form is not feasible; transfer to the oral form as soon as possible, *to decrease the potential for severe adverse effects.*

- Titrate the dose to the smallest amount needed to achieve control of the arrhythmia, *to decrease the risk of severe adverse effects.*
- Consult with the prescriber to reduce the dosage in patients with renal or hepatic dysfunction; reduced dosage may be needed *to ensure therapeutic effects without increased risk of toxic effects.*
- Establish safety precautions, including siderails, lighting, and noise control, if CNS effects occur, *to ensure patient safety.*
- Arrange for periodic monitoring of cardiac rhythm when the patient is receiving long-term therapy, *to evaluate effects on cardiac status.*
- Provide comfort measures, *to help the patient tolerate drug effects.* These include small, frequent meals; access to bathroom facilities; bowel program as needed; food with drug if GI upset is severe; environmental controls; orientation; and appropriate skin care as needed.
- Provide thorough patient teaching, including the name of the drug, dosage prescribed, measures to avoid adverse effects, and warning signs of problems as well as the need for periodic monitoring and evaluation, *to enhance patient knowledge about drug therapy and promote compliance with the drug regimen.*
- Offer support and encouragement, *to help the patient deal with the diagnosis and the drug regimen.*

Evaluation

- Monitor patient response to the drug (stabilization of cardiac rhythm and output).
- Monitor for adverse effects (sedation, hypotension, cardiac arrhythmias, respiratory depression, CNS effects).
- Evaluate the effectiveness of the teaching plan (patient can name drug, dosage, adverse effects to watch for, specific measures to avoid adverse effects, and the importance of continued follow-up).
- Monitor the effectiveness of comfort measures and compliance to the regimen (see Critical Thinking Scenario 45-1).

Class II Antiarrhythmics

The class II antiarrhythmics are beta-adrenergic blockers that block beta receptors, causing a depression of phase 4 of the action potential (Figure 45.8). In this way, these drugs slow the recovery of the cells, leading to a slowing of conduction and decreased automaticity. Several beta-adrenergic blockers are used as antiarrhythmics (Table 45.2).

Acebutolol (*Sectral*), an oral drug also used as an antihypertensive, is especially effective in the treatment of PVCs. Esmolol (*Brevibloc*), an IV drug, is used for the short-term management of supraventricular tachycardia and tachycardia that is not responding to other measures. Propranolol (*Inderal*) is used as an antihypertensive, antianginal, and antimigraine headache drug and as an antiarrhythmic to treat supraventricular tachycardias caused by digoxin or catecholamines.

Therapeutic Actions and Indications

The class II antiarrhythmics competitively block beta-receptor sites in the heart and kidneys, thereby decreasing heart rate, cardiac excitability, and cardiac output; slowing conduction through the AV node; and decreasing the release of renin. These effects stabilize excitable cardiac tissue and decrease blood pressure, which decreases the heart's workload and may further stabilize hypoxic cardiac tissue. These drugs are indicated for the treatment of supraventricular tachycardias and PVCs.

Pharmacokinetics

These drugs are absorbed from the GI tract and undergo hepatic metabolism. Food has been found to increase the bioavailability of propranolol, although this effect has not been found with other beta-adrenergic blocking agents. Because these drugs are excreted in urine, caution is required in patients with renal impairment. Teratogenic effects have occurred in animal studies with all of these drugs. The use of any beta-adrenergic blocker during pregnancy should be reserved for situations in which the benefit to the mother outweighs the risk to the fetus. In general, they should not be used during lactation because of the potential for adverse effects on the baby. The safety and efficacy for use of these drugs in children has not been established.

Contraindications and Cautions

The use of these drugs is contraindicated in the presence of sinus bradycardia (rate less than 45 beats/min) and AV block, *which could be exacerbated by the effects of these drugs;* with cardiogenic shock, CHF, asthma, or respiratory depression, *which could be made worse by the blocking of beta receptors;* and with pregnancy and lactation, *because of the potential for adverse effects on the fetus or neonate.*

Caution should be used in patients with diabetes and thyroid dysfunction, *which could be altered by the blockade of the beta receptors,* and with renal and hepatic dysfunction, *which could alter the metabolism and excretion of these drugs.*

Adverse Effects

The adverse effects associated with class II antiarrhythmics are related to the effects of blocking beta receptors in the sympathetic nervous system. CNS effects include dizziness, insomnia, dreams, and fatigue. Cardiovascular symptoms

CRITICAL THINKING SCENARIO 45-1

Recognizing Quinidine Toxicity

The Situation

R.A., a 56-year-old post–myocardial infarction patient with a documented duodenal ulcer, has felt highly "stressed" lately. He called the nurse with complaints of dizziness, confusion, headaches, nausea, vomiting, and a very slow pulse. The nurse requested that R.A. come in immediately to be evaluated. On examination, his pulse was 52 beats/min, and an electrocardiogram (ECG) showed second-degree heart block with occasional escape beats. His blood pressure was 82/60 mm Hg. He reported that he was still taking quinidine, which had been started after the myocardial infarction, to regulate arrhythmias. He stated that he had been taking *Mylanta* (an antacid) for ulcer pain, about 12 tablets a day, and that he has been drinking a lot of orange juice to treat a cold.

Critical Thinking

Based on your knowledge of the drug quinidine and the symptoms reported by R.A., what do you think happened?

If R.A. is found to be quinidine toxic, what should be done to alleviate his signs and symptoms and to return him to his normal cardiac rhythm?

What teaching points will be essential to convey to R.A. before he goes home?

Should any other problems be addressed while R.A. is being evaluated at this time?

Discussion

R.A. has many signs and symptoms of quinidine toxicity—slow pulse, atrioventricular heart block, hypotension, nausea, vomiting, dizziness, headache, confusion. The initial treatment for this condition includes withholding all medications, ordering blood drawn for a serum quinidine level determination, and careful monitoring of R.A., with emergency life support equipment on standby in case his condition deteriorates. (This equipment should include sodium lactate, which blocks the drug's effects on the myocardium, and adrenergic stimulants, which can increase blood pressure, pulse rate, and cardiac output.)

R.A. stabilized rapidly, and patient teaching on the current drug therapy was initiated. The effects of foods and drugs on urine pH and on quinidine excretion were stressed, and R.A. received a written list of foods and antacids that cause alkaline urine (e.g., citrus juices, milk, vegetables). Alkaline urine prevents quinidine excretion, thereby leading to a buildup of toxic quinidine levels. The combination of the orange juice and the numerous doses of antacid probably made R.A.'s urine quite alkaline, leading to increased serum levels of quinidine and a toxic response to the drug. The signs and symptoms of quinidine toxicity should be reviewed with R.A., as well as precautionary measures that he should take. He should be told that he did the correct thing in calling and should be encouraged to do so again if he has further problems. The teaching program should be directed at preventing future problems.

While R.A. is within the health care system, it is important to offer him support and encouragement. His ulcer can be evaluated at this time, as well as his feelings of stress. R.A. may need to ventilate his feelings and explore new ways of coping with or avoiding stressful situations. The effects of stress on the heart can be reviewed with R.A. to help him realize the importance of stress management. It would also be helpful to review the problems of self-medication for various complaints while taking a prescription drug. R.A. should receive all information in writing for future reference. Eventually, he may be re-evaluated to determine the actual need for continuing this medication. In the meantime, good patient education can help prevent serious complications while he is using the drug.

Nursing Care Guide for R.A.: Quinidine and Antiarrhythmic Agents

Assessment: History and Examination

Assess the patient's health history for allergies to quinidine and other antiarrhythmics, renal or hepatic dysfunction, heart block, congestive heart failure, shock, hypotension, electrolyte disturbances

Focus the physical examination on the following areas:

CV: blood pressure, pulse, perfusion

Neuro (CNS): orientation, affect, reflexes, vision

Skin: color, lesions, texture

Resp: respiratory rate and character, adventitious sounds

GI: abdominal examination, bowel sounds

Laboratory tests: liver and renal function tests, CBC

(continued)

Recognizing Quinidine Toxicity *(continued)*

Nursing Diagnoses

Disturbed Sensory Perception related to CNS effects

High Risk for Injury related to CNS effects

Decreased Cardiac Output related to CV effects

Deficient Knowledge regarding drug therapy

Implementation

Continually monitor cardiac rhythm when initiating or changing doses.

Provide comfort and safety measures: have life support equipment on standby; use parenteral form only if oral form cannot be used; titrate dose to smallest needed for therapeutic effects; reduce dosage with renal or hepatic dysfunction; lower dose with renal, hepatic impairment; use siderails, environmental controls as needed for safety; provide small frequent meals, access to bathroom facilities, skin care.

Provide support and reassurance to deal with drug effects.

Provide patient teaching regarding drug, dosage, adverse effects, what to report, and safety precautions.

Evaluation

Evaluate drug effects: stabilization of cardiac rhythm and output.

Monitor for adverse effects: sedation, dizziness, insomnia; cardiac arrhythmias; GI upset; respiratory depression.

Monitor for drug–drug interactions as indicated for each drug.

Evaluate effectiveness of patient teaching program and comfort and safety measures.

Patient Teaching For R.A.

- ☐ An antiarrhythmic drug, such as quinidine, acts to stop irregular rhythm in the heart, helping it to beat more regularly and therefore more efficiently. The drug may work by making the heart less irritable and by slowing it down to a more effective rate.
- ☐ When taking quinidine, plan to limit your intake of certain foods (e.g., citrus juices, milk, vegetables) and avoid over-the-counter drugs (e.g., antacids) that make your urine alkaline. If your urine becomes alkaline, you may develop signs of an overdose of quinidine, which may be signaled by very slow pulse. It is helpful to take your pulse on a regular basis. You should count the number of beats in 1 minute and determine whether your pulse is regular or irregular. Your usual resting heart rate is _____. Record your pulse on your calendar for easy reference.
- ☐ Quinidine and disopyramide may be taken with food if gastrointestinal upset occurs.
- ☐ If you are taking procainamide, remember to take it around the clock. You will need to have an alarm clock at night to awaken you to take your medication. It should be taken on an empty stomach. The best times for you to take procainamide are _____, _____, _____, _____.
- ☐ If you are taking the antiarrhythmic verapamil, take it on an empty stomach, 1 hour before or 2 hours after a meal.
- ☐ Some of the following adverse effects may occur:
  - *Tiredness, weakness:* Space your activities throughout the day and take periodic rest periods to help conserve your energy and rest your heart.
  - *Nausea, vomiting, loss of appetite:* These problems may pass over time; taking the drug with meals, if appropriate, or eating small, frequent meals may help.
  - *Sensitivity to light* (more pronounced with disopyramide): Avoid prolonged exposure to ultraviolet light or sunlight.
  - *Constipation or diarrhea:* These reactions are very common; if either occurs and becomes too uncomfortable, consult your health care provider.
  - Report any of the following to your health care provider: *chest pain, difficulty breathing, ringing in the ears, swelling in the ankles or legs, unusually slow pulse rate* (<35 beats/min), *unusually fast pulse rate* (>15 beats/min above your normal rate), *suddenly irregular pulse rate, fever, rash.*
- ☐ Tell any doctor, nurse, or other health care provider involved in your care that you are taking this drug.
- ☐ Keep this drug, and all medications, out of the reach of children.
- ☐ Avoid using over-the-counter medications while you are taking this drug. If you feel that you need one of these, consult with your health care provider for the best choice. Many of these drugs can interfere with the effects of your medication.
- ☐ Schedule regular medical appointments while you are on this drug, to evaluate your heart rhythm and your response to the drug.
- ☐ Do not stop taking this medication. If you have to stop the medication for any reason, contact your health care provider immediately.

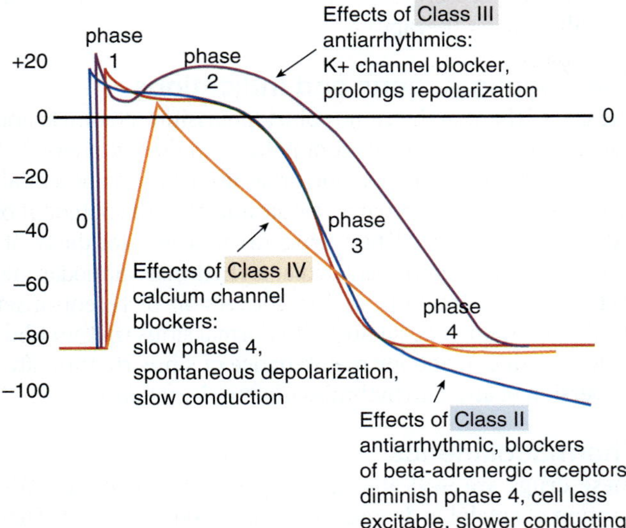

FIGURE 45.8 The cardiac action potentials, showing the effects of class II, III, and IV antiarrhythmics.

can include hypotension, bradycardia, AV block, arrhythmias, and alterations in peripheral perfusion. Respiratory effects can include bronchospasm and dyspnea. GI problems frequently include nausea, vomiting, anorexia, constipation, and diarrhea. Other effects to anticipate include a loss of libido, decreased exercise tolerance, and alterations in blood glucose levels.

Clinically Important Drug–Drug Interactions

The risk of adverse effects increases if these drugs are taken with verapamil; if this combination is used, dosage adjustment will be needed.

There is a possibility of increased hypoglycemia if these drugs are combined with insulin; patients should be monitored closely.

Other specific drug interactions may occur with each drug; check a drug reference before combining these drugs with any others.

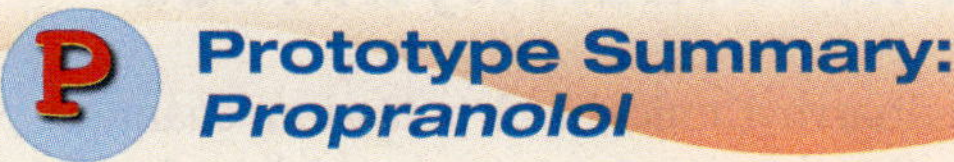

Prototype Summary: Propranolol

Indications: Treatment of cardiac arrhythmias, especially supraventricular tachycardia; treatment of ventricular tachycardia induced by digitalis or catecholamines

Actions: Competitively blocks beta-adrenergic receptors in the heart and kidney; has a membrane-stabilizing effect and decreases the influence of the sympathetic nervous system

Pharmacokinetics:

Route	Onset	Peak	Duration
Oral	20–30 min	60–90 min	6–12 h
IV	Immediate	1 min	4–6 h

$T_{1/2}$: 3–5 hours; metabolized in the liver and excreted in urine

Adverse effects: Bradycardia, CHF, cardiac arrhythmias, heart blocks, cerebrovascular accident (CVA), pulmonary edema, gastric pain, flatulence, nausea, vomiting, diarrhea, impotence, decreased exercise tolerance, antinuclear antibody (ANA) development

Nursing Considerations for Patients Receiving Class II Antiarrhythmics

The nursing considerations for patients taking any antiarrhythmic drug are outlined in the section on class I antiarrhythmics.

Table 45.2 DRUGS IN FOCUS

Class II Antiarrhythmics

Drug Name	Usual Dosage	Usual Indications
acebutolol (*Sectral*)	200–600 mg PO b.i.d., based on patient response; use lower doses with older patients; decrease dose by 50% with renal or hepatic impairment	Management of premature ventricular contractions in adults; intraoperative and postoperative tachycardia
esmolol (*Brevibloc*)	Loading dose of 500 mcg/kg/min IV, then 50 mcg/kg/min for 4 min, maintain with 100 mcg/kg/min IV infusion	Short-term management of supraventricular tachycardia in adults
P propranolol (*Inderal*)	10–30 mg PO t.i.d. to q.i.d.; 1–3 mg IV for life-threatening arrhythmias, may repeat in 2 min, then do not repeat for 4 h	Treatment of supraventricular tachycardias caused by digoxin or catecholamines in adults; treatment of hypertension, angina, migraine, situational anxiety

Class III Antiarrhythmics

The class III antiarrhythmics block potassium channels, prolonging phase 3 of the action potential, which prolongs repolarization and slows the rate and conduction of the heart (see Figure 45.8). Class III antiarrhythmics include a number of agents (Table 45.3).

- Amiodarone (*Cordarone*) is available as an oral or an IV drug. It should be used only to treat documented life-threatening arrhythmias, because it has been associated with serious and even fatal toxic reactions. In 2005, the American Heart Association issued new guidelines for Advanced Cardiac Life Support (ACLS) that named amiodarone the drug of choice for treating ventricular fibrillation or pulseless ventricular tachycardia in cardiac arrest situations.
- Bretylium (generic), which is administered IV or IM, is indicated for the short-term treatment of ventricular fibrillation or ventricular arrhythmias that do not respond to other drugs.
- Ibutilide (*Corvert*) is given IV to rapidly convert atrial fibrillation or atrial flutter of recent onset; it is most effective if the duration of atrial fibrillation/flutter is less than 90 days.
- A newer drug, dofetilide (*Tikosyn*) is used orally to convert atrial fibrillation or flutter to normal sinus rhythm and to maintain normal sinus rhythm after conversion.
- Sotalol (*Betapace, Betapace AF*) is an oral drug that is indicated for the treatment of documented life-threatening arrhythmias and for the maintenance of normal sinus rhythm after conversion of atrial arrhythmias. Because it is known to be proarrhythmic, patients should be monitored very closely at the initiation of therapy and periodically during therapy.

Therapeutic Actions and Indications

The class III antiarrhythmics block potassium channels and slow the outward movement of potassium during phase 3 of the action potential. This action prolongs the action potential. All of these drugs are proarrhythmic and have the potential of inducing arrhythmias. These drugs are indicated for the treatment of life-threatening ventricular arrhythmias (amiodarone, bretylium, and sotalol), for the conversion of recent-onset atrial fibrillation or atrial flutter to normal sinus rhythm (ibutilide, dofetilide), and for maintenance of sinus rhythm after conversion of atrial arrhythmias (dofetilide, sotalol).

Pharmacokinetics

These drugs are well absorbed and widely distributed. Absorption of sotalol is decreased by the presence of food. They are metabolized in the liver and excreted in urine. There are no well-controlled studies of effects during pregnancy, so use during pregnancy should be limited to those situations in which the benefit to the mother far outweighs any potential risk to the fetus. There is little good information about use during lactation. Because of the potential for adverse effects on the neonate, another method of feeding the baby should be used if the mother requires one of these drugs during lactation.

Contraindications and Cautions

When these drugs are used to treat life-threatening arrhythmias for which no other drug has been effective, there are no contraindications. Ibutilide and dofetilide should not be used in the presence of AV block, *which could be exacerbated by the drug.* Caution should be used with all of these drugs in the presence of shock, hypotension, or respiratory depres-

Table 45.3 DRUGS IN FOCUS

Class III Antiarrhythmics

Drug Name	Usual Dosage	Usual Indications
amiodarone (*Cordarone*)	800–1600 mg/day PO in divided doses for 1–3 wk, then 600–800 mg/day PO for 1 mo, reduce to 400 mg/day PO if rhythm is stable; 1000 mg IV over 24 h; then 540 mg IV at 0.5 mg/min for 18–96 h	Treatment of life-threatening ventricular arrhythmias not responding to any other drug; for use in adults only; preferred antiarrhythmic in Advanced Cardiac Life Support protocol
bretylium (generic)	Adult: 5 mg/kg IV bolus, then 1–2 mg/min by continuous IV infusion; 5–10 mg/kg IM repeated at intervals of 6–8 h Pediatric: 5 mg/kg per dose IV followed by 10 mg/kg at intervals of 15–30 min, maintain at 5–10 mg/kg per dose IV q6h	Treatment of ventricular fibrillation and ventricular tachycardias not responsive to other drugs
dofetilide (*Tikosyn*)	125–500 mcg PO b.i.d. based on creatinine clearance	Conversion of atrial fibrillation/flutter to normal sinus rhythm, maintenance of normal sinus rhythm after conversion for adults
ibutilide (*Corvert*)	1 mg infused IV over 1 min, may be repeated in 10 min if needed	Conversion of recent-onset atrial fibrillation/flutter in adults
P sotalol (*Betapace*)	80 mg/day PO, may be titrated to 240–320 mg/day PO, reduce dosage with renal impairment	Treatment of life-threatening ventricular arrhythmias not responding to any other drug; for use with adults
(*Betapace AF*)	80–120 mg PO daily to b.i.d. based on patient response	Maintenance of sinus rhythm after conversion in adults

sion; with a prolonged QTc interval, *which could be made worse by the depressive effects on action potentials;* and with renal or hepatic disease, *which could alter the biotransformation and excretion of these drugs.*

Adverse Effects

The adverse effects associated with these drugs are related to the changes they cause in action potentials. Nausea, vomiting, and GI distress; weakness and dizziness; and hypotension, CHF, and arrhythmia are common. Amiodarone has been associated with a potentially fatal liver toxicity, ocular abnormalities, and the development of very serious cardiac arrhythmias.

Clinically Important Drug–Drug Interactions

These drugs can cause serious toxic effects if they are combined with digoxin or quinidine.

Other specific drug–drug interactions have been reported with individual drugs; a drug reference should always be consulted when adding a new drug to a regimen containing any of these agents.

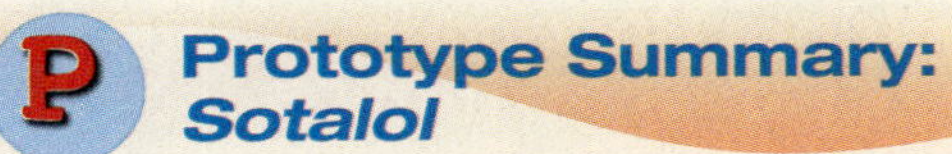

Prototype Summary: *Sotalol*

Indications: Treatment of life-threatening ventricular arrhythmias; maintenance of sinus rhythm to delay the time to recurrence of atrial fibrillation/flutter in patients with symptomatic atrial fibrillation/flutter who are currently in sinus rhythm

Actions: Blocks beta-adrenergic receptors in the heart, as well as potassium channels, prolonging phase 3 of the action potential, which prolongs repolarization and slows the rate and conduction of the heart

Pharmacokinetics:

Route	Onset	Peak	Duration
Oral	Varies	3–4 h	8–12 h

$T_{1/2}$: 12 hours; largely excreted unchanged in urine

Adverse effects: Laryngospasm, respiratory distress, CHF, cardiac arrhythmias, heart blocks, CVA, pulmonary edema, gastric pain, flatulence, constipation, diarrhea, nausea, vomiting, impotence, decreased exercise tolerance, ANA development

Nursing Considerations for Patients Receiving Class III Antiarrhythmics

The nursing considerations for patients taking any antiarrhythmic agent are outlined in the section on class I antiarrhythmics.

Class IV Antiarrhythmics

The class IV antiarrhythmics act to block calcium channels in the cell membrane, leading to a depression of depolarization and a prolongation of phases 1 and 2 of repolarization, which slows automaticity and conduction (see Figure 45.8). The calcium channel blockers are used as antihypertensives (see Chapter 43) and to treat angina (see Chapter 46). The two calcium channel blockers that seem to have special effects on the heart muscle are diltiazem (*Cardizem*), which is administered IV to treat paroxysmal supraventricular tachycardia, and verapamil (*Calan, Covera-HS*), which is used parenterally to treat supraventricular tachycardia and to temporarily control the rapid ventricular response to atrial flutter or fibrillation (Table 45.4).

Therapeutic Actions and Indications

The class IV antiarrhythmics block the movement of calcium ions across the cell membrane, depressing the generation of action potentials, delaying phases 1 and 2 of repolarization, and slowing conduction through the AV node. They are indicated for the treatment of supraventricular tachycardia and to control the ventricular response to rapid atrial rates. They are given IV for these purposes.

Table 45.4 DRUGS IN FOCUS

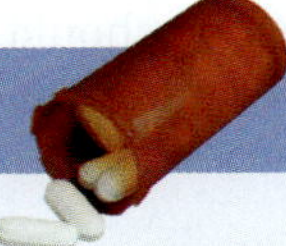

Class IV Antiarrhythmics

Drug Name	Usual Dosage	Usual Indications
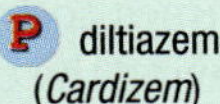 diltiazem (*Cardizem*)	0.25 mg/kg IV bolus, then a second bolus of 0.35 mg/kg IV if needed; maintain with continuous infusion of 5–10 mg/h for up to 24 h	IV to treat paroxysmal supraventricular tachycardia in adults
verapamil (*Calan, Covera-HS*)	Adult: 5–10 mg IV over 2 min, may repeat with 10 mg in 30 min if needed Pediatric: 0.1–0.3 mg/kg IV over 2 min, do not exceed 5 mg per dose; may repeat in 30 min if needed	IV to treat paroxysmal supraventricular tachycardia; slow the ventricular response to rapid atrial rates

Pharmacokinetics

These drugs are well absorbed, highly protein bound, and metabolized in the liver. They are excreted in the urine. They cross the placenta and have been associated with fetal abnormalities in animal studies. They should not be used in pregnancy unless the benefit to the mother clearly outweighs the risk to the fetus. They enter breast milk, and if they are needed by a lactating mother, another method of feeding the baby should be used because of the risk of adverse effects on the neonate.

Contraindications and Cautions

These drugs are contraindicated with known allergy to any calcium channel blocker; with sick sinus syndrome or heart block (unless an artificial pacemaker is in place), *because the block could be exacerbated by these drugs;* with pregnancy or lactation, *because of the potential for adverse effects on the fetus or neonate;* and with CHF or hypotension, *because of the hypotensive effects of these drugs.* Caution should be used with idiopathic hypertrophic subaortic stenosis (IHSS), *which could be exacerbated,* or with impaired renal or liver function, *which could affect the metabolism or excretion of these drugs.*

Adverse Effects

The adverse effects associated with these drugs are related to their vasodilation of blood vessels throughout the body. CNS effects include dizziness, weakness, fatigue, depression, and headache. GI upset, nausea, and vomiting can occur. Hypotension, CHF, shock, arrhythmias, and edema have also been reported.

Clinically Important Drug–Drug Interactions

Verapamil has been associated with many drug–drug interactions, including increased risk of cardiac depression with beta blockers; additive AV slowing with digoxin; increased serum levels and toxicity of digoxin, carbamazepine, prazosin, and quinidine; increased respiratory depression with atracurium, gallamine, pancuronium, tubocurarine, and vecuronium; and decreased effects if combined with calcium products or rifampin.

There is a risk of severe cardiac effects if these drugs are given IV within 48 hours of IV beta-adrenergic drugs. The combination should be avoided.

Diltiazem can increase the serum levels and toxicity of cyclosporine if both drugs are taken concurrently.

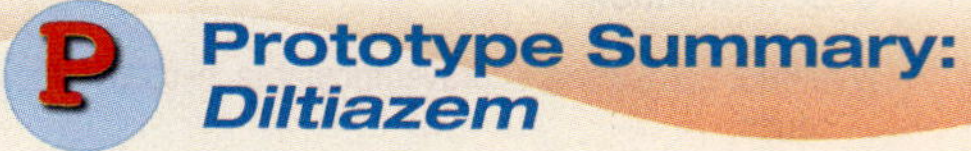

Prototype Summary: Diltiazem

Indications: Treatment of paroxysmal supraventricular tachycardia, atrial fibrillation, atrial flutter

Actions: Blocks the movement of calcium ions across the cell membrane, depressing the generation of action potentials, delaying phases 1 and 2 of repolarization, and slowing conduction through the AV node

Pharmacokinetics:

Route	Onset	Peak	Duration
Oral	30–60 min	2–3 h	6–8 h
IV	Immediate	2–3 min	Unknown

$T_{1/2}$: 3.5–6 hours; metabolized in the liver and excreted in urine

Adverse effects: Dizziness, light-headedness, headache, asthenia, peripheral edema, bradycardia, AV block, flushing, nausea, hepatic injury

Nursing Considerations for Patients Receiving Class IV Antiarrhythmics

The nursing considerations for patients taking any antiarrhythmic are outlined in the section on class I antiarrhythmics.

Other Drugs Used to Treat Arrhythmias

Adenosine (*Adenocard*) is another antiarrhythmic agent that is used to convert supraventricular tachycardia to sinus rhythm if vagal maneuvers have been ineffective. It is often the drug of choice for terminating supraventricular tachycardias, including those associated with the use of alternative conduction pathways around the AV node (e.g., Wolff–Parkinson–White syndrome), for two reasons: (1) it has a very short duration of action (about 15 seconds), after which it is picked up by circulating red blood cells and cleared through the liver; and (2) it is associated with very few adverse effects (headache, flushing, and dyspnea of short duration). This drug slows conduction through the AV node, prolongs the refractory period, and decreases automaticity in the AV node. It is given IV with continuous monitoring of the patient.

Digoxin (see Chapter 44) is also used at times to treat arrhythmias. This drug slows calcium from leaving the cell, prolonging the action potential and slowing conduction and heart rate. Digoxin is effective in the treatment of atrial arrhythmias. The drug is also positively inotropic, leading to increased cardiac output, which increases perfusion of the

Table 45.5 DRUGS IN FOCUS

Other Antiarrhythmics

Drug Name	Usual Dosage	Usual Indications
adenosine (*Adenocard*)	6 mg IV as a rapid bolus over 1–2 sec; may repeat with 12 mg IV bolus after 1–2 min if needed, may be repeated a second time if needed	Treatment of supraventricular tachycardias, including those caused by the use of alternate conduction pathways in adults
digoxin (*Lanoxin, Lanoxicaps*)	Adult: 0.75–1.25 mg PO loading dose, then 0.125–0.25 mg/day PO or 0.125–0.25 mg IV loading dose and then 0.125–0.25 mg/day PO Pediatric: 10–50 mcg/kg loading dose PO or 8–50 mcg/kg loading dose IV, based on age; then maintenance dose of 25%–35% of loading dose	Treatment of atrial flutter, atrial fibrillation, paroxysmal atrial tachycardia

coronary arteries and may eliminate the cause of some arrhythmias as hypoxia is resolved and waste products are removed more effectively (Table 45.5).

Table 45.6 provides a summary of the types of arrhythmias and the specific drugs used to treat each type.

Nursing Considerations for Patients Receiving Other Antiarrhythmics

The nursing considerations for patients taking any of these antiarrhythmics are outlined in the section on class I antiarrhythmics.

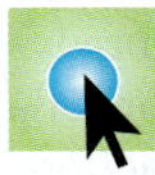

WEB LINKS

Patients and health care providers may want to consult the following Internet sources:

http://www.nscardiology.com/factsarrhythmia.htm Information on arrhythmias, drug therapy, and current research, from the National Heart, Lung and Blood Institute.

http://www.nhlbi.nih.gov Patient information on patient teaching, therapy, research, supports, and other educational programs.

http://www.americanheart.org Patient information, support groups, research information on heart disease, and scientific programs.

Table 45.6 Types of Arrhythmias and Drugs of Choice for Treatment

Arrhythmia	Antiarrhythmic Drugs
Atrial	
Flutter or fibrillation	Class Ia: quinidine* (long-term) Class III: ibutilide* (conversion of recent onset), dofetilide (conversion and maintenance)
Paroxysmal atrial tachycardia (PAT)	Other: digoxin
Supraventricular tachycardia (SVT)	Class Ic: flecainide, propafenone* Class II: esmolol* (short-term), propranolol Class IV: diltiazem (IV), verapamil (IV) Other: adenosine* (SVT, including those caused by using alternate conduction pathways)
Ventricular	
Premature ventricular contractions (PVCs)	Class Ib: lidocaine* Class II: acebutolol
Tachycardia or fibrillation	Class Ib: lidocaine* Class III: bretylium
Life-threatening ventricular arrhythmias	Class Ia: disopyramide, moricizine (X), procainamide Class Ib: mexiletine Class Ic: flecainide (X), propafenone Class III: amiodarone*, sotalol (X)

*drug of choice
(X) not drug of choice; proarrhythmic

Points to Remember

- Disruptions in the normal rate or rhythm of the heart are called arrhythmias (also known as dysrhythmias).
- Cardiac rate and rhythm are normally determined by the heart's specialized conduction system, starting with the SA node and progressing through the atria to the AV node, through the bundle of His into the ventricles, and down the bundle branches to the fibers of the Purkinje system.
- The cardiac cells possess the property of automaticity, which allows them to generate an action potential and to stimulate the cardiac muscle without stimulation from external sources.
- Disruptions in the automaticity of the cells or in the conduction of the impulse that result in arrhythmias can be caused by changes in heart rate (tachycardias or bradycardias); stimulation from ectopic foci in the atria or ventricles that cause an uncoordinated muscle contraction; or blocks in the conduction system (e.g., AV heart block, bundle branch blocks) that alter the normal movement of the impulse through the system.
- Arrhythmias can arise because of changes to the automaticity or the conductivity of the heart cells caused by electrolyte disturbances; decreases in the oxygen delivered to the cells, leading to hypoxia or anoxia; structural damage that changes the conduction pathway; acidosis or the accumulation of waste products; or drug effects.
- Arrhythmias cause problems because they alter the hemodynamics of the cardiovascular system. They can cause a decrease in cardiac output related to the uncoordinated pumping action of the irregular rhythm, leading to lack of filling time for the ventricles. Any of these effects can interfere with the delivery of blood to the brain, to other tissues, or to the heart muscle itself.
- Antiarrhythmics are drugs that alter the action potential of the heart cells and interrupt arrhythmias. The CAST study found that the long-term treatment of arrhythmias may actually cause cardiac death, so these drugs are now indicated only for the short-term treatment of potentially life-threatening ventricular arrhythmias.
- Class I antiarrhythmics block sodium channels, depress phase 0 of the action potential, and generally prolong the action potential, leading to a slowing of conduction and automaticity.
- Class II antiarrhythmics are beta-adrenergic receptor blockers that prevent sympathetic stimulation.
- Class III antiarrhythmics block potassium channels and prolong phase 3 of the action potential.
- Class IV antiarrhythmics are calcium channel blockers that shorten the action potential, disrupting ineffective rhythms and rates.
- A patient receiving an antiarrhythmic drug needs to be constantly monitored while being stabilized and during the use of the drug to detect the development of arrhythmias or other adverse effects associated with alteration of the action potentials of other muscles or nerves.

CHECK YOUR UNDERSTANDING

Answers to the questions in this chapter may be found in the Answer Key in the back of the book.

Multiple Choice

Select the best response to the following.

1. Cardiac contraction and relaxation are controlled by
   a. the brain.
   b. the sympathetic nervous system.
   c. the autonomic nervous system.
   d. impulses that arise spontaneously with the heart itself.

2. Antiarrhythmic drugs alter the action potential of the cardiac cells. Because they alter the action potential, antiarrhythmic drugs often
   a. cause congestive heart failure.
   b. alter blood flow to the kidney.
   c. cause new arrhythmias.
   d. cause electrolyte disturbances.

3. Because of the results of the CAST study,
   a. antiarrhythmics are now more widely used.
   b. antiarrhythmics are used as prophylactic measures in situations that might lead to an arrhythmia.
   c. antiarrhythmics are no longer used in the United States.
   d. antiarrhythmics are reserved for use in cases of life-threatening arrhythmias.

4. Ibutilide (*Corvert*) is a class III antiarrhythmic drug that is used for
   a. sedation during electrocardioversion.
   b. conversion of recent-onset atrial fibrillation and flutter.

c. treatment of life-threatening ventricular arrhythmias.
d. treatment of arrhythmias complicated by CHF.

5. The drug of choice for the treatment of a supraventricular tachycardia associated with Wolff–Parkinson–White syndrome is
a. digoxin.
b. verapamil.
c. lidocaine.
d. adenosine.

6. A patient who is receiving an antiarrhythmic drug needs
a. constant cardiac monitoring until stabilized.
b. frequent blood tests including drug levels.
c. an antidepressant drug to deal with the psychological depression.
d. changes in diet and exercise programs to prevent irritation of the heart muscle.

7. A patient is brought into the emergency room with a potentially life-threatening ventricular arrhythmia. Immediate treatment would include
a. a loading dose of digoxin.
b. injection of quinidine.
c. bolus and titrated intravenous doses of lidocaine.
d. loading dose of propafenone.

8. A client stabilized on quinidine for the regulation of atrial fibrillation would be cautioned to
a. avoid foods high in potassium.
b. avoid foods high in tyrosine.
c. avoid foods high in sodium content.
d. avoid foods that alkalinize the urine.

Multiple Response

Select all that apply.

1. The conduction system of the heart would include which of the following?
a. The sinoatrial node
b. The sinuses of Valsalva
c. The atrial bundles
d. The Purkinje fibers
e. The coronary sinus
f. The bundle of His

2. Arrhythmias or dysrhythmias can be caused by which of the following?
a. Lack of oxygen to the heart muscle cells
b. Acidosis near a cell
c. Structural damage in the conduction pathway through the heart
d. Vasodilation in the myocardial vascular bed
e. Thyroid hormone imbalance
f. Electrolyte imbalances

Fill in the Blanks

1. Arrhythmias can be caused by changes in heart rate, either ____________________ or ____________________.

2. Arrhythmias can cause a decrease in ____________________ ____________________, leading to a decrease in the amount of blood being pumped to the brain and periphery.

3. Antiarrhythmics alter the ____________________ of the heart cells and interfere with conduction, blocking arrhythmias.

4. Long-term treatment of arrhythmias is no longer considered prudent because of the results of the ____________________.

5. Cardiac cells possess the property of ____________________, which allows them to generate an action potential but also makes them susceptible to arrhythmias.

6. Class II antiarrhythmics are ____________________ blockers.

7. A commonly used cardiotonic agent that is used to slow the heart rate and treat atrial arrhythmias is ____________________.

8. ____________________ can be used to treat ventricular arrhythmias in emergency situations and is also a commonly used local anesthetic.

Word Scramble

Unscramble the following letters to form the names of commonly used antiarrhythmic agents.

1. namedooria ____________________
2. moolesl ____________________
3. bytermiul ____________________
4. apevirmal ____________________
5. moperacnidia ____________________
6. pdolproran ____________________
7. inifledeca ____________________
8. onidigx ____________________

Bibliography and References

Epstein, A. E., et al. (1993). Mortality following ventricular arrhythmic suppression: The original design concept of the CAST study. *Journal of the American Medical Association, 270,* 2451–2455.

Fang, M. C., et al. (2004). National trends in antiarrhythmic and antithrombotic medication use in atrial fibrillation. *Archives of Internal Medicine 164,* 55–60.

Gilman, A., Hardman, J. G., & Limbird, L. E. (Eds.). (2006). *Goodman and Gilman's the pharmacological basis of therapeutics* (11th ed.). New York: McGraw-Hill.

Karch, A. M. (2006). *2007 Lippincott's nursing drug guide.* Philadelphia: Lippincott Williams & Wilkins.

McEvoy, B. R. (2006). *Facts and comparisons 2004.* St. Louis: Facts and Comparisons.

The medical letter on drugs and therapeutics. (2006). New Rochelle, NY: Medical Letter.

Porth, C. M. (2005). *Pathophysiology: Concepts of altered health states* (7th ed.). Philadelphia: Lippincott Williams & Wilkins.

CHAPTER 46

Antianginal Agents

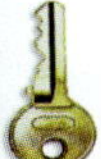

KEY TERMS

angina pectoris
atheromas
atherosclerosis
coronary artery disease (CAD)
myocardial infarction
nitrates
Prinzmetal's angina
pulse pressure

LEARNING OBJECTIVES

Upon completion of this chapter, you will be able to:

1. Describe the nature of coronary artery disease and the identified risk factors associated with the development of the disease and the clinical presentation of the disease.
2. Describe the therapeutic actions, indications, pharmacokinetics, contraindications, most common adverse reactions, and important drug–drug interactions associated with the nitrates, beta-blockers, and calcium channel blockers used to treat angina.
3. Discuss the use of antianginal agents across the lifespan.
4. Compare and contrast the prototype drugs nitroglycerin, metoprolol, and diltiazem with other agents used to treat angina.
5. Outline the nursing considerations, including important teaching points, for patients receiving drugs used to treat angina.

NITRATES

amyl nitrate
isosorbide dinitrate
isosorbide mononitrate
P nitroglycerin

BETA-BLOCKERS

P metoprolol
nadolol
propranolol

CALCIUM CHANNEL BLOCKERS

amlodipine
P diltiazem
nicardipine
nifedipine
verapamil

Coronary artery disease (CAD) has, for many years, been the leading cause of death in the United States and most Western nations. Despite great strides in understanding of the contributing causes of this disease and ways to prevent it, CAD claims more lives than any other disease. The drugs discussed in this chapter are used to prevent myocardial death when the coronary vessels are already seriously damaged and are having trouble maintaining the blood flow to the heart muscle. Chapters 47 and 48 discuss drugs that are used to prevent the blocking of the coronary arteries before they become narrowed and damaged or to restore blood flow through narrowed vessels.

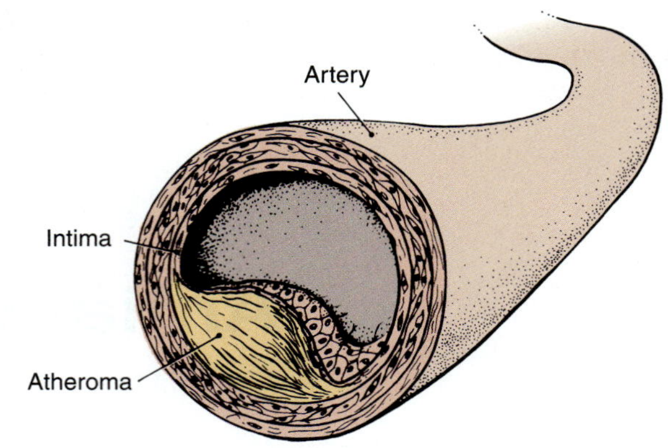

FIGURE 46.1 Schematic illustration of atheromatous plaque.

Coronary Artery Disease

The myocardium, or heart muscle, must receive a constant supply of blood in order to have the oxygen and nutrients needed to maintain a constant pumping action. The myocardium receives all of its blood from two coronary arteries that exit the sinuses of Valsalva at the base of the aorta. These vessels divide and subdivide to form the capillaries that deliver oxygen to heart muscle fibers.

Unlike other tissues in the body, the heart muscle receives its blood supply during diastole, while it is at rest. This is important because when the heart muscle contracts, it becomes tight and clamps the blood vessels closed, rendering them unable to receive blood during systole, which is when all other tissues receive fresh blood. The openings in the sinuses of Valsalva, which are the beginnings of the coronary arteries, are positioned so that they can be filled when the blood flows back against the aortic valve when the heart is at rest. The pressure that fills these vessels is the **pulse pressure** (the systolic pressure minus the diastolic pressure)—the pressure of the column of blood falling back onto the closed aortic valve. The heart has just finished contracting and using energy and oxygen. The acid and carbon dioxide built up in the muscle causes a local vasodilation, and the blood flows freely through the coronary arteries and into the muscle cells.

In CAD, the lumens of the blood vessels become narrowed so that blood is no longer able to flow freely to the muscle cells. The narrowing of the vessels is caused by the development of **atheromas**, or fatty tumors in the intima of the vessels (Figure 46.1). This is a process called **atherosclerosis**. These fatty deposits cause damage to the intimal lining of the vessels, attracting platelets and immune factors and causing swelling and the development of a larger deposit. Over time, these deposits severely decrease the size of the vessel. While the vessel is being narrowed by the deposits in the intima, it is also losing its natural elasticity and becoming unable to respond to the normal stimuli to dilate or constrict to meet the needs of the tissues.

The person with atherosclerosis has a classic supply-and-demand problem. The heart may do just fine until there is increased activity or other stresses that put a demand on it to beat faster or harder. The normal heart would stimulate the vessels to deliver more blood when this occurs, but the narrowed vessels are not able to respond and cannot supply the blood needed by the working heart (Figure 46.2). The heart muscle then becomes hypoxic. As a result, the heart demands increased blood supply in order to function properly, but the supply cannot be delivered. This happens with **angina pectoris**, literally "suffocation of the chest." If the supply-and-demand issue becomes worse, or if a vessel becomes so narrow that it occludes, the cells in the myocardium may actually become necrotic and die from lack of oxygen. This is called a **myocardial infarction**.

Stable Angina

The body's response to a lack of oxygen in the heart muscle is pain. Although the heart muscle does not have any pain fibers, a substance called factor P is released from ischemic myocardial cells, and pain is felt wherever substance P reacts

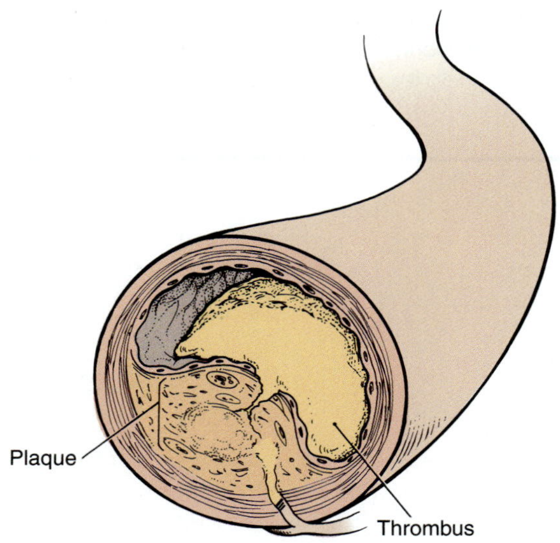

FIGURE 46.2 Thrombosis of atherosclerotic plaque. It may partially or completely occlude the lumen of the vessel.

with a pain receptor. For many people this is the chest, and for others it is the left arm; still others have pain in the jaw and teeth. The basic response to this type of pain is to stop whatever one is doing and to wait for the pain to go away. In cases of minor limitations to the blood flow through vessels, stopping activity may bring the supply and demand for blood back into balance. This condition is called stable angina. There is no damage to heart muscle, and the basic reflexes surrounding the pain restore blood flow to the heart muscle.

Unstable Angina

If the narrowing of the coronary arteries becomes more pronounced, the heart may experience episodes of ischemia even when the patient is at rest. This condition is called unstable angina or preinfarction angina. Though there is still no damage to heart muscle, the person is at great risk of a complete cutting off of the blood supply to the heart muscle if the heart should have to work hard or increase demand.

Prinzmetal's Angina

Prinzmetal's angina is an unusual form of angina because it seems to be caused by spasm of the blood vessels and not just by vessel narrowing. The person with this type of angina has angina at rest, often at the same time each day, and usually with an associated electrocardiogram (ECG) pattern change.

Acute Myocardial Infarction

If a coronary vessel becomes completely occluded and is unable to deliver blood to the cardiac muscle, the area of muscle that depends on that vessel for oxygen becomes ischemic, and then necrotic. This is called a myocardial infarction (MI). The pain associated with this event can be excruciating; nausea and a severe sympathetic stress reaction may also be present. A serious danger of an MI is that arrhythmias can develop in nearby tissue that is ischemic and very irritable. Most of the deaths caused by MI occur as a result of fatal arrhythmias. If the heart muscle has a chance to heal, within 6 to 10 weeks the dead area will be replaced with a scar and the muscle will compensate for the injury. If the area of the muscle that is damaged is very large, however, the muscle may not be able to compensate for the loss, and congestive heart failure and even cardiogenic shock may occur. These conditions can be fatal or can leave a person severely limited by the weakened heart muscle.

FOCUS POINTS

- In the United States and most Western nations, CAD is the leading cause of death in adults.
- CAD involves changes in the coronary vessels that promote atheromas (tumors), which narrow the coronary arteries and decrease their elasticity and responsiveness to normal stimuli.
- Angina pectoris occurs when the narrowed vessels cannot accommodate the myocardial demand for oxygen.
- Stable angina occurs when the heart muscle is perfused adequately except during exertion or increased demand.
- Unstable or preinfarction angina occurs when the vessels are so narrow that the myocardial cells are deprived of sufficient oxygen even at rest.
- Prinzmetal's angina is a spasm of a coronary vessel that decreases the flow of blood through the narrowed lumen.
- When a coronary vessel is completely occluded, the cells that depend on that vessel for oxygen become ischemic, then necrotic, and die. The result is known as an MI.

Antianginal Drugs

In early cases of angina, avoidance of exertion or stressful situations may be sufficient to prevent anginal pain. Antianginal drugs are used to help restore the supply-and-demand ratio in oxygen delivery to the myocardium when rest is not enough. These drugs can work to improve blood delivery to the heart muscle in one of two ways: (1) by dilating blood vessels (i.e., increasing the supply of oxygen) or (2) by decreasing the work of the heart (i.e., decreasing the demand for oxygen). Nitrates, beta-adrenergic blockers, and calcium channel blockers are used to treat angina (Figure 46.3). They are all effective and are sometimes used in combination to achieve good control of the anginal pain. The type of drug that is best for a patient is determined by

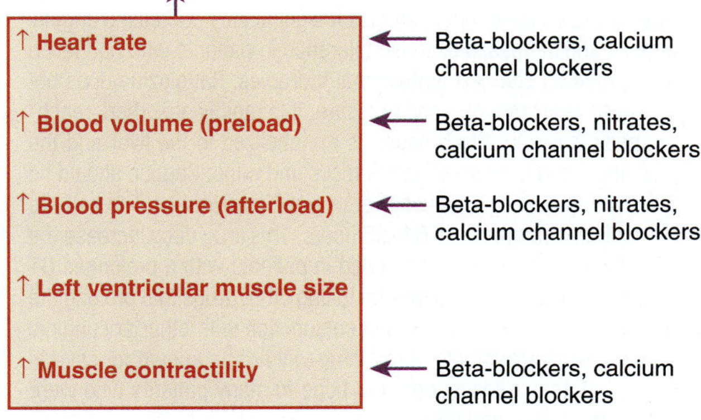

FIGURE 46.3 Factors affecting myocardial oxygen demand and points where antianginal drugs have their effects.

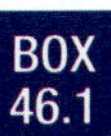

BOX 46.1 DRUG THERAPY ACROSS THE LIFESPAN

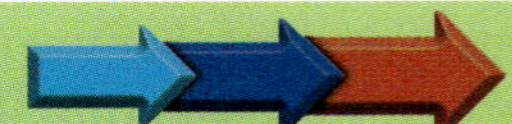

Antianginal Agents

CHILDREN

The antianginals are not indicated for any condition commonly found in children. In some situations, particularly congenital heart defects or cardiac surgery, nitroglycerin may be used. The dosage of the drug should be determined by considering age and weight. The child should be very carefully monitored for adverse reactions, including potentially dangerous changes in blood pressure.

ADULTS

Adults who receive these drugs should be instructed in their proper administration, particularly if varying forms of nitroglycerin are used. Patients should also be encouraged to determine what activities or situations tend to precipitate an anginal attack so that they can take measures to avoid those particular circumstances or take an antianginal agent before the event occurs.

With nitroglycerin use, it is important that the patient know how to store the drug, how to determine whether it is still effective, and how much to take before seeking emergency medical care.

Patients should know that regular medical follow-up is important and should be instructed in nonpharmacological measures—weight loss, smoking cessation, activity changes, diet changes—that could decrease their risk of coronary artery disease and improve the effectiveness of the antianginal therapy.

The safety for the use of these drugs during pregnancy has not been established. There is a significant potential for adverse effects on the fetus related to blood flow changes and direct drug effects when the drugs cross the placenta. The drugs do enter breast milk, and it is advised that another method of feeding the baby be used if one of these drugs is prescribed during lactation.

OLDER ADULTS

Older adults frequently are prescribed one of these drugs. Older adults are more likely to develop adverse effects associated with the use of these drugs—arrhythmias, hypotension, and congestive heart disease. Safety measures may be needed if these effects occur and interfere with the patient's mobility and balance.

The older adults are also more likely to have renal and/or hepatic impairment related to underlying medical conditions, which could interfere with the metabolism and excretion of these drugs. The dosage for older adults should be started at a lower level than that recommended for younger adults. The patient should be monitored very closely and dosage adjusted based on patient response.

If other drugs are added or removed from the drug regimen, appropriate dosage adjustments may need to be made. If the patient is using a different form of nitroglycerin, special care should be taken to make sure that the proper administration, storage, and timing of use are understood.

tolerance of adverse effects and response to the drug. The use of antianginal agents with different age groups is discussed in Box 46.1.

In 2006, a new class of drugs was introduced to treat chronic angina (see Box 46.2).

BOX 46.2 New Drug Approved for Treating Chronic Angina

In late January 2006, the Food and Drug Administration approved the first new drug in over 10 years for treating chronic angina. Ranolazine (*Ranexa*) is available in an extended-release tablet for oral use. The usual dose is 500 to 1000 mg b.i.d. The mechanisms of action of this drug are not known, but in studies it significantly decreased anginal attacks and increased exercise tolerance in patients who had failed to improve on standard antianginal therapies. Ranolazine does not decrease heart rate or blood pressure. It is rapidly absorbed, reaching peak levels in 2 to 5 hours; is metabolized in the liver and the intestines; and is excreted in the feces and urine. Caution should be used with patients who have liver or renal impairment. The half-life of ranolazine ranges from 6 to 22 hours. This drug does increase the QT interval and should not be used in patients with a prolonged QT interval or in patients who may be taking other drugs that prolong the QT interval. This drug is taken in conjunction with other antianginal drugs. Long-term effects of this drug will not be known for several years, but at its release it offered hope to many patients who were not responding to traditional therapy.

Nitrates

Nitrates (Table 46.1) are drugs that act directly on smooth muscle to cause relaxation and to depress muscle tone. Because the action is direct, it does not have to influence any nerve or other activity. The response to this type of drug is usually quite fast. The nitrates relax and dilate veins, arteries, and capillaries, allowing increased blood flow through these vessels and lowering systemic blood pressure because of a drop in resistance. Because CAD causes a stiffening and lack of responsiveness in the coronary arteries, the nitrates probably have very little effect on increasing blood flow through these arteries. They do increase blood flow through healthy coronary arteries, so there will be an increased supply of blood through any healthy vessels in the heart, and that could help the heart to compensate somewhat.

The main effect of nitrates, however, seems to be related to the drop in blood pressure that occurs. The vasodilation causes blood to pool in veins and capillaries, decreasing the volume of blood that the heart has to pump around (the preload), while the relaxation of the vessels decreases the resistance the heart has to pump against (the afterload). The combination of these effects greatly reduces the cardiac workload and the demand for oxygen, thus bringing the supply-and-demand ratio back into balance.

Nitroglycerin (*Nitro-Bid, Nitrostat,* and others) is the nitrate of choice in an acute anginal attack. It can be given

Table 46.1 DRUGS IN FOCUS

Nitrates

Drug Name	Usual Dosage	Usual Indications
amyl nitrate (generic)	0.3 mL by inhalation of vapor, may repeat in 3–5 min	Relief of acute anginal pain in adults
isosorbide dinitrate (*Isordil*)	2.5–5 mg SL; 5-mg chewable tablet; 5–20 mg PO; maintenance 10–40 mg PO q6h or 40–80 mg PO sustained release q8–12h Acute prophylaxis: 5–10 mg SL or chewable tablets q2–3h	Prevention and treatment of angina in adults
isosorbide mononitrate (*ISMO, Imdur*)	2.5–5 mg SL; 5-mg chewable tablet; 5–20 mg PO; maintenance 10–40 mg PO q6h or 40–80 mg PO sustained release q8–12h Acute prophylaxis: 5–10 mg SL or chewable tablets q2–3h	Prevention and treatment of angina in adults
P nitroglycerin (*Nitro-Bid, Nitrostat, others*)	5 mcg/min via IV infusion pump every 3–5 min; one tablet SL every 5 min for acute attack, up to three tablets in 15 min; 0.4-mg metered dose translingual, up to three doses in 15 min for acute attacks Prevention: one tablet SL 5–10 min before activities that might precipitate an attack; 2.5–2.6 mg PO t.i.d. to q.i.d.; sustained-release tablets, doses as high as 26 mg PO q.i.d. have been used; 0.5 in q8h for topical application, up to 4–5 in (60–75 mg) have been used; one pad transdermal system per day; 1 mg q3–5h while awake for transmucosal system	Treatment of acute angina attack; prevention of anginal attacks

sublingually, as a translingual spray, intravenously (IV), transdermally, topically, or as a transmucosal agent. It is rapidly absorbed and has an onset of action within minutes. It can be carried with the patient, who can use it when the need arises. It can also be used for prevention of anginal attacks in the slow-release forms. Other nitrates also are available for treating angina. Amyl nitrate (generic) is inhaled and has an onset of action of about 30 seconds. It comes as a capsule that has to be broken and waved under the patient's nose. The administration is somewhat awkward and usually requires a person other than the patient to give it properly. Isosorbide dinitrate (*Isordil* and others) and isosorbide mononitrate (*Imdur, Monoket*), both oral drugs, have a slower onset of action but may last up to 4 hours. They are taken before chest pain begins in situations in which exertion or stress can be anticipated. They are not drugs of choice during an acute attack.

Therapeutic Actions and Indications

The nitrates cause direct relaxation of smooth muscle with a resultant decrease in venous return and decrease in arterial pressure, effects that reduce cardiac workload and decrease myocardial oxygen consumption. They are indicated for the prevention and treatment of attacks of angina pectoris.

Pharmacokinetics

These drugs are very rapidly absorbed, metabolized in the liver, and excreted in urine. They cross the placenta and enter breast milk. Because of the potential for serious adverse effects related to blood flow changes on the fetus and neonate, they are not recommended for use during pregnancy or lactation.

Contraindications and Cautions

Nitrates are contraindicated in the presence of any allergy to nitrates. These drugs also are contraindicated in the following conditions: severe anemia, *because the decrease in cardiac output could be detrimental;* head trauma or cerebral hemorrhage, *because the relaxation of cerebral vessels could cause intracranial bleeding;* and pregnancy or lactation, *because of potential adverse effects on the neonate and ineffective blood flow to the fetus.*

Caution should be used in patients with hepatic or renal disease, *which could alter the metabolism and excretion of these drugs.* Caution also is required with hypotension, hypovolemia, and conditions that limit cardiac output (e.g., tamponade, low ventricular filling pressure, low pulmonary capillary wedge pressure), *because these conditions could be exacerbated, resulting in serious adverse effects.*

Adverse Effects

The adverse effects associated with these drugs are related to the vasodilation and decrease in blood flow that occurs. Central nervous system (CNS) effects include headache, dizziness, and weakness. Gastrointestinal (GI) symptoms can include nausea, vomiting, and incontinence. Cardiovascular problems include hypotension, which can be severe and must be monitored; reflex tachycardia that occurs when blood pressure falls; syncope; and angina. Skin-related effects include flushing, pallor, and increased perspiration. With the transdermal preparation, there is a risk of contact dermatitis and local hypersensitivity reactions.

Clinically Important Drug–Drug Interactions

There is a risk of hypertension and decreased antianginal effects if these drugs are given with ergot derivatives. There

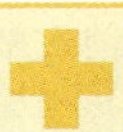

FOCUS ON **PATIENT SAFETY**

Errors have been reported with inappropriate use of nitroglycerin patches (transdermal systems) and with nitroglycerin paste. Patients have presented with severe hypotension and related physical findings after they neglected to remove the old nitroglycerin patch before putting on a new one; one patient presented with 20 patches on the body, not able to find a spot for a new one. It is very important, even if it seems silly, to teach patients to remove the old transdermal system and to wash the area before placing a new system.

Errors have also been reported when patients mistook nitroglycerin paste for hand cream and inadvertently applied a toxic dose of the drug. Patients given tubes of nitroglycerin paste need to be urged to label it clearly in large letters and to store it safely away from other people in a secure place.

is also a risk of decreased therapeutic effects of heparin if these drugs are given together with heparin; if this combination is used, the patient should be monitored and appropriate dosage adjustments made.

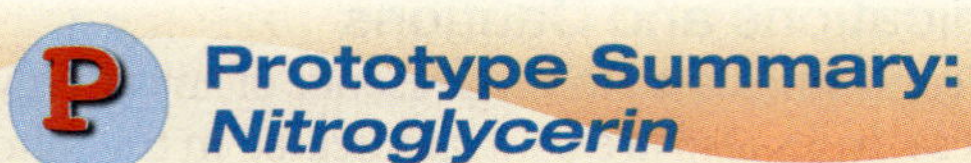

Prototype Summary: *Nitroglycerin*

Indications: Treatment of acute angina, prophylaxis of angina, intravenous treatment of angina unresponsive to beta-blockers or organic nitrates, perioperative hypertension, congestive heart failure (CHF) associated with acute MI; to produce controlled hypotension during surgery

Actions: Relaxes vascular smooth muscle with a resultant decrease in venous return and decrease in arterial blood pressure, reducing the left ventricular workload and decreasing myocardial oxygen consumption

Pharmacokinetics:

Route	Onset	Duration
IV	1–2 min	3–5 min
Sublingual	1–3 min	30–60 min
Translingual spray	2 min	30–60 min
Transmucosal tablet	1–2 min	3–5 min
Oral, SR tablet	20–45 min	8–12 h
Topical ointment	30–60 min	4–8 h
Transdermal	30–60 min	24 h

$T_{1/2}$: 1–4 min; metabolized in the liver and excreted in urine

Adverse effects: Hypotension, headache, dizziness, tachycardia, rash, flushing, nausea, vomiting, sweating, chest pain

Nursing Considerations for Patients Receiving Nitrates

Assessment: History and Examination

Screen for the following conditions, *which could be cautions or contraindications to use of the drug:* any known allergies to nitrates; impaired liver or kidney function, *which could alter the metabolism and excretion of the drug;* any condition that could be exacerbated by the hypotension and change in blood flow caused by these drugs (e.g., early MI, head trauma, cerebral hemorrhage, hypotension, hypovolemia, anemia, low cardiac output states); and pregnancy or lactation, *because of the potential adverse effects on the fetus or neonate.*

Include screening *for baseline status before beginning therapy and for any potential adverse effects.* Assess the following: skin color, lesions, and temperature; affect, orientation, and reflexes; pulse, blood pressure, perfusion, and baseline ECG; respirations and adventitious sounds; liver and renal function tests; complete blood count; and hemoglobin level.

Nursing Diagnoses

The patient receiving a nitrate may have the following nursing diagnoses related to drug therapy:

- Decreased Cardiac Output related to hypotensive effects
- Risk for Injury related to CNS or cardiovascular effects
- Ineffective Tissue Perfusion (Total Body) related to hypotension or change in cardiac output
- Deficient Knowledge regarding drug therapy

Implementation With Rationale

- Give sublingual preparations under the tongue or in the buccal pouch, and encourage the patient not to swallow, *to ensure that therapeutic effectiveness is achieved* (Box 46.3).
- Ask the patient if the tablet "fizzles" or burns, which indicates potency. Always check the expiration date on the bottle and protect the medication from heat and light, *because these drugs are volatile and lose their potency.*
- Give sustained-release (SR) forms with water, and caution the patient not to chew or crush them, *because these preparations need to reach the GI tract intact.*
- Rotate the sites of topical forms, *to decrease the risk of skin abrasion and breakdown;* monitor for signs of skin breakdown *to arrange for appropriate skin care as needed.*

BOX 46.3 FOCUS ON **CLINICAL SKILLS**

Sublingual and Transbuccal Administration of Nitroglycerin

Nitroglycerin can be given by several routes; sublingual administration is one of the most common. Patients often prefer to administer this themselves, even in the institutional setting. It is important for the nurse to make sure that the drug is given correctly:

- Check under the tongue to make sure there are no lesions or abrasions that could interfere with the absorption of the drug. Have the patient take a sip of water to moisten the mucous membranes so the tablet will dissolve quickly. Then instruct the patient to place the tablet under the tongue, close the mouth, and wait until the tablet has dissolved.
- Caution the patient not to swallow the tablet; its effectiveness would be lost if the tablet entered the stomach. If the patient uses translingual drugs often, encourage the patient to alternate sides of the tongue—placing it under the left side for one dose, and under the right side for the other dose.
- Here's a tip to help administer sublingual medications to patients who cannot do it themselves or who cannot open their mouths: Use a tongue depressor to move the tongue aside and place the tablet, or slide the tablet down through a straw to the underside of the tongue.

Transbuccal administration is also possible for nitroglycerin. Make sure that the tablet the patient is going to use is designed for buccal administration.

- Check the inside of the cheeks to be sure there are no ulcerations or abrasions that could interfere with the absorption of the drug. Have the patient place the tablet between his or her gums and cheek pocket; then hold it in place until the tablet dissolves.
- Again, caution the patient not to swallow the tablet, and to rotate the site of placement from side to side with each dose.

- Make sure that translingual spray is used under the tongue and not inhaled, *to ensure that the therapeutic effects can be achieved.*
- Break an amyl nitrate capsule and wave it under the nose of the angina patient *to provide rapid relief using the inhalation form of the drug;* this may be repeated with another capsule in 3 to 5 minutes if needed.
- Provide life support equipment on a standby basis, *in case of severe reaction to the drug or myocardial infarction.*
- Taper the dosage gradually (over 4 to 6 weeks) after long-term therapy, *because abrupt withdrawal could cause a severe reaction, including MI.*
- Provide comfort measures *to help the patient tolerate drug effects.* These include small, frequent meals; access to bathroom facilities if GI upset is severe; environmental controls; safety precautions; orientation; and appropriate skin care as needed.
- Provide thorough patient teaching, including the name of the drug, dosage prescribed, proper administration, measures to avoid adverse effects, warning signs of problems, and the importance of periodic monitoring and evaluation, *to enhance patient knowledge about drug therapy and promote compliance to the drug regimen.*
- Offer support and encouragement, *to help the patient deal with the diagnosis and the drug regimen.*

Evaluation

- Monitor patient response to the drug (alleviation of signs and symptoms of angina, prevention of angina).
- Monitor for adverse effects (hypotension, cardiac arrhythmias, GI upset, skin reactions, headache).
- Evaluate the effectiveness of the teaching plan (patient can name drug, dosage, proper administration, adverse effects to watch for, specific measures to avoid adverse effects, and the importance of continued follow-up).
- Monitor the effectiveness of comfort measures and compliance to the regimen (see Critical Thinking Scenario 46-1).

Beta-Blockers

As discussed in Chapter 31, beta-adrenergic blockers are used to block the stimulatory effects of the sympathetic nervous system. These drugs block beta-adrenergic receptors and vasoconstriction (thereby stopping an increase in blood pressure) and prevent the increase in heart rate and increased intensity of myocardial contraction that occur with sympathetic stimulation such as exertion or stress. These effects decrease the cardiac workload and the demand for oxygen.

These drugs are sometimes used in combination with nitrates to increase exercise tolerance. Beta-blockers have many adverse effects associated with the blockade of the sympathetic nervous system. The dose that is used to prevent angina is lower than doses used to treat hypertension, so there is a decreased incidence of adverse effects associated with this specific use of beta-blockers. These drugs are not recommended for use in patients with diabetes, peripheral vascular disease, or chronic obstructive pulmonary disease (COPD), because the effects on the sympathetic nervous system could exacerbate these problems. The beta-blockers that are recommended for use in angina are metoprolol (*Toprol, Toprol XL*), propranolol (*Inderal*), and nadolol (*Corgard*) (Table 46.2).

(text continues on page 756)

CRITICAL THINKING SCENARIO 46-1

Handling an Angina Attack

The Situation

S.W. is a 48-year-old white woman with a 2-year history of angina pectoris. She was given sublingual nitroglycerin to use when she had chest pain. For the past 6 months, she has been stable, experiencing little chest pain. This morning after her exercise class, S.W. had an argument with her daughter and experienced severe chest pain that was unrelieved by four nitroglycerin tablets taken over a 20-minute period. S.W.'s daughter rushed her to the hospital, where she was given oxygen through nasal prongs and placed on a cardiac monitor, which showed a sinus tachycardia of 110 beats/min. A 12-lead electrocardiogram (ECG) showed no changes from her previous ECG of 7 months ago.

S.W. did not have elevated troponin levels. The chest pain subsided within 3 minutes after she received another sublingual nitroglycerin. It was decided that S.W. should stay in the emergency room (ER) for a few hours for observation. The diagnosis of angina attack was made.

Critical Thinking

What nursing interventions are appropriate for S.W. while she is still in the ER? *Consider the progression of coronary artery disease (CAD) and the ways in which that progression can be delayed and chest pain avoided.* What teaching points should be stressed with this patient?

What type of guilt may the daughter experience after the disagreement with S.W.? *What interventions would be useful in dealing with mother and daughter during this crisis?*

Should any further tests or treatments be addressed with S.W. when discussing her heart disease?

Discussion

S.W.'s vital signs should be monitored closely while she is in the ER. If her attack subsides, she will be discharged and teaching points about CAD will be reviewed with her. It would be a good time to discuss angina with S.W. and her daughter, explaining the pathophysiology of the disease and ways to avoid upsetting the supply-and-demand ratio in the heart muscle.

Because S.W. took four nitroglycerin tablets with no effect before coming to the ER, it would be important to find out the age and potency of her drug. Review the storage requirements for the drug, ways to tell whether it is potent, and the importance of replacing the pills at least every 6 months.

S.W. and her daughter should be encouraged to air their feelings about this episode; for example, guilt or anger may be precipitated by this scare. They should have the opportunity to explore other ways of handling their problems, try to pace activities to avoid excessive demand for oxygen, and plan what to do if this happens again. They should both receive support and encouragement to cope with the angina and its implications.

Written information, including drug information, should be given to S.W. Once her condition is stabilized, further studies may be indicated to monitor the progress of her disease. The use of hormone therapy in this patient may be explored, as well as dietary interventions, avoidance of smoking as appropriate, blood pressure control, and monitoring of activity.

Nursing Care Guide for S.W.: Antianginal Nitrates

Assessment: History and Examination

Assess S.W. for allergies to any nitrates, renal or hepatic dysfunction, pregnancy and lactation (if appropriate), early MI, head trauma, hypotension, hypovolemia

Focus the physical examination on the following areas:

CV: blood pressure, pulse, perfusion, ECG

Neuro (CNS): orientation, affect, reflexes, vision

Skin: color, lesions, texture

Resp: respiratory rate and character, adventitious sounds

GI: abdominal examination, bowel sounds

Laboratory tests: liver and renal function tests, CBC, hemoglobin

Nursing Diagnoses

Decreased Cardiac Output related to hypotension

Risk for injury related to CNS, CV effects

Ineffective Tissue Perfusion (Total Body) related to CV effects

Deficient Knowledge regarding drug therapy

Implementation

Ensure proper administration of drug and protect drug from heat and light.

Handling an Angina Attack *(continued)*

Provide comfort and safety measures:

- Rotate transdermal sites.
- Offer environmental control for headaches.
- Give drug with food if GI upset occurs.
- Provide skin care as needed.
- Taper dosage after long-term use.

Provide support and reassurance to deal with drug effects.

Provide patient teaching regarding drug, dosage, adverse effects, what to report, safety precautions.

Evaluation

Evaluate drug effects: relief of signs and symptoms of angina, prevention of angina.

Monitor for adverse effects: headache, dizziness; arrhythmias; GI upset; skin reactions; hypotension, and CV effects.

Monitor for drug–drug interactions as indicated for each drug.

Evaluate effectiveness of patient teaching program and comfort and safety measures.

Patient Teaching for S.W.

☐ A nitrate is given to patients with chest pain that occurs because the heart muscle is not receiving enough oxygen. The nitrates act by decreasing the heart's workload, and thus its need for oxygen, which it uses for energy. This relieves the pain of angina.

☐ Besides taking the drug as prescribed, you can also help your heart by decreasing the work that it must do. For example, you can

- Reduce weight, if necessary.
- Decrease or avoid the use of coffee, cigarettes, or alcoholic beverages.
- Avoid going outside in very cold weather; if this can't be avoided, dress warmly and avoid exertion while outside.
- Avoid stressful activities, especially in combination. For example, if you eat a big meal, do not drink coffee or alcoholic beverages with that meal. If you have just eaten a big meal, do not climb stairs; rest for a while.
- Determine which social interactions are stressful or anxiety producing; then find ways to limit or avoid these situations.
- Determine ways to ventilate your feelings (e.g., throwing things, screaming, diversions).
- Learn to slow down, rest periodically, and schedule your activities to allow your heart to pace its use of energy throughout the day and to help you to maintain your activities without pain.

☐ Nitroglycerin tablets are taken sublingually. Place one tablet under your tongue. Do not swallow until the tablet has dissolved. The tablet should burn slightly or "fizzle" under your tongue; if this does not occur, the tablet is not effective and you should get a fresh supply of tablets.

☐ Ideally, take the nitroglycerin before your chest pain begins. If you know that a certain activity usually causes pain (e.g., eating a big meal, attending a business meeting, engaging in sexual intercourse), take the tablet before undertaking the particular activity.

☐ Dermal patches should be applied daily. They may be placed on the chest, upper arm, upper thigh, or back. They should be placed on an area that is free of body hair. The site of the application should be changed slightly each day to avoid excess irritation to the skin.

☐ Sublingual nitroglycerin is a very unstable compound. Do not buy large quantities at a time, because it does not store well. Keep the drug in a dark, dry place and in a dark-colored glass container, not a plastic bottle, with a tight lid. Leave it in its own bottle. Do not combine it with other drugs.

☐ Some of the following adverse effects may occur:

- *Dizziness, light-headedness:* This often passes as you adjust to the drug. Use great care if you are taking sublingual or transmucosal forms of the drug. Sit or lie down to avoid dizziness or falls. Change position slowly to help decrease the dizziness.
- *Headache:* This is a common problem. Over-the-counter headache remedies often provide no relief for the pain. Lying down in a cool environment and resting may help alleviate some of the discomfort.
- *Flushing of the face and neck:* This is usually a very minor problem that passes as the drug's effects pass.
- Report any of the following to your health care provider: *blurred vision, persistent or severe headache, skin rash, more frequent or more severe angina attacks, fainting.*

☐ Sublingual nitroglycerin usually relieves chest pain within 3 to 5 minutes. If pain is not relieved within 5 minutes, take another tablet. If pain continues, take

(continued)

Handling an Angina Attack *(continued)*

another tablet in 5 minutes. A total of _____ tablets may be used, spaced every 5 minutes. If the pain is not relieved after that time, call your health care provider or go to a hospital emergency room as soon as possible.

- ☐ Tell any doctor, nurse, or other health care provider involved in your care that you are taking this drug.
- ☐ Keep this drug, and all medications, out of the reach of children.
- ☐ Avoid taking over-the-counter medications while you are taking this drug. If you feel that you need one of these, consult with your health care provider for the best choice. Many of these drugs can change the effects of this drug and cause problems.
- ☐ Avoid alcohol while you are taking this drug because the combination can cause serious problems.
- ☐ If you are taking this drug for a prolonged period of time, do not stop taking it suddenly. Your body will need time to adjust to the loss of the drug. The dosage must be gradually reduced to prevent serious problems from developing.

Therapeutic Actions and Indications

The beta-blockers competitively block beta-adrenergic receptors in the heart and juxtaglomerular apparatus, decreasing the influence of the sympathetic nervous system on these tissues and thereby decreasing the excitability of the heart, decreasing cardiac output, decreasing cardiac oxygen compensation, and lowering blood pressure. They are indicated for the long-term management of angina pectoris caused by atherosclerosis. They are not indicated for the treatment of Prinzmetal's angina, because they could cause vasospasm when they block beta-receptor sites. Propranolol is also used to prevent reinfarction in stable patients 1 to 4 weeks after an MI. This effect is thought to be caused by the suppression of myocardial oxygen demand for a prolonged period.

Pharmacokinetics

These drugs are absorbed from the GI tract and undergo hepatic metabolism. Food has been found to increase the bioavailability of propranolol, but this effect has not been found with other beta-adrenergic blocking agents. These drugs are excreted in urine, necessitating caution in patients with renal impairment. Teratogenic effects have occurred in animal studies with all of these drugs. The use of any beta-adrenergic blocker during pregnancy should be reserved for situations in which the benefit to the mother outweighs the risk to the fetus. In general, they should not be used during lactation because of the potential for adverse effects on the baby. The safety and efficacy of the use of these drugs in children has not been established.

Contraindications and Cautions

The beta-blockers are contraindicated in patients with bradycardia, heart block, cardiogenic shock, asthma, or COPD *because their blocking of the sympathetic response could exacerbate these diseases.* They also are contraindicated with pregnancy and lactation, *because of the potential for adverse effects on the fetus or neonate.*

Caution should be used in patients with diabetes, peripheral vascular disease, or thyrotoxicosis, *because the blockade of the sympathetic response blocks normal reflexes that are necessary for maintaining homeostasis in patients with these diseases.*

Adverse Effects

The adverse effects associated with these drugs are related to their blockade of the sympathetic nervous system. CNS effects

Table 46.2 DRUGS IN FOCUS

Beta-Blockers

Drug Name	Usual Dosage	Usual Indications
P metoprolol (*Toprol, Toprol XL*)	100 mg/day PO as single dose, extended-release tablet; 100–400 mg/day PO in two divided doses regular release	Treatment of angina in adults; prevention of reinfarction within 3–10 days after myocardial infarction (MI)
nadolol (*Corgard*)	40–80 mg/day PO	Long-term management of angina in adults
propranolol (*Inderal*)	10–20 mg PO t.i.d. to q.i.d., titrate based on patient response, 160 mg/day is often needed for maintenance	Long-term management of angina and prevention of reinfarction in patients 1–4 wk after MI in adults

include dizziness, fatigue, emotional depression, and sleep disturbances. GI problems include gastric pain, nausea, vomiting, colitis, and diarrhea. Cardiovascular effects can include congestive heart failure, reduced cardiac output, and arrhythmias. Respiratory symptoms can include bronchospasm, dyspnea, and cough. Decreased exercise tolerance and malaise are also common complaints.

Clinically Important Drug–Drug Interactions

A paradoxical hypertension occurs when clonidine is given with beta-blockers, and an increased rebound hypertension with clonidine withdrawal may also occur; it is best to avoid this combination.

A decreased antihypertensive effect occurs when beta-blockers are given with nonsteroidal anti-inflammatory drugs; if this combination is used, the patient should be monitored closely and a dosage adjustment made.

An initial hypertensive episode followed by bradycardia occurs if these drugs are given with epinephrine, and a possibility of peripheral ischemia exists if beta-blockers are taken in combination with ergot alkaloids.

There also is a potential for a change in blood glucose levels if these drugs are given with insulin or antidiabetic agents, and the patient will not have the usual signs and symptoms of hypoglycemia or hyperglycemia to alert him or her to potential problems. If this combination is used, the patient should monitor blood glucose frequently throughout the day and should be alert to new warnings about glucose imbalance.

P Prototype Summary: *Metoprolol*

Indications: Treatment of stable angina pectoris; also used for treatment of hypertension, prevention of reinfarction in MI patients, and treatment of stable, symptomatic CHF

Actions: Competitively blocks beta-adrenergic receptors in the heart and kidneys, decreasing the influence of the sympathetic nervous system on these tissues and the excitability of the heart; decreases cardiac output and the release of renin, which results in a lowered blood pressure and decreased cardiac workload

Pharmacokinetics:

Route	Onset	Peak	Duration
Oral	15 min	90 min	15–19 h
IV	Immediate	60–90 min	15–19 h

$T_{1/2}$: 3–4 hours; metabolized in the liver and excreted in urine

Adverse effects: Dizziness, vertigo, CHF, arrhythmias, gastric pain, flatulence, diarrhea, vomiting, impotence, decreased exercise tolerance

Nursing Considerations for Patients Receiving Beta-Blockers

See Chapter 31 for the nursing considerations associated with beta-blockers.

Calcium Channel Blockers

The calcium channel blockers prevent the movement of calcium into the cardiac and smooth muscle cells when the cells are stimulated, interfering with their ability to contract. This leads to a loss of smooth muscle tone, vasodilation, and decreased peripheral resistance. These effects decrease venous return (preload) and the resistance the heart muscle has to pump against (afterload), which in turn decrease cardiac workload and oxygen consumption. The drug of choice depends on the patient's diagnosis and ability to tolerate adverse drug effects (Table 46.3).

Therapeutic Actions and Indications

Calcium channel blockers inhibit the movement of calcium ions across the membranes of myocardial and arterial muscle cells, altering the action potential and blocking muscle cell contraction. These effects depress myocardial contractility, slow cardiac impulse formation in the conductive tissues, and relax and dilate arteries, causing a fall in blood pressure and a decrease in venous return. These effects decrease the workload of the heart and myocardial oxygen consumption and, in Prinzmetal's angina, relieve the vasospasm of the coronary artery, increasing blood flow to the muscle cells. Research also indicates that these drugs block the proliferation of cells in the endothelial layer of the blood vessel, slowing the progress of the atherosclerosis. These drugs are indicated for the treatment of Prinzmetal's angina, chronic angina, effort-associated angina, and hypertension. Verapamil (*Calan, Isoptin*) is also used to treat rapid cardiac arrhythmias, because it slows conduction more than the other calcium channel blockers do.

Pharmacokinetics

These drugs are generally well absorbed, metabolized in the liver, and excreted in urine. These drugs cross the placenta and enter breast milk. Fetal toxicity has been reported in animal studies. Although there are no well-defined studies about effects during pregnancy, these drugs should not be used during pregnancy unless the benefit to the mother clearly outweighs any potential risk to the fetus. Because of the potential for serious adverse effects on the baby, another method of feeding the infant should be used if these drugs are required during lactation.

Contraindications and Cautions

These drugs are contraindicated in the presence of allergy to any of these drugs; with heart block or sick sinus syndrome,

Table 46.3 DRUGS IN FOCUS

Calcium Channel Blockers Used to Treat Angina

Drug Name	Usual Dosage	Usual Indications
amlodipine (*Norvasc*)	5 mg/day PO; reduce dosage with hepatic impairment or with geriatric patients	Treatment of chronic, stable angina and of Prinzmetal's angina in adults
P diltiazem (*Cardizem, Cardizem SR*)	180–360 mg/day PO in three or four divided doses; 120–180 mg PO b.i.d. sustained release	Treatment of angina in adults
nicardipine (*Cardene*)	20–40 mg PO t.i.d.; use immediate release only	Treatment of angina in adults
nifedipine (*Adalat, Procardia*)	10–20 mg PO t.i.d.	Treatment of angina in adults
verapamil (*Calan, Isoptin*)	320–480 mg/day PO	Treatment of angina in adults

which could be exacerbated by the conduction-slowing effects of these drugs; with renal or hepatic dysfunction, *which could alter the metabolism and excretion of these drugs;* and with pregnancy or lactation, *because of the potential for adverse effects on the fetus or neonate.*

Adverse Effects

The adverse effects associated with these drugs are related to their effects on cardiac output and on smooth muscle. CNS effects include dizziness, light-headedness, headache, and fatigue. GI effects can include nausea and hepatic injury related to direct toxic effects on hepatic cells. Cardiovascular effects include hypotension, bradycardia, peripheral edema, and heart block. Skin effects include flushing and rash.

Clinically Important Drug–Drug Interactions

Drug–drug interactions vary with each of the calcium channel blockers. Potentially serious effects to keep in mind include increased serum levels and toxicity of cyclosporine if taken with diltiazem and increased risk of heart block and digoxin toxicity if combined with verapamil (because verapamil increases digoxin serum levels). Both drugs depress myocardial conduction. If any combinations of these drugs must be used, the patient should be monitored very closely and appropriate dosage adjustments made. Verapamil has also been associated with serious respiratory depression when given with general anesthetics or as an adjunct to anesthesia.

P Prototype Summary: Diltiazem

Indications: Treatment of Prinzmetal's angina, effort-associated angina, chronic stable angina; also used to treat essential hypertension, paroxysmal supraventricular tachycardia

Actions: Inhibits the movement of calcium ions across the membranes of myocardial and arterial muscle cells, altering the action potential and blocking muscle cell contraction, which depresses myocardial contractility; slows cardiac impulse formation in the conductive tissues, and relaxes and dilates arteries, causing a fall in blood pressure and a decrease in venous return; decreases the workload of the heart and myocardial oxygen consumption and, in Prinzmetal's angina, also relieves the vasospasm of the coronary artery, increasing blood flow to the muscle cells

Pharmacokinetics:

Route	Onset	Peak
Oral	30–60 min	2–3 h
SR, ER	30–60 min	6–11 h
IV	Immediate	2–3 min

$T_{1/2}$: 3.5–6 hours (SR), 5–7 hours (ER) metabolized in the liver and excreted in urine

Adverse effects: Dizziness, light-headedness, headache, asthenia, peripheral edema, bradycardia, atrioventricular block, flushing, rash, nausea

Nursing Considerations for Patients Receiving Calcium Channel Blockers

Assessment: History and Examination

Screen for the following conditions, *which could be cautions or contraindications to use of the drug:* known allergies to any of these drugs; impaired liver or kidney function, *which could alter the metabolism and excretion of the drug;* heart block, *which could be exacerbated by the conduction depression of these drugs;* and pregnancy or lactation, *because of the potential adverse effects on the fetus or neonate.*

Include screening *for baseline status before beginning therapy and for any potential adverse effects.* Assess the following: skin color, lesions, and temperature; affect, orientation, and reflexes; pulse, auscultation, blood pressure, perfusion, and baseline ECG; respirations and adventitious sounds; and liver and renal function tests.

Nursing Diagnoses

The patient receiving a calcium channel blocker may have the following nursing diagnoses related to drug therapy:

- Decreased Cardiac Output related to hypotension
- Risk for Injury related to CNS or cardiovascular effects
- Ineffective Tissue Perfusion (Total Body) related to hypotension or change in cardiac output
- Deficient Knowledge regarding drug therapy

Implementation With Rationale

- Monitor the patient carefully (blood pressure, cardiac rhythm, cardiac output) while the drug is being titrated or dosage is being changed, *to ensure early detection of potentially serious adverse effects.*
- Monitor blood pressure very carefully if the patient is also taking nitrates, *because there is an increased risk of hypotensive episodes.*
- Periodically monitor blood pressure and cardiac rhythm while the patient is using these drugs, *because of the potential for adverse cardiovascular effects.*
- Provide comfort measures *to help the patient tolerate drug effects.* These include small, frequent meals; access to bathroom facilities if GI upset is severe; environmental controls; and safety precautions.
- Provide thorough patient teaching, including the name of the drug, dosage prescribed, proper administration, measures to avoid adverse effects, warning signs of problems, and the need for periodic monitoring and evaluation, *to enhance patient knowledge about drug therapy and to promote compliance with the drug regimen.*
- Offer support and encouragement, *to help the patient deal with the diagnosis and the drug regimen.*

Evaluation

- Monitor patient response to the drug (alleviation of signs and symptoms of angina, prevention of angina).
- Monitor for adverse effects (hypotension, cardiac arrhythmias, GI upset, skin reactions, headache).
- Evaluate the effectiveness of the teaching plan (patient can name drug, dosage, proper administration, adverse effects to watch for, specific measures to avoid adverse effects, and the importance of continued follow-up).
- Monitor the effectiveness of comfort measures and compliance to the regimen.

WEB LINKS

Patients and health care providers may want to explore information from the following Internet sources:

http://www.nhlbi.nih.gov/index.htm National Heart, Lung, and Blood Institute information on angina, drug therapy, and current research.

http://www.cardioassoc.com Information on patient teaching, supports, and other educational programs.

http://www.nscardiology.com

http://www.americanheart.org Patient information, support groups, research information on heart disease, and scientific programs.

http://heartdisease.miningco.com/mbody.htm?PID-2370&COB-home Information on diet, exercise, drug therapy, cardiac rehabilitation, and prevention of CAD.

Points to Remember

- CAD is the leading cause of death in the United States and most Western nations.
- CAD develops when changes in the intima of coronary vessels lead to the development of atheromas or fatty tumors, accumulation of platelets and debris, and a thickening of arterial muscles, resulting in a loss of elasticity and responsiveness to normal stimuli.
- Narrowing of the coronary arteries secondary to the atheroma buildup is called atherosclerosis.
- Narrowed coronary arteries eventually become unable to deliver all the blood that is needed by the myocardial cells, causing a problem of supply and demand.
- Angina pectoris, or "suffocation of the chest," occurs when the myocardial demand for oxygen cannot be met by the narrowed vessels. Pain, anxiety, and fatigue develop when the supply-and-demand ratio is upset.
- Stable angina occurs when the heart muscle is perfused adequately except during exertion or increased demand.

People usually respond to the pain of angina by stopping all activity and resting, which decreases the demand for oxygen and restores the supply-and-demand balance.

- Unstable or preinfarction angina occurs when the vessels are so narrowed that the myocardial cells are low on oxygen even at rest.
- Prinzmetal's angina occurs as a result of a spasm of a coronary vessel, leading to decreased blood flow through the narrowed lumen.
- MI occurs when a coronary vessel is completely occluded and the cells that depend on that vessel for oxygen become ischemic, then necrotic, and die.
- Angina can be treated by drugs that either increase the supply of oxygen or decrease the heart's workload, which decreases the demand for oxygen.
- Nitrates and beta-blockers are used to cause vasodilation and to decrease venous return and arterial resistance, effects that decrease cardiac workload and oxygen consumption.
- Calcium channel blockers block muscle contraction in smooth muscle and decrease the heart's workload, relax spasm in Prinzmetal's angina, and possibly block the proliferation of the damaged endothelium in coronary vessels.

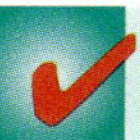

CHECK YOUR UNDERSTANDING

Answers to the questions in this chapter may be found in the Answer Key in the back of the book.

Multiple Choice

Select the best answer to the following.

1. Coronary artery disease results in
   a. an imbalance in the supply and the demand for oxygen in the heart muscle.
   b. delivery of blood to the heart muscle during systole.
   c. increased pulse pressure.
   d. a decreased workload on the heart.

2. Angina
   a. causes death of heart muscle cells.
   b. is pain associated with lack of oxygen to heart muscle cells.
   c. only occurs with vigorous exercise.
   d. is not treatable.

3. Nitrates are commonly used antianginal drugs that act to
   a. increase the preload on the heart.
   b. increase the afterload on the heart.
   c. dilate coronary vessels to increase the delivery of oxygen through those vessels.
   d. decrease venous return to the heart, thereby decreasing the myocardial workload.

4. Calcium channel blockers are effective in treating angina because they
   a. prevent any cardiovascular exercise, preventing strain on the heart.
   b. block strong muscle contractions and cause vasodilation, decreasing the work of the heart.
   c. alter the electrolyte balance of the heart and prevent arrhythmias.
   d. increase the heart rate, making it more efficient.

5. Verapamil has been associated with potentially serious adverse effects if given with
   a. oral contraceptives.
   b. cyclosporine.
   c. digoxin.
   d. barbiturate anesthetics.

6. Prinzmetal's angina occurs as a result of
   a. electrolyte imbalance.
   b. a spasm of a coronary vessel.
   c. decreased venous return to the heart.
   d. a ventricular arrhythmia.

Multiple Response

Select all that apply.

1. Risk factors for the development of atherosclerosis would include which of the following?
   a. A high-fat diet
   b. Increasing age
   c. Female gender
   d. A sedentary lifestyle
   e. Diabetes mellitus
   f. Hypertension

2. An acute myocardial infarction is usually associated with which of the following?
   a. Permanent injury to the heart muscle
   b. Potentially serious arrhythmias
   c. Pain, nausea, and sympathetic stress reaction
   d. The development of hypertension
   e. Loss of consciousness
   f. Sweating and a feeling of anxiety

3. Antianginal drugs work to do which of the following?
   a. Decrease the workload on the heart
   b. Increase the supply of oxygen to the heart

c. Change the metabolic pathway in the heart muscle to remove the need for oxygen
d. Restore the supply-and-demand balance of oxygen in the heart
e. Decrease venous return to the heart
f. Alter the coronary artery filling pathway

4. A client who has nitroglycerin to avert an acute anginal attack would need to be taught
   a. to take five or six tablets and then seek medical help if no relief occurs.
   b. to buy the tablets in bulk to decrease the cost.
   c. to protect tablets from light and to discard them if they do not fizzle when placed under the tongue.
   d. to store the tablets in a clearly marked, clear container in open view, where they can easily be found if they are needed.
   e. to use the nitroglycerin before an event or activity that will most likely precipitate an anginal attack.
   f. that a headache may occur after taking the nitroglycerin.

Matching

Match the word with the appropriate definition.

1. ____________________ CAD
2. ____________________ pulse pressure
3. ____________________ atheroma
4. ____________________ atherosclerosis
5. ____________________ angina pectoris
6. ____________________ Prinzmetal's angina
7. ____________________ myocardial infarction
8. ____________________ nitrates

A. "Suffocation of the chest"
B. Drop in blood flow through the coronary arteries caused by a vasospasm in the artery
C. Coronary artery disease
D. End result of vessel blockage in the heart
E. Fatty tumor in the intima of a coronary artery
F. Filling pressure of the coronary arteries
G. Narrowing of the arteries caused by buildup of atheromas
H. Drugs used to cause direct relaxation of smooth muscle

True or False

Indicate whether the following statements are true (T) or false (F).

_____ 1. Coronary artery disease (CAD) is second to cancer as the leading cause of death in the United States and most Western nations.

_____ 2. CAD develops when changes in the intima of coronary vessels lead to the development of atheromas, or fatty tumors.

_____ 3. Narrowing of the coronary arteries secondary to the atheroma buildup is called angina.

_____ 4. Angina pectoris, or "suffocation of the chest," occurs when the narrowed vessels cannot meet the myocardial demand for oxygen.

_____ 5. Stable angina occurs when the heart muscle is perfused adequately except at rest.

_____ 6. Unstable or preinfarction angina occurs when the vessels are so narrowed that the myocardial cells are low on oxygen during exertion.

_____ 7. Prinzmetal's angina occurs as a result of a spasm of a coronary vessel.

_____ 8. Myocardial infarction occurs when a coronary vessel is completely occluded.

Bibliography and References

Drug facts and comparisons. (2006). St. Louis: Facts and Comparisons.

Gilman, A., Hardman, J. G., & Limbird, L. E. (Eds.). (2006). *Goodman and Gilman's the pharmacological basis of therapeutics* (11th ed.). New York: McGraw-Hill.

Karch, A. M. (2006). *2007 Lippincott's nursing drug guide.* Philadelphia: Lippincott Williams & Wilkins.

The medical letter on drugs and therapeutics. (2006). New Rochelle, NY: Medical Letter.

Porth, C. M. (2005). *Pathophysiology: Concepts of altered health states* (7th ed.). Philadelphia: Lippincott Williams & Wilkins.

CHAPTER
47

Lipid-Lowering Agents

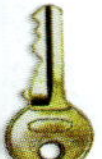

KEY TERMS

bile acids
cholesterol
chylomicron
high-density lipoprotein (HDL)
HMG-CoA reductase
hyperlipidemia
low-density lipoprotein (LDL)
risk factors

LEARNING OBJECTIVES

Upon completion of this chapter, you will be able to:

1. Outline the mechanisms of fat metabolism in the body and discuss the role of hyperlipidemia as a risk factor for coronary artery disease.
2. Describe the therapeutic actions, indications, pharmacokinetics, contraindications, most common adverse reactions, and important drug–drug interactions associated with the bile acid sequestrants, HMG-CoA inhibitors, cholesterol absorption inhibitors, and other agents used to lower lipid levels.
3. Discuss the use of drugs that lower lipid levels across the lifespan.
4. Compare and contrast the prototype drugs cholestyramine, atorvastatin, and ezetimibe with other agents used to lower lipid levels.
5. Outline the nursing considerations, including important teaching points, for patients receiving drugs used to lower lipid levels.

BILE ACID SEQUESTRANTS

P cholestyramine
colesevelam
colestipol

HMG-CoA REDUCTASE INHIBITORS

P atorvastatin
fluvastatin
lovastatin
pravastatin
rosuvastatin
simvastatin

CHOLESTEROL ABSORPTION INHIBITOR

P ezetimibe

OTHER ANTIHYPERLIPIDEMIC AGENTS

fenofibrate
gemfibrozil
niacin

The drugs discussed in this chapter lower serum levels of cholesterol and lipids. There is mounting evidence that the incidence of coronary artery disease (CAD), the leading killer of adults in the Western world, is higher among people with high serum lipid levels. The cause of CAD is poorly understood, but some evidence indicates that cholesterol and fat play a major role in disease development.

Coronary Artery Disease

As explained in Chapter 46, CAD is characterized by the progressive growth of atheromatous plaques, or atheromas, in the coronary arteries. These plaques, which begin as fatty streaks in the endothelium, eventually injure the endothelial lining of the artery, causing an inflammatory reaction. This inflammatory process triggers the development of characteristic foam cells, containing fats and white blood cells that further injure the endothelial lining. Over time, platelets, fibrin, other fats, and remnants collect on the injured vessel lining and cause the atheroma to grow, further narrowing the interior of the blood vessel and limiting blood flow.

The injury to the vessel also causes scarring and a thickening of the vessel wall. As the vessel thickens, it becomes less distensible and less reactive to many neurological and chemical stimuli that would ordinarily dilate or constrict it. As a result, the coronary vessels no longer are able to balance the myocardial demand for oxygen with increased blood supply. More recent evidence indicates that the makeup of the core of the atheroma may be a primary determinant of which atheromas might rupture and cause acute blockage of a vessel. The softer, more lipid-filled atheromas appear to be more likely to rupture than stable, harder cores.

Risk Factors

Strong evidence exists that atheroma development occurs more quickly in patients with elevated cholesterol and lipid levels. Patients who consume high-fat diets are more likely to develop high lipid levels. However, patients without increased lipid levels can also develop atheromas leading to CAD, so other factors evidently contribute to this process. Although the exact mechanism of atherogenesis (atheroma development) is not understood, certain **risk factors** increase the likelihood that a person will develop CAD.

The following is a list of unmodifiable and modifiable risk factors (see also Critical Thinking Scenario 47-1):

Unmodifiable Risk Factors

Genetic predispositions: CAD is more likely to occur in people who have a family history of the disease.

Age: The incidence of CAD increases with age.

Gender: Men are more likely than premenopausal women to have CAD; however, the incidence is almost equal in men and postmenopausal women, a possible link to a protective effect of estrogens (see Box 47.1).

Modifiable Risk Factors

Gout: Increased uric acid levels seem to injure vessel walls.

Cigarette smoking: Nicotine causes vasoconstriction and may have an effect on the endothelium of blood vessels; over time, smoking can lower oxygen levels in the blood.

Sedentary lifestyle: Exercise increases the levels of chemicals that seem to protect the coronary arteries.

High stress levels: Constant sympathetic reactions increase the myocardial oxygen demand while causing vasoconstriction and may contribute to a remodeling of the blood vessel endothelium, leading to an increased susceptibility to atheroma development.

Hypertension: High pressure in the arteries causes endothelial injury and increases afterload and myocardial oxygen demand.

Obesity: This may reflect altered fat metabolism, which increases the heart's workload.

Diabetes: Diabetics have a capillary membrane thickening, which accelerates the effects of atherosclerosis, and an abnormal fat metabolism.

Other factors that, if untreated, may contribute to CAD include bacterial infections (*Chlamydia* infections have been correlated with onset of CAD, and treatment with tetracycline and fluororoentgenography has been associated with decreased incidence of CAD, indicating a possible bacterial link) and autoimmune processes (some plaques contain antibodies and other products of immune reactions, making autoimmune reactions a possibility). Different ethnic groups also have different risk factors, as discussed in Box 47.2.

Treatment

Because an exact cause of CAD is not known, successful treatment involves manipulating a number of these risk factors (Table 47.1). Overall treatment and prevention of CAD should include the following measures: decreasing dietary fats (a decrease in total fat intake and limiting saturated fats seems to have the most impact on serum lipid levels); losing weight; eliminating smoking; increasing exercise levels; decreasing stress; and treating hypertension, diabetes, and gout.

Fats and Biotransformation (Metabolism)

Fats are taken into the body as dietary fats, then broken down in the stomach to fatty acids, lipids, and cholesterol (Figure 47.1). The presence of these products in the duodenum stimulates contraction of the gallbladder and the release

CRITICAL THINKING SCENARIO 47-1

Treating Hyperlipidemia

The Situation

M.M., a 55-year-old white businessman, was seen for a routine insurance physical examination. He was found to be obese and borderline hypertensive, with a nonfasting low-density lipoprotein (LDL) level of 325 mg/dL (very high). M.M. reported smoking two packs of cigarettes a day and noted in his family history that both of his parents died of heart attacks before age 50. He described himself as a "workaholic" with no time to exercise and a tendency to eat most of his meals in restaurants. The primary medical regimen suggested for M.M. included ceasing or decreasing smoking, weight loss, dietary changes to eliminate saturated fats, and decreased stress. On a return visit after 4 weeks, M.M. had lost 7 pounds and reported a decrease in smoking, but his LDL levels were unchanged. The use of an antihyperlipidemic drug was discussed.

Critical Thinking

What nursing interventions are appropriate at this point? *Consider all of the known risk factors for coronary artery disease (CAD), then rank M.M's risk based on those factors.*

What lifestyle changes can help M.M. reduce his risk of heart disease?

What support services should be consulted to help M.M.?

Should other tests be done before considering any drug therapy for M.M.? *Think about the kind of patient teaching that would help M.M. cope with the overwhelming lifestyle changes that have been suggested, yet remain compliant to his medical regimen.*

Discussion

M.M.'s description of himself as a workaholic should alert the nurse to the possibility that he will have trouble adapting to any prescribed lifestyle changes. (Workaholics tend to be very organized, goal-driven, and somewhat controlling individuals). M.M. should first receive extensive teaching about CAD, his risk factors, and his options. The benefits of decreasing or eliminating risk factors should be discussed. M.M. may be more compliant if he exercises some control over his situation, so he should be invited to suggest possible lifestyle changes or adaptations. M.M. also should be encouraged to set short-range goals that are achievable, to help him feel successful.

Referral to a dietitian and to an exercise program may help M.M. select foods and exercises that fit into his lifestyle. A stress test, angiogram, or both may be ordered to evaluate the actual state of M.M.'s coronary arteries. The results of these tests could serve as powerful teaching tools and motivators.

M.M. needs to understand that antihyperlipidemic drugs can cause dizziness, headaches, gastrointestinal upset, and constipation. Because of his busy lifestyle, M.M. may have trouble coping with these adverse effects. M.M.'s health care provider may need to try a variety of different drugs or combinations of drugs to find ones that are effective but do not cause unacceptable adverse effects.

The American Heart Association (AHA) has numerous booklets, diets, support groups, and counselors who can help M.M. as he tries to adapt to his medical regimen. He can contact the AHA online at http://www.americanheart.org for a quick reference and referrals to other sources. M.M. will benefit from having a consistent health care provider who can offer him encouragement, answer any questions, and allow him to vent his feelings. This health care provider can help to coordinate all of his various referrals and activities and act as a consistent base for reassurance and questions. Many times, lifestyle changes are the most difficult part of this medical regimen, so M.M. will need constant support.

Nursing Care Guide for M.M.: HMG-CoA Reductase Inhibitors

Assessment: History And Examination

Assess M.M.'s health history for allergies to any HMG-CoA reductase inhibitor or fungal byproducts; hepatic dysfunction, pregnancy, lactation, endocrine disorders

Focus the physical examination on the following areas:

CV: blood pressure, pulse, perfusion

Neuro (CNS): orientation, affect, reflexes, vision

Skin: color, lesions, texture

Resp: rate, adventitious sounds

GI: abdominal examination, bowel sounds

Laboratory tests: liver and renal function tests, serum lipids

(continued)

Treating Hyperlipidemia *(continued)*

Nursing Diagnoses

Disturbed Sensory Perception related to CNS effects

Risk for Injury related to CNS, liver, renal effects

Acute Pain related to headache, myalgia, and GI effects

Deficient Knowledge regarding drug therapy

Implementation

Administer drug at bedtime.

Monitor serum lipids prior to therapy.

Provide comfort and safety measures: Give small meals.

Arrange for periodic ophthalmic exams to screen for cataracts.

Give drug with food if GI upset occurs

Institute bowel program as needed

Provide safety measures if needed

Monitor liver function and arrange to stop drug if liver impairment occurs.

Provide support and reassurance to deal with drug effects and need to make lifestyle, diet, and exercise changes.

Provide patient teaching regarding drug, dosage, adverse effects, what to report, safety precautions.

Evaluation

Evaluate drug effects: lowering of serum cholesterol and lipid levels, prevention of first myocardial infarction, slowed progression of CAD.

Monitor for adverse effects: sedation, dizziness, headache, cataracts, GI upset; hepatic or renal dysfunction; rhabdomyolysis.

Monitor for drug–drug interactions as indicated for each drug.

Evaluate effectiveness of patient teaching program.

Evaluate effectiveness of comfort and safety measures.

Patient Teaching for M.M.

- ☐ An HMG-CoA reductase inhibitor, or "statin," is an antihyperlipidemic agent, which means it works to decrease the levels of certain lipids, or fats, in your blood. An increase in serum lipid levels has been associated with the development of many blood vessel disorders, including coronary artery disease, which can lead to a heart attack. This drug must be used in conjunction with a low-calorie, low-saturated-fat diet and an exercise program.
- ☐ Some of the following adverse effects may occur:
  - *Headache, blurred vision, nervousness, insomnia:* Avoid driving or performing hazardous or delicate tasks that require concentration; these effects may pass with time.
  - *Nausea, vomiting, flatulence, constipation:* Small, frequent meals may help. If constipation becomes a problem, consult with your health care provider for appropriate interventions.
  - Report any of the following to your health care provider: *severe GI upset, vision changes, unusual bleeding, dark urine, or light-colored stools.*
- ☐ You will need to have regular medical examinations to monitor the effectiveness of this drug on your lipid levels and to detect any adverse effects. These examinations will include blood tests and eye examinations.
- ☐ Tell any doctor, nurse, or other health care provider that you are taking this drug.
- ☐ Keep this drug, and all medications, out of the reach of children.
- ☐ To help decrease your risk of heart disease, follow these guidelines; adhere to a diet that is low in calories and saturated fat, exercise regularly, stop smoking, and reduce stress.

of bile. **Bile acids**, which contain high levels of **cholesterol** (fat), act like a detergent in the small intestine, breaking up fats. (Imagine ads for dishwashing detergents that break up the grease and fats in the dishwashing water; bile acids do much the same thing.)

Bile acids break down the fats into small units, called micelles, that can be absorbed into the wall of the small intestine. The bile acids are then reabsorbed and recycled to the gallbladder, where they remain until the gallbladder is again stimulated to release them to facilitate fat absorption.

Because fats and water do not mix, the fats cannot be absorbed directly into the plasma but need to be transported on a plasma protein. To allow absorption, micelles are carried on a **chylomicron**, a package of fats and proteins. This packaging is done by brush enzymes in all of the small intestine. The chylomicrons pass through the wall of the small intestine, where they are picked up by the lymphatic system surrounding the intestines. The chylomicrons travel through the lymphatic system to the heart and then are sent out into circulation. The proteins that are exposed on the chylomicron, called apoproteins, determine the fate of the lipids or fats

BOX 47.1 Gender Considerations: Women and Heart Disease

Until the late 1990s, heart disease was considered to be a condition that primarily affected men. Because of that belief, women were seldom screened for heart disease, and when they did experience acute cardiac events, they were not treated promptly or adequately. However, recent research has shown that heart disease is the leading cause of death among women, surpassing such diseases as breast and colon cancers. This finding has led to further research, still ongoing, about women and heart disease.

Women enjoy a protective hormone effect against the development of coronary artery disease (CAD) until menopause, when estrogen loss seems to rapidly increase the production of atheromas and the development of CAD. In several studies, women who received hormone replacement therapy (HRT) at menopause had a significantly reduced risk of CAD and myocardial infarction (MI) in the first few years after the onset of menopause. Research showed, however, that after 5 years of HRT the incidence of MI and stroke rose sharply, leading to an early closure of the study. Studies have found that women experience different symptoms of heart disease—jaw and neck pain, fatigue, and insomnia—and sometimes these are overlooked.

HRT is not recommended as a means of reducing risk of heart disease or stroke, although it is still recommended for the treatment of severe menopausal symptoms in the first few years after menopause. Women should be advised to reduce other cardiac risk factors by eating a diet low in saturated fats, exercising regularly, not smoking, controlling weight, managing stress, and seeking treatment for gout, hypertension, and diabetes.

Clearly, heart disease is not just a disease of men. Research will continue to offer health care professionals new information on preventing and treating heart disease in women.

being carried. For example, some of these packages are broken down in the tissues to be used for energy, some are stored in fat deposits for future use as energy, and some continue to the liver, where they are further processed into lipoproteins.

The lipoproteins produced in the liver that have well-known clinical implications are the **low-density lipoproteins (LDL)** and the **high-density lipoproteins (HDL)**. LDLs enter circulation as tightly packed cholesterol, triglycerides, and lipids—all of which are carried by proteins that enter circulation to be broken down for energy or stored for future use as energy. When an LDL package is broken down, many remnants or leftovers need to be returned to the liver for recycling. If a person has many of these remnants in the blood vessels, it is thought that the inflammatory process is initiated to help remove this debris. Some experts believe that this is the underlying process involved in atherogenesis.

HDLs enter circulation as loosely packed lipids that are used for energy and to pick up remnants of fats and cholesterol that are left in the periphery by LDL breakdown. HDLs serve a protective role in cleaning up remnants in blood vessels. It is known that HDL levels increase during exercise, which could explain why people who exercise regularly lower their risk of CAD. HDL levels also increase in response to estrogen, which could explain some of the protective effect of estrogen before menopause.

BOX 47.2 CULTURAL CONSIDERATIONS FOR DRUG THERAPY

Variations in Coronary Artery Disease Risk Among Cultures

Despite the fact that white Americans have the highest incidence of coronary artery disease, certain known risk factors may place other ethnic groups at greater risk. For example, hypertension and diabetes occur more frequently among African Americans and Native Americans than among whites. Regardless of race, all adults should be screened both for risk factors and for signs and symptoms of coronary artery disease.

Cultural variations in key parameters:

- Serum cholesterol levels: Whites > African Americans, Native Americans
- High-density lipoprotein (HDL) levels: African Americans, Asian Americans > Whites; Mexican Americans > Whites
- Low-density lipoprotein (LDL) levels: African Americans < Whites
- HDL:cholesterol ratio: African Americans < Whites

Rosuvastatin, the newest of the HMG Co-A inhibitors, reaches higher serum levels in Asian Americans than in other populations. Because of the risk of rhabdomyolysis with high serum levels, it is recommended that this drug not be used in Asian American patients until a safety record can be established.

Cholesterol

The body needs fats, particularly cholesterol, to maintain normal function. Cholesterol is the base unit for the formation of the steroid hormones (the sex hormones as well as the adrenal cortical hormones). It is also a basic unit in the formation and maintenance of cell membranes. Cholesterol is usually provided through the diet and the fat metabolism process just described. If dietary cholesterol falls off, the body is prepared to produce cholesterol to ensure that the cell membranes and the endocrine system are intact. Every cell in the body has the metabolic capability of producing cholesterol. The enzyme hydroxymethylglutaryl–coenzyme A reductase **(HMG-CoA reductase)** regulates the early, rate-limiting step in the cellular synthesis of cholesterol. If dietary cholesterol is severely limited, the cellular synthesis of cholesterol will increase (Figure 47.2).

Table 47.1 Risk Factors for Coronary Artery Disease

Unmodifiable Risks	Modifiable Risks	Suggested Modifications
Family history	Sedentary lifestyle	Exercise
Age	High-fat diet	Low-fat diet (polyunsaturated and monounsaturated fats)
Gender	Smoking	Smoking cessation
	Obesity	Weight loss
	High stress levels	Stress management
	Bacterial infections	Antibiotic treatment
	Diabetes	Control of blood glucose levels
	Hypertension	Control of blood pressure
	Gout	Control of uric acid levels
	Menopause	Hormone replacement therapy (first few years of menopause only)

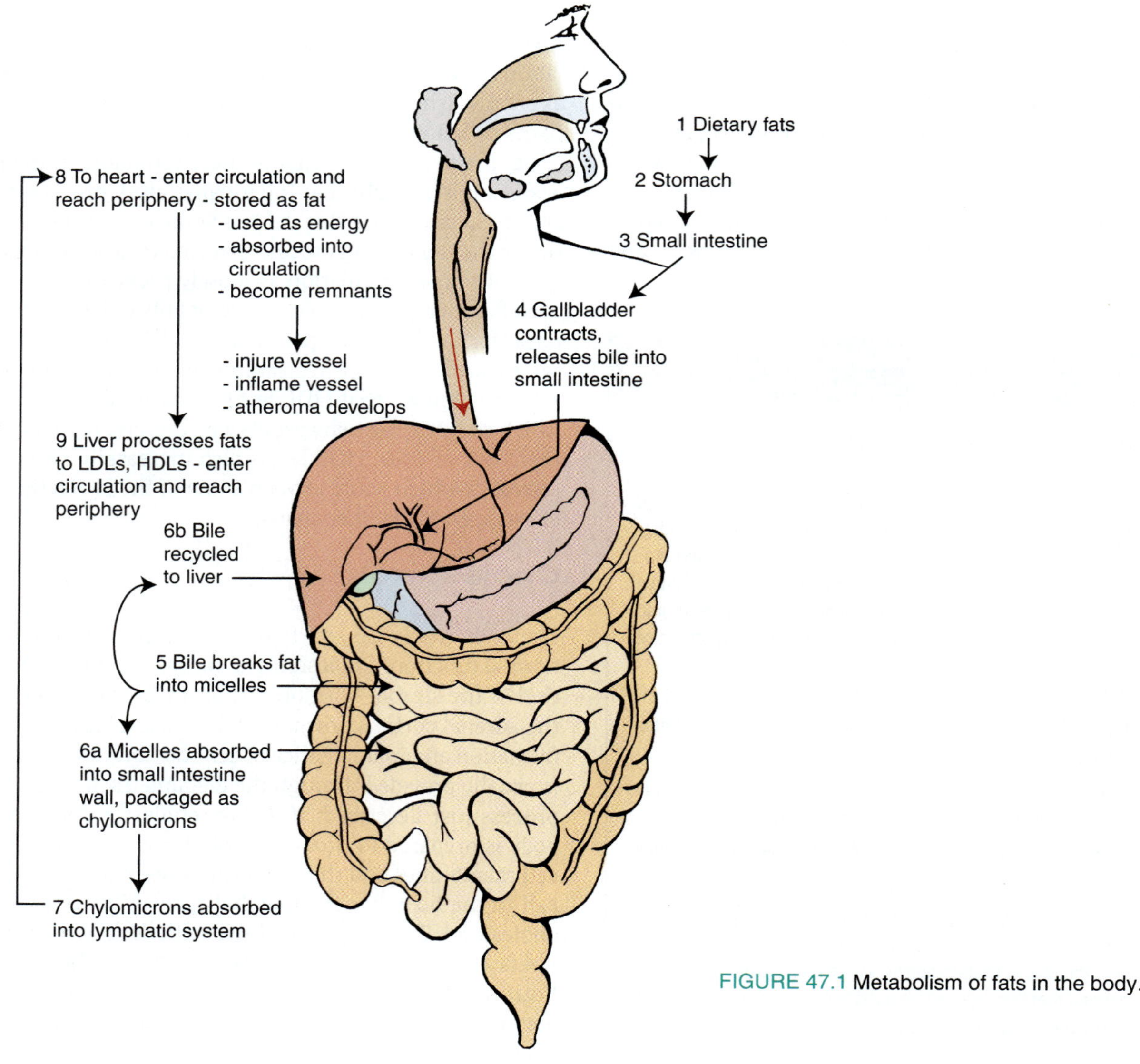
1 Dietary fats
2 Stomach
3 Small intestine
4 Gallbladder contracts, releases bile into small intestine
5 Bile breaks fat into micelles
6a Micelles absorbed into small intestine wall, packaged as chylomicrons
6b Bile recycled to liver
7 Chylomicrons absorbed into lymphatic system
8 To heart - enter circulation and reach periphery - stored as fat
- used as energy
- absorbed into circulation
- become remnants
- injure vessel
- inflame vessel
- atheroma develops
9 Liver processes fats to LDLs, HDLs - enter circulation and reach periphery

FIGURE 47.1 Metabolism of fats in the body.

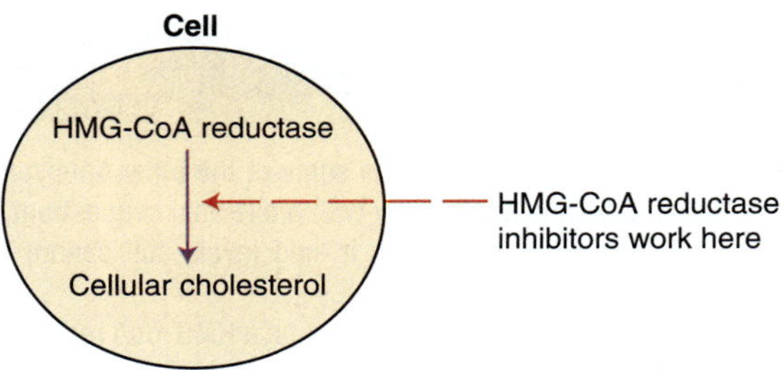

FIGURE 47.2 Cellular production of cholesterol.

Hyperlipidemias

Hyperlipidemia, an increase in the level of lipids in the blood, increases a person's risk for the development of CAD. Though the exact role that lipids play is not completely understood, the levels of lipids that contribute to CAD risk have been established (Table 47.2). Hyperlipidemia can result from excessive dietary intake of fats or from genetic alterations in fat metabolism leading to a variety of elevated fats in the blood (e.g., hypercholesterolemia, hypertriglyceridemia, alterations in LDL and HDL concentrations). Dietary modifications are often successful in treating hyperlipidemia that is caused by excessive dietary intake of fats. Drug therapy is needed if the cause is genetically linked alterations in lipid levels or if dietary limits do not decrease the serum lipid levels to an acceptable range.

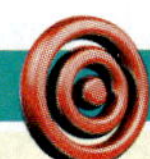

FOCUS POINTS

- CAD is associated with arterial atheromas or plaques, narrowed arterial lumens, and hardening of the artery wall, all of which lead to impaired contraction and vascular dilation.
- Risk factors for CAD include increasing age, male gender, genetic predisposition, high-fat diet, sedentary lifestyle, smoking, obesity, high stress levels, bacterial infections, diabetes, hypertension, gout, and menopause.
- CAD prevention and treatment aim at decreasing risk factors to delay disease or decrease its progress.
- Bile acids act like detergents to break down or metabolize fats into small molecules called micelles. Micelles are absorbed into the intestinal wall and combined with proteins to become chylomicrons, which can be transported throughout the circulatory system.
- Cholesterol is a fat that is used to make bile acids; all cells can produce cholesterol, which is the base for steroid hormones and cell membrane structure.
- The enzyme HMG-CoA reductase controls the final step that produces cellular cholesterol; HMG-CoA is active in every cell.

Antihyperlipidemic Agents

Drugs that are used to treat hyperlipidemia include bile acid sequestrants, HMG-CoA inhibitors, fibrates, niacin, cholesterol absorption inhibitors, and, in some cases, hormones (in women). These drugs are often used in combination and should be part of an overall health care regimen that includes exercise, dietary restrictions, and lifestyle changes to decrease the risk of CAD. (See Box 47.3 for their use in various age groups.)

Bile Acid Sequestrants

Bile acid sequestrants bind with bile acids, leading to their excretion in the feces. The resulting low levels of bile acids re-entering hepatic circulation stimulate the production of more bile acids in the liver. Bile acids contain cholesterol. Because the liver must use cholesterol to manufacture bile

Table 47.2 Lipid Blood Level Classifications

	Serum Concentration (mg/dL)					
Lipid type	*Low*	*Optimal*	*Normal or desirable*	*Borderline high*	*High*	*Very high*
Total cholesterol	—	—	<200	200–239	≥240	—
LDL cholesterol	—	<100	100–129	130–159	160–189	≥190
HDL cholesterol	<40	—	—	—	≥60	—
Triglycerides	—	—	<150	150–199	200–499	≥500

Patients with other risk factors (e.g., diabetes, hypertension) should be advised to strive for the lower end of cholesterol, LDL, and triglyceride levels.
Source: Third Report of the National Cholesterol Education Program (NCEP) Expert Panel. (September 2002). Bethesda, MD: NIH Publication No. 02-5215. National Institutes of Health. National Heart, Lung and Blood Institute.

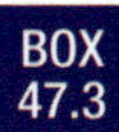

BOX 47.3 **DRUG THERAPY ACROSS THE LIFESPAN**

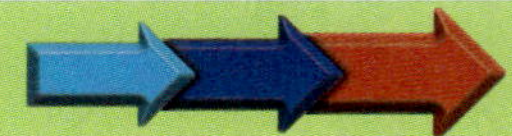

Hyperlipidemic Agents

CHILDREN

Familial hypercholesterolemia may be seen in children. Because of the importance of lipids in the developing nervous system, treatment is usually restricted to tight dietary restrictions to limit fats and calories.

Clofibrate has been used to treat genetic hypercholesterolemia that is unresponsive to dietary restrictions. The HMG-CoA inhibitors lovastatin, simvastatin, and atorvastatin can be used in postmenarchal girls and boys 10–17 years of age for treating familial hypercholesterolemia. Pravastatin has been approved for use in children >8 years of age, but these children should be monitored very closely.

ADULTS

Lifestyle changes including dietary restrictions, exercise, smoking cessation, and stress reduction should be tried before any antihyperlipidemic drug is used.

HMG-CoA reductase inhibitors are the first drug of choice in the treatment of hypercholesterolemia in patients who are at risk for, or who have already developed, coronary artery disease. The drugs are well tolerated and less expensive than some of the other antihyperlipidemic drugs. Combination therapy with a bile acid sequestrant, a fibrate, or niacin may be necessary if lipid levels still cannot be reduced.

Women of child-bearing age should not take HMG-CoA reductase inhibitors, which are pregnancy category X. Bile acid sequestrants are the drug of choice for these women if a lipid-lowering agent is needed.

OLDER ADULTS

No outcome data are available to prove the impact of lipid-lowering agents in decreasing the incidence of myocardial infarction or cardiac death in the older population.

Lifestyle changes including dietary restrictions, exercise, smoking cessation, and stress reduction should be tried before any antihyperlipidemic drug is used.

Lower doses of HMG-CoA reductase inhibitors should be used in elderly patients and in any patient with renal dysfunction. Care must be taken with those drugs that cannot be cut, crushed, or chewed. Alert patients about these restrictions.

acids, the hepatic intracellular cholesterol level falls, leading to an increased absorption of cholesterol-containing LDL segments from circulation to replenish the cell's cholesterol. The end result is a decrease in plasma cholesterol levels. Three bile acid sequestrants are currently in use (Table 47.3).

Cholestyramine (*Questran*) is a powder that must be mixed with liquids and taken up to six times a day. Colestipol (*Colestid*), available in both powder and tablet form, is taken only four times a day. Colesevelam (*Welchol*) is available in tablet form and is taken once or twice a day.

Therapeutic Actions and Indications

Bile acid sequestrants bind with bile acids in the intestine to form a complex that is excreted in the feces (Figure 47.3). As a result, the liver must use cholesterol to make more bile acids. The serum levels of cholesterol and LDL decrease as the circulating cholesterol is used to provide the cholesterol the liver needs to make bile acids. These drugs are used to reduce serum cholesterol in patients with primary hypercholesterolemia (manifested by high cholesterol and high LDLs) as an adjunct to diet and exercise. Cholestyramine is also used to treat pruritus associated with partial biliary obstruction.

Pharmacokinetics

The bile acid sequestrants are resins that bind with bile acids in the intestine to form an insoluble complex that is then excreted in feces. These drugs are not absorbed systemically.

Table 47.3 DRUGS IN FOCUS

Bile Acid Sequestrants

Drug Name	Usual Dosage	Usual Indications
P cholestyramine (*Questran*)	4 g PO one to two times per day, maximum dose 24 g/day; must be mixed with water or other noncarbonated fluids	Adjunctive treatment of primary hypercholesterolemia; pruritus associated with partial biliary obstruction
colesevelam (*Welchol*)	Three 625-mg tablets taken twice a day with meals, or six tablets taken once daily with a meal	Adjunctive therapy with diet and exercise to reduce low-density lipoproteins in patients with familial hypercholesterolemia; may be combined with an HMG-CoA reductase inhibitor
colestipol (*Colestid*)	Granule form: 5–30 g/day PO; may be taken in divided doses; must be mixed in water or other liquid Tablet form: 2–16 g/day PO taken once or in divided doses; tablets must not be cut, crushed, or chewed	Adjunctive treatment of primary hypercholesterolemia

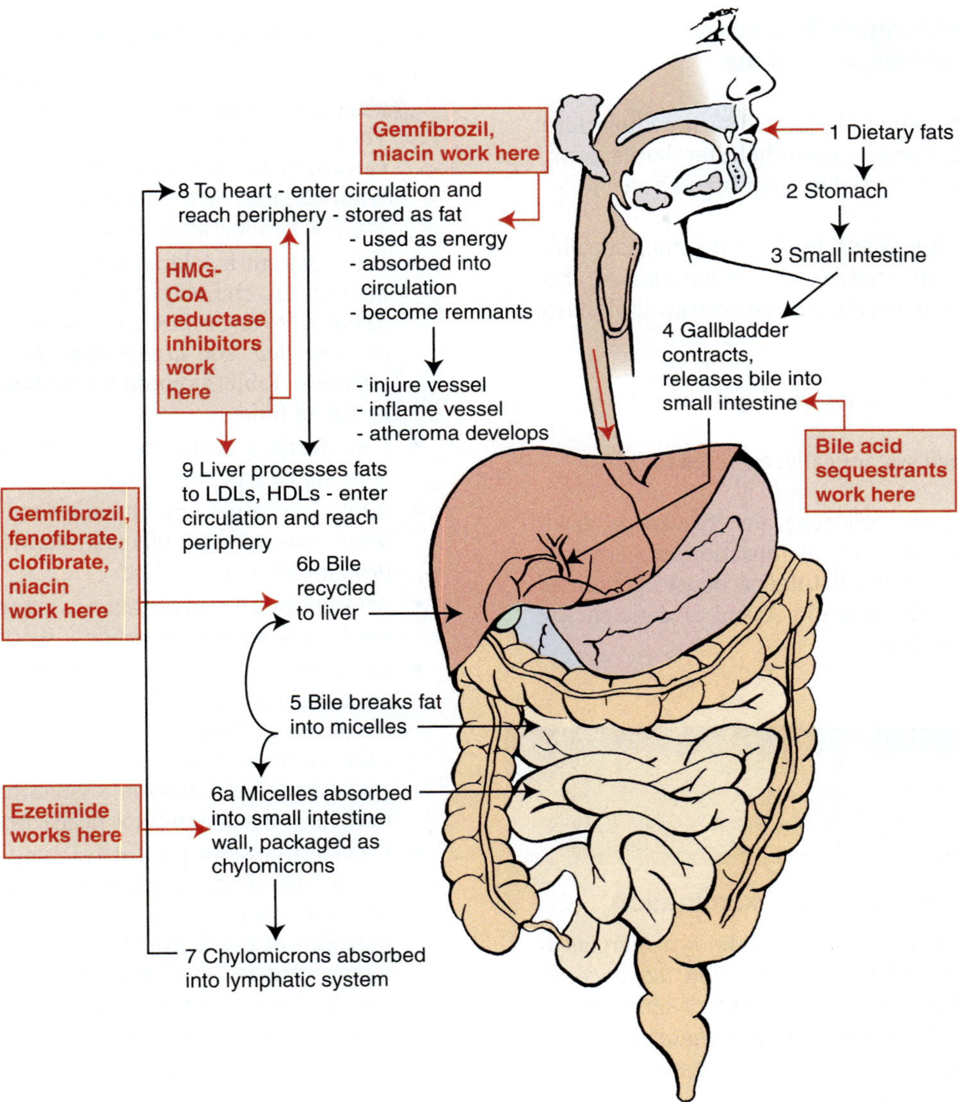

Gemfibrozil, niacin work here
8 To heart - enter circulation and reach periphery - stored as fat
- used as energy
- absorbed into circulation
- become remnants
HMG-CoA reductase inhibitors work here
- injure vessel
- inflame vessel
- atheroma develops
9 Liver processes fats to LDLs, HDLs - enter circulation and reach periphery
Gemfibrozil, fenofibrate, clofibrate, niacin work here
6b Bile recycled to liver
5 Bile breaks fat into micelles
Ezetimide works here
6a Micelles absorbed into small intestine wall, packaged as chylomicrons
7 Chylomicrons absorbed into lymphatic system
1 Dietary fats
2 Stomach
3 Small intestine
4 Gallbladder contracts, releases bile into small intestine
Bile acid sequestrants work here

FIGURE 47.3 Sites of action of lipid-lowering agents.

Their action is limited to their effects while they are present in the intestine.

Contraindications and Cautions

Bile acid sequestrants are contraindicated in the presence of allergy to any bile acid sequestrant. These drugs also are contraindicated in the following conditions: complete biliary obstruction, *which would prevent bile from being secreted into the intestine;* abnormal intestinal function, *which could be aggravated by the presence of these drugs;* and pregnancy or lactation, *because the potential decrease in the absorption of fat and fat-soluble vitamins could have a detrimental effect on the fetus or neonate.*

Adverse Effects

Adverse effects associated with the use of these drugs include headache, anxiety, fatigue, and drowsiness, which could be related to changes in serum cholesterol levels. Direct gastrointestinal (GI) irritation, including nausea and constipation that may progress to fecal impaction, and aggravation of hemorrhoids may occur. Other effects include increased bleeding times related to a decreased absorption of vitamin K and consequent decreased production of clotting factors; vitamin A and D deficiencies related to decreased absorption of fat-soluble vitamins; rash; and muscle aches and pains.

Clinically Important Drug–Drug Interactions

Malabsorption of fat-soluble vitamins occurs when they are combined with these drugs. These drugs decrease or delay the absorption of thiazide diuretics, digoxin, warfarin, thyroid hormones, and corticosteroids. Consequently, any of these drugs should be taken 1 hour before or 4 to 6 hours after the bile acid sequestrant.

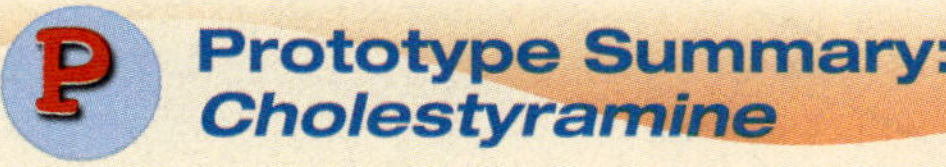

Prototype Summary: Cholestyramine

Indications: Reduction of elevated serum cholesterol in patients with primary hypercholesterolemia, pruritus associated with partial biliary obstruction

Actions: Binds bile acids in the intestine, allowing excretion in feces instead of reabsorption, causing cholesterol to be iodized in the liver and serum cholesterol levels to fall

Pharmacokinetics: Not absorbed systemically

$T_{1/2}$: Not absorbed systemically, excreted in feces

Adverse effects: Rash, headache, anxiety, vertigo, dizziness, constipation due to fecal impaction, exacerbation of hemorrhoids, cramps, flatulence, nausea, increased bleeding tendencies, vitamin A and D deficiencies, muscle and joint pain

Nursing Considerations for Patients Receiving Bile Acid Sequestrants

Assessment: History and Examination

Screen for the following conditions: known allergies to these drugs; impaired intestinal function, *which could be exacerbated by these drugs;* biliary obstruction, *which could block the effectiveness of these drugs;* and pregnancy and lactation, *which are contraindications.*

Include screening *for baseline status before beginning therapy and for any potential adverse effects.* Assess the following: body temperature and weight; skin color, lesions, and temperature; pulse and blood pressure; affect, orientation, and reflexes; bowel sounds and abdominal examination; and serum cholesterol and lipid levels.

Nursing Diagnoses

The patient receiving a bile acid sequestrant may have the following nursing diagnoses related to drug therapy:

- Acute Pain related to central nervous system (CNS) and GI effects
- Constipation related to GI effects
- Decreased Cardiac Output related to increased bleeding
- Deficient Knowledge regarding drug therapy

Implementation With Rationale

- Do not administer powdered agents in dry form; *these drugs must be mixed in fluids to be effective.* They may be mixed with fruit juices, soups, liquids, cereals, or pulpy fruits. Colestipol, but not cholestyramine, may be mixed with carbonated beverages. Stir and swallow all of the dose.
- If the patient is taking tablets, ensure that tablets are not cut, chewed, or crushed, *because they are designed to be broken down in the GI tract; if they are crushed, the active ingredients will not be effective.* Tablets should be swallowed whole with plenty of fluid.
- Give the drug before meals, *to ensure that the drug is in the GI tract with food.*
- Administer other oral medications 1 hour before or 4 to 6 hours after the bile sequestrant, *to avoid drug–drug interactions.*
- Arrange for a bowel program as appropriate *to effectively deal with constipation if it occurs.*
- Provide comfort measures *to help the patient tolerate the drug effects.* These include small, frequent meals; access to bathroom facilities; safety precautions to prevent injury if bleeding is a problem; replacement of fat-soluble vitamins; skin care as needed; and analgesics for headache.
- Provide thorough patient teaching, including the name of the drug, dosage prescribed, proper administration, measures to avoid adverse effects, warning signs of problems, the importance of periodic monitoring and evaluation, and the need to avoid overdose and poisoning, *to enhance patient knowledge about drug therapy and promote compliance with the drug regimen.*
- Offer support and encouragement, *to help the patient deal with the diagnosis and the drug regimen and lifestyle changes that may be necessary;* refer the patient to services that might help with the high cost of these drugs.

Evaluation

- Monitor patient response to the drug as appropriate (reduction in serum cholesterol levels).
- Monitor for adverse effects (headache, vitamin deficiency, increased bleeding times, constipation, nausea, rash).
- Evaluate the effectiveness of the teaching plan (patient can name drug, dosage, adverse effects to watch for, specific measures to avoid adverse effects; patient understands importance of continued follow-up).
- Monitor the effectiveness of comfort measures and compliance with the regimen.

HMG-CoA Reductase Inhibitors

The early rate-limiting step in the synthesis of cellular cholesterol involves the enzyme HMG-CoA reductase. If this enzyme is blocked, serum cholesterol and LDL levels decrease, because more LDLs are absorbed by the cells for processing into cholesterol. In contrast, HDL levels increase slightly with this alteration in fat metabolism. HMG-CoA reductase inhibitors block HMG-CoA reductase from completing the synthesis of cholesterol. Most of these drugs are chemical modifications of compounds produced by fungi. As a group, they are frequently referred to as "statins."

The HMG-CoA reductase inhibitors include the following (Table 47.4):

- Atorvastatin (*Lipitor*) is associated with severe liver complications but can be used to lower cholesterol levels in children 10 to 17 years of age who meet specific criteria.
- Fluvastatin (*Lescol*) is actually a fungal product and should not be used with any known allergies to fungal byproducts.
- Lovastatin (*Mevacor*), one of the oldest HMG-CoA drugs available, is very long-acting and is not associated with some of the severe liver toxicity that is seen with the other agents; it too can be used with adolescents who meet specific criteria. The risk of rhabdomyolysis (an acute, sometimes fatal disease characterized by destruction of the muscles, often associated with renal failure as myoglobin builds up in the kidneys) seems to be greater with this agent.
- Pravastatin (*Pravachol*) is the only statin with outcome data to show that it is effective in decreasing CAD and the incidence of MI. It is used to prevent a first MI even in patients who do not have a documented increased cholesterol concentration, an effect that may be related to blocking of the formation of foam cells in injured arteries, which can decrease the risk of MI. It is also used with children 8 years of age or older who meet specific criteria. This drug is not associated with the severe liver toxicities of some of the other statins.
- Rosuvastatin (*Crestor*) is the newest statin; it was approved for marketing in late 2003. It appears to lower LDL and raise HDL slightly better than the other statins, and at a lower price. Some concern has been raised that it appears to pose a higher risk for the development of rhabdomyolysis in Asian patients, so it is recommended that this drug be reserved for use in non-Asian patients.
- Simvastatin (*Zocor*) is indicated for lowering cholesterol and preventing MI in patients with known hypercholesterolemia and CAD; this drug is not associated with the severe liver toxicities of some of the other statins. It is also approved for use in children 10 to 17 years of age who meet specific criteria.

Table 47.4 DRUGS IN FOCUS

HMG-CoA Reductase Inhibitors

Drug Name	Usual Dosage	Usual Indications
P atorvastatin (*Lipitor*)	10 mg/day PO with a possible dosage range of 10–80 mg/day; may be taken at any time of day Children (10–17 yr): 10 mg/day PO, maximum dose 20 mg/day	Adjunctive therapy for reduction of increased cholesterol and low-density lipoprotein (LDL) levels, triglycerides; prevention of coronary artery disease (CAD) in adults with multiple risk factors
fluvastatin (*Lescol*)	20–80 mg PO, taken at bedtime; >2 h after a bile acid sequestrant, if this combination is being used	Adjunctive therapy for reduction of increased cholesterol and LDL levels; to slow the progression of CAD in patients with known CAD; reduction of the risk of undergoing revascularization procedures
lovastatin (*Mevacor*)	20 mg/day PO taken with the evening meal; maximum dose 80 mg/day; do not exceed 20 mg/day if patient is taking immunosuppressives or has renal impairment Boys and girls 1 yr postmenarche: 20 mg/day PO, may increase to 80 mg/day	Adjunctive therapy for reduction of increased cholesterol and LDL levels; to slow the progression of CAD; primary prevention of CAD in patients with elevated lipid levels
pravastatin (*Pravachol*)	10–40 mg/day PO taken at bedtime; start with 10 mg/day in elderly patients and those with hepatic or renal impairment Children (8–13 yr): 20 mg/day PO, (14–18 yr): 40 mg/day PO	Prevention of first myocardial infarction (MI) even in patients who do not have a documented increased cholesterol level, slowing of the progression of CAD; adjunctive therapy for reduction of increased cholesterol and LDL levels
simvastatin (*Zocor*)	5–80 mg/day PO taken once a day in the evening; start with 5 mg/day in elderly patients and those with hepatic or renal impairment Children (10–17 yr): 10 mg/day PO, up to 40 mg/day based on response	Prevention of first MI in patients with known hypercholesterolemia and CAD; adjunctive therapy for reduction of increased cholesterol and LDL levels
rosuvastatin (*Crestor*)	10 mg/day PO initial dose range; 5–40 mg/day	Adjunctive therapy for reduction of increased cholesterol and LDL levels, triglycerides

Therapeutic Actions and Indications

HMG-CoA reductase inhibitors block the formation of cellular cholesterol, leading to a decrease in serum cholesterol and a decrease in serum LDLs, with a slight increase or no change in the levels of HDLs (see Figure 47.2). Because these drugs undergo a marked first-pass effect in the liver, most of their effects are seen in the liver. These drugs may also have some effects on the process that generates atheromas in vessel walls. That exact mechanism of action is not understood. These drugs are indicated as adjuncts with diet and exercise for the treatment of increased cholesterol and LDL levels that are unresponsive to dietary restrictions alone; to slow the progression of CAD in patients with documented CAD (pravastatin, lovastatin, and simvastatin); and to prevent first MI in patients who are at risk for MI (pravastatin, atorvastatin, lovastatin, and simvastatin).

Pharmacokinetics

The statins are all absorbed from the GI tract and undergo first-pass metabolism in the liver. They are excreted through feces and urine. Atorvastatin levels are not affected by renal disease, but patients with renal impairment who are taking other statins must be monitored closely. The peak effect of these drugs is usually seen within 2 to 4 weeks. These drugs cross the placenta and have been associated with skeletal malformations of the fetus. The effects of these drugs on cholesterol pathways can cause serious harm to the developing fetus, and they should be avoided by women of child-bearing age who might become pregnant. These drugs are labeled pregnancy category X. Most of these drugs have been found to cross into breast milk, and, because of their effect on cholesterol synthesis, they could pose a threat to the neonate. Nursing mothers who need this drug should find another way to feed the baby.

Contraindications and Cautions

These drugs are contraindicated in the presence of allergy to any of the statins or to fungal byproducts or compounds. They also are contraindicated with active liver disease or a history of alcoholic liver disease, *which could be exacerbated, leading to severe liver failure,* and with pregnancy or lactation, *because of the potential for adverse effects on the fetus or neonate.* Caution should be used in patients with impaired endocrine function *because of the potential alteration in the formation of steroid hormones.*

Adverse Effects

The most common adverse effects associated with these drugs reflect their effects on the GI system: flatulence, abdominal pain, cramps, nausea, vomiting, and constipation. CNS effects can include headache, dizziness, blurred vision, insomnia, fatigue, and cataract development and may reflect changes in the cell membrane and synthesis of cholesterol. Increased concentrations of liver enzymes commonly occur, and acute liver failure has been reported with the use of atorvastatin and fluvastatin. Rhabdomyolysis, a breakdown of muscles whose waste products can injure the glomerulus and cause acute renal failure, has also occurred with the use of lovastatin, atorvastatin, fluvastatin, and rosuvastatin.

Clinically Important Drug–Drug Interactions

The risk of rhabdomyolysis increases if any of these drugs is combined with erythromycin, cyclosporine, gemfibrozil, niacin, or antifungal drugs; such combinations should be avoided.

Increased serum levels and resultant toxicity can occur if these drugs are combined with digoxin or warfarin; if this combination is used, serum digoxin levels and/or clotting times should be monitored carefully and the prescriber consulted for appropriate dosage changes.

Increased estrogen levels can occur if these drugs are taken with oral contraceptives; the patient should be monitored carefully if this combination is used.

Serum levels and the risk of toxicity increase if these drugs are combined with grapefruit juice; this combination should be avoided.

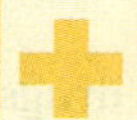

FOCUS ON **PATIENT SAFETY**

Patients who are taking HMG-CoA inhibitors need to be cautioned to avoid using grapefruit juice while taking these drugs. Grapefruit juice alters the metabolism of the drugs, leading to an increased serum level of drug and increased risk for adverse effects, such as the potentially fatal rhabdomyolysis with renal failure. The effects may last for several days, so just drinking the grapefruit juice at a different time of day does not protect the patient from risk.

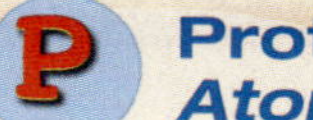

Prototype Summary: *Atorvastatin*

Indications: Adjunct to diet in the treatment of elevated cholesterol, triglycerides, and LDL; to increase HDL cholesterol in patients with primary hypercholesterolemia; treatment of boys and postmenarchal girls age 10 to 17 years with familial hypercholesterolemia and two or more risk factors for CAD

Actions: Inhibits HMG-CoA, causing a decrease in serum cholesterol levels, LDLs, and triglycerides and an increase in HDL levels

Pharmacokinetics:

Route	Onset	Peak	Duration
Oral	Slow	1–2 h	20–30 h

$T_{1/2}$: 14 hours; metabolized in the liver and cells and excreted in bile

Adverse effects: Headache, flatulence, abdominal pain, cramps, constipation, rhabdomyolysis with acute renal failure

Nursing Considerations for Patients Receiving HMG-CoA Reductase Inhibitors

Assessment: History and Examination

Screen for the following conditions, *which could be cautions or contraindications to use of the drug:* any known allergies to these drugs or to fungal byproducts; active liver disease or history of alcoholic liver disease, *which could be exacerbated by the effects of these drugs;* pregnancy or lactation, *because of potential adverse effects on the fetus or neonate;* and impaired endocrine function, *which could be exacerbated by effects on steroid hormones.*

Include screening *for baseline status before beginning therapy and for any potential adverse effects.* Assess the following: body temperature and weight; skin color, lesions, and temperature; affect, orientation, and reflexes; pulse, blood pressure, and perfusion; respirations and adventitious sounds; bowel sounds and abdominal examination; renal and liver function tests; and serum lipid levels.

Nursing Diagnoses

The patient receiving an HMG-CoA reductase inhibitor may have the following nursing diagnoses related to drug therapy:

- Disturbed Sensory Perception (Visual, Kinesthetic, Gustatory) related to CNS effects
- Risk for Injury related to CNS, liver, and renal effects
- Acute Pain related to headache, myalgia, and GI effects
- Deficient Knowledge regarding drug therapy

Implementation With Rationale

- Administer the drug at bedtime, *because the highest rates of cholesterol synthesis occur between midnight and 5 AM* (atorvastatin can be taken at any time during the day), and the drug should be taken when it will be most effective.
- Monitor serum cholesterol and LDL levels before and periodically during therapy, *to evaluate the effectiveness of this drug.*
- Arrange for periodic ophthalmic examinations, *to monitor for cataract development.*
- Monitor liver function tests before and periodically during therapy, *to monitor for liver damage;* consult with the prescriber to discontinue the drug if the aspartate aminotransferase (AST) or alanine aminotransferase (ALT) level increases to three times normal.
- Ensure that the patient has attempted a cholesterol-lowering diet and exercise program for at least 3 to 6 months before beginning therapy, *to ensure the need for drug therapy.*
- Encourage the patient to make the lifestyle changes necessary *to decrease the risk of CAD and to increase the effectiveness of drug therapy.*
- Withhold lovastatin, atorvastatin, or fluvastatin in any acute, serious medical condition (e.g., infection, hypotension, major surgery or trauma, metabolic endocrine disorders, seizures) *that might suggest myopathy or serve as a risk factor for the development of renal failure.*
- Suggest the use of barrier contraceptives for women of child-bearing age, *because there is a risk of severe fetal abnormalities if these drugs are taken during pregnancy.*
- Provide comfort measures *to help the patient tolerate drug effects.* These include small, frequent meals; access to bathroom facilities; bowel program as needed; food with the drug if GI upset is severe; environmental controls; safety precautions; and orientation as needed.
- Provide thorough patient teaching, including the name of the drug, dosage prescribed, measures to avoid adverse effects, warning signs of problems, and the need for periodic monitoring and evaluation, *to enhance the patient's knowledge of drug therapy and to promote compliance with the drug regimen.*
- Offer support and encouragement, *to help the patient deal with the diagnosis, needed lifestyle changes, and the drug regimen.*

Evaluation

- Monitor patient response to the drug (lowering of serum cholesterol and LDL levels, prevention of first MI, slowing of progression of CAD).
- Monitor for adverse effects (headache, dizziness, blurred vision, cataracts, GI upset, liver failure, rhabdomyolysis).
- Evaluate the effectiveness of the teaching plan (patient can name drug, dosage, adverse effects to watch for, specific measures to avoid adverse effects; patient understands importance of continued follow-up).
- Monitor the effectiveness of comfort measures and compliance with the regimen.

Cholesterol Absorption Inhibitors

The first of a new class of drugs to lower cholesterol levels was approved in 2003. This class of drugs localizes in the brush border of the small intestine and inhibits the absorption of cholesterol from the small intestine. As a result, less dietary cholesterol is delivered to the liver, and the liver increases the clearance of cholesterol from the serum to make up for the drop in dietary cholesterol, causing the total serum cholesterol level to drop. Ezetimibe (*Zetia*) is the first drug of this class to be approved (Table 47.5).

Therapeutic Actions and Indications

Ezetimibe works in the brush border of the small intestine to decrease the absorption of dietary cholesterol, leading to a drop in serum cholesterol levels. It is indicated as an adjunct to diet and exercise to lower cholesterol levels as monotherapy or as part of combination therapy with an HMG-CoA inhibitor or a bile acid sequestrant; in combination with atorvastatin or simvastatin as a treatment for homozygous familial hypercholesterolemia; and as adjunctive therapy to diet for the treatment of homozygous sitosterolemia to reduce elevated sitosterol and campesterol levels.

Pharmacokinetics

Ezetimibe is absorbed well after oral administration, reaching peak levels in 4 to 6 hours. It is metabolized in the liver and the small intestine, with a 22-hour half-life. Excretion is through feces and urine. It is not known whether the drug crosses the placenta or enters breast milk, so use in pregnant or lactating women should be reserved for those situations in which the benefits outweigh any potential risk to the fetus or neonate.

Contraindications and Cautions

Ezetimibe is contraindicated with allergy to any component of the drug. If it is used in combination with a statin, it should not be used during pregnancy or lactation or with severe liver disease *because of the known effects of statins, including possible liver problems and renal failure.*

The drug should be used with caution as monotherapy during pregnancy or lactation, *because the effects on the fetus or neonate are not known,* and with elderly patients or patients with liver disease *because of the potential for adverse reactions.*

Adverse Effects

The most common adverse effects associated with ezetimibe are mild abdominal pain and diarrhea. It is not associated with the bloating and flatulence that occurs with the bile acid sequestrants and the fibrates. Other adverse effects that have been reported include headache, dizziness, fatigue, upper respiratory tract infection (URI), back pain, and muscle aches and pains.

Clinically Important Drug–Drug Interactions

The risk of elevated serum levels of ezetimibe increases if it is given with cholestyramine, fenofibrate, gemfibrozil, or antacids. If these drugs are used in combination, ezetimibe should be taken at least 2 hours before or 4 hours after the other drugs.

The risk of toxicity also increases if ezetimibe is combined with cyclosporine. If this combination cannot be avoided, the patient should be monitored very closely.

If ezetimibe is combined with any fibrate, the risk of cholethiasis increases. The patient should be monitored closely.

Warfarin levels increase in a patient who is also taking ezetimibe; if this combination is used, the patient should be monitored very closely.

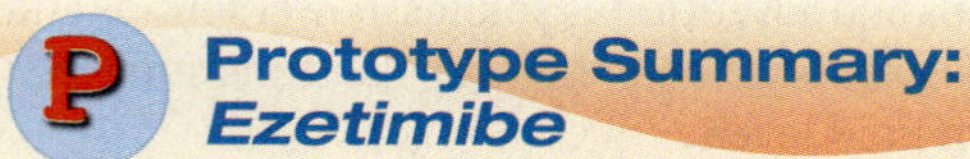

Indications: Adjunct to diet and exercise to lower serum cholesterol levels; in combination with atorvastatin or simvastatin for the treatment of homozygous familial hypercholesterolemia; with diet for the treatment of homozygous sitosterolemia to lower sitosterol and campesterol levels

Actions: Works in the brush border of the small intestine to inhibit the absorption of cholesterol

Pharmacokinetics:

Route	Onset	Peak
Oral	Moderate	4–12 h

$T_{1/2}$: 22 hours; metabolized in the liver and small intestine and excreted in feces and urine

Adverse effects: Headache, dizziness, abdominal pain, diarrhea, URI, back pain, myalgia, arthralgia

Table 47.5 DRUGS IN FOCUS

Cholesterol Absorption Inhibitor

Drug Name	Usual Dosage	Usual Indications
P ezetimibe (*Zetia*)	10 mg/day PO	Adjunct to diet and exercise to reduce cholesterol as monotherapy or combined with a statin; adjunct to diet to reduce elevated sitosterol and campesterol levels in homozygous sitosterolemia

Nursing Considerations for Patients Receiving Cholesterol Absorption Inhibitors

Assessment: History and Examination

Screen for the following conditions, *which could be cautions or contraindications to use of the drug:* any known allergies to any component of the drug; pregnancy or lactation, *because the possible effects on the fetus or neonate are not known;* or liver dysfunction or advanced age, *because the processing of the drug may differ from the norm.*

Include screening *for baseline status before beginning therapy and for any potential adverse effects.* Assess the following: skin color and lesions; affect, orientation, and reflexes; respirations and adventitious sounds; bowel sounds and abdominal examination; liver function tests; and serum lipid levels.

Nursing Diagnoses

The patient receiving a cholesterol absorption inhibitor may have the following nursing diagnoses related to drug therapy:

- Disturbed Sensory Perception (Visual, Kinesthetic, Gustatory) related to CNS effects
- Acute Pain related to headache, myalgia, and GI effects
- Deficient Knowledge regarding drug therapy

Implementation With Rationale

- Monitor serum cholesterol, triglyceride, and LDL levels before and periodically during therapy, *to evaluate the effectiveness of this drug.*
- Monitor liver function tests before and periodically during therapy *to detect possible liver damage;* consult with the prescriber *to discontinue drug use* if the AST or ALT level increases to three times normal.
- Ensure that the patient has attempted a cholesterol-lowering diet and exercise program for at least several months before beginning therapy, *to ensure the need for drug therapy.*
- Encourage the patient to make the lifestyle changes necessary *to decrease the risk of CAD and to increase the effectiveness of drug therapy.*
- Suggest the use of barrier contraceptives for women of child-bearing age if the drug is being used in combination with a statin, *because there is a risk of severe fetal abnormalities if these drugs are taken during pregnancy.*
- Provide comfort measures *to help the patient tolerate drug effects.* These include small, frequent meals; access to bathroom facilities; safety precautions; orientation as needed; and analgesics for headache and muscle aches if appropriate.
- Provide thorough patient teaching, including the name of the drug, dosage prescribed, measures to avoid adverse effects, warning signs of problems, and the need for periodic monitoring and evaluation, *to enhance the patient's knowledge of drug therapy and to promote compliance with the drug regimen.*
- Offer support and encouragement, *to help the patient deal with the diagnosis, needed lifestyle changes, and drug regimen.*

Evaluation

- Monitor patient response to the drug (lowering of serum cholesterol and LDL levels, lowering of sitosterol and campesterol levels).
- Monitor for adverse effects (headache, dizziness, GI pain, muscle aches and pains, URI).
- Evaluate the effectiveness of the teaching plan (patient can name drug, dosage, adverse effects to watch for, specific measures to avoid adverse effects; patient understands importance of continued follow-up).
- Monitor the effectiveness of comfort measures and compliance with the regimen.

Other Drugs Used to Affect Lipid Levels

Other drugs that are used to affect lipid levels do not fall into any of the classes discussed previously. They include the fibrates (derivatives of fibric acid) and the vitamin, niacin (Table 47.6).

The fibrates stimulate the breakdown of lipoproteins from the tissues and their removal from the plasma. They lead to a decrease in lipoprotein and triglyceride synthesis and secretion. The fibrates are absorbed from the GI tract and are metabolized in the liver and excreted in urine. Fibrates in use today include the following agents:

- Fenofibrate (*Tricor* and others) inhibits triglyceride synthesis in the liver, resulting in reduction of LDL levels; increases uric acid secretion; and may stimulate triglyceride breakdown. It is used for adults with very high triglyceride levels that are not responsive to strict dietary measures and who are at risk for pancreatitis. Peak effects are usually seen within 4 weeks, and the patient's serum lipid levels should be re-evaluated at that time.
- Gemfibrozil (*Lopid*) inhibits peripheral breakdown of lipids, reduces production of triglycerides and LDLs, and increases HDL concentrations. It is associated with GI and muscle discomfort. This drug should not be combined

Table 47.6 DRUGS IN FOCUS

Other Antihyperlipidemic Drugs

Drug Name	Dosage/Route	Usual Indications
fenofibrate (*Tricor*)	67 mg/day PO given with a meal; may be increased up to 67 mg PO t.i.d. as needed; monitor patients with impaired renal function and the elderly very carefully	Treatment of very high triglyceride levels in adults who are at risk for pancreatitis if not responsive to dietary measures
gemfibrozil (*Lopid*)	1200 mg/day PO divided into two doses and taken before the morning and evening meals	Treatment of very high triglyceride levels with abdominal pain and potential pancreatitis in adults
niacin (*Niaspan*)	1.5–2 g/day PO in divided doses for tablets; 500–2000 mg/day PO for ER tablets taken at bedtime	Treatment of hyperlipidemia not responding to diet and weight loss; to slow progression of coronary artery disease when combined with a bile acid sequestrant

with statins. There is an increased risk of rhabdomyolysis from 3 weeks to several months after therapy if this combination is used. If this combination cannot be avoided, the patient should be monitored very closely.

Vitamin B_3, known as niacin (*Niaspan*) or nicotinic acid, inhibits release of free fatty acids from adipose tissue, increases the rate of triglyceride removal from plasma, and generally reduces LDL and triglyceride levels and increases HDL levels. It may also decrease levels of apoproteins needed to form chylomicrons. The initial effect on lipid levels is usually seen within 5 to 7 days, with the maximum effect occurring in 3 to 5 weeks. Niacin is associated with intense cutaneous flushing, nausea, and abdominal pain, making its use somewhat limited. It also increases serum levels of uric acid and may predispose patients to the development of gout. Niacin is often combined with bile acid sequestrants for increased effect. It is given at bedtime to make maximum use of nighttime cholesterol synthesis, and it must be given 4 to 6 hours after the bile sequestrant to ensure absorption.

Combination Therapy

Frequently, if the patient shows no response to strict dietary modification, exercise, and lifestyle changes and the use of one lipid-lowering agent, combination therapy may be initiated to achieve desirable serum LDL and cholesterol levels. For example, a bile acid sequestrant might be combined with niacin; the combination would decrease the synthesis of LDLs while lowering the serum levels of LDLs. This combination is thought to help slow the progression of CAD. Box 47.4 dis-

BOX 47.4 Combination Therapy for Lowering Cholesterol Levels

In 2002, the U.S. Food and Drug administration approved *Advicor,* a fixed combination of extended-release niacin and lovastatin, for reducing the risk of atherosclerosis in patients with multiple risk factors. It was thought that the convenience of taking one tablet each day in the evening would improve patient compliance with the lipid-lowering therapy.

The drug is not intended as initial therapy. It should be used only after the patient has been stabilized on lovastatin and extended-release niacin and found to tolerate the combination and to have acceptable lower cholesterol levels.

The drug is available in three strengths: 500 mg niacin/20 mg lovastatin, 750 mg niacin/20 mg lovastatin, and 1000 mg niacin/20 mg lovastatin. The contraindications and cautions for both niacin and lovastatin apply to this drug, and patient teaching should incorporate the same warnings about adverse effects that are used with both agents.

Newer Combination Drugs for Treating CAD

Two new combination products became available in late 2003 and early 2004 for the prevention of coronary artery disease (CAD) in patients at risk for developing CAD.

- *Pravigard* is a combination of 81 or 325 mg buffered aspirin, packaged with 20, 40, or 80 mg pravastatin. The combination adds the protective effect of low-dose aspirin with the lipid-lowering effects of the pravastatin. The usual adult dose is 40 mg pravastatin with 81 or 325 mg aspirin. Dosage can be adjusted based on lipid levels.
- *Caduet* is a combination of amlodipine 5 or 10 mg and atorvastatin 10, 20, 40, or 80 mg. The patient should first be stabilized on the individual drugs before the correct combination is selected. The combination provides the blood pressure-lowering and antianginal effect of the amlodipine with the lipid-lowering effects of the atorvastatin. The usual adult dose is 5–10 mg amlodipine with 10–80 mg atorvastatin, based on patient response. The recommended pediatric dosage in children 10–17 years of age is 2.5–5 mg amlodipine with 10–20 mg atorvastatin.

In 2005, *Vytorin*, a combination of ezetimibe and simvastatin, was approved to help lower lipid levels in patients who did not have good results with single drug therapy. Ezetimibe decreases the absorption of cholesterol and simvastatin decreases the body's production of cholesterol. The drug is available in tablets that contain 10 mg ezetimibe and 10, 20, 40, or 80 mg simvastatin. Dosage should be determined based on lipid levels.

cusses fixed combination therapies that are available. However, care must be taken not to combine agents that increase the risk of rhabdomyolysis. For example, HMG-CoA reductase inhibitors are not usually combined with niacin or gemfibrozil.

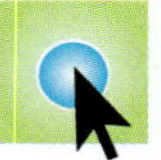

WEB LINKS

Patients and health care providers may want to consult the following Internet sources:

http://www.fda.gov/hearthealth Information on products used to prevent, diagnose, and treat cardiovascular disease.

http://www.heartcenteronline.com Information on diet, exercise, drug therapy, and cardiac rehabilitation.

http://www.my.webmd.com Patient information on the latest resources, diets, and programs.

http://www.americanheart.org Patient information, support groups, diet, exercise, and research information on heart disease.

http://www.nhlbi.nih.gov/health Specific information on exercise programs and safety.

Points to Remember

- CAD is the leading cause of death in the Western world. It is associated with the development of atheromas or plaques in arterial linings that lead to narrowing of the lumen of the artery and hardening of the artery wall, with loss of distensibility and responsiveness to stimuli for contraction or dilation.
- The cause of CAD is not known, but many contributing risk factors have been identified, including increasing age, male gender, genetic predisposition, high-fat diet, sedentary lifestyle, smoking, obesity, high stress levels, bacterial infections, diabetes, hypertension, gout, and menopause.
- Treatment and prevention of CAD is aimed at manipulating the known risk factors to decrease CAD development and progression.
- Fats are metabolized with the aid of bile acids, which act as a detergent to break fats into small molecules called micelles. Micelles are absorbed into the intestinal wall and combined with proteins to become chylomicrons, which can be transported throughout the circulatory system.
- Some fats are used immediately for energy or are stored in adipose tissue; others are processed in the liver to LDLs, which are associated with the development of CAD. LDLs are broken down in the periphery and leave many remnants (e.g., fats) that must be removed from blood vessels. This process involves the inflammatory reaction and may initiate or contribute to atheroma production.
- Some fats are processed into HDLs, which are able to absorb fats and remnants from the periphery and offer a protective effect against the development of CAD.
- Cholesterol is an important fat that is used to make bile acids. It is the base for steroid hormones and provides necessary structure for cell membranes. All cells can produce cholesterol.
- HMG-CoA reductase is an enzyme that controls the final step in production of cellular cholesterol. Blockade of this enzyme results in lower serum cholesterol levels, a resultant breakdown of LDLs, and a slight increase in HDLs.
- Bile acid sequestrants bind with bile acids in the intestine and lead to their excretion in feces. This results in lower bile acid levels as the liver uses cholesterol to produce more bile acids. The end result is a decrease in serum cholesterol and LDL levels as the liver changes its metabolism of these fats to meet the need for more bile acids.
- The cholesterol absorption inhibitor, ezetimibe, works in the brush border of the small intestine to prevent the absorption of dietary cholesterol, which leads to increased clearance of cholesterol by the liver and a resultant fall in serum cholesterol.
- Overall treatment of patients taking lipid-lowering drugs should include diet, exercise, and lifestyle changes to reduce the risk of CAD. Such lifestyle changes include stopping smoking; managing stress; and treating hypertension, gout, diabetes, estrogen deficiencies, and bacterial infections (particularly chlamydial infections).

CHECK YOUR UNDERSTANDING

Answers to the questions in this chapter may be found in the Answer Key in the back of the book.

Multiple Choice

Select the best answer to the following.

1. The body uses cholesterol in many ways, including
   a. the production of water-soluble vitamins.
   b. the formation of steroid hormones.
   c. the mineralization of bones.
   d. the development of dental plaques.

2. The formation of atheromas in blood vessels precedes the signs and symptoms of
   a. hepatitis.
   b. coronary artery disease.
   c. diabetes mellitus.
   d. COPD.

3. High cholesterol levels are considered to be
   a. a normal finding in adult males.
   b. related to stress levels.
   c. a treatable risk factor for the development of heart disease.
   d. a side effect of cigarette smoking.

4. The bile acid sequestrants
   a. are absorbed into the liver.
   b. take several weeks to show an effect.
   c. have no associated adverse effects.
   d. work in the small intestine to prevent bile salts from being reabsorbed.

5. HMG-CoA reductase works in the
   a. process of bile secretion.
   b. process of formation of cholesterol within the cell.
   c. intestinal wall to block fat absorption.
   d. kidney to block fat excretion.

6. Patients taking HMG-CoA reductase inhibitors
   a. will not have a heart attack.
   b. will not develop CAD.
   c. may develop cataracts as a result.
   d. may stop absorbing fat-soluble vitamins.

7. A patient who has high lipid levels and cannot take fibrates or HMG-CoA reductase inhibitors may be able to take
   a. nicotine.
   b. vitamin C.
   c. niacin.
   d. bran fiber products.

8. Rhabdomyolysis is a very serious adverse effect that can be seen with HMG-CoA reductase inhibitors; to detect it, patients taking these drugs would be monitored for
   a. flatulence and abdominal bloating.
   b. increased bleeding.
   c. the development of cataracts.
   d. muscle pain and weakness.

Multiple Response

Select all that apply.

1. Bile acid sequestrants would be a drug of choice for a client who has which of the following?
   a. A high LDL concentration
   b. A high triglyceride concentration
   c. Biliary obstruction
   d. Vitamin K deficiency
   e. A high HDL concentration
   f. Intolerance to statins

2. A client presents with high cholesterol and high LDL levels. Teaching for this client should include which of the following?
   a. The importance of exercise
   b. The need for dietary changes to alter cholesterol levels
   c. That taking a statin will allow a full, unrestricted diet
   d. That drug therapy is always needed when these levels are elevated
   e. The importance of controlling blood pressure and blood glucose levels
   f. That stopping smoking may also help lower lipid levels

Web Exercise

R.K. is a 46-year-old man who is diagnosed with hypertension and elevated LDLs during a routine insurance physical examination. He has a strong family history of heart disease and is concerned about the findings. He is referred to the nurse for appropriate teaching. Use the Internet to obtain the most recent information that might be useful for R.K., then prepare a teaching program for him.

Word Scramble

Unscramble the following letters to form words related to lipid-lowering therapy.

1. leolroehtcs ______________________________

2. boretaclif ______________________________

3. nniica ______________________________

4. hypipdeermliia ______________________________

5. cpoolleits ______________________________

6. vastraottina ______________________________

7. fizemiglrob ______________________________

8. lebi scaid ______________________________

9. ppooiilntre ______________________________

10. statviolna ______________________________

Bibliography and References

Abramowicz, M. (1996). Choice of lipid-lowering drugs. *Medical Letter, 38,* 67–70.

Drug facts and comparisons. (2006). St. Louis: Facts and Comparisons.

Gilman, A., Hardman, J. G., & Limbird, L. E. (Eds.). (2006). *Goodman and Gilman's the pharmacological basis of therapeutics* (11th ed.). New York: McGraw-Hill.

Karch, A. M. (2006). *2007 Lippincott's nursing drug guide.* Philadelphia: Lippincott Williams & Wilkins.

Knopp, R. H. (1999). Drug treatment of lipid disorders. *New England Journal of Medicine, 341,* 498–511.

The medical letter on drugs and therapeutics. (2006). New Rochelle, NY: Medical Letter.

Porth, C. M. (2005). *Pathophysiology: Concepts of altered health states* (7th ed.). Philadelphia: Lippincott Williams & Wilkins.

CHAPTER 48

Drugs Affecting Blood Coagulation

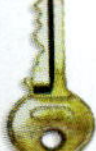

KEY TERMS

anticoagulants
clotting factors
coagulation
extrinsic pathway
Hageman factor
hemorrhagic disorders
hemostatic drugs
intrinsic pathway
plasminogen
platelet aggregation
thromboembolic disorders
thrombolytic drugs

LEARNING OBJECTIVES

Upon completion of this chapter, you will be able to:

1. Outline the mechanisms by which blood clots dissolve in the body, correlating this information with the actions of drugs used to affect blood clotting.
2. Describe the therapeutic actions, indications, pharmacokinetics, contraindications, most common adverse reactions, and important drug–drug interactions associated with antiplatelet agents, anticoagulants, low-molecular-weight heparins, thrombolytic agents, antihemophilic agents, and hemostatic agents.
3. Discuss the use of drugs that affect blood coagulation across the lifespan.
4. Compare and contrast the prototype drugs aspirin, heparin, streptokinase, antihemophilic factor, and aminocaproic acid with other agents used to affect blood coagulation.
5. Outline the nursing considerations, including important teaching points, for patients receiving drugs used to affect blood coagulation.

ANTICOAGULANTS

Antiplatelet Drugs

abciximab
anagrelide
P aspirin
cilostazol
clopidogrel
dipyridamole
eptifibatide
sulfinpyrazone
ticlopidine
tirofiban

Anticoagulants

antithrombin
argatroban
bivalirudin
desirudin
P heparin
warfarin

Low-Molecular-Weight Heparins

dalteparin
enoxaparin
tinzaparin

Anticoagulant Adjunctive Therapy

lepirudin
protamine sulfate
vitamin K

Hemorrheologic Agent

pentoxifylline

Thrombolytic Agents

alteplase
reteplase
P streptokinase
tenecteplase
urokinase

DRUGS USED TO CONTROL BLEEDING

Antihemophilic Agents

P antihemophilic factor
coagulation factor VIIa
factor IX complex

Systemic Hemostatic Agents

P aminocaproic acid
aprotinin

Topical Hemostatic Agents

absorbable gelatin
microfibrillar collagen
thrombin

The cardiovascular system is a closed system, and blood remains in a fluid state while in it. Because the blood is trapped in a closed space, it maintains the difference in pressures required to keep the system moving along. If the vascular system is injured—from a cut, a puncture, or capillary destruction—the fluid blood could leak out, causing the system to lose pressure and potentially to shut down entirely.

To deal with the problem of blood leaking and potentially shutting down the system, blood that is exposed to an injury in a vessel almost immediately forms into a solid state, or clot, which plugs the hole in the system and keeps the required pressure differences intact. These little injuries to the blood vessels occur all the time (e.g., coughing too hard with a cold, knocking into the corner of the desk when sitting down). Consequently, the system must maintain an intricate balance between the tendency to clot or form a solid state, called **coagulation**, and the need to "unclot" or reverse coagulation to keep the vessels open and the blood flowing. If a great deal of vascular damage occurs, such as with a major cut or incision, the balance in the area shifts to a procoagulation mode and a large clot is formed. At the same time, the enzymes in the plasma work to dissolve this clot before blood flow to tissues is lost, with resultant hypoxia and potential cell death.

Drugs that affect blood coagulation work at various steps in the blood clotting and clot-dissolving processes to restore the balance that is needed to maintain the cardiovascular system. Box 48.1 discusses the uses of these drugs in various age groups.

Blood Coagulation

Blood coagulation is a complex process that involves vasoconstriction, platelet clumping or aggregation, and a cascade of **clotting factors** produced in the liver that eventually react to break down fibrinogen (a protein also produced in the liver) into insoluble fibrin threads. When a clot is formed, plasmin (another blood protein) acts to break it down. Blood

BOX 48.1 DRUG THERAPY ACROSS THE LIFESPAN

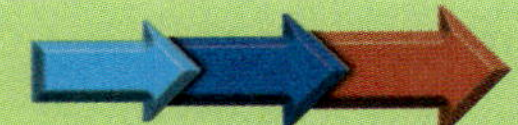

Drugs Affecting Coagulation

CHILDREN

Little research is available on the use of anticoagulants in children. If they are used, the child needs to be monitored very carefully to avoid excessive bleeding related to drug interactions or alterations in gastrointestinal or liver function. People who interact with the child need to understand the importance of preventing injuries and providing safety precautions and should be aware of what to do if the child is injured and begins to bleed.

If heparin is used, the dosage should be carefully calculated based on weight and age and checked by another person before the drug is administered.

Warfarin is used with children who are to undergo cardiac surgery. Again, the dosage must be determined based on weight and age and the child should be monitored closely.

The safety of low-molecular-weight heparins has not been established in children.

At this time, there are no indications for the use of antiplatelet or thrombolytic drugs with children.

ADULTS

Adults receiving these drugs need to be instructed in ways to prevent injury—such as using an electric razor instead of a straight razor, using a soft-bristled toothbrush to protect the gums, avoiding contact sports—and instructed in what to do if bleeding does occur (apply constant, firm pressure and contact a health care provider). They should receive a written list of signs of bleeding to watch for and to report to their health care provider.

Because so many drugs and alternative therapies are known to interact with these agents, it is very important that these patients be urged to report the use of this drug to any other health care provider and to consult with one before using any over-the-counter drugs or alternative therapies.

It is prudent to advise any patient using one of these drugs in the home setting to carry or wear a Medic-Alert notification in case of emergency.

The patient also needs to understand the importance of regular, periodic blood tests to evaluate the effects of the drug.

Because of the many risks associated with increased bleeding or increased blood clotting during pregnancy, these drugs should not be used during pregnancy unless the benefit to the mother clearly outweighs the potential risk to the fetus and to the mother at delivery. Risks of altered blood clotting in the neonate makes these drugs generally inadvisable for use during lactation.

OLDER ADULTS

Older adults may have many underlying medical conditions that require the need for drugs that alter blood clotting (e.g., coronary artery disease, cerebrovascular accident, peripheral vascular disease, transient ischemic attacks). Statistically, older adults also take more medications, making them more likely to encounter drug–drug interactions associated with these drugs. The older adult is also more likely to have impaired liver and kidney function, conditions that can alter the metabolism and excretion of these drugs.

The older adult should be carefully evaluated for liver and kidney function, use of other medications, and ability to follow through with regular blood testing and medical evaluation before therapy begins. Therapy should be started at the lowest possible level and adjusted accordingly after the patient response has been noted.

Careful attention needs to be given to the patient's total drug regimen. Starting, stopping, or changing the dosage of another drug may alter the body's metabolism of the drug that is being used to affect coagulation, leading to increased risk of bleeding or ineffective anticoagulation.

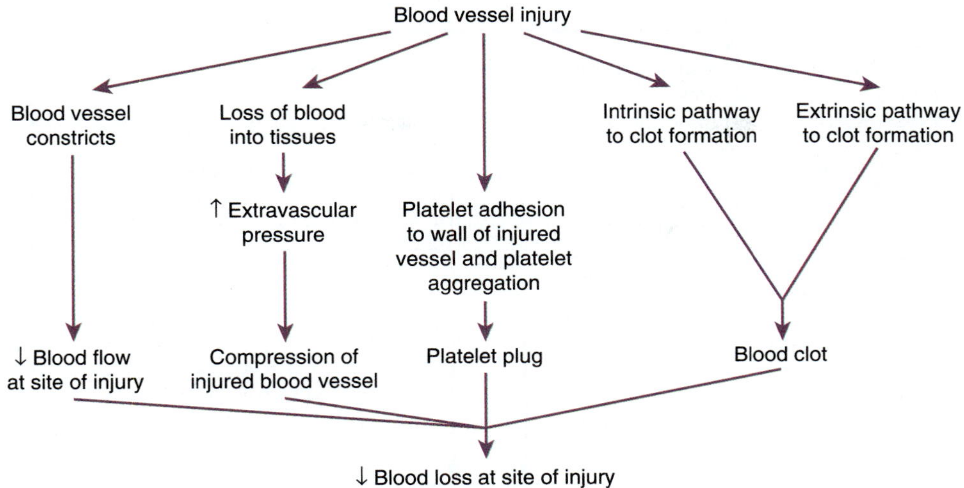

FIGURE 48.1 Process of blood coagulation.

coagulation can be affected at any step in this complicated process to alter the way that blood clotting occurs.

Vasoconstriction

The first reaction to a blood vessel injury is local vasoconstriction (Figure 48.1). If the injury to the blood vessel is very small, this vasoconstriction can seal off any break and allow the area to heal.

Platelet Aggregation

Injury to a blood vessel exposes blood to the collagen and other substances under the endothelial lining of the vessel. This exposure causes platelets in the circulating blood to stick or adhere to the site of the injury. Once they stick, the platelets release adenosine diphosphate (ADP) and other chemicals that attract other platelets, causing them to gather or aggregate and to stick as well. ADP is also a precursor of the prostaglandins, from which thromboxane A_2 is formed. Thromboxane A_2 causes local vasoconstriction and further **platelet aggregation** and adhesion. This series of events forms a platelet plug at the site of the vessel injury. In many injuries, the combination of vasoconstriction and platelet aggregation is enough to seal off the injury and keep the cardiovascular system intact (Figure 48.2).

Intrinsic Pathway

As blood comes in contact with the exposed collagen of the injured blood vessel, one of the clotting factors, **Hageman factor** (also called factor XII), a chemical substance that is found circulating in the blood, is activated. (Clotting factors are often known by a name and by a Roman numeral. When one of these factors becomes activated, the lowercase letter "a" is added; for example, activated Hageman factor is also called factor XIIa.) The activation of Hageman factor starts a number of reactions in the area: The clot formation process is activated, the clot-dissolving process is activated, and the inflammatory response is started (see Chapter 15). The activation of Hageman factor first activates clotting factor XI (plasma thromboplastin antecedent, or PTA) and then

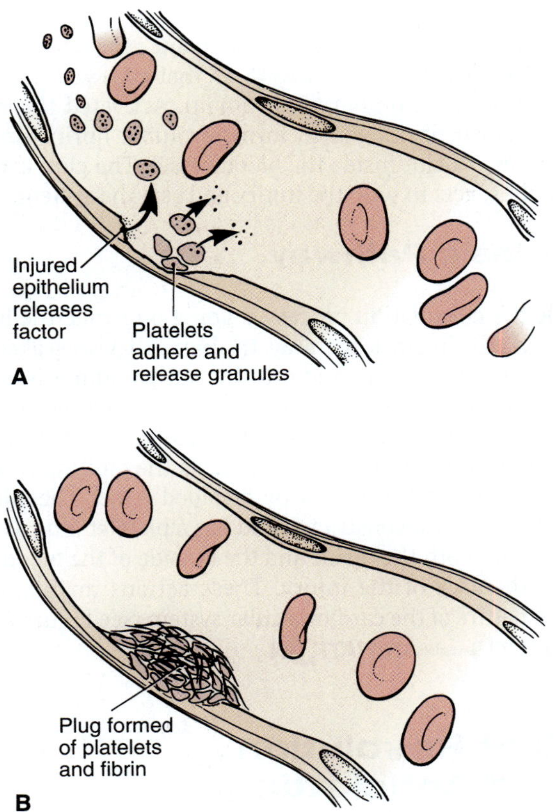

FIGURE 48.2 **(A)** Damaged vessel endothelium is a stimulus to circulating platelets, causing platelet adhesion. Platelets release mediators **(B)** and platelet aggregation results.

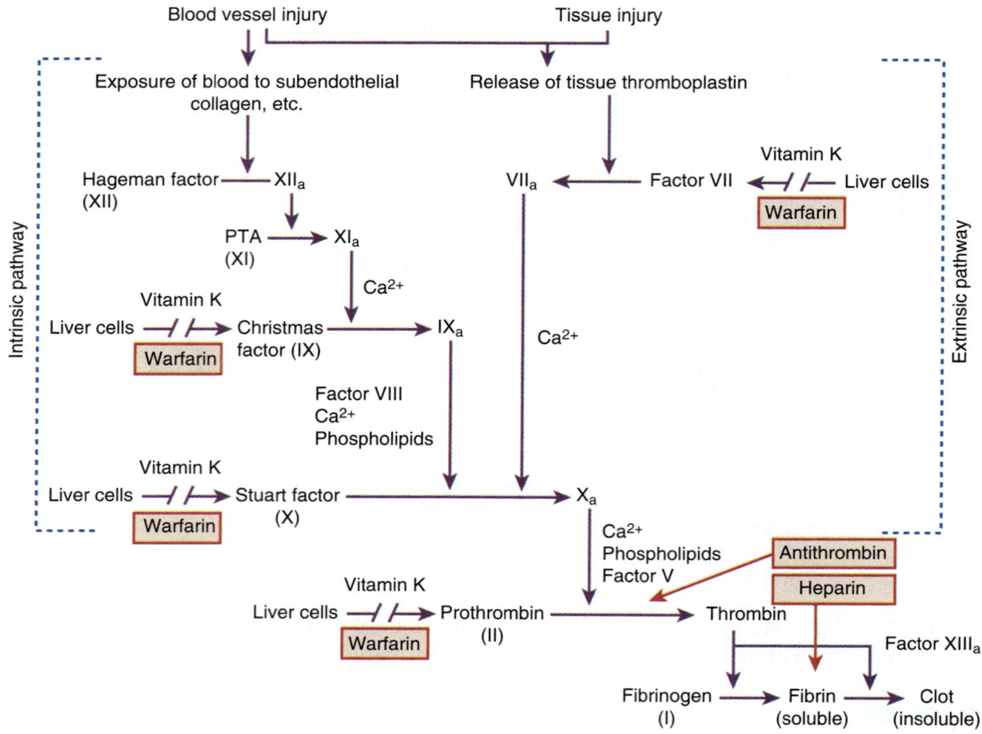

FIGURE 48.3 Details of the intrinsic and extrinsic clotting pathways. The sites of action of some of the drugs that can influence these processes are shown in red.

activates a cascading series of coagulant substances, called the **intrinsic pathway** (Figure 48.3), that ends with the conversion of prothrombin to thrombin. Activated thrombin breaks down fibrinogen to form insoluble fibrin threads, which form a clot inside the blood vessel. The clot, called a thrombus, acts to plug the injury and seal the system.

Extrinsic Pathway

While the coagulation process is going on inside the blood vessel via the intrinsic pathway, the blood that has leaked out of the vascular system and into the surrounding tissues is caused to clot by the **extrinsic pathway**. Injured cells release a substance called tissue thromboplastin, which activates clotting factors in the blood and starts the clotting cascade to form a clot on the outside of the blood vessel. The injured vessel is now vasoconstricted and has a platelet plug as well as a clot on both the inside and the outside of the blood vessel in the area of the injury. These actions maintain the closed nature of the cardiovascular system (see Figure 48.3).

CONCEPTS in action **ANIMATION**

Clot Resolution and Anticlotting

Blood plasma also contains anticlotting substances that inhibit clotting reactions that might otherwise lead to an obstruction of blood vessels by blood clots. For example, antithrombin III prevents the formation of thrombin, thus stopping the breakdown of the fibrin threads.

Another substance in the plasma, called plasmin or fibrinolysin, dissolves clots to ensure free movement of blood through the system. Plasmin is a protein-dissolving substance that breaks down the fibrin framework of blood clots and opens up vessels. Its precursor, called **plasminogen**, is found in the plasma. The conversion of plasminogen to plasmin begins with the activation of Hageman factor and is facilitated by a number of other factors, including antidiuretic hormone (ADH), epinephrine, pyrogens, emotional stress, physical activity, and the chemicals urokinase and streptokinase. Plasmin helps keep blood vessels open and functional. Very high levels of plasmin are found in the lungs (which contain millions of tiny, easily injured capillaries) and in the uterus (which in pregnancy must maintain a constant blood flow for the developing fetus). The action of plasmin is evident in the female menstrual flow in that clots do not form rapidly when the lining of the uterus is shed; the blood oozes slowly over a period of days (Figure 48.4).

Thromboembolic Disorders

Medical conditions that involve the formation of thrombi result in decreased blood flow through or total occlusion of a blood vessel. These conditions are marked by the signs and

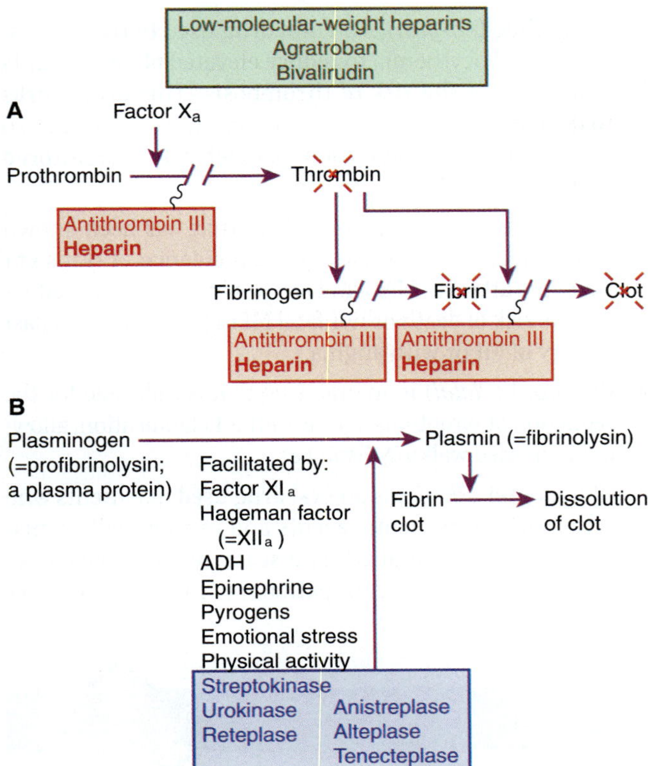

FIGURE 48.4 **(A)** Anticlotting process. Antithrombin III (in plasma) inhibits the activity of Stuart factor (factor X_a) and thrombin; the drug, heparin, enhances the activity of antithrombin III. Steps in clot formation that are inhibited by heparin are shown in red. **(B)** Fibrinolytic process: Clots are dissolved. The step that is facilitated by the clot-dissolving drugs and by other agents is shown in blue.

symptoms of hypoxia, anoxia, or even necrosis in areas affected by the decreased blood flow. In some of these disorders, pieces of the thrombus, called emboli, can break off and travel through the cardiovascular system until they become lodged in a tiny vessel, plugging it up.

Conditions that predispose a person to the formation of clots and emboli are called **thromboembolic disorders**. Coronary artery disease (CAD) involves a narrowing of the coronary arteries caused by damage to the endothelial lining of these vessels. Thrombi tend to form along the damaged endothelial lining. As the damage builds up, the lumen of the vessels become narrower and narrower. Over time, the coronary arteries are unable to deliver enough blood to meet the needs of the heart muscle, and hypoxia develops. If a vessel becomes so narrow that a tiny clot occludes it completely, the blood supply to that area is cut off and anoxia occurs, followed by infarction and necrosis. With age, many of the vessels in the body can be damaged and develop similar problems with narrowing and blood delivery. These disorders are treated with drugs that interfere with the normal coagulation process to prevent the formation of clots in the system.

Hemorrhagic Disorders

Hemorrhagic disorders, in which excess bleeding occurs, are less common than thromboembolic disorders. These disorders include hemophilia, in which there is a genetic lack of clotting factors; liver disease, in which clotting factors and proteins needed for clotting are not produced; and bone marrow disorders, in which platelets are not formed in sufficient quantity to be effective. These disorders are treated with clotting factors and drugs that promote the coagulation process.

FOCUS POINTS

- The transformation of fluid blood into a solid state to seal breaks in the vascular system is known as coagulation.
- The coagulation process involves vasoconstriction, platelet aggregation to form a plug, and intrinsic and extrinsic clot formation initiated by Hageman factor to plug any breaks in the system.
- The conversion of prothrombin to thrombin, which results in insoluble fibrin threads, is the final step of clot formation.
- To prevent the occlusion of blood vessels and the denying of blood to the tissues, a formed clot must be dissolved.
- The base of the clot-dissolving system is the conversion of plasminogen to plasmin (fibrinolysin) by several factors, including Hageman factor. Plasmin dissolves fibrin threads and resolves the clot.

Anticoagulants

Anticoagulants are drugs that interfere with the normal coagulation process. They can affect the process at any step to slow or prevent clot formation. (Box 48.2 discusses the interaction of herbal remedies with these drugs.) Antiplatelet drugs alter the formation of the platelet plug. Anticoagulants interfere with the clotting cascade and thrombin formation. **Thrombolytic drugs** break down the thrombus that has been formed by stimulating the plasmin system

Antiplatelet Drugs

Antiplatelet drugs decrease the formation of the platelet plug by decreasing the responsiveness of the platelets to stimuli that would cause them to stick and aggregate on a vessel wall. These drugs are used effectively to treat cardiovascular diseases that are prone to produce occluded vessels; for the maintenance of venous and arterial grafts; to prevent cerebrovascular occlusion; and as adjuncts to thrombolytic therapy in the treatment of myocardial infarction (MI) and the prevention of reinfarction. The prescriber's choice of drug

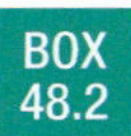

BOX 48.2 HERBAL AND ALTERNATIVE THERAPIES

Many herbal therapies can cause problems when used with drugs that affect blood coagulation. Patients taking these drugs should be cautioned to avoid angelica, cat's claw, chamomile, chondroitin, feverfew, garlic, ginkgo, goldenseal, grape seed extract, green leaf tea, horse chestnut seed, psyllium, and turmeric. If a patient who is taking an anticoagulant presents with increased bleeding and no other interaction or cause is found, question the patient about the possibility of use of herbal therapies.

depends on the intended use and the patient's tolerance of the associated adverse effects. Antiplatelet drugs that are available for use include the following (Table 48.1):

- Abciximab (*ReoPro*) is an intravenous (IV) drug used in conjunction with heparin and aspirin to prevent acute cardiac events during transluminal coronary angioplasty and as early treatment of unstable angina and non–Q-wave MI.
- Anagrelide (*Agrylin*) is an oral drug used to treat essential thrombocythemia to reduce elevated platelet counts and decrease the risk of thrombosis. This drug works to decrease the bone marrow production of platelets, so patients need to have their platelet count monitored regularly.
- Aspirin (generic) is an oral drug that has been shown to be effective in decreasing the incidence of transient ischemic attacks (TIAs) and strokes in men and in reducing the risk of death or nonfatal MI in patients with a past history of MI or with angina.
- Cilostazol (*Pletal*) is an oral drug that is indicated for the reduction of symptoms of intermittent claudication, allowing increased walking distance.
- Clopidogrel (*Plavix*) is an oral drug used in patients who are at risk for ischemic events and in those with a history of MI, peripheral artery disease, or ischemic stroke and for the treatment of patients with acute coronary syndrome.

Table 48.1 DRUGS IN FOCUS

Antiplatelet Drugs

Drug Name	Usual Dosage	Usual Indications
abciximab (*ReoPro*)	0.25 mg/kg IV bolus 10–60 min before procedure, then continuous infusion of 10 mcg/kg/min for 12 h Angina: 0.25 mg/kg by IV bolus, then 10 mcg/kg/min IV for 18–24 h	In conjunction with heparin and aspirin to prevent acute cardiac events during transluminal coronary angioplasty; early treatment of unstable angina
anagrelide (*Agrylin*)	0.5 mg PO q.i.d. or 1 mg PO b.i.d., may increase by 0.5 mg/day each wk; maximum dose—10 mg/day or 2.5 mg as a single dose	Treatment of essential thrombocythemia to reduce elevated platelet count and the risk of thrombosis
P aspirin (*generic*)	1300 mg/day PO to decrease TIAs; 300–325 mg/day PO to reduce MI risk	Reduction of the incidence of transient ischemic attacks (TIAs) and strokes in men and reduction of the risk of death or nonfatal myocardial infarction (MI) in patients with a past history of MI or with angina
cilostazol (*Pletal*)	100 mg PO b.i.d.	Reduction of symptoms of intermittent claudication, allowing increased walking distance in adults
clopidogrel (*Plavix*)	75 mg/day PO	Treatment of patients who are at risk for ischemic events; patients with a history of MI, peripheral artery disease, or ischemic stroke; and patients with acute coronary syndrome
dipyridamole (*Persantine*)	50 mg PO t.i.d. for angina; 75–100 mg PO q.i.d. for heart valve patients; 0.142 mg/kg/min IV over 4 min for diagnosis	In combination with warfarin to prevent thromboembolism in patients with artificial heart valves; diagnosis of coronary artery disease in patients who cannot exercise; treatment of angina
eptifibatide (*Integrelin*)	180 mcg/kg IV over 1–2 min, then 2 mcg/kg/min IV for up to 72 h for acute coronary syndrome; 135 mcg/kg IV bolus before procedure, then 0.5 mcg/kg/min IV for 20–24 h	Treatment of acute coronary syndrome; prevention of ischemic episodes in patients undergoing percutaneous coronary interventions
sulfinpyrazone (*Anturane*)	200 mg PO t.i.d. or q.i.d.	Prevention of reinfarction after MI; reduction of incidence of systemic emboli in patients with rheumatic mitral stenosis
ticlopidine (*Ticlid*)	250 mg PO b.i.d.	Reduction of the risk of thrombotic stroke in patients with TIAs or history of stroke who are intolerant to aspirin therapy
tirofiban (*Aggrastat*)	0.4 mcg/kg/min IV over 30 min, then continuous infusion of 0.1 mcg/kg/min	In combination with heparin to treat acute coronary syndrome and prevent cardiac ischemic events during percutaneous coronary intervention

- Dipyridamole (*Persantine*) is used orally in combination with warfarin to prevent thromboembolism in patients with artificial heart valves, as well as IV to aid diagnosis of CAD in patients who cannot exercise. This drug previously was used for long-term treatment of angina, but it was found to be only "possibly effective" by the U.S. Food and Drug Administration.
- Eptifibatide (*Integrilin*) is an IV drug used to treat acute coronary syndrome and to prevent ischemic episodes in patients undergoing percutaneous coronary interventions.
- Sulfinpyrazone (*Anturane*) is an oral drug used to prevent reinfarction after MI and to decrease the incidence of systemic emboli in patients with rheumatic mitral stenosis. It is also an antigout agent.
- Ticlopidine (*Ticlid*) is an oral drug used in patients who are intolerant to aspirin therapy to decrease the risk of thrombotic stroke in patients with TIAs or history of stroke.
- Tirofiban (*Aggrastat*) is an IV drug used in combination with heparin to treat acute coronary syndrome and prevent cardiac ischemic events during percutaneous coronary intervention.

Therapeutic Actions and Indications

The antiplatelet drugs inhibit platelet adhesion and aggregation by blocking receptor sites on the platelet membrane, preventing platelet–platelet interaction or the interaction of platelets with other clotting chemicals. One drug, anagrelide, blocks the production of platelets in the bone marrow. These drugs are used to decrease the risk of fatal MI, to prevent reinfarction after MI, to prevent thromboembolic stroke, and to maintain the patency of grafts; in addition, an unlabeled use is the treatment of other thromboembolic disorders.

Pharmacokinetics

These drugs are generally well absorbed and highly bound to plasma proteins. They are metabolized in the liver and excreted in urine. There are no adequate studies of these drugs in pregnancy, but, because of the potential for increased bleeding, they should be used during pregnancy only if the benefits to the mother clearly outweigh the potential risks to the fetus. These drugs tend to enter breast milk. If they are needed by a breast-feeding mother, she should find another method of feeding the baby.

Contraindications and Cautions

Antiplatelet drugs are contraindicated in the presence of allergy to the specific drug and also with pregnancy or lactation, *because of the potential adverse effects on the fetus or neonate.* Caution should be used in the following conditions: the presence of any known bleeding disorder, *because of the risk of excessive blood loss;* recent surgery, *because of the risk of increased bleeding in unhealed vessels;* and closed head injuries, *because of the risk of bleeding from the injured vessels in the brain.*

Adverse Effects

The most common adverse effect seen with these drugs is bleeding, which often occurs as increased bruising and bleeding while brushing the teeth. Other common problems include headache, dizziness, and weakness; the cause of these reactions is not understood. Nausea and gastrointestinal (GI) distress may occur because of direct irritating effects of the oral drug on the GI tract. Skin rash, another common effect, may be related to direct drug effects on the dermis.

Clinically Important Drug–Drug Interactions

The risk of excessive bleeding increases if any of these drugs is combined with another drug that affects blood clotting.

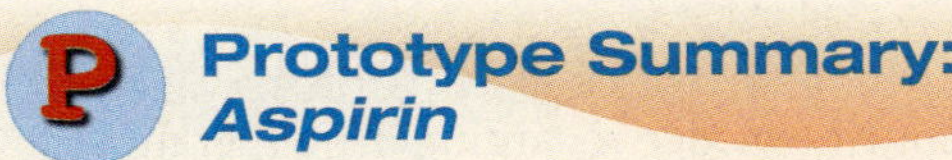

Prototype Summary: Aspirin

Indications: Reduction of risk of recurrent TIAs or strokes in males with a history of TIA due to fibrin or platelet emboli; reduction of death or nonfatal MI in patients with a history of infarction or unstable angina; MI prophylaxis; also used for its anti-inflammatory, analgesic, and antipyretic effects

Actions: Inhibits platelet aggregation by inhibiting platelet synthesis of thromboxane A_2

Pharmacokinetics:

Route	Onset	Peak	Duration
Oral	5–30 min	0.25–2 h	3–6 h

$T_{1/2}$: 15 min–12 hours; metabolized in the liver and excreted in urine

Adverse effects: Acute aspirin toxicity with hyperpnea, possibly leading to fever, coma, and cardiovascular collapse; nausea, dyspepsia, heartburn, epigastric discomfort, GI bleeding, occult blood loss, dizziness, tinnitus, difficulty hearing, anaphylactoid reaction

Nursing Considerations for Patients Receiving Antiplatelet Drugs

Assessment: History and Examination

Screen for the following conditions, *which could be cautions or contraindications to use of the drug:* any known allergies to these drugs; pregnancy or lactation, *because of the potential adverse effects on the fetus or neonate;* and bleeding disorders, recent surgery, or closed head injury, *because of the potential for excessive bleeding.* Include screening *for baseline status before beginning therapy and for any potential adverse effects:* body temperature; skin color, lesions, and temperature; affect, orientation, and reflexes; pulse, blood pressure, and perfusion; respirations and adventitious sounds; complete blood count (CBC); and clotting studies.

Nursing Diagnoses

The patient receiving antiplatelet drugs may have the following nursing diagnoses related to drug therapy:

- Risk for Injury related to bleeding effects or CNS effects
- Acute Pain related to GI or CNS effects
- Deficient Knowledge regarding drug therapy

Implementation With Rationale

- Provide small, frequent meals *to relieve GI discomfort* if GI upset is a problem.
- Provide comfort measures and analgesia for headache, *to relieve pain and improve patient compliance to the drug regimen.*
- Suggest safety measures, including the use of an electric razor and avoidance of contact sports, *to decrease the risk of bleeding.*
- Provide increased precautions against bleeding during invasive procedures; use pressure dressings and ice *to decrease excessive blood loss caused by anticoagulation.*
- Mark the chart of any patient receiving this drug, *to alert medical staff that there is a potential for increased bleeding.*
- Provide thorough patient teaching, including the name of the drug, dosage prescribed, measures to avoid adverse effects, warning signs of problems, the need for periodic monitoring and evaluation, and the need to wear or carry a Medic-Alert notification, *to enhance patient knowledge about drug therapy and to promote compliance with the drug regimen.*
- Offer support and encouragement, *to help the patient deal with the diagnosis and the drug regimen.*

Evaluation

- Monitor patient response to the drug (increased bleeding time, prevention of occlusive events).
- Monitor for adverse effects (bleeding, GI upset, dizziness, headache).
- Evaluate the effectiveness of the teaching plan (patient can name drug, dosage, adverse effects to watch for, specific measures to avoid adverse effects; patient understands importance of continued follow-up).
- Monitor the effectiveness of comfort measures and compliance to the regimen.

Anticoagulants

Anticoagulants interfere with the coagulation process by interfering with the clotting cascade and thrombin formation. Drugs in this class include warfarin, heparin, antithrombin, argatroban, bivalirudin, and desirudin (Table 48.2). These drugs can be used orally (warfarin) or parenterally (heparin, antithrombin, argatroban, and bivalirudin).

- Warfarin (*Coumadin*), an oral drug, is used to maintain a state of anticoagulation in situations in which the patient is susceptible to potentially dangerous clot formation. Warfarin works by interfering with the formation of vitamin K–dependent clotting factors in the liver. The eventual effect is a depletion of these clotting factors and a prolongation of clotting times. Warfarin is readily absorbed through the GI tract, metabolized in the liver, and excreted in urine and feces. Warfarin's onset of action is about 3 days; its effects last for 4 to 5 days. Because of the time delay, warfarin is not the drug of choice in an acute situation, but it is convenient and useful for prolonged effects. It is used to treat patients with atrial fibrillation, artificial heart valves, or valvular damage that makes them susceptible to thrombus and embolus formation. It also is used to treat and prevent venous thrombosis and embolization after acute MI or pulmonary embolism. It is not used during pregnancy or lactation because of the risk of bleeding complications for the mother and the fetus or baby.
- Heparin (generic) is a naturally occurring substance that inhibits the conversion of prothrombin to thrombin, thus blocking the conversion of fibrinogen to fibrin—the final step in clot formation. It is injected IV or subcutaneously (Sub-Q) and has an almost immediate onset of action. It is excreted in urine. Heparin does not cross the placenta (although some adverse fetal effects have been reported with its use during pregnancy) and does not enter breast milk, so it would be the anticoagulant of choice if one is needed during lactation. Its usual indications include acute treatment and prevention of venous thrombosis and pulmonary embolism; treatment of atrial fibrillation with embolization; prevention of clotting in blood samples and in dialysis and venous tubing; and diagnosis and treatment of disseminated intravascular coagulation (DIC) (Box 48.3). It is also used as an adjunct in the treatment of MI and stroke. Because heparin must be injected, it is often not the drug of choice for outpatients, who would

Table 48.2 DRUGS IN FOCUS

Anticoagulants

Drug Name	Usual Dosage	Usual Indications
antithrombin (*Thrombate III*)	Dosage must be calculated using body weight and baseline levels, given q2–8 days	Replacement in antithrombin III deficiency; treatment of patients with this deficiency who are to undergo surgery or obstetrical procedures
argatroban (*Acova*)	2 mcg/kg/min IV until the desired effect is seen; then dosage is adjusted	Treatment of thrombosis in heparin-induced thrombocythemia
bivalirudin (*Angiomax*)	1 mg/kg IV bolus, then 2.5 mg/kg/h IV for 4 h and 0.2 mg/kg/h IV as a low-dose infusion	With aspirin to prevent ischemic events in patients undergoing transluminal coronary angioplasty
desirudin (*Iprivask*)	15 mg by Sub-Q injection q12h beginning 5–15 min before surgery and continuing for 9–12 days	Prevention of deep vein thrombosis in patients undergoing elective hip replacement
P heparin (*generic*)	10,000–20,000 units Sub-Q, then 8,000–10,000 units q8h; 5,000–10,000 units IV q4–6h Pediatric: 50 units/kg IV bolus, then 100 units/kg IV q4h	Prevention and treatment of venous thrombosis, pulmonary embolus, clotting in blood samples and venous lines; diagnosis and treatment of disseminated intravascular coagulation
warfarin (*Coumadin*)	10–15 mg/day PO then 2–10 mg/day PO based on PT ratio or INR, use lower doses with geriatric patients	Prevention and treatment of venous thrombosis, pulmonary embolus, embolus with atrial fibrillation, systemic emboli after myocardial infarction

INR, international normalized ratio; PT, prothrombin time.

be responsible for injecting the drug several times during the day. Patients may be started on heparin in the acute situation, then switched to the oral drug warfarin.

- Antithrombin (*Thrombate III*) is a naturally occurring anticoagulant. The body handles it in the same way that it handles naturally occurring antithrombin. It has been used without reported adverse effects during pregnancy and lactation. It is given IV to patients with hereditary antithrombin III deficiencies who are undergoing surgery or obstetrical procedures that might put them at risk for thromboembolism. It also is used for replacement therapy in congenital antithrombin III deficiency.
- Argatroban (*Acova*) is an IV thrombin-inhibiting drug that is used to treat thrombosis in heparin-induced thrombocythemia.
- Bivalirudin (*Angiomax*), an IV drug that inhibits thrombin. It is used with aspirin to prevent ischemic events in patients undergoing transluminal coronary angioplasty.
- Desirudin (*Iprivask*) is a thrombin-inhibiting drug that is given by Sub-Q injection to prevent deep venous thrombosis (DVT) in patients undergoing elective hip replacement.

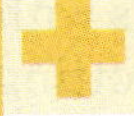

FOCUS ON **PATIENT SAFETY**

Injectable vitamin K is used to reverse the effects of warfarin. Vitamin K is responsible for promoting the liver synthesis of several clotting factors. When these pathways have been inhibited by warfarin, clotting time is increased. If an increased level of vitamin K is provided, more of these factors are produced, and the clotting time can be brought back within a normal range. Because of the way in which vitamin K exerts its effects on clotting, there is a delay of at least 24 hours from the time the drug is given until some change can be seen. This occurs because there is no direct effect on the warfarin itself, but rather an increased stimulation of the liver, which must then produce the clotting factors. The usual dosage for the treatment of anticoagulant-induced prothrombin deficiency is 2.5 to 10 mg intramuscularly (IM) or subcutaneously (Sub-Q) or, rarely, 25 mg IM or Sub-Q. Oral doses can be used if injection is not feasible. A prothrombin time (PT) response within 6 to 8 hours after parenteral doses or 12 to 48 hours after oral doses will determine the need for a repeat dose. If a response is not seen and the patient is bleeding excessively, fresh-frozen plasma or an infusion of whole blood may be needed.

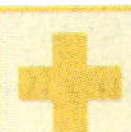

FOCUS ON **PATIENT SAFETY**

In cases of a heparin overdose, the antidote is protamine sulfate (generic). This strongly basic protein drug forms stable salts with heparin as soon as the two drugs come in contact, immediately reversing heparin's anticoagulant effects. Paradoxically, if protamine is given to a patient who has not received heparin, it has anticoagulant effects. The dosage is determined by the amount of heparin that was given and the time that elapsed since then. A dose of 1 mg IV protamine neutralizes 90 USP of heparin derived from lung tissue or 110 USP of heparin derived from intestinal mucosa. The drug must be administered very slowly, not to exceed 50 mg IV in any 10-minute period. Care must be taken to calculate the amount of heparin that has been given to the patient. Potentially fatal anaphylactic reactions have been reported with the use of protamine sulfate, so life support equipment should be readily available when it is used (Box 48.4).

BOX 48.3 **Understanding Disseminated Intravascular Coagulation**

Disseminated intravascular coagulation (DIC) is a syndrome in which bleeding and thrombosis are found together. It can occur as a complication of many problems, including severe infection with septic shock, traumatic childbirth or missed abortion, and massive injuries. In these disorders, local tissue damage causes the release of coagulation-stimulating substances into circulation. These substances then stimulate the coagulation process, causing fibrin clot formation in small vessels in the lungs, kidneys, brain, and other organs. This continuing reaction consumes excessive amounts of fibrinogen, other clotting factors, and platelets. The end result is increased bleeding. In essence, the patient clots too much, resulting in the possibility of bleeding to death.

The first step in treating this disorder is to control the problem that initially precipitated it. For example, treating the infection, performing dilation and curettage to clear the uterus, or stabilizing injuries can help stop this continuing process. Whole-blood infusions or the infusion of fibrinogen may be used to buy some time until the patient is stable and can form clotting factors again. There are associated problems with giving whole blood (e.g., development of hepatitis or AIDS), and there is a risk that fibrinogen may set off further intravascular clotting. Paradoxically, the treatment of choice for DIC is the anticoagulant heparin. Heparin prevents the clotting phase from being completed, thus inhibiting the breakdown of fibrinogen. It may also help avoid hemorrhage by preventing the body from depleting its entire store of coagulation factors.

Because heparin is usually administered to prevent blood clotting, and the adverse effects that are monitored with heparin therapy include signs of bleeding, it can be a real challenge for the nursing staff to feel comfortable administering heparin to a patient who is bleeding to death. Understanding of the disease process can help alleviate any doubts about the treatment.

Therapeutic Actions and Indications

As noted previously, the anticoagulants interfere with the normal cascade of events involved in the clotting process. Warfarin causes a decrease in the production of vitamin K–dependent clotting factors in the liver. Heparin, argatroban, and bivalirudin block the formation of thrombin from prothrombin. Antithrombin interferes with the formation of thrombin from prothrombin. These drugs are used to treat thromboembolic disorders such as atrial fibrillation, MI, pulmonary embolus, and evolving stroke and to prevent the formation of thrombi in such disorders.

Pharmacokinetics

Pharmacokinetic parameters are different for each drug (see earlier discussions).

Contraindications and Cautions

The anticoagulants are contraindicated in the presence of known allergy to the drugs. They also should not be used with any conditions *that could be compromised by increased bleeding tendencies,* including hemorrhagic disorders, recent trauma, spinal puncture, GI ulcers, recent surgery, intrauterine device placement, tuberculosis, presence of indwelling catheters, and threatened abortion. In addition, anticoagulants are contraindicated in pregnancy, *because fetal injury and death have occurred;* in lactation (use of heparin is suggested if an anticoagulant is needed during lactation); and in renal or hepatic disease, *which could interfere with the metabolism and effectiveness of these drugs.*

Caution should be used in patients with congestive heart failure (CHF), thyrotoxicosis, senility, or psychosis, *because of the potential for unexpected effects,* and in those with diarrhea or fever, *which could alter the normal clotting process by, respectively, loss of vitamin K from the intestine or activation of plasminogen.*

Adverse Effects

The most commonly encountered adverse effect of the anticoagulants is bleeding, ranging from bleeding gums with tooth brushing to severe internal hemorrhage. Clotting times should be monitored closely to avoid these problems. Nausea, GI upset, diarrhea, and hepatic dysfunction also may occur secondary to direct drug toxicity. Warfarin has been associated with alopecia and dermatitis as well as bone marrow depression and, less frequently, prolonged and painful erections.

Clinically Important Drug–Drug Interactions

Increased bleeding can occur if heparin is combined with oral anticoagulants, salicylates, penicillins, or cephalosporins. Decreased anticoagulation can occur if heparin is combined with nitroglycerin.

Warfarin has documented drug–drug interactions with a vast number of other drugs (Table 48.3). It is a wise practice never to add or take away a drug from the regimen of a patient receiving warfarin without careful patient monitoring and adjustment of the warfarin dosage to prevent serious adverse effects.

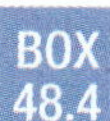

Lepirudin: Treating Heparin Allergy

Lepirudin (*Refludan*) is an intravenous (IV) drug that was developed to treat a rare allergic reaction to heparin. In some patients, an allergy to heparin precipitates a heparin-induced thrombocythemia with associated thromboembolic disease. Lepirudin directly inhibits thrombin, blocking the thromboembolic effects of this reaction.

A 0.4 mg/kg initial IV bolus followed by a continuous infusion of 0.15 mg/kg for 2 to 10 days is the usual treatment. The patient needs to be monitored for bleeding from any site and for the development of direct hepatic injury.

Table 48.3 Clinically Important Drug–Drug Interactions With Warfarin

↑Bleeding Effects	↓Anticoagulation	↑Activity and Effects of Other Drug
salicylates	barbiturates	phenytoin
chloral hydrate	griseofulvin	
phenylbutazone	rifampin	
clofibrate	phenytoin	
disulfiram	glutethimide	
chloramphenicol	carbamazepine	
metronidazole	vitamin K	
cimetidine	vitamin E	
ranitidine	cholestyramine	
cotrimoxazole	aminoglutethimide	
sulfinpyrazone	ethchlorvynol	
quinidine		
quinine		
oxyphenbutazone		
thyroid drugs		
glucagon		
danazol		
erythromycin		
androgens		
amiodarone		
cefamandole		
cefoperazone		
cefotetan		
moxalactam		
cefazolin		
cefoxitin		
ceftriaxone		
meclofenamate		
mefenamic acid		
famotidine		
nizatidine		
nalidixic acid		

P Prototype Summary: Heparin

Indications: Prevention and treatment of venous thrombosis and pulmonary emboli; treatment of atrial fibrillation with embolization; diagnosis and treatment of DIC; prevention of clotting in blood samples and heparin lock sets

Actions: Inhibits thrombus and clot production by blocking the conversion of prothrombin to thrombin and fibrinogen to fibrin

Pharmacokinetics:

Route	Onset	Peak	Duration
IV	Immediate	Min	2–6 h
Sub-Q	20–60 min	2–4 h	8–12 h

$T_{1/2}$: 30–180 min; metabolized in the cells and excreted in urine

Adverse effects: Loss of hair, bruising, chills, fever, osteoporosis, suppression of renal function (with long-term use)

Nursing Considerations for Patients Receiving Anticoagulants

Assessment: History and Examination

Screen for any known allergies to these drugs. Also screen for conditions *that could be exacerbated by increased bleeding tendencies,* including hemorrhagic disorders, recent trauma, spinal puncture, GI ulcers, recent surgery, intrauterine device placement, tuberculosis, presence of indwelling catheters, and threatened abortion. Also screen for pregnancy, *because fetal injury and death have occurred;* lactation (use of heparin is suggested if an anticoagulant is needed during lactation); renal or hepatic disease, *which could interfere with the metabolism and effectiveness of these drugs;* CHF; thyrotoxicosis; senility or psychosis, *because of the potential for unexpected effects;* and diarrhea or fever, *which could alter the normal clotting process.*

Include screening *for baseline status before beginning therapy and for any potential adverse effects.* Assess the following: body temperature; skin color, lesions, and temperature; affect, orientation, and reflexes; pulse, blood pressure, and perfusion; respirations and adventitious sounds; clotting studies, renal and hepatic function tests, CBC, and stool guaiac; and electrocardiogram (ECG), if appropriate.

Nursing Diagnoses

The patient receiving an anticoagulant may have the following nursing diagnoses related to drug therapy:

- Risk for Injury related to bleeding effects and bone marrow depression
- Disturbed Body Image related to alopecia and skin rash
- Ineffective Tissue Perfusion (Total Body) related to blood loss
- Deficient Knowledge regarding drug therapy

Implementation With Rationale

- Evaluate for therapeutic effects of warfarin—prothrombin time (PT) 1.5 to 2.5 times the control value or ratio of PT to INR (international normalized ratio) of 2 to 3—*to evaluate the effectiveness of the drug dose.*
- Evaluate for therapeutic effects of heparin—whole blood clotting time (WBCT) 2.5 to 3 times control or activated partial thromboplastin time (APTT) 1.5 to 3 times the control value—*to evaluate the effectiveness of the drug dose.*
- Evaluate the patient regularly for any sign of blood loss (petechiae, bleeding gums, bruises, dark-colored stools, dark-colored urine) *to evaluate the effectiveness of the drug dose and to consult with the prescriber if bleeding becomes apparent.*
- Establish safety precautions, *to protect the patient from injury.*
- Provide safety measures, such as use of an electric razor and avoidance of contact sports, *to decrease the risk of bleeding.*
- Provide increased precautions against bleeding during invasive procedures; use pressure dressings; avoid intramuscular injections; and do not rub Sub-Q injection sites, *because the state of anticoagulation increases the risk of blood loss.*
- Mark the chart of any patient receiving this drug, *to alert the medical staff that there is a potential for increased bleeding.*
- Maintain antidotes on standby (protamine sulfate for heparin, vitamin K for warfarin), *in case of overdose.*
- Monitor the patient carefully when any drug is added to or withdrawn from the drug regimen of a patient taking warfarin, *because of the risk of drug–drug interactions that would change the effectiveness of the anticoagulant.*
- Make sure that the patient receives regular follow-up and monitoring, including measurement of clotting times, *to ensure maximum therapeutic effects.*
- Provide thorough patient teaching, including the name of the drug, dosage prescribed, measures to avoid adverse effects, warning signs of problems, the need for periodic monitoring and evaluation, and the need to wear or carry a Medic-Alert notification, *to enhance patient knowledge about drug therapy and to promote compliance with the drug regimen.*
- Offer support and encouragement, *to help the patient deal with the diagnosis and the drug regimen.*

Evaluation

- Monitor patient response to the drug: increased bleeding time (warfarin, PT 1.5 to 2.5 times the control value or PT/INR ratio of 2 to 3; heparin, WBCT of 2.5 to 3 times the control value or APTT of 1.5 to 3 times control).
- Monitor for adverse effects (bleeding, bone marrow depression, alopecia, GI upset, rash).
- Evaluate the effectiveness of the teaching plan (patient can name drug, dosage, adverse effects to watch for, specific measures to avoid adverse effects; patient understands importance of continued follow-up).
- Monitor the effectiveness of comfort measures and compliance to the regimen (Critical Thinking Scenario 48-1).

Low-Molecular-Weight Heparins

In the late 1990s, a series of low-molecular-weight heparins were developed (Table 48.4). These drugs inhibit thrombus and clot formation by blocking factors Xa and IIa. Because of the size and nature of their molecules, these drugs do not greatly affect thrombin, clotting, or the PT; therefore, they cause fewer systemic adverse effects. They have also been found to block angiogenesis, the process that allows cancer cells to develop new blood vessels. They are being studied as possible adjuncts to cancer chemotherapy. These drugs are indicated for very specific uses in the prevention of clots and emboli formation after certain surgeries or prolonged bed rest; however, each is being studied for use after additional types of surgery (Box 48.5). The nursing care of a patient receiving one of these drugs is similar to that of a patient receiving heparin. The drug is given just before (or just after) the surgery, then is continued for 7 to 14 days during the postoperative recovery process. Caution must be used to avoid combining these drugs with standard heparin therapy; serious bleeding episodes and deaths have been reported when this combination was inadvertently used.

Thrombolytic Agents

If a thrombus has already formed in a vessel (e.g., during an acute MI), it may be necessary to dissolve that clot to open the vessel and restore blood flow to the dependent tissue. All of the drugs that are available for this purpose work to activate the natural anticlotting system, conversion of plasminogen to plasmin. The activation of this system breaks down fibrin threads and dissolves any formed clot. The thrombolytic drugs are effective only if the patient has plasminogen in the plasma. Thrombolytic agents include the following (Table 48.5):

CRITICAL THINKING SCENARIO 48-1

Oral Anticoagulant Therapy

The Situation

G.R. is a 68-year-old woman with a history of severe mitral valve disease. For the last several years, she has been able to manage her condition with digoxin, a diuretic, and a potassium supplement. However, on a recent visit to her physician she disclosed that she had been experiencing periods of breathlessness, palpitations, and dizziness. Tests showed that she was having frequent periods of atrial fibrillation (AF), with a heart rate of up to 140 beats/min. Because of the danger of emboli as a result of her valve disease and the bouts of AF, warfarin therapy was begun.

Critical Thinking

What nursing interventions should be done at this point?

Why do people with mitral valve disease frequently develop AF? *Think about why emboli form when the atria fibrillate.*

Stabilizing G.R. on warfarin may take several weeks of blood tests and dosage adjustments. How can this process be made easier?

What patient teaching points should be covered with G.R. to ensure that she is protected from emboli and does not experience excessive bleeding?

Discussion

G.R.'s situation is complex. She has a progressive degenerative valve disease that usually leads to congestive heart failure (CHF) and frequently to other complications, such as AF and emboli formation. Her digoxin and potassium levels should be checked to determine whether her CHF is stabilized or the digoxin is causing the AF because of excessive doses or potassium imbalance. If these tests are within normal limits, G.R. may be experiencing AF because of irritation to the atrial cells caused by the damaged mitral valve and associated swelling and scarring. If this is the case, an anticoagulant will help protect G.R. against emboli, which form in the auricles when blood pools there while the atria are fibrillating. There is less chance of emboli formation if clotting is slowed.

G.R. will need extensive teaching about warfarin, including the need for frequent blood tests, the list of potential drug–drug interactions, the importance of being alert to the many factors that can affect dosage needs (including illness and diet), and how to monitor for subtle blood loss. This can also be a good opportunity to review teaching about valvular disease and CHF and to answer any questions that she might have about how all of these things interrelate. If possible, it would be useful to teach G.R. or a responsible caregiver how to take a pulse so that G.R. can be alerted to potential arrhythmias and avert problems before they begin. It also would be a good idea to check on support services for G.R., to ensure that her blood tests can be done and that her response to the drug is monitored carefully.

Nursing Care Guide for G.R.: Warfarin

Assessment: History and Examination

Assess G.R.'s health history for allergies to warfarin, subacute bacterial endocarditis (SBE), hemorrhagic disorders, tuberculosis, renal or hepatic dysfunction, gastric ulcers, thyroid disease, uncontrolled hypertension, severe trauma, or a long-term indwelling catheter (which increases the risk of bleeding). Also assess concurrent use of numerous drugs and herbal therapies

Focus the physical examination on the following areas:

CV: blood pressure, pulse, perfusion, baseline electrocardiogram (ECG)

Neuro (CNS): orientation, affect, reflexes, vision

Skin: color, lesions, texture

Resp: respiratory rate and character, adventitious sounds

GI: abdominal examination, guaiac stool test results (for occult blood)

Laboratory tests: liver and renal function tests, prothrombin time (PT), international normalized ratio (INR)

Nursing Diagnoses

Ineffective Tissue Perfusion (Total Body) related to alteration in clotting effects

Risk for Injury related to anticoagulant effects

Disturbed Body Image related to alopecia, skin rash

Deficient Knowledge regarding drug therapy

Implementation

Ensure proper administration of drug.

Provide comfort and safety measures, such as small meals, protection from injury during invasive and other procedures, bowel program as needed, standby antidotes (e.g., vitamin K), and careful skin care.

(continued)

Oral Anticoagulant Therapy *(continued)*

Provide support and reassurance to deal with drug effects.

Provide patient teaching regarding drug, dosage, adverse effects, what to report, safety precautions.

Evaluation

Evaluate drug effects: increased bleeding times, PT 1.5–2.5 times control or PT/INR ratio of 2:3.

Monitor for adverse effects: bleeding, alopecia, rash, GI upset, excessive bleeding.

Monitor for drug–drug interactions (numerous).

Evaluate effectiveness of patient teaching program comfort and safety measures.

Patient Teaching for G.R.

- ☐ An anticoagulant slows the body's normal blood clotting processes to prevent harmful blood clots from forming. This type of drug is often called a "blood thinner"; however, it cannot dissolve any clots that have already formed.
- ☐ *Never* change any medication that you are taking—such as adding or stopping another drug, taking a new over-the-counter medication, or stopping one that you have been taking regularly—without consulting with your health care provider. Many other drugs affect the way that your anticoagulant works; starting or stopping another drug can cause excessive bleeding or interfere with the desired effects of the drug.
- ☐ Some of the following adverse effects may occur:
  - *Stomach bloating, cramps:* These problems often pass with time; consult your health care provider if they persist or become too uncomfortable.
  - *Loss of hair, skin rash:* These problems can be very frustrating; you may wish to discuss these with your health care provider.
  - *Orange-yellow discoloration of the urine:* This can be frightening, but it may just be an effect of the drug. If you are concerned that this might be blood, simply add vinegar to your urine; the color should disappear. If the color does not disappear, it may be caused by blood and you should contact your health care provider.
  - Report any of the following to your health care provider: *unusual bleeding (when brushing your teeth, excessive bleeding from an injury, excessive bruising); black or tarry stools; cloudy or dark urine; sore throat, fever, or chills; severe headache or dizziness.*
- ☐ Tell any doctor, nurse, or other health care provider involved in your care that you are taking this drug. You should carry or wear medical identification stating that you are taking this drug, to alert emergency medical personnel that you are at increased risk for bleeding.
- ☐ Avoid situations in which you could be easily injured—for example, engaging in contact sports or games with children or using a straight razor.
- ☐ Keep this drug, and all medications, out of the reach of children.
- ☐ Avoid the use of over-the-counter medications while you are taking this drug. If you feel that you need one of these, consult with your health care provider for the best choice. Many of these drugs can interfere with your anticoagulant.
- ☐ Schedule regular, periodic blood tests while you are taking this drug to monitor the effects of the drug on your body and adjust your dosage as needed.

- Alteplase (*Activase*) is used for treatment of MI, acute pulmonary embolism, and acute ischemic stroke. It is given IV, and the patient needs to be monitored closely for bleeding.
- Reteplase (*Retavase*) is given IV for the treatment of coronary artery thrombosis associated with an acute MI.
- Streptokinase (*Streptase, Kabikinase*) is used IV to treat coronary artery thrombosis, pulmonary embolism, DVT, and arterial thrombosis or embolism, and to open an occluded atrioventricular cannula.
- Tenecteplase (*TNKase*) is given IV to reduce mortality associated with acute MI. The timing of administration is critical to the success of the therapy.
- Urokinase (*Abbokinase*) is used IV to lyse pulmonary emboli, to treat coronary thrombosis, and to clear occluded IV catheters.

Box 48.6 discusses pentoxifylline (*Trental*), a hemorrheologic agent. Box 48.7 discusses drotrecogin alfa (*Xigris*), a drug that affects coagulation and was recently approved for the treatment of severe sepsis.

Therapeutic Actions and Indications

The thrombolytic agents work by activating plasminogen to plasmin, which in turn breaks down fibrin threads in a clot to dissolve a formed clot. They are indicated for the treatment of acute MI (to dissolve the clot and prevent further tissue damage, if used within 6 hours after the onset of symptoms);

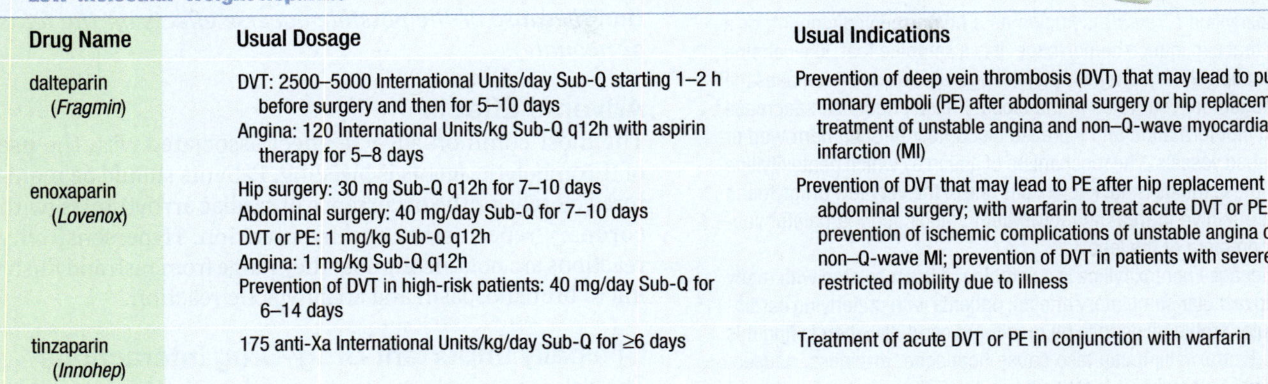

Table 48.4 DRUGS IN FOCUS

Low-Molecular-Weight Heparins

Drug Name	Usual Dosage	Usual Indications
dalteparin (*Fragmin*)	DVT: 2500–5000 International Units/day Sub-Q starting 1–2 h before surgery and then for 5–10 days Angina: 120 International Units/kg Sub-Q q12h with aspirin therapy for 5–8 days	Prevention of deep vein thrombosis (DVT) that may lead to pulmonary emboli (PE) after abdominal surgery or hip replacement; treatment of unstable angina and non–Q-wave myocardial infarction (MI)
enoxaparin (*Lovenox*)	Hip surgery: 30 mg Sub-Q q12h for 7–10 days Abdominal surgery: 40 mg/day Sub-Q for 7–10 days DVT or PE: 1 mg/kg Sub-Q q12h Angina: 1 mg/kg Sub-Q q12h Prevention of DVT in high-risk patients: 40 mg/day Sub-Q for 6–14 days	Prevention of DVT that may lead to PE after hip replacement or abdominal surgery; with warfarin to treat acute DVT or PE; prevention of ischemic complications of unstable angina or non–Q-wave MI; prevention of DVT in patients with severely restricted mobility due to illness
tinzaparin (*Innohep*)	175 anti-Xa International Units/kg/day Sub-Q for ≥6 days	Treatment of acute DVT or PE in conjunction with warfarin

to treat pulmonary emboli and ischemic stroke; and to open clotted IV catheters.

BOX 48.5 Specific Factor Xa Inhibitor to Prevent Deep Venous Thrombosis

Fondaparinux (*Arixtra*), a specific blocker of factor Xa, was approved in 2002 for the prevention of venous thromboembolic events in patients undergoing surgery for hip fracture, hip replacement, or knee replacement. The usual dosage of fondaparinux is 2.5 mg/day Sub-Q starting 6–8 h after surgical closure and continuing for 5–9 days. It is supplied in prefilled syringes, making it convenient for patients who will be self-administering the drug at home. As with other drugs that affect coagulation, bleeding is the most common and potentially the most serious adverse effect that can occur with the use of this drug. Patients need teaching about administration, disposal of the syringes, and signs of bleeding to watch for. Periodic blood tests will be needed to assess the effects of the drug on the body.

Pharmacokinetics

These drugs must be injected and are cleared from the body after liver metabolism. They cross the placenta and have been associated with adverse fetal effects. These drugs should not be used during pregnancy unless the benefits to the mother clearly outweigh the potential risks to the fetus. It is not known whether these drugs enter breast milk. Caution should be used during lactation because of the potential risk for bleeding effects.

Contraindications and Cautions

The use of thrombolytic agents is contraindicated in the presence of allergy to any of these drugs. They also should

Table 48.5 DRUGS IN FOCUS

Thrombolytic Agents

Drug Name	Usual Dosage	Usual Indications
alteplase (*Activase*)	100 mg IV given over 2 h	Treatment of myocardial infarction (MI), acute pulmonary embolism (PE), and acute ischemic stroke; restoration of function in occluded central venous access devices
reteplase (*Retavase*)	10 International Units + 10 International Units double-bolus IV, each over 2 min, 30 min apart	Treatment of coronary artery thrombosis associated with an acute MI
P streptokinase (*Streptase, Kabikinase*)	Total dose of 140,000 International Units over 60 min for coronary artery thrombosis; 250,000 International Units over 30 min and then 100,000 International Units/h IV for 24–72 h for PE, DVT, arterial thrombosis, or embolism; 250,000 International Units in 2-mL IV solution to clear cannula	Treatment of coronary artery thrombosis, PE, deep venous thrombosis (DVT), arterial thrombosis, or embolism, and to open occluded atrioventricular cannula
tenecteplase (*TNKase*)	30–50 mg IV over 5 sec	Reduction of mortality associated with acute MI
urokinase (*Abbokinase*)	4400–10,000 units/min for up to 2 h, based on clinical response	Lysis of pulmonary emboli, to treat coronary thrombosis, and to clear occluded intravenous catheters

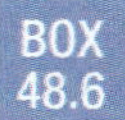

BOX 48.6

Pentoxifylline: Hemorrheologic Agent

Pentoxifylline (*Trental*) is known as a hemorrheologic agent, or a drug that can induce hemorrhage. It is a xanthine that, like caffeine and theophylline, decreases platelet aggregation and decreases the fibrinogen concentration in the blood. These effects can decrease blood clot formation and increase blood flow through narrowed or damaged vessels. The mechanism of action by which pentoxifylline does these things is not known. It is one of the very few drugs found to be effective in treating intermittent claudication, a painful vascular problem of the legs.

Because pentoxifylline is a xanthine, it is associated with many cardiovascular stimulatory effects; patients with underlying cardiovascular problems need to be monitored carefully when taking this drug. Pentoxifylline can also cause headache, dizziness, nausea, and upset stomach. It is taken orally three times a day for at least 8 weeks to evaluate its effectiveness.

not be used with any condition *that could be worsened by the dissolution of clots,* including recent surgery, active internal bleeding, cerebrovascular accident (CVA) within the last 2 months, aneurysm, obstetrical delivery, organ biopsy, recent serious GI bleeding, rupture of a noncompressible blood vessel, recent major trauma (including cardiopulmonary resuscitation), known blood clotting defects, cerebrovascular disease, uncontrolled hypertension, liver disease (*which could affect normal clotting factors and the production of plasminogen*), and pregnancy or lactation (*because of the possible adverse effects on the fetus or neonate*).

BOX 48.7

First Drug Approved for Treating Severe Sepsis Alters Coagulation Processes

In late 2001, the U.S. Food and Drug Administration approved the first drug for treatment of severe sepsis. Patients with severe sepsis suffer multiple organ failure and often death. The processes that lead to this state can be caused by infection from a number of sources leading to shock and vascular shutdown. Drotrecogin alfa (*Xigris*) is a human activated protein C that exerts an antithrombotic effect by inhibiting factors Va and VIIIa. It may also have indirect profibrinolytic activity, activating fibrinolysin to dissolve clots. It is thought that it also may exert an anti-inflammatory effect in the body by inhibiting human necrosis factor production by monocytes, blocking leukocyte adhesion to cells, and limiting thrombin-induced inflammatory responses within the microvascular endothelium.

The mechanism of action of drotrecogin alfa in severe sepsis is not completely understood, but it is thought to be a combination of all of these effects that leads to lessened swelling and inflammation in blood vessels, decreased clotting within the injured vessels, and improved blood flow to the organs before necrosis and cell death occurs. Overall, this would cause a decrease in the complex organ failure associated with sepsis. The drug is approved for use only in adults at a dose of 24 mcg/kg/h by IV infusion for a total of 96 h, not to exceed 24 mcg/kg/h. Increased risk of bleeding is the most common adverse reaction to the drug, and the patient must be monitored closely for any signs of increased bleeding. As more is learned about the minute, intravascular processes in the body, more drugs of this type may be developed.

Adverse Effects

The most common adverse effect associated with the use of thrombolytic agents is bleeding. Patients should be monitored closely for the occurrence of cardiac arrhythmias (with coronary reperfusion) and hypotension. Hypersensitivity reactions are not uncommon; they range from rash and flushing to bronchospasm and anaphylactic reaction.

Clinically Important Drug–Drug Interactions

The risk of hemorrhage increases if thrombolytic agents are used with any anticoagulant or antiplatelet drug.

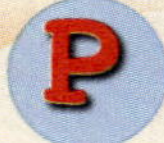

Prototype Summary: *Streptokinase*

Indications: Coronary artery thrombosis; management of acute evolving transmural MI; lysis of pulmonary emboli; treatment of DVT, arterial thrombosis, and embolism; opening of occluded atriovenous cannulae

Actions: Converts endogenous plasminogen to plasmin, which breaks down fibrin clots, fibrinogen, and other plasma proteins; lyses thrombi and emboli

Pharmacokinetics:

Route	Onset	Peak	Duration
IV	Immediate	30–60 min	4–12 h

$T_{1/2}$: 23 min; metabolized in the cells; excretion method unknown

Adverse effects: Headache, angioneurotic edema, hypotension, skin rash, bleeding, breathing difficulties, pain, fever, anaphylactic shock

Nursing Considerations for Patients Receiving Thrombolytic Agents

Assessment: History and Examination

Screen for any known allergies to these drugs. Also screen for any conditions *that could be worsened by the dissolution of clots,* including recent surgery, active internal bleeding, CVA within the last 2 months, aneurysm, obstetrical delivery, organ biopsy, recent serious GI bleeding, rupture of a noncompressible blood vessel, recent major trauma (including cardiopulmonary resuscitation), known blood clotting defects, cerebrovascular disease, uncontrolled hypertension, liver disease (*which could affect normal clotting factors and the production of plasminogen*), and pregnancy or lactation (*because of the possible adverse effects on the neonate*).

Include screening *for baseline status before beginning therapy and for any potential adverse effects.* Assess the following: body temperature; skin color, lesions, and temperature; affect, orientation, and reflexes; pulse, blood pressure, and perfusion; respirations and adventitious sounds; and clotting studies, renal and hepatic function tests, CBC, guaiac test for occult blood in stool, and ECG.

Nursing Diagnoses

The patient receiving a thrombolytic drug may have the following nursing diagnoses related to drug therapy:

- Risk for Injury related to clot-dissolving effects
- Ineffective Tissue Perfusion (Total Body) related to possible blood loss
- Decreased Cardiac Output related to bleeding and arrhythmias
- Deficient Knowledge regarding drug therapy

Implementation With Rationale

- Discontinue heparin if it is being given before administration of a thrombolytic agent, unless specifically ordered for coronary artery infusion, *to prevent excessive loss of blood.*
- Evaluate the patient regularly for any sign of blood loss (petechiae, bleeding gums, bruises, dark-colored stools, dark-colored urine) *to evaluate drug effectiveness and to consult with the prescriber if blood loss becomes apparent.*
- Monitor coagulation studies regularly; consult with the prescriber *to adjust the drug dose appropriately.*
- Institute treatment within 6 hours after the onset of symptoms of acute MI, *to achieve optimum therapeutic effectiveness.*
- Arrange to type and cross-match blood, *in case of serious blood loss that requires whole-blood transfusion.*
- Monitor cardiac rhythm continuously if being given for acute MI, *because of the risk of alteration in cardiac function;* have life support equipment on standby as needed.
- Provide increased precautions against bleeding during invasive procedures; use pressure dressings and ice; avoid intramuscular injections; and do not rub Sub-Q injection sites, *because of the risk of increased blood loss in the anticoagulated state.*
- Mark the chart of any patient receiving this drug, *to alert medical staff that there is a potential for increased bleeding.*
- Provide thorough patient teaching, including the name of the drug, dosage prescribed, measures to avoid adverse effects, warning signs of problems, and the need for periodic monitoring and evaluation, *to enhance patient knowledge about drug therapy and to promote compliance with the drug regimen.*
- Offer support and encouragement, *to help the patient deal with the diagnosis and the drug regimen.*

Evaluation

- Monitor patient response to the drug (dissolution of the clot and return of blood flow to the area).
- Monitor for adverse effects (bleeding, arrhythmias, hypotension, hypersensitivity reaction).
- Evaluate the effectiveness of the teaching plan (patient can name drug, adverse effects to watch for, specific measures to avoid adverse effects).
- Monitor the effectiveness of comfort measures and compliance with the regimen.

FOCUS POINTS

- To keep blood from coagulating, anticoagulants block blood aggregates or interfere with the mechanisms that cause blood to clot.
- Thrombolytic drugs activate the plasminogen system to dissolve clots naturally.

Drugs Used to Control Bleeding

On the other end of the spectrum of coagulation problems are various bleeding disorders. These include the following:

Hemophilia, in which there is a genetic lack of clotting factors that leaves the patient vulnerable to excessive bleeding with any injury

Liver disease, in which clotting factors and proteins needed for clotting are not produced

Bone marrow disorders, in which platelets are not formed in sufficient quantity to be effective

These disorders are treated with clotting factors and drugs that promote the coagulation process.

Antihemophilic Agents

The drugs used to treat hemophilia are replacement factors for the specific clotting factors that are genetically missing in that particular type of hemophilia. These drugs include the following (Table 48.6):

- Antihemophilic factor (*Bioclate, ReFacto,* and others) is factor VIII, the clotting factor that is missing in classic hemophilia (hemophilia A). It is used to correct or prevent bleeding episodes or to allow necessary surgery.
- Coagulation factor VIIa (*NovoSeven*) is a preparation made from mouse, hamster, and bovine proteins that contains variable amounts of preformed clotting factors. It is used to treat bleeding episodes in patients with hemophilia A or B.
- Factor IX complex (*Benefix, Profilnine SD,* and others) contains plasma fractions of many of the clotting factors and increases blood levels of factors II, VII, IX, and X. It is given intravenously to prevent or treat hemophilia B (Christmas disease, a deficiency of factor IX), to control bleeding episodes in hemophilia A, and to control bleeding episodes in cases of factor VII deficiency.

Therapeutic Actions and Indications

The antihemophilic drugs replace clotting factors that are either genetically missing or low in a particular type of hemophilia. They are used to prevent blood loss from injury or surgery and to treat bleeding episodes. The drug of choice depends on the particular hemophilia that is being treated.

Pharmacokinetics

These agents replace normal clotting factors and are processed as such by the body. They should be used during pregnancy only if the benefit to the mother clearly outweighs the potential risk to the fetus. It is recommended that another method of feeding the baby be used if these drugs are needed during lactation because of the potential for adverse effects on the baby.

Contraindications and Cautions

Antihemophilic factor is contraindicated in the presence of known allergy to mouse proteins. Factor IX is contraindicated in the presence of liver disease with signs of intravascular coagulation or fibrinolysis. Coagulation factor VIIa is contraindicated with known allergies to mouse, hamster, or bovine products. These drugs are not recommended for use during lactation, and caution should be used during pregnancy *because of the potential for adverse effects on the baby or fetus.* Because these drugs are used to prevent serious bleeding problems or to treat bleeding episodes, there are few contraindications to their use.

Adverse Effects

The most common adverse effects associated with antihemophilic agents involve risks associated with the use of blood products (e.g., hepatitis, AIDS). Headache, flushing, chills, fever, and lethargy may occur as a reaction to the injection of a foreign protein. Nausea and vomiting may also occur, as may stinging, itching, and burning at the site of the injection.

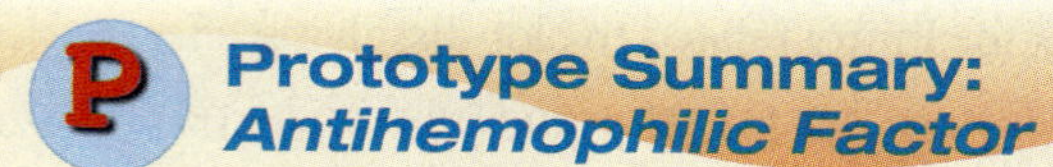

Indications: Treatment of classic hemophilia to provide temporary replacement of clotting factors to correct or prevent bleeding episodes or to allow necessary surgery

Actions: Normal plasma protein that is needed for the transformation of prothrombin to thrombin, the final step in the clotting pathway

Pharmacokinetics:

Route	Onset	Peak	Duration
IV	Immediate	Unknown	Unknown

$T_{1/2}$: 12 hours; cleared from the body by normal protein metabolism

Table 48.6 DRUGS IN FOCUS

Antihemophilic Agents

Drug Name	Usual Dosage	Usual Indications
P antihemophilic factor (*Bioclate, others*)	IV dosage based on level of antihemophilic factor, weight, and patient response	Treatment of hemophilia A; to correct bleeding episodes or to allow surgery
coagulation factor VIIa (*NovoSeven*)	90 mcg/kg IV q2h until hemostasis is achieved	Treatment of bleeding episodes in patients with hemophilia A or B
factor IX complex (*Benefix, others*)	IV dosage based on factor levels, weight, and desired response	Treatment of hemophilia B; treatment of bleeding episodes in patients with factor VII and factor VIII deficiencies

Adverse effects: Allergic reaction, stinging at injection site, headache, rash, chills, nausea, hepatitis, AIDS (risks associated with the use of blood products)

Nursing Considerations for Patients Receiving Antihemophilic Agents

Assessment: History and Examination

Screen for the following conditions, *which could be cautions or contraindications to use of the drug:* any known allergies to these drugs or to mouse proteins with antihemophilic factor; liver disease.

Include screening *for baseline status before beginning therapy and for any potential adverse effects.* Assess the following: body temperature; skin color, lesions, and temperature; affect, orientation, and reflexes; pulse, blood pressure, and perfusion; respirations and adventitious sounds; clotting studies; and hepatic function tests.

Nursing Diagnoses

The patient receiving an antihemophilic drug may have the following nursing diagnoses related to drug therapy:

- Ineffective Tissue Perfusion (Total Body) related to changes in coagulation
- Acute Pain related to GI, CNS, or skin effects
- Anxiety or Fear related to the diagnosis and use of blood-related products
- Deficient Knowledge regarding drug therapy

Implementation With Rationale

- Administer by the IV route only, *to ensure therapeutic effectiveness.*
- Monitor clinical response and clotting factor levels regularly, *in order to arrange to adjust dosage as needed.*
- Monitor the patient for any sign of thrombosis, *to arrange to use comfort and support measures as needed* (e.g., support hose, positioning, ambulation, exercise).
- Decrease the rate of infusion if headache, chills, fever, or tingling occurs, *to prevent severe drug reaction;* in some individuals the drug will need to be discontinued.
- Arrange to type and cross-match blood *in case of serious blood loss that will require whole-blood transfusion.*
- Mark the chart of any patient receiving this drug, *to alert medical staff that there is a potential for increased bleeding.*
- Provide thorough patient teaching, including the name of the drug, dosage prescribed, measures to avoid adverse effects, warning signs of problems, and the need for periodic monitoring and evaluation, *to enhance patient knowledge about drug therapy and to promote compliance with the drug regimen.*
- Offer support and encouragement, *to help the patient deal with the diagnosis and the drug regimen.*

Evaluation

- Monitor patient response to the drug (control of bleeding episodes, prevention of bleeding episodes).
- Monitor for adverse effects (thrombosis, CNS effects, nausea, hypersensitivity reaction, hepatitis, AIDS).
- Evaluate the effectiveness of the teaching plan (patient can name drug, dosage of drug, adverse effects to watch for, specific measures to avoid adverse effects, warning signs to report).
- Monitor the effectiveness of comfort measures and compliance to the regimen.

Systemic Hemostatic Agents

Some situations result in a fibrinolytic state with excessive plasminogen activity and risk of bleeding from clot dissolution. For example, patients undergoing repeat coronary artery bypass graft (CABG) surgery are especially prone to excessive bleeding and may require blood transfusion. **Hemostatic drugs** are used to stop bleeding. The hemostatic drugs that are used systemically include the following (Table 48.7):

- Aprotinin (*Trasylol*), an IV drug derived from bovine lung tissue, forms complexes with kinins, plasmin, and other clot-dissolving factors to block the activation of the plasminogen system. It is used during repeat CABG surgery and in certain unusual cases of first-time CABG surgery in which the patient is at increased risk of bleeding. Aprotinin is widely distributed after IV injection and is excreted primarily by the kidneys with a half-life of 150 minutes. Degradation appears to be accomplished by lysosomal enzymes. Its safety for use during pregnancy and lactation has not been established, and it should be used only if the benefits to the mother clearly outweigh the potential risks to the fetus.
- Aminocaproic acid (*Amicar*) inhibits plasminogen-activating substances and has some antiplasmin activity. It is available in oral and IV forms and is used to

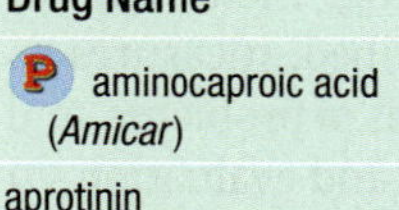

Table 48.7 DRUGS IN FOCUS

Systemic Hemostatic Agents

Drug Name	Usual Dosage	Usual Indications
P aminocaproic acid (*Amicar*)	5 mg PO or IV, then 1–1.25 g/h; do not exceed 30 g in 24 h	Treatment of excessive bleeding in hyperfibrinolytic states; prevention of recurrence of bleeding with subarachnoid hemorrhage
aprotinin (*Trasylol*)	1–2 million KIU IV into pump primer volume, then 250,000–500,000 KIU/h while on the pump	Prevention of blood loss and need for transfusion after repeat coronary artery bypass graft (CABG) surgery; in rare instances, for first CABG surgery in patients prone to bleeding

KIU, kallikrein inactivation units.

limit excessive bleeding in hyperfibrinolysis states, to prevent recurrence of subarachnoid hemorrhage, and, at times, to treat attacks of hereditary angioedema. When taking the oral form, the patient may need to take 10 tablets in the first hour and then continue taking the drug around the clock. This drug is rapidly absorbed and widely distributed throughout the body. It is excreted largely unchanged in urine, with a half-life of 2 hours. Safety for use during pregnancy and lactation has not been established, and it should be used only if the benefits to the mother clearly outweigh the potential risks to the fetus or neonate.

Therapeutic Actions and Indications

The systemic hemostatic agents stop the natural plasminogen clot-dissolving mechanism by blocking its activation or by directly inhibiting plasmin. These drugs are used to prevent or treat excess bleeding in hyperfibrinolytic states, including repeat CABG surgery.

Pharmacokinetics

Pharmacokinetic parameters are different for each drug (see earlier discussions).

Contraindications and Cautions

Systemic hemostatic agents are contraindicated in the presence of allergy to these drugs and with acute DIC *because of the risk of tissue necrosis.* Caution should be used in the following conditions: cardiac disease, *because of the risk of arrhythmias;* renal and hepatic dysfunction, *which could alter the excretion of these drugs and the normal clotting processes;* and pregnancy and lactation, *because of the potential for adverse effects on the neonate.*

Adverse Effects

The most common adverse effect associated with systemic hemostatic agents is excessive clotting. CNS effects can include hallucinations, drowsiness, dizziness, headache, and psychotic states, all of which could be related to changes in cerebral blood flow associated with changes in clot dissolution. GI effects, including nausea, cramps, and diarrhea, may be related to excessive clotting in the GI tract, causing reflex GI stimulation. Weakness, fatigue, malaise, and muscle pain can occur as small clots build up in muscles. Intrarenal obstruction and renal dysfunction have also been reported.

Aprotinin has been associated with cardiac arrhythmias, MI, CHF, and hypotension. These effects may be related to the fact that this drug is used during CABG surgery. Anaphylactic and respiratory reactions have also been reported with aprotinin, possibly related to immune reactions to the bovine protein.

Clinically Important Drug–Drug Interactions

The risk of bleeding increases if these drugs are given with heparin.

Aminocaproic acid is associated with the development of hypercoagulation states if it is combined with oral contraceptives or estrogens.

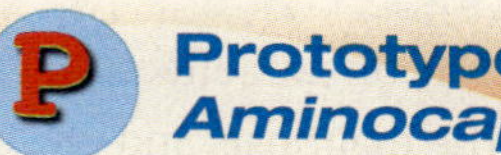

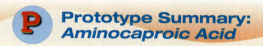

Prototype Summary: *Aminocaproic Acid*

Indications: Treatment of excessive bleeding resulting from hyperfibrinolysis; also used to prevent recurrence of subarachnoid hemorrhage, for management of megakaryocytic thrombocytopenia, to decrease the need for platelet administration, to abort and treat attacks of hereditary angioneurotic edema

Actions: Inhibits plasminogen activator substances and has antiplasmin activity that inhibits fibrinolysis and prevents the breakdown of clots

Pharmacokinetics:

Route	Onset	Peak	Duration
Oral	Rapid	2 h	Unknown
IV	Immediate	Minutes	2–3 h

$T_{1/2}$: 2 hours; excreted unchanged in urine

Adverse effects: Dizziness, tinnitus, headache, weakness, hypotension, nausea, cramps, diarrhea, fertility problems, malaise, elevated serum creatine phosphokinase (CPK)

Nursing Considerations for Patients Receiving Systemic Hemostatic Agents

Assessment: History and Examination

Screen for the following conditions, *which could be cautions or contraindications to use of the drug:* any known allergies to these drugs; acute DIC, *because of the risk of tissue necrosis;* cardiac disease, *because of the risk of arrhythmias;* renal and hepatic dysfunction, *which could alter the excretion of these drugs and the normal clotting processes;* and lactation, *because of the potential for adverse effects on the neonate.*

Include screening *for baseline status before beginning therapy and for any potential adverse effects.* Assess the following: body temperature; skin color, lesions, and temperature; affect, orientation, and reflexes; pulse, blood pressure, and perfusion; respirations and adventitious sounds; bowel sounds and normal output; urinalysis and clotting studies; and renal and hepatic function tests.

Nursing Diagnoses

The patient receiving a systemic hemostatic drug may have the following nursing diagnoses related to drug therapy:

- Disturbed Sensory Perception related to CNS effects
- Acute Pain related to GI, CNS, or muscle effects
- Risk for Injury related to CNS or blood-clotting effects
- Deficient Knowledge regarding drug therapy

Implementation With Rationale

- Monitor clinical response and clotting factor levels regularly, *in order to arrange to adjust dosage as needed.*
- Monitor the patient for any sign of thrombosis, *in order to arrange to use comfort and support measures as needed* (e.g., support hose, positioning, ambulation, exercise).
- Orient patient and offer support and safety measures if hallucinations or psychoses occur, *to prevent patient injury.*
- Offer comfort measures, *to help the patient deal with the effects of the drug.* These include small, frequent meals; mouth care; environmental controls; and safety measures.
- Provide thorough patient teaching, including the name of the drug, dosage prescribed, measures to avoid adverse effects, warning signs of problems, and the need for periodic monitoring and evaluation, *to enhance patient knowledge about drug therapy and to promote compliance with the drug regimen.*
- Offer support and encouragement, *to help the patient deal with the diagnosis and the drug regimen.*

Evaluation

- Monitor the patient response to the drug (control of bleeding episodes).
- Monitor for adverse effects (thrombosis, CNS effects, nausea, hypersensitivity reaction).
- Evaluate the effectiveness of the teaching plan (patient can name drug, dosage of drug, adverse effects to watch for, specific measures to avoid adverse effects, warning signs to report).
- Monitor the effectiveness of comfort measures and compliance to the regimen.

Topical Hemostatic Agents

Some surface injuries involve so much damage to the small vessels in the area that clotting does not occur and blood is slowly and continually lost. For these situations, topical or local hemostatic agents are often used (Table 48.8).

Absorbable gelatin (*Gelfoam*) and microfibrillar collagen (*Avitene*) are available in sponge form and are applied directly to the injured area until the bleeding stops. Use of these products can pose a risk of infection, because bacteria can become trapped in the vascular area when the sponge is applied. Immediate removal of the sponge and cleaning of the area can help to decrease this risk.

Thrombin (*Thrombinar, Thrombostat*), which is derived from bovine sources, is applied topically and mixed in with the blood. Because this drug comes from animal sources, it may precipitate an allergic response; the patient needs to be carefully monitored for such a reaction.

The use of these drugs is incorporated into the care of the wound or decubitus ulcer as adjunctive therapy. The drug of choice depends on the nature of the injury and the prescriber's personal preference.

WEB LINKS

Health care providers and patients may want to explore the following Internet sources:

http://www.heartcenteronline.com Information on thrombosis—process, interventions, and pathology.

http://www.e-mds.com/healthinfo view/drug/ Information designed for patients and families regarding the home use of warfarin.

Table 48.8 DRUGS IN FOCUS

Topical Hemostatic Agents

Drug Name	Usual Dosage	Usual Indications
absorbable gelatin (*Gelfoam*)	Smear or press onto surface; do not remove, will be absorbed	Control of bleeding from surface cuts or injury
microfibrillar collagen (*Avitene*)	Use dry; apply to area and apply pressure for 3–5 min	Control of bleeding from surface cuts or injury
thrombin (*Thrombostat, Thrombinar*)	100–1000 units/mL freely mixed with blood	Control of bleeding from surface cuts or injury **Special considerations:** Use caution with allergy to bovine products

http://www.nlm.nih.gov/medlineplus/druginfo/uspdi/202280.html Information on heparin—use, research, and complications.

Points to Remember

- Coagulation is the transformation of fluid blood into a solid state to plug up breaks in the vascular system.
- Coagulation involves several processes, including vasoconstriction, platelet aggregation to form a plug, and intrinsic and extrinsic clot formation initiated by Hageman factor to plug any breaks in the system.
- The final step of clot formation is the conversion of prothrombin to thrombin, which breaks down fibrinogen to form insoluble fibrin threads.
- Once a clot is formed, it must be dissolved to prevent the occlusion of blood vessels and loss of blood supply to tissues.
- Plasminogen is the basis of the clot-dissolving system. It is converted to plasmin (fibrinolysin) by several factors, including Hageman factor. Plasmin dissolves fibrin threads and resolves the clot.
- Anticoagulants block blood coagulation by interfering with one or more of the steps involved, such as blocking platelet aggregation or inhibiting the intrinsic or extrinsic pathways to clot formation.
- Thrombolytic drugs dissolve clots or thrombi that have formed. They activate the plasminogen system to stimulate natural clot dissolution.
- Hemostatic drugs are used to stop bleeding. They may replace missing clotting factors or prevent the plasminogen system from dissolving formed clots.
- Hemophilia, a genetic lack of essential clotting factors, results in excessive bleeding. It is treated by replacing missing clotting factors.

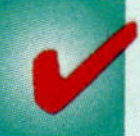

CHECK YOUR UNDERSTANDING

Answers to the questions in this chapter may be found in the Answer Key in the back of the book.

Multiple Choice

Select the best answer to the following.

1. Blood coagulation is a complex reaction that involves
   a. vasoconstriction, platelet aggregation, and plasminogen action.
   b. vasodilation, platelet aggregation, and activation of the clotting cascade.
   c. vasoconstriction, platelet aggregation, and conversion of prothrombin to thrombin.
   d. vasodilation, platelet inhibition, and action of the intrinsic and extrinsic clotting cascades.

2. Warfarin, an oral anticoagulant, acts
   a. to directly prevent the conversion of prothrombin to thrombin.
   b. to decrease the production of vitamin K clotting factors in the liver.
   c. as a catalyst in the conversion of plasminogen to plasmin.
   d. immediately, so it is the drug of choice in emergency situations.

3. Heparin reacts to prevent the conversion of prothrombin to thrombin. Heparin
   a. is available in oral and parenteral forms.
   b. takes about 72 hours to cause a therapeutic effect.
   c. effects are reversed with the administration of protamine sulfate.
   d. effects are reversed with the injection of vitamin K.

4. The low-molecular-weight heparin of choice for preventing deep venous thrombosis after hip replacement therapy would be
   a. tinzaparin.
   b. dalteparin.
   c. heparin.
   d. enoxaparin.

5. A thrombolytic agent could be safely used in
   a. CVA within the last 2 months.
   b. acute MI within the last 3 hours.
   c. recent, serious GI bleeding.
   d. obstetrical delivery.

6. Antihemophilic agents are used to replace missing clotting factors to prevent severe blood loss. The most common side effects associated with the use of these drugs are
   a. bleeding.
   b. dark stools and urine.
   c. hepatitis, AIDS.
   d. constipation.

Multiple Response

Select all that apply.

1. Hageman factor is known to activate which of the following?
   a. The clotting cascade
   b. The anticlotting process
   c. The inflammatory response
   d. Platelet aggregation
   e. Thromboxane A_2
   f. Troponin coupling

2. Plasminogen is converted to plasmin, a clot-dissolving substance, by which of the following?
   a. Nicotine
   b. Hageman factor
   c. Streptokinase
   d. Pyrogens
   e. Thrombin
   f. Christmas factor

3. Antiplatelet drugs block the aggregation of platelets and keep vessels open. These drugs would be useful in which of the following?
   a. Maintaining the patency of grafts
   b. Decreasing the risk of fatal MI
   c. Preventing reinfarction after MI
   d. Dissolving a pulmonary embolus and improving oxygenation
   e. Decreasing damage in a subarachnoid bleed
   f. Preventing thromboembolic strokes

4. Evaluating a client who is taking an anticoagulant for blood loss would usually include assessing for which of the following?
   a. The presence of petechiae
   b. Bleeding gums while brushing the teeth
   c. Dark-colored urine
   d. Yellow color to the sclera or skin
   e. The presence of ecchymotic areas
   f. Loss of hair

True or False

Indicate whether the following statements are true (T) or false (F).

______ 1. Coagulation is the transformation of fluid blood to a solid state.

______ 2. Coagulation involves vasodilation, platelet aggregation, and intrinsic and extrinsic clot formation.

______ 3. Coagulation is initiated by Hageman factor to plug up any holes in the cardiovascular system.

______ 4. The final step of clot formation is the conversion of prothrombin to thrombin, which breaks down fibrinogen to form soluble fibrin threads.

______ 5. Once a clot is formed, it must be dissolved to prevent the occlusion of blood vessels and loss of blood supply to tissues.

______ 6. Plasminogen is the basis of the coagulation system.

______ 7. Plasmin dissolves fibrin threads and resolves the clot.

______ 8. Anticoagulants dissolve clots that have formed.

______ 9. Thrombolytic drugs block coagulation and prevent the formation of clots.

______ 10. Hemophilia is a genetic lack of essential clotting factors that results in excessive bleeding situations.

Web Exercise

You are discharging a patient to home with a prescription for warfarin (*Coumadin*). The patient and his family have many questions and concerns about the continued use of this anticoagulant. Go online and find information to prepare a teaching pamphlet for the patient, including things to avoid, signs and symptoms to watch for, when to call the doctor, and when blood tests should be done. To get started, you might want to go to http://www.ptinr.com.

Bibliography and References

Drug facts and comparisons. (2006). St. Louis: Facts and Comparisons.

Gilman, A., Hardman, J. G., & Limbird, L. E. (Eds.). (2006). *Goodman and Gilman's the pharmacological basis of therapeutics* (11th ed.). New York: McGraw-Hill.

Karch, A. M. (2006). *2007 Lippincott's nursing drug guide.* Philadelphia: Lippincott Williams & Wilkins.

The medical letter on drugs and therapeutics. (2006). New Rochelle, NY: Medical Letter.

Porth, C. M. (2005). *Pathophysiology: Concepts of altered health states* (7th ed.). Philadelphia: Lippincott Williams & Wilkins.

CHAPTER

49

Drugs Used to Treat Anemias

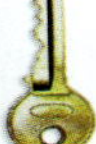

KEY TERMS

anemia
erythrocytes
erythropoiesis
erythropoietin
iron deficiency anemia
megaloblastic anemia
pernicious anemia
plasma
reticulocyte

LEARNING OBJECTIVES

Upon completion of this chapter, you will be able to:

1. Explain the process of erythropoiesis and use this information to discuss the development of three types of anemias.
2. Describe the therapeutic actions, indications, pharmacokinetics, contraindications, most common adverse reactions, and important drug–drug interactions associated with erythropoietic agents, iron preparations, folic acid derivatives, and vitamin B_{12}.
3. Discuss the use of drugs used to treat anemias across the lifespan.
4. Compare and contrast the prototype drugs epoetin alfa, ferrous sulfate, folic acid, and hydroxocobalamin with other agents in their class.
5. Outline the nursing considerations, including important teaching points, for patients receiving drugs used to treat anemias.

ERYTHROPOIETIN

darbepoetin alfa
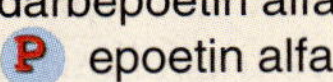
P epoetin alfa

IRON PREPARATIONS

ferrous fumarate
ferrous gluconate
P ferrous sulfate
ferrous sulfate exsiccated
iron dextran
iron sucrose
sodium ferric gluconate complex

FOLIC ACID DERIVATIVES

P folic acid
leucovorin

VITAMIN B_{12}

cyanocobalamin
P hydroxocobalamin

The cardiovascular system exists to pump blood to all of the body's cells. Blood is essential for cell survival because it contains oxygen and nutrients and removes waste products that could be toxic to the tissues. It also contains clotting factors that help maintain the vascular system and keep it sealed. In addition, blood contains the important components of the immune system that protect the body from infection. This chapter discusses drugs that are used to treat anemias, which are disorders that involve too few red blood cells (RBCs) or ineffective RBCs that can alter the blood's ability to carry oxygen.

Blood Components

Blood is composed of liquid and formed elements. The liquid part of blood is called **plasma**. Plasma is mostly water, but it also contains proteins that are essential for the immune response and for blood clotting. The formed elements of the blood include leukocytes (white blood cells), which are an important part of the immune system (see Chapter 15); **erythrocytes** (RBCs), which carry oxygen to the tissues and remove carbon dioxide for delivery to the lungs; and platelets, which play an important role in coagulation (see Chapter 48).

Erythropoiesis

Erythropoiesis is the process of RBC production. RBCs are produced in the myeloid tissue of the bone marrow. The rate of RBC production is controlled by the glycoprotein **erythropoietin**, which is released from the kidneys in response to decreased blood flow or decreased oxygen tension in the kidneys. Under the influence of erythropoietin, an undifferentiated cell in the bone marrow becomes a hemocytoblast. This cell uses certain amino acids, lipids, carbohydrates, vitamin B_{12}, folic acid, and iron to turn into an immature RBC. In the last phase of RBC production, the cell loses its nucleus and enters circulation. This cell, called a **reticulocyte**, finishes its maturing process in circulation (Figure 49.1).

Although the mature RBC has no nucleus, it does have a vast surface area to improve its ability to transport oxygen and carbon dioxide. Because it lacks a nucleus, the RBC cannot reproduce or maintain itself, so it will eventually wear out. The average lifespan of an RBC is about 120 days. At that time, the elderly RBC is lysed in the liver, spleen, or bone marrow. The building blocks of the RBC (e.g., iron, vitamin B_{12}) are then recycled and returned to the bone marrow for the production of new RBCs (see Figure 49.1). The only part of the RBC that cannot be recycled is the toxic pigment bilirubin, which is conjugated in the liver, passed into the bile, and excreted from the body in the feces or the urine. Bilirubin is what gives color to both of these excretions. Erythropoiesis is a constant process, wherein about 1% of the body's RBCs are destroyed and replaced each day.

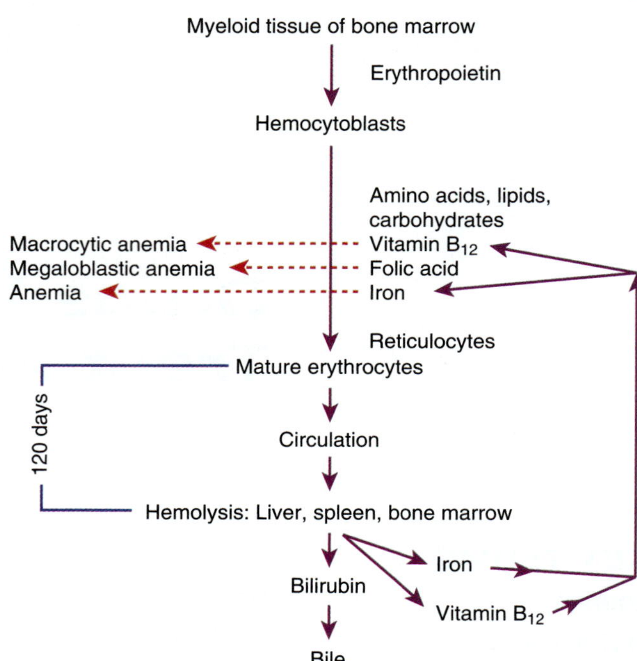

FIGURE 49.1 Erythropoiesis. Red blood cells are produced in the myeloid tissue of the bone marrow in response to the hormone erythropoietin. The hemocytoblasts require various essential factors to produce mature erythrocytes. A lack of any one of these can result in an anemia of the type indicated opposite each factor. Mature erythrocytes survive for about 120 days and are then lysed in the liver, spleen, or bone marrow.

Anemia

Anemia, a decrease in the number of RBCs, can occur if erythropoietin levels are low. This is seen in renal failure, when the kidneys are no longer able to produce erythropoietin. It can also occur if the body does not have enough of the building blocks necessary to form RBCs. To produce healthy RBCs, the bone marrow must have the following:

- Adequate amounts of iron, which is used in forming hemoglobin rings to carry the oxygen
- Minute amounts of vitamin B_{12} and folic acid, to form a strong supporting structure that can survive being battered through blood vessels for 120 days
- Essential amino acids and carbohydrates, to complete the hemoglobin rings, cell membrane, and basic structure

See Box 49.1, for information about differences in hemoglobin and other hematological values in African Americans, and Box 49.2, on issues involving different age groups.

Normally, an individual's diet supplies adequate amounts of all of these substances, which are absorbed from the gastrointestinal (GI) tract and transported to the bone marrow. But when the diet cannot supply enough of a nutrient, or enough of the nutrient cannot be absorbed, the person can

BOX 49.1 CULTURAL CONSIDERATIONS FOR DRUG THERAPY

Hematological Laboratory Test Variations

There are racial variations in hematological laboratory test results:

Hemoglobin/hematocrit—African Americans are generally 1 g lower than other groups.

Serum transferrin levels (children age 1–3.5 yr)—The mean value for African American children is 22 mg/100 mL higher than for white children. (This may be because African Americans have lower hematocrit and hemoglobin; transferrin levels increase normally in the presence of anemia.)

Because of these variations, the diagnosis and treatment of anemia in African Americans should be based on a different norm than with other groups of patients.

develop a deficiency anemia. Fewer RBCs are produced, and the ones that are produced are not mature and are not efficient iron carriers. The person with this type of anemia, a deficiency anemia, may complain of being tired because there is insufficient oxygen delivery to the tissues.

Another type of anemia is **megaloblastic anemia**, a condition in which the bone marrow contains a large number of megaloblasts, or large, immature RBCs. Because these RBCs are so large, they become crowded in the bone marrow and fewer RBCs are produced. There is an increase in these immature cells in circulation. Overall, fewer RBCs are produced, and those that are produced are ineffective and do not usually survive for the 120 days that is normal for the life of an RBC. Patients with megaloblastic anemia usually have a lack of vitamin B_{12} or folic acid. (See Box 49.3 for information on sickle cell anemia.)

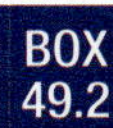

BOX 49.2 DRUG THERAPY ACROSS THE LIFESPAN

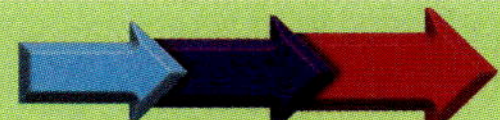

Drugs Used to Treat Anemias

CHILDREN

Proper nutrition should be established for children to provide the essential elements needed for formation of red blood cells (RBCs). The cause of the anemia should be determined to avoid prolonged problems.

The safety and efficacy of epoetin alfa use has not been established for children. If the drug is used, careful dosage calculation should be done based on weight and age, and the child should be monitored very closely for response, iron levels, and nutrition.

Iron doses for replacement therapy are determined by age. If a liquid solution is being used, the child should drink it through a straw to avoid staining of the teeth. Periodic blood counts should be performed; it may take 4–6 mo of oral therapy to reverse an iron deficiency. Remember that iron can be toxic to children, and iron supplements should be kept out of their reach and administration monitored.

Maintenance doses for folic acid have been established for children, based on age. Nutritional means should be used to establish folic acid levels whenever possible.

Children with pernicious anemia will require a monthly injection of vitamin B_{12}; the nasal form has not been approved for use with children.

ADULTS

The underlying cause of the anemia should be established and appropriate steps taken to reverse the cause if possible. Adults receiving epoetin alfa or darbapoetin alfa should be monitored closely for response, for the need for iron or other RBC building blocks, and for the possibility of development of pure red cell aplasia.

Advertised heavily in the mass media, epoetin is often requested by adults to help return energy. Careful patient teaching about the drug, and how and why it is administered, may be needed.

Adults receiving iron replacement may experience gastrointestinal upset and frequently experience constipation. Appropriate measures to maintain bowel function may be needed.

Adults also need to know that periodic blood tests will be needed to evaluate response.

Adults being treated for pernicious anemia may opt for the nasal vitamin B_{12}. These patients need to receive careful instructions about the proper administration of the drug and should have nasal mucous membranes evaluated periodically.

Proper nutrition during pregnancy and lactation is often still not an adequate way to meet the increased demands of those states. Prenatal vitamins contain iron and folic acid and are usually prescribed for pregnant women. Use of epoetin alfa or darbapoetin alfa is not recommended during pregnancy or lactation because of the potential for adverse effects on the fetus or baby. Iron replacement is frequently needed postpartum to provide the iron lost during delivery. The new mother should be reminded to keep the drug out of the reach of children and not to combine prescribed iron with an over-the-counter preparation containing high levels of iron.

Women maintained on vitamin B_{12} before pregnancy should continue the treatment during pregnancy. Increased doses may be needed due to changes associated with the pregnancy.

OLDER ADULTS

Older adults may have nutritional problems related to age and may lose more iron through cellular sloughing. Older adults should be assessed for anemia, and possible causes should be evaluated.

Replacement therapy in the older adult can cause the same adverse effects as are seen in the younger person. Bowel training programs may be needed to prevent severe constipation.

Use of nasal vitamin B_{12} may not be practical. If the patient desires to use this administration technique, nasal mucous membranes should be evaluated before and periodically during treatment.

BOX 49.3 CULTURAL CONSIDERATIONS FOR DRUG THERAPY

Sickle Cell Anemia

Sickle cell anemia is a chronic hemolytic anemia that occurs almost exclusively in blacks. (Hemolytic anemias involve a lysing of red blood cells [RBCs] because of genetic factors or from exposure to toxins.) Sickle cell anemia is characterized by a genetically inherited hemoglobin S, which gives the RBCs a sickle-shaped appearance. The patient with sickle cell anemia produces fewer than normal RBCs, and the RBCs produced are unable to carry oxygen efficiently. The patient may be of short stature with stubby fingers and toes; these characteristics are related to the body's response to the inability to deliver oxygen to the tissues.

The sickle-shaped RBCs can become lodged in tiny blood vessels, where they stack up on one another and occlude the vessel. This occlusion leads to anoxia and infarction of the tissue in that area, which is characterized by severe pain and an acute inflammatory reaction—a condition often called sickle cell crisis. (The patient may have ulcers on the extremities as a result of such occlusions.) Severe, acute episodes of sickling with vessel occlusion may be associated with acute infections and the body's reactions to the immune and inflammatory responses.

In the past, the only treatment for sickle cell anemia was pain medication and support of the patient. Now hydroxyurea (*Hydrea*) has been found to effectively treat this disease. Hydroxyurea is a cytotoxic antineoplastic agent that is used to treat leukemia, ovarian cancer, and melanoma. It has been shown that it increases the amount of fetal hemoglobin produced in the bone marrow and dilutes the formation of the abnormal hemoglobin S in patients with sickle cell anemia. The process takes several months, but, once effective, it prevents the clogging of small vessels and the painful, anoxic effects of RBC sickling. Because this drug is associated with several uncomfortable adverse effects—including gastrointestinal problems, rash, headache, and possible bone marrow depression—the decision to use it is not made lightly. However, it has been found to be effective in preventing the painful crises of sickle cell anemia.

Iron Deficiency Anemias

All cells in the body require some amount of iron, but iron can be very toxic to cells, especially neurons. To maintain the needed iron levels and avoid toxic levels, the body has developed a system for controlling the amount of iron that can enter the body through intestinal absorption. Only enough iron is absorbed to replace the amount of iron that is lost each day. Once iron is absorbed, it is carried by a plasma protein called transferrin, a beta-globulin. This protein carries iron to various tissues to be stored and transports iron from RBC lysis back to the bone marrow for recycling.

Only about 1 mg of iron is actually lost each day in sweat, in sloughed skin, and from GI and urinary tract linings. Because of the body's efficient iron recycling, very little iron is usually needed in the diet, and most diets quite adequately replace the iron that is lost. However, in situations in which blood is being lost, such as internal bleeding or heavy menstrual flow, a negative iron balance might occur, and the patient could develop **iron deficiency anemia**. This can also occur in certain GI diseases in which the patient is unable to absorb iron from the GI tract. These conditions are usually treated with iron replacement therapy.

Megaloblastic Anemias

Megaloblastic anemias occur when there is not sufficient folic acid or vitamin B_{12} to adequately create the stromal structure needed in a healthy RBC. The lack of these two chemicals causes a slowing of nuclear DNA synthesis in human cells. This effect is seen in other rapidly dividing cells, not just bone marrow cells. For example, cells in the GI tract are often affected, resulting in the appearance of a characteristic red and glossy tongue and diarrhea.

Folic Acid Deficiency

Folic acid is essential for cell division in all types of tissue. Deficiencies in folic acid are noticed first in rapidly growing cells, such as those in cancerous tissues, in the GI tract, and in the bone marrow. Most people can get all the folic acid they need from their diet. For example, folic acid is found in green leafy vegetables, milk, eggs, and liver. Deficiency in folic acid may occur in certain malabsorption states, such as sprue and celiac diseases. Malnutrition that accompanies alcoholism is also a common cause of folic acid deficiency. Repeated pregnancies and extended treatment with certain antiepileptic medications can also contribute to folic acid deficiency. This disorder is treated by the administration of folic acid or folate.

Vitamin B_{12} Deficiency

Vitamin B_{12} is used in minute amounts by the body and is stored for use if dietary intake falls. It is necessary not only for the health of the RBCs but also for the formation and maintenance of the myelin sheath in the central nervous system (CNS). It is found in the diet in meats, seafood, eggs, and cheese. Strict vegetarians who eat nothing but vegetables may develop a vitamin B_{12} deficiency. Such individuals with a dietary insufficiency of vitamin B_{12} typically respond to vitamin B_{12} replacement therapy to reverse their anemia.

The most common cause of this deficiency, however, is inability of the GI tract to absorb the needed amounts of the vitamin. Gastric mucosal cells produce a substance called intrinsic factor, which is necessary for the absorption of vitamin B_{12} by the upper intestine.

Pernicious anemia occurs when the gastric mucosa cannot produce intrinsic factor and vitamin B_{12} cannot be absorbed. The person with pernicious anemia will complain of fatigue and lethargy and will also have CNS effects because of damage to the myelin sheath. Patients will complain of numbness, tingling, and eventually lack of coordination and motor activity. Pernicious anemia was once a fatal disease, but it is now treated with injections of vitamin B_{12} to replace the amount that can no longer be absorbed.

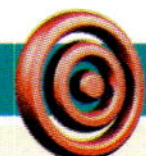

FOCUS POINTS

- RBCs are produced in the bone marrow in a process called erythropoiesis, which is controlled by the glycoprotein erythropoietin, produced in the kidneys.
- The bone marrow uses iron, amino acids, carbohydrates, folic acid, and vitamin B_{12} to produce healthy, efficient RBCs.
- Anemia is a state of too few RBCs. Anemia can be caused by a lack of erythropoietin, or a lack of the components needed to produce RBCs may cause anemia, a disorder marked by too few RBCs.
- Iron deficiency anemia results from inadequate iron intake or an inability to absorb iron from the GI tract.
- Folic acid and vitamin B_{12} are the building blocks of RBCs; without them, a person is at risk for megaloblastic anemia.
- Pernicious anemia, caused by the deficient production of intrinsic factor by gastric cells, is a lack of vitamin B_{12} and causes neurological changes as well as fatigue and signs of decreased oxygen delivery.

Erythropoietins

Patients who are no longer able to produce enough erythropoietin in the kidneys may benefit from treatment with erythropoietin (EPO), which is available as the drugs epoetin alfa (*Epogen, Procrit*) and darbepoetin alfa (*Aranesp*) (see also Table 49.1).

Epogen is used to treat anemia associated with renal failure (including patients on dialysis). It is also used to decrease the need for blood transfusions in patients undergoing surgery and to treat anemias related to treatment for AIDS. It is not approved to treat severe anemia associated with other causes, and it is not meant to replace whole blood for emergency treatment of anemia. There is a risk of decreasing the normal levels of erythropoietin if this drug is given to patients who have normal renal functioning and adequate levels of erythropoietin. A negative feedback occurs with the renal cells, and less endogenous erythropoietin is produced if exogenous erythropoietin is given. Administration of this drug to an anemic patient with normal renal function can actually cause a more severe anemia if the endogenous levels fall and no longer stimulate RBC production. *Procrit* is also used to treat severe anemia related to chemotherapy in cancer patients, in whom bone marrow is depressed and kidneys may be affected by the toxic drugs (Figure 49.2).

Darbepoetin alfa is an erythropoietin-like protein produced in Chinese hamster ovary cells with the use of recombinant DNA technology. It is used to treat anemia associated with chronic renal failure, including patients on dialysis, and to treat cancer chemotherapy-induced anemia. It has the advantage of once-weekly administration, compared with two to three times a week, as with epoetin. This drug gained negative publicity after it was used by athletes to increase their RBC count in the hope that it would give them more endurance and strength. Many athletic groups now screen for the presence of darbepoetin among other banned drugs.

Therapeutic Actions and Indications

Epoetin alfa acts like the natural glycoprotein erythropoietin to stimulate the production of RBCs in the bone marrow (Figure 49.3). It is indicated in the treatment of anemia associated with renal failure and for patients on dialysis. It is also used to decrease the need for blood transfusions in patients undergoing surgery, for the treatment of anemia associated with AIDS therapy, and for the treatment of anemia associated with cancer chemotherapy (*Procrit* only). Darbepoetin alfa is indicated only for the treatment of anemia associated

Table 49.1 DRUGS IN FOCUS

Erythropoietin

Drug Name	Usual Dosage	Usual Indications
darbepoetin alfa (*Aranesp*)	0.45 mcg/kg IV or Sub-Q once per week; 2.25 mcg/kg/wk Sub-Q (with chemotherapy)	Treatment of anemia associated with chronic renal failure, including in dialysis patients; treatment of chemotherapy-induced anemia
P epoetin alfa (*Epogen*)	50–100 units/kg IV or Sub-Q three times per week; 300 units/kg/day Sub-Q for 15 days (reduction of need for blood transfusions)	Treatment of anemia associated with renal failure; reduction in need for transfusions in surgical patients; treatment of anemia associated with AIDS therapy
(*Procrit*)	150 units/kg Sub-Q three times per week	Treatment of anemia associated with cancer chemotherapy

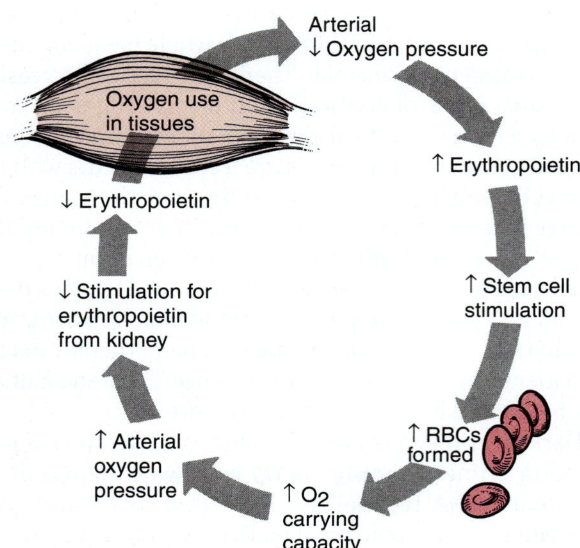

FIGURE 49.2 Erythropoiesis controls the rate of blood cell production.

with chronic renal failure and for anemia induced by cancer chemotherapy.

Pharmacokinetics

Epoetin alfa is metabolized through the normal kinetic processes, with a half-life of 4 to 13 hours. Darbepoetin alfa has a half-life of 21 hours after intravenous administration or 49 hours after subcutaneous administration. There are no adequate studies in pregnancy, so use should be limited to those situations in which the benefit to the mother clearly outweighs the potential risk to the fetus. It is not known whether epoetin alfa enters into breast milk, Darbepoetin alfa does cross into breast milk. Caution should be used if the drug is needed by a nursing mother.

Contraindications and Cautions

Epoetin alfa and darbepoetin alfa are contraindicated in the presence of uncontrolled hypertension, *because of the risk of even further hypertension when RBC numbers increase and the pressure within the vascular system increases;* with allergy to mammalian cell–derived products or to human albumin; and with lactation, *because of the potential for allergic-type reactions with the neonate.*

Adverse Effects

The adverse effects most commonly associated with these drugs include the CNS effects of headache, fatigue, asthenia, and dizziness, and the potential for serious seizures. These effects may be the result of a cellular response to the glycoprotein. Nausea, vomiting, and diarrhea also are common effects. Cardiovascular symptoms can include hypertension, edema, and possible chest pain and may be related to the increase in RBC numbers changing the balance within the cardiovascular system. Patients receiving intravenous administration must also be monitored for possible clotting of the access line related to direct cellular effects of the drug. In 2005, postmarketing studies showed that pure red cell aplasia associated with erythropoietin neutralizing antibodies could occur with all of these products (see Focus on Patient Safety).

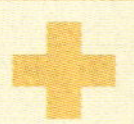

FOCUS ON PATIENT SAFETY

In late 2005, the makers of epoetin and darbepoetin sent out warning letters to health care professionals to bring attention to serious adverse effects that had been noted in postmarketing studies. Cases of pure red cell aplasia and severe anemias, with or without cytopenias, had been reported. These cases were associated with

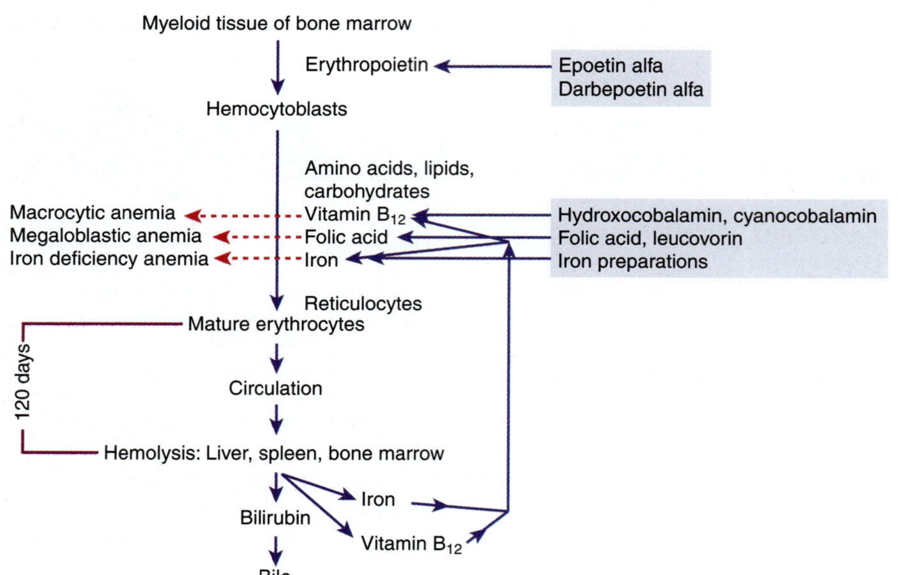

FIGURE 49.3 Sites of action of drugs used to treat anemia.

the development of neutralizing antibodies to erythropoietin. Use of any therapeutic protein brings with it the risk of antibody production. All of the erythropoietic proteins (*Aranesp, Epogen, Procrit*) will now carry a warning about the potential for this problem. If a patient is being treated with one of these drugs and develops a sudden loss of response, accompanied by severe anemia and low reticulocyte count, the patient should be assessed for the possible causes. Assays for binding and neutralizing antibodies should be done. If an antibody-mediated anemia is confirmed, the drug should be permanently stopped and the patient should not be switched to another erythropoietic protein because cross-reaction could occur. Most of the patients in the reported cases had chronic renal failure and were being treated with subcutaneous injections. It is now recommended that patients on hemodialysis receive the drug intravenously and not subcutaneously. If the drug is started and there is no response or if a patient fails to maintain a response, the dosage should not be increased and red blood cell aplasia should be suspected. The patient should be evaluated with the appropriate tests and supported.

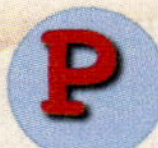

Prototype Summary: Epoetin Alfa

Indications: Treatment of anemia associated with chronic renal failure, related to treatment of HIV infection or to chemotherapy in cancer patients; to reduce the need for allogenic blood transfusions in surgical patients

Actions: Natural glycoprotein that stimulates RBC production in the bone marrow

Pharmacokinetics:

Route	Onset	Peak	Duration
Sub-Q	7–14 days	5–24 h	24 h

$T_{1/2}$: 4–13 hours; metabolized in serum and excreted in urine

Adverse effects: Headache, arthralgias, fatigue, asthenia, dizziness, hypertension, edema, chest pain, nausea, vomiting, diarrhea

Nursing Considerations for Patients Receiving Erythropoietins

Assessment: History and Examination

Screen for the following conditions, *which could be cautions or contraindications to use of the drug:* any known allergies to this drug, to mammalian cell–derived products, or to human albumin; severe hypertension, *which could be exacerbated;* and lactation, *because of potential adverse effects on the neonate.*

Include screening *for baseline status before beginning therapy and for any potential adverse effects.* Assess the following: affect, orientation, and reflexes; pulse, blood pressure, and perfusion; respirations and adventitious breath sounds; and renal function tests, complete blood count (CBC), hematocrit, iron concentration, and electrolytes.

Nursing Diagnoses

The patient receiving erythropoietins may have the following nursing diagnoses related to drug therapy:

- Nausea, Diarrhea related to GI effects
- Risk for Injury related to CNS effects
- Risk for Imbalanced Fluid Volume related to cardiovascular effects
- Deficient Knowledge regarding drug therapy

Implementation With Rationale

- Confirm the chronic, renal nature of the patient's anemia before administering the drug, *to ensure proper use of the drug.*
- Give epoetin alfa three times per week, either intravenously or subcutaneously, *to achieve appropriate therapeutic drug levels.* Darbepoetin alfa is given once per week, subcutaneously or intravenously. The patient should receive a calendar of marked days *to increase compliance with the drug regimen.*
- Do not mix with any other drug solution, *to avoid potential incompatibilities.*
- Monitor access lines for clotting and *arrange to clear line as needed.*
- Arrange for hematocrit reading before drug administration *to determine correct dosage.* If the patient does not respond within 8 weeks, re-evaluate the cause of anemia.
- Evaluate iron stores before and periodically during therapy, *because supplemental iron may be needed as the patient makes more RBCs.*
- Maintain seizure precautions on standby, *in case seizures occur as a reaction to the drug.*
- Provide comfort measures, *to help the patient tolerate the drug effects.* These include small, frequent meals; access to bathroom facilities; and analgesia for headache or arthralgia.
- Provide thorough patient teaching, including the name of the drug, dosage prescribed, measures to avoid adverse effects, warning signs of problems, and the need for periodic monitoring and evaluation, *to enhance patient knowledge about drug therapy and to promote compliance with the drug regimen.*
- Offer support and encouragement, *to help the patient deal with the diagnosis and the drug regimen.*

Evaluation

- Monitor patient response to the drug (alleviation of anemia).
- Monitor for adverse effects (headache, hypertension, nausea, vomiting, seizures, dizziness).
- Evaluate the effectiveness of the teaching plan (patient can name drug, dosage, adverse effects to watch for, specific measures to avoid adverse effects; patient understands importance of continued follow-up).
- Monitor the effectiveness of comfort measures and compliance to the regimen.

Iron Preparations

Although most people get all the iron they need through diet, in some situations diet alone may not be adequate. Iron deficiency anemia is a relatively common problem in certain groups, including the following:

- Menstruating women, who lose RBCs monthly
- Pregnant and nursing women, who have increased demands for iron
- Rapidly growing adolescents, especially those who do not have a nutritious diet
- Persons with GI bleeding, including individuals with slow bleeding associated with use of nonsteroidal anti-inflammatory drugs (NSAIDs)

Oral iron preparations are often used to help these patients regain a positive iron balance; these preparations need to be supplemented with adequate dietary intake of iron. Ferrous fumarate (*Feostat*), ferrous gluconate (*Fergon*), ferrous sulfate (*Feosol*), and ferrous sulfate exsiccated (*Feratab, Slow FE*) are the oral iron preparations that are available for use (see Table 49.2). Most of the drug that is taken is lost in the feces, but slowly some of the metal is absorbed into the intestine and transported to the bone marrow. It can take 2 to 3 weeks to see improvement and up to 6 to 10 months to return to a stable iron level once a deficiency exists. The drug of choice depends on the prescriber's personal preference and experience, and often on what kinds of samples are available to give the patient.

Iron dextran (*InFeD*) is a parenteral form of iron that may be used if the oral form cannot be given or cannot be tolerated. Patients with severe GI absorption problems may require this form of iron. If given intramuscularly, it must be given by the Z-track method, because it can stain the tissues brown and can be very painful (see Box 49.4). Patients should be switched to the oral form if at all possible. Severe hypersensitivity reactions have been associated with the parenteral form of iron. Iron sucrose (*Venofer*) and sodium ferric gluconate complex (*Ferrlecit*) are given intravenously, specifically for patients who are undergoing chronic hemodialysis or who are in renal

Table 49.2 DRUGS IN FOCUS

Iron Preparations

Drug Name	Usual Dosage	Usual Indications
ferrous fumarate (*Feostat*)	100–200 mg/day PO Children 2–12 yr: 50–100 mg/day PO Children 6 mo–2 yr: 6 mg/kg/day PO Infants: 10–25 mg/day PO	Treatment of iron deficiency anemia
ferrous gluconate (*Fergon*)	100–200 mg/day PO Children 2–12 yr: 50–100 mg/day PO Children 6 mo–2 yr: 6 mg/kg/day PO Infants: 10–25 mg/day PO	Treatment of iron deficiency anemia
P ferrous sulfate (*Feosol*)	100–200 mg/day PO Children 2–12 yr: 50–100 mg/day PO Children 6 mo–2 yr: 6 mg/kg/day PO Infants: 10–25 mg/day PO	Treatment of iron deficiency anemia
ferrous sulfate exsiccated (*Ferralyn Lanacaps, Slow FE*)	100–200 mg/day PO Children 2–12 yr: 50–100 mg/day PO Children 6 mo–2 yr: 6 mg/kg/day PO Infants: 10–25 mg/day PO	Treatment of iron deficiency anemia
iron dextran (*InFeD*)	mg iron = 0.3 × (weight in lb) × {[100 – (hemoglobin in g/dL) ×100] / 14.8} Given IM, using Z-track technique	Parenteral treatment of iron deficiency anemia
iron sucrose (*Venofer*)	100 mg one to three times per week given IV during dialysis sessions, slowly over 1 min	Treatment of iron deficiency in patients undergoing chronic hemodialysis or nondialysis patients with renal failure who are also receiving supplemental erythropoietin therapy
sodium ferric gluconate complex (*Ferrlecit*)	10 mL diluted in 100 mL 0.9% sodium chloride for injection over 60 min; initially eight doses given at separate dialysis sessions, then give periodically to maintain hematocrit	Treatment of iron deficiency in patients undergoing chronic hemodialysis who are also receiving supplemental erythropoietin therapy

BOX 49.4 FOCUS ON **CLINICAL SKILLS**

Z-Track Injections

The Z-track method is used when injecting iron to reduce the risk of subcutaneous staining and irritation. It is a good idea to review the method of giving Z-track injections before giving one. The area to be injected is prepped for the injection. Place your gloved finger on the skin surface and pull the skin and the subcutaneous layers out of alignment with the muscle lying beneath. Try to move the skin about 1 cm, or ½ inch. Insert the needle at a 90-degree angle at the point where you originally placed your finger. Inject the drug and then withdraw the needle. Remove your finger from the skin, which will allow the layers to slide back into their normal position. The track that the needle made when inserting into the muscle is now broken by the layers, and the drug is trapped in the muscle.

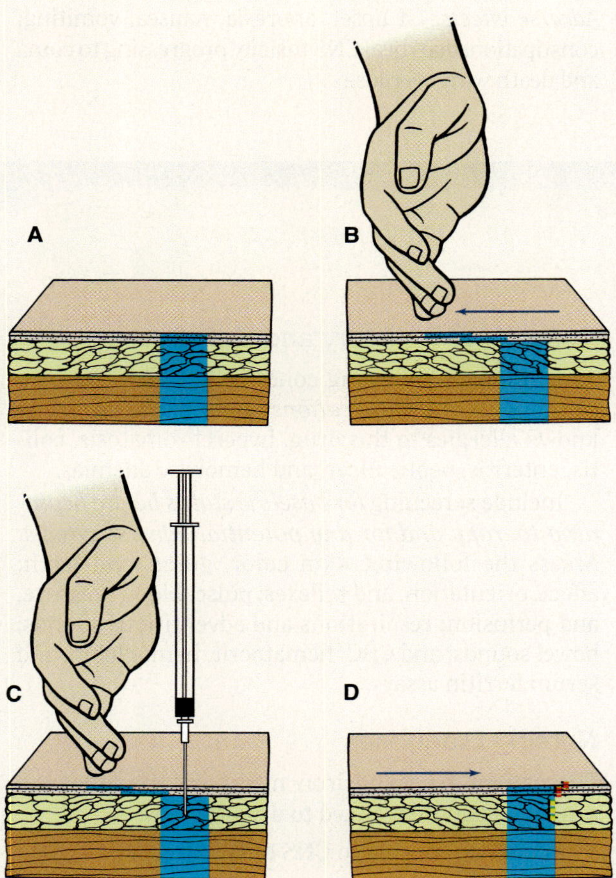

Use the Z-track, or zigzag, technique for injections. **(A)** Normal skin and tissues. **(B)** Move the skin to one side. **(C)** Insert needle at a 90-degree angle and aspirate for blood. **(D)** Withdraw the needle and allow the displaced tissue to return to normal position, thereby keeping the solution from leaving the muscle tissue (with permission from Taylor, C., Lillis, C., LeMone, P. [2005]. *Fundamentals of nursing: The art and science of nursing care,* 5th ed. Philadelphia: Lippincott Williams & Wilkins).

failure but not on dialysis and who are also receiving supplemental erythropoietin therapy.

Therapeutic Actions and Indications

Iron preparations elevate the serum iron concentration (see Figure 49.3). They are then either converted to hemoglobin or trapped in reticuloendothelial cells for storage and eventual release and conversion into a useable form of iron for RBC production. They are indicated for the treatment of iron deficiency anemias and may also be used as adjunctive therapy in patients receiving epoetin alfa.

Pharmacokinetics

Iron is primarily absorbed from the small intestine by an active transport system. It is transported in the blood, bound to transferrin. Small amounts are lost daily in the sweat, urine, sloughing of skin and mucosal cells, and sloughing of intestinal cells, as well as in the menstrual flow of women. It is used during pregnancy and lactation to help the mother meet the increased demands for iron that occur at those times.

Contraindications and Cautions

These drugs are contraindicated for patients with known allergy to any of these preparations. They also are contraindicated in the following conditions: hemochromatosis (excessive iron); hemolytic anemias, *which may increase serum iron levels and cause toxicity;* normal iron balance, *because the drug will not be absorbed and will just pass through the body;* and peptic ulcer, colitis, or regional enteritis, *because the drug can be directly irritating to these tissues and can cause exacerbation of the diseases.*

Adverse Effects

The most common adverse effects associated with oral iron are related to direct GI irritation; these include GI upset, anorexia, nausea, vomiting, diarrhea, dark stools, and constipation. With increasing serum levels, iron can be directly CNS toxic, causing coma and even death. (Box 49.5 discusses iron toxicity and drugs that are used to counteract this effect.) Parenteral iron is associated with severe anaphylactic reactions, local irritation, staining of the tissues, and phlebitis.

Clinically Important Drug–Drug Interactions

Iron absorption decreases if iron preparations are taken with antacids, tetracyclines, or cimetidine; if these drugs must be used, they should be spaced at least 2 hours apart.

Anti-infective response to ciprofloxacin, norfloxacin, or ofloxacin can decrease if these drugs are taken with iron, because of a decrease in absorption; they also should be taken at least 2 hours apart.

BOX 49.5 Chelating Agents

Heavy metals, including iron, lead, arsenic, mercury, copper, and gold, can cause toxicity in the body by their ability to tie up chemicals in living tissues that need to be free in order for the cell to function normally. When these vital substances (thiols, sulfurs, carboxyls, and phosphoryls) are bound to the metal, certain cellular enzyme systems become deactivated, resulting in failure of cellular function and eventual cell death. Drugs that have been developed to counteract metal toxicity are called chelating agents (from the Greek word for "claw").

Chelating agents grasp and hold a toxic metal so that it can be carried out of the body before it has time to harm the tissues. The chelating agent binds the molecules of the metal, preventing it from damaging the cells within the body. The complex that is formed by the chelating agent and the metal is nontoxic and is excreted by the kidneys.

Chelating Agent	Toxic Metal	Notes
calcium disodium edetate	lead	Given IM or IV; monitor renal and hepatic function, because serious and even fatal toxicity can occur
deferoxamine mesylate (*Desferal*)	iron	Given IM, Sub-Q, or IV; rash and vision changes are common
dimercaprol (*BAL in Oil*)	arsenic, gold, mercury	Given IM only for 7–10 days; cardiovascular toxicity may occur; push fluids and alkalinize urine to increase excretion
succimer (*Chemet*)	lead	Children with lead poisoning: 10 mg/kg or 350 mg/m² q8h PO for 5 days; reduce to 10 mg/kg or 350 mg/m² q12h PO for 2 wk; make sure patient is well hydrated

Increased iron levels occur if iron preparations are taken with chloramphenicol; patients receiving this combination should be monitored closely for any sign of iron toxicity. The effects of levodopa may decrease if it is taken with iron preparations; patients receiving both of these drugs should take them at least 2 hours apart.

Clinically Important Drug–Food Interactions

Iron is not absorbed if taken with antacids, eggs, milk, coffee, or tea. These substances should not be administered concurrently.

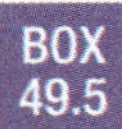

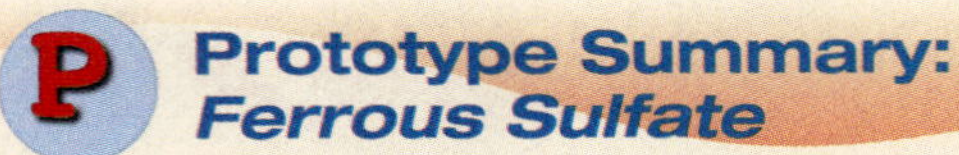

Prototype Summary: *Ferrous Sulfate*

Indications: Prevention and treatment of iron deficiency anemia; dietary supplement for iron

Actions: Elevates the serum iron concentration and is then converted to hemoglobin or stored for eventual conversion to a usable form of iron

Pharmacokinetics:

Route	Onset	Peak	Duration
Oral	4 days	7–10 days	2–4 mo

$T_{1/2}$: Not known; recycled for use, not excreted

Adverse effects: GI upset, anorexia, nausea, vomiting, constipation, diarrhea, CNS toxicity progressing to coma and death with overdose

Nursing Considerations for Patients Receiving Iron Preparations

Assessment: History and Examination

Screen for the following conditions, *which could be cautions or contraindications to use of the drug:* any known allergies to this drug, hyperchromatosis, colitis, enteritis, peptic ulcer, and hemolytic anemias.

Include screening *for baseline status before beginning therapy and for any potential adverse effects.* Assess the following: skin color, gums, and teeth; affect, orientation, and reflexes; pulse, blood pressure, and perfusion; respirations and adventitious sounds; bowel sounds; and CBC, hematocrit, hemoglobin, and serum ferritin assays.

Nursing Diagnoses

The patient receiving iron may have the following nursing diagnoses related to drug therapy:

- Acute Pain related to CNS or GI effects
- Disturbed Body Image related to drug staining
- Risk for Injury related to CNS effects
- Deficient Knowledge regarding drug therapy

Implementation With Rationale

- Confirm iron deficiency anemia before administering drugs, *to ensure proper use of the drug.*
- Consult with the physician to arrange for treatment of the underlying cause of anemia if possible,

because iron replacement will not correct the cause of the iron loss.

- Administer with meals (avoiding eggs, milk, coffee, and tea), *to relieve GI irritation if GI upset is severe.* Have patient drink solutions through a straw *to prevent staining of teeth.*
- Caution the patient that stool may be dark or green, *to prevent undue alarm if this occurs.*
- Administer intramuscularly only by Z-track technique, *to ensure proper administration and to avoid staining.*
- Arrange for hematocrit and hemoglobin measurements before administration and periodically during therapy, *to monitor drug effectiveness.*
- Provide comfort measures, *to help the patient tolerate drug effects.* These include small, frequent meals and access to bathroom facilities.
- Provide thorough patient teaching, including the name of the drug, dosage prescribed, measures to avoid adverse effects, warning signs of problems, and the need for periodic monitoring and evaluation, *to enhance patient knowledge about drug therapy and to promote compliance with drug regimen* (see Critical Thinking Scenario 49-1).
- Offer support and encouragement, *to help the patient deal with the diagnosis and the drug regimen.*

Evaluation

- Monitor patient response to the drug (alleviation of anemia).
- Monitor for adverse effects (GI upset and reaction, CNS toxicity, coma).
- Evaluate the effectiveness of the teaching plan (patient can name drug, dosage, adverse effects to watch for, specific measures to avoid adverse effects; patient understands importance of continued follow-up).
- Monitor the effectiveness of comfort measures and compliance to the regimen.

Folic Acid Derivatives and Vitamin B_{12}

Megaloblastic anemia is treated with folic acid and vitamin B_{12}. Folate deficiencies usually occur secondary to increased demand (as in pregnancy or growth spurts); as a result of absorption problems in the small intestine; because of drugs that cause folate deficiencies; or secondary to the malnutrition of alcoholism. Vitamin B_{12} deficiencies can result from poor diet or increased demand, but the usual cause is lack of intrinsic factor in the stomach, which is necessary for absorption. The drugs are usually given together to ensure that the problem is addressed and the blood cells can be formed properly (Table 49.3).

Folic acid (*Folvite*) can be given in oral, intramuscular, intravenous, and subcutaneous forms. The parenteral drugs are preferred for patients with potential absorption problems; all other patients should be given the oral form if at all possible. Leucovorin (*Wellcovorin*) is a reduced form of folic acid that is available for oral, intramuscular, and intravenous use. (It is used for the "leucovorin rescue" of patients receiving high doses of methotrexate for osteocarcinoma, allowing noncancerous cells to survive the chemotherapy. It is also used with fluorouracil for palliative treatment of colorectal cancer—see Chapter 14.)

Hydroxocobalamin (*Hydro-Crysti 12*) is the traditional treatment for pernicious anemia and vitamin B_{12} deficiency. It must be given intramuscularly every day for 5 to 10 days to build up levels, then once a month for life. It cannot be taken orally, because the problem with pernicious anemia is the inability to absorb vitamin B_{12} secondary to low levels of intrinsic factor. It can be used in states of increased demand (e.g., pregnancy, growth spurts) or dietary deficiency, but oral vitamins are preferred in most of those cases. Cyanocobalamin (*Nascobal*) is not as tightly bound to proteins and does not last in the body as long as hydroxocobalamin does. It is available as an intranasal gel that allows vitamin B_{12} absorption directly through the nasal mucosa. *Nascobal* is used once a week as an intranasal spray in one nostril.

Therapeutic Actions and Indications

Folic acid and vitamin B_{12} are essential for cell growth and division and for the production of a strong stroma in RBCs (see Figure 49.3). Vitamin B_{12} is also necessary for maintenance of the myelin sheath in nerve tissue. Both are given as replacement therapy for dietary deficiencies; as replacement in high-demand states such as pregnancy and lactation; and to treat megaloblastic anemia. Folic acid is used as a rescue drug for cells exposed to some toxic chemotherapeutic agents.

Pharmacokinetics

These vitamins are well absorbed after injection, metabolized mainly in the liver, and excreted in urine. Much of the hydroxocobalamin is highly protein bound and slowly released for use in the body. Cyanocobalamin is primarily stored in the liver and slowly released as needed for metabolic functions. These vitamins are considered essential during pregnancy and lactation because of the increased demands of the mother's metabolism.

(text continues on page 820)

CRITICAL THINKING SCENARIO 49-1

Iron Preparations and Toxicity

The Situation

L.L., a 28-year-old woman, suffered a miscarriage 6 weeks ago. She lost a great deal of blood during the miscarriage and underwent a dilation and curettage to control the bleeding. On her 6-week routine follow-up visit, she was found to have recovered physically from the event but was still depressed over her loss. Her hematocrit was 31%, and she admitted feeling tired and weak. She was offered emotional support and given a supply of ferrous sulfate tablets, with instructions to take one tablet three times a day.

At home, L.L. transferred the pills to a decorative bottle that had once held vitamins and left it on her table as a reminder to take the tablets. The next day, she discovered her 2-year-old daughter eating the tablets and punished her for getting into them. About 1 hour later, the toddler complained of a really bad "tummy ache" and started vomiting. She then became lethargic and L.L. called the pediatrician, who told them to go immediately to the emergency department and bring the remaining tablets with them. The toddler was found to have a weak, rapid pulse (156 beats/min); rapid, shallow respirations (32 per minute); and a low blood pressure (60/42 mm Hg). When a diagnosis of acute iron toxicity was made, L.L. became distraught. She said she had no idea that iron could be dangerous because it can be bought over the counter (OTC) in so many preparations. She had not read the written information given to her because it was "just iron."

Critical Thinking

What nursing interventions should be done at this point?

What sort of crisis intervention would be most appropriate for L.L.? *Think about the combined depression from the miscarriage, fear and anxiety related to this crisis, and L.L.'s iron-depleted state.*

What kind of reserve does she have for dealing with this crisis? Which measures would be appropriate for helping the mother cope with this crisis, and for treating the toddler?

Discussion

The first priority is to support and detoxify the child in iron toxicity. In cases of acute iron poisoning, the patient should be induced to vomit and given eggs and milk to bind the iron and prevent absorption. Gastric lavage, using a 1% sodium bicarbonate solution, can be done in a medical facility. This procedure is safe for about the first hour after ingestion. After that time, there is an increased risk of gastric erosion caused by the corrosive iron, making the lavage very dangerous. Because this toddler is well beyond the first hour, other measures will be needed. Supportive measures to deal with shock, dehydration, and gastrointestinal damage will be necessary. In addition, an iron-chelating agent such as deferoxamine mesylate may be tried.

During this crisis, L.L. will need a great deal of support, including a responsible relative or friend or other person who can stay with her. She also will need reassurance and a place to rest. After the situation is stabilized, L.L. will need teaching and additional support. For example, she should be reassured that most people do not take OTC drugs seriously, and many do not even read the labels. However, the nurse can use this opportunity to stress the importance of reading all of the labels and following the directions that come with OTC drugs. L.L. also should be commended for calling the pediatrician and getting medical care for the toddler quickly. Finally, she should receive a review of the iron teaching information and be encouraged to ask questions.

This case is a good example for a staff in-service program, stressing not only the dangers of iron toxicity but also the vital importance of providing good patient education before sending a patient home with a new drug. Simply giving a patient written information is often not enough.

Nursing Care Guide For L.L.: Iron Preparations

Assessment: History And Examination

Assess L.L.'s health history for allergies to any iron preparation, colitis, enteritis, hepatic dysfunction, peptic ulcer.

Then focus the physical examination on the following areas:

CV: blood pressure, pulse, perfusion

Neuro (CNS): orientation, affect, reflexes, vision

Skin: color, lesions, gums, teeth

Resp: respiratory rate and character, adventitious sounds

GI: abdominal examination, bowel sounds

Laboratory tests: complete blood count, hemoglobin, hematocrit, serum ferritin assays

Iron Preparations and Toxicity *(continued)*

Nursing Diagnoses

Acute Pain related to GI, CNS effects

Risk for Injury related to CNS effects

Disturbed Body Image related to drug staining

Deficient Knowledge regarding drug therapy

Implementation

Confirm iron deficiency anemia before administering the drug.

Provide comfort and safety measures, for example, give small meals; ensure access to bathroom facilities; use Z-track method for IM injections; give drug with food if GI upset occurs; and institute bowel program as needed.

Arrange for treatment of underlying cause of anemia.

Provide support and reassurance to deal with drug effects.

Provide patient teaching regarding drug, dosage, adverse effects, what to report, safety precautions.

Evaluation

Evaluate drug effects (relief of signs and symptoms of anemia, hematocrit within normal limits).

Monitor for adverse effects: GI upset, CNS toxicity, coma.

Monitor hematocrit and hemoglobin periodically.

Monitor for drug–drug interactions as indicated for each drug.

Evaluate effectiveness of patient teaching program and comfort and safety measures.

Patient Teaching For L.L.

☐ Iron is a naturally occurring mineral found in many foods. It is used by the body to make red blood cells, which carry oxygen to all parts of the body. Supplemental iron needs to be taken when the body does not have enough iron available to make healthy red blood cells, a condition called anemia.

☐ Iron is a toxic substance if too much is taken. You must avoid self-medicating with over-the-counter preparations containing iron while you are taking this drug.

☐ You will need to return for regular medical checkups while taking this drug to determine its effectiveness.

☐ Take your medication as follows, depending on the specific iron preparation that has been prescribed:

- Dissolve *ferrous salts* in orange juice to improve the taste.
- Take *liquid iron preparations* with a straw, to prevent the iron from staining teeth.
- Place iron drops on the back of the tongue to prevent staining of the teeth.

☐ Some of the following adverse effects may occur:

- *Dark, tarry, or green stools:* The iron preparations stain the stools; the color remains as long as you are taking the drug and should not cause concern.
- *Constipation:* This is a common problem; if it becomes too uncomfortable, consult with your health care provider for an appropriate remedy.
- *Nausea, indigestion, vomiting:* This problem can often be solved by taking the drug with food, making sure to avoid the foods listed earlier.
- Report any of the following to your health care provider: *severe diarrhea, severe abdominal pain or cramping, unusual tiredness or weakness, bluish tint to the lips or fingernail beds.*

☐ Tell any doctor, nurse, or other health care provider that you are taking this drug.

☐ Keep this drug, and all medications, out of the reach of children. Because iron can be very toxic, seek emergency medical help immediately if you suspect that a child has taken this preparation unsupervised.

☐ Because iron can interfere with the absorption of some drugs, do not take iron at the same time as *tetracycline* or *antacids.* These drugs must be taken during intervals when iron is not in the stomach.

Table 49.3 DRUGS IN FOCUS

Folic Acid Derivatives and Vitamin B_{12}

Drug Name	Usual Dosage	Usual Indications
Folic Acid Derivatives		
P folic acid (*Folvite*)	1 mg/day PO, IM, Sub-Q, or IV	Replacement therapy and treatment of megaloblastic anemia
leucovorin (*Wellcovorin*)	1 mg/day IM for replacement; 12–15 g/m² PO, then 10 g/m² PO q6h for 72 h for rescue	Replacement therapy and treatment of megaloblastic anemia; rescue after chemotherapy
Vitamin B_{12}		
P hydroxocobalamin (*Hydro-Crysti 12*)	30 mcg/day IM for 5–10 days, then 100–200 mcg/mo IM Pediatric: 1–5 mg IM over 2 or more wk, then 30–50 mcg IM every 4 wk	Replacement therapy; treatment of megaloblastic anemia, pernicious anemia
cyanocobalamin (*Nascobal*)	One spray (500 mcg) in one nostril once a week	Replacement therapy; treatment of megaloblastic anemia

Contraindications and Cautions

These drugs are contraindicated in the presence of known allergies to these drugs or to their components. They should be used cautiously in patients who are pregnant or lactating or who have other anemias. Nasal cyanocobalamin should be used with caution in the presence of nasal erosion or ulcers.

Adverse Effects

These drugs have relatively few adverse effects because they are used as replacement for required chemicals. Pain and discomfort can occur at injection sites. Nasal irritation can occur with the use of intranasal spray.

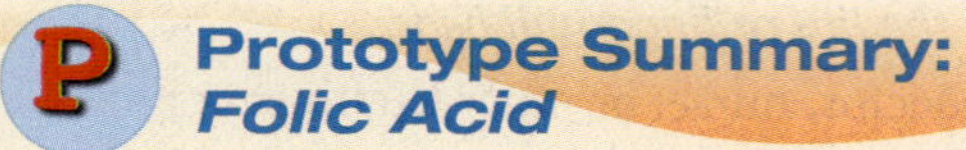

Prototype Summary: Folic Acid

Indications: Treatment of megaloblastic anemia due to sprue, nutritional deficiency

Actions: Reduced form of folic acid, required for nucleoprotein synthesis and maintenance of normal erythropoiesis

Pharmacokinetics:

Route	Onset	Peak
Oral, IM, Sub-Q, IV	Varies	30–60 min

$T_{1/2}$: Unknown; metabolized in the liver and excreted in urine

Adverse effects: Allergic reactions, pain and discomfort at injection site

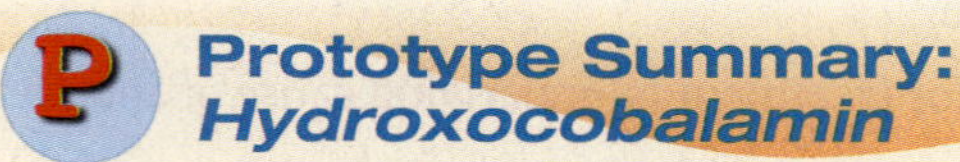

Prototype Summary: Hydroxocobalamin

Indications: Treatment of vitamin B_{12} deficiency; to meet increased vitamin B_{12} requirements related to disease, pregnancy, or blood loss

Actions: Essential for nucleic acid and protein synthesis; used for growth, cell reproduction, hematopoiesis, and nucleoprotein and myelin synthesis

Pharmacokinetics:

Route	Onset	Peak
IM	Intermediate	60 min

$T_{1/2}$: 24–36 hours; metabolized in the liver and excreted in urine

Adverse effects: Itching, transitory exanthema, mild diarrhea, anaphylactic reaction, CHF, pulmonary edema, hypokalemia, pain at injection site

Nursing Considerations for Patients Receiving Folic Acid Derivatives or Vitamin B_{12}

Assessment: History and Examination

Screen for the following conditions, *which could be cautions or contraindications to use of the drug:* any known allergies to these drugs or drug components, other anemias, pregnancy, lactation, and nasal erosion.

Include screening *for baseline status before beginning therapy and for any potential adverse effects.* Assess the following: affect, orientation, and reflexes; pulse, blood pressure, and perfusion; respirations and adventitious sounds; and renal function tests, CBC, hematocrit, iron levels, and electrolytes.

Nursing Diagnoses

The patient receiving folic acid/vitamin B_{12} may have the following nursing diagnoses related to drug therapy:

- Acute Pain related to injection or nasal irritation
- Risk for Fluid Volume Imbalance related to cardiovascular effects
- Deficient Knowledge regarding drug therapy

Implementation With Rationale

- Confirm the nature of the megaloblastic anemia, *to ensure that the proper drug regimen is being used.*
- Give both types of drugs in cases of pernicious anemia, *to ensure therapeutic effectiveness.*
- Parenteral vitamin B_{12} must be given intramuscularly each day for 5 to 10 days and then once a month for life, *if used to treat pernicious anemia.*
- Arrange for nutritional consultation, *to ensure a well-balanced diet.*
- Monitor for the possibility of hypersensitivity reactions; *have life support equipment on standby in case reactions occur.*
- Arrange for hematocrit readings before and periodically during therapy, *to monitor drug effectiveness.*
- Provide comfort measures, *to help the patient tolerate drug effects.* These include small, frequent meals, access to bathroom facilities, and analgesia for muscle or nasal pain.
- Provide thorough patient teaching, including the name of the drug, dosage prescribed, measures to avoid adverse effects, warning signs of problems, and the need for periodic monitoring and evaluation, *to enhance patient knowledge about drug therapy and to promote compliance with the drug regimen.*
- Offer support and encouragement, *to help the patient deal with the diagnosis and the drug regimen.*

Evaluation

- Monitor patient response to the drug (alleviation of anemia).
- Monitor for adverse effects (nasal irritation, pain at injection site, nausea).
- Evaluate the effectiveness of the teaching plan (patient can name drug, dosage, adverse effects to watch for, specific measures to avoid adverse effects; patient understands importance of continued follow-up).
- Monitor the effectiveness of comfort measures and compliance to the regimen.

WEB LINKS

Health care providers and patients may want to explore the following Internet sources:

http://www.aplastic.org Information on various forms of anemias—causes, characteristics, diagnosis, and treatment.

http://www.anemia.com Information designed for patients and families regarding anemias.

http://www.ansci.cornell.edu/courses/as625/1998term/Adams/iron.html Information on iron toxicity—treatment, diagnosis, and complications—for patients and health care providers.

http://www.ich.ucl.ac.uk/factsheets/misc/erythropoietin_epo Information on erythropoietin—action and uses.

Points to Remember

- The cardiovascular system exists to pump blood to all of the body's cells.
- Blood contains oxygen and nutrients that are essential for cell survival; it delivers these to the cells and removes waste products from the tissues.
- Blood is composed of a liquid plasma (containing water, proteins, glucose, and electrolytes) and formed components including white blood cells, RBCs, and platelets.
- RBCs are produced in the bone marrow in a process called erythropoiesis, which is controlled by the glycoprotein erythropoietin, produced by the kidneys.
- RBCs do not have a nucleus, and their lifespan is about 120 days, at which time they are lysed and their building blocks are recycled to make new RBCs.
- The bone marrow uses iron, amino acids, carbohydrates, folic acid, and vitamin B_{12} to produce healthy, efficient RBCs.
- An insufficient number or immaturity of RBCs results in low oxygen levels in the tissues, with tiredness, fatigue, and loss of reserve.
- Anemia is a state of too few RBCs. Anemia can be caused by a lack of erythropoietin or by a lack of the components needed to produce RBCs.
- Iron deficiency anemia occurs when there is inadequate iron intake in the diet or an inability to absorb iron from the GI tract. Iron is needed to produce hemoglobin, which

carries oxygen. Iron deficiency anemia is treated with iron replacement.

- Iron is a very toxic mineral at high levels. The body controls the absorption of iron and carefully regulates its storage and movement in the body.
- Folic acid and vitamin B_{12} are needed to produce a strong supporting structure in the RBC so that it can survive 120 days of being propelled through the vascular system. These are usually found in adequate amounts in the diet.
- A dietary lack of or inability to absorb folic acid, vitamin B_{12}, or both will produce a megaloblastic anemia, in which the RBCs are large and immature and have a short lifespan.
- Pernicious anemia is a lack of vitamin B_{12}, which is also used by the body to maintain the myelin sheath on nerve axons. If vitamin B_{12} is lacking, these neurons will degenerate and cause many CNS effects.
- Pernicious anemia is caused by the deficient production of intrinsic factor by gastric cells.
- Intrinsic factor is needed to allow the body to absorb vitamin B_{12}. If intrinsic factor is lacking, vitamin B_{12} must be given parenterally or intranasally for life to ensure absorption.

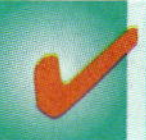

CHECK YOUR UNDERSTANDING

Answers to the questions in this chapter may be found in the Answer Key in the back of the book.

Multiple Choice

Select the best answer to the following.

1. The rate of red blood cell production is controlled by
   a. iron.
   b. folic acid.
   c. erythropoietin.
   d. vitamin B_{12}.

2. Red blood cells must be continually produced by the body because
   a. the iron within the RBC wears out.
   b. with no nucleus, the RBC cannot maintain itself and wears out over time.
   c. there is continual loss of RBCs from the gastrointestinal tract of healthy adults.
   d. RBCs are processed into bile salts and must be replaced.

3. Anemia is
   a. a decreased number of red blood cells.
   b. a lack of iron in the body.
   c. a lack of vitamin B_{12} in the body.
   d. an excessive number of platelets.

4. Megaloblastic anemia is a result of insufficient folic acid or vitamin B_{12}, and it affects
   a. white blood cell production.
   b. vegetarians.
   c. all cells in the body that are rapidly turning over.
   d. slow-growing cells.

5. *Epogen* (epoetin alfa) would be the drug of choice
   a. for acute blood loss during surgery.
   b. to replace blood loss from traumatic injury.
   c. for treatment of anemia during lactation.
   d. for the treatment of anemia associated with renal failure.

6. A patient with anemia who is given iron salts could expect to show a therapeutic increase in hematocrit
   a. within 72 hours.
   b. within 2 to 3 weeks.
   c. over 6 to 10 months.
   d. within 1 to 2 weeks.

7. Iron is not absorbed from the gastrointestinal tract if it is taken with
   a. protein.
   b. anticoagulants.
   c. dairy products.
   d. any other drugs.

8. A patient with pernicious anemia would be advised to take vitamin B_{12}
   a. orally with breakfast.
   b. orally at bedtime.
   c. subcutaneously every day.
   d. intramuscularly every 5 to 10 days.

Multiple Response

Select all that apply.

1. Clients are often given iron pills by their clinic. Instructions in giving these pills should include
   a. taking the drug with milk to avoid gastrointestinal problems.
   b. the potential for constipation.
   c. keeping these potentially toxic pills away from children.

d. taking the drug with antacids to alleviate the gastrointestinal upset.
e. having periodic blood tests to evaluate the drug effect.
f. being aware that stools may be colored green.

2. In a healthy person, very little iron is needed on a daily basis. Loss of iron is associated with which of the following?
   a. Heavy menstrual flow
   b. Bile duct obstruction
   c. Internal bleeding
   d. Traumatic injury and loss of blood
   e. Bone marrow suppression
   f. Alcoholic cirrhosis

Word Scramble

Unscramble the following letters to form words related to anemias.

1. tryhertyesco ________________________________
2. laamsp ________________________________
3. gamelasticbo ________________________________
4. sinpicroue ________________________________
5. tipnoee ________________________________
6. cloif dica ________________________________
7. maneai ________________________________
8. eproyitehsrios ________________________________
9. coryetteucil ________________________________
10. fineccediy ________________________________

True or False

Indicate whether the following statements are true (T) or false (F).

_____ 1. Blood is composed of a liquid plasma (containing water, proteins, glucose, and electrolytes) and formed components including white blood cells, red blood cells, and platelets.

_____ 2. RBCs are produced in the bone marrow in a process called erythropoiesis, which is controlled by intrinsic factor.

_____ 3. RBCs have a small nucleus, and their lifespan is about 120 days.

_____ 4. An insufficient number or maturity of RBCs results in low oxygen levels in the tissues, with tiredness, fatigue, and loss of reserve.

_____ 5. Anemia can be caused by a lack of erythropoietin or by a lack of the components needed to produce RBCs.

_____ 6. Iron is needed to produce hemoglobin, which carries the oxygen.

_____ 7. Folic acid and vitamin B_6 are needed to produce a strong supporting structure in the RBC.

_____ 8. Pernicious anemia is a lack of vitamin B_{12}, which is also used by the body to maintain the myelin sheath on nerve axons.

Bibliography and References

Drug facts and comparisons. (2006). St. Louis: Facts and Comparisons.

Gilman, A., Hardman, J. G., & Limbird, L. E. (Eds.). (2006). *Goodman and Gilman's the pharmacological basis of therapeutics* (11th ed.). New York: McGraw-Hill.

Karch, A. M. (2006). *2007 Lippincott's nursing drug guide.* Philadelphia: Lippincott Williams & Wilkins.

The medical letter on drugs and therapeutics. (2006). New Rochelle, NY: Medical Letter.

Porth, C. M. (2005). *Pathophysiology: Concepts of altered health states* (7th ed.). Philadelphia: Lippincott Williams & Wilkins.

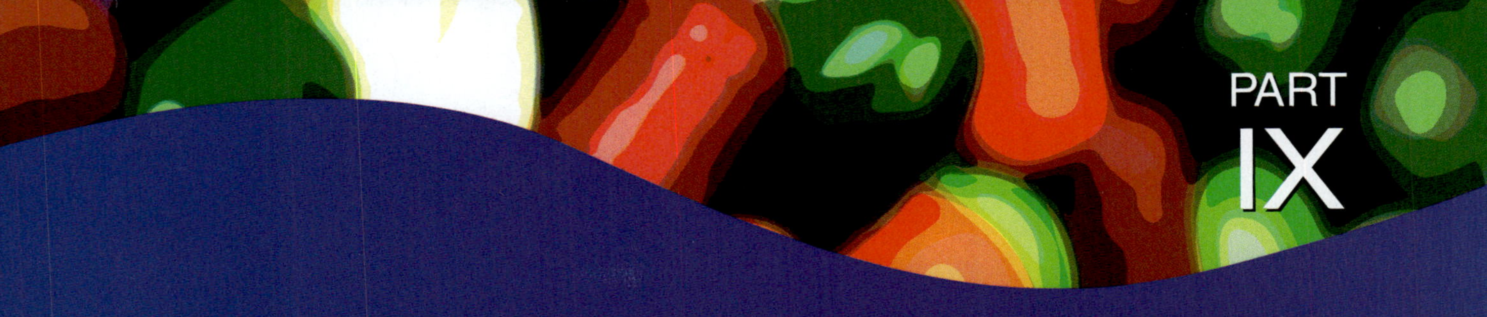

PART IX

Drugs Acting on the Renal System

CHAPTER

50

Introduction to the Kidneys and the Urinary Tract

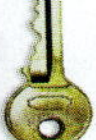

KEY TERMS

aldosterone

antidiuretic hormone (ADH)

carbonic anhydrase

countercurrent mechanism

filtration

glomerulus

nephron

prostate gland

reabsorption

renin–angiotensin system

secretion

LEARNING OBJECTIVES

Upon completion of this chapter, you will be able to:

1. Review the anatomy of the kidney and, using a diagram of the nephron, explain the basic processes of the kidney and where these activities occur.
2. Explain the control of calcium, sodium, potassium, and chloride in the nephron.
3. Discuss the countercurrent mechanism and the control of urine concentration and dilution, and apply its effects to various clinical scenarios.
4. Describe the renin–angiotensin–aldosterone system, including controls and clinical situations where this system is active.
5. Discuss the metabolic roles of the kidney/acid–base balance, calcium regulation, and red blood cell production, and use this information to explain the clinical manifestations of renal failure.

The renal system is composed of the kidneys and the structures of the urinary tract: the ureters, the urinary bladder, and the urethra. This system has four major functions in the body:

- Maintaining the volume and composition of body fluids within normal ranges, which includes clearing nitrogenous wastes from protein metabolism, maintaining acid–base balance and electrolyte levels, and excreting various drugs and drug metabolites
- Regulating vitamin D activation, which helps to maintain and regulate calcium levels
- Regulating blood pressure through the renin–angiotensin system
- Regulating red blood cell production through the production and secretion of erythropoietin.

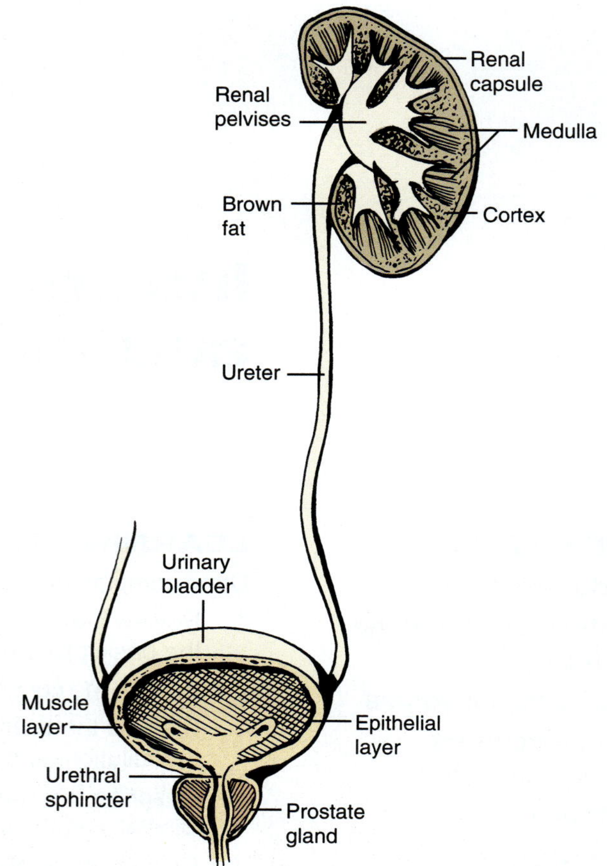

FIGURE 50.1 The kidney and organs of the urinary tract.

The Kidneys

The kidneys are two small organs that make up about 0.5% of total body weight but receive about 25% of the cardiac output. Approximately 1600 L of blood flows through these two small organs each day for cleansing. Most of the fluid that is filtered out by the kidneys is returned to the body, and the waste products that remain are excreted in a relatively small amount of water as urine.

The kidneys are located under the ribs, for protection from injury, and have three protective layers that make up the renal capsule: a fiber layer, a perirenal or brown fat layer, and the renal parietal layer. The capsule contains pain fibers, which are stimulated if the capsule is stretched secondary to an inflammatory process. The kidneys have three identifiable regions: the outer cortex, the inner medulla, and the renal pelvises. The renal pelvises drain the urine into the ureters. The ureters are muscular tubes that lead into the urinary bladder, where urine is stored until it is excreted (Figure 50.1).

The functional unit of the kidneys is called the **nephron**. There are approximately 2.4 million nephrons in an adult. All of the nephrons filter fluid and make urine, but only the medullary nephrons can concentrate or dilute urine. It is estimated that only about 25% of the total number of nephrons are necessary to maintain healthy renal function. That means that the renal system is well protected from failure with a large backup system. However, it also means that by the time a patient has signs and symptoms of renal failure, extensive kidney damage has already occurred.

The nephron is basically a tube (Figure 50.2). It begins with Bowman's capsule, which has a fenestrated or "windowed" epithelium that works like a sieve or a strainer to allow fluid to flow through but keeps large components (e.g., proteins) from entering. The nephron then curls around in a section called the proximal convoluted tubule. From there, it narrows to form the descending and ascending loop of Henle, widens as the distal convoluted tubule, then flows into the collecting ducts, which meet at the renal pelvises. Each section of the tubule functions in a slightly different manner to maintain fluid and electrolyte balance in the body.

The blood flow to the nephron is unique. The renal arteries come directly off the aorta and enter each kidney. As a renal artery enters each of the kidneys, it divides to form interlobar arteries, which become smaller arcuate (bowed) arteries, then afferent arterioles. The afferent arterioles branch to form the **glomerulus** inside Bowman's capsule. The glomerulus is like a tuft of blood vessels with a capillary-like endothelium that allows easy passage of fluid and waste products. The efferent arteriole exits from the glomerulus and branches into the peritubular capillary system, which returns fluid and electrolytes that have been reabsorbed from the tubules to the bloodstream. These capillaries flow into the vasa recta, which flows into intralobar veins, which in turn drain into the inferior vena cava. The two arterioles around the glomerulus work together to closely regulate the flow of fluid into the glomerulus, increasing or decreasing pressure on either side of the glomerulus as needed.

A small group of cells, called the juxtaglomerular apparatus, connects the afferent arteriole to the distal convoluted tubule; this is where erythropoietin and renin are produced. Because of their proximity to the afferent arteriole, these cells are especially sensitive to the volume and quality of blood

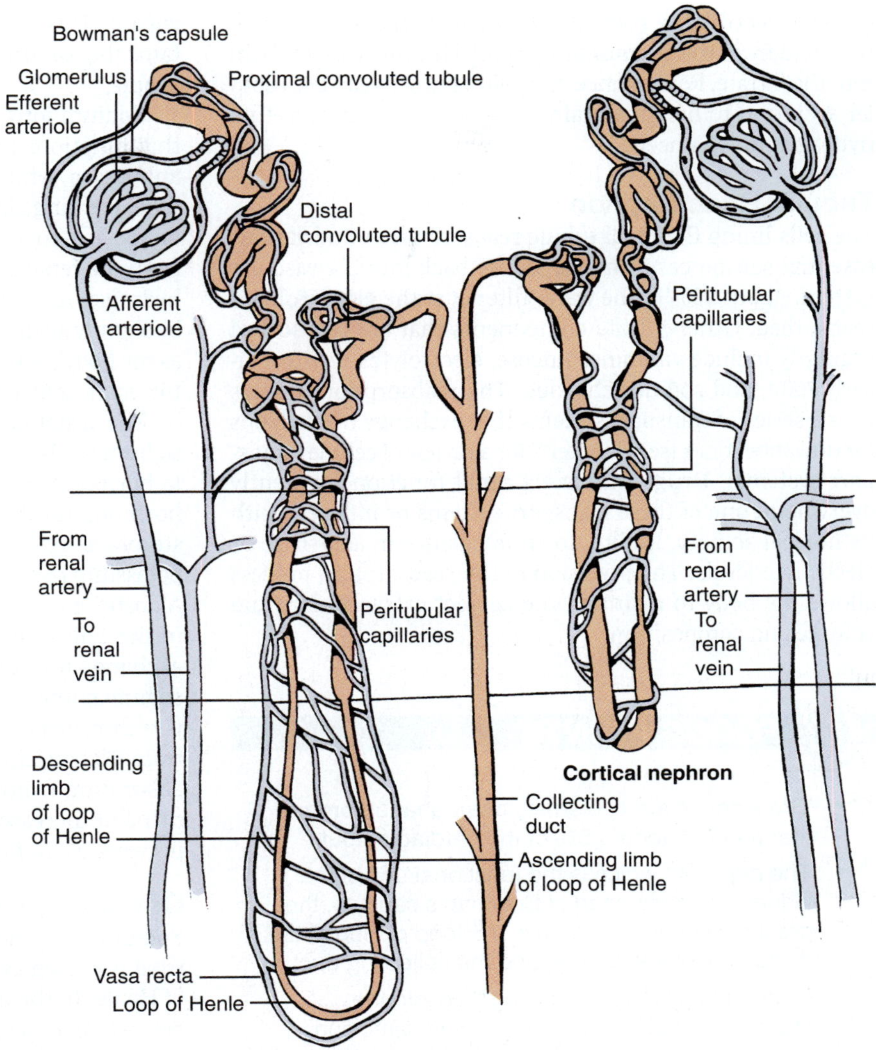

FIGURE 50.2 The nephron, the functional unit of the kidneys. Secretion and reabsorption of water, electrolytes, and other solutes in the various segments of the renal tubule, the loop of Henle, and the collecting duct can be influenced by diuretics, other drugs, and endogenous substances, including certain hormones. In the kidneys, the distal convoluted tubule wraps around and is actually next to the afferent arteriole.

flow into the glomerulus. Surrounding the nephrons is an area called the macula densa, which is full of immune system cells and chemicals that can respond quickly to any cellular damage or injury.

Renal Processes

The nephrons function by using three basic processes: glomerular **filtration** (straining fluid into the nephron), tubular **secretion** (actively removing components from the capillary system and depositing them into the tubule), and tubular **reabsorption** (removing components from the tubule to return them to the capillary system and circulation).

Glomerular Filtration

The glomerulus acts as an ultrafine filter for all of the blood that flows into it. The semipermeable membrane keeps blood cells, proteins, and lipids inside the vessel, whereas the hydrostatic pressure from the blood pushes water and smaller components of the plasma into the tubule. A clinical sign of renal damage is blood cells or protein in the urine. This can happen if the semipermeable membrane is scarred, swollen, or damaged, allowing the larger plasma components to escape into the filtrate. The large size of these components prevents them from being reabsorbed by the tubule, and they are lost in the urine.

Approximately 125 mL of fluid is filtered out each minute, or 180 L/day. About 99% of the filtered fluid is returned to the bloodstream as the filtrate progresses through the renal tubule. Approximately 1% of the filtrate, less than 2 L of fluid, is excreted each day in the form of urine.

Tubular Secretion

The epithelial cells that line the renal tubule can secrete substances from the blood into the tubular fluid. This is an energy-using process that allows active transport systems to remove electrolytes, some drugs and drug metabolites, and uric acid from the surrounding capillaries and secrete them into the filtrate. For instance, the epithelial cells can use tubular secretion to help maintain acid–base levels by secreting hydrogen ions as needed.

Tubular Reabsorption

The cells lining the renal tubule reabsorb water and various essential substances from the filtrate back into the vascular system. About 99% of the water filtered at the glomerulus is reabsorbed. Other filtrate components that are reabsorbed regularly include vitamins, glucose, electrolytes, sodium bicarbonate, and sodium chloride. The reabsorption process uses a series of transport systems that exchange needed ions for unwanted ones (see Chapter 7 for a review of cellular transport systems). Drugs that affect renal function frequently overwhelm one of these transport systems or interfere with its normal activity, leading to an imbalance in acid–base or electrolyte levels. The precision of the reabsorption process allows the body to maintain the correct extracellular fluid volume and composition.

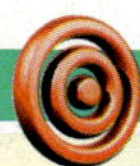

FOCUS POINTS

- The kidneys are two small, bean-shaped organs that receive about 25% of the cardiac output.
- The nephron, which is the functional unit of the kidneys, is composed of Bowman's capsule, the proximal convoluted tubule, the loop of Henle, the distal convoluted tubule, and the collecting duct.
- Glomerular filtration (straining fluid into the nephron), tubular secretion (actively removing components from the capillary system and depositing them into the tubule), and tubular reabsorption (removing components from the tubule to return them to the capillary system and circulation) are the three basic processes of the nephron.

Maintenance of Volume and Composition of Body Fluids

The kidneys regulate the composition of body fluids by balancing the levels of the key electrolytes, secreting or absorbing these electrolytes to maintain the desired levels. The volume of body fluids is controlled by diluting or concentrating the urine.

Sodium Regulation

Sodium is one of the body's major cations (positively charged ions). It filters through the glomerulus and enters the renal tubule, then is actively reabsorbed in the proximal convoluted tubule to the peritubular capillaries. As sodium is actively moved out of the filtrate, it takes chloride ions and water with it. This occurs by passive diffusion as the body maintains the osmotic and electrical balances on both sides of the tubule.

Sodium ions are also reabsorbed via a transport system that functions under the influence of the catalyst **carbonic anhydrase**, which allows carbon dioxide and water to combine, forming carbonic acid. The carbonic acid immediately dissociates to form sodium bicarbonate, using a sodium ion from the renal tubule and a free hydrogen ion (an acid). The hydrogen ion is then left in the filtrate, causing the urine to be slightly acidic. The bicarbonate is stored in the renal tubule as the body's alkaline reserve, for use when the body becomes too acidic and a buffer is needed.

The distal convoluted tubule acts to further adjust the sodium levels in the filtrate under the influence of **aldosterone** (a hormone produced by the adrenal gland) and natriuretic hormone (probably produced by the hypothalamus). Aldosterone is released into the circulation in response to high potassium levels, sympathetic stimulation, or angiotensin III. Aldosterone stimulates a sodium–potassium exchange pump in the cells of the distal tubule, which reabsorbs sodium in exchange for potassium (see Chapter 7 for a review of the sodium pump). As a result of aldosterone stimulation, sodium is reabsorbed into the system and potassium is lost in the filtrate. Natriuretic hormone causes a decrease in sodium reabsorption from the distal tubules with a resultant dilute urine or increased volume. Natriuretic hormone is released in response to fluid overload or hemodilution.

Countercurrent Mechanism

Sodium is further regulated in the medullary nephrons in what is known as the **countercurrent mechanism** in the loop of Henle. In the descending loop of Henle, the cells are freely permeable to water and sodium. Sodium is actively reabsorbed into the surrounding peritubular tissue, and water flows out of the tubule into this sodium-rich tissue to maintain osmotic balance. The filtrate at the end of the descending loop of Henle is concentrated in comparison to the rest of the filtrate.

In contrast, the ascending loop of Henle is impermeable to water, so water that remains in the tubule is trapped there. Chloride is actively transported out of the tubule using energy in a process that is referred to as the chloride pump; sodium leaves with the chloride to maintain electrical neutrality. As a result, the fluid in the ascending loop of Henle becomes hypotonic in comparison to the hypertonic situation in the peritubular tissue.

Antidiuretic hormone (ADH), which is produced by the hypothalamus and stored in the posterior pituitary gland, is important in maintaining fluid balance. ADH is released in response to falling blood volume, sympathetic stimulation, or rising sodium levels (a concentration that is sensed by the osmotic cells of the hypothalamus).

If ADH is present at the distal convoluted tubule and the collecting duct, the permeability of the membrane to water is increased. Consequently, the water remaining in the tubule rapidly flows into the hypertonic tissue surrounding the loop of Henle, where it either is absorbed by the peritubular capillaries or re-enters the descending loop of Henle in a countercurrent style. The resulting urine is hypertonic and of small volume. If ADH is not present, the tubule remains impermeable to water. The water that has been trapped in the ascending loop of Henle passes into the collection duct, resulting in a hypotonic urine of greater volume. This countercurrent mechanism allows the body to finely regulate fluid volume by regulating the control of sodium and water (Figure 50.3).

Potassium Regulation

Potassium is another cation that is vital to proper functioning of the nervous system, muscles, and cell membranes. About 65% of the potassium that is filtered at the glomerulus is reabsorbed at Bowman's capsule and the proximal convoluted tubule. Another 25% to 30% is reabsorbed in the ascending loop of Henle. The fine tuning of potassium levels occurs in the distal convoluted tubule, where aldosterone activates the sodium–potassium exchange, leading to a loss of potassium. If potassium levels are very high, the retention of sodium in exchange for potassium also leads to a retention of water and a dilution of blood volume, which further decreases the potassium concentration (see Figure 50.3).

Chloride Regulation

Chloride is an important negatively charged ion that helps to maintain electrical neutrality with the movement of cations across the cell membrane. Chloride is primarily reabsorbed in the loop of Henle, where it promotes the movement of sodium out of the cell.

Regulation of Vitamin D Activation

Calcium is another important cation that is regulated by the kidneys. The absorption of calcium from the gastrointestinal (GI) tract is regulated by vitamin D, which is taken in as part of the diet and then must be activated in the kidneys to a form that will promote calcium absorption. Once absorbed from the GI tract, calcium levels are maintained within a very tight range by the activity of parathyroid hormone (PTH) and calcitonin.

Calcium Regulation

Calcium is important in muscle function, blood clotting, bone formation, contraction of cell membranes, and muscle movement. Calcium is filtered at the glomerulus and mostly reabsorbed in the proximal convoluted tubule and ascending loop of Henle. Fine tuning of calcium reabsorption occurs in the distal convoluted tubule, where the presence of PTH stimulates reabsorption of calcium to increase serum calcium levels when they are low (see Figure 50.3 and Chapter 37).

Blood Pressure Control: Renin–Angiotensin System

The fragile nephrons require a constant supply of blood and are equipped with a system to ensure that they are perfused. This mechanism, called the **renin–angiotensin system** (sometimes called the renin–angiotensin–aldosterone system), involves a total body reaction to decreased blood flow to the nephrons.

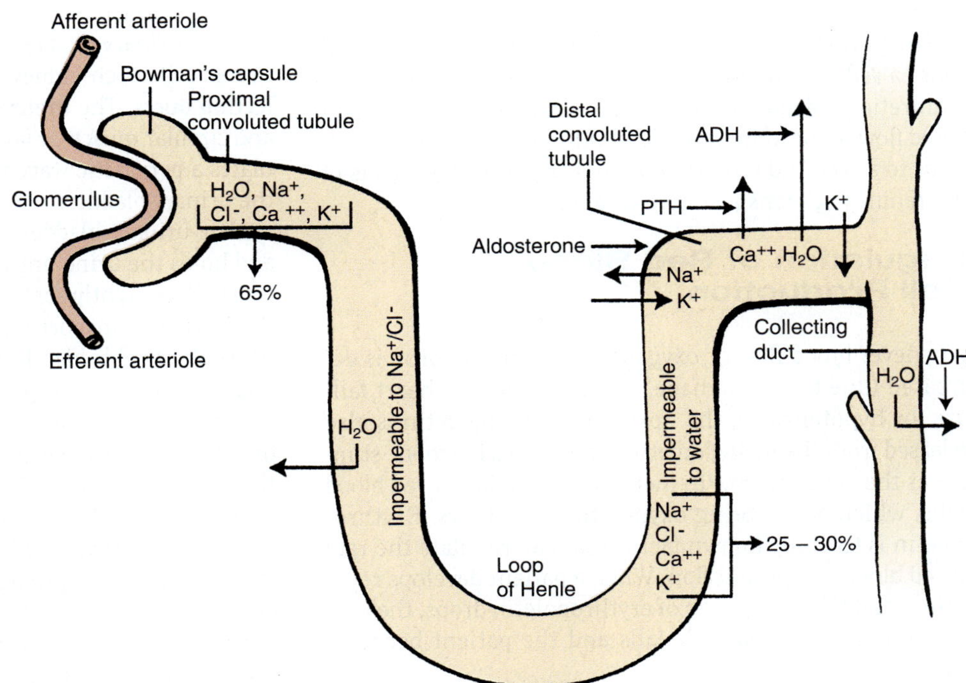

FIGURE 50.3 Nephron and points of regulation of sodium, chloride, potassium, calcium, and water. ADH, antidiuretic hormone; PTH, parathyroid hormone.

Whenever blood flow or oxygenation to the nephron is decreased (due to hemorrhage, shock, congestive heart failure, or hypotension), renin is released from the juxtaglomerular cells. (These cells, which are positioned next to the glomerulus, are stimulated by decreased stretch and decreased oxygen levels.) The released renin immediately is absorbed into the capillary system and enters circulation.

The released renin activates angiotensinogen, a substrate produced in the liver, which becomes angiotensin I. Angiotensin I is then converted to angiotensin II by a converting enzyme found in the lungs and some vessels. Angiotensin II is a very powerful vasoconstrictor, reacting with angiotensin II receptor sites in blood vessels to cause vasoconstriction. This powerful vasoconstriction raises blood pressure and should increase blood flow to the kidneys.

Angiotensin II is converted in the adrenal gland to angiotensin III, which stimulates the release of aldosterone from the adrenal gland. Aldosterone acts on the renal tubules to retain sodium and therefore water. This increases blood volume and further increases blood pressure, which should increase blood flow to the kidneys. The osmotic center in the brain senses the increased sodium levels and releases ADH, leading to a further retention of water and a further increase in blood volume and pressure, which should again increase blood flow to the kidneys.

The renin–angiotensin system constantly works to maintain blood flow to the kidneys. For example, an individual rising from a lying position experiences a drop in blood flow to the kidneys as blood pools in the legs because of gravity. This causes a massive release of renin and activation of this system to ensure that blood pressure is maintained and the kidneys are perfused. Blood loss from injury or during surgery also activates this system to increase blood flow through the kidneys.

Drugs that interfere with any aspect of this system will cause a reflex response. For instance, taking a drug such as a diuretic to decrease fluid volume can lead to decreased blood flow to the kidneys as blood volume drops. This in turn leads to a rebound retention of fluid as part of the effects of the renin–angiotensin system (Figure 50.4).

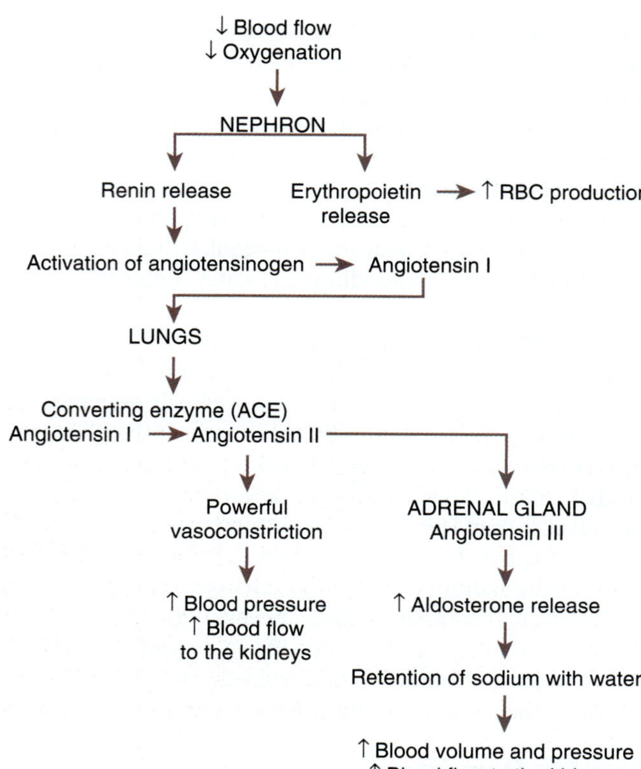

FIGURE 50.4 The renin–angiotensin system for reflex maintenance of blood pressure control.

Regulation of Red Blood Cell Production

Whenever blood flow or oxygenation to the nephron is decreased (due to hemorrhage, shock, congestive heart failure, or hypotension), the hormone erythropoietin is also released from the juxtaglomerular cells. This hormone stimulates the bone marrow to increase production of red blood cells, which act to bring oxygen to the kidneys. Erythropoietin is the only known factor that can regulate the rate of red blood cell production. When a patient develops renal failure and the production of erythropoietin drops, the production of red blood cells falls and the patient becomes anemic.

The Urinary Tract

As noted previously, the urinary tract is composed of the ureters, urinary bladder, and urethra (see Figure 50.1). One ureter exits each kidney, draining the filtrate from the collecting ducts. The ureters have a smooth endothelial lining and circular muscular layers. Urine entering the ureter stimulates a peristaltic wave that pushes the urine down toward the urinary bladder.

The urinary bladder is a muscular pouch that stretches and holds the urine until it is excreted from the body. Urine is usually a slightly acidic fluid; this acidity helps to maintain the normal transport systems and to destroy bacteria that may enter the bladder. In the female, the urethra is very short and leads to an area populated by normal flora including *Escherichia coli,* which can cause frequent bladder infections or cystitis. In the male, the urethra is much longer and passes through the **prostate gland**, a small gland that produces an acidic fluid that is important in maintaining the sperm and lubricating the tract. Enlargement and infection in the prostate gland are often problems in older males. Control of bladder emptying is learned control over the urethral sphincter; once it is established, a functioning nervous system is necessary to maintain control.

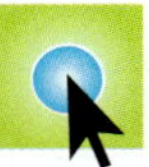

WEB LINK

To explore the virtual kidneys and urinary tract, visit the following Internet source:
http://www.InnerBody.com

Points to Remember

- The kidneys are two small organs that receive about 25% of the cardiac output.
- The functional unit of the kidneys is called the nephron; it is composed of Bowman's capsule, the proximal convoluted tubule, the loop of Henle, the distal convoluted tubule, and the collecting duct.
- The blood flow to the nephron is unique, allowing autoregulation of blood flow through the glomerulus.
- The nephrons function by using three basic processes: glomerular filtration (straining fluid into the nephron), tubular secretion (actively removing components from the capillary system and depositing them into the tubule), and tubular reabsorption (removing components from the tubule to return them to the capillary system and circulation).
- Sodium levels are regulated throughout the tubule by active and passive movement and are fine-tuned by the presence of aldosterone in the distal tubule.
- The countercurrent mechanism in the medullary nephrons allows for the concentration or dilution of urine under the influence of ADH secreted by the hypothalamus.
- Potassium concentration is regulated throughout the tubule, with aldosterone being the strongest influence for potassium loss.
- The kidneys play a key role in the regulation of calcium by activating vitamin D to allow GI calcium reabsorption and by reabsorbing or excreting calcium from the tubule under the influence of parathyroid hormone (PTH).
- The kidneys influence blood pressure control, releasing renin to activate the renin–angiotensin system, which leads to increased blood pressure and volume and a resultant increased blood flow to the kidney. The balance of this reflex system can lead to water retention or excretion and has an impact on drug therapy that promotes water or sodium loss.
- The ureters, urinary bladder, and urethra make up the rest of the urinary tract. The longer male urethra passes through the prostate gland, which may enlarge or become infected, a problem often associated with advancing age.

CHECK YOUR UNDERSTANDING

Answers to the questions in this chapter may be found in the Answer Key in the back of the book.

Multiple Choice

Select the best answer to the following.

1. During severe exertion, a man may lose up to 4 L of hypotonic sweat per hour. This loss would result in
   a. decreased plasma volume.
   b. decreased plasma osmolarity.
   c. decreased circulating levels of ADH.
   d. return of body fluid balance to normal after ingestion of 100 mL of water.

2. Urine passes through the ureter by
   a. osmosis.
   b. air pressure.
   c. filtration.
   d. gravity and peristalsis.

3. Renal reabsorption
   a. is the movement of substances from the renal tubule into the blood.
   b. is the movement of substances from the blood into the renal tubule.
   c. of water is increased in the absence of ADH.
   d. of sodium occurs only in the proximal tubule.

4. The major reason older adults should monitor their intake of fluids is that
   a. older people have decreased levels of ADH.
   b. older people do not exercise, so fluids do not shift between compartments easily.
   c. total body water decreases with age and restoration of homeostasis is slower.
   d. older people lose more fluid through the skin as it becomes thinner.

5. Blood flow to the nephron differs from blood flow to other tissues in that
   a. the venous system is not involved.
   b. there are no capillaries in the nephron.
   c. efferent and afferent arterioles allow for autoregulation of blood flow through the glomerulus.
   d. the capillary bed has a fenestrated membrane.

6. Concentration and dilution of urine is controlled by
   a. afferent arterioles.
   b. the renin–angiotensin system.
   c. aldosterone release.
   d. the countercurrent mechanism in medullary nephrons.

7. Women tend to have more problems with bladder infections than men because
   a. women have *E. coli* in the urinary tract.
   b. the female has a short urethra, making access to the bladder easier for bacteria.
   c. the prostate gland secretes a substance that protects men from bladder infections.
   d. women are more acidotic, encouraging the growth of bladder bacteria.

Multiple Response

Select all that apply.

1. Considering the metabolic functions of the kidneys, renal failure would be expected to cause which of the following?
   a. Anemia
   b. Loss of calcium regulation
   c. Urea buildup on the skin
   d. Respiratory alkalosis
   e. Metabolic acidosis
   f. Changes in the function of blood cells

2. During severe diarrhea, there is a loss of water, bicarbonate, and sodium from the gastrointestinal tract. Physiological compensation for this would probably include which of the following?
   a. Increased alveolar ventilation
   b. Decreased hydrogen ion secretion by the renal tubules
   c. Decreased urinary excretion of sodium and water
   d. Increased renin secretion
   e. Increased hydrogen ion secretion by the renal tubules
   f. Increased ADH levels

3. Maintenance of blood pressure is important in maintaining the fragile nephrons. Reflex systems that work to ensure blood flow to the kidneys include
   a. the renin–angiotensin system causing vasoconstriction.
   b. baroreceptor monitoring of the renal artery.
   c. aldosterone release secondary to angiotensin stimulation.
   d. ADH release in response to decreased blood volume with increased osmolarity.
   e. release of erythropoietin.
   f. local response of the afferent arterioles.

Word Scramble

Unscramble the following letters to form words associated with the renal system.

1. rumsoulgel ____________________
2. nattrofili ____________________
3. tonisceer ____________________
4. enrootladse ____________________
5. proberostani ____________________
6. ubluetu ____________________
7. niner ____________________
8. streatpo ____________________

Fill in the Blanks

1. The kidneys are two small organs that receive approximately __________ of the cardiac output.

2. The functional unit of the kidney is called the __________, which is composed of __________, the proximal convoluted tubule, the __________, the distal convoluted tubule, and the __________.

3. The nephrons function by using three basic processes: __________, __________, __________, and __________ __________.

4. Sodium levels are regulated throughout the tubule by active and passive movement and are fine-tuned by the presence of __________ in the distal tubule.

5. The countercurrent mechanism in the medullary nephrons allows for the __________ or __________ of urine under the influence of antidiuretic hormone (ADH) secreted by the hypothalamus.

6. Potassium concentration is regulated throughout the tubule, with __________ being the strongest influence for potassium loss.

7. The kidneys play a key role in the regulation of calcium by activating __________ ___.

8. The kidneys have an important role in blood pressure control, releasing __________ to activate the renin–angiotensin system.

Bibliography and References

Fox, S. (1991). *Perspectives on human biology.* Dubuque, IA: Wm. C. Brown.

Ganong, W. (1999). *Review of medical physiology* (19th ed.). Norwalk, CT: Appleton & Lange.

Gilman, A., Hardman, J. G., & Limbird, L. E. (Eds.). (2006). *Goodman and Gilman's the pharmacological basis of therapeutics* (11th ed.). New York: McGraw-Hill.

Guyton, A., & Hall, J. (2004). *Textbook of medical physiology.* Philadelphia: W. B. Saunders.

CHAPTER 51

Diuretic Agents

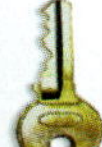

KEY TERMS

alkalosis
edema
fluid rebound
high-ceiling diuretics
hyperaldosteronism
hypokalemia
osmotic pull

LEARNING OBJECTIVES

Upon completion of this chapter, you will be able to:

1. Define the term diuretic and list four types of diuretic drugs.
2. Describe the therapeutic actions, indications, pharmacokinetics, contraindications, most common adverse reactions, and important drug–drug interactions associated with thiazide and thiazide-like diuretics, loop diuretics, carbonic anhydrase inhibitors, potassium-sparing diuretics, and osmotic diuretics.
3. Discuss the use of diuretic agents across the lifespan.
4. Compare and contrast the prototype drugs hydrochlorothiazide, furosemide, acetazolamide, spironolactone, and mannitol with other agents in their class.
5. Outline the nursing considerations, including important teaching points, for patients receiving diuretic agents.

THIAZIDE DIURETICS

bendroflumethiazide
chlorothiazide
P hydrochlorothiazide
hydroflumethiazide
methyclothiazide

THIAZIDE-LIKE DIURETICS

chlorthalidone
indapamide
metolazone

LOOP DIURETICS

bumetanide
ethacrynic acid
P furosemide
torsemide

CARBONIC ANHYDRASE INHIBITORS

P acetazolamide
methazolamide

POTASSIUM-SPARING DIURETICS

amiloride
P spironolactone
triamterene

OSMOTIC DIURETICS

glycerin
isosorbide
P mannitol
urea

There are five classes of diuretics, each working at a slightly different site in the nephron or using a different mechanism. Diuretic classes include the thiazide and thiazide-like diuretics, the loop diuretics, the carbonic anhydrase inhibitors, the potassium-sparing diuretics, and the osmotic diuretics. For the most part, the overall nursing care of a patient receiving any diuretic is similar (however, see Box 51.1 for differences across the lifespan). The diuretic classes are discussed in this chapter, starting with the most frequently used drugs.

Diuretic Agents

Diuretic agents are commonly thought of simply as drugs that increase the amount of urine produced by the kidneys. Most diuretics do increase the volume of urine produced to some extent, but the greater clinical significance of diuretics is their ability to increase sodium excretion.

Therapeutic Actions and Indications

Diuretics prevent the cells lining the renal tubules from reabsorbing an excessive proportion of the sodium ions in the glomerular filtrate. As a result, sodium and other ions (and the water in which they are dissolved) are lost in the urine instead of being returned to the blood, where they would cause increased intravascular volume and therefore increased hydrostatic pressure, which could result in leaking of fluids at the capillary level.

Diuretics are indicated for the treatment of **edema** associated with congestive heart failure (CHF), acute pulmonary edema, liver disease (including cirrhosis), and renal disease and for the treatment of hypertension. They are also used to decrease fluid pressure in the eye (intraocular pressure), which is useful in treating glaucoma. Diuretics that decrease potassium levels may also be indicated in the treatment of conditions that cause hyperkalemia.

CHF can cause edema as a result of several factors. The failing heart muscle does not pump sufficient blood to the kidneys, causing activation of the renin–angiotensin system and resulting in increases in blood volume and sodium retention. Because the failing heart muscle cannot respond to the usual reflex stimulation, the increased volume is slowly pushed out into the capillary level as venous pressure increases because the blood is not being pumped effectively (see Chapter 44).

Pulmonary edema, or left-sided CHF, develops when the increased volume of fluids backs up into the lungs. The fluid pushed out into the capillaries in the lungs interferes with gas exchange. If this condition develops rapidly, it can be life-threatening.

BOX 51.1 **DRUG THERAPY ACROSS THE LIFESPAN**

Diuretic Agents

CHILDREN

Diuretics are often used in children to treat edema associated with heart defects, to control hypertension, and to treat edema associated with renal and pulmonary disorders.

Hydrochlorothiazide and chlorothiazide have established pediatric dosing guidelines. Furosemide is often used when a stronger diuretic is needed; care should be taken not to exceed 6 mg/kg/day when using this drug. Ethacrynic acid may be used orally in some situations but should not be used in infants. Bumetanide, although not recommended for use in children, may be used for children who are taking other ototoxic drugs, including antibiotics, and may cause less hypokalemia, making it preferable to furosemide for children also taking digoxin. Spironolactone is the only potassium-sparing diuretic that is recommended for use in children, but, as with adults, it should not be used in the presence of severe renal impairment.

Because of the size and rapid metabolism of children, the effects of diuretics may be rapid and adverse effects may occur suddenly. The child receiving a diuretic should be monitored for serum electrolyte changes; for evidence of fluid volume changes; for rapid weight gain or loss, which could reflect fluid volume; and for signs of ototoxicity.

ADULTS

Adults may be taking diuretics for prolonged periods and need to be aware of the signs and symptoms of fluid imbalance to report to their health care provider. Adults receiving chronic diuretic therapy should weigh themselves on the same scale, in the same clothes, and at the same time each day to monitor for fluid retention or sudden fluid loss. They should be alerted to situations that could aggravate fluid loss, such as diarrhea, vomiting, or excessive heat and sweating, which could change their need for the diuretic. They should also be urged to maintain their fluid intake to help balance their body's compensatory mechanisms and to prevent fluid rebound.

Patients taking potassium-losing diuretics should be encouraged to eat foods that are high in potassium and to have their serum potassium levels checked periodically. Patients taking potassium-sparing diuretics should be cautioned to avoid those same foods.

The use of diuretics to change the fluid shifts associated with pregnancy is not appropriate. Women maintained on these drugs for underlying medical reasons should not stop taking the drug, but they need to be aware of the potential for adverse effects on the fetus. Women who are nursing and need a diuretic should find another method of feeding the baby because of the potential for adverse effects on the baby as well as the lactating mother.

OLDER ADULTS

Older adults often have conditions that are treated with diuretics. They are also more likely to have renal or hepatic impairment, which requires cautious use of these drugs.

Older adults should be started on the lowest possible dose of the drug, and the dosage should be titrated slowly based on patient response. Frequent serum electrolyte measurements should be done to monitor for adverse reactions.

The intake and activity level of the patient can alter the effectiveness and need for the diuretic. High-salt diets and inactivity can aggravate conditions that lead to edema, and patients should be encouraged to follow activity and dietary guidelines if possible.

Patients with liver failure and cirrhosis often present with edema and ascites. This is caused by (1) reduced plasma protein production, which results in less oncotic pull in the vascular system and fluid loss at the capillary level, and (2) obstructed blood flow through the portal system, which is caused by increased pressure from congested hepatic vessels.

Renal disease produces edema because of the loss of plasma proteins into the urine when there is damage to the glomerular basement membrane. Other types of renal disease produce edema because of activation of the renin–angiotensin system as a result of decreasing volume (associated with the loss of fluid into the urine), which causes a drop in blood pressure, or because of failure of the renal tubules to regulate electrolytes effectively.

Hypertension is predominantly an idiopathic disorder; in other words, the underlying pathology is not known. Treatment of hypertension is aimed at reducing the higher-than-normal blood pressure, which can damage end organs and lead to serious cardiovascular disorders. Diuretics were once the key element in antihypertensive therapy, the goal of which was to decrease volume and sodium, which would then decrease pressure in the system. Now several other classes of drugs, including angiotensin-converting enzyme (ACE) inhibitors, angiotensin receptor blockers (ARBs), beta-blockers, and calcium channel blockers, are also used for the initial treatment of hypertension; however, some studies have found that the use of diuretics is still the most effective way of treating initial hypertension. Diuretics are also often used as an adjunct to improve the effectiveness of these other drugs.

Glaucoma is an eye disease characterized by increased pressure in the eye—known as intraocular pressure (IOP)—which can cause optic nerve atrophy and blindness. Diuretics are used to provide osmotic pull to remove some of the fluid from the eye, which decreases the IOP, or as adjunctive therapy to reduce fluid volume and pressure in the cardiovascular system, which also decreases pressure in the eye somewhat.

Contraindications and Cautions

Diuretic use is contraindicated in the presence of allergy to any of the drugs given. Other conditions in which diuretics are contraindicated include fluid and electrolyte imbalances, *which can be potentiated by the fluid and electrolyte changes caused by the diuretics,* and severe renal disease, *which may prevent the diuretic from working or could be pushed into a crisis stage by the blood flow changes brought about by the diuretic.*

Caution should be used with the following conditions: systemic lupus erythematosus (SLE), *which frequently causes glomerular changes and renal dysfunction that could precipitate renal failure in some cases;* glucose tolerance abnormalities or diabetes mellitus, *which is worsened by the glucose-elevating effects of many diuretics;* gout, *which reflects an abnormality in normal tubule reabsorption and secretion;* liver disease, *which could interfere with the normal metabolism of the drugs, leading to an accumulation of the drug or toxicity;* and pregnancy and lactation, *which are conditions that could be jeopardized by changes in fluid and electrolyte balance.*

Adverse Effects

Adverse effects associated with diuretics are specific to the particular class used. For details, see the section on adverse effects for each class of diuretics discussed in this chapter, and refer to Table 51.1. The most common adverse effects seen with diuretics include gastrointestinal (GI) upset, fluid and electrolyte imbalances (Box 51.2), hypotension, and electrolyte disturbances.

Clinically Important Drug–Drug Interactions

When diuretics are used, there is a potential for interactions with drugs that depend on a particular electrolyte balance for their therapeutic effects (e.g., antiarrhythmics such as digoxin), with drugs that depend on urine alkalinity for proper excretion (e.g., quinidine), and with drugs that depend on normal reflexes to balance their effects (e.g., antihypertensives, antidiabetic agents), because these factors are altered by the actions of diuretics.

Other specific drug–drug interactions that might relate to the chemical makeup of a particular diuretic are noted in the sections for each drug.

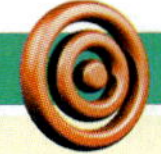

FOCUS POINTS

- Diuretics increase sodium excretion, and therefore water excretion, from the kidneys.
- Diuretics help relieve edema associated with CHF and pulmonary edema, liver failure and cirrhosis, and various types of renal disease. They are also used in treating hypertension.
- Diuretics must be used cautiously whenever changes in fluid and electrolyte balance could exacerbate a disorder.
- Electrolyte imbalance (potassium, sodium, chloride), hypotension and hypovolemia, hypoglycemia, and metabolic alkalosis are all potential adverse effects of diuretic therapy.

Thiazide and Thiazide-Like Diuretics

Hydrochlorothiazide (*HydroDIURIL*), the most frequently used of the thiazide diuretics, is often used in combination with other drugs for the treatment of hypertension. It can be used in small doses because it is more potent than chlorothiazide (*Diuril*), which is the oldest drug of this class, and it is considered the prototype. Other thiazides

Table 51.1 Comparison of Diuretics

Diuretic Class	Major Site of Action	Usual Indications	Major Adverse Effects
Thiazide, thiazide-like	Distal convoluted tubule	Edema of CHF, liver and renal disease Adjunct for hypertension	GI upset, CNS complications, hypovolemia
Loop	Loop of Henle	Acute CHF Acute pulmonary edema Hypertension Edema of CHF, renal and liver disease	Hypokalemia, volume depletion, hypotension, CNS effects, GI upset, hyperglycemia
Carbonic anhydrase inhibitors	Proximal tubule	Glaucoma Diuresis in CHF Mountain sickness Epilepsy	GI upset, urinary frequency
Potassium-sparing	Distal tubule and collecting duct	Adjunct for edema of CHF, liver and renal disease Treatment of hypokalemia Adjunct for hypertension Hyperaldosteronism	Hyperkalemia, CNS effects, diarrhea
Osmotic	Glomerulus, tubule	Reduction of intracranial pressure Prevention of oliguric phase of renal failure Reduction of intraocular pressure Renal clearance of toxic substances	Hypotension, GI upset, fluid and electrolyte imbalances

include bendroflumethiazide (*Naturetin*), hydroflumethiazide (*Saluron*), and methyclothiazide (*Enduron*) (Table 51.2).

The thiazide-like diuretics include chlorthalidone (*Hygroton*), indapamide (*Lozol*), and metolazone (*Mykrox*). All of these drugs are used less often than hydrochlorothiazide and are typically chosen according to the prescriber's personal preference.

BOX 51.2 FOCUS ON CLINICAL SKILLS

Explaining Fluid Rebound

Care must be taken when using diuretics to avoid **fluid rebound**, which is associated with fluid loss. If a patient stops taking in water and takes the diuretic, the result will be a concentrated plasma of smaller volume. The decreased volume is sensed by the nephrons, which activate the renin–angiotensin cycle. When the concentrated blood is sensed by the osmotic center in the brain, antidiuretic hormone (ADH) is released to hold water and dilute the blood. The result can be a "rebound" edema as fluid is retained.

Many patients who are taking a diuretic markedly decrease their fluid intake so as to decrease the number of trips to the bathroom. The result is a rebound of water retention after the diuretic effect. This effect can also be seen in many diets that promise "immediate results"; they frequently contain a key provision to increase fluid intake to 8 to 10 full glasses of water daily. The reflex result of diluting the system with so much water is a drop in ADH release and fluid loss.

Some people can lose 5 lb in a few days by doing this. However, the body's reflexes soon kick in, causing rebound retention of fluid to re-establish fluid and electrolyte balance. Most people get frustrated at this point and give up the fad diet.

It is important to be able to explain this effect. Teaching patients about balancing the desired diuretic effect with the actions of the normal reflexes is a clinical skill.

Therapeutic Actions and Indications

The thiazide diuretics belong to a chemical class of drugs called the sulfonamides. Thiazide-like diuretics have a slightly different chemical structure but work in the same way that thiazide diuretics do. Their action is to block the chloride pump. Chloride is actively pumped out of the tubule by cells lining the ascending limb of the loop of Henle and the distal tubule. Sodium passively moves with the chloride to maintain an electrical neutrality. (Chloride is a negative ion, and sodium is a positive ion.) Blocking of the chloride pump keeps the chloride and the sodium in the tubule to be excreted in the urine, thus preventing the reabsorption of both chloride and sodium in the vascular system (Figure 51.1). Because these segments of the tubule are impermeable to water, there is little increase in the volume of urine produced, but it will be sodium rich, a saluretic effect. Thiazides are considered to be mild diuretics compared with the more potent loop diuretics.

Thiazide and thiazide-like diuretics are usually indicated for the treatment of edema associated with CHF or with liver or renal disease. These drugs also are used as monotherapy or as adjuncts for the treatment of hypertension.

Pharmacokinetics

These drugs are well absorbed from the GI tract, with onset of action ranging from 1 to 3 hours. They are metabolized in

Table 51.2 DRUGS IN FOCUS

Thiazide Diuretics

Drug Name	Usual Dosage	Usual Indications
Thiazide Diuretics		
bendroflumethiazide (*Naturetin*)	2.5–5 mg/day PO for edema; 2.5–15 mg/day PO for hypertension	All of the thiazide diuretics are indicated for the treatment of edema caused by congestive heart failure (CHF), liver disease, or renal disease, and for adjunctive treatment of hypertension
chlorothiazide (*Diuril*)	Adult: 0.5–2 g PO or IV, daily to b.i.d. for edema; 0.5–2 g/day PO for hypertension Pediatric (<6 mo): up to 33 mg/kg/day PO Pediatric (>6 mo): 22 mg/kg/day PO in two divided doses	
P hydrochlorothiazide (*HydroDIURIL*)	Adult: 25–100 mg/day PO or intermittently, up to 200 mg/day maximum for edema; 25–100 mg/day PO for hypertension Pediatric (<6 mo): up to 3.3 mg/kg/day PO in two divided doses Pediatric (6 mo–2 yr): 12.5–37.5 mg/day PO in two divided doses Pediatric (2–12 yr): 37.6–100 mg/day PO in two divided doses	
hydroflumethiazide (*Saluron*)	25–200 mg PO b.i.d. for edema; 50–100 mg/day PO for hypertension	
methyclothiazide (*Enduron*)	2.5–10 mg/day PO for edema; 2.5–5 mg/day PO for hypertension	
Thiazide-like Diuretics		
chlorthalidone (*Hygroton*)	50–100 mg/day PO for edema; 25–100 mg/day PO for hypertension	All of the thiazide-like diuretics are indicated for the treatment of edema caused by CHF or by liver or renal disease, and for adjunctive treatment of hypertension
indapamide (*Lozol*)	2.5–5 mg/day PO for edema or hypertension, based on patient response	
metolazone (*Mykrox, Zaroxolyn*)	*Mykrox:* 0.5–1 mg/day PO for mild hypertension *Zaroxolyn:* 2.5–5 mg/day PO for hypertension; 5–20 mg/day PO for edema, based on patient response	

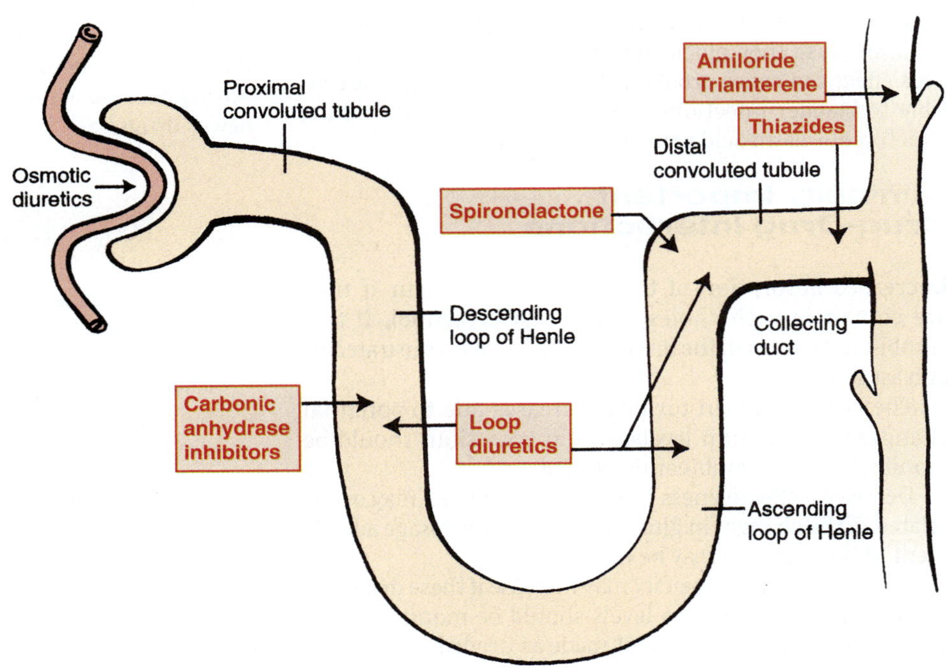

FIGURE 51.1 Sites of action of diuretics in the nephrons.

the liver and excreted in the urine. These diuretics cross the placenta and enter breast milk. Routine use during pregnancy is not appropriate; these drugs should be reserved for situations in which the mother has pathological reasons for use, not pregnancy manifestations or complications, and only if the benefit to the mother clearly outweighs the risk to the fetus. If one of these drugs is needed during lactation, another method of feeding the baby should be used, because of the potential for adverse effects on fluid and electrolyte changes in the baby.

Contraindications and Cautions

Thiazide and thiazide-like diuretics are contraindicated with allergy to thiazides or sulfonamides, fluid or electrolyte imbalances, and renal and liver disease. Additional cautions include gout, systemic lupus erythematosus, diabetes, hyperparathyroidism, bipolar disorder, pregnancy, and lactation.

Adverse Effects

Adverse effects of thiazide use are related to interference with the normal regulatory mechanisms of the nephron. Potassium is lost at the distal tubule because of the actions on the pumping mechanism, and **hypokalemia** (low blood levels of potassium) may result. Signs and symptoms of hypokalemia include weakness, muscle cramps, and arrhythmias. Another adverse effect is decreased calcium excretion, which leads to increased calcium levels. Uric acid excretion also is decreased, because the thiazides interfere with its secretory mechanism. High levels of uric acid can result in a condition called gout.

If these drugs are used over a prolonged period, blood glucose levels may increase. This may result from the change in potassium levels (which keeps glucose out of the cells), or it may relate to some other mechanism of glucose control.

Urine will be slightly alkalinized when the thiazides are used, because they block the reabsorption of bicarbonate. This effect can cause problems for patients who are susceptible to bladder infections and for those taking quinidine, which requires an acid urine for excretion.

Clinically Important Drug–Drug Interactions

Decreased absorption of these drugs may occur if they are combined with cholestyramine or colestipol. If this combination is used, the drugs should be taken separated by at least 2 hours.

The risk of digoxin toxicity increases due to potential changes in potassium levels; serum potassium should be monitored if this combination is used.

Decreased effectiveness of antidiabetic agents may occur related to the changes in glucose metabolism; dosage adjustment of those agents may be needed.

The risk of lithium toxicity may increase if these drugs are combined. Serum lithium levels should be monitored and appropriate dosage adjustment made as needed.

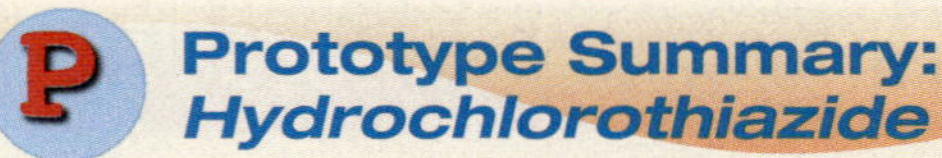

Prototype Summary: Hydrochlorothiazide

Indications: Adjunctive therapy for edema associated with CHF, cirrhosis, corticosteroid or estrogen therapy, and renal dysfunction; treatment of hypertension as monotherapy or in combination with other antihypertensives

Actions: Inhibits reabsorption of sodium and chloride in distal renal tubules, increasing the excretion of sodium, chloride, and water by the kidneys

Pharmacokinetics:

Route	Onset	Peak	Duration
Oral	2 h	4–6 h	6–12 h

$T_{1/2}$: 5.6–14 hours; metabolized in the liver and excreted in urine

Adverse effects: Dizziness, vertigo, orthostatic hypotension, nausea, anorexia, vomiting, dry mouth, diarrhea, polyuria, nocturia, muscle cramps or spasms

Loop Diuretics

Loop diuretics are so named because they work in the loop of Henle. Four loop diuretics are currently available (Table 51.3). Furosemide (*Lasix*), the most commonly used loop diuretic, is less powerful than the new loop diuretics, bumetanide (*Bumex*) and torsemide (*Demadex*), and therefore has a larger margin of safety for home use (see Critical Thinking Scenario 51-1). Ethacrynic acid (*Edecrin*), the first loop diuretic introduced, is used less frequently in the clinical setting because of the improved potency and reliability of the newer drugs.

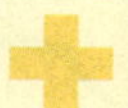

FOCUS ON **PATIENT SAFETY**

Name confusion has been reported between furosemide and torsemide; the dosage and strength of effect of these two drugs are very different. Use extreme caution to make sure you are using the prescribed drug and dosage.

Therapeutic Actions and Indications

Loop diuretics are also referred to as **high-ceiling diuretics** because they cause a greater degree of diuresis than other diuretics do. These drugs block the chloride pump in the

Table 51.3 DRUGS IN FOCUS

Loop Diuretics

Drug Name	Usual Dosage	Usual Indications
bumetanide (*Bumex*)	0.5–2 mg/day PO as a single dose repeated to a maximum of 10 mg; 0.5–1 mg IM or IV given over 1–2 min, may be repeated in 2–3 h, do not exceed 10 mg/day Geriatric or renal-impaired patient: 12 mg by continuous IV infusion over 12 h may be most effective and least toxic	All of the loop diuretics are indicated for the treatment of acute congestive heart failure (CHF); acute pulmonary edema; hypertension; and edema of CHF, renal disease, or liver disease
ethacrynic acid (*Edecrin*)	50–200 mg/day PO based on patient response; 0.5–1 mg/kg IV slowly Pediatric: 25 mg PO with slow titration up as needed; do not use with infants	
P furosemide (*Lasix*)	20–80 mg/day PO, up to 600 mg/day may be given; 20–40 mg IM or IV given slowly; 40 mg IV over 1–2 min for acute pulmonary edema, increase to 80 mg after 1 h if response is not adequate; 40 mg PO b.i.d. for hypertension Geriatric or renal-impaired patient: 2–2.5 g/day PO Pediatric: 2 mg/kg/day PO for hypertension, do not exceed 6 mg/kg/day; 1 mg/kg IV or IM for edema, increase by 1 mg/kg as needed; do not exceed 6 mg/kg	
torsemide (*Demadex*)	10–20 mg/day PO for IV for CHF or chronic renal failure; 5–10 mg/day PO for hypertension	

ascending loop of Henle, where normally 30% of all filtered sodium is reabsorbed. This action decreases the reabsorption of sodium and chloride. The loop diuretics have a similar effect in the descending loop of Henle and in the distal convoluted tubule, resulting in the production of a copious amount of sodium-rich urine. These drugs work even in the presence of acid–base disturbances, renal failure, electrolyte imbalances, or nitrogen retention.

Because they can produce a loss of fluid of up to 20 lb/day, loop diuretics are the drugs of choice when a rapid and extensive diuresis is needed. In cases of severe edema or acute pulmonary edema, it is important to remember that these drugs can have an effect only on the blood that reaches the nephrons. A rapid diuresis occurs, producing a more hypertonic intravascular fluid. In pulmonary edema, this fluid then circulates back to the lungs, pulls fluid out of the interstitial spaces by its oncotic pull, and delivers this fluid to the kidneys, where the water is pulled out, completing the cycle. In the treatment of pulmonary edema, it can sometimes take hours to move all of the fluid out of the lungs, because the fluid must be pulled out of the interstitial spaces in the lungs before it can be circulated to the kidneys for removal. Remembering how the drugs work and the way in which fluid moves in the vascular system will make it easier to understand the effects to anticipate.

Loop diuretics are commonly indicated for the treatment of acute CHF, acute pulmonary edema, edema associated with CHF or with renal or liver disease, and hypertension. Box 51.3 describes nesiritide, a recombinant form of natriuretic peptide that was approved in 2001 for the treatment of CHF and that can cause diuresis.

Pharmacokinetics

These drugs are metabolized and excreted primarily through urine. There are no well-controlled studies of the effects of these drugs during pregnancy. They have been associated with fetal and maternal deaths in animal studies, and they should not be used during pregnancy unless the benefit to the mother far outweighs the potential risk. These drugs enter breast milk; if one of these drugs is needed during lactation, a decision should be made about whether to discontinue nursing or to discontinue the drug. Safety for use in children younger than 18 years of age has not been established. If one of these drugs is used for a child, careful monitoring of the child's fluid and electrolyte balance is needed, and emergency support measures should be on standby.

Contraindications and Cautions

Among the contraindications to these drugs are allergy to a loop diuretic, electrolyte depletion, anuria, severe renal failure, hepatic coma, and pregnancy and lactation. Cautious use is recommended for patients with SLE, gout, or diabetes mellitus.

Adverse Effects

Adverse effects are related to the imbalance in electrolytes and fluid that these drugs cause. Hypokalemia is a very common adverse effect, because potassium is lost when the transport systems in the tubule try to save some of the sodium being lost. **Alkalosis**, or a drop in serum pH to an

CRITICAL THINKING SCENARIO 51-1

Using Furosemide (*Lasix*) in Congestive Heart Failure

The Situation

M.R. is a 68-year-old woman with rheumatic mitral valve heart disease. She has refused any surgical intervention and has developed progressively worsening congestive heart failure (CHF). Recently furosemide (*Lasix*), 40 mg/d PO, was prescribed for her along with digoxin. After 10 days with the new prescription, M.R. calls to tell you that she is allergic to the new medicine and can't take it any more. She reports extensive ankle swelling and difficulty breathing. You refer her to a cardiologist for immediate review.

Critical Thinking

Think about the physiology of mitral valve disease and the progression of CHF in this patient. How does furosemide work in the body?

What additional activities will be important to help maintain some balance in this patient's cardiac status?

What is the nature of M.R.'s reported allergy, and what other options could be tried?

Discussion

Over time, an incompetent mitral valve leads to an enlarged and overworked left ventricle as the backup of blood "waiting to be pumped" continues to progress. Drug therapy for a patient with this disorder is usually aimed at decreasing the workload of the heart as much as possible to maintain cardiac output. Digoxin increases the contractility of the heart muscle, which should lead to better perfusion of the kidneys. Furosemide, a loop diuretic, acts on the loop of Henle to block the reabsorption of sodium and water and lead to a diuresis, which decreases the volume of blood the heart needs to pump and makes the blood that is pumped more efficient. This blood then has an oncotic pull to move fluid from the tissue into circulation, where it can be acted on by the kidney, leading to further diuresis.

M.R. should be encouraged to maintain fluid intake and to engage in activity as much as possible, but to take frequent rest periods. Her potassium level should be monitored regularly (this is especially important because she is also taking digoxin, which is very sensitive to potassium levels), her edematous limbs should be elevated periodically during the day, and she should monitor her sodium intake.

When M.R. was questioned about her reported allergy, it was discovered that her "allergic reaction" was actually increased urination (a therapeutic effect). M.R. needs to learn about the actions of the drug. She also needs information about the timing of administration so that the resultant diuresis will not interfere with rest or with her daily activities. CHF is a progressive, incurable disease, so patient education is a very important part of the overall management regimen.

Nursing Care Guide For M.R.: Diuretic Agents

Assessment: History and Examination

Assess M.R.'s health history including allergies to diuretics, fluid or electrolyte disturbances, gout, glucose tolerance abnormalities, liver disease, systemic lupus erythematosus, pregnancy and breast-feeding.

Focus the physical examination on the following areas:

Neuro: orientation, reflexes, strength

Skin: color, texture, edema

CV: blood pressure, pulse, cardiac auscultation

GI: liver evaluation

GU: urinary output

Laboratory tests: hematology; serum electrolytes, glucose, uric acid; liver function tests

Nursing Diagnoses

Risk for Deficient Fluid Volume related to diuretic effect

Impaired Urinary Elimination

Imbalanced Nutrition: Less than Body Requirements, related to GI upset and metabolic changes

Deficient Knowledge regarding drug therapy

Implementation

Obtain daily weights, and monitor urine output.

Provide comfort and safety measures: sugarless lozenges, mouth care, safety precautions, skin care, nutrition.

Administer drug with food, early in day.

Provide support and reassurance to deal with drug effects and lifestyle changes.

Provide patient teaching regarding drug name, dosage, side effects, precautions, warnings to report, daily weighing, and recording dietary changes as needed.

Using Furosemide (*Lasix*) in Congestive Heart Failure *(continued)*

Evaluation

Evaluate drug effects: urinary output, weight changes, status of edema, blood pressure changes.

Monitor for adverse effects: hypotension, hypokalemia hyperkalemia, hypocalcemia, hypercalcemia, hyperglycemia, increased uric acid levels.

Monitor for drug–drug interactions as indicated.

Evaluate effectiveness of patient teaching program and comfort and safety measures.

Patient Teaching For M.R.

- ☐ A diuretic, or "water pill," such as furosemide (*Lasix*) will help to reduce the amount of fluid that is in your body by causing the kidneys to pass larger amounts of water and salt into your urine. By removing this fluid, the diuretic helps to decrease the work of the heart, lower blood pressure, and get rid of edema or swelling in your tissues.
- ☐ This drug can be taken with food, which may eliminate possible stomach upset. When taking a diuretic, you should maintain your usual fluid intake and try to avoid excessive intake of salt.
- ☐ Furosemide is a diuretic that causes potassium loss, so you should eat foods that are high in potassium (e.g., orange juice, raisins, bananas). If your diuretic is one that causes potassium retention, you should avoid foods high in potassium as well as salt substitutes, as appropriate. You also may be asked to take a potassium substitute.
- ☐ Weigh yourself each day, at the same time of day and in the same clothing. Record these weights on a calendar. Report any loss or gain of 3 lb or more in 1 day.
- ☐ Common effects of this drug include the following.
  - *Increased volume and frequency of urination:* Have ready access to bathroom facilities. Once you are used to the drug, you will know how long the effects last for you.
  - *Dizziness, feeling faint on arising, drowsiness:* Loss of fluid can lower blood pressure and cause these feelings. Change positions slowly; if you feel drowsy, avoid driving or other dangerous activities. These feelings are often increased if alcohol is consumed; avoid this combination or take special precautions if you combine them.
  - *Increased thirst:* As fluid is lost, you may experience a feeling of thirst. Sucking on sugarless lozenges and frequent mouth care might help alleviate this feeling. Do not drink an excessive amount of fluid while taking a diuretic. Try to maintain your usual fluid intake.
  - Report any of the following to your health care provider: *muscle cramps or pain, loss or gain of more than 3 lb in one day, swelling in your fingers or ankles, nausea or vomiting, unusual bleeding or bruising, trembling or weakness.*
- ☐ Avoid the use of any over-the-counter (OTC) medication without first checking with your health care provider. Several OTC medications can interfere with the effectiveness of this drug.
- ☐ Tell any doctor, nurse, or other health care provider involved in your care that you are taking this drug.
- ☐ Keep this drug, and all medications, out of the reach of children.

alkaline state, may occur as bicarbonate is lost in the urine. Calcium is also lost in the tubules along with the bicarbonate, which may result in hypocalcemia and tetany. The fast loss of fluid can result in hypotension and dizziness if it causes a rapid imbalance in fluid levels. Long-term use of these drugs may also result in hyperglycemia because of the diuretic effect on blood glucose levels, so susceptible patients need to be monitored for this effect. Ototoxicity and even deafness have been reported with these drugs, but the loss of hearing is usually reversible after the drug is stopped. This may be an effect of electrolyte changes on the conduction of fragile nerves in the central nervous system.

Clinically Important Drug–Drug Interactions

The risk of ototoxicity increases if loop diuretics are combined with aminoglycosides or cisplatin. Anticoagulation effects may increase if these drugs are given with anticoagulants. There may also be a decreased loss of sodium and decreased antihypertensive effects if these drugs are combined with indomethacin, ibuprofen, salicylates, or other nonsteroidal anti-inflammatory agents; the patient receiving this combination should be monitored closely and appropriate dosage adjustments should be made.

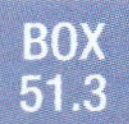

BOX 51.3 Hormone-like Treatment for Congestive Heart Failure

The U.S. Food and Drug Administration recently approved nesiritide (*Natrecor*), a recombinant form of natriuretic peptide. This drug acts like natriuretic hormone, a natural substance, probably produced by the hypothalamus, which causes a decrease in sodium reabsorption from the distal renal tubules with a resultant dilute urine or increased volume. Natriuretic hormone is normally released in response to fluid overload or hemodilution. In studies, this drug was effective in the treatment congestive heart failure (CHF), reducing volume and cardiac workload.

Nesiritide is given as an IV bolus of 2 mcg/kg followed by a continuous infusion of 0.01 mcg/kg/min for up to 48 hours. It is approved for the treatment of patients with acutely decompensated CHF who have dyspnea at rest or with minimal activity. After therapy with nesiritide, patients reported increased activity tolerance and easier breathing at rest.

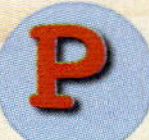

Prototype Summary: Furosemide

Indications: Treatment of edema associated with CHF, acute pulmonary edema, hypertension

Actions: Inhibits the reabsorption of sodium and chloride from the proximal and distal renal tubules and the loop of Henle, leading to a sodium-rich diuresis

Pharmacokinetics:

Route	Onset	Peak	Duration
Oral	60 min	60–120 min	6–8 h
IV, IM	5 min	30 min	2 h

$T_{1/2}$: 120 min; metabolized in the liver and excreted in urine

Adverse effects: Dizziness, vertigo, paresthesias, blurred vision, orthostatic hypotension, thrombophlebitis, photosensitivity, rash, urticaria, nausea, anorexia, vomiting, constipation, glycosuria, urinary bladder spasm, leukopenia, anemia, thrombocytopenia, muscle cramps, and spasms

Carbonic Anhydrase Inhibitors

The carbonic anhydrase inhibitors are relatively mild diuretics. Most often, they are used to treat glaucoma, because the inhibition of carbonic anhydrase results in decreased secretion of aqueous humor of the eye. Available agents include acetazolamide (*Diamox*) and methazolamide (generic) (Table 51.4).

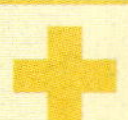

FOCUS ON **PATIENT SAFETY**

Name confusion has occurred between acetazolamide and acetohexamide—an antidiabetic agent—and between *Diamox* (acetazolamide) and *Dymelor* (acetohexamide). Use caution if either of these drugs is prescribed for your patient; make sure that the diagnosis and the treatment are appropriate.

Therapeutic Actions and Indications

The enzyme carbonic anhydrase is a catalyst for the formation of sodium bicarbonate, which is stored as the alkaline reserve in the renal tubule, and for the excretion of hydrogen, which results in a slightly acidic urine. Diuretics that block the effects of carbonic anhydrase slow down the movement of hydrogen ions; as a result, more sodium and bicarbonate are lost in the urine.

These drugs are used as adjuncts to other diuretics when a more intense diuresis is needed. Acetazolamide is used to treat glaucoma, in conjunction with other drugs to treat epilepsy, and to treat mountain sickness. Methazolamide is used primarily for the treatment of glaucoma.

Pharmacokinetics

These drugs are rapidly absorbed and widely distributed. They are excreted in urine. Some of these agents have been associated with fetal abnormalities, and they should not be used during pregnancy. Because of the potential for adverse effects on the baby, another method of feeding the infant should be used if one of these drugs is needed during lactation.

Table 51.4 DRUGS IN FOCUS

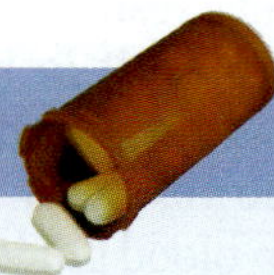

Carbonic Anhydrase Inhibitors

Drug Name	Usual Dosage	Usual Indications
P acetazolamide (*Diamox*)	500 mg IV repeated in 2–4 h, then 250 mg–1 g/day in divided doses q6–8h for glaucoma; 8–30 mg/kg/day in divided doses for epilepsy	Treatment of glaucoma; adjunctive treatment of epilepsy, mountain sickness
methazolamide (*generic*)	50–100 mg PO b.i.d. to t.i.d.	Treatment of glaucoma

Contraindications and Cautions

Allergy to the drug, or to antibacterial sulfonamides or thiazides, or chronic noncongestive angle closure glaucoma are contraindications for use. Cautious use is recommended in patients who are breast-feeding or who have fluid or electrolyte imbalances, renal or hepatic disease, adrenocortical insufficiency, respiratory acidosis, or chronic obstructive pulmonary disease.

Adverse Effects

Adverse effects of carbonic anhydrase inhibitors are related to the disturbances in acid–base and electrolyte balances. Metabolic acidosis is a relatively common and potentially dangerous effect that occurs when bicarbonate is lost. Hypokalemia is also common, because potassium excretion is increased as the tubule loses potassium in an attempt to retain some of the sodium that is being excreted. Patients also complain of paresthesias (tingling) of the extremities, confusion, and drowsiness, all of which are probably related to the neural effect of the electrolyte changes.

Clinically Important Drug–Drug Interactions

There may be an increased excretion of salicylates and lithium if they are combined with these drugs. Caution should be used to monitor serum levels of patients taking lithium.

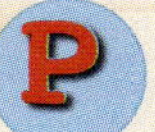

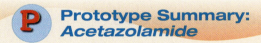

Prototype Summary: *Acetazolamide*

Indications: Adjunctive treatment of open-angle glaucoma, secondary glaucoma; preoperative use in acute angle-closure glaucoma when delay of surgery is indicated; edema caused by CHF, drug-induced edema; centrencephalic epilepsy; prophylaxis and treatment of acute altitude sickness

Actions: Inhibits carbonic anhydrase, which decreases aqueous humor formation in the eye, intraocular pressure, and hydrogen secretion by the renal tubules

Pharmacokinetics:

Route	Onset	Peak	Duration
Oral	1 h	2–4 h	6–12 h
Sustained-release oral	2 h	8–12 h	18–24 h
IV	1–2 min	15–18 min	4–5 h

$T_{1/2}$: 5–6 hours; excreted unchanged in urine

Adverse effects: Weakness, fatigue, rash, anorexia, nausea, urinary frequency, renal calculi, bone marrow suppression, weight loss

Potassium-Sparing Diuretics

The potassium-sparing diuretics include amiloride (*Midamor*), spironolactone (*Aldactone*), and triamterene (*Dyrenium*) (Table 51.5). These diuretics are used for patients who are at high risk for hypokalemia associated with diuretic use (e.g., patients receiving digitalis, patients with cardiac arrhythmias). They are not as powerful as the loop diuretics, but they retain potassium instead of wasting it.

Therapeutic Actions and Indications

Certain diuretics cause a loss of sodium while retaining potassium. Spironolactone acts as an aldosterone antagonist, blocking the actions of aldosterone in the distal tubule. Amiloride and triamterene block potassium secretion through the tubule. The diuretic effect of these drugs comes from the balance achieved in losing sodium to offset potassium retained.

Potassium-sparing diuretics are often used as adjuncts with thiazide or loop diuretics or in patients who are especially at risk if hypokalemia develops, such as patients taking certain antiarrhythmics or digoxin and those who have particular neurological conditions. Spironolactone, the most frequently prescribed of these drugs, is the drug of choice for treating **hyperaldosteronism**, a condition seen in cirrhosis of the liver and nephrotic syndrome.

Pharmacokinetics

These drugs are well absorbed, protein bound, and widely distributed. They are metabolized in the liver and primarily excreted in urine. These diuretics cross the placenta and enter breast milk. Routine use during pregnancy is not appropriate, and they should be saved for situations in which the mother has pathological reasons for use, not pregnancy manifestations or complications, and the benefit to the mother clearly outweighs the risk to the fetus. If one of these drugs is needed during lactation, another method of feeding the baby should be used, because of the potential for adverse effects on fluid and electrolyte changes in the baby.

Contraindications and Cautions

These drugs are contraindicated for use in patients with allergy to the drug, hyperkalemia, renal disease, or anuria. They are also contraindicated in patients taking amiloride or triamterene. They are given cautiously during pregnancy and lactation.

Adverse Effects

The most common adverse effect of potassium-sparing diuretics is hyperkalemia, which can cause lethargy, confusion, ataxia, muscle cramps, and cardiac arrhythmias. Patients taking these drugs need to be evaluated regularly for signs of

Table 51.5 DRUGS IN FOCUS

Potassium-Sparing Diuretics

Drug Name	Usual Dosage	Usual Indications
amiloride (*Midamor*)	15–20 mg/day PO with monitoring of electrolytes	All of the potassium-sparing diuretics are indicated for the adjunctive treatment of edema caused by congestive heart failure, liver disease, or renal disease; hypertension; hyperkalemia; and hyperaldosteronism **Special considerations:** Not for use in children
P spironolactone (*Aldactone*)	100–200 mg/day PO for edema;100–400 mg/day PO for hyperaldosteronism; 50–100 mg/day PO for hypertension Pediatric: 3.3 mg/kg/day PO	**Special considerations:** Can be used in children with careful monitoring of electrolytes
triamterene (*Dyrenium*)	100 mg/day PO b.i.d.	**Special considerations:** Not for use in children

increased potassium and informed about the signs and symptoms to watch for. They also should be advised to avoid foods that are high in potassium (Box 51.4).

Clinically Important Drug–Drug Interactions

The diuretic effect decreases if potassium-sparing diuretics are combined with salicylates. Dosage adjustment may be necessary to achieve therapeutic effects.

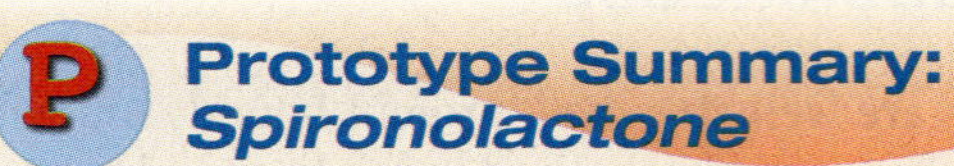

Prototype Summary: *Spironolactone*

Indications: Primary hyperaldosteronism, adjunctive therapy in the treatment of edema associated with CHF, nephritic syndrome, hepatic cirrhosis; treatment of hypokalemia or prevention of hypokalemia in patients at high risk if hypokalemia occurs; essential hypertension

Actions: Competitively blocks the effects of aldosterone in the renal tubule, causing loss of sodium and water and retention of potassium

Pharmacokinetics:

Route	Onset	Peak	Duration
Oral	24–48 h	48–72 h	48–72 h

$T_{1/2}$: 20 hours; metabolized in the liver and excreted in urine

Adverse effects: Dizziness, headache, drowsiness, rash, cramping, diarrhea, hyperkalemia, hirsutism, gynecomastia, deepening of the voice, irregular menses

BOX 51.4 Potassium-Rich Foods

avocados	bananas	broccoli	cantaloupe	dried fruits
grapefruit	lima beans	nuts	navy beans	oranges
peaches	potatoes	prunes	rhubarb	*Sanka* coffee
sunflower seeds	spinach	tomatoes	watermelon	

Osmotic Diuretics

Osmotic diuretics pull water into the renal tubule without sodium loss. They are the diuretics of choice in cases of increased cranial pressure or acute renal failure due to shock, drug overdose, or trauma. The osmotic diuretics include two mild agents, glycerin (*Osmoglyn*) and isosorbide (*Ismotic*), and two powerful ones, mannitol (*Osmitrol*) and urea (*Ureaphil*) (Table 51.6). Glycerin can be given intravenously to treat elevated intracranial pressure and is used orally to treat glaucoma. Isosorbide is available only in oral form and is a preferred drug for the treatment of glaucoma. Mannitol, which is available only for intravenous use, is the mainstay for treatment of elevated intracranial pressure and acute renal failure. Urea also is available only for intravenous use; it is indicated for reduction of intracranial pressure and in the treatment of acute glaucoma.

Therapeutic Actions and Indications

Some nonelectrolytes are used intravenously to increase the volume of fluid produced by the kidneys. Mannitol, for example, is a sugar that is not well reabsorbed by the tubules; it

Table 51.6 DRUGS IN FOCUS

Osmotic Diuretics

Drug Name	Usual Dosage	Usual Indications
glycerin (*Osmoglyn*)	1–1.5 mg/kg PO for glaucoma	Treatment of elevated intracranial pressure (IV); glaucoma (PO)
isosorbide (*Ismotic*)	1.5 g/kg PO b.i.d. to q.i.d.	Treatment of glaucoma
P mannitol (*Osmitrol*)	50–100 g IV for oliguria; 1.5–2 g/kg IV to reduce intracranial pressure; dosage not established for children <12 yr	Treatment of elevated intracranial pressure; renal failure; acute glaucoma
urea (*Ureaphil*)	1–1.5 g/kg IV, do not exceed 120 g/day Pediatric: 0.5–1.5 mg/kg IV; as little as 0.1 mg/kg may be sufficient in children <2 yr	Treatment of elevated intracranial pressure; acute glaucoma

acts to pull large amounts of fluid into the urine by the **osmotic pull** of the large sugar molecule. Because the tubule is not able to reabsorb all of the sugar pulled into it, large amounts of fluid are lost in the urine. The effects of these osmotic drugs are not limited to the kidneys, because the injected substance pulls fluid into the vascular system from extravascular spaces, including the aqueous humor. Therefore, these drugs are often used in acute situations when it is necessary to decrease intraocular pressure before eye surgery or during acute attacks of glaucoma. Mannitol is also used to decrease intracranial pressure, to prevent the oliguric phase of renal failure, and to promote the movement of toxic substances through the kidneys.

Pharmacokinetics

These drugs are freely filtered at the renal glomerulus, poorly reabsorbed by the renal tubule, not secreted by the tubule, and resistant to metabolism. Their action depends on the concentration of the osmotic activity in the solution. It is not known whether these drugs can cause fetal harm, so their use during pregnancy should be limited to situations in which the benefit to the mother outweighs the potential risk to the fetus. Effects of these drugs during lactation are not well understood; because of the potential for risk to the neonate or changes in the fluid balance of the mother, caution should be used if one of these drugs is needed during lactation.

Contraindications and Cautions

Renal disease and anuria from severe renal disease, pulmonary congestion, intracranial bleeding, dehydration, and CHF are contraindications to use.

Adverse Effects

The most common and potentially dangerous adverse effect related to osmotic diuretics is the sudden drop in fluid levels. Nausea, vomiting, hypotension, light-headedness, confusion, and headache can be accompanied by cardiac decompensation and even shock. Patients receiving these drugs should be closely monitored for fluid and electrolyte imbalance.

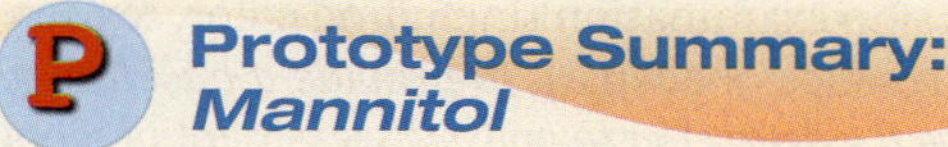

Prototype Summary: Mannitol

Indications: Prevention and treatment of oliguric phase of renal failure; reduction of intracranial pressure and treatment of cerebral edema; reduction of elevated intraocular pressure; promotion of urinary excretion of toxic substances; diagnostic use for measurement of glomerular filtration rate; irrigant in transurethral prostatic resection and other transurethral procedures

Actions: Elevates the osmolarity of the glomerular filtrate, leading to a loss of water, sodium, and chloride; creates an osmotic gradient in the eye, reducing intraocular pressure; creates an osmotic effect that decreases swelling after transurethral surgery

Pharmacokinetics:

Route	Onset	Peak	Duration
IV	30–60 min	1 h	6–8 h
Irrigant	Rapid	Rapid	Short

$T_{1/2}$: 15–100 min; excreted unchanged in urine

Adverse effects: Dizziness, headache, hypotension, rash, nausea, anorexia, dry mouth, thirst, diuresis, fluid and electrolyte imbalances

Nursing Considerations for Patients Receiving Diuretics

Assessment: History and Examination

Screen for the following conditions, *which could be cautions or contraindications to use of the drug:* any known allergies to diuretics; fluid or electrolyte disturbances, *which could be exacerbated by the diuretic or render the diuretic ineffective;* gout, *which reflects an abnormal tubule function and could be worsened by the diuretic or reflect a condition that would render the diuretic ineffective;* glucose tolerance abnormalities, *which may be exacerbated by the glucose-elevating effects of some diuretics;* liver disease, *which could alter the metabolism of the diuretic, leading to toxic levels;* systemic lupus erythematosus, *which frequently affects the glomerulus and could be exacerbated by the use of a diuretic;* and pregnancy or lactation, *which could be affected by the change in fluid and electrolyte balance.*

Physical assessment should include the following: thorough skin examination (including color, texture, and the presence of edema), *to provide a baseline as a reference for drug effectiveness;* assessment of blood pressure, pulse, and cardiac auscultation, *to provide a baseline for effects on blood pressure and volume;* assessment of body weight, *to provide a baseline to monitor fluid load;* liver evaluation, *to determine potential problems in drug metabolism;* check of urinary output, *to establish a baseline of renal function;* and evaluation of blood tests, *to provide a baseline reference for electrolyte balance, glucose levels, uric acid levels, and liver function tests.*

Nursing Diagnoses

The patient receiving a diuretic may have the following nursing diagnoses related to drug therapy:

- Risk for Deficient Fluid Volume related to diuretic effect
- Impaired Urinary Elimination related to diuretic effect
- Imbalanced Nutrition: Less Than Body Requirements related to GI upset and metabolic changes
- Deficient Knowledge regarding drug therapy

Implementation With Rationale

- Administer oral drug with food or milk, *to buffer the drug effect on the stomach lining if GI upset is a problem.*
- Administer intravenous drug slowly, *to prevent severe changes in fluid and electrolytes;* protect the drug from light, *because disintegration can occur;* discard diluted drug after 24 hours, *to prevent contamination or ineffective drug use.*
- Continuously monitor urinary output, cardiac response, and heart rhythm of patients receiving intravenous diuretics, *to monitor for rapid fluid switch and potential electrolyte disturbances leading to cardiac arrhythmia.* Switch to the oral form, *which is less potent and easier to monitor,* as soon as possible.
- Administer early in the day, *so that increased urination will not interfere with sleep.*
- Monitor the dose carefully and reduce the dosage of one or both drugs if given with antihypertensive agents; *loss of fluid volume can precipitate hypotension.*
- Monitor the patient response to the drug (e.g., blood pressure, urinary output, weight, serum electrolytes, hydration, periodic blood glucose monitoring), *to evaluate the effectiveness of the drug and monitor for adverse effects.*
- Provide comfort measures, including skin care and nutrition consultation, *to increase compliance to drug therapy and decrease severity of adverse effects;* provide safety measures if dizziness and weakness are a problem.
- Provide potassium-rich or potassium-poor diet as appropriate for drug being given, *to maintain electrolyte balance and replace lost potassium.*
- Provide thorough patient teaching, including measures to avoid adverse effects and warning signs of problems and ways to incorporate the diuretic's effect in planning the day's activities, *to enhance patient knowledge about drug therapy and to promote compliance.*

Evaluation

- Monitor patient response to the drug (weight, urinary output, edema changes, blood pressure).
- Monitor for adverse effects (electrolyte imbalance, orthostatic hypotension, rebound edema, hyperglycemia, increased uric acid levels, acid–base disturbances, dizziness).
- Evaluate the effectiveness of the teaching plan (patient can name drug, dosage, adverse effects to watch for, specific measures to avoid adverse effects).
- Monitor the effectiveness of comfort measures and compliance to the regimen

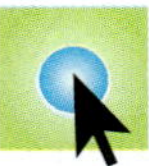

WEB LINKS

Health care providers and patients may want to consult the following Internet sources:

http://www.tmc.edu/thi/diurmeds.html Information on diuretics, good teaching guides and aids.

http://www.americanheart.org and http://www.nhlbi.nih.gov Information on CHF, pathophysiology, treatment, and research.

http://cpmcnet.columbia.edu/dept/gi/other.html Information on liver disease and related treatment.

Points to Remember

- Diuretics are drugs that increase the excretion of sodium, and therefore water, from the kidneys.
- Diuretics are used in the treatment of edema associated with CHF and pulmonary edema, liver failure and cirrhosis, and various types of renal disease, and as adjuncts in the treatment of hypertension.
- Diuretics must be used cautiously in any condition that would be exacerbated by changes in fluid and electrolyte balance.
- Adverse effects associated with diuretics include electrolyte imbalance (potassium, sodium, chloride); hypotension and hypovolemia; hypoglycemia; and metabolic alkalosis.
- Classes of diuretics differ in their site of action and intensity of effects. Thiazide diuretics work to block the chloride pump in the distal convoluted tubule. This effect leads to a loss of sodium and potassium and a minor loss of water. Thiazides are frequently used alone or in combination with other drugs to treat hypertension. They are considered to be mild diuretics.
- Loop diuretics work in the loop of Henle and have a powerful diuretic effect, leading to the loss of water, sodium, and potassium. These drugs are the most potent diuretics and are used in acute situations as well as chronic conditions not responsive to milder diuretics.
- Carbonic anhydrase inhibitors work to block the formation of carbonic acid and bicarbonate in the renal tubule. These drugs can cause an alkaline urine and loss of the bicarbonate buffer. Carbonic anhydrase inhibitors are used in combination with other diuretics when a stronger diuresis is needed, and they are frequently used to treat glaucoma because they decrease the amount of aqueous humor produced in the eye.
- Potassium-sparing diuretics are mild diuretics that act to spare potassium in exchange for the loss of sodium and water in the urine. These diuretics are preferable if potassium loss could be detrimental to a patient's cardiac or neuromuscular condition. Patients must be careful not to become hyperkalemic while taking these drugs.
- Osmotic diuretics use hypertonic pull to remove fluid from the intravascular spaces and to deliver large amounts of water into the renal tubule. There is a danger of sudden change of fluid volume and massive fluid loss with some of these drugs. These drugs are used to decrease intracranial pressure, to treat glaucoma, and to help push toxic substances through the kidney.
- Patients receiving diuretics need to be monitored for fluid loss and retention (daily weights, blood pressure, skin evaluation, urinary output); have periodic electrolyte evaluations and blood glucose determinations; and have evaluations of the effectiveness of their teaching program.

CHECK YOUR UNDERSTANDING

Answers to the questions in this chapter may be found in the Answer Key in the back of the book.

Multiple Choice

Select the best answer to the following.

1. Most diuretics act in the body to cause
   a. loss of water.
   b. loss of sodium.
   c. retention of potassium.
   d. retention of chloride.

2. Diuretics cause a loss of blood volume in the body. The drop in volume activates compensatory mechanisms to restore the volume, including
   a. suppression of ADH release.
   b. suppression of aldosterone release.
   c. activation of the renin–angiotensin system with increased ADH and aldosterone.
   d. stimulation of the countercurrent mechanism.

3. Thiazide diuretics are considered mild diuretics because
   a. they block the sodium pump in the loop of Henle.
   b. they block the chloride pump, which causes loss of sodium and chloride but little water.

c. they do not cause a fluid rebound when they work in the kidneys.
d. they have no effect on electrolytes.

4. A loop diuretic would be the drug of choice in treating
a. hypertension.
b. shock.
c. pulmonary edema.
d. fluid retention of pregnancy.

5. Any patient receiving a loop diuretic needs to have regular monitoring of
a. sodium levels.
b. bone marrow function.
c. calcium levels.
d. potassium levels.

6. The diuretic of choice for treating hyperaldosteronism would be
a. spironolactone.
b. furosemide.
c. hydrochlorothiazide.
d. acetazolamide.

7. A patient with severe glaucoma who is about to undergo eye surgery would benefit from a decrease in intraocular fluid. This is often best accomplished by giving the patient
a. a loop diuretic.
b. a thiazide diuretic.
c. a carbonic anhydrase inhibitor.
d. an osmotic diuretic.

8. Patients receiving diuretics should be taught to report
a. yellow vision.
b. weight loss of 1 lb/day.
c. muscle pain or cramping.
d. increased urination.

Multiple Response

Select all that apply.

1. Diuretics are currently recommended for the treatment of which of the following?
a. Hypertension
b. Renal disease
c. Obesity
d. Severe liver disease
e. Fluid retention of pregnancy
f. Congestive heart failure

2. Routine nursing care of a client receiving a diuretic would include which of the following?
a. Daily weights
b. Tight fluid restrictions
c. Periodic electrolyte evaluations
d. Monitoring of urinary output
e. Regular intraocular pressure testing
f. Teaching the patient to report muscle cramping

Definitions

Define the following terms.

1. edema ____________________
2. fluid rebound ____________________
3. thiazide diuretic ____________________
4. hypokalemia ____________________
5. high-ceiling diuretics ____________________
6. alkalosis ____________________
7. hyperaldosteronism ____________________
8. osmotic pull ____________________

Matching

Match the diuretic with the appropriate class. (Some classes will be used more than once.)

1. ____________ glycerin
2. ____________ acetazolamide
3. ____________ furosemide
4. ____________ benzthiazide
5. ____________ indapamide
6. ____________ mannitol
7. ____________ spironolactone
8. ____________ hydrochlorothiazide
9. ____________ amiloride
10. ____________ bumetanide

A. Osmotic
B. Thiazide
C. Loop
D. Potassium-sparing
E. Carbonic anhydrase inhibitor

Bibliography and References

Drug facts and comparisons. (2006). St. Louis: Facts and Comparisons.

Gilman, A., Hardman, J. G., & Limbird, L. E. (Eds.). (2006). *Goodman and Gilman's the pharmacological basis of therapeutics* (11th ed.). New York: McGraw-Hill.

Karch, A. M. (2006). *2007 Lippincott's nursing drug guide.* Philadelphia: Lippincott Williams & Wilkins.

Porth, C. M. (2005). *Pathophysiology: Concepts of altered health states* (7th ed.). Philadelphia: Lippincott Williams & Wilkins.

Professional's guide to patient drug facts. (2006). St. Louis: Facts and Comparisons.

CHAPTER 52

Drugs Affecting the Urinary Tract and the Bladder

KEY TERMS

acidification
antispasmodics
benign prostatic hyperplasia (BPH)
cystitis
dysuria
interstitial cystitis
nocturia
pyelonephritis
urgency
urinary frequency

LEARNING OBJECTIVES

Upon completion of this chapter, you will be able to:

1. Describe four common problems associated with the urinary tract and the clinical manifestations of these problems.
2. Describe the therapeutic actions, indications, pharmacokinetics, contraindications, most common adverse reactions, and important drug–drug interactions associated with urinary tract antispasmodics, anti-infectives, and analgesics and bladder protectants and drugs used to treat BPH.
3. Discuss the use of drugs affecting the urinary tract and bladder across the lifespan.
4. Compare and contrast the prototype drugs norfloxacin, oxybutynin, and doxazosin with other agents in their class.
5. Outline the nursing considerations, including important teaching points, for patients receiving drugs affecting the urinary tract and bladder.

URINARY TRACT ANTI-INFECTIVES

cinoxacin
fosfomycin
methenamine
methylene blue
nalidixic acid
nitrofurantoin
P norfloxacin

URINARY TRACT ANTISPASMODICS

darifenacin
flavoxate
P oxybutynin
solifenacin
tolterodine
trospium

URINARY TRACT ANALGESIC

phenazopyridine

BLADDER PROTECTANT

pentosan polysulfate sodium

DRUGS USED TO TREAT BENIGN PROSTATIC HYPERPLASIA

alfuzosin
P doxazosin
dutasteride
finasteride
tamsulosin
terazosin

Acute urinary tract infections (UTIs) occur second in frequency only to respiratory tract infections in the American population. Females, with shorter urethras, are particularly vulnerable to repeated bladder and even kidney infections. (Children also may have frequent problems—see Box 52.1.) Patients with indwelling catheters or intermittent catheterizations often are affected by bladder infections or **cystitis**, which can result from bacteria introduced into the bladder by these devices. Blockage anywhere in the urinary tract can lead to backflow problems and the spread of bladder infections into the kidney.

The signs and symptoms of a UTI are uncomfortable and include **urinary frequency**; **urgency**; burning on urination (associated with cystitis); and chills, fever, flank pain, and tenderness (associated with acute **pyelonephritis**). To treat these infections, clinicians use antibiotics (see Chapter 9), as well as specific agents that reach antibacterial levels only in the kidney and bladder and are thought to sterilize the urinary tract.

Drugs also are available to block spasms of the urinary tract muscles, decrease urinary tract pain, protect the cells of the bladder from irritation, and treat enlargement of the prostate gland in men. All of these agents are discussed in this chapter. Table 52.1 provides a summary of urinary tract problems and the drugs of choice to treat them.

Urinary Tract Anti-infectives

Urinary tract anti-infectives are of two types (Table 52.2). One type is the antibiotics, which include the following:

- Cinoxacin (*Cinobac*) interferes with DNA replication in gram-negative bacteria. This drug is rapidly absorbed, undergoes hepatic metabolism, and is excreted in urine. It is used in lower doses in the presence of renal impairment because it is not excreted properly. It should be used with caution during pregnancy and lactation because it does cross the placenta and enter breast milk.
- Norfloxacin (*Noroxin*), a newer and more broad-spectrum drug, is effective against even more gram-negative strains than is cinoxacin. This drug is rapidly absorbed and undergoes hepatic metabolism and renal excretion. Dosage must be reduced in the presence of renal impairment. This drug crosses the placenta and enters breast milk and should not be used during pregnancy or lactation unless the benefit to the mother clearly outweighs the potential risk to the fetus or neonate.
- Fosfomycin (*Monurol*) has the convenience of only one dose. It is not recommended for children younger than 18 years of age. It is rapidly absorbed, undergoes slow hepatic metabolism, and is excreted in urine and feces. It might be a drug of choice for cystitis during pregnancy

BOX 52.1 **DRUG THERAPY ACROSS THE LIFESPAN**

Urinary Tract Agents

CHILDREN

Children often have cystitis and need to be treated with a urinary tract agent. Some children, because of congenital problems or indwelling catheters, require other urinary tract agents. The older anti-infectives—nalidixic acid, nitrofurantoin, and methenamine—have established pediatric guidelines.

Children need to be instructed in proper hygiene and should not be given bubble baths if urinary tract infections occur. They should be encouraged to avoid the alkaline ash juices and urged to drink lots of water.

If an antispasmodic is needed, oxybutynin is indicated for children >5 yr of age, and flavoxate can be used in children >12 yr. Phenazopyridine is indicated as a urinary tract analgesic for children 6–12 yr of age.

The child should be cautioned about the change in urine color, which might be frightening if the child is not expecting it.

ADULTS

Adults need to be cautioned about the various measures that can be used to decrease the likelihood of urinary tract infections. They should be encouraged to drink plenty of fluids to maintain bladder health.

If taking an anticholinergic to block spasm, adult patients need to be advised of other precautions to take when the parasympathetic system is blocked.

Adult men being treated for benign prostatic hyperplasia need to be aware of the possibility of decreased sexual function, as well as fatigue, lethargy, and the potential for dizziness, which could interfere with working or activities of daily living.

The use of urinary tract agents during pregnancy should be approached with caution. If an antibiotic is needed, the one-dose fosfomycin might be a drug of choice because of the limited exposure to the drug. Women who are nursing should use these agents with caution because of the potential for adverse effects on the baby, or they should find another method of feeding the baby.

OLDER ADULTS

Older adults often have conditions that are treated with the urinary tract agents. They are also more likely to have renal or hepatic impairment, which requires caution in the use of these drugs. Older adults should be started on the lowest possible dose of the drug, and it should be titrated slowly based on patient response. Special precautions to monitor cardiac function, intraocular pressure, blood pressure, and bladder emptying need to be taken when using alpha-adrenergic blockers with these patients. Older patients may have a difficult time maintaining fluid intake and might benefit from extra encouragement to drink fluids, including cranberry juice, and to avoid alkaline ash drinks.

Table 52.1 Drugs Used to Treat Urinary Tract Problems

Urinary Tract Problem	Drugs of Choice
Infection	Urinary tract anti-infectives: fosfomycin, cinoxacin, methenamine, nalidixic acid, methylene blue, nitrofurantoin, norfloxacin
Spasm	Antispasmodics: flavoxate, oxybutynin, tolterodine
Pain	Urinary tract analgesic: phenazopyridine Bladder protectant for interstitial cystitis: pentosan
Benign prostatic hyperplasia	Alpha-adrenergic blockers: doxazosin, tamsulosin, terazosin, alfuzosin Testosterone inhibitor: finasteride

or lactation because of the short exposure to the drug. Unpleasant gastrointestinal (GI) effects limit its usefulness in some patients.

- Nalidixic acid (*NegGram*) is an older drug that is not effective against as many strains of gram-negative bacteria as the other antibiotics used for UTIs. This drug is rapidly absorbed, metabolized in the liver, and excreted in urine. It has a short half-life—1 to 2.5 hours. It is known to cross the placenta and to enter breast milk, so it should not be used during pregnancy or lactation. It is available in a suspension form and has an established dosage for children ages 3 months to 12 years.
- Nitrofurantoin (*Furadantin*) is another older drug with a very short half-life (20 to 60 minutes). It is not effective against as many gram-negative bacteria as the newer drugs are, but it has been successfully used for suppression therapy in adults and children with chronic UTIs. It is metabolized in the liver and excreted in urine. It is not recommended during pregnancy or lactation because of the potential for adverse effects on the neonate or baby.

The other type of urinary tract anti-infective works to acidify the urine, killing bacteria that might be in the bladder. This group includes two drugs:

- Methenamine (*Hiprex*) undergoes metabolism in the liver and is excreted in urine. It crosses the placenta and enters breast milk and should not be used during pregnancy or lactation. Methenamine has established dosage guidelines for children and comes in a suspension form.
- Methylene blue (*Urolene Blue*) is widely distributed, metabolized in the tissues, and excreted in urine, bile, and feces. This drug stains the tissues and can cause GI upset. It is not recommended during pregnancy or lactation.

Table 52.2 DRUGS IN FOCUS

Urinary Tract Anti-infectives

Drug Name	Usual Dosage	Usual Indications
cinoxacin (*Cinobac*)	1 g/day PO for 7–14 days; 250 mg/day PO at bedtime for prevention; reduce dosage with impaired renal function	Treatment of urinary tract infections caused by susceptible bacteria in patients >12 yr
fosfomycin (*Monurol*)	One packet (3 g) dissolved in water PO	Treatment of urinary tract infections caused by susceptible bacteria (one-dose drug) in patients >18 yr
methenamine (*Hiprex*)	1 g b.i.d. to q.i.d. PO Pediatric (6–12 yr): 0.5–1 g PO b.i.d. to q.i.d. Pediatric (<6 yr): 0.25–0.5 mg/kg/day PO in divided doses	Suppression or elimination of bacteriuria associated with urinary tract infections and anatomical abnormalities
methylene blue (*Urolene Blue*)	65–130 mg PO t.i.d.	Suppression or elimination of bacteriuria associated with urinary tract infections and anatomical abnormalities
nalidixic acid (*NegGram*)	1 g PO q.i.d. for 1–2 wk, reduce to 2 g/day for prolonged use Pediatric (<12 yr): 55 mg/kg/day PO in four divided doses, for prolonged therapy reduce to 33 mg/kg/day	Treatment of urinary tract infections caused by susceptible bacteria
nitrofurantoin (*Furadantin*)	50–100 mg PO q.i.d. for 10–14 days; 50–100 mg PO at bedtime for chronic suppressive therapy Pediatric: 5–7 mg/kg/day in four divided doses; 1 mg/kg/day PO at bedtime for chronic suppressive therapy	Treatment of urinary tract infections caused by susceptible bacteria
P norfloxacin (*Noroxin*)	400 mg q12h PO, length of therapy dependent on site and intensity of infection	Treatment of urinary tract infections caused by susceptible bacteria (broad-spectrum agent)

Therapeutic Actions and Indications

Urinary tract anti-infectives act specifically within the urinary tract to destroy bacteria, either through a direct antibiotic effect or through **acidification** of the urine. They do not generally have an antibiotic effect systemically, being activated or effective only in the urinary tract (Figure 52.1). They are used to treat chronic UTIs, as adjunctive therapy in acute cystitis and pyelonephritis, and as prophylaxis with urinary tract anatomical abnormalities and residual urine disorders. Fosfomycin, a relatively new agent, is a one-dose-only antibacterial. Ease of treatment makes this a very desirable agent; however, many patients experience unpleasant adverse effects, especially GI effects, with this drug.

Pharmacokinetics

Because these drugs are from several different chemical classes, the pharmacokinetic data are different for each drug. See discussions above or consult a nursing drug guide for additional details.

Contraindications and Cautions

These drugs are contraindicated in the presence of any known allergy to any of these drugs. They should be used with caution in the presence of renal dysfunction, *which could interfere with the excretion and action of these drugs,* and with pregnancy and lactation *because of the potential for adverse effects on the fetus or neonate.*

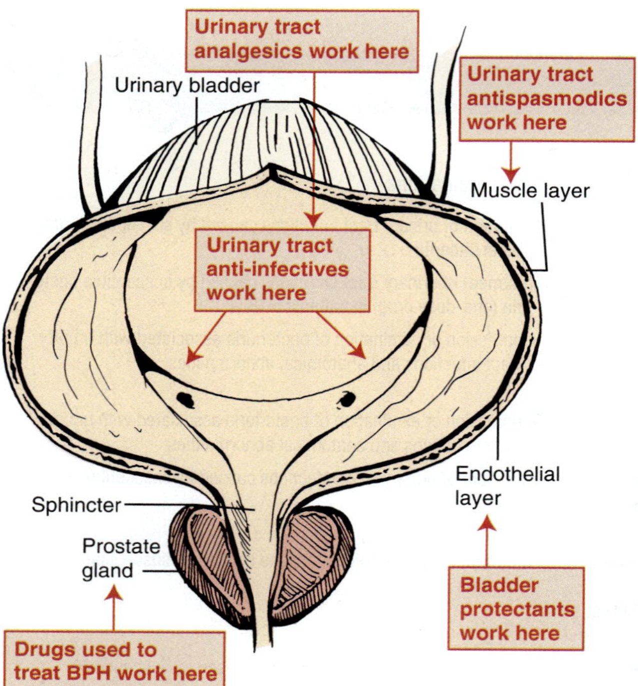

FIGURE 52.1 Sites of action of drugs acting on the urinary tract.

Adverse Effects

Adverse effects associated with these drugs include nausea, vomiting, diarrhea, anorexia, bladder irritation, and dysuria. Infrequent symptoms include pruritus, urticaria, headache, dizziness, nervousness, and confusion. These effects may result from GI irritation caused by the agent, which may be somewhat alleviated if the drug is taken with food, or from a systemic reaction to the urinary tract irritation.

Clinically Important Drug–Drug Interactions

Because these drugs are from several different chemical classes, the drug–drug interactions that can occur are very specific to the drug being used. Consult a nursing drug guide for specific interactions.

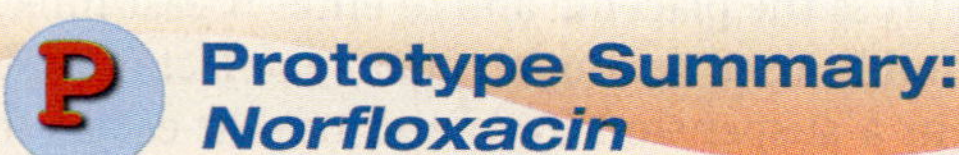

Prototype Summary: *Norfloxacin*

Indications: Treatment of adults with UTIs caused by susceptible strains of bacteria; uncomplicated urethral and cervical gonorrhea; prostatitis caused by *Escherichia coli*

Actions: Interferes with DNA replication in susceptible gram-negative bacteria, leading to cell death

Pharmacokinetics:

Route	Onset	Peak	Duration
Oral	Varies	2–3 h	12 h

$T_{1/2}$: 3–4.5 hours; metabolized in the liver and excreted in urine

Adverse effects: Headache, dizziness, nausea, vomiting, dry mouth, fever, rash, photosensitivity

Nursing Considerations for Patients Receiving Urinary Tract Anti-infectives

Assessment: History and Examination

Screen for the following conditions, *which could be cautions or contraindications to use of the drug:* any history of allergy to antibacterials; liver or renal dysfunction *that might interfere with the drug's metabo-*

lism and excretion; and pregnancy and lactation, *which are contraindications to the use of these drugs.*

Physical assessment should be done *to establish baseline data for assessing the effectiveness of the drug and the occurrence of any adverse effects associated with drug therapy.* Assess for the following: skin, *to evaluate for the development of rash or hypersensitivity reactions;* orientation and reflexes, *to evaluate any central nervous system (CNS) effects of the drug;* and renal and hepatic function tests, *to determine baseline function of these organs.*

Nursing Diagnoses

The patient receiving a urinary tract anti-infective may have the following nursing diagnoses related to drug therapy:

- Acute Pain related to GI, CNS, or skin effects of drug
- Disturbed Sensory Perception (Kinesthetic, Tactile, Visual) related to CNS effects
- Deficient Knowledge regarding drug therapy

Implementation With Rationale

- Ensure that culture and sensitivity tests are performed before therapy begins and repeated if the response is not as expected *to ensure appropriate treatment of the infection.*
- Administer the drugs with food *to decrease GI adverse effects if they occur.*
- Institute safety precautions if the patient experiences CNS effects *to prevent patient injury.*
- Advise patients to continue the full course of the drug ordered and not to stop taking it as soon as the uncomfortable signs and symptoms pass *to ensure eradication of the infection and prevent the emergence of resistant strains of bacteria.*
- Encourage the patient to drink lots of fluids (unless contraindicated by other conditions) *to flush the bladder and urinary tract frequently and decrease the opportunity for bacteria growth.*
- Educate patients with chronic UTIs about additional activities that can facilitate an acidic urine *to increase the effectiveness of urinary tract anti-infectives.* For example, all patients should:

  Avoid foods that cause an alkaline ash and produce an alkaline urine (e.g., citrus juices, fruits, antacids).

  Drink high-acid cranberry juice.

  Void immediately after sexual intercourse, to help clear any invading organisms.

  In addition, women should:

  Avoid baths if possible, especially bubble baths (because the bubbles act as transport agents to deliver bacteria through the short urethra) and

  Wipe front to back and never back to front, which introduces *E. coli* and other agents to the urethra.
- Provide thorough patient teaching, including the drug name and prescribed dosage, measures to help avoid adverse effects, warning signs that may indicate problems, and the need for periodic monitoring and evaluation, *to enhance patient knowledge about drug therapy and to promote compliance.*

Evaluation

- Monitor patient response to the drug (resolution of UTI and relief of signs and symptoms); repeat culture and sensitivity tests are recommended for evaluation of the effectiveness of all of these drugs.
- Monitor for adverse effects (skin evaluation, orientation and reflexes, GI effects).
- Evaluate the effectiveness of the teaching plan (patient can name drug, dosage, adverse effects to watch for, specific measures to avoid adverse effects, and measures to take to increase the effectiveness of the drug).
- Monitor the effectiveness of comfort and safety measures and compliance with the therapeutic regimen (Critical Thinking Scenario 52-1).

Urinary Tract Antispasmodics

Urinary tract **antispasmodics** block the spasms of urinary tract muscles caused by various conditions. Flavoxate (*Urispas*) prevents smooth muscle spasm specifically in the urinary tract, but it is associated with CNS effects (blurred vision, dizziness, confusion) that make it less desirable to use in certain patients.

Oxybutynin (*Ditropan*) is a potent urinary antispasmodic, but it has numerous anticholinergic effects, making it undesirable in certain conditions or situations that might be aggravated by decreased sweating, urinary retention, tachycardia, and changes in GI activity. It is available in an oral as well as a dermal patch form for the treatment of overactive bladder.

Tolterodine (*Detrol, Detrol LA*), darifenacin (*Enablex*), and solifenacin (*VESIcare*) are newer agents that block muscarinic receptors, preventing bladder contraction and spasm. They are indicated for the treatment of overactive bladder in patients who exhibit urinary frequency, urgency, or incontinence. *Detrol* has been widely marketed directly to the consumer.

Trospium (*Sanctura*) is the newest drug approved to block urinary tract spasms. It also specifically blocks muscarinic receptors and reduces the muscle tone of the bladder. It is

CRITICAL THINKING SCENARIO 52-1

Teaching About Cystitis Treatment

The Situation

J.K. is a 6-year-old girl with a history of repeated urinary tract infections (UTIs). She is seen with complaints of dysuria, frequency, urgency, and a low-grade fever. A urine sample is sent for culture and sensitivity testing. The physician prescribes methenamine (*Hiprex*), 500 mg q.i.d., and refers J.K. and her mother to the nurse for teaching.

Critical Thinking

What is the best approach for this patient?

What key teaching points (at least five) should be emphasized to assist the pharmacological therapy in treating this infection? *Think about the following points: what the drug is doing, how does it work, and how does it work best.*

Discussion

Cystitis is very difficult to treat in young girls and can become a chronic problem. Patient and parent education is very important for trying to block the growth of bacteria and cure the infection. Teaching points should emphasize activities that will decrease the number of bacteria introduced into the bladder, acidify the urine to make the bladder an inhospitable environment for bacterial growth, and flush the bladder to prevent stagnant urine from encouraging bacterial growth.

To decrease the number of bacteria introduced into the bladder, patient education should cover the following hygiene measures: always wipe from front to back and never from back to front, to avoid the introduction of intestinal bacteria into the urethra; avoid baths, particularly bubble baths, which facilitate the entry of bacteria into the urethra on the bubbles; and wear dry, cotton underwear to discourage bacterial growth.

Patient education also should stress the importance of avoiding alkaline ash foods (e.g., citrus fruits, certain vegetables) and encouraging foods that acidify the urine. Cranberry juice is often recommended as a choice for fruit juice because it helps to acidify the bladder and destroy bacteria. Fluid intake, especially water, should be encouraged as much as possible to keep the bladder flushed. Finally, the patient should be encouraged to complete the full course of medication prescribed and not to stop taking the drug when symptoms disappear.

Nursing Care Guide for J.K.: Urinary Tract Anti-infective Methenamine

Assessment: History And Examination

Assess J.K.'s health history, particularly any allergies to antibacterial medications, and liver or renal dysfunction. (If J.K. were of childbearing age, you would assess pregnancy and breast-feeding status.)

Focus the physical examination on the following areas:

Neurological: orientation, reflexes, strength

Skin: color, texture, edema

GI: liver evaluation

GU: urinary output

Laboratory tests: liver function tests, urinalysis, urine culture, and sensitivity testing

Nursing Diagnoses

Acute Pain related to GI, CNS, skin effects of drug

Disturbed Sensory Perception related to CNS effects

Deficient Knowledge regarding drug therapy

Implementation

Obtain urine sample for culture and sensitivity test.

Provide comfort and safety measures: safety precautions, skin care, nutrition.

Encourage eating acidifying foods and drinking lots of fluids.

Teach hygiene measures.

Administer medication with food if GI upset is a problem.

Provide support and reassurance to deal with drug effects and lifestyle changes.

Provide patient teaching to J.K. and her parents or caregivers regarding drug name, dosage, adverse effects, precautions, warnings to report, hygiene measures, and dietary changes as needed.

Evaluation

Evaluate drug effects: relief of symptoms, resolution of infection.

Monitor for adverse effects: GI upset, headache, dizziness, confusion, dysuria, pruritus, urticaria.

Monitor for drug–drug interactions as indicated for each drug.

Teaching About Cystitis Treatment *(continued)*

Evaluate effectiveness of patient teaching program and comfort and safety measures.

Patient Teaching for J.K.

- ☐ A urinary tract anti-infective, such as methenamine, treats UTIs by destroying bacteria and by helping produce an environment that is not conducive to bacterial growth.
- ☐ If this drug causes stomach upset, it can be taken with food. It is important to avoid foods that alkalinize the urine, such as citrus fruits and milk, because they decrease the effectiveness of the drug. Cranberry juice is one juice that can be used. As much fluid as possible (8–10 eight-ounce glasses of water a day) should be taken to help treat the infection.
- ☐ Avoid using any over-the-counter (OTC) medication that might contain sodium bicarbonate (e.g., antacids, baking soda) because these drugs alkalinize the urine and interfere with the ability of methenamine to treat the infection. If you question the use of any OTC drug, check with your health care provider.
- ☐ Take the full course of your prescription. Do not use this drug to self-treat any other infection.
- ☐ Common adverse effects of this drug may include:
  - *Stomach upset, nausea:* Taking the drug with food or eating small, frequent meals may help.
  - *Painful urination:* If this occurs, report it to your health care provider. A dosage adjustment may be needed.
  - Report any of the following to your health care provider: *skin rash or itching, severe GI upset, GI upset that prevents adequate fluid intake, very painful urination* (and pregnancy in older female patients).
- ☐ The following activities can help to decrease UTIs:
  - Avoid bubble baths.
  - Void whenever you feel the urge; try not to wait.
  - *For men and women:* Always try to void after sexual intercourse to flush the urethra.
  - *For women only:* Always wipe from front to back, never from back to front.
- ☐ Tell any doctor, nurse, or other health care provider involved in your care that you are taking this drug.

specifically indicated for the treatment of overactive bladder with symptoms of urge urinary incontinence, urgency, and urinary frequency. (See Table 52.3 for a list of these drugs.)

Therapeutic Actions and Indications

Inflammation in the urinary tract, such as cystitis, prostatitis, urethritis, and urethrocystitis/urethrotrigonitis, causes smooth muscle spasms along the urinary tract. Irritation of the urinary tract leading to muscle spasm also occurs in patients with neurogenic bladder. These spasms lead to the uncomfortable effects of **dysuria** (pain or discomfort with urination), urgency, incontinence, **nocturia** (recurrent nighttime urination), and suprapubic pain. The urinary tract antispasmodics relieve these spasms by blocking parasympathetic activity and relaxing the detrusor and other urinary tract muscles (see Figure 52.1).

Pharmacokinetics

These drugs are rapidly absorbed, widely distributed, metabolized in the liver, and excreted in urine. Caution should be used in the presence of hepatic or renal impairment because of the potential of alterations in metabolism or excretion of the drugs. They cross the placenta and are found in breast milk, so they should be used during pregnancy and lactation only if the benefit to the mother clearly outweighs the potential risk to the fetus or neonate.

Contraindications and Cautions

These drugs are contraindicated in the presence of known allergy to the drugs; with pyloric or duodenal obstruction or recent surgery *because the anticholinergic effects can cause serious complications;* with obstructive urinary tract problems, *which could be further aggravated by the blocking of muscle activity;* and with glaucoma, myasthenia gravis, or acute hemorrhage, *which could all be exacerbated by the anticholinergic effects of these drugs.* Caution should be used in patients with renal or hepatic dysfunction, *which could alter the metabolism and excretion of the drugs;* and in pregnant and lactating patients *because of potential adverse effects on the fetus or neonate secondary to the anticholinergic effects of the drugs.*

Table 52.3 DRUGS IN FOCUS

Urinary Tract Antispasmodics

Drug Name	Usual Dosage	Usual Indications
darifenacin (*Enablex*)	7.5 mg/day PO; may be increased to 15 mg/day	Treatment of overactive bladder in patients with urinary urgency, incontinence, or frequency
flavoxate (*Urispas*)	100–200 mg PO t.i.d. to q.i.d.; reduce dosage when patient improves	Symptomatic relief of urinary bladder spasm in patients >12 yr
P oxybutynin (*Ditropan, Oxytrol*)	5 mg PO t.i.d. to q.i.d.; ER tablets—5 mg/day PO up to a maximum 30 mg/day Transdermal patch: apply to dry, intact skin q3–4 days Pediatric (>5 yr): 5 mg PO b.i.d., up to a maximum 5 mg PO t.i.d.	Symptomatic relief of urinary bladder spasm
solifenacin (*VESIcare*)	5–10 mg/day PO	Treatment of overactive bladder in patients with urinary urgency, incontinence, or frequency
tolterodine (*Detrol, Detrol LA*)	1–2 mg PO b.i.d.; ER capsules—4 mg/day; reduce dosage with hepatic impairment to 1 mg PO b.i.d.	Treatment of overactive bladder in patients with urinary urgency, frequency, or incontinence
trospium (*Sanctura*)	20 mg PO b.i.d. at least 1 h before meals; reduce dosage with renal or hepatic impairment	Symptomatic relief of overactive bladder

Adverse Effects

Adverse effects of urinary tract antispasmodics are related to the blocking of the parasympathetic system and include nausea, vomiting, dry mouth, nervousness, tachycardia, and vision changes.

Clinically Important Drug–Drug Interactions

Decreased effectiveness of phenothiazines and haloperidol has been associated with the combination of these drugs with oxybutynin. If any such combinations must be used, the patient should be monitored closely and appropriate dosage adjustments made.

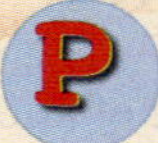

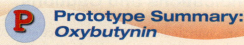

Prototype Summary: Oxybutynin

Indications: Relief of symptoms of bladder instability associated with uninhibited neurogenic and reflex neurogenic bladder; treatment of signs and symptoms of overactive bladder

Actions: Acts directly to relax smooth muscle in the bladder; inhibits the effects of acetylcholine at muscarinic receptors

Pharmacokinetics:

Route	Onset	Peak	Duration
Oral	30–60 min	3–6 h	6–10 h

$T_{1/2}$: Unknown; metabolized in the liver and excreted in urine

Adverse effects: Drowsiness, dizziness, blurred vision, tachycardia, dry mouth, nausea, urinary hesitancy, decreased sweating

Nursing Considerations for Patients Receiving Urinary Tract Antispasmodics

Assessment: History and Examination

Screen for the following conditions, *which could be cautions or contraindications to use of the drug:* any history of allergy to these drugs; pyloric or duodenal obstruction or other GI lesions or obstructions, *which could be dangerously exacerbated by these drugs;* obstructions of the lower urinary tract, *which also could be exacerbated by these drugs;* glaucoma, *which requires caution because of the blockage of the parasympathetic nervous system and the potential for increased intraocular pressure;* and pregnancy or lactation, *which require caution if using these drugs.*

Physical assessment should be done *to establish baseline data for assessing the effectiveness of the drug and the occurrence of any adverse effects associated with drug therapy.* Assess the following: skin, *to evaluate for the development of rash or hypersen-*

sitivity reactions; orientation and reflexes, *to evaluate any CNS effects of the drug;* ophthalmological examination including intraocular pressure, *to assess for any developing glaucoma;* and pulse, *to establish a baseline for evaluating the extent of parasympathetic blockade.*

Nursing Diagnoses

The patient receiving a urinary tract antispasmodic may have the following nursing diagnoses related to drug therapy:

- Acute Pain related to GI, CNS, or ophthalmological effects of drug
- Disturbed Sensory Perception (Visual) related to CNS or ophthalmological effects
- Deficient Knowledge regarding drug therapy

Implementation With Rationale

- Arrange for appropriate treatment of any underlying UTI, *which may be causing the spasm.*
- Arrange for an ophthalmological examination at the beginning of therapy and periodically during long-term treatment *to evaluate drug effects on intraocular pressure so that the drug can be stopped if intraocular pressure increases.*
- Institute safety precautions if the patient experiences CNS effects *to prevent patient injury.*
- Encourage the patient to continue treatment for the underlying cause of the spasm *to treat the cause and prevent the return of the signs and symptoms.*
- Provide thorough patient teaching, including the drug name and prescribed dosage, measures to help avoid adverse effects, warning signs that may indicate problems, and the need for periodic monitoring and evaluation *to enhance patient knowledge about drug therapy and to promote compliance.*
- Offer support and encouragement *to help the patient deal with the discomfort of the drug therapy.*

Evaluation

- Monitor patient response to the drug (resolution of urinary tract spasms and relief of signs and symptoms); repeat culture and sensitivity tests are recommended for evaluation of the effectiveness of all of these drugs.
- Monitor for adverse effects (skin evaluation, orientation and reflexes, intraocular pressure).
- Evaluate the effectiveness of the teaching plan (patient can name drug, dosage, adverse effects to watch for, specific measures to avoid adverse effects).
- Monitor the effectiveness of comfort and safety measures and compliance with the regimen.

FOCUS POINTS

- In the United States, only respiratory tract infections occur more frequently than acute urinary tract infections (UTIs)
- Urinary tract anti-infectives kill urinary tract bacteria by acidifying the urine, making the tract a poor host for bacterial growth, or by killing the bacteria outright.
- Hygiene measures, proper diet, and extra hydration are activities that help decrease harmful bacteria in the urinary tract, which promotes the effect of urinary tract anti-infective agents.
- Smooth muscle spasms affecting the urinary tract may be caused by inflammation and irritation; effects of the spasms include dysuria, urinary urgency, incontinence, nocturia, and suprapubic pain.

Urinary Tract Analgesic

Urinary tract pain can be very uncomfortable and lead to urinary retention and increased risk of infection. The agent phenazopyridine (*Azo-Standard, Baridium,* and others) is a dye that is used to relieve that pain (Table 52.4).

Table 52.4 DRUGS IN FOCUS

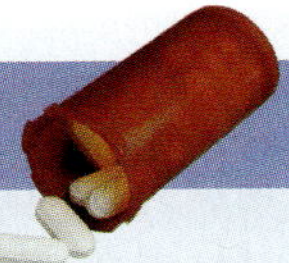

Urinary Tract Analgesic

Drug Name	Usual Dosage	Usual Indications
phenazopyridine (*Azo-Standard, Baridium, Pyridium*)	200 mg PO t.i.d. for up to 2 days Pediatric (6–12 yr): 12 mg/kg/day or 350 mg/m²/day PO, divided into three doses, do not exceed 2 days	Symptomatic relief of the discomforts associated with urinary tract trauma or infection

Therapeutic Actions and Indications

When phenazopyridine is excreted in urine, it exerts a direct, topical analgesic effect on the urinary tract mucosa (see Figure 52.1). It is used to relieve symptoms (burning, urgency, frequency, pain, discomfort) related to urinary tract irritation from infection, trauma, or surgery.

Pharmacokinetics

Phenazopyridine is rapidly absorbed and has a very rapid onset of action. It is widely distributed, crossing the placenta and entering breast milk. It is metabolized in the liver and excreted in urine. Effects during pregnancy and lactation are not well documented, so use during pregnancy and lactation should be reserved for those situations in which the benefit to the mother clearly outweighs any potential risk to the fetus or neonate.

Contraindications and Cautions

Phenazopyridine is contraindicated in the presence of known allergy to the drug and with serious renal dysfunction, *which would interfere with the excretion and effectiveness of the drug.* Caution should be used with pregnancy and lactation *because of the potential for adverse effects on the fetus or neonate.*

Adverse Effects

Adverse effects associated with this drug include GI upset, headache, rash, and a reddish-orange coloring of the urine, all of which are related to the drug's chemical actions in the system. There also is a potential for renal or hepatic toxicity. This drug should not be used for longer than 2 days because the toxic effects may be increased.

Clinically Important Drug–Drug Interactions

The risk of toxic effects of this drug increases if it is combined with antibacterial agents used for treating UTIs. If this combination is used, the phenazopyridine should not be used for longer than 2 days.

Nursing Considerations for Patients Receiving a Urinary Tract Analgesic

Assessment: History and Examination

Screen for the following conditions, *which could be cautions or contraindications to use of the drug:* history of allergy to these drugs or renal insufficiency, *which are contraindications to the use of this drug;* pregnancy or lactation, *which require caution if using this drug.*

Physical assessment should be done *to establish baseline data for assessing the effectiveness of the drug and the occurrence of any adverse effects associated with drug therapy.* Assess for the following: skin, *to evaluate for the development of rash or hypersensitivity reactions;* normal GI function and liver evaluation, *to establish baseline data to assess adverse effects of the drug;* renal and hepatic function tests, *to assess for any underlying condition that might affect the metabolism or excretion of this drug;* and urinalysis, *to assess for underlying infection or renal problems.*

Nursing Diagnoses

The patient receiving a urinary tract analgesic may have the following nursing diagnoses related to drug therapy:

- Acute Pain related to GI effects of drug and headache
- Deficient Knowledge regarding drug therapy

Implementation With Rationale

- Arrange for appropriate treatment of any underlying UTI, *which may be causing the pain.*
- Caution the patient that urine may be reddish-brown and may stain fabrics, *to prevent undue anxiety when this adverse effect occurs.*
- Administer the drug with food *to alleviate GI irritation if GI upset is a problem.*
- Teach the patient to discontinue use of the drug and contact his/her health care provider if sclera or skin become yellowish—*a sign of drug accumulation in the body and a possible sign of hepatic toxicity.*
- Provide thorough patient teaching, including the drug name and prescribed dosage, measures to help avoid adverse effects, warning signs that may indicate problems, and the need for periodic monitoring and evaluation, *to enhance patient knowledge about drug therapy and to promote compliance.*

Evaluation

- Monitor patient response to the drug (resolution of urinary tract pain).
- Monitor for adverse effects (skin evaluation, GI upset and complaints, headache).
- Evaluate the effectiveness of the teaching plan (patient can name drug, dosage, adverse effects to watch for, specific measures to avoid adverse effects).
- Monitor the effectiveness of comfort measures and compliance with the regimen.

Bladder Protectant

The bladder protectant pentosan polysulfate sodium (*Elmiron*) is used to coat or adhere to the bladder mucosal wall and protect it from irritation related to solutes in urine (Table 52.5).

Therapeutic Actions and Indications

Pentosan polysulfate sodium is a heparin-like compound that has anticoagulant and fibrinolytic effects. This drug adheres to the bladder wall mucosal membrane and acts as a buffer to control cell permeability, preventing irritating solutes in the urine from reaching the bladder wall cells (see Figure 52.1). It is used specifically to decrease the pain and discomfort associated with **interstitial cystitis**.

Pharmacokinetics

Very little of this drug is absorbed (3%). It is distributed to the GI tract, liver, spleen, skin, bone marrow, and periosteum. It undergoes metabolism in the liver and spleen and is excreted in urine. There are no adequate studies of the effects of pentosan during pregnancy or lactation. Use should be limited to those situations in which the benefit to the mother outweighs the potential risk to the fetus or neonate.

Contraindications and Cautions

Pentosan should not be used with any condition that involves an increased risk of bleeding (surgery, pregnancy, anticoagulation, hemophilia) *because of its heparin-like effects.* It is also contraindicated in the presence of a history of heparin-induced thrombocytopenia, *which could recur with use of this drug.*

Caution should be used in patients with hepatic or splenic dysfunction, *which could be affected by the heparin-like actions of the drug,* and in pregnant or lactating women *because of the potential for adverse effects on the fetus or neonate.*

Adverse Effects

Adverse effects associated with pentosan use include bleeding that may progress to hemorrhage (related to the drug's heparin effects), headache, alopecia (seen with heparin-type drugs), and GI disturbances related to local irritation of the GI tract with administration.

Clinically Important Drug–Drug Interactions

There is a potential for increased bleeding risks if this drug is combined with anticoagulants, aspirin, or nonsteroidal anti-inflammatory drugs. If such a combination is used, the patient should be monitored very closely for any signs of bleeding, and appropriate dosage adjustments should be made.

Nursing Considerations for Patients Receiving a Bladder Protectant

Assessment: History and Examination

Screen for the following conditions, *which could be cautions or contraindications to use of the drug:* history of allergy to this drug; history of bleeding abnormalities, splenic disorders, or hepatic dysfunction, *which could result in bleeding when combined with the heparin-like effect of this drug;* and pregnancy and lactation, *which require cautious use of this drug.*

Physical assessment should be initiated *to establish baseline data for assessing the effectiveness of the drug and the occurrence of any adverse effects associated with drug therapy.* Assess the following: skin, *to evaluate for the development of rash or hypersensitivity reactions;* orientation, affect, and reflexes, *to establish a baseline to evaluate CNS effects of the drug;* and liver function tests and bleeding times, *to establish a baseline to monitor safe use of the drug and the occurrence of adverse effects.*

Nursing Diagnoses

The patient receiving a bladder protectant may have the following nursing diagnoses related to drug therapy:

- Ineffective Tissue Perfusion related to bleeding secondary to heparin effects of the drug

Table 52.5 DRUGS IN FOCUS

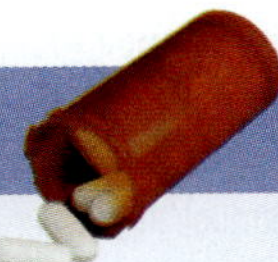

Bladder Protectant

Drug Name	Usual Dosage	Usual Indications
pentosan polysulfate sodium (*Elmiron*)	100 mg PO t.i.d.	Relief of bladder pain or discomfort associated with interstitial cystitis

- Acute Pain related to headache, CNS effects, and GI effects of the drug
- Risk for Injury related to bleeding and CNS effects
- Deficient Knowledge regarding drug therapy

Implementation With Rationale

- Establish the presence of interstitial cystitis by biopsy or cystoscopy before beginning therapy *to ensure that appropriate therapy is being used.*
- Administer the drug on an empty stomach, 1 hour before or 2 hours after meals, *to relieve GI discomfort and improve absorption.*
- Monitor bleeding times periodically during therapy *to assess for excessive heparin effect.*
- Arrange for a wig or appropriate head covering *if alopecia develops as a result of drug therapy.*
- Provide thorough patient teaching, including the drug name and prescribed dosage, measures to help avoid adverse effects, warning signs that may indicate problems, and the need for periodic monitoring and evaluation, *to enhance patient knowledge about drug therapy and to promote compliance.*

Evaluation

- Monitor patient response to the drug (relief of bladder pain and discomfort).
- Monitor for adverse effects (skin evaluation, GI upset and complaints, headache, bleeding time).
- Evaluate the effectiveness of the teaching plan (patient can name drug, dosage, adverse effects to watch for, specific measures to avoid adverse effects).
- Monitor the effectiveness of comfort measures and compliance with the regimen.

Drugs for Treating Benign Prostatic Hyperplasia

Two types of drugs are currently used to relieve the symptoms of **benign prostatic hyperplasia (BPH)**, which is also called benign prostatic hypertrophy or enlarged prostate (Table 52.6). Alpha-adrenergic blockers doxazosin (*Cardura*), tamsulosin (*Flomax*), alfuzosin (*Uroxatral*), and terazosin (*Hytrin*) are used to block the dilation of arterioles in the bladder and urinary tract. Tamsulosin was developed specifically for the treatment of BPH and is not associated with as many adverse adrenergic-blocking effects as the other agents. Finasteride (*Proscar*) is specifically used to treat BPH by blocking testosterone production and is associated with more androgen-blocking effects than the other drugs are. Dutasteride (*Avodart*) is the newest androgen hormone inhibitor used to treat BPH. (Box 52.2 discusses an alternative therapy used to treat BPH.)

Therapeutic Actions and Indications

BPH is a common problem in men, and it increases in incidence with age. This enlargement of the gland surrounding the urethra leads to discomfort, difficulty in initiating a stream of urine, feelings of bloating, and an increased incidence of cystitis. Alpha-adrenergic blockers are indicated for the treatment of symptomatic BPH. These drugs block postsynaptic alpha$_1$-adrenergic receptors, which results in a dilation of arterioles and veins and a relaxation of sympathetic effects on the bladder and urinary tract. These drugs are also indicated for treating hypertension (see Chapter 43).

Finasteride and dutasteride inhibit the intracellular enzyme that converts testosterone to a potent androgen dihydrotestosterone (DHT), which the prostate gland depends on for its development and maintenance (see Figure 52.1). They are used for long-term therapy to shrink the prostate and relieve the symptoms of hyperplasia. Finasteride (*Propecia*)

Table 52.6 DRUGS IN FOCUS

Drugs Used to Treat Benign Prostatic Hyperplasia (BPH)

Drug Name	Usual Dosage	Usual Indications
alfuzosin (*Uroxatral*)	10 mg/day PO, take after the same meal each day	Relief of symptoms of BPH
P doxazosin (*Cardura*)	1 mg PO daily with titration up to 8 mg/day if needed; not for use in children	Relief of symptoms of BPH; hypertension
dutasteride (*Avodart*)	0.5 mg/day PO	Treatment of symptomatic BPH
finasteride (*Proscar, Propecia*)	5 mg/day PO for BPH, 1 mg/day PO for male pattern baldness (*Propecia*)	Relief of symptoms of BPH; prevention of male-pattern baldness
tamsulosin (*Flomax*)	0.4–0.8 mg/day PO, 30 min after the same meal each day	Treatment of BPH
terazosin (*Hytrin*)	1–20 mg/day PO based on patient response	Relief of symptoms of BPH; hypertension

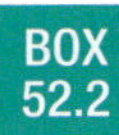

BOX 52.2 HERBAL AND ALTERNATIVE THERAPIES

Saw palmetto is an herbal therapy that has been used very successfully for the relief of symptoms associated with BPH. Patients with BPH should be cautioned not to combine saw palmetto with finasteride because serious toxicity can occur. Patients should also be cautioned that random studies of various saw palmetto products have shown a huge variation in contents and activity of the tablets. If patients choose to use this alternative therapy, they should be cautioned to check products carefully and to avoid switching products once they have success with one.

is also used to prevent male pattern baldness in patients with a strong family history.

When any of these drugs are used, it is important to make sure that the prostate enlargement is benign and not caused by cancer, infection, stricture, or hypotonic bladder. Patients receiving long-term therapy need to be reassessed periodically.

Pharmacokinetics

The alpha$_1$-selective adrenergic blocking agents are well absorbed and undergo extensive hepatic metabolism. Therefore, they must be used with caution in patients with hepatic impairment. They are excreted in urine. Finasteride and dutasteride are rapidly absorbed from the GI tract, undergo hepatic metabolism, and are excreted in feces and urine. They have no indications for women and are rated pregnancy category X because of androgen effects. Women must be cautioned not to touch finasteride or dutasteride because of the risk of absorption through the skin.

Contraindications and Cautions

These drugs are contraindicated in patients who are allergic to the drugs. Caution should be used in patients with hepatic or renal dysfunction, *which could alter the metabolism and excretion of the drugs.* The adrenergic blockers should be used with caution in patients with congestive heart failure or known coronary disease.

Adverse Effects

Adverse effects of alpha-adrenergic blockers include headache, fatigue, dizziness, postural dizziness, lethargy, tachycardia, hypotension, GI upset, and sexual dysfunction, all of which are effects seen with blockade of the alpha receptors. Finasteride and dutasteride are associated with decreased libido, impotence, and sexual dysfunction, all of which are related to decreased levels of DHT. Patients using either of these drugs cannot donate blood for 6 months after the last dose to protect potential blood recipients.

Clinically Important Drug–Drug Interactions

There is a possibility of decreased theophylline levels if it is combined with these drugs. The patient should be monitored and appropriate dosage adjustments made if this combination is used.

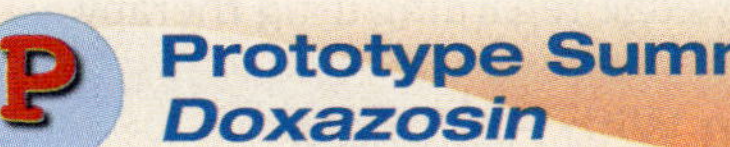

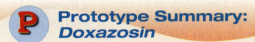

Prototype Summary: *Doxazosin*

Indications: Treatment of benign prostatic hypertrophy

Actions: Blocks postsynaptic alpha$_1$-adrenergic receptors, which results in a dilation of arterioles and veins and a relaxation of sympathetic effects on the bladder and urinary tract.

Pharmacokinetics:

Route	Onset	Peak
Oral	Varies	2–3 h

$T_{1/2}$: 22 hours; metabolized in the liver and excreted in urine, bile, and feces

Adverse effects: Headache, fatigue, dizziness, postural dizziness, lethargy, vertigo, tachycardia, palpitations, nausea, dyspepsia, diarrhea, sexual dysfunction, rash

Nursing Considerations for Patients Receiving Drugs to Treat Benign Prostatic Hypertrophy

Assessment: History and Examination

Screen for the following conditions, *which could be cautions or contraindications to the use of the drug:* history of allergy to this drug; history of congestive heart failure; and renal or hepatic failure, *which would require caution when using these drugs.*

Physical assessment should be done *to establish baseline data for assessing the effectiveness of the drug and the occurrence of any adverse effects associated with drug therapy.* Assess the following: skin, *to evaluate for the development of rash or hypersensitivity reactions;* blood pressure, pulse, auscultation, and perfusion, *to evaluate the cardiovascular effects of alpha-adrenergic blockade;* urinalysis and normal urinary function; prostate palpation; and appropriate tests, including prostate-specific antigen (PSA) levels, *to evaluate prostate problems.*

Nursing Diagnoses

The patient receiving a drug to treat BPH may have the following nursing diagnoses related to drug therapy:

- Sexual Dysfunction related to drug effects
- Acute Pain related to headache, CNS effects, and GI effects of the drug
- Deficient Knowledge regarding drug therapy

Implementation With Rationale

- Determine the presence of BPH and periodically evaluate through prostate examination and measurement of PSA levels *to reconfirm that no other problem is occurring.*
- Administer the drug without regard to meals, but give with meals *if GI upset is a problem.*
- Provide thorough patient teaching, including the drug name and prescribed dosage, measures to help avoid adverse effects, warning signs that may indicate problems, and the need for periodic monitoring and evaluation, *to enhance patient knowledge about drug therapy and to promote compliance.*
- Offer support and encouragement *to help the patient cope with potential decreases in sexual functioning.*

Evaluation

- Monitor patient response to the drug (relief of signs and symptoms of BPH, improved urine flow, decrease in discomfort).
- Monitor for adverse effects (skin evaluation, GI upset and complaints, headache, cardiovascular effects).
- Evaluate the effectiveness of the teaching plan (patient can name drug, dosage, adverse effects to watch for, specific measures to avoid adverse effects).
- Monitor the effectiveness of comfort measures and compliance with the regimen.

WEB LINKS

Health care providers and patients may want to consult the following Internet sources:

http://www.pslgroup.com/ENLARGPROST.HTM Information on benign prostatic hyperplasia (BPH), support groups, research, and treatment for patients.

http://www.uro.com/bph.htm Information on BPH research and medical information.

http://www.nlm.nih.gov/medlineplus/ency/article/000754.htm Information on neurogenic bladder.

http://www.ichelp.org Information on interstitial cystitis.

http://search.nlm.nih.gov/medlineplus/interstitialcystitis.html Information on interstitial cystitis—research, prevention, treatment, and pathology.

Points to Remember

- Acute urinary tract infections (UTIs) are second in frequency to respiratory tract infections in the American population.
- Urinary tract anti-infectives are drugs used to kill bacteria in the urinary tract by producing an acidic urine, which is undesirable to bacteria growth, or by acting to destroy bacteria in the urinary tract.
- Many activities are necessary to help decrease the bacteria in the urinary tract (e.g., hygiene measures, proper diet, forcing fluids), to facilitate the treatment of UTIs and help the urinary tract anti-infectives be more effective.
- Inflammation and irritation of the urinary tract can cause smooth muscle spasms along the urinary tract. These spasms lead to the uncomfortable effects of dysuria, urgency, incontinence, nocturia, and suprapubic pain.
- The urinary tract antispasmodics act to relieve spasms of the urinary tract muscles by blocking parasympathetic activity and relaxing the detrusor and other urinary tract muscles.
- The urinary tract analgesic phenazopyridine is used to provide relief of symptoms (burning, urgency, frequency, pain, discomfort) related to urinary tract irritation resulting from infection, trauma, or surgery.
- Pentosan polysulfate sodium is a heparin-like compound that has anticoagulant and fibrinolytic effects and adheres to the bladder wall mucosal membrane to act as a buffer to control cell permeability. This action prevents irritating solutes in the urine from reaching the cells of the bladder wall. It is used specifically to decrease the pain and discomfort associated with interstitial cystitis.
- Benign prostatic hyperplasia (BPH) is a common enlargement of the prostate gland in older men.
- Drugs frequently used to relieve the signs and symptoms of prostate enlargement include alpha-adrenergic blockers, which relax the sympathetic effects on the bladder and sphincters, and finasteride, which blocks the body's production of a powerful androgen. The prostate is dependent on testosterone for its maintenance and development; blocking the androgen leads to shrinkage of the gland and relief of symptoms.

CHECK YOUR UNDERSTANDING

Answers to the questions in this chapter may be found in the Answer Key in the back of the book.

Multiple Choice

Select the best answer to the following.

1. Methylene blue is a urinary tract anti-infective that acts by
   a. interfering with bacterial cell wall formation.
   b. interfering with bacterial cell division.
   c. alkalinizing the urine, which kills bacteria.
   d. acidifying the urine, which kills bacteria.

2. The antibiotic of choice for a patient with cystitis who has great difficulty following medical regimens would be
   a. cinoxacin.
   b. fosfomycin.
   c. nitrofurantoin.
   d. norfloxacin.

3. Urinary tract antispasmodics block the pain and discomfort associated with spasm in the smooth muscle of the urinary tract. The numerous adverse effects associated with these drugs are related to
   a. their blockade of sympathetic beta-receptors.
   b. their stimulation of cholinergic receptors.
   c. their stimulation of sympathetic receptors.
   d. their blockade of cholinergic receptors.

4. BPH is a very common diagnosis in older men. Two types of drugs have been developed to treat the signs and symptoms of this disorder:
   a. alpha-adrenergic blockers and anticholinergic drugs.
   b. alpha-adrenergic blockers and testosterone production blockers.
   c. anticholinergic drugs and adrenergic stimulators.
   d. testosterone production blockers and adrenal androgens.

5. The drug of choice for treatment of BPH in a man with known hypotension might be
   a. doxazosin.
   b. terazosin.
   c. tamsulosin.
   d. propranolol.

6. Before administering a drug for the treatment of BPH, the nurse should ensure that
   a. the patient has had a prostate examination and measurement of the PSA level.
   b. the patient has not had a vasectomy.
   c. the patient is still sexually active.
   d. the patient is hypertensive and will tolerate the blood pressure-lowering effects.

7. A male who is very concerned about his hair loss and who is being treated for BPH might prefer treatment with
   a. doxazosin.
   b. finasteride.
   c. tamsulosin.
   d. terazosin.

8. After bladder surgery, many patients experience burning, urgency, frequency, and pain related to the urinary tract irritation. Such patients would benefit from treatment with
   a. methylene blue.
   b. fosfomycin.
   c. phenazopyridine.
   d. flavoxate.

Multiple Response

Select all that apply.

1. In evaluating a client for the presence of a bladder infection, one would expect to find reports of which of the following?
   a. Frequency of urination
   b. Painful urination
   c. Edema of the fingers and hands
   d. Urgency of urination
   e. Feelings of abdominal bloating
   f. Itching, scaly skin

2. Important educational points for clients with cystitis would include which of the following?
   a. Avoidance of bubble baths
   b. Voiding immediately after sexual intercourse
   c. Always wiping from back to front
   d. Avoidance of foods high in alkaline ash
   e. Tight fluid restriction
   f. Always wiping from front to back

Web Exercise

H.H. and his wife are referred to you for teaching after a diagnosis of benign prostatic hyperplasia (BPH) is made on a routine physical. They do not understand the problem and are somewhat shy talking about it. Go to the Internet to get information for them about the disease, treatment, and research.

True or False

Indicate whether the following statements are true (T) or false (F).

_____ 1. Acute urinary tract infections are second in frequency to respiratory tract infections in the American population.

_____ 2. Urinary tract anti-infectives are used to kill bacteria in the urinary tract by producing alkaline urine or by destroying bacteria in the urinary tract.

_____ 3. There is nothing that can be done to help decrease the bacteria in the urinary tract.

_____ 4. Inflammation and irritation of the urinary tract can cause smooth muscle spasms, leading to the uncomfortable effects of dysuria, urgency, incontinence, nocturia, and suprapubic pain.

_____ 5. The urinary tract antispasmodics relieve spasms of the urinary tract muscles by blocking sympathetic activity.

_____ 6. Pentosan polysulfate sodium is a heparin-like compound that has anticoagulant and fibrinolytic effects and is used specifically to decrease the pain and discomfort associated with interstitial cystitis.

_____ 7. BPH is a rare condition that involves enlargement of the prostate gland in older males.

_____ 8. Drugs commonly used to relieve the signs and symptoms of prostate enlargement include alpha-adrenergic blockers, which relax the sympathetic effects on the bladder and sphincters, and finasteride and dutasteride, which block the body's production of a powerful androgen.

Bibliography and References

Drug facts and comparisons. (2006). St. Louis: Facts and Comparisons.

Gilman, A., Hardman, J. G., & Limbird, L. E. (Eds.). (2006). *Goodman and Gilman's the pharmacological basis of therapeutics* (11th ed.). New York: McGraw-Hill.

Karch, A. M. (2006). *2007 Lippincott's nursing drug guide.* Philadelphia: Lippincott Williams & Wilkins.

The medical letter on drugs and therapeutics. (2006). New Rochelle, NY: Medical Letter.

Porth, C. M. (2005). *Pathophysiology: Concepts of altered health states* (7th ed.). Philadelphia: Lippincott Williams & Wilkins.

Professional's guide to patient drug facts. (2006). St. Louis: Facts and Comparisons.

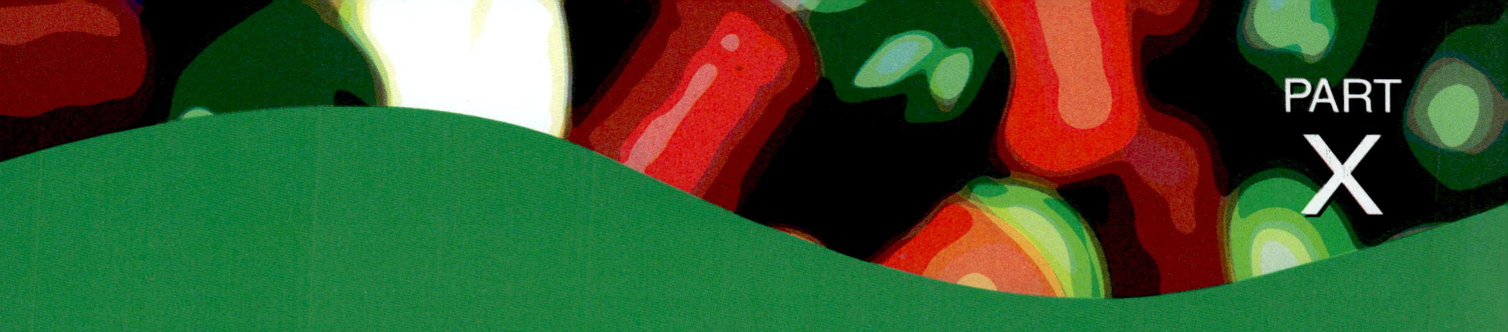

Drugs Acting on the Respiratory System

CHAPTER 53

Introduction to the Respiratory System

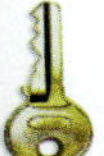

KEY TERMS

alveoli
asthma
bronchial tree
chronic obstructive pulmonary disease (COPD)
cilia
common cold
cough
cystic fibrosis
larynx
lower respiratory tract
pneumonia
respiration
respiratory distress syndrome (RDS)
respiratory membrane
seasonal rhinitis
sinuses
sinusitis
sneeze
surfactant
trachea
upper respiratory tract
ventilation

LEARNING OBJECTIVES

Upon completion of this chapter, you will be able to:

1. Describe the parts of the respiratory system and explain the role of each part in respiration.
2. Describe the process of respiration and give clinical examples of problems that can arise with alterations in the respiratory membrane.
3. Differentiate between the common conditions that affect the upper respiratory system.
4. Identify three conditions involving the lower respiratory tract, including the clinical presentations of these conditions.
5. Discuss the process involved in obstructive respiratory diseases and correlate this to the signs and symptoms of these diseases.

The respiratory system is essential for survival. It brings oxygen into the body, allowing for the exchange of gases and expelling carbon dioxide and other waste products. The normal functioning of the respiratory system depends on an intricate balance of the nervous, cardiovascular, and musculoskeletal systems. The respiratory system consists of two parts: the **upper respiratory tract** and the **lower respiratory tract**. The upper portion, or conducting airways, is composed of the nose, mouth, pharynx, larynx, trachea, and the upper **bronchial tree** (Figure 53.1). The lower portion is made up of the smallest bronchi and the **alveoli** (respiratory sacs), which make up the lungs.

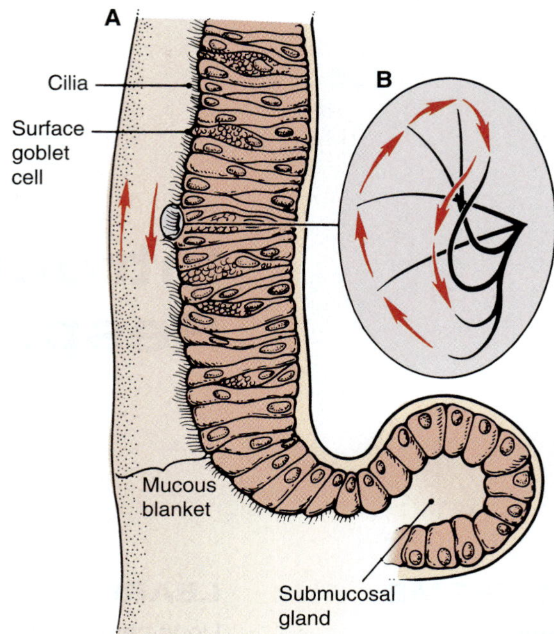

FIGURE 53.2 **(A)** The mucociliary escalator. **(B)** Conceptual scheme of ciliary movement, which allows forward motion to move the viscous gel layer and backward motion to occur entirely within the less viscous sol layer of the mucous blanket.

The Upper Respiratory Tract

Air usually moves into the body through the nose and into the nasal cavity. The nasal hairs catch and filter foreign substances that may be present in the inhaled air. The air is warmed and humidified as it passes by blood vessels close to the surface of the epithelial lining in the nasal cavity. The epithelial lining contains goblet cells that produce mucus, which traps dust, microorganisms, pollen, and any other foreign substances. The epithelial cells of this lining contain **cilia**—microscopic, hair-like projections of the cell membrane—which are constantly moving and directing the mucus and any trapped substances down toward the throat (Figure 53.2).

Pairs of **sinuses** (air-filled passages through the skull) open into the nasal cavity. Because the epithelial lining of the nasal passage is continuous with the lining of the sinuses, the mucus produced in the sinuses drains into the nasal cavity. From there, the mucus drains into the throat and is swallowed into the gastrointestinal tract, where stomach acid destroys foreign materials.

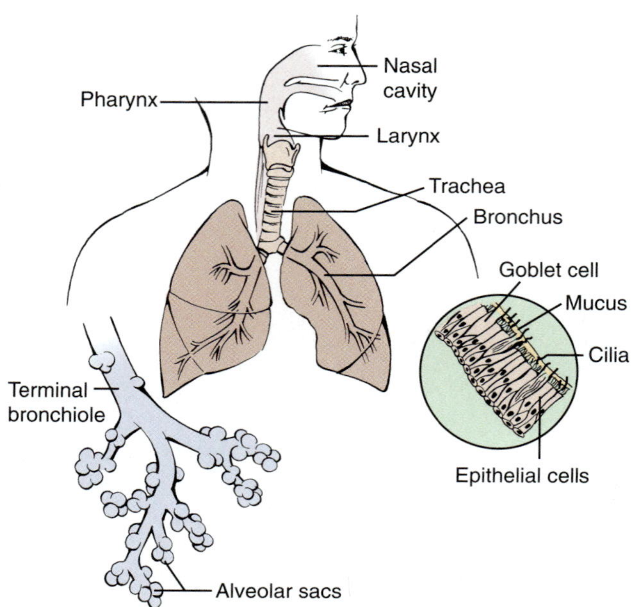

FIGURE 53.1 The respiratory tract.

Air moves from the nasal cavity into the pharynx and **larynx**. The larynx contains the vocal chords and the epiglottis, which close during swallowing to protect the lower respiratory tract from any foreign particles. From the larynx, air proceeds to the **trachea**, the main conducting airway into the lungs. The trachea bifurcates, or divides, into two main bronchi, which further divide into smaller and smaller branches. All of these tubes contain mucus-producing goblet cells and cilia to entrap any particles that may have escaped the upper protective mechanisms. The cilia in these tubes move the mucus up the trachea and into the throat, where again it is swallowed.

The bronchial tubes are composed of three layers: cartilage, muscle, and epithelial cells. The cartilage keeps the tube open and becomes progressively less abundant as the bronchi divide and get smaller. The muscles keep the bronchi open; the muscles in the bronchi become smaller and less abundant, with only a few muscle fibers remaining in the terminal bronchi and alveoli. The epithelial cells are very similar in structure and function to the epithelial cells in the nasal passage.

The walls of the trachea and conducting bronchi are highly sensitive to irritation. When receptors in the walls are stimulated, a central nervous system reflex is initiated and a **cough** results. The cough causes air to be pushed through the bronchial tree under tremendous pressure, cleaning out any foreign irritant. This reflex, along with the similar **sneeze** reflex (which is initiated by receptors in the nasal cavity), forces foreign materials directly out of the system, opening it for more efficient flow of gas.

Throughout the airways, many macrophage scavengers freely move about the epithelium and destroy invaders. Mast cells are present in abundance and release histamine, serotonin, adenosine triphosphate (ATP), and other chemicals to ensure a rapid and intense inflammatory reaction to any cell injury. The end result of these various defense mechanisms is that the lower respiratory tract is virtually sterile—an important protection against respiratory infection that could interfere with essential gas exchange.

The Lower Respiratory Tract

The lower respiratory tract (i.e., the respiratory airways) is composed of the smallest bronchioles and the alveoli (see Figure 53.1). These structures are the functional units of the lungs. Within the lungs are a network of bronchi, alveoli, and blood vessels. The lung tissue receives its blood supply from the bronchial artery, which branches directly off the aorta. The alveoli receive unoxygenated blood from the right ventricle via the pulmonary artery. The delivery of this blood to the alveoli is referred to as perfusion.

Gas exchange occurs in the alveoli. In this process, carbon dioxide is lost from the blood and oxygen is transferred to the blood. The exchange of gases at the alveolar level is called **ventilation**. The alveolar sac holds the gas, allowing needed oxygen to diffuse across the **respiratory membrane** into the capillary while carbon dioxide, which is more abundant in the capillary blood, diffuses across the membrane and enters the alveolar sac to be expired.

The respiratory membrane is made up of the capillary endothelium, the capillary basement membrane, the interstitial space, the alveolar basement membrane, the alveolar epithelium, and the surfactant layer (Figure 53.3). The sac is able to stay open because the surface tension of the cells is decreased by the lipoprotein **surfactant**. Absence of surfactant leads to alveolar collapse. Surfactant is produced by the type II cells in the alveoli. These cells have other metabolic functions, including the conversion of angiotensin I to angiotensin II, the degradation of serotonin, and possibly the metabolism of various hormones.

The oxygenated blood is returned to the left atrium via the pulmonary veins; from there it is pumped throughout the body to deliver oxygen to the cells and to pick up waste products.

Respiration

Respiration, or the act of breathing, is controlled by the central nervous system. The inspiratory muscles—diaphragm, external intercostals, and abdominal muscles—are stimulated to contract by the respiratory center in the medulla.

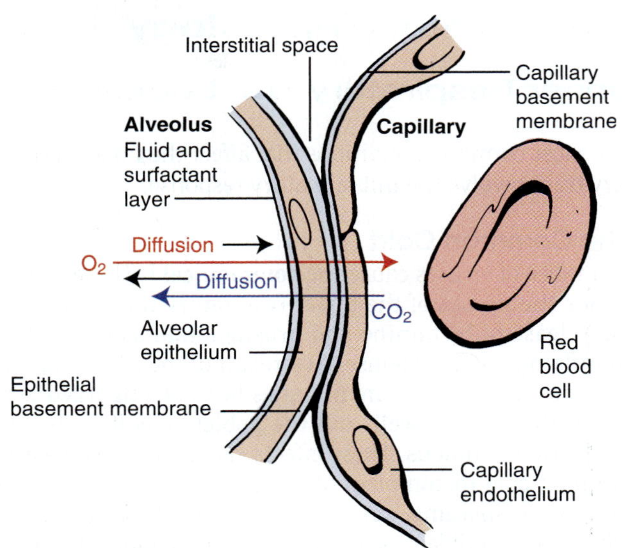

FIGURE 53.3 The respiratory membrane.

The medulla receives input from chemoreceptors (neuroreceptors sensitive to carbon dioxide and acid levels) and increases the rate and/or depth of respiration to maintain homeostasis in the body.

The vagus nerve, a predominantly parasympathetic nerve, plays a key role in stimulating diaphragm contraction and inspiration. Vagal stimulation also leads to a bronchoconstriction or tightening. The sympathetic system also innervates the respiratory system. Stimulation of the sympathetic system leads to increased rate and depth of respiration and dilation of the bronchi to allow freer flow of air through the system.

CONCEPTS in action ANIMATI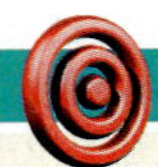N

FOCUS POINTS

- The respiratory system has two parts: the upper respiratory tract, or conducting airways, and the lower respiratory tract, or the alveoli, which make up the lungs.
- The hairs, mucus producing goblet cells, cilia, the superficial blood supply of the upper respiratory tract, and the cough and sneeze reflexes all work to protect the fragile alveoli and promote gas exchange.
- Gas exchange occurs across the respiratory membrane in the alveolar sac. The alveoli produce surfactant, which reduces surface tension among other functions.
- The medulla controls respiration, which depends on a functioning muscular system and a balance between the sympathetic and parasympathetic systems.

Respiratory Pathology

Upper Respiratory Tract Conditions

The most common conditions that affect the upper respiratory tract involve the inflammatory response.

The Common Cold

A number of viruses cause the **common cold**. These viruses invade the tissues of the upper respiratory tract, initiating the release of histamine and prostaglandins and causing an inflammatory response. As a result of the inflammatory response, the mucous membranes become engorged with blood, the tissues swell, and the goblet cells increase the production of mucus. These effects cause the person with a common cold to complain of sinus pain, nasal congestion, runny nose, sneezing, watery eyes, scratchy throat, and headache. In susceptible people, this swelling can block the outlet of the eustachian tube, which drains the inner ear and equalizes pressure across the tympanic membrane. If this outlet becomes blocked, feelings of ear stuffiness and pain can occur, and the individual is more likely to develop an ear infection (otitis media).

Seasonal Rhinitis

A similar condition that afflicts many people is allergic or **seasonal rhinitis** (an inflammation of the nasal cavity), commonly called hay fever. This condition occurs when the upper airways respond to a specific antigen (e.g., pollen, mold, dust) with a vigorous inflammatory response, resulting again in nasal congestion, sneezing, stuffiness, and watery eyes.

Sinusitis

Other areas of the upper respiratory tract can become irritated or infected, with a resultant inflammation of that particular area. **Sinusitis** occurs when the epithelial lining of the sinus cavities becomes inflamed. The resultant swelling often causes severe pain because the bony cavity cannot stretch, and the swollen tissue pushes against the bone and blocks the sinus passage. The danger of a sinus infection is that, if it is left untreated, microorganisms can move up the sinus passages and into brain tissue.

Pharyngitis and Laryngitis

Pharyngitis and laryngitis are infections of the pharynx and larynx, respectively. These infections are frequently caused by common bacteria or viruses. Pharyngitis and laryngitis are frequently seen with influenza, which is caused by a variety of different viruses and produces uncomfortable respiratory symptoms or other inflammations along with a fever, muscle aches and pains, and malaise.

Lower Respiratory Tract Conditions

A number of disorders affect the lower respiratory tract, including atelectasis, **pneumonia** (bacterial, viral, or aspiration), bronchitis or inflammation of the bronchi (acute and chronic), bronchiectasis, and the obstructive disorders—**asthma**, chronic obstructive pulmonary disease (COPD), cystic fibrosis, and respiratory distress syndrome (RDS). Tuberculosis, discussed in Chapter 9, is a bacterial infection. Once known as consumption, this disease has been responsible for many respiratory deaths throughout the centuries. All of these disorders involve, to some degree, an alteration in the ability to move gases in and out of the respiratory system.

Atelectasis

Atelectasis, the collapse of once-expanded lung tissue, can occur as a result of outside pressure against the alveoli—for example, from a pulmonary tumor, a pneumothorax (air in the pleural space exerting high pressure against the alveoli), or a pleural effusion. Atelectasis most commonly occurs as a result of airway blockage, which prevents air from entering the alveoli, keeping the lung expanded. This occurs when a mucous plug, edema of the bronchioles, or a collection of pus or secretions occludes the airway and prevents the movement of air. Patients may experience atelectasis after surgery, when the effects of anesthesia, pain, and decreased coughing reflexes can lead to a decreased tidal volume and accumulation of secretions in the lower airways. Patients may present with rales, dyspnea, fever, cough, hypoxia, and changes in chest wall movement. Treatment may involve clearing the airways, delivering oxygen, and assisting ventilation. In the case of a pneumothorax, treatment would also involve insertion of a chest tube to restore the negative pressure to the space between the pleura.

Pneumonia

Pneumonia is an inflammation of the lungs caused either by bacterial or viral invasion of the tissue or by aspiration of foreign substances into the lower respiratory tract. The rapid inflammatory response to any foreign presence in the lower respiratory tract leads to a localized swelling, engorgement, and exudation of protective sera. The respiratory membrane is affected, resulting in decreased gas exchange. Patients complain of difficulty breathing and fatigue, and they present with fever, noisy breath sounds, and poor oxygenation.

Bronchitis

Acute bronchitis occurs when bacteria, viruses, or foreign materials infect the inner layer of the bronchi. The person with bronchitis may have a narrowed airway during the inflammation; this condition can be very serious in a person with obstructed or narrowed airflow. Chronic bronchitis is an inflammation of the bronchi that does not clear.

Bronchiectasis

Bronchiectasis is a chronic disease that involves the bronchi and bronchioles. It is characterized by dilation of the bronchial tree and chronic infection and inflammation of the bronchial passages. With chronic inflammation, the bronchial epithelial cells are replaced by a fibrous scar tissue. The loss of the protective mucus and ciliary movement of the epithelial cell membranes, combined with the dilation of the bronchial tree, leads to chronic infections in the now unprotected lower areas of the lung tissue. Patients with bronchiectasis often have an underlying medical condition that makes them more susceptible to infections (e.g., immune suppression, acquired immune deficiency syndrome, chronic inflammatory conditions). Patients present with the signs and symptoms of acute infection, including fever, malaise, myalgia, arthralgia, and a purulent, productive cough.

Obstructive Pulmonary Diseases

As noted previously, the obstructive pulmonary diseases include asthma, cystic fibrosis, COPD, and RDS.

Asthma

Asthma is characterized by reversible bronchospasm, inflammation, and hyperactive airways (Figure 53.4). The hyperactivity is triggered by allergens or nonallergic inhaled irritants or by factors such as exercise and emotions. The triggers cause an immediate release of histamine, which results in bronchospasm in about 10 minutes. The later response (3 to 5 hours) is cytokine-mediated inflammation, mucus production, and edema contributing to obstruction. Appropriate treatment depends on understanding the early and late responses. The extreme case of asthma is called status asthmaticus; this is a life-threatening bronchospasm that does not respond to usual treatment and occludes air flow into the lungs.

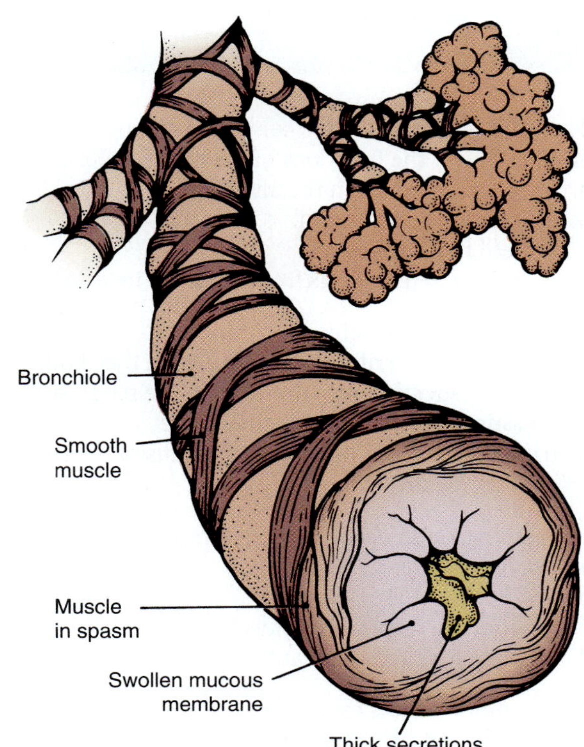

FIGURE 53.4 Asthma. The bronchiole is obstructed on expiration, particularly by muscle spasm, edema of the mucosa, and thick secretions.

Chronic Obstructive Pulmonary Disease (COPD)

Chronic obstructive pulmonary disease (COPD) is a permanent, chronic obstruction of airways, often related to cigarette smoking. It is caused by two related disorders, emphysema and chronic bronchitis, both of which result in airflow obstruction on expiration, as well as by overinflated lungs and poor gas exchange. Emphysema is characterized by loss of the elastic tissue of the lungs, destruction of alveolar walls, and a resultant hyperinflation and tendency to collapse with expiration. Chronic bronchitis is a permanent inflammation of the airways with mucus secretion, edema, and poor inflammatory defenses. Characteristics of both disorders often are present in the person with COPD (Figure 53.5).

Cystic Fibrosis

Cystic fibrosis is a hereditary disease that results in the accumulation of copious amounts of very thick secretions in the lungs. Eventually, the secretions obstruct the airways, leading to destruction of the lung tissue. Treatment is aimed at keeping the secretions fluid and moving and maintaining airway patency as much as possible.

Respiratory Distress Syndrome

Respiratory distress syndrome (RDS) is frequently seen in premature babies who are delivered before their lungs have fully developed and while surfactant levels are still very low. Surfactant is necessary for lowering the surface tension in the alveoli so that they can stay open to allow the flow of gases. Treatment is aimed at instilling surfactant to prevent atelectasis and to allow the lungs to expand. Adult respiratory distress syndrome (ARDS) is characterized by progressive loss of lung compliance and increasing hypoxia. This syndrome occurs as a result of a severe insult to the body, such as cardiovascular collapse, major burns, severe trauma,

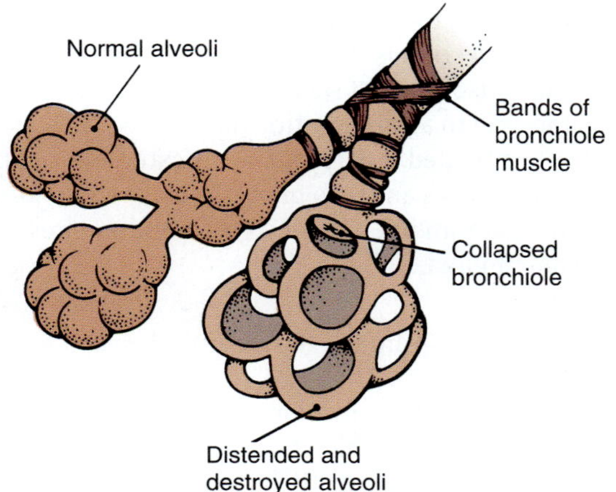

FIGURE 53.5 Distended and destroyed alveoli versus normal alveoli.

or rapid depressurization. Treatment of ARDS involves reversal of the underlying cause of the problem combined with ventilatory support.

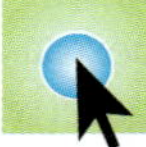

WEB LINK

To explore the virtual respiratory tract, refer to the following Internet source:
http://www.InnerBody.com

Points to Remember

- The respiratory system is composed of the upper respiratory tract, or conducting airways (nose, mouth, pharynx, larynx, trachea, and the bronchial tree), and the lower respiratory tract, containing alveoli (respiratory sacs), which make up the lungs.
- The respiratory system is essential for survival; it brings oxygen into the body, allowing for the exchange of gases (ventilation) and the expelling of carbon dioxide and other waste products.
- The upper airways have many features to protect the fragile alveoli: hairs filter the air; goblet cells produce mucus to trap material; cilia move the trapped material toward the throat for swallowing; the blood supply close to the surface warms the air and adds humidity to improve gas movement and gas exchange; and the cough and sneeze reflexes clear the airways.
- The alveolar sac is where gas exchange occurs across the respiratory membrane. The alveoli produce surfactant to decrease surface tension within the sac and have other metabolic functions.
- Respiration is controlled through the medulla in the central nervous system and depends on a balance between the sympathetic and parasympathetic systems and a functioning muscular system.
- Inflammation of the upper respiratory tract is seen in many uncomfortable disorders, including the common cold, seasonal rhinitis, sinusitis, pharyngitis, and laryngitis.
- Inflammation of the lower respiratory tract can result in serious disorders that interfere with gas exchange, including bronchitis and pneumonia.
- Obstructive disorders interfere with the ability to deliver gases to the alveoli because of obstructions in the conducting airways and eventually in the respiratory airways. These disorders include asthma, chronic obstructive pulmonary disease (COPD), cystic fibrosis, and respiratory distress syndrome (RDS).

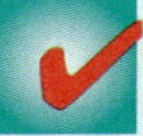

CHECK YOUR UNDERSTANDING

Answers to the questions in this chapter may be found in the Answer Key in the back of the book.

Multiple Choice

Select the best answer to the following.

1. Sinusitis needs to be taken very seriously. The danger of a sinus infection is that
   a. it can cause a loss of sleep and exhaustion.
   b. it can lead to a painful otitis media.
   c. if left untreated, microorganisms can move up the sinus passages and into brain tissue.
   d. drainage from infected sinus membranes often leads to pneumonia.

2. Diffusion of CO_2 from the tissues into the capillary blood
   a. occurs if the concentration of CO_2 in the tissues is greater than in the blood.
   b. decreases as blood acidity increases.
   c. increases in the absence of carbonic anhydrase.
   d. is accompanied by a decrease in plasma bicarbonate.

3. The walls of the alveoli are composed of type I and type II cells. One of the functions of the type II cells is
   a. to replace mucous in the alveoli.
   b. production of serotonin.
   c. secretion of surfactant.
   d. protection of the lungs from bacterial invasion.

4. A patient who coughs has
   a. inflammation irritating the sinuses in the skull
   b. irritants affecting receptor sites in the nasal cavity
   c. pressure against the eustachian tube
   d. irritation to receptor sites in the walls of the trachea, conducting bronchi

5. For respiration to occur, a person must have
   a. low levels of oxygen.
   b. low levels of CO_2.
   c. functioning inspiratory muscles.
   d. an actively functioning autonomic system.

6. The common cold is caused by
   a. bacteria that grow best in the cold.
   b. allergens in the environment.
   c. irritation of the delicate mucous membrane.
   d. a number of different viruses.

7. A patient with COPD would have
   a. a viral infection.
   b. loss of the protective respiratory mechanisms after prolonged irritation or damage.
   c. localized swelling and inflammation within the lungs.
   d. inflammation or swelling of the sinus membranes over a prolonged period.

Multiple Response

Select all that apply.

1. Inflammation of the upper respiratory tract usually causes which of the following?
   a. A runny nose
   b. Laryngitis
   c. Sneezing
   d. Hypoxia
   e. Rales
   f. Wheezing

2. In order for gas exchange to occur in the lungs, oxygen must pass through which of the following?
   a. 17 divisions of conducting airways
   b. The alveolar epithelium
   c. The pleural fluid
   d. The interstitial alveolar wall
   e. The capillary basement membrane
   f. The interstitial space

3. The nose performs which of the following functions in the respiratory system?
   a. Serves as a passageway for air movement
   b. Warms and humidifies the air
   c. Cleanses the air using hair fibers
   d. Stimulates surfactant release from the alveoli
   e. Initiates the cough reflex
   f. Initiates the sneeze reflex

Matching

Match the word with the appropriate definition.

1. ______________________ upper respiratory tract
2. ______________________ bronchial tree
3. ______________________ lower respiratory tract
4. ______________________ alveoli
5. ______________________ cilia
6. ______________________ sinuses
7. ______________________ larynx
8. ______________________ trachea
9. ______________________ cough
10. ______________________ ventilation
11. ______________________ respiratory membrane
12. ______________________ surfactant

A. Air-filled passages through the skull
B. The area where gas exchange takes place
C. The vocal chords and the epiglottis
D. The conducting airways leading into the alveoli
E. Microscopic hair-like projections of the epithelial cell membrane
F. The exchange of gases at the alveolar level
G. The main conducting airway leading into the lungs
H. Lipoprotein that reduces surface tension in the alveoli
I. The surface through which gas exchange must occur
J. The respiratory sacs
K. The nose, mouth, pharynx, larynx, trachea, and upper bronchial tree area through which gas exchange must be made
L. Reflex response in the respiratory membrane; results in forced air expelled through the mouth

Web Exercise

Your patient is asking you to explain the process that is occurring when he has a common cold. Why are his eyes red? Why is his nose runny? Why do his ears hurt? Go online and find information to prepare a teaching program about the common cold, including illustrations to help the patient understand what is going on in the body.

Bibliography and References

Ganong, W. (1999). *Review of medical physiology* (19th ed.). Norwalk, CT: Appleton & Lange.

Gilman, A., Hardman, J. G., & Limbird, L. E. (Eds.). (2006). *Goodman and Gilman's the pharmacological basis of therapeutics* (11th ed.). New York: McGraw-Hill.

Guyton, A., & Hall, J. (2004). *Textbook of medical physiology.* Philadelphia: W. B. Saunders.

Porth, C. M. (2005). *Pathophysiology: Concepts of altered health states* (7th ed.). Philadelphia: Lippincott Williams & Wilkins.

CHAPTER 54

Drugs Acting on the Upper Respiratory Tract

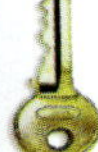

KEY TERMS

antihistamines
antitussives
decongestants
expectorants
mucolytics
rebound congestion
rhinitis medicamentosa

LEARNING OBJECTIVES

Upon completion of this chapter, you will be able to:

1. Outline the underlying physiological events that occur with upper respiratory disorders.
2. Describe the therapeutic actions, indications, pharmacokinetics, contraindications, most common adverse reactions, and important drug–drug interactions associated with antitussives, decongestants, topical nasal steroids, antihistamines, expectorants, and mucolytics.
3. Discuss the use of drugs that act on the upper respiratory tract across the lifespan.
4. Compare and contrast the prototype drugs dextromethorphan, ephedrine, flunisolide, diphenhydramine, guaifenesin, and acetylcysteine with other agents in their class and with other classes of drugs that act on the upper respiratory tract.
5. Outline the nursing considerations, including important teaching points, for patients receiving drugs acting on the upper respiratory tract.

ANTITUSSIVES

benzonatate
codeine
P dextromethorphan
hydrocodone

DECONGESTANTS

Topical Nasal Decongestants

P ephedrine
oxymetazoline
phenylephrine
tetrahydrozoline
xylometazoline

Oral Decongestants

pseudoephedrine

Topical Nasal Steroid Decongestants

beclomethasone
budesonide
dexamethasone
P flunisolide
fluticasone
triamcinolone

ANTIHISTAMINES

azelastine
brompheniramine
buclizine
cetirizine
chlorpheniramine
clemastine
cyclizine
cyproheptadine
desloratadine
dexchlorpheniramine
dimenhydrinate
P diphenhydramine
fexofenadine
hydroxyzine
loratadine
meclizine
promethazine

EXPECTORANT

P guaifenesin

MUCOLYTICS

P acetylcysteine
dornase alfa

Drugs that affect the respiratory system work to keep the airways open and gases moving efficiently. The classes discussed in this chapter mainly act on the upper respiratory tract and include the following:

- **Antitussives**, which block the cough reflex
- **Decongestants**, which decrease the blood flow to the upper respiratory tract and decrease the overproduction of secretions
- **Antihistamines**, which block the release or action of histamine, a chemical released during inflammation that increases secretions and narrows airways
- **Expectorants**, which increase productive cough to clear the airways
- **Mucolytics**, which increase or liquefy respiratory secretions to aid the clearing of the airways

Figure 54.1 displays the sites of action of these drugs. Box 54.1 discusses the use of these agents in various age groups.

Antitussives

Antitussives are drugs that suppress the cough reflex. Many disorders of the respiratory tract, including the common cold, sinusitis, pharyngitis, and pneumonia, are accompanied by an uncomfortable, unproductive cough. Persistent coughing can be exhausting and can cause muscle strain and further irritation of the respiratory tract. A cough that occurs without the presence of any active disease process or persists after treatment may be a symptom of another disease process and should be investigated before any medication is given to alleviate it.

Therapeutic Actions and Indications

The traditional antitussives (Table 54.1), including codeine (generic only), hydrocodone (*Hycodan*), and dextromethorphan (*Benylin* and many others), act directly on the medullary cough center of the brain to depress the cough reflex. Because they are centrally acting, they are not the drugs of choice for anyone who has a head injury or who could be impaired by central nervous system (CNS) depression. These drugs are rapidly absorbed, metabolized in the liver, and excreted in the urine. They cross the placenta and enter breast milk and should not be used during pregnancy or lactation because of the potential for CNS depressive effects on the fetus or neonate.

Other antitussives have a direct effect on the respiratory tract. Benzonatate (*Tessalon*) acts as a local anesthetic on the respiratory passages, lungs, and pleurae, blocking the effectiveness of the stretch receptors that stimulate a cough reflex. This drug is metabolized in the liver and excreted in the urine. It should be avoided in pregnancy and lactation because of the potential for adverse effects on the fetus or

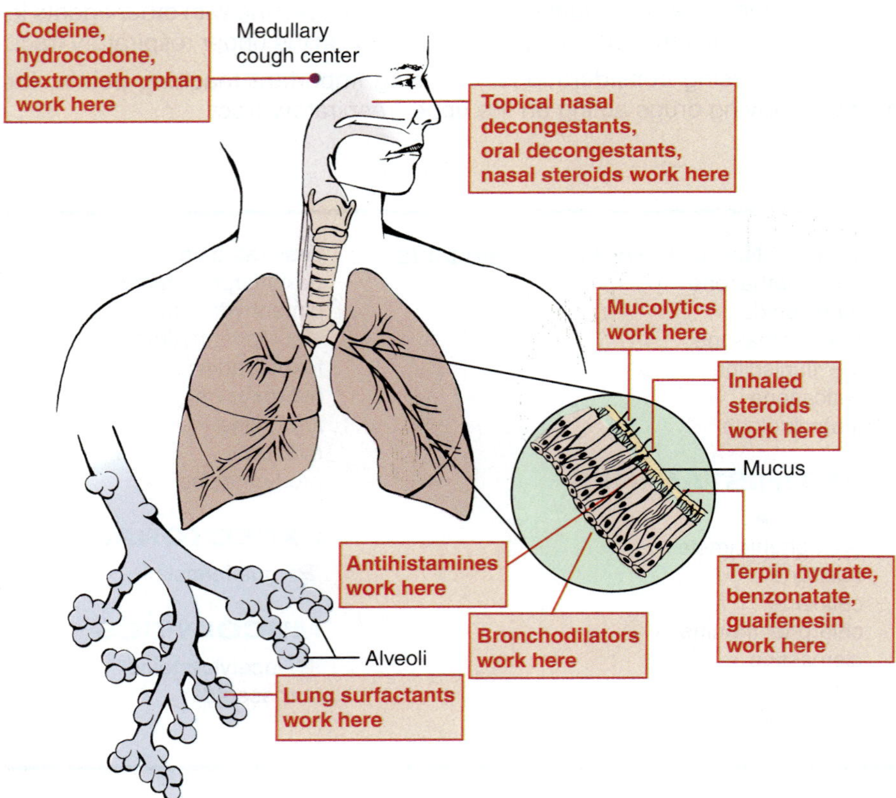

FIGURE 54.1 Sites of action of drugs acting on the upper respiratory tract.

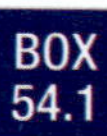

BOX 54.1 **DRUG THERAPY ACROSS THE LIFESPAN**

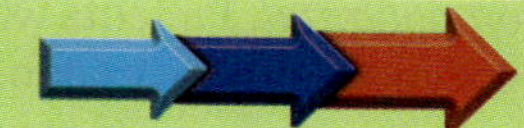

Upper Respiratory Tract Agents

CHILDREN

These drugs are used frequently with children. Most of these agents have established pediatric guidelines. Care must be taken when these drugs are used with children because the risk of adverse effects—including sedation, confusion, and dizziness—are more common with children.

Because many of these agents are available in over-the-counter (OTC) cold, flu, and allergy remedies, it is very important to educate parents about reading labels and following dosing guidelines to avoid potentially serious accidental overdose. Parents should always be asked specifically whether they are giving the child an OTC or herbal remedy.

Parents should also be encouraged to implement nondrug measures to help the child cope with the upper respiratory problem—drink plenty of fluids, use a humidifier, avoid smoke-filled areas, avoid contact with known allergens or irritants, and wash hands frequently during the cold and flu season.

ADULTS

Adults may inadvertently overdose on these agents when taking multiple OTC preparations to help them get through the misery of a cold or flu. They need to be questioned specifically about the use of OTC or herbal remedies before any of these drugs are advised or administered. Adults can also be encouraged to use nondrug measures to help them cope with the signs and symptoms.

The safety for the use of these drugs during pregnancy and lactation has not been established. There is a potential for adverse effects on the fetus related to blood flow changes and direct drug effects when the drugs cross the placenta. The drugs may enter breast milk and also may alter fluid balance and milk production. It is advised that caution be used if one of these drugs is prescribed during lactation.

OLDER ADULTS

Older adults frequently are prescribed one of these drugs. Older adults are more likely to develop adverse effects associated with the use of these drugs, including sedation, confusion, and dizziness. Safety measures may be needed if these effects occur and interfere with the patient's mobility and balance.

Older adults are also more likely to have renal and/or hepatic impairment related to underlying medical conditions, which could interfere with the metabolism and excretion of these drugs. The dosage for older adults should be started at a lower level than recommended for younger adults. The patient should be monitored very closely, and dosage adjustment should be based on the patient's response.

These patients also need to be alerted to the potential for toxic effects when using OTC preparations and should be advised to check with their health care provider before beginning any OTC drug regimen.

baby. All of these drugs are indicated for the treatment of nonproductive cough.

Contraindications and Cautions

Antitussives are contraindicated in patients who need to cough to maintain the airways (e.g., postoperative patients and those who have undergone abdominal or thoracic surgery). Careful use is recommended for patients with asthma and emphysema *because cough suppression in these patients could lead to an accumulation of secretions and a loss of respiratory reserve.* Caution should also be used in patients who are hypersensitive to or have a history of addiction to narcotics (codeine, hydrocodone). *Codeine is a narcotic and has*

Table 54.1 DRUGS IN FOCUS

Antitussives

Drug Name	Usual Dosage	Usual Indications
benzonatate (*Tessalon*)	Adult and pediatric (>10 yr): 100–200 mg PO t.i.d.	All of the antitussives are indicated for treatment of nonproductive cough
codeine (*generic*)	Adult: 10–20 mg PO q4–6h Pediatric (6–12 yr): 5–10 mg PO q4–6h Pediatric (2–6 yr): 2.5–5 mg PO q4–6h	
P dextromethorphan (*Benylin* and others)	Adult: 10–30 mg PO q4–8h; 60 mg PO b.i.d. for sustained action Pediatric (6–12 yr): 5–10 mg PO q4h; 30 mg PO b.i.d. for sustained action Pediatric (2–6 yr): 2.5–7.5 mg PO q4–8h; 15 mg PO b.i.d. for sustained action	
hydrocodone (*Hycodan*)	Adult: 5–10 mg PO q4–6h Pediatric (2–12 yr): 1.25–5 mg PO q4–6h	

addiction potential. Patients who need to drive or to be alert should use codeine, hydrocodone, and dextromethorphan with extreme caution *because these drugs can cause sedation and drowsiness.*

Adverse Effects

Traditional antitussives have a drying effect on the mucous membranes and can increase the viscosity of respiratory tract secretions. Because they affect centers in the brain, these antitussives are associated with CNS adverse effects, including drowsiness and sedation. Their drying effect can lead to nausea, constipation, and complaints of dry mouth. The locally acting antitussives are associated with gastrointestinal (GI) upset, headache, feelings of congestion, and sometimes dizziness.

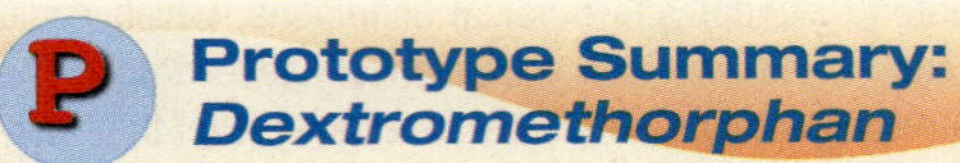

Prototype Summary: Dextromethorphan

Indications: Control of nonproductive cough

Actions: Depresses the cough center in the medulla to control cough spasms

Pharmacokinetics:

Route	Onset	Peak	Duration
Oral	25–30 min	2 h	3–6 h

$T_{1/2}$: 2–4 hours; metabolized in the liver and excreted in urine

Adverse effects: Dizziness, respiratory depression, dry mouth

Nursing Considerations for Patients Receiving Antitussives

Assessment: History and Examination

Screen for the following conditions, *which could be cautions or contraindications to use of the drug:* any history of allergy to any component of the drug or drug vehicle; cough that persists longer than 1 week or is accompanied by other signs and symptoms; and pregnancy or lactation.

Physical assessment should be done *to establish baseline data for assessing the effectiveness of the drug and the occurrence of any adverse effects associated with drug therapy.* Assess the following: temperature, *to evaluate for possible underlying infection;* respirations and adventitious sounds, *to assess drug effectiveness and to monitor for accumulation of secretions;* and orientation and affect, *to monitor for CNS effects of the drug.*

Nursing Diagnoses

The patient receiving an antitussive may have the following nursing diagnoses related to drug therapy:

- Ineffective Airway Clearance related to excessive drug effects
- Disturbed Sensory Perception related to CNS effects
- Deficient Knowledge regarding drug therapy

Implementation With Rationale

- Ensure that the drug is not taken any longer than recommended *to prevent serious adverse effects and increased respiratory tract problems.*
- Arrange for further medical evaluation for coughs that persist or are accompanied by high fever, rash, or excessive secretions *to detect the underlying cause of the cough and to arrange for appropriate treatment of the underlying problem.*
- Provide other measures *to help relieve cough* (e.g., humidity, cool temperatures, fluids, use of topical lozenges) as appropriate.
- Provide thorough patient teaching, including the drug name and prescribed dosage, measures to help avoid adverse effects, warning signs that may indicate problems, and the need for periodic monitoring and evaluation, *to enhance patient knowledge about drug therapy and to promote compliance.*
- Offer support and encouragement *to help the patient cope with the disease and the drug regimen.*

Evaluation

- Monitor patient response to the drug (control of nonproductive cough).
- Monitor for adverse effects (respiratory depression, dizziness, sedation).
- Evaluate the effectiveness of the teaching plan (patient can name drug, dosage, adverse effects to watch for, specific measures to avoid adverse effects, measures to take to increase the effectiveness of the drug).
- Monitor effectiveness of other measures to relieve cough.

Decongestants

Decongestants are drugs, usually adrenergics or sympathomimetics, that cause local vasoconstriction and therefore decrease the blood flow to the irritated and dilated capillaries of the mucous membranes lining the nasal passages and sinus cavities. This vasoconstriction leads to a shrinking of swollen membranes and tends to open clogged nasal passages, providing relief from the discomfort of a blocked nose and promoting drainage of secretions and improved air flow. An adverse effect that accompanies frequent or prolonged use of these drugs is a rebound congestion, officially called **rhinitis medicamentosa**. The reflex reaction to vasoconstriction is a rebound vasodilation, which often leads to prolonged overuse of decongestants.

Topical steroids are also used as decongestants. Topical steroids act to directly block the effects of inflammation on the nasal mucous membranes. This blocks the swelling, congestion, and increased secretions that accompany inflammation. The end result is an opening of the nasal passages and an increase in air flow. These drugs take several weeks to be really effective and are more often used in cases of chronic rhinitis.

Topical Nasal Decongestants

The topical nasal decongestants include ephedrine (*Pretz-D*), oxymetazoline (*Afrin, Allerest,* and others), phenylephrine (*Coricidin* and many others), tetrahydrozoline (*Tyzine*), and xylometazoline (*Otrivin*) (Table 54.2). Many of these are available as over-the-counter (OTC) preparations. The choice of a topical nasal decongestant is individual. Some patients may have no response to one and respond very well to another.

Therapeutic Actions and Indications

Topical decongestants are sympathomimetics, meaning that they imitate the effects of the sympathetic nervous system to cause vasoconstriction, leading to decreased edema and inflammation of the nasal membranes. Because these drugs are applied topically, the onset of action is almost immediate and there is less chance of systemic effects. They are available as nasal sprays that are used to relieve the discomfort of nasal congestion that accompanies the common cold, sinusitis, and allergic rhinitis. These drugs can also be used when dilation of the nares is desired to facilitate medical examination or to relieve the pain and congestion of otitis media. Opening the nasal passage allows better drainage of the eustachian tube, relieving pressure in the middle ear.

Pharmacokinetics

Although they are not generally absorbed systemically, any portion of these topical decongestants that is absorbed is metabolized in the liver and excreted in urine. There are no studies regarding the effects of these topical drugs in pregnancy or lactation. As with any drug used during pregnancy or lactation, caution should be used.

Contraindications and Cautions

Caution should be used when there is any lesion or erosion in the mucous membranes *that could lead to systemic absorption.* Caution should also be used in patients with any condition that might be exacerbated by sympathetic activity, such as glaucoma, hypertension, diabetes, thyroid disease, coronary disease, or prostate problems, *because these agents have adrenergic properties.*

Adverse Effects

Adverse effects associated with topical decongestants include local stinging and burning, which may occur the first few times the drug is used. If the sensation does not pass, the drug should be discontinued, because it may indicate lesions or erosion of the mucous membranes. Use for longer than 3 to 5 days can lead to a rebound congestion. (**Rebound congestion** occurs when the nasal passages become congested

Table 54.2 DRUGS IN FOCUS

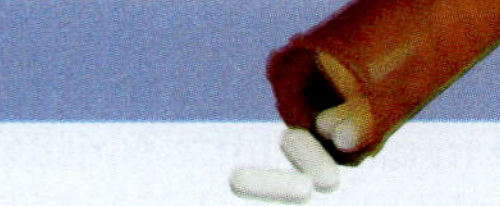

Topical Nasal Decongestants

Drug Name	Usual Dosage	Usual Indications
P ephedrine (*Pretz-D*)	Instill solution in each nostril q4h, do not use for children <6 yr unless advised by physician	Relief of the discomfort of nasal congestion associated with the common cold, sinusitis, allergic rhinitis; relief of pressure of otitis media
oxymetazoline (*Afrin, Allerest*)	Adult and pediatric (>6 yr): two to three sprays or drops in each nostril b.i.d. Pediatric (2–5 yr): two to three drops of 0.05% solution in each nostril b.i.d.	Relief of the discomfort of nasal congestion associated with the common cold, sinusitis, allergic rhinitis
phenylephrine (*Coricidin*)	Adult and pediatric (>6 yr): one to two sprays in each nostril q3–4h Pediatric (2–6 yr): two to three drops of 0.125% solution in each nostril q4h PRN	Relief of the discomfort of nasal congestion associated with the common cold, sinusitis, allergic rhinitis
tetrahydrozoline (*Tyzine*)	Adult and pediatric (>6 yr): two to four drops in each nostril t.i.d. to q.i.d. Pediatric (2–6 yr): two to three drops of 0.05% solution in each nostril q4–6h	Relief of the discomfort of nasal congestion associated with the common cold, sinusitis, allergic rhinitis; relief of pressure of otitis media
xylometazoline (*Otrivin*)	Adult: two to three sprays or two to three drops in each nostril q8–10h (0.17% solution) Pediatric (2–12 yr): two to three drops of 0.05% solution q8–12h	Relief of the discomfort of nasal congestion associated with the common cold, sinusitis, allergic rhinitis; relief of pressure of otitis media

as the drug effect wears off. As a result, patients tend to use more drug to decrease the congestion, thus initiating a vicious cycle of congestion–drug–congestion, which leads to abuse of the decongestant.) Sympathomimetic effects (e.g., increased pulse, blood pressure; urinary retention) should be monitored because some systemic absorption may occur, although these effects are less likely with topical administration than with other routes.

Clinically Important Drug–Drug Interactions

The use of topical nasal decongestants is contraindicated with concurrent use of cyclopropane or halothane anesthesia because serious cardiovascular effects could occur. Combined use with any other sympathomimetic drug or sympathetic-blocking drug could result in toxic or noneffective responses. Monitor the use of these combinations carefully.

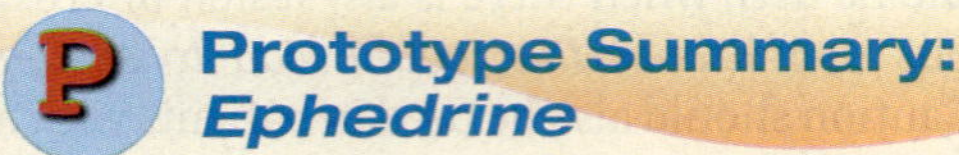

Prototype Summary: Ephedrine

Indications: Symptomatic relief of nasal and nasopharyngeal mucosal congestion due to the common cold, hay fever, or other respiratory allergies; adjunctive therapy of middle ear infections to decrease congestion around the eustachian ostia

Actions: Sympathomimetic effects, partly due to release of norepinephrine from nerve terminals; vasoconstriction leads to decreased edema and inflammation of the nasal membranes

Pharmacokinetics:

Route	Onset	Duration
Topical (nasal spray)	Immediate	4–6 h

$T_{1/2}$: 0.4–0.7 hours; metabolized in the liver and excreted in urine; little is usually absorbed for systemic metabolism

Adverse effects: Disorientation, confusion, lightheadedness, nausea, vomiting, fever, dyspnea, rebound congestion

Nursing Considerations for Patients Receiving Topical Nasal Decongestants

Assessment: History and Examination

Screen for the following conditions, *which could be cautions or contraindications to use of the drug:* any history of allergy to the drug or a component of the drug vehicle; glaucoma, hypertension, diabetes, thyroid disease, coronary disease, and prostate problems, *all of which could be exacerbated by the sympathomimetic effects;* and pregnancy or lactation, *which require cautious use of the drug.*

Physical assessment should be done *to establish baseline data for assessing the effectiveness of the drug and the occurrence of any adverse effects associated with drug therapy.* Assess the following: skin color and temperature, *to assess sympathetic response;* orientation and reflexes, *to evaluate CNS effects of the drug;* pulse, blood pressure, and cardiac auscultation, *to monitor cardiovascular and sympathomimetic effects;* respirations and adventitious breath sounds, *to assess effectiveness of drug and potential excess effect;* bladder percussion, *to monitor for urinary retention related to sympathomimetic effects;* and nasal mucous membrane evaluation, *to monitor for lesions that could lead to systemic absorption and to evaluate decongestant effect.*

Nursing Diagnoses

The patient receiving a topical nasal decongestant may have the following nursing diagnoses related to drug therapy:

- Acute Pain related to GI, CNS, or local effects of drug
- Disturbed Sensory Perception (Kinesthetic) related to CNS effects (less likely with this route of administration)
- Deficient Knowledge regarding drug therapy

Implementation With Rationale

- Teach the patient the proper administration of the drug *to ensure therapeutic effect* (Box 54.2). The patient should be instructed to clear the nasal passages before use, to tilt the head back when applying the drops or spray, and to keep it tilted back for a few seconds after administration. This technique *helps ensure contact with the affected mucous membranes and decreases the chances of letting the drops trickle down the back of throat, which may lead to more systemic effects.*
- Caution patients not to use the drug for longer than 5 days and to seek medical care if signs and symptoms persist after that time *to facilitate detection of underlying medical conditions that may require treatment.*
- Caution patients that these drugs are found in many OTC preparations and that care should be taken not to inadvertently combine drugs with the same ingredients, *leading to overdose.*

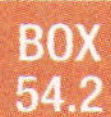

BOX 54.2 FOCUS ON **CLINICAL SKILLS**

Administering Nasal Medications

Proper administration technique is very important for assuring that drugs given nasally have the desired therapeutic effect. It is important to periodically check the nares for any signs of erosion or lesions, which could allow systemic absorption of the drug. Most patients prefer to self-administer nasal drugs, so patient teaching is very important. Explain the technique and then observe the patient using the technique.

Nasal Spray

Teach the patient to sit upright and press a finger over one nares to close it. Hold the spray bottle upright and place the tip of the bottle about ½ inch into the open nares. Firmly squeeze the bottle to deliver the drug. Caution the patient not to squeeze too forcefully, which could send the drug up into the sinuses, causing more problems. Repeat with the other nares.

Nasal Aerosol

Teach the patient to place the medication cartridge into the plastic nasal adapter and shake it well. Remove the plastic cap from the applicator and place the tip inside the nostril. Have the patient sit upright and tilt the head back. The patient should firmly press on the canister once to deliver the drug; inhale; and hold his or her breath for a few seconds. Then exhale. The patient should be encouraged to keep the head titled back for a few minutes and reminded not to blow his or her nose for at least 2 minutes.

- Provide safety measures if dizziness or sedation occur as a result of drug therapy *to prevent patient injury.*
- Institute other measures *to help relieve the discomfort of congestion* (e.g., humidity, increased fluid intake, cool environment, avoidance of smoke-filled areas) as appropriate.
- Provide thorough patient teaching, including the drug name and prescribed dosage, measures to help avoid adverse effects, warning signs that may indicate problems, and the need for periodic monitoring and evaluation, *to enhance patient knowledge about drug therapy and to promote compliance.*
- Offer support and encouragement *to help the patient cope with the disease and the drug regimen.*

Evaluation

- Monitor patient response to the drug (relief of nasal congestion).
- Monitor for adverse effects (local burning and stinging; adrenergic effects such as increased pulse, blood pressure, urinary retention, cool and clammy skin).
- Evaluate the effectiveness of the teaching plan (patient can name drug, dosage, adverse effects to watch for, specific measures to avoid adverse effects, measures to take to increase the effectiveness of the drug, proper administration technique).
- Monitor the effectiveness of comfort and safety measures and compliance with the regimen.

Oral Decongestants

Oral decongestants are drugs that are taken orally to decrease nasal congestion related to the common cold, sinusitis, and allergic rhinitis. They are also used to relieve the pain and congestion of otitis media. Opening of the nasal passage allows better drainage of the eustachian tube, relieving pressure in the middle ear. The only oral decongestant currently available for use is pseudoephedrine (*Dorcol, Decofed,* and others) (Table 54.3).

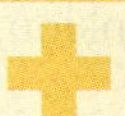

FOCUS ON **PATIENT SAFETY**

In late 2000, the U.S. Food and Drug Administration removed the oral decongestant phenylpropanolamine (PPA) from the market. This drug, which had been the center of controversy for many years, was found to be associated with an increased number of strokes in young women who took the drug. The drug had been an ingredient in many over-the-counter cold, allergy, and flu remedies. After a short absence, most of these products reappeared on the market with the drug pseudoephedrine taking the place of PPA. This drug, a sympathomimetic, is also known to cause sympathetic effects, including increased blood pressure and increased heart rate. Close follow-up of the effects of this drug will be done to monitor for any increased risk associated with its use.

Therapeutic Actions and Indications

Oral decongestants shrink the nasal mucous membrane by stimulating the alpha-adrenergic receptors in the nasal mucous membranes. This shrinkage results in a decrease in membrane size, promoting drainage of the sinuses and improving air flow. Because this drug is taken systemically, adverse effects related to the sympathomimetic effects (e.g., cardiac stimulation, feelings of anxiety) are more likely to occur.

Pharmacokinetics

Pseudoephedrine is generally well absorbed and reaches peak levels quickly—in 20 to 45 minutes. It is widely distributed in the body, metabolized in the liver, and primarily excreted in urine. There are no adequate studies about its use during pregnancy and lactation, and such use should be reserved for situations in which the benefit to the mother outweighs any potential risk to the fetus or neonate.

Table 54.3 DRUGS IN FOCUS

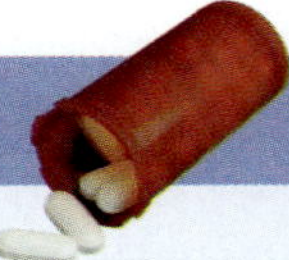

Oral Decongestant

Drug Name	Usual Dosage	Usual Indications
pseudoephedrine (*Sudafed, Decofed*)	Adult: 60 mg PO q4–6h Pediatric: 6–12 yr—30 mg PO q4–6h; 2–5 yr—15 mg PO q4–6h; 1–2 yr—0.02 mL/kg PO q4–6h; 3–12 mo—three drops/kg PO q4–6h	Decrease nasal congestion associated with the common cold, allergic rhinitis; relief of pain and congestion of otitis media

Contraindications and Cautions

Because pseudoephedrine has adrenergic properties, caution should be used in patients with any condition *that might be exacerbated by sympathetic activity,* such as glaucoma, hypertension, diabetes, thyroid disease, coronary disease, and prostate problems.

Adverse Effects

Adverse effects associated with pseudoephedrine include rebound congestion. Sympathetic effects include feelings of anxiety, tenseness, restlessness, tremors, hypertension, arrhythmias, sweating, and pallor.

Clinically Important Drug–Drug Interactions

Many OTC products, including cold remedies, allergy medications, and flu remedies, may contain pseudoephedrine. Taking many of these products concurrently can cause serious adverse effects. Teach patients to read the OTC labels to avoid inadvertent overdose.

Nursing Considerations for Patients Receiving an Oral Decongestant

Assessment: History and Examination

Screen for the following conditions, *which could be cautions or contraindications to use of the drug:* any history of allergy to the drug and pregnancy or lactation, *which are contraindications to drug use;* hypertension or coronary artery disease, *which require cautious use;* and hyperthyroidism, diabetes mellitus, or prostate enlargement, *all of which could be exacerbated by these drugs.*

Physical assessment should be done *to establish baseline data for assessing the effectiveness of the drug and the occurrence of any adverse effects associated with drug therapy.* Assess the following: skin color and lesions, *to monitor for adverse reactions;* orientation, reflexes, and affect, *to monitor CNS effects of the drug;* blood pressure, pulse, and auscultation, *to monitor cardiovascular stimulations;* respiration and adventitious sounds, *to monitor drug effectiveness;* and urinary output, *to evaluate for urinary retention.*

Nursing Diagnoses

The patient receiving an oral decongestant may have the following nursing diagnoses related to drug therapy:

- Acute Pain related to GI, CNS, or skin effects of drug
- Increased Cardiac Output related to sympathomimetic actions of the drug
- Disturbed Sensory Perception (Kinesthetic) related to CNS effects
- Deficient Knowledge regarding drug therapy

Implementation With Rationale

- Note that this drug is found in many OTC products, especially combination cold and allergy preparations; *care should be taken to prevent inadvertent overdose or excessive adverse effects.*
- Provide safety measures as needed if CNS effects occur, *to prevent patient injury.*
- Monitor pulse, blood pressure, and cardiac response to the drug, especially in patients who are at risk for cardiac stimulation, *to detect adverse effects early and arrange to reduce dosage or discontinue the drug.*
- Encourage the patient not to use this drug for longer than 1 week and to seek medical evaluation if symptoms persist after that time *to encourage the detection of underlying medical conditions that could be causing these symptoms and to arrange for appropriate treatment.*
- Provide thorough patient teaching, including the drug name and prescribed dosage, measures to help avoid adverse effects, warning signs that may indicate problems, and the need for periodic monitoring and evaluation, *to enhance patient knowledge about drug therapy and to promote compliance.*
- Offer support and encouragement *to help the patient cope with the disease and the drug regimen.*

Evaluation

- Monitor patient response to the drug (improvement in nasal congestion).
- Monitor for adverse effects (sympathomimetic reactions including increased pulse, blood pressure, pallor, sweating, arrhythmias, feelings of anxiety, tension, dry skin).
- Evaluate the effectiveness of the teaching plan (patient can name drug, dosage, adverse effects to watch for, specific measures to avoid adverse effects, measures to take to increase the effectiveness of the drug).
- Monitor the effectiveness of comfort and safety measures and compliance with the regimen.

Topical Nasal Steroid Decongestants

Topical nasal steroid decongestants are currently very popular for the treatment of allergic rhinitis. They have been found to be effective in patients who are no longer getting a response with other decongestants. The topical nasal steroid decongestants include beclomethasone (*Beclovent* and others), budesonide (*Pulmicort*), dexamethasone (*Decadron* and others), flunisolide (*AeroBid* and others), fluticasone (*Flovent*), and triamcinolone (*Azmacort*) (Table 54.4).

Therapeutic Actions and Indications

The exact mechanism of action of topical steroids is not known. Their anti-inflammatory action results from their ability to produce a direct local effect that blocks many of the complex reactions responsible for the inflammatory response. Because they are applied topically, there is less of a chance of systemic absorption and associated adverse effects. The onset of action is not immediate, and they may actually require up to a week to cause any changes. If no effects are seen after 3 weeks, the drug should be discontinued. Topical nasal steroidal preparations are used to treat seasonal allergic rhinitis for patients who are not getting any response from other decongestant preparations. They are frequently used to relieve inflammation after the removal of nasal polyps.

Pharmacokinetics

Because these drugs are not generally absorbed systemically, their pharmacokinetics are not reported. If they were to be absorbed systemically, they would have the same pharmacokinetics as other steroids (see Chapter 36).

Contraindications and Cautions

Because nasal steroids block the inflammatory response, their use is contraindicated in the presence of acute infections. Increased incidence of *Candida albicans* infection has been reported with their use, related to the anti-inflammatory and anti-immune activities associated with steroids. Caution should be used in any patient who has an active infection, including tuberculosis, *because systemic absorption would interfere with the inflammatory and immune responses.* Patients using nasal steroids should avoid exposure to any airborne infection, such as chickenpox or measles.

Adverse Effects

The most common adverse effects associated with the use of topical nasal steroids are local burning, irritation, stinging,

Table 54.4 DRUGS IN FOCUS

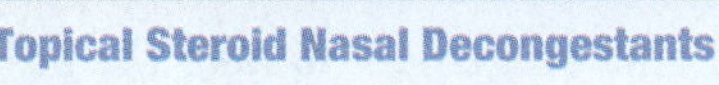
Topical Steroid Nasal Decongestants

Drug Name	Usual Dosage	Usual Indications
beclomethasone (*Beclovent*)	Adult: one to two inhalations in each nostril b.i.d. Pediatric (6–11 yr): one inhalation in each nostril b.i.d.	All of the topical steroid nasal decongestants are indicated for treatment of seasonal allergic rhinitis in patients who are not obtaining a response with other decongestants or preparations and for relief of inflammation after the removal of nasal polyps
budesonide (*Pulmicort*)	Adult and pediatric (>6 yr): two sprays in each nostril morning and evening or four sprays in each nostril in the morning	
dexamethasone (*Decadron*)	Adult: two sprays in each nostril b.i.d. to t.i.d. Pediatric: one to two sprays in each nostril b.i.d.	
P flunisolide (*AeroBid*)	Adult: two sprays in each nostril b.i.d. Pediatric (6–14 yr): one spray in each nostril t.i.d. to two sprays in each nostril b.i.d.	
fluticasone (*Flovent*)	Adult and pediatric (4–11 yr): two sprays in each nostril daily	
triamcinolone (*Azmacort*)	Adult: two sprays in each nostril every day	

dryness of the mucosa, and headache. Because healing is suppressed by steroids, patients who have recently experienced nasal surgery or trauma should be monitored closely until healing has occurred.

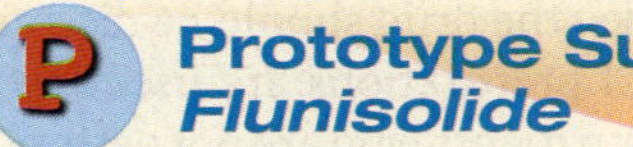

Prototype Summary: Flunisolide

Indications: Treatment of seasonal allergic rhinitis for patients who are not getting any response from other decongestant preparations; relief of inflammation after the removal of nasal polyps.

Actions: Anti-inflammatory action, which results from the ability to produce a direct local effect that blocks many of the complex reactions responsible for the inflammatory response

Pharmacokinetics:

Route	Onset	Peak	Duration
Topical (nasal spray)	Immediate	10–30 min	4–6 h

$T_{1/2}$: Not generally absorbed systemically

Adverse effects: Local burning, irritation, stinging, dryness of the mucosa, headache, increased risk of infection

Nursing Considerations for Patients Receiving Topical Steroid Nasal Decongestants

Assessment: History and Examination

Screen for the following conditions, *which could be cautions or contraindications to use of the drug:* any history of allergy to steroid drugs or any components of the drug vehicle, *which would be a contraindication,* and acute infection, *which would require cautious use.*

Physical assessment should be done *to establish baseline data for assessing the effectiveness of the drug and the occurrence of any adverse effects associated with drug therapy.* Intranasal examination should be performed *to determine the presence of any lesions that would increase the risk of systemic absorption of drug.* Assess the following: respiration and adventitious sounds, *to evaluate drug effectiveness;* and temperature, *to monitor for the possibility of acute infection.*

Nursing Diagnoses

The patient receiving topical steroid nasal decongestants may have the following nursing diagnoses related to drug therapy:

- Acute Pain related to local effects of the drug
- Risk for Injury related to suppression of inflammatory reaction
- Deficient Knowledge regarding drug therapy

Implementation With Rationale

- Teach the patient how to administer these drugs properly, *which is very important to ensure effectiveness and prevent systemic effects.* A variety of preparations are available (e.g., sprays, aerosols, powder disks). Advise the patient about the proper administration technique for whichever preparation is recommended.
- Have the patient clear nasal passages before using the drug, *to improve the effectiveness of the drug.*
- Encourage the patient to continue using the drug regularly, even if results are not seen immediately, *because benefits may take 2 to 3 weeks to appear.*
- Monitor the patient for the development of acute infection that would require medical intervention. Encourage the patient to avoid areas where airborne infections could be a problem *because steroid use decreases the effectiveness of the immune and inflammatory responses.*
- Provide thorough patient teaching, including the drug name and prescribed dosage, measures to help avoid adverse effects, warning signs that may indicate problems, and the need for periodic monitoring and evaluation, *to enhance patient knowledge about drug therapy and to promote compliance.*
- Offer support and encouragement *to help the patient cope with the disease and the drug regimen.*

Evaluation

- Monitor patient response to the drug (relief of nasal congestion).
- Monitor for adverse effects (local burning and stinging).
- Evaluate the effectiveness of the teaching plan (patient can name drug, dosage, adverse effects to watch for, specific measures to avoid adverse effects, measures to take to increase the effectiveness of the drug).
- Monitor the effectiveness of comfort and safety measures and compliance with the regimen.

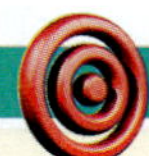

FOCUS POINTS

- Antitussive drugs suppress the cough reflex by acting centrally, to suppress the medullary cough center, or locally, as an anesthetic or to increase secretion and buffer irritation.
- Decongestants cause local vasoconstriction, thereby reducing blood flow to the mucous membranes of the nasal passages and sinus cavities.
- Rebound vasodilation (rhinitis medicamentosa) is an adverse effect of excessive or long-term decongestant use.
- Topical nasal decongestants are preferred for patients who need to avoid systemic adrenergic effects associated with oral decongestants.
- Topical nasal steroid decongestants block the inflammatory response and are preferred for patients with allergic rhinitis for whom systemic steroid therapy is undesirable.

Antihistamines

Antihistamines are found in multiple OTC preparations that are designed to relieve respiratory symptoms and to treat allergies. These agents block the effects of histamine, bringing relief to patients suffering from itchy eyes, swelling, congestion, and drippy nose.

Numerous antihistamines are available, including first- and second-generation agents (Table 54.5). First-generation antihistamines have greater anticholinergic effects, with resultant drowsiness. These drugs include azelastine (*Astelin*), brompheniramine (*Bidhist* and others), buclizine (*Bucladin-S*), cetirizine (*Zyrtec*), chlorpheniramine (*Aller-Chlor* and others), clemastine (*Tavist*), cyclizine (*Marezine*), cyproheptadine (generic), dexchlorpheniramine (generic), dimenhydrinate (*Dimentabs* and others), diphenhydramine (*Benadryl* and others), hydroxyzine (*Vistaril* and others), meclizine (*Antivert*), and promethazine (*Phenergan* and others). Second-generation antihistamines, including desloratadine (*Clarinex*), fexofenadine (*Allegra*), and loratadine (*Claritin*), have fewer anticholinergic effects than do first-generation agents.

When choosing an antihistamine, the individual patient's reaction to the drug is usually the governing factor. If a person needs to be alert, one of the second-generation, nonsedating antihistamines would be the drug of choice. Because of their OTC availability, these drugs are often misused to treat colds and influenza.

Therapeutic Actions and Indications

The antihistamines selectively block the effects of histamine at the histamine-1 receptor sites, decreasing the allergic response. They also have anticholinergic (atropine-like) and antipruritic effects. Antihistamines are used for the relief of symptoms associated with seasonal and perennial allergic rhinitis, allergic conjunctivitis, uncomplicated urticaria, and angioedema. They are also used for amelioration of allergic reactions to blood or blood products, for relief of discomfort associated with dermographism, and as adjunctive therapy in anaphylactic reactions. Other uses that are being explored include relief of exercise- and hyperventilation-induced asthma and histamine-induced bronchoconstriction in asthmatics. They are most effective if used before the onset of symptoms.

Pharmacokinetics

The oral antihistamines are well absorbed orally, with an onset of action ranging from 1 to 3 hours. They are generally metabolized in the liver, with excretion in feces and urine. These drugs cross the placenta and enter breast milk, so their use should be avoided in pregnancy and lactation unless the benefit to the mother outweighs the potential risk to the fetus or baby.

Contraindications and Cautions

Antihistamines are contraindicated during pregnancy or lactation. They should be used with caution in renal or hepatic impairment, *which could alter the metabolism and excretion of the drug.* Special care should be taken when these drugs are used by any patient with a history of arrhythmias or prolonged Q-T intervals *because fatal cardiac arrhythmias have been associated with the use of certain antihistamines and drugs that increase Q-T intervals, including erythromycin.*

Adverse Effects

The adverse effects most often seen with antihistamine use are drowsiness and sedation (Critical Thinking Scenario 54-1), although second-generation antihistamines are less sedating in many people. The anticholinergic effects that can be anticipated include drying of the respiratory and GI mucous membranes, GI upset and nausea, arrhythmias, dysuria, urinary hesitancy, and skin eruption and itching associated with dryness.

Drug–Drug Interactions

Drug–drug interactions vary among the antihistamines; for example, anticholinergic effects may be prolonged if diphenhydramine is taken with a monoamine inhibitor and the interaction of fexofenadine with ketoconazole or erythromycin may raise fexofenadine concentrations to toxic levels. For more information, consult a nursing drug handbook or package insert for individual details.

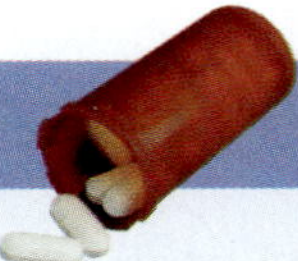

Table 54.5 DRUGS IN FOCUS

Antihistamines

Drug Name	Usual Dosage	Usual Indications
First-Generation		
azelastine (*Astelin*)	Two sprays per nostril b.i.d.	Relief of symptoms of seasonal and perennial allergic rhinitis
brompheniramine (*Bidhist*)	Adult and pediatric (>12 yr): 6–12 mg PO q12h Pediatric (6–12 yr): 6 mg/day PO	Relief of symptoms of seasonal and perennial allergic rhinitis
buclizine (*Bucladin-S*)	50–150 mg/day PO; use caution with elderly patients	Relief of nausea and vomiting associated with motion sickness
cetirizine (*Zyrtec*)	Adult and pediatric (>12 yr): 5–10 mg/day PO; use 5 mg with hepatic or renal impairment Pediatric (6–11 yr): 5 or 10 mg/day PO Pediatric (6 mo–5 yr): 2.5 mg PO q12h or 5 mg/day PO	Relief of symptoms of seasonal and perennial allergic rhinitis; management of chronic urticaria
chlorpheniramine (*Aller-Chlor*, others)	Adult and pediatric (>12 yr): 4 mg PO q4–6h; 8–12 mg at bedtime for sustained release; use caution in elderly patients Pediatric (6–12 yr): 2 mg PO q4–6h Pediatric (2–5 yr): 1 mg PO q4–6h Sustained release: 6–12 yr—8 mg PO at bedtime; <6 yr—not recommended	Relief of symptoms of seasonal and perennial allergic rhinitis; allergic conjunctivitis; uncomplicated urticaria and angioedema; amelioration of allergic reactions; relief of discomfort associated with dermographism; and as an adjunctive therapy in anaphylactic reactions
clemastine (*Tavist*)	Adult and pediatric (>12 yr): 1.34 mg PO b.i.d.; use caution with elderly patients Pediatric (6–12 yr): 0.67 mg PO b.i.d. Pediatric (<6 yr): not recommended	Relief of symptoms of seasonal and perennial allergic rhinitis; allergic conjunctivitis; uncomplicated urticaria and angioedema; amelioration of allergic reactions; relief of discomfort associated with dermographism; and as an adjunctive therapy in anaphylactic reactions
cyclizine (*Marezine*)	Adult: 50 mg PO q4–6h; use caution with elderly patients Pediatric (6–12 yr): 25 mg PO t.i.d.	Relief of nausea and vomiting associated with motion sickness
cyproheptadine (*generic*)	Adult: 4–20 mg/day PO in divided doses Pediatric (7–14 yr): 4 mg PO b.i.d. to t.i.d. Pediatric (2–6 yr): 2 mg PO b.i.d. to t.i.d.	Relief of symptoms of seasonal and perennial allergic rhinitis; allergic conjunctivitis; uncomplicated urticaria and angioedema; amelioration of allergic reactions; relief of discomfort associated with dermographism; and as an adjunctive therapy in anaphylactic reactions
dexchlorpheniramine (*generic*)	Adult and pediatric (>12 yr): 4–6 mg PO at bedtime or q8–10h during the day Pediatric (6–12 yr): 4 mg/day PO at bedtime	Relief of symptoms of seasonal and perennial allergic rhinitis; allergic conjunctivitis; uncomplicated urticaria and angioedema; amelioration of allergic reactions; relief of discomfort associated with dermographism; and as an adjunctive therapy in anaphylactic reactions
dimenhydrinate (*Dimentabs*, others)	Adult and pediatric (>12 yr): 50–100 mg PO q4–6h or 50 mg IM as needed Pediatric: <2 yr—1.25 mg/kg IM q.i.d.; 2–6 yr—25 mg PO q6–8h; 6–12 yr—25–50 mg PO q6–8h	Relief of nausea and vomiting associated with motion sickness
P diphenhydramine (*Benadryl*, others)	Adult: 25–50 mg PO q4–6h or 10–50 mg IM or IV Pediatric: 12.5–25 mg PO t.i.d. to q.i.d. or 5 mg/kg/day IM or IV Geriatric: use caution	Relief of symptoms of seasonal and perennial allergic rhinitis; allergic conjunctivitis; uncomplicated urticaria and angioedema; amelioration of allergic reactions; relief of discomfort associated with dermographism; and as an adjunctive therapy in anaphylactic reactions; sleeping aid; parkinsonism
hydroxyzine (*Vistaril*, others)	Adult: 25–100 mg PO t.i.d. to q.i.d. or 25–100 mg IM q4–6h Pediatric (>6 yr): 50–100 mg/day PO in divided doses Pediatric (<6 yr): 50 mg/day PO in divided doses or 1.1 mg/kg per dose IM	Relief of symptoms of seasonal and perennial allergic rhinitis; allergic conjunctivitis; uncomplicated urticaria and angioedema; amelioration of allergic reactions; relief of discomfort associated with dermographism; and as an adjunctive therapy in anaphylactic reactions; sedation

Table 54.5 DRUGS IN FOCUS *(Continued)*

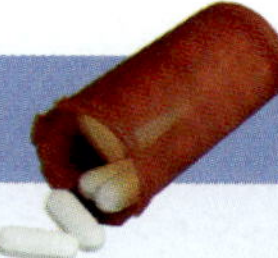

Antihistamines

Drug Name	Usual Dosage	Usual Indications
meclizine (*Antivert*)	Adult and pediatric (>12 yr): 25–100 mg/day PO; use caution with elderly patients	Relief of nausea and vomiting associated with motion sickness
promethazine (*Phenergan*)	Adult: 25 mg PO, PR, IM, or IV Pediatric: 6.25–25 mg PO or PR	Relief of symptoms of seasonal and perennial allergic rhinitis; allergic conjunctivitis; uncomplicated urticaria and angioedema; amelioration of allergic reactions; relief of discomfort associated with dermographism; and as an adjunctive therapy in anaphylactic reactions; sedation
Second-Generation (Nonsedating)		
desloratadine (*Clarinex*)	Adult and pediatric (>12 yr): 5 mg/day PO Pediatric: 6–11 yr—1 tsp, 2.5 mg/5 mL/day PO; 12 mo–5 yr—½ tsp, 1.25 mg/2.5 mL/day PO; 6–11 mo—1 mg/day PO Hepatic or renal impairment: 5 mg PO every other day	Relief of symptoms of seasonal allergic rhinitis; chronic idiopathic urticaria
fexofenadine (*Allegra*)	Adult and pediatric (>12 yr): 60 mg PO b.i.d. Pediatric (6–11 yr): 30 mg PO b.i.d. Geriatric or renal-impaired patient: 60 mg PO every day Pediatric (6–11 yr): 30 mg PO b.i.d.	Relief of symptoms of seasonal and perennial allergic rhinitis
loratadine (*Claritin*)	Adult and pediatric (>6 yr): 10 mg/day PO Geriatric or hepatic-impaired patient: 10 mg PO every other day Pediatric (2–5 yr): 5 mg/day PO (syrup)	Relief of symptoms of seasonal and perennial allergic rhinitis; allergic conjunctivitis; uncomplicated urticaria and angioedema; amelioration of allergic reactions; relief of discomfort associated with dermographism; and as an adjunctive therapy in anaphylactic reactions

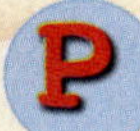

Prototype Summary: *Diphenhydramine*

Indications: Symptomatic relief of perennial and seasonal rhinitis, vasomotor rhinitis, allergic conjunctivitis, urticaria, and angioedema; also used for treating motion sickness and parkinsonism, and as a nighttime sleep aid and to suppress coughs

Actions: Competitively blocks the effects of histamine at H1-receptor sites; has atropine-like antipruritic and sedative effects

Pharmacokinetics:

Route	Onset	Peak	Duration
Oral	15–30 min	1–4 h	4–7 h
IM	20–30 min	1–4 h	4–8 h
IV	Rapid	30–60 min	4–8 h

$T_{1/2}$: 2.5–7 hours; metabolized in the liver and excreted in urine

Adverse effects: Drowsiness, sedation, dizziness, epigastric distress, thickening of bronchial secretions, urinary frequency, rash, bradycardia

Nursing Considerations for Patients Receiving Antihistamines

Assessment: History and Examination

Screen for the following conditions, *which could be cautions or contraindications to use of the drug:* any history of allergy to antihistamines; pregnancy or lactation; and prolonged Q-T interval, *which are contraindications to the use of the drug;* and renal or hepatic impairment, *which requires cautious use of the drug.*

Physical assessment should be done *to establish baseline data for assessing the effectiveness of the drug and the occurrence of any adverse effects associated with drug therapy.* Assess the following: skin color, texture, and lesions, *to monitor for anticholinergic effects or allergy;* orientation, affect, and reflexes, *to monitor for changes due to CNS effects;* respirations and adventitious sounds, *to monitor drug effects;* and serum liver and renal function tests, *to monitor for factors that could affect the metabolism or excretion of the drug.*

CRITICAL THINKING SCENARIO 54-1

Dangers of Self-Medicating for Seasonal Rhinitis

The Situation

K.E. is a 46-year-old businessman who has been self-treating for seasonal rhinitis and a cold. His wife calls the physician's office; she is concerned that her husband is dizzy, has lost his balance several times, and is very drowsy. He is unable to drive to work or to stay awake. She wants to take him to the emergency department of the local hospital.

Critical Thinking

What is the best approach for this patient?

What crucial patient history questions should you ask before proceeding any further?

If you do not know this patient, given his presenting story, what medical conditions would need to be ruled out before proceeding further?

If K.E. is self-medicating for the signs and symptoms of seasonal rhinitis, what could be causing his drowsiness and dizziness?

What teaching points should be emphasized with this patient and his wife?

Discussion

The first impression of K.E.'s condition is that it is a neurologic disorder. K.E. should be evaluated by a health care provider to rule out significant neurologic problems. However, after a careful patient history and physical examination, K.E.'s condition seemed to be related to high levels of over-the-counter (OTC) medications.

There are a multitude of OTC cold and allergy remedies, most of which contain the same ingredients in varying proportions. A patient may be taking one to stop his nasal drip, another to help his cough, another to relieve his congestion, and so on. By combining OTC medications like this, a patient is at great risk for inadvertently overdosing or at least allowing the medication to reach toxic levels.

In this situation, the first thing to determine is exactly what medication is being taken and how often. K.E. seems to have received toxic levels of antihistamines, decongestants, or other upper respiratory tract agents. The nurse should encourage K.E.—and all patients—to check the labels of any OTC medications being taken and to check with the health care provider if there are any questions. K.E. and his wife should receive written information about the drugs that K.E. is taking. They also should be shown how to read OTC bottles or boxes for information on the contents of various preparations. In addition, they should be encouraged to use alternative methods to relieve the discomfort of seasonal rhinitis (e.g., using a humidifier, drinking lots of liquids, avoiding smoky areas) to allay the belief that many OTC drugs are needed. Finally, K.E. and his wife should be advised to check with their health care provider if they have any questions about OTC or prescription drugs, or if they have continued problems coping with seasonal allergic reactions. Other prescription medication may prove more effective.

Nursing Care Guide for K.E.: Antihistamines

Assessment: History And Examination

Assess K.E.'s health history for allergies and GI stenosis or obstruction, bladder obstruction, narrow-angle glaucoma, benign prostatic hypertrophy and concurrent use of monoamine oxidase inhibitors and OTC allergy or cold products.

Focus the physical examination on the following areas:

Neurological: orientation, reflexes, affect, coordination

Skin: lesions

CV: blood pressure, pulse, peripheral perfusion

GI: bowel sounds, abdominal exam

Hematological: CBC

Respiratory: respiratory rate and character, nares, adventitious sounds

GU: urinary output

Nursing Diagnoses

Acute Pain related to GI effects or dry mouth

Decreased Cardiac Output

Impaired Sensory Perception (Kinesthetic)

Impaired Urinary Elimination related to thickening mucus

Deficient Knowledge regarding drug therapy

Dangers of Self-Medicating for Seasonal Rhinitis *(continued)*

Implementation

Provide comfort and safety measures, e. g., give drug with meals; teach about mouth care; increase humidity; institute safety measures if dizziness occurs.

Provide support and reassurance to deal with drug effects and allergy.

Provide patient teaching regarding drug name, dosage, adverse effects, precautions, and warning signs to report.

Evaluation

Evaluate drug effects, i. e., relief of respiratory symptoms.

Monitor for adverse effects: CNS effects, thickening of secretions, urinary retention, glaucoma.

Monitor for drug–drug interactions as indicated.

Evaluate effectiveness of support and encouragement strategies, patient teaching program, and comfort and safety measures.

Patient Teaching For K.E.

☐ Antihistamines are commonly used to treat the signs and symptoms of various allergic reactions. Because these drugs work throughout the body, many systemic effects can occur with their use (e.g., dry mouth, dizziness, drowsiness).

☐ Take this drug only as prescribed. Do not increase the dosage if symptoms are not relieved. Instead, consult your health care provider.

☐ Common effects of this drug include:

- *Drowsiness, dizziness:* Do not drive or operate dangerous machinery if this occurs. Use caution to prevent injury.
- *Gastrointestinal upset, nausea, vomiting, heartburn:* Taking the drug with food may help this problem.
- *Dry mouth:* Frequent mouth care and sucking sugarless lozenges may help.
- *Thickening of the mucus, difficulty coughing, tightening of the chest:* Use a humidifier or, if you do not have one, place pans of water throughout the house to increase the humidity of the room air; avoid smoke-filled areas; drink plenty of fluids.
- Report any of the following to your health care provider: *difficulty breathing, rash, hives, difficulty in voiding, abdominal pain, visual changes, disorientation or confusion.*

☐ Avoid the use of alcoholic beverages while you are taking this drug. Serious drowsiness or sedation can occur if these are combined.

☐ Avoid the use of any over-the-counter medication without first checking with your health care provider. Several of these medications contain drugs that can interfere with the effectiveness of this drug or they can contain very similar drugs and you could experience toxic effects.

☐ Tell any doctor, nurse, or other health care provider involved in your care that you are taking this drug.

☐ Take this drug only as prescribed. Do not give this drug to anyone else, and do not take similar preparations that have been prescribed for someone else. Keep this drug, and all medications, out of the reach of children.

Nursing Diagnoses

The patient receiving antihistamines may have the following nursing diagnoses related to drug therapy:

- Acute Pain related to GI, CNS, or skin effects of the drug
- Disturbed Sensory Perception (Kinesthetic) related to CNS effects
- Deficient Knowledge regarding drug therapy

Implementation With Rationale

- Administer the drug on an empty stomach, 1 hour before or 2 hours after meals, *to increase the absorption of the drug;* the drug may be given with meals if GI upset is a problem.
- Note that a patient may have poor response to one of these agents but a very effective response to another; the prescriber may need to try several different agents *to find the one that is most effective.*
- Because of the drying nature of antihistamines, patients often experience dry mouth, which may lead to nausea and anorexia; suggest sugarless candies or lozenges *to relieve some of this discomfort.*
- Provide safety measures as appropriate, if CNS effects occur, *to prevent patient injury.*

- Increase humidity and push fluids *to decrease the problem of thickened secretions and dry nasal mucosa.*
- Have the patient void before each dose *to decrease urinary retention if this is a problem.*
- Provide skin care as needed if skin dryness and lesions become a problem *to prevent skin breakdown.*
- Caution the patient to avoid excessive dosage and to check OTC drugs for the presence of antihistamines, *which are found in many OTC preparations and which could cause toxicity.*
- Caution the patient to avoid alcohol while taking these drugs *because serious sedation can occur.*
- Provide thorough patient teaching, including the drug name and prescribed dosage, measures to help avoid adverse effects, warning signs that may indicate problems, and the need for periodic monitoring and evaluation, *to enhance patient knowledge about drug therapy and to promote compliance.*
- Offer support and encouragement *to help the patient cope with the disease and the drug regimen.*

Evaluation

- Monitor patient response to the drug (relief of the symptoms of allergic rhinitis).
- Monitor for adverse effects (skin dryness, GI upset, sedation and drowsiness, urinary retention, thickened secretions, glaucoma).
- Evaluate the effectiveness of the teaching plan (patient can name drug, dosage, adverse effects to watch for, specific measures to avoid adverse effects, measures to take to increase the effectiveness of the drug).
- Monitor the effectiveness of comfort and safety measures and compliance with the regimen.

Expectorants

Expectorants liquefy the lower respiratory tract secretions, reducing the viscosity of these secretions and making it easier for the patient to cough them up. Expectorants are available in many OTC preparations, making them widely available to the patient without advice from a health care provider. The only available expectorant is guaifenesin (*Mucinex* and others) (Table 54.6).

Therapeutic Actions and Indications

Guaifenesin enhances the output of respiratory tract fluids by reducing the adhesiveness and surface tension of these fluids, allowing easier movement of the less viscous secretions. The result of this thinning of secretions is a more productive cough and thus decreased frequency of coughing. Expectorants are used for the symptomatic relief of respiratory conditions characterized by a dry, nonproductive cough, including the common cold, acute bronchitis, and influenza.

Pharmacokinetics

Guaifenesin is rapidly absorbed with an onset of 30 minutes and a duration of 4 to 6 hours. Sites of metabolism and excretion have not been reported.

Adverse Effects

The most common adverse effects associated with expectorants are GI symptoms (e.g., nausea, vomiting, anorexia). Some patients experience headache, dizziness, or both; occasionally, a mild rash develops. The most important consideration in the use of these drugs is discovering the cause of the underlying cough. Prolonged use of the OTC preparations could result in the masking of important symptoms of a serious underlying disorder. These drugs should not be used for more than 1 week; if the cough persists, encourage the patient to seek health care.

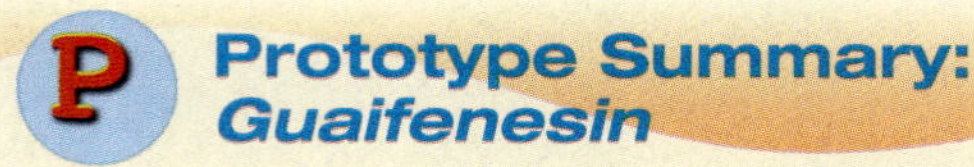

Indications: Symptomatic relief of respiratory conditions characterized by dry, nonproductive cough and in the presence of mucus in the respiratory tract

Table 54.6 DRUGS IN FOCUS

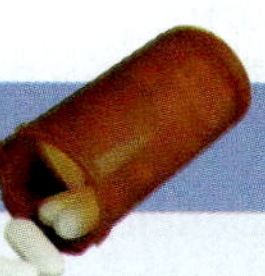

Expectorant

Drug Name	Usual Dosage	Usual Indications
P guaifenesin (*Mucinex*, others)	Adult and pediatric (>12 yr): 200–400 mg PO q4h Pediatric (6–12 yr): 100–200 mg PO q4h Pediatric (2–6 yr): 50–100 mg PO q4h	Symptomatic relief of dry, nonproductive cough

Actions: Enhances the output of respiratory tract fluid by reducing the adhesiveness and surface tension of the fluid, facilitating the removal of viscous mucus

Pharmacokinetics:

Route	Onset	Peak	Duration
Oral	30 min	Unknown	4–6 h

$T_{1/2}$: Unknown; metabolism and excretion are also unknown

Adverse effects: Nausea, vomiting, headache, dizziness, rash

Nursing Considerations for Patients Receiving Expectorants

Assessment: History and Examination

Screen for the following conditions, *which could be cautions or contraindications to use of the drug:* any history of allergy to the drug; persistent cough due to smoking, asthma, or emphysema, *which would be cautions to the use of the drug;* and very productive cough, *which would indicate an underlying problem that should be evaluated.*

Physical assessment should be done *to establish baseline data for assessing the effectiveness of the drug and the occurrence of any adverse effects associated with drug therapy.* Assess the following: skin, *for presence of lesions and color (to monitor for any adverse reaction);* temperature (*to monitor for an underlying infection*); respirations and adventitious sounds (*to evaluate the respiratory response to the drug effects*); and orientation and affect (*to monitor CNS effects of the drug*).

Nursing Diagnoses

The patient receiving an expectorant may have the following nursing diagnoses related to drug therapy:

- Acute Pain related to GI, CNS, or skin effects of the drug
- Disturbed Sensory Perception (Kinesthetic) related to CNS effects
- Deficient Knowledge regarding drug therapy

Implementation With Rationale

- Caution the patient not to use these drugs for longer than 1 week and to seek medical attention if the cough still persists after that time *to evaluate for any underlying medical condition and to arrange for appropriate treatment.*
- Advise the use of small, frequent meals *to alleviate some of the GI discomfort associated with these drugs.*
- Advise the patient to avoid driving or performing dangerous tasks if dizziness and drowsiness occur *to prevent patient injury.*
- Alert the patient that these drugs may be found in OTC preparations and that care should be taken *to avoid excessive dosage.*
- Provide thorough patient teaching, including the drug name and prescribed dosage, measures to help avoid adverse effects, warning signs that may indicate problems, and the need for periodic monitoring and evaluation, *to enhance patient knowledge about drug therapy and to promote compliance.*
- Offer support and encouragement *to help the patient cope with the disease and the drug regimen.*

Evaluation

- Monitor patient response to the drug (improved effectiveness of cough).
- Monitor for adverse effects (skin rash, GI upset, CNS effects).
- Evaluate the effectiveness of the teaching plan (patient can name drug, dosage, adverse effects to watch for, specific measures to avoid adverse effects, measures to take to increase the effectiveness of the drug).
- Monitor the effectiveness of comfort and safety measures and compliance with the regimen.

Mucolytics

Mucolytics work to break down mucus in order to aid the high-risk respiratory patient in coughing up thick, tenacious secretions. The medication may be administered by nebulization or by direct instillation into the trachea via an endotracheal tube or tracheostomy. The mucolytics include acetylcysteine (*Mucomyst* and others) and dornase alfa (*Pulmozyme*) (Table 54.7).

Therapeutic Actions and Indications

Mucolytics are usually reserved for patients who have difficulty mobilizing and coughing up secretions, such as individuals with chronic obstructive pulmonary disease (COPD), cystic fibrosis, pneumonia, or tuberculosis. These drugs are also indicated for patients who develop atelectasis because of thick mucus secretions. They can be used during diagnostic bronchoscopy to clear the airway and to facilitate the removal

Table 54.7 DRUGS IN FOCUS

Mucolytics

Drug Name	Usual Dosage	Usual Indications
P acetylcysteine (*Mucomyst*)	By nebulization, 2–20 mL of 10% solution q2–6h; by direct instillation, 1–2 mL of 10–20% solution q1–4h; 140 mg/kg PO loading dose, then 17 doses of 70 mg/kg PO q4h as an antidote	Liquefaction of secretions in patients who have difficulty moving secretions; clearing of secretions for diagnostic tests; postoperatively to facilitate clearing of secretions; orally to protect liver from acetaminophen toxicity
dornase alfa (*Pulmozyme*)	2.5 mg inhaled through nebulizer, may increase to 2.5 mg b.i.d. if needed	To relieve the buildup of secretions in cystic fibrosis to keep airways open longer

of secretions, as well as postoperatively and in patients with tracheostomies to facilitate airway clearance and suctioning.

Acetylcysteine is used orally to protect liver cells from being damaged during episodes of acetaminophen toxicity because it normalizes hepatic glutathione levels and binds with a reactive hepatotoxic metabolite of acetaminophen. Acetylcysteine affects the mucoproteins in the respiratory secretions by splitting apart disulfide bonds that are responsible for holding the mucus material together. The result is a decrease in the tenacity and viscosity of the secretions. Acetylcysteine is metabolized in the liver and excreted somewhat in urine. It is not known whether it crosses the placenta or enters breast milk.

Dornase alfa is a mucolytic prepared by recombinant DNA techniques that selectively break down respiratory tract mucus by separating extracellular DNA from proteins. It has a long duration of action, and its fate in the body is not known. There are no data on its effects in pregnancy or lactation. This drug is used to relieve the buildup of secretions in cystic fibrosis, to help keep the airways open and functioning longer.

Contraindications and Cautions

Caution should be used in cases of acute bronchospasm, peptic ulcer, and esophageal varices *because the increased secretions could aggravate the problem.*

Adverse Effects

Adverse effects most commonly associated with mucolytic drugs include GI upset, stomatitis, rhinorrhea, bronchospasm, and occasionally a rash.

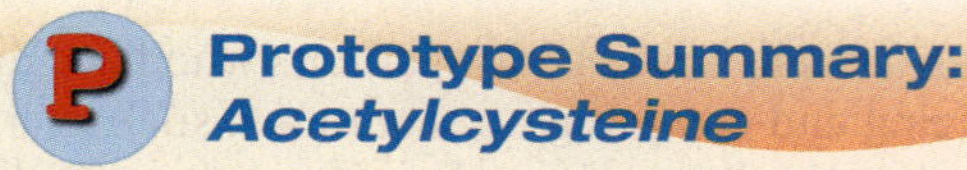

Prototype Summary: Acetylcysteine

Indications: Mucolytic adjunctive therapy for abnormal, viscid, or inspissated mucous secretions in acute and chronic bronchopulmonary disorders; to lessen hepatic injury in cases of acetaminophen toxicity

Actions: Splits links in the mucoproteins contained in the respiratory mucus secretions, decreasing the viscosity of the secretions; protects liver cells from acetaminophen effects

Pharmacokinetics:

Route	Onset	Peak	Duration
Instillation inhalation	1 min	5–10 min	2–3 h
Oral	30–60 min	1–2 h	Unknown

$T_{1/2}$: 6.25 hours; metabolized in the liver and excreted in urine

Adverse effects: Nausea, stomatitis, urticaria, bronchospasm, rhinorrhea

Nursing Considerations for Patients Receiving Mucolytics

Assessment: History and Examination

Screen for the following conditions, *which could be cautions or contraindications to use of the drug:* any history of allergy to the drug and the presence of acute bronchospasm, *which are contraindications to the use of these drugs;* and peptic ulcer and esophageal varices, *which would require careful monitoring and cautious use.*

Physical assessment should be done *to establish baseline data for assessing the effectiveness of the drug and the occurrence of any adverse effects associated with drug therapy.* Assess the following: skin color and lesions, *to monitor for adverse reactions;* blood pressure and pulse, *to evaluate cardiac response to drug treatment;* and respirations and adventitious sounds, *to monitor drug effectiveness.*

Nursing Diagnoses

The patient receiving a mucolytic may have the following nursing diagnoses related to drug therapy:

- Acute Pain related to GI, CNS, or skin effects of the drug
- Disturbed Sensory Perception (Kinesthetic) related to CNS effects
- Ineffective Airway Clearance related to bronchospasm
- Deficient Knowledge regarding drug therapy

Implementation With Rationale

- Avoid combining with other drugs in the nebulizer *to avoid the formation of precipitates and potential loss of effectiveness of either drug.*
- Dilute the concentrate with sterile water for injection *if buildup becomes a problem that could impede drug delivery.*
- Note that patients receiving acetylcysteine by face mask should have the residue wiped off the face mask and off their face with plain water *to prevent skin breakdown.*
- Review the use of the nebulizer with patients receiving dornase alfa at home *to ensure the most effective use of the drug.* Patients should be cautioned to store the drug in the refrigerator, protected from light.
- Caution cystic fibrosis patients receiving dornase alfa about the need to continue all therapies for their cystic fibrosis *because dornase alfa is only a palliative therapy that improves respiratory symptoms, and other therapies are still needed.*
- Provide thorough patient teaching, including the drug name and prescribed dosage, measures to help avoid adverse effects, warning signs that may indicate problems, and the need for periodic monitoring and evaluation, *to enhance patient knowledge about drug therapy and to promote compliance.*
- Offer support and encouragement, *to help the patient cope with the disease and the drug regimen.*

Evaluation

- Monitor patient response to the drug (improvement of respiratory symptoms, loosening of secretions).
- Monitor for adverse effects (CNS effects, skin rash, bronchospasm, GI upset).
- Evaluate the effectiveness of the teaching plan (patient can name drug, dosage, adverse effects to watch for, specific measures to avoid adverse effects, measures to take to increase the effectiveness of the drug).
- Monitor the effectiveness of comfort and safety measures and compliance with the regimen.

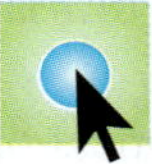

WEB LINKS

Health care providers and patients may want to consult the following Internet sources:

http://www.rhinitisinfo.com Information on allergic rhinitis and seasonal rhinitis, including support groups, research, and treatment.

http://www.healthy.net Information on education programs, research, and other information related to allergies and seasonal rhinitis.

http://www.niaid.nih.gov/research.htm Information about allergy research and treatment.

http://allergy.mcg.edu/media/rhinit.html Information for patients, including special pediatric information on seasonal allergies and hay fever, resources, and references.

http://www.cff.org Information on cystic fibrosis, including research, treatments, and resources:

Points to Remember

- The classes of drugs that affect the upper respiratory system work to keep the airways open and gases moving efficiently.
- Antitussives are drugs that suppress the cough reflex. They can act centrally, to suppress the medullary cough center, or locally, to increase secretion and buffer irritation or to act as local anesthetics. These drugs should not be used longer than 1 week; patients with persistent cough after that time should seek medical evaluation.
- Decongestants are drugs that cause local vasoconstriction and therefore decrease the blood flow to the irritated and dilated capillaries of the mucous membranes lining the nasal passages and sinus cavities.
- An adverse effect that accompanies frequent or prolonged use of decongestants is rebound vasodilation, called rhinitis medicamentosa. The reflex reaction to vasoconstriction is a rebound vasodilation, which often leads to prolonged overuse of decongestants.
- Topical nasal decongestants are preferable in patients who need to avoid systemic adrenergic effects. Oral deconges-

tants are associated with systemic adrenergic effects and require caution in patients with cardiovascular disease, hyperthyroidism, or diabetes mellitus.

- Topical nasal steroid decongestants block the inflammatory response from occurring. These drugs, which take several days to weeks to reach complete effectiveness, are preferred for patients with allergic rhinitis who need to avoid the complications of systemic steroid therapy.
- The antihistamines selectively block the effects of histamine at the histamine-1 receptor sites, decreasing the allergic response. Antihistamines are used for the relief of symptoms associated with seasonal and perennial allergic rhinitis, allergic conjunctivitis, uncomplicated urticaria, or angioedema.
- Patients taking antihistamines may react to dryness of the skin and mucous membranes. The nurse should encourage them to drink plenty of fluids, to use a humidifier if possible, to avoid smoke-filled rooms, and to use good skin care and moisturizers.
- Antihistamines should be avoided with any patient who has a prolonged Q-T interval because serious cardiac complications and even death have occurred.
- Expectorants are drugs that liquefy the lower respiratory tract secretions. They are used for the symptomatic relief of respiratory conditions characterized by a dry, nonproductive cough.
- Mucolytics work to break down mucus in order to aid high-risk respiratory patients in coughing up thick, tenacious secretions.
- Many of the drugs that act on the upper respiratory tract are found in various OTC cough and allergy preparations. Patients need to be advised to always read the labels carefully to avoid inadvertent overdose and toxicity.

CHECK YOUR UNDERSTANDING

Answers to the questions in this chapter may be found in the Answer Key in the back of the book.

Multiple Choice

Select the best answer to the following.

1. A patient with sinus pressure and pain related to a seasonal rhinitis would benefit from taking
   a. an antitussive.
   b. an expectorant.
   c. a mucolytic.
   d. a decongestant.
2. Antitussives are useful in blocking the cough reflex and preserving the energy associated with prolonged, nonproductive coughing. Antitussives are best used with
   a. postoperative patients.
   b. asthma patients.
   c. patients with a dry, irritating cough.
   d. COPD patients who tire easily.
3. Patients with seasonal rhinitis experience irritation and inflammation of the nasal passages and passages of the upper airways. Treatment for these patients might include
   a. systemic corticosteroids.
   b. mucolytic agents.
   c. an expectorant.
   d. topical nasal steroids.
4. A patient taking an OTC cold medication and an OTC allergy medicine is found to be taking double doses of pseudoephedrine. As a result, the patient might exhibit
   a. ear pain.
   b. restlessness, tenseness, tremors, and palpitations.
   c. sinus pressure.
   d. an irritating cough.
5. Antihistamines should be used very cautiously in patients with
   a. a history of arrhythmias or prolonged Q-T intervals because fatal cardiac arrhythmias can occur.
   b. COPD.
   c. asthma.
   d. angioedema.
6. A patient is not getting a response to the antihistamine that was prescribed. Appropriate action might include
   a. switching to a decongestant.
   b. stopping the drug and increasing fluids.
   c. trying a different antihistamine.
   d. switching to a corticosteroid.
7. Dornase alfa (*Pulmozyme*), because of its mechanism of action, is reserved for use in
   a. clearing secretions before diagnostic tests.
   b. facilitating removal of secretions postoperatively.
   c. protecting the liver from acetaminophen toxicity.
   d. relieving the buildup of secretions in cystic fibrosis.

Multiple Response

Select all that apply.

1. Common adverse effects associated with the use of topical nasal steroids would include which of the following?
   a. Local burning and stinging
   b. Dryness of the mucosa
   c. Headache
   d. Constipation and urinary retention
   e. Fungal infections
   f. Osteonecrosis

2. An antihistamine would be the drug of choice for treating which of the following?
   a. Itchy eyes
   b. Irritating cough
   c. Nasal congestion
   d. Drippy nose
   e. Idiopathic urticaria
   f. Thick, tenacious secretions

3. Additional nursing interventions for clients receiving antihistamines probably would include which of the following?
   a. Using a humidifier
   b. Advising client to suck sugarless lozenges to help relieve the dry mouth
   c. Limiting fluid intake to decrease swelling
   d. Providing safety measures to prevent falls or injury
   e. Encouraging pushing fluids, if allowed
   f. Leaving bowls of water around the house to increase humidity

Web Exercise

R.W. recently moved to the area and has developed seasonal rhinitis. He had asthma as a child and is concerned that it might be returning. He asks for up-to-date information on the two disorders and how to survive the discomfort. Go to the Internet and find information that would be useful in preparing a teaching program for R.W.

Word Scramble

Unscramble the following letters to form the names of drugs commonly used to treat upper respiratory tract problems.

1. mactelseni ______________________________
2. extramodernphhot ______________________________
3. inpeerhed ______________________________
4. hatzooterylriden ______________________________
5. heednoripesuepd ______________________________
6. dobnudesie ______________________________
7. catflunisoe ______________________________
8. mazetileso ______________________________

Bibliography and References

Drug facts and comparisons. (2006). St. Louis: Facts and Comparisons.

Gilman, A., Hardman, J. G., & Limbird, L. E. (Eds.). (2006). *Goodman and Gilman's the pharmacological basis of therapeutics* (11th ed.). New York: McGraw-Hill.

Karch, A. M. (2006). *2007 Lippincott's nursing drug guide.* Philadelphia: Lippincott Williams & Wilkins.

The medical letter on drugs and therapeutics. (2006). New Rochelle, NY: Medical Letter.

Professional's guide to patient drug facts. (2006). St. Louis: Facts and Comparisons.

CHAPTER

55

Drugs Used to Treat Obstructive Pulmonary Disorders

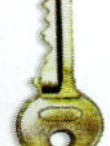

KEY TERMS

bronchodilators

Cheyne–Stokes respiration

leukotriene receptor antagonists

mast cell stabilizers

respiratory distress syndrome (RDS)

sympathomimetics

xanthines

LEARNING OBJECTIVES

Upon completion of this chapter, you will be able to:

1. Describe the underlying pathophysiology involved in obstructive pulmonary disease and correlate this information with the presenting signs and symptoms.
2. Describe the therapeutic actions, indications, pharmacokinetics, contraindications, most common adverse reactions, and important drug–drug interactions associated with xanthines, sympathomimetic bronchodilators, anticholinergic bronchodilators, inhaled steroids, leukotriene receptor antagonists, lung surfactants, and mast cell stabilizers.
3. Discuss the use of drugs used to treat obstructive pulmonary disorders across the lifespan.
4. Compare and contrast the prototype drugs theophylline, epinephrine, ipratropium, budesonide, zafirlukast, beractant, and cromolyn with other agents in their class and with other classes of drugs used to treat obstructive pulmonary disorders.
5. Outline the nursing considerations, including important teaching points, for patients receiving drugs used to treat obstructive pulmonary disorders.

BRONCHODILATORS/ ANTIASTHMATICS, XANTHINES

aminophylline
caffeine
dyphylline
P theophylline

SYMPATHOMIMETICS

albuterol
bitolterol
ephedrine
P epinephrine
formoterol
isoetharine
isoproterenol
levalbuterol
metaproterenol
pirbuterol
salmeterol
terbutaline

ANTICHOLINERGICS

P ipratropium
tiotropium

INHALED STEROIDS

beclomethasone
P budesonide
fluticasone
triamcinolone

LEUKOTRIENE RECEPTOR ANTAGONISTS

montelukast
P zafirlukast
zileuton

LUNG SURFACTANTS

P beractant
calfactant
poractant

MAST CELL STABILIZERS

P cromolyn
nedocromil

Pulmonary obstructive diseases include asthma and chronic obstructive pulmonary disease (COPD), which includes emphysema. These diseases cause obstruction of the major airways. The obstruction of asthma, emphysema, and COPD can be related to inflammation that results in narrowing of the interior of the airway and to muscular constriction that results in narrowing of the conducting tube (Figure 55.1). With chronic inflammation, muscular and cilial action is lost, and complications related to the loss of these protective processes can occur, such as infections, pneumonia, and movement of inhaled substances deep into the respiratory system. In severe COPD, air is trapped in the lower respiratory tract, the alveoli degenerate and fuse together, and the exchange of gases is greatly impaired.

Reducing environmental exposure to irritants—stopping smoking, filtering allergens from the air, avoiding exposure to known irritants and allergens—is the first step in treating these conditions. If these efforts are not sufficient to prevent problems, treatment is aimed at either opening the conducting airways through muscular bronchodilation or decreasing the effects of inflammation on the lining of the airway. See Table 55.1 for guidelines for maintenance treatment of asthma.

Another obstructive disease, **respiratory distress syndrome (RDS)**, causes obstruction at the alveolar level. The obstruction of RDS in the neonate is related to a lack of the lipoprotein surfactant, which leads to an inability to maintain an open alveolus. Surfactant is essential in decreasing the surface tension in the tiny alveolus, allowing it to expand and remain open. If surfactant is lacking, the alveoli collapse and gas exchange cannot occur. Pharmacological therapy for this condition involves instilling surfactant into the alveoli.

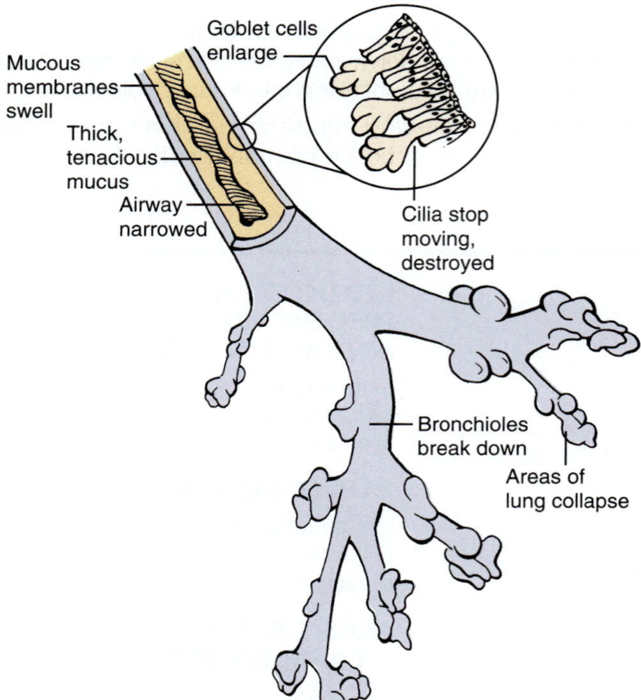

FIGURE 55.1 Changes in the airways with chronic obstructive pulmonary disease.

Adult respiratory distress syndrome (ARDS) is characterized by progressive loss of lung compliance and increasing hypoxia. This syndrome occurs as a result of a severe insult to the body, such as cardiovascular collapse, major burns, severe trauma, and rapid depressurization. Treatment of ARDS involves reversal of the underlying cause of the problem combined with ventilatory support.

Bronchodilators/ Antiasthmatics

Bronchodilators, or antiasthmatics, are medications used to facilitate respirations by dilating the airways. They are helpful in symptomatic relief or prevention of bronchial asthma and for bronchospasm associated with COPD. Several of the bronchodilators are administered orally and absorbed systemically, giving them the potential for many systemic adverse effects. Other medications are administered directly into the airways by nebulizers. These medications have the advantage of fewer systemic adverse reactions. Box 55.1 discusses the use of these drugs with different age groups. A new type of drug used to treat alpha$_1$-protease deficiency, *Zemaira,* is discussed in Box 55.2.

Xanthines

The **xanthines**, including caffeine and theophylline, come from a variety of naturally occurring sources. These drugs were once the main treatment choices for asthma and bronchospasm. However, because they have a relatively narrow margin of safety, and they interact with many other drugs, they are no longer considered the first-choice bronchodilators. Xanthines used to treat respiratory disease include aminophylline (*Truphylline*), caffeine (*Caffedrine* and others), dyphylline (*Dilor* and others), and theophylline (*Slo-Bid, Theo-Dur*) (Table 55.2).

Therapeutic Actions and Indications

The xanthines have a direct effect on the smooth muscles of the respiratory tract, both in the bronchi and in the blood vessels (Figure 55.2). Although the exact mechanism of action is not known, one theory suggests that xanthines work by directly affecting the mobilization of calcium within the cell. They do this by stimulating two prostaglandins, result-

Table 55.1 Guidelines for Maintenance Treatment of Asthma*

Treatment	Intermittent Asthma (symptoms less than once a week, no symptoms between attacks)		Mild Persistent Asthma (symptoms at least once a week but less than once a day)		Moderate Persistent Asthma (daily symptoms and treatment, attacks affect activities)		Severe Asthma (continuous symptoms, limited physical activity, frequent exacerbations)	
	Prevention	*Acute*	*Prevention*	*Acute*	*Prevention*	*Acute*	*Prevention*	*Acute*
Short-acting inhaled beta-agonist[†]		X		X		X		X
Inhaled corticosteroids[†]			X		X		X	
Mast cell stabilizer			X[‡]					
Leukotriene receptor agonist			X					
Long-acting bronchodilators					X		X	
Inhaled beta-agonists[†]								
Sustained-release theophylline			X[§]					
Long-acting oral beta-agonist								
Corticosteroids							X[‖]	

*Effective treatment depends on patient response; a combination of therapies may be required to achieve good control.[†] Considered drug of choice.[‡] May be preferred treatment in children older than 2 years.[§] Not a preferred treatment.[‖] Wean to inhaled preparation as soon as possible.

ing in smooth muscle relaxation, which increases the vital capacity that has been impaired by bronchospasm or air trapping. Xanthines also inhibit the release of slow-reacting substance of anaphylaxis (SRSA) and histamine, decreasing the bronchial swelling and narrowing that occurs as a result of these two chemicals.

Xanthines are indicated for the symptomatic relief or prevention of bronchial asthma and for reversal of bronchospasm associated with COPD. Unlabeled uses include stimulation of respirations in **Cheyne–Stokes respiration** and the treatment of apnea and bradycardia in premature infants.

Pharmacokinetics

The xanthines are rapidly absorbed from the gastrointestinal (GI) tract, reaching peak levels within 2 hours. They are widely distributed and metabolized in the liver and excreted in urine. Xanthines cross the placenta and enter breast milk. They have been associated with fetal abnormalities and breathing difficulties at birth in animal studies. Although no clear studies are available in human pregnancy, use should be limited to situations in which the benefit to the mother clearly outweighs the potential risk to the fetus. Because the xanthines enter breast milk and could affect the baby, another method of feeding the baby should be selected if these drugs are needed during lactation.

Contraindications and Cautions

Caution should be taken with any patient with GI problems, coronary disease, respiratory dysfunction, renal or hepatic disease, alcoholism, or hyperthyroidism *because these conditions can be exacerbated by the systemic effects of xanthines.* Xanthines are available for oral and parenteral use; the parenteral drug should be switched to the oral form as soon as possible *because the systemic effects of the oral form are less acute and more manageable.*

Adverse Effects

Adverse effects associated with xanthines are related to theophylline levels in the blood (Critical Thinking Scenario 55-1). Therapeutic theophylline levels are from 10 to 20 mcg/mL. With increasing levels, predictable adverse effects are seen, ranging from GI upset, nausea, irritability, and tachycardia to seizures, brain damage, and even death (Table 55.3).

Clinically Important Drug–Drug Interactions

Because of the mechanism of xanthine metabolism in the liver, many drugs interact with xanthines. The list of interacting drugs should be checked any time a drug is added or removed from a drug regimen.

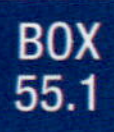

BOX 55.1 **DRUG THERAPY ACROSS THE LIFESPAN**

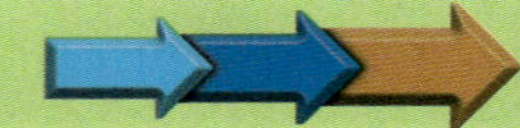

Lower Respiratory Tract Agents

CHILDREN

Antiasthmatics are frequently used in children. The incidence of asthma in children has been rapidly increasing in the 21st century. The leukotriene receptor antagonists have been found to be especially effective for long-term prophylaxis in children. Acute episodes are best treated with a beta-agonist and then a long-acting inhaled steroid or a mast cell stabilizer.

Parents need to be encouraged to take measures to prevent acute attacks, including avoidance of known allergens, smoke-filled rooms, and crowded or dusty areas. Parents should be cautioned about the proper way to measure liquid preparations to avoid inadvertent toxic doses or lack of therapeutic effects.

Theophylline has been used in children, but because of its many adverse effects and the better control afforded by newer agents, its use is reserved for cases that do not respond to other therapies.

As the child grows and matures, the disease will need to be re-evaluated and dosage adjustments made to meet the needs of the growing child. Teenagers need to learn the proper administration and use of inhaled steroids for prevention of exercise-induced asthma.

As with other classes of medications, children may be more susceptible to the adverse effects associated with these drugs and need to be carefully monitored and evaluated. Over-the-counter (OTC) drugs and herbal remedies should be avoided if possible; if they are used, they should be reported to the health care provider so that appropriate dosage adjustments can be made where needed.

The parents of premature babies undergoing surfactant therapy will require consistent support and education to help them to cope with the stress of this event.

ADULTS

Adults may be able to manage their asthma quite well with the use of inhalers and avoidance of aggravating situations. Periodic review of the proper use of the various inhalers should be part of routine evaluation of these patients. Periodic spirometry readings should be done to evaluate the effectiveness of the therapy.

The safety of these drugs during pregnancy and lactation has not been established. There is a potential for adverse effects of the fetus related to blood flow changes and direct drug effects when the drugs cross the placenta. Use should be reserved for those situations in which the benefit to the mother outweighs the potential risk to the fetus. The drugs may enter breast milk and also may alter fluid balance and milk production. It is advised that caution be used if one of these drugs is prescribed during lactation.

OLDER ADULTS

Older adults frequently are prescribed one or more of these drugs. Older adults are more likely to develop adverse effects associated with the use of these drugs, such as sedation, confusion, dizziness, urinary retention, and cardiovascular effects. Safety measures may be needed if these effects occur and interfere with the patient's mobility and balance.

Older adults are also more likely to have renal and/or hepatic impairment related to underlying medical conditions, which could interfere with the metabolism and excretion of these drugs. The dosage for older adults should be started at a lower level than recommended for young adults. Patients should be monitored very closely and dosage adjustment based on patient response.

These patients also need to be alerted to the potential for toxic effects when using OTC preparations and should be advised to check with their health care provider before beginning any OTC drug regimen. Older adults with progressive chronic obstructive pulmonary disease may be taking many combined drugs to help them maintain effective respirations. These patients should have an overall treatment plan involving complex pulmonary toilet, positioning, fluids, nutrition, humidified air, rest, and activity plans, as well as a complicated drug regimen to deal with the impact of this disease.

Nicotine increases the metabolism of xanthines in the liver; xanthine dosage must be increased in patients who continue to smoke while using xanthines. In addition, extreme caution must be used if the patient decides to decrease or discontinue smoking because severe xanthine toxicity can occur.

BOX 55.2 **Focus on Enzyme Therapy: Alpha$_1$-Protease Inhibitor (Human)**

An alpha$_1$-protease inhibitor, *Zemaira,* was approved in 2003 for the treatment of alpha$_1$-protease deficiency, a chronic, hereditary, autosomal dominant disorder that presents as progressive, severe emphysema, usually during a person's 30s or 40s. Alpha$_1$-protease inhibitor is normally present in the lungs and acts to neutralize neutrophil elastase, which is increased by smoking or lung infection. Patients who do not produce enough alpha$_1$-protease inhibitor are at risk for progressive lung tissue destruction with smoking or lung infection. This type of emphysema and COPD does not respond well to the drug therapy usually associated with COPD. *Zemaira* is infused during a period of 15 minutes once each week at a dose of 60 mg/kg and provides protection from tissue destruction.

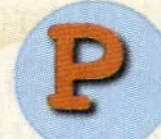

Prototype Summary: *Theophylline*

Indications: Symptomatic relief or prevention of bronchial asthma and reversible bronchospasm associated with chronic bronchitis and emphysema

Actions: Directly relaxes bronchial smooth muscle, causing bronchodilation and increasing vital capacity; also inhibits the release of SRSA and histamine

Pharmacokinetics:

Route	Onset	Peak	Duration
Oral	Varies	2 h	Varies

$T_{1/2}$: 3–15 hours (nonsmoker), 4–5 hours (smoker); metabolized in the liver and excreted in urine

Adverse effects: Irritability, restlessness, dizziness, palpitations, life-threatening arrhythmias, loss of appetite, proteinuria, respiratory arrest, fever, flushing

Table 55.2 DRUGS IN FOCUS

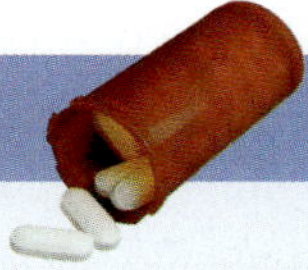

Xanthine Bronchodilators

Drug Name	Usual Dosage	Usual Indications
aminophylline (*Truphylline*)	Adult: 6 mg/kg PO loading dose, then 3.8 mg/kg q4h × three doses Maintenance: 3 mg/kg q6h Range: 600–1600 mg/day PO in three to four divided doses Rectal: 500 mg q6–8h *Geriatric or impaired: reduce dosage and monitor* closely Pediatric: 6 mg/kg PO loading dose, then 4 mg/kg (6 mo–9 yr) or 3 mg/kg (9–16 yr) q4h for three doses, then maintain at same dose q6h Range: 12 mg/kg/day PO Base all doses on patient response and serum levels	All of the xanthine bronchodilators are indicated for symptomatic relief or prevention of bronchial asthma and reversal of bronchospasm associated with COPD
caffeine (*generic*)	Adult: 500–1000 mg IM, do not exceed 2.5 g/day Pediatric: 10 mg/kg IV followed by 2.5 mg/kg/day for neonatal apnea	
dyphylline (*Dilor*)	Adult: up to 15 mg/kg PO q.i.d. or 250–500 mg injected slowly IM Geriatric or impaired adult: use caution	
P theophylline (*Slo-bid, Theo-Dur*)	Dosage varies widely based on preparation and patient response Adult: 6 mg/kg PO loading dose followed by 3 mg/kg PO q4h × three doses, then 3 mg/kg PO q6h Chronic therapy: 400 mg/day PO in divided doses Rectal: 500 mg q6–8h Pediatric: 6 mg/kg PO loading dose, then 4 mg/kg (6 mo–9 yr) or 3 mg/kg (9–16 yr) PO q4h × three doses, then the same dose q6h Chronic therapy: 400 mg/day PO in divided doses	

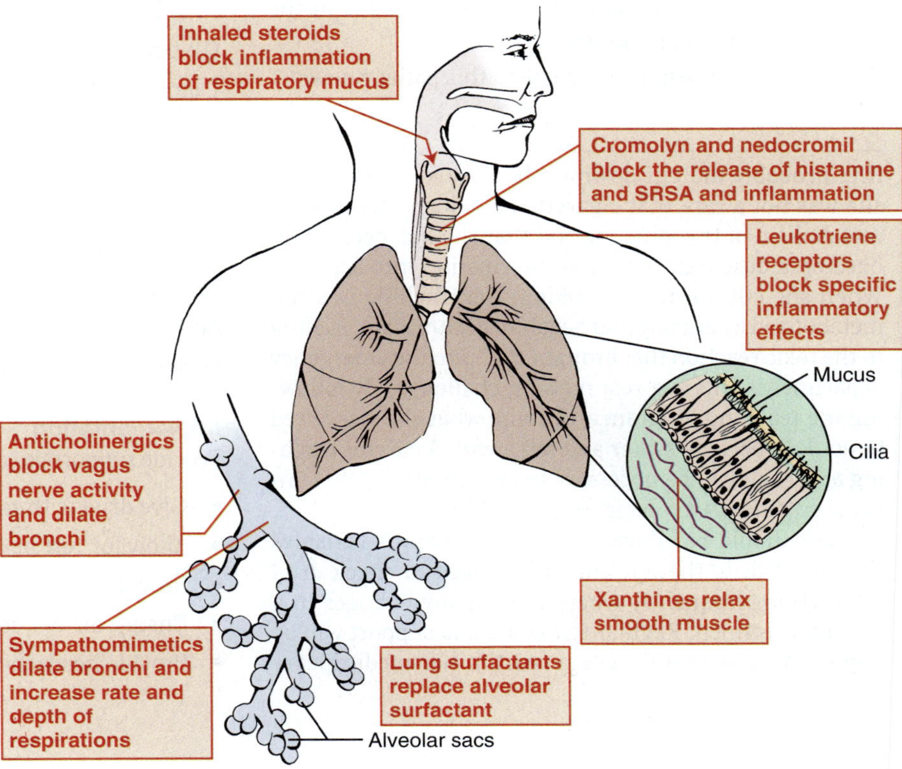

FIGURE 55.2 Sites of action of drugs used to treat obstructive pulmonary disorders.

CRITICAL THINKING SCENARIO 55-1

Toxic Reaction to Theophylline

The Situation

R.P. has a medical diagnosis of chronic bronchitis and has been stabilized on theophylline for the past 3 years. She has been labeled as noncompliant with medical therapy because she continues to smoke cigarettes (more than three packs per day), knowing that she has a progressive pulmonary disease. R.P. was referred to a student nurse for teaching. After several sessions, in which the student presented posters and pictures and gave R.P. a great deal of personal attention and encouragement, it was determined that R.P. had a good understanding of her problem and would stop or at least cut down on her smoking. Three days later, R.P. presented to the emergency department with complaints of dizziness, nausea, vomiting, confusion, grouchiness, and palpitations. Her admission heart rate was 96 beats/min with occasional to frequent premature ventricular contractions.

Critical Thinking

What probably happened to R.P.?

What information should the student have known before conducting the teaching program?

How could that information have been included in the patient teaching program?

What would the best approach be to this patient now?

Discussion

R.P. probably did cut down on her smoking. However, she was not aware that cigarette smoking increases the metabolism of theophylline and that she had been stabilized on a dose that took that information into account. When she cut down on smoking, theophylline was not metabolized as quickly and began to accumulate, leading to the toxic reaction that brought R.P. into the emergency department. This is a real nursing challenge. By following the teaching program and doing what she was asked to do, R.P. became sicker and felt awful. A careful teaching approach will be necessary to encourage R.P. to continue cutting down on cigarette smoking.

Staff should be educated on the numerous variables that affect drug therapy and encouraged to check drug interactions frequently when making any changes in a patient's regimen. Regular follow-up and support will be important to help R.P. regain trust in her medical care providers and continue her progress in cutting down smoking. Frequent checks of theophylline levels should be done while R.P. is cutting back, and dosage adjustments should be made by her prescriber to maintain therapeutic levels of theophylline and avoid toxic levels.

Nursing Care Guide For R.P.: Xanthines

Assessment: History and Examination

Assessment parameters include a health history focused particularly on allergies, peptic ulcer, gastritis, renal or hepatic dysfunction, coronary disease, cigarette use, pregnancy, and lactation, as well as concurrent use of cimetidine, erythromycin, troleandomycin, ciprofloxacin, hormonal contraceptives, ticlodipine, ranitidine, rifampin, barbiturates, phenytoin, benzodiazepines, and beta blockers.

Focus the physical examination on the following areas:

Neurological: orientation, reflexes, affect, coordination

Respiratory: respiratory rate and character, adventitious sounds

Skin: color, lesions

CV: blood pressure, pulse, peripheral perfusion, baseline EKG

GI: bowel sounds, abdominal exam

Laboratory tests: serum theophylline levels, renal, hepatic function tests

Nursing Diagnoses

Acute Pain related to GI effects or dry mouth

Decreased Cardiac Output

Impaired Sensory Perception (Kinesthetic, Visual)

Activity Intolerance

Deficient Knowledge regarding drug therapy

Implementation

Provide supportive care with comfort and safety measures:

- Give drug with meals.
- Allow for rest periods.
- Provide a quiet environment.
- Ensure dietary control of caffeine.
- Provide headache therapy as needed.

Toxic Reaction to Theophylline *(continued)*

Provide reassurance to deal with drug effects and lifestyle changes.

Provide patient teaching regarding drug name, dosage, adverse effects, precautions, warnings to report, dietary cautions, and need for follow-up.

Evaluation

Evaluate drug effects: relief of respiratory difficulty, improvement of air movement.

Monitor for adverse effects: GI upset, CNS effects, cardiac arrhythmias; monitor for drug–drug interactions as appropriate.

Evaluate effectiveness of patient teaching program and comfort and safety measures.

Patient Teaching For R.P.

- ☐ The drug that has been prescribed for you, theophylline, is called a bronchodilator. Bronchodilators work by relaxing the airways, helping to make breathing easier and to decrease wheezes and shortness of breath. To be effective, this drug must be taken exactly as prescribed.
- ☐ This drug should be taken on an empty stomach with a full 8-oz glass of water. If GI upset is severe, you can take the drug with food. Do not chew the enteric-coated or time-release capsules or tablets—they must be swallowed whole to be effective.
- ☐ Common effects of this drug include:
  - *Gastrointestinal upset, nausea, vomiting, heartburn:* Taking the drug with food may help this problem.
  - *Restlessness, nervousness, difficulty in sleeping:* The body often adjusts to these effects over time. Avoiding other stimulants, such as caffeine, may help decrease some of these symptoms.
  - *Headache:* This often goes away with time. If headaches persist or become worse, notify your health care provider.
  - Report any of the following to your health care provider: *vomiting, severe abdominal pain, pounding or fast heart beat, confusion, unusual tiredness, muscle twitching, skin rash, hives.*
- ☐ Many foods can change the way that your drug works; if you decide to change your diet, consult with your health care provider.
- ☐ Adverse effects of the drug can be avoided by avoiding foods that contain caffeine or other xanthine derivatives (coffee, cola, chocolate, tea) or by using them in moderate amounts. This is especially important if you experience nervousness, restlessness, or sleeplessness.
- ☐ Cigarette smoking affects the way your body uses this drug. If you decide to change your smoking habits, such as increasing or decreasing the number of cigarettes you smoke each day, consult with your health care provider regarding the possible need to adjust your dosage.
- ☐ Avoid the use of any over-the-counter medication without first checking with your health care provider. Several of these medications can interfere with the effectiveness of this drug.
- ☐ Tell any doctor, nurse, or other health care provider involved in your care that you are taking this drug.
- ☐ Keep this drug, and all medications, out of the reach of children.

Table 55.3 Adverse Effects Associated with Various Serum Levels of Theophylline

Serum Level	Adverse Effects
≤20 (mcg/mL)	Uncommon
>20–25 (mcg/mL)	Nausea, vomiting, diarrhea, insomnia, headache, irritability
>30–35 (mcg/mL)	Hyperglycemia, hypotension, cardiac arrhythmias, tachycardia, seizures, brain damage, death

Nursing Considerations for Patients Receiving Xanthines

Assessment: History and Examination

Screen for the following conditions, *which could be cautions or contraindications to use of the drug:* any known allergies; cigarette use, *which would affect the metabolism of the drug;* peptic ulcer, gastritis, renal or hepatic dysfunction, and coronary disease, *all of which require cautious use;* and pregnancy and lactation, *which are contraindications.*

Physical assessment should be performed *to establish baseline data for assessing the effectiveness of the drug and the occurrence of any adverse effects associated with drug therapy.* Perform the following assessments: thorough skin examination including color and the presence of lesions, *to provide a baseline as a reference for drug effectiveness;* blood pressure, pulse, cardiac auscultation, peripheral perfusion, and baseline electrocardiogram (ECG), *to provide a baseline for effects on the cardiovascular system;* and bowel sounds, liver evaluation, and blood tests, *to provide a baseline for renal and hepatic function tests.* In addition, evaluate serum theophylline levels *to provide a baseline reference and identify conditions that may require caution in the use of xanthines.*

Nursing Diagnoses

The patient receiving a xanthine bronchodilator may have the following nursing diagnoses related to drug therapy:

- Acute Pain related to headache and GI upset
- Disturbed Sensory Perception (Kinesthetic, Visual) related to central nervous system (CNS) effects
- Deficient Knowledge regarding drug therapy

Implementation With Rationale

- Administer oral drug with food or milk *to relieve GI irritation, if GI upset is a problem.*
- Monitor patient's response to the drug (e.g., relief of respiratory difficulty, improved air flow) *to determine the effectiveness of the drug dosage and to adjust dosage as needed.*
- Provide comfort measures, including rest periods, quiet environment, dietary control of caffeine, and headache therapy as needed, *to help the patient cope with the effects of drug therapy.*
- Provide periodic follow-up, including blood tests, *to monitor serum theophylline levels.*
- Provide thorough patient teaching, including the drug name and prescribed dosage, measures to help avoid adverse effects, warning signs that may indicate problems, and the need for periodic monitoring and evaluation, *to enhance patient knowledge about drug therapy and to promote compliance.*

Evaluation

- Monitor patient response to the drug (improved air flow, ease of respirations).
- Monitor for adverse effects (CNS effects, cardiac arrhythmias, GI upset, local irritation).
- Monitor for potential drug–drug interactions; consult with the prescriber to adjust dosages as appropriate.
- Evaluate the effectiveness of the teaching plan (patient can name drug, dosage, adverse effects to watch for, specific measures to avoid adverse effects).
- Monitor effectiveness of comfort measures and compliance with the regimen.

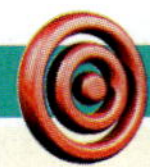

FOCUS POINTS

- Asthma, emphysema, chronic obstructive pulmonary disease (COPD), and respiratory distress syndrome (RDS) are pulmonary obstructive diseases. All but RDS involve obstruction of the major airways; RDS obstructs the alveoli.
- Drug treatment of asthma and COPD aims to relieve inflammation and promote bronchial dilation.
- Xanthine-derived drugs affect the smooth muscles of the respiratory tract—both in the bronchi and in the blood vessels.
- The effects of the xanthines are directly related to blood levels of theophylline. Excessive or toxic levels can lead to coma and death.

Sympathomimetics

Sympathomimetics are drugs that mimic the effects of the sympathetic nervous system. One of the actions of the sympathetic nervous system is dilation of the bronchi with increased rate and depth of respiration. This is the desired effect when selecting a sympathomimetic as a bronchodilator. Sympathomimetics that are used as bronchodilators include the following (Table 55.4):

- Albuterol (*Proventil* and others) is long-acting and available in inhaled and oral forms for patients older than 2 years of age.
- Bitolterol (*Tornalate*) is long-acting and inhaled; it is preferred for prophylaxis of bronchospasm in patients older than 12 years of age.
- Ephedrine (generic) is used parenterally for acute bronchospasm in adults and children, although epinephrine is the drug of choice.
- Epinephrine (*Sus-Phrine, EpiPen,* and others) is the drug of choice in adults and children for the treatment of acute bronchospasm, including that caused by anaphylaxis; it is also available for inhalation. Because epinephrine is associated with systemic sympathomimetic effects, it is not the drug of choice for patients with cardiac conditions.

Table 55.4 DRUGS IN FOCUS

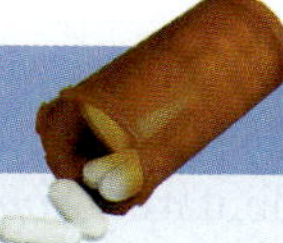

Sympathomimetic Bronchodilators

Drug Name	Usual Dosage	Usual Indications
albuterol (*Proventil*)	Adult: 2–4 mg PO t.i.d. to q.i.d. *or* two inhalations q4–6h *or* two inhalations 15 min before exercise Pediatric: >12 yr—adult dosage; 6–12 yr—2 mg t.i.d. to q.i.d. oral tablets; 6–14 yr—2 mg t.i.d. to q.i.d. PO oral syrup; 2–6 yr to 0.1 mg/kg PO t.i.d. oral syrup (2–12 yr inhalation):—1.25–2.5 mg; for prevention of exercise-induced bronchospasm, 200-mcg capsule inhaled 15 min before exercise	Treatment and prophylaxis of bronchospasm; prevention of exercise-induced bronchospasm
bitolterol (*Tornalate*)	Adult: two inhalations q8h for prevention, at intervals of 1–3 min for treatment; use special caution if >60 yr Pediatric (>12 yr): as adult Pediatric (<12 yr): not recommended	Treatment and prophylaxis for bronchospasm
ephedrine (*generic*)	Adult: 25–50 mg IM, Sub-Q, or IV Pediatric: 25–100 mg/m² IM or Sub-Q divided into four to six doses	Treatment of acute bronchospasm
P epinephrine (*Sus-Phrine*)	Adult: 0.1–0.3 mL Sub-Q q20min for 4 h as needed, may also be given by aerosol inhalation or nebulization Pediatric: 0.01–0.3 mL/m² Sub-Q q20min for 4 h as needed	Drug of choice for treatment of acute bronchospasm
formoterol (*Foradil*)	Adult and pediatric (≥5 yr) for asthma maintenance: 12-mcg capsule q12h, inhaled using the *Aerolizer inhaler* Adult and pediatric (≥12 yr): 12-mcg capsule inhaled using the *Aerolizer inhaler,* at least 15 min before exercising, do not use additional doses for 12 h	Maintenance treatment of asthma and prevention of bronchospasm in patients ≥5 yr of age with reversible obstructive airway disease; prevention of exercise-induced bronchospasm in patients ≥12 yr of age **Special considerations:** If taking the drug for asthma maintenance, do not use additional doses of drug for exercise-induced asthma.
isoetharine (*generic*)	Adult: four inhalations from handheld nebulizers or 1–2 mL over 15–20 min with oxygen aerosolization; use caution if >60 yr	Treatment and prophylaxis of bronchospasm
isoproterenol (*Isuprel*)	Adult: 0.01–0.02 mg IV during anesthesia; 1:200 solution with 5–15 deep inhalations for acute bronchial asthma, or 5–15 inhalations using nebulizer for COPD-related bronchospasm Pediatric: 0.25 mL or the 1:200 solution for each 10–15 min of nebulization	Treatment of bronchospasm during anesthesia and prophylaxis of bronchospasm
levalbuterol (*Xopenex*)	Adult and pediatric (>12 yr): 0.63 mg q6–8h by nebulization Pediatric (6–11 yr): 0.31 mg t.i.d. by nebulizer	Treatment and prevention of bronchospasm
metaproterenol (*Alupent*)	Adult: Two to three inhalations q3–4h; use caution if >60 yr Pediatric (>12 yr): inhalation, same as adult Pediatric (6–12 yr): nebulizer, 0.1–0.2 mL in saline	Treatment of prophylaxis of bronchospasm and acute asthma attacks in children ≤6 yr of age
pirbuterol (*Maxair*)	Adult and pediatric (>12 yr): 0.4 mg (two inhalations) q4–6h, do not exceed 12 inhalations per day	Treatment and prophylaxis of bronchospasm
salmeterol (*Serevent*)	Adult and pediatric (≥12 yr): two puffs q12h; or two puffs 30–60 min before exercise Pediatric (4–12 yr): one inhalation b.i.d. at least 12 h apart; one inhalation ≥30 min before exercising	Prophylaxis of bronchospasm and prevention of exercise-induced asthma
terbutaline (*Brethaire*)	Adult and pediatric (>15 yr): 5 mg PO q6h while awake; 0.25 mg Sub-Q repeat in 15 min as needed; two inhalations separated by 60 sec q4–6h Pediatric (12–15 yr): 2.5 mg PO t.i.d.; two inhalations separated by 60 sec q4–6h as needed	Treatment and prophylaxis of bronchospasm

- Formoterol (*Foradil*) is an inhaled drug used for maintenance treatment of asthma and prevention of bronchospasm in patients older than 5 years of age who have reversible obstructive airway disease, and for prevention of exercise-induced bronchospasm in patients older than 12 years of age.
- Isoetharine (generic) is an inhaled drug used for prophylaxis and treatment of bronchospasm. Dosage guidelines for children have not been established.
- Isoproterenol (*Isuprel* and others) is used for treatment of bronchospasm during anesthesia and as an inhalant for treatment of bronchospasm in adults and children;

it is associated with more cardiac side effects than some other drugs.

- Levalbuterol (*Xopenex*) is an inhaled agent used to treat and prevent bronchospasm in patients older than 6 years of age who have reversible obstructive pulmonary disease.
- Metaproterenol (*Alupent*) is an inhaled agent and is used for both treatment and prophylaxis of bronchospasm in patients older than 6 years of age.
- Pirbuterol (*Maxair*) is an inhaled drug used for both treatment and prophylaxis of bronchospasm in patients older than 12 years of age.

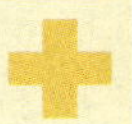

FOCUS ON PATIENT SAFETY

Name confusion has been reported between *Maxair* (pirbuterol), a sympathomimetic agent used for the treatment of asthma, and *Maxalt* (rizatriptan), a triptan used for the treatment of migraine headaches. Serious adverse effects have occurred when these drugs were inadvertently confused. Use caution if you have a patient on either of these drugs.

- Salmeterol (*Serevent*) is an inhaled drug successfully used to prevent exercise-induced asthma and for prophylaxis of bronchospasm in selected patients older than 4 years of age. (See Box 55.3 for important information regarding African Americans taking this drug.)
- Terbutaline (*Brethaire* and others) can be used orally, parenterally, and by inhalation for both prophylaxis and treatment of bronchospasm in patients older than 12 years of age

Therapeutic Actions and Indications

Most of the sympathomimetics used as bronchodilators are beta$_2$-selective adrenergic agonists. That means that at therapeutic levels their actions are specific to the beta$_2$-receptors found in the bronchi (see Chapter 30). This specificity is lost at higher levels. Other systemic effects of sympathomimetics include increased blood pressure, increased heart rate, vasoconstriction, and decreased renal and GI blood flow—all actions of the sympathetic nervous system. These overall effects limit the systemic usefulness of these drugs in certain patients.

The sympathomimetic epinephrine is given by injection during acute asthma attacks, when the need for bronchodilation outweighs the risk of adverse effects. Other sympathomimetics are used in the treatment of bronchospasm in reversible obstructive airway disease (e.g., acute or chronic asthma, chronic bronchitis). They have also been effective in preventing exercise-induced bronchospasm (see Figure 55.2).

BOX 55.3 CULTURAL CONSIDERATIONS FOR DRUG THERAPY

As a result of postmarketing studies, the boxed warning label on the asthma drug salmeterol (*Serevent*) was changed to warn of a small but significant increase in the risk of life-threatening asthma episodes in patients using salmeterol. In the study, which involved 13,000 patients each in a salmeterol treatment group and a control group, there were 13 asthma-related deaths in a 28-week period in the salmeterol group compared with 4 asthma-related deaths in the control group. The study showed that African American patients had a greater risk of asthma-related deaths than did other groups. The FDA agreed that the benefit of using salmeterol for the treatment of asthma was greater than the risk that the drug poses, but cautioned health care professionals to be cautious when prescribing these drugs.

Pharmacokinetics

These drugs are rapidly distributed after injection; they are transformed in the liver to metabolites that are excreted in the urine. The half-life of these drugs is relatively short, less than 1 hour. These drugs should be used during pregnancy and lactation only if the benefits to the mother clearly outweigh potential risks to the fetus or neonate because they are known to cross the placenta and to enter breast milk. The inhaled drugs are rapidly absorbed into the lung tissue. Any absorbed drug will still be metabolized in the liver and excreted in urine.

Contraindications and Cautions

These drugs are contraindicated or should be used with caution, depending on the severity of the underlying condition, *in conditions that would be aggravated by the sympathetic stimulation,* including cardiac disease, vascular disease, arrhythmias, diabetes, hyperthyroidism, pregnancy, and lactation.

Adverse Effects

Adverse effects of these drugs, which can be attributed to sympathomimetic stimulation, include CNS stimulation, GI upset, cardiac arrhythmias, hypertension, bronchospasm, sweating, pallor, and flushing.

Clinically Important Drug–Drug Interactions

Special precautions should be taken to avoid the combination of sympathomimetic bronchodilators with the general anesthetics cyclopropane and halogenated hydrocarbons. Because these drugs sensitize the myocardium to catecholamines, serious cardiac complications could occur.

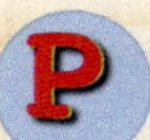

Prototype Summary: *Epinephrine*

Indications: Treatment of anaphylactic reactions, acute asthmatic attacks; relief from respiratory distress of COPD and bronchial asthma

Actions: Reacts at alpha- and beta-receptor sites in the sympathetic nervous system to cause bronchodilation, increased heart rate, increased respiratory rate, and increased blood pressure

Pharmacokinetics:

Route	Onset	Peak	Duration
Sub-Q	5–10 min	20 min	20–30 min
IM	5–10 min	20 min	20–30 min
IV	Instant	20 min	20–30 min
Inhalation	3–5 min	20 min	1–3 h

$T_{1/2}$: Unknown; metabolized by normal neural pathways

Adverse effects: Fear, anxiety, restlessness, headache, nausea, decreased renal formation, pallor, palpitation, tachycardia, local burning and stinging, rebound congestion with nasal inhalation

Nursing Considerations for Patients Receiving Sympathomimetic Bronchodilators

Assessment: History and Examination

Screen for the following conditions, *which could be cautions or contraindications to use of the drug:* allergy to any sympathomimetic or drug vehicle; pregnancy or lactation, *which would require cautious use of the drug;* cardiac disease, vascular disease, arrhythmias, diabetes, and hyperthyroidism, *which may be exacerbated by sympathomimetic effects;* and use of the general anesthetics cyclopropane and halogenated hydrocarbons, *which sensitize the myocardium to catecholamines and could cause serious cardiac complications if used with these drugs.*

Physical assessment should be performed *to establish baseline data for assessing the effectiveness of the drug and the occurrence of any adverse effects associated with drug therapy.* Assess the following: reflexes and orientation, *to evaluate CNS effects of the drug;* respirations and adventitious sounds, *to establish a baseline for drug effectiveness and possible adverse effects;* pulse, blood pressure, and, in certain cases, a baseline ECG, *to monitor the cardiovascular effects of sympathetic stimulation;* and liver function tests, *to assess for changes that could interfere with metabolism of the drug and require dosage adjustment.*

Nursing Diagnoses

The patient receiving a sympathomimetic bronchodilator may have the following nursing diagnoses related to drug therapy:

- Increased Cardiac Output related to sympathomimetic effects
- Acute Pain related to CNS, GI, or cardiac effects of the drug
- Disturbed Thought Processes related to CNS effects
- Deficient Knowledge related to drug therapy

Implementation With Rationale

- Reassure the patient that the drug of choice will vary with each individual. *These sympathomimetics are slightly different chemicals and are prepared in a variety of delivery systems.* A patient may have to try several different sympathomimetics before the most effective one is found.
- Advise patients to use the minimal amount needed for the shortest period necessary *to prevent adverse effects and accumulation of drug levels.*
- Teach patients who use one of these drugs for exercise-induced asthma to use it 30 to 60 minutes before exercising *to ensure peak therapeutic effects when they are needed.*
- Provide safety measures as needed if CNS effects become a problem *to prevent patient injury.*
- Provide small, frequent meals and nutritional consultation if GI effects interfere with eating *to ensure proper nutrition.*
- Carefully teach the patient about the proper use of the prescribed delivery system. Review that procedure periodically *because improper use may result in ineffective therapy* (Box 55.4.)
- Provide thorough patient teaching, including the drug name and prescribed dosage, measures to help avoid adverse effects, warning signs that may indicate problems, and the need for periodic monitoring and evaluation, *to enhance patient knowledge about drug therapy and to promote compliance.*
- Offer support and encouragement, *to help the patient cope with the disease and the drug regimen.*

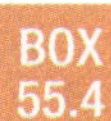

BOX 55.4 FOCUS ON **CLINICAL SKILLS**

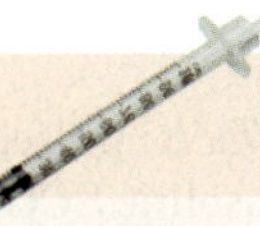

Teaching Patients to Self-administer Medication

It is important to deliver inhaled drugs into the lungs to achieve a rapid reaction and decrease the occurrence of systemic adverse effects. Patients who are self-administering inhaled drugs may be using an inhaler or a nebulizer.

Inhalers

An inhaler is a device that allows a canister containing the drug to be inserted into a metered-dose device that will deliver a specific amount of the drug when the patient compresses the canister. The inhaler has a mouthpiece and may also have a spacer, which is used to hold the dose of the drug while the patient inhales. This is advantageous if the patient has difficulty compressing the canister and inhaling at the same time, or if inhaling is difficult.

Have the patient shake the canister, exhale, and then place the spacer in his or her mouth. (If a spacer is not being used, he or she should hold the device about 1 inch from the open mouth.) The patient should then compress the canister while inhaling, hold his or her breath as long as possible, and then exhale through pursed lips. The patient should then rinse his or her mouth and wash the spacer (if used). Some drugs come with a very specific inhaling device designed just for that drug. If the patient is using one of those drugs, the manufacturer's instructions should be consulted.

Nebulizers

A nebulizer uses compressed air to change a liquid drug into a fine mist for inhalation. If a patient is using a handheld device or a mask, he or she should sit upright or in a semi-Fowler's position and place the correct amount of liquid (drug dose) in the nebulizer chamber, which is attached to a compressed gas system. The patient should breathe slowly and deeply during the treatment. After the liquid is gone, the patient should rinse his or her mouth and clean the mask or device.

Patients may use these devices for several years. It is important to check their administration techniques periodically to ensure that the patient is getting a therapeutic dose of the drug.

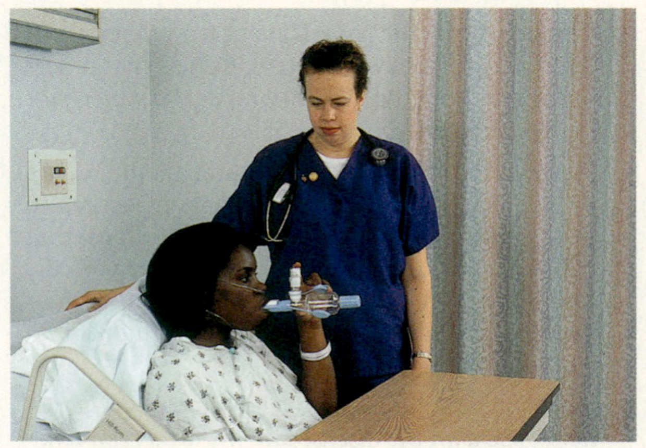

Teaching a patient to use a metered-dose inhaler. © B Proud.

Evaluation

- Monitor patient response to the drug (improved breathing).
- Monitor for adverse effects (CNS effects, increased pulse and blood pressure, GI upset).
- Evaluate the effectiveness of the teaching plan (patient can name drug, dosage, adverse effects to watch for, specific measures to avoid adverse effects, measures to take to increase the effectiveness of the drug).
- Monitor the effectiveness of other measures to ease breathing.

Anticholinergic Bronchodilators

Patients who cannot tolerate the sympathetic effects of the sympathomimetics might respond to the anticholinergic drugs ipratropium (*Atrovent*) or tiotropium (*Spiriva*) (Table 55.5). These drugs are not as effective as the sympathomimetics but can provide some relief to those patients who cannot tolerate the other drugs. Tiotropium was the first drug approved for once-daily maintenance treatment of bronchospasm associated with COPD.

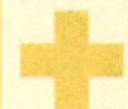

FOCUS ON **PATIENT SAFETY**

The propellant used to make ipratropium an inhaled drug has a cross-sensitivity to the antigen that causes peanut allergies. Patients who are started on inhaled ipratropium, or the combination drug *Combivent,* should be questioned about the possibility of peanut allergies, which would make this drug contraindicated. With the number of reported peanut allergies growing each year, it is an important safety reminder to check with patients about food allergies, as well as known drug allergies.

Therapeutic Actions and Indications

Anticholinergics are used as bronchodilators because of their effect on the vagus nerve, which is to block or antagonize the action of the neurotransmitter acetylcholine at vagal-mediated receptor sites (see Figure 55.2). Normally, vagal stimulation results in a stimulating effect on smooth muscle, causing contraction. By blocking the vagal effect, relaxation of smooth muscle in the bronchi occurs, leading to bronchodilation. Ipratropium is the only anticholinergic recommended for bronchodilation. It is indicated for the maintenance treatment of patients with COPD, including bronchospasm and emphysema.

Table 55.5 DRUGS IN FOCUS

Anticholinergic Bronchodilators

Drug Name	Usual Dosage	Usual Indications
 ipratropium (*Atrovent*)	36 mcg (two inhalations) four times per day, up to 12 inhalations if needed	Maintenance treatment of adults with COPD
tiotropium (*Spiriva*)	18 mcg/day (one capsule) using the *Handihaler* inhalation device	Long-term, once-daily maintenance treatment of bronchospasm associated with COPD

Pharmacokinetics

Ipratropium has an onset of action of 15 minutes when inhaled. Its peak effects occur in 1 to 2 hours, and it has a duration of effect of 3 to 4 hours. Little is known about its fate in the body. It is generally not absorbed systemically. Tiotropium has a rapid onset of action and a long duration, with a half-life of 5 to 6 days. It is excreted unchanged in urine.

Contraindications and Cautions

Caution should be used in any condition *that would be aggravated by the anticholinergic or atropine-like effects of the drug,* such as narrow-angle glaucoma (*drainage of the vitreous humor can be blocked by smooth muscle relaxation*), bladder neck obstruction, or prostatic hypertrophy (*relaxed muscle causes decreased bladder tone*), and conditions aggravated by dry mouth and throat. The use of ipratropium or tiotropium is contraindicated in the presence of known allergy to the drug.

Adverse Effects

Adverse effects are related to the anticholinergic effects of the drug if it is absorbed systemically. These effects include dizziness, headache, fatigue, nervousness, dry mouth, sore throat, palpitations, and urinary retention.

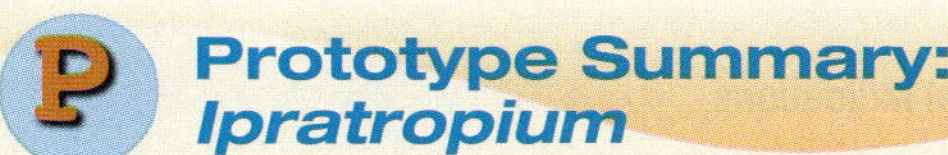

Prototype Summary: Ipratropium

Indications: Maintenance treatment of bronchospasm associated with COPD

Actions: Anticholinergic that blocks vagally mediated reflexes by antagonizing the action of acetylcholine

Pharmacokinetics:

Route	Onset	Peak	Duration
Inhalation	15 min	1–2 h	3–4 h

$T_{1/2}$: Unknown; metabolized by neural pathways

Adverse effects: Nervousness, dizziness, headache, nausea, GI distress, cough, palpitations

Nursing Considerations for Patients Receiving an Anticholinergic Bronchodilator

Assessment: History and Examination

Screen for the following conditions, *which could be cautions or contraindications to use of the drug:* allergy to atropine or other anticholinergics; acute bronchospasm, *which would be a contraindication;* narrow-angle glaucoma (*drainage of the vitreous humor can be blocked by smooth muscle relaxation*), bladder neck obstruction or prostatic hypertrophy (*relaxed muscle causes decreased bladder tone*), and conditions aggravated by dry mouth and throat, *all of which could be exacerbated by the use of this drug;* and pregnancy and lactation, *which would require cautious use.*

Physical assessment should be done *to establish baseline data for assessing the effectiveness of the drug and the occurrence of any adverse effects associated with drug therapy.* Assess the following: skin color and lesions, *to assess for dryness or allergic reaction;* orientation, affect, and reflexes, *to evaluate CNS effects;* pulse and blood pressure, *to monitor cardiovascular effects of the drug;* respirations and adventitious sounds, *to monitor drug effectiveness and possible adverse effects;* and urinary output and prostate palpation as appropriate, *to monitor anticholinergic effects.*

Nursing Diagnoses

The patient receiving an anticholinergic bronchodilator may have the following nursing diagnoses related to drug therapy:

- Acute Pain related to CNS, GI, or respiratory effects of the drug
- Imbalanced Nutrition: Less Than Body Requirements, related to dry mouth and GI upset
- Deficient Knowledge regarding drug therapy

Implementation With Rationale

- Ensure adequate hydration and provide environmental controls, such as the use of a humidifier, *to make the patient more comfortable.*
- Encourage the patient to void before each dose of medication *to prevent urinary retention related to drug effects.*
- Provide safety measures if CNS effects occur *to prevent patient injury.*
- Provide small, frequent meals and sugarless lozenges *to relieve dry mouth and GI upset.*
- Review use of the inhalator with the patient; caution the patient not to exceed 12 inhalations in 24 hours *to prevent serious adverse effects.*
- Advise the patient not to drive or use hazardous machinery if nervousness, dizziness, and drowsiness occur with this drug *to prevent injury.*
- Provide thorough patient teaching, including the drug name and prescribed dosage, measures to help avoid adverse effects, warning signs that may indicate problems, and the need for periodic monitoring and evaluation, *to enhance patient knowledge about drug therapy and to promote compliance.*
- Offer support and encouragement *to help the patient cope with the disease and the drug regimen.*

Evaluation

- Monitor patient response to the drug (improved breathing).
- Monitor for adverse effects (CNS effects, increased pulse or blood pressure, GI upset, dry skin and mucous membranes).
- Evaluate the effectiveness of the teaching plan (patient can name drug, dosage, adverse effects to watch for, specific measures to avoid adverse effects, measures to take to increase the effectiveness of the drug).
- Monitor the effectiveness of other measures to ease breathing.

Inhaled Steroids

Inhaled steroids have been found to be a very effective treatment for bronchospasm. Agents approved for this use include beclomethasone (*Beclovent* and others), budesonide (*Pulmicort*), fluticasone (*Flovent*), and triamcinolone (*Azmacort* and others) (Table 55.6). The drug of choice depends on the individual patient's response; a patient may have little response to one agent and do very well on another. It is usually useful to try another preparation if one is not effective within 2 to 3 weeks.

Fixed-combination drugs are also available using some of these drugs (Box 55.5).

Therapeutic Actions and Indications

Inhaled steroids are used to decrease the inflammatory response in the airway. In an airway that is swollen and

Table 55.6 DRUGS IN FOCUS

Inhaled Steroids

Drug Name	Usual Dosage	Usual Indications
beclomethasone (*Beclovent*)	Adult: 84–168 mcg t.i.d. to q.i.d. (two inhalations) Pediatric (6–12 yr): one to two inhalations t.i.d. to q.i.d., do not exceed 10 inhalations per day	All of the inhaled steroids are used for the prevention and treatment of asthma; for treatment of chronic steroid-dependent bronchial asthma; and as adjunctive therapy for asthma patients who do not respond to traditional bronchodilators
P budesonide (*Pulmicort*)	Adult and pediatric (>6 y): 200–400 mcg b.i.d. (two inhalations), maximum dose 800 mcg b.i.d. Pediatric (>6 yr): 200 mcg b.i.d.	
fluticasone (*Flovent*)	Adult: 88–440 mcg b.i.d. by inhalation Pediatric (4–11 yr): 50–100 mcg b.i.d. by inhalation	
triamcinolone (*Azmacort*)	Adult: two inhalations (200 mcg) t.i.d. to q.i.d. Pediatric (6–12 yr): one to two inhalations t.i.d. to q.i.d.	

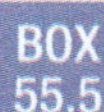

BOX 55.5 Fixed-Combination Respiratory Drugs

The benefit of combining different classes of drugs for the treatment of asthma has resulted in the availability of fixed-combination drugs.

- Advair Diskus *is a combination of fluticasone (a steroid) and salmeterol (a sympathetic agent). It is approved for managing asthma in patients 4 years of age and older.*
- *Combivent* is a combination of ipratropium (an anticholinergic agent) and albuterol (a sympathetic agent).

Patients should be stabilized on each drug separately before switching to the fixed-combination drug. Once the switch has been made, the dosing is cut in half and most patients find it easier to be compliant with drug therapy.

narrowed by inflammation and swelling, this action will increase air flow and facilitate respiration. Inhaling the steroid tends to decrease the numerous systemic effects that are associated with steroid use. When administered into the lungs by inhalation, steroids decrease the effectiveness of the inflammatory cells. This has two effects: decreased swelling associated with inflammation and promotion of beta-adrenergic receptor activity, which may promote smooth muscle relaxation and inhibit bronchoconstriction (see Figure 55.2).

These drugs are used for the prevention and treatment of asthma, to treat chronic steroid-dependent bronchial asthma, and as adjunct therapy for patients whose asthma is not controlled by traditional bronchodilators. These drugs are rapidly absorbed but take from 2 to 3 weeks to reach effective levels.

Pharmacokinetics

These drugs are absorbed well from the respiratory tract. They are metabolized by natural systems, mostly within the liver, and are excreted in the urine. The glucocorticoids are known to cross the placenta and to enter breast milk; they should be used during pregnancy and lactation only if the benefits to the mother clearly outweigh the potential risks to the fetus or neonate.

Contraindications and Cautions

Inhaled corticosteroids are not for emergency use and not for use during an acute asthma attack or status asthmaticus. They should not be used during pregnancy or lactation. These preparations should be used with caution in any patient who has an active infection of the respiratory system *because the depression of the inflammatory response could result in serious illness.*

Adverse Effects

Adverse effects are limited because of the route of administration. Sore throat, hoarseness, coughing, dry mouth, and pharyngeal and laryngeal fungal infections are the most common side effects encountered. If a patient does not administer the drug appropriately or develops lesions that allow absorption of the drug, the systemic side effects associated with steroids may occur.

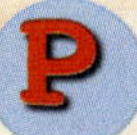

Prototype Summary: Budesonide

Indications: Prevention and treatment of asthma; to treat chronic steroid-dependent bronchial asthma; as adjunct therapy for patients whose asthma is not controlled by traditional bronchodilators

Actions: Decreases the inflammatory response in the airway; this action will increase air flow and facilitate respiration in an airway narrowed by inflammation

Pharmacokinetics:

Route	Onset	Peak	Duration
Inhalation	Slow	Rapid	8–12 h

$T_{1/2}$: 2–3 hours; metabolized in the liver and excreted in urine

Adverse effects: Irritability, headache, rebound congestion, epistaxis, local infection

Nursing Considerations for Patients Receiving Inhaled Steroids

Assessment: History and Examination

Screen for the following conditions, *which could be cautions or contraindications to use of the drug:* acute asthmatic attacks, allergy to the drugs, and pregnancy and lactation, *which are contraindications,* and systemic infections, *which require cautious use.*

Physical assessment should be done *to establish baseline data for assessing the effectiveness of the drug and the occurrence of any adverse effects associated with drug therapy.* Assess the following: temperature, *to monitor for possible infections;* blood pressure, pulse, and auscultation, *to evaluate cardiovascular response;* and respirations and adventitious sounds, *to monitor drug effectiveness.* In addition, conduct an examination of the nares *to evaluate for any lesions that might lead to systemic absorption of the drug.*

Nursing Diagnoses

The patient receiving an inhaled steroid may have the following nursing diagnoses related to drug therapy:

- Risk for Injury related to immunosuppression
- Acute Pain related to local effects of the drug
- Deficient Knowledge regarding drug therapy

Implementation With Rationale

- Do not administer the drug to treat an acute asthma attack or status asthmaticus *because these drugs are not intended for treatment of acute attack.*
- Taper systemic steroids carefully during the transfer to inhaled steroids; *deaths have occurred from adrenal insufficiency with sudden withdrawal.*
- Have the patient use decongestant drops before using the inhaled steroid *to facilitate penetration of the drug if nasal congestion is a problem.*
- Have the patient rinse the mouth after using the inhaler *because this will help to decrease systemic absorption and decrease GI upset and nausea.*
- Monitor the patient for any sign of respiratory infection; *continued use of steroids during an acute infection can lead to serious complications related to the depression of the inflammatory and immune responses.*
- Provide thorough patient teaching, including the drug name and prescribed dosage, measures to help avoid adverse effects, warning signs that may indicate problems, and the need for periodic monitoring and evaluation, *to enhance patient knowledge about drug therapy and to promote compliance.*
- Offer support and encouragement *to help the patient cope with the disease and the drug regimen.*

Evaluation

- Monitor patient response to the drug (improved breathing).
- Monitor for adverse effects (nasal irritation, fever, GI upset).
- Evaluate the effectiveness of the teaching plan (patient can name drug, dosage, adverse effects to watch for, specific measures to avoid adverse effects, measures to take to increase the effectiveness of the drug).
- Monitor the effectiveness of other measures to ease breathing.

Leukotriene Receptor Antagonists

A newer class of drugs, the **leukotriene receptor antagonists**, was developed to act more specifically at the site of the problem associated with asthma. Zafirlukast (*Accolate*) was the first drug of this class to be developed. Montelukast (*Singulair*) and zileuton (*Zyflo*) are the other drugs currently available in this class (see Table 55.7). Because this class is relatively new, long-term effects and the benefits of one drug over another have not yet been determined.

Therapeutic Actions and Indications

Leukotriene receptor antagonists selectively and competitively block (zafirlukast, montelukast) or antagonize (zileuton) receptors for the production of leukotrienes D_4 and E_4, components of SRSA. As a result, these drugs block many of the signs and symptoms of asthma, such as neutrophil and eosinophil migration, neutrophil and monocyte aggregation, leukocyte adhesion, increased capillary permeability,

Table 55.7 DRUGS IN FOCUS

Leukotriene Receptor Antagonists

Drug Name	Usual Dosage	Usual Indications
montelukast (*Singulair*)	Adult and pediatric (>15 yr): 10 mg PO daily in the evening Pediatric (12–23 mo): 4-mg granules PO in the evening Pediatric (2–5 yr): 4-mg chewable tablet PO in the evening Pediatric (6–14 yr): 5-mg chewable tablet PO in the evening	Prophylaxis and chronic treatment of bronchial asthma
P zafirlukast (*Accolate*)	Adult and pediatric (>12 yr): 20 mg PO b.i.d. Pediatric (5–11 yr): 10 mg PO b.i.d.	Prophylaxis and chronic treatment of bronchial asthma
zileuton (*Zyflo*)	Adult and pediatric (≥12 yr): 600 mg PO q.i.d. for a total of 2400 mg/day	Prophylaxis and chronic treatment of bronchial asthma in patients ≥12 yr of age

and smooth muscle contraction. These factors contribute to inflammation, edema, mucus secretion, and bronchoconstriction seen in patients with asthma. The leukotriene receptor antagonists are indicated for the prophylaxis and chronic treatment of bronchial asthma in adults and in patients younger than 12 years of age. They are not indicated for the treatment of acute asthmatic attacks (see Figure 55.2).

Pharmacokinetics

These drugs are rapidly absorbed from the GI tract. Zafirlukast and montelukast are extensively metabolized in the liver by the cytochrome P450 system and are primarily excreted in feces. Zileuton is metabolized and cleared through the liver. These drugs cross the placenta and enter breast milk. Fetal toxicity has been reported in animal studies, so these drugs should be used during pregnancy only if the benefit to the mother clearly outweighs the potential risks to the fetus. No adequate studies have been done on the effects on the baby if these drugs are used during lactation; caution should be used.

Contraindications and Cautions

These drugs should be used cautiously in patients with hepatic or renal impairment *because these conditions can affect the drug's metabolism and excretion* and during pregnancy and lactation *because of the potential for adverse effects on the fetus or neonate.*

Adverse Effects

Adverse effects associated with leukotriene receptor antagonists include headache, dizziness, myalgia, nausea, diarrhea, abdominal pain, elevated liver enzyme concentrations, vomiting, generalized pain, fever, and myalgia.

Clinically Important Drug–Drug Interactions

Use caution if propranolol, theophylline, terfenadine, or warfarin is taken with these drugs because increased toxicity can occur. Toxicity may also occur if these drugs are combined with calcium channel blockers, cyclosporine, or aspirin; decreased dosage of either drug may be necessary.

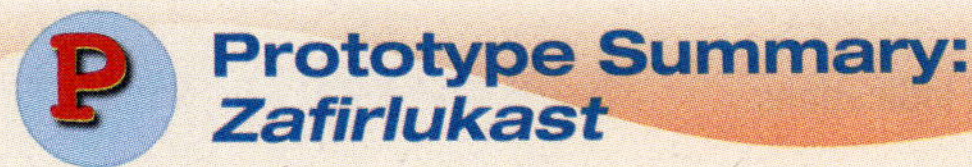

Prototype Summary: *Zafirlukast*

Indications: Prevention and long-term treatment of asthma in adults and children 5 years of age or older

Actions: Specifically blocks receptors for leukotrienes, which are components of SRSA, blocking airway edema and processes of inflammation in the airway

Pharmacokinetics:

Route	Onset	Peak	Duration
Oral	Rapid	3 h	Unknown

$T_{1/2}$: 10 hours; metabolized in the liver and excreted in urine and feces

Adverse effects: Headache, dizziness, nausea, generalized pain and fever, infection

Nursing Considerations for Patients Receiving Leukotriene Receptor Antagonists

Assessment: History and Examination

Screen for the following conditions, *which could be cautions or contraindications to use of the drug:* allergy to the drug, pregnancy or lactation, and acute bronchospasm or asthmatic attack, *all of which would be contraindications to the use of the drug;* and impaired renal or hepatic function, *which could alter the metabolism and excretion of the drug and might require a dosage adjustment.*

Physical assessment should be done *to establish baseline data for assessing the effectiveness of the drug and the occurrence of any adverse effects associated with drug therapy.* Assess the following: temperature, *to monitor for underlying infection;* orientation and affect, *to monitor for CNS effects of the drug;* respirations and adventitious breath sounds, *to monitor the effectiveness of the drug;* liver and renal function tests, *to assess for impairments;* and abdominal evaluation, *to monitor GI effects of the drug.*

Nursing Diagnoses

The patient receiving a leukotriene receptor antagonist may have the following nursing diagnoses related to drug therapy:

- Acute Pain related to headache, GI upset, or myalgia
- Risk for Injury related to CNS effects
- Deficient Knowledge regarding drug therapy

Implementation With Rationale

- Administer the drug on an empty stomach, 1 hour before or 2 hours after meals; *the bioavailability of these drugs is decreased markedly by the presence of food.*
- Caution the patient that these drugs are not to be used during an acute asthmatic attack or bron-

chospasm; *instead, regular emergency measures will be needed.*

- Caution the patient to take the drug continuously and not to stop the medication during symptom-free periods *to ensure that therapeutic levels are maintained.*
- Provide appropriate safety measures if dizziness occurs *to prevent patient injury.*
- Urge the patient to avoid over-the-counter preparations containing aspirin, *which might interfere with the effectiveness of these drugs.*
- Provide thorough patient teaching, including the drug name and prescribed dosage, measures to help avoid adverse effects, warning signs that may indicate problems, and the need for periodic monitoring and evaluation, *to enhance patient knowledge about drug therapy and to promote compliance.*
- Offer support and encouragement *to help the patient cope with the disease and the drug regimen.*

Evaluation

- Monitor patient response to the drug (improved breathing).
- Monitor for adverse effects (drowsiness, headache, abdominal pain, myalgia).
- Evaluate the effectiveness of the teaching plan (patient can name drug, dosage, adverse effects to watch for, specific measures to avoid adverse effects, measures to take to increase the effectiveness of the drug).
- Monitor the effectiveness of other measures to ease breathing.

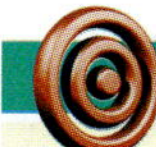

FOCUS POINTS

- Sympathomimetics replicate the effects of the sympathetic nervous system; they dilate the bronchi and increase the rate and depth of respiration.
- Anticholinergics affect the vagus nerve to relax bronchial smooth muscle and thereby promote bronchodilation.
- Corticosteroids decrease the inflammatory response. The inhalable form is associated with many fewer systemic effects than are the other steroid formulations.
- To block various signs and symptoms of asthma, the leukotriene receptor antagonists block or antagonize receptors for the production of leukotrienes D_4 and E_4.

Lung Surfactants

Lung surfactants are naturally occurring compounds or lipoproteins containing lipids and apoproteins that reduce the surface tension within the alveoli, allowing expansion of the alveoli for gas exchange. Three lung surfactants currently available for use are beractant (*Survanta*), calfactant (*Infasurf*), and the newest drug, poractant (*Curosurf*) (Table 55.8). Poractant is being tried in the treatment of adult RDS and with adults after near-drowning.

Therapeutic Actions and Indications

These drugs are used to replace the surfactant that is missing in the lungs of neonates with RDS (see Figure 55.2). They are indicated for the rescue treatment of infants who have developed RDS. They are also used for prophylactic treatment of infants at high risk for RDS—those with a birth weight of less than 1350 g and those with a birth weight greater than 1350 g who have evidence of respiratory immaturity.

Table 55.8 DRUGS IN FOCUS

Lung Surfactants

Drug Name	Usual Dosage	Usual Indications
P beractant (*Survanta*)	4 mL/kg birth weight, instilled intratracheally, may repeat up to four times in 48 h	Rescue treatment of infants who have respiratory distress syndrome (RDS); prophylactic treatment of infants at high risk for development of RDS
calfactant (*Infasurf*)	3 mg/kg birth weight as soon as possible for prophylaxis; 3 mg/kg birth weight divided into two doses, repeat up to a total of three doses 12 h apart for rescue	Rescue treatment of infants who have RDS; prophylactic treatment of infants at high risk for RDS
poractant (*Curosurf*)	2.5 mL/kg birth weight intratracheally, half in each bronchus, may repeat with up to two 1.25-mL/kg doses at 12-h intervals	Rescue treatment of infants who have RDS

Pharmacokinetics

These drugs begin to act immediately on instillation into the trachea. They are metabolized in the lungs by the normal surfactant metabolic pathways. They are not indicated for use in pregnancy or lactation and are not categorized.

Contraindications and Cautions

Because lung surfactants are used as emergency drugs, there are no contraindications.

Adverse Effects

Adverse effects that are associated with the use of lung surfactants include patent ductus arteriosus, hypotension, intraventricular hemorrhage, pneumothorax, pulmonary air leak, hyperbilirubinemia, and sepsis. These effects may be related to the immaturity of the patient, the invasive procedures used, or reactions to the lipoprotein.

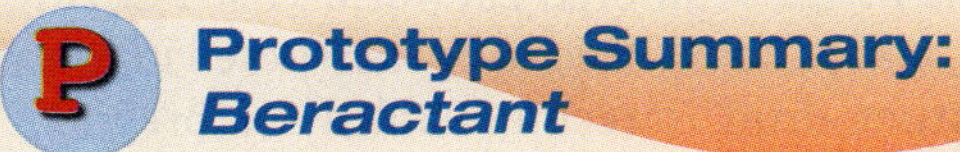

Prototype Summary: *Beractant*

Indications: Prophylactic treatment of infants at high risk for developing RDS; rescue treatment of infants who have developed RDS

Actions: Natural bovine compound of lipoproteins that reduce the surface tension and allow expansion of the alveoli; replaces the surfactant that is missing in infants with RDS

Pharmacokinetics:

Route	Onset	Peak
Intratracheal	Immediate	Hours

$T_{1/2}$: Unknown; metabolized by surfactant pathways

Adverse effects: Patent ductus arteriosus, intraventricular hemorrhage, hypotension, bradycardia, pneumothorax, pulmonary air leak, pulmonary hemorrhage, apnea, sepsis, infection

Nursing Considerations for Patients Receiving Lung Surfactants

Assessment: History and Examination

Screen for time of birth and exact weight *to determine appropriate dosages.* Because this drug is used as an emergency treatment, there are no contraindications to screen for.

Physical assessment should be done *to establish baseline data for assessing the effectiveness of the drug and the occurrence of any adverse effects associated with drug therapy.* Assess the following: skin temperature and color, *to evaluate perfusion;* respirations, adventitious sounds, endotracheal tube placement and patency, and chest movements, *to evaluate the effectiveness of the drug and drug delivery;* blood pressure, pulse, and arterial pressure, *to monitor the status of the infant;* blood gases and oxygen saturation, *to monitor drug effectiveness;* and temperature and complete blood count, *to monitor for sepsis.*

Nursing Diagnoses

The patient receiving a lung surfactant may have the following nursing diagnoses related to drug therapy:

- Decreased Cardiac Output related to cardiovascular and respiratory effects of the drug
- Risk for Injury related to prematurity and risk of infection
- Ineffective Airway Clearance related to the possibility of mucous plugs
- Deficient Knowledge regarding drug therapy (for parents)

Implementation With Rationale

- Monitor the patient continuously during administration and until stable *to provide life support measures as needed.*
- Ensure proper placement of the endotracheal tube with bilateral chest movement and lung sounds *to provide adequate delivery of the drug.*
- Have staff view the manufacturer's teaching video before regular use *to review the specific technical aspects of administration.*
- Suction the infant immediately before administration, but do not suction for 2 hours after administration unless clinically necessary, *to allow the drug time to work.*
- Provide support and encouragement to parents of the patient, explaining the use of the drug in the teaching program, *to help them cope with the diagnosis and treatment of their infant.*
- Continue other supportive measures related to the immaturity of the infant *because this is only one aspect of medical care needed for premature infants.*

Evaluation

- Monitor patient response to the drug (improved breathing, alveolar expansion).

- Monitor for adverse effects (pneumothorax, patent ductus arteriosus, bradycardia, sepsis).
- Evaluate the effectiveness of the teaching plan and support parents as appropriate.
- Monitor the effectiveness of other measures to support breathing and stabilize the patient.
- Evaluate effectiveness of other supportive measures related to the immaturity of the infant.

Mast Cell Stabilizers

Two other drugs that are often used in the treatment of asthma and allergy are cromolyn (*Intal*) and nedocromil (*Tilade, Alocril*) (Table 55.9). These drugs are **mast cell stabilizers**. They prevent the release of inflammatory and bronchoconstricting substances when the mast cells are stimulated to release these substances because of irritation or the presence of an antigen.

Therapeutic Actions and Indications

Cromolyn works at the cellular level to inhibit the release of histamine (released from mast cells in response to inflammation or irritation) and inhibits the release of SRSA (see Figure 55.2). By blocking these chemical mediators of the immune reaction, cromolyn prevents the allergic asthmatic response when the respiratory tract is exposed to the offending allergen. It is inhaled from a capsule and may not reach its peak effect for 1 week. It is recommended for the treatment of chronic bronchial asthma, exercise-induced asthma, and allergic rhinitis.

Nedocromil inhibits the mediators of a variety of inflammatory cells, including eosinophils, neutrophils, macrophages, and mast cells (see Figure 55.2). By blocking these effects, nedocromil decreases the release of histamine and blocks the overall inflammatory response. This drug is indicated for the management of patients with mild to moderate bronchial asthma who are older than 12 years of age. This drug should be taken continually for best results and is often used concomitantly with corticosteroids.

Pharmacokinetics

Cromolyn is primarily active in the lungs, and most of the inhaled dose is excreted during exhalation or, if swallowed, excreted in urine and feces. Nedocromil, when absorbed, is excreted primarily unchanged in urine. Safety for use in pregnancy and lactation has not been established. Use should be reserved for those situations when the benefit to the mother greatly outweighs any potential risk to the fetus or neonate.

Contraindications and Cautions

Both drugs are contraindicated in the presence of known allergy to the drug. Cromolyn cannot be used during an acute attack, and patients need to be instructed in this precaution. Neither drug is recommended for pregnant or nursing women. Cromolyn is not recommended for children younger than 2 years of age, and nedocromil is not recommended before 12 years of age.

Adverse Effects

Few adverse effects have been reported with the use of cromolyn; those that do occur on occasion include swollen eyes, headache, dry mucosa, and nausea. Careful patient management (avoidance of dry or smoky environments, analgesics, use of proper inhalation technique, use of a humidifier, and pushing fluids as appropriate) can help to make drug-related discomfort tolerable. Adverse effects associated with nedocromil include headache, dizziness, fatigue, tearing, GI upset, and cough; this drug should not be discontinued abruptly.

Table 55.9 DRUGS IN FOCUS

Mast Cell Stabilizers

Drug Name	Usual Dosage	Usual Indications
P cromolyn (*Intal*)	Adult and pediatric (>5 yr): 20 mg inhaled q.i.d. Adult and pediatric (>2 yr): 20 mg q.i.d. via nebulizer Adult and pediatric (>6 yr): one spray of nasal solution in each nostril three to six times per day Adult: two ampules PO q.i.d. Pediatric (2–12 yr): one ampule PO q.i.d.	Treatment of chronic bronchial asthma, exercise-induced asthma, and allergic rhinitis
nedocromil (*Tilade, Alocril*)	Adult and pediatric (>12 yr): two inhalations q.i.d. at regular intervals	Management of mild to moderate bronchial asthma

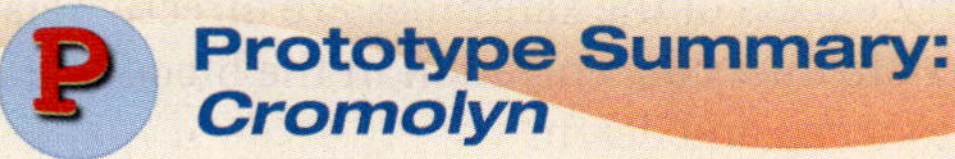

Indications: Prophylaxis of severe bronchial asthma; prevention of exercise-induced asthma

Actions: Inhibits the allergen-triggered release of histamine, SRSA, and leukotrienes from mast cells; decreases the overall allergic response in the airways

Pharmacokinetics:

Route	Onset	Peak	Duration
Inhaled	Slow	15 min	6–8 h

$T_{1/2}$: 80 min; metabolized in the liver and excreted via exhalation

Adverse effects: Headache, dizziness, nausea, sore throat, dysuria, cough, nasal congestion

Nursing Considerations for Patients Receiving Mast Cell Stabilizers

Assessment: History and Examination

Screen for the following conditions, *which could be cautions or contraindications to use of the drug:* allergy to cromolyn or nedocromil; impaired renal or hepatic function, *which could interfere with the metabolism or excretion of the drug, leading to a need for dosage adjustment;* and pregnancy or lactation, *which require very cautious administration.*

Physical assessment should be done *to establish baseline data for assessing the effectiveness of the drug and the occurrence of any adverse effects associated with drug therapy.* Assess the following: skin color and lesions, *to monitor for adverse effects of the drug;* respirations and adventitious sounds, *to evaluate drug effectiveness;* patency of nares, *to determine efficacy of inhaled preparations;* orientation, *to monitor adverse effects and headache;* and liver and renal function tests, *to assess for potential problems with drug metabolism or excretion.*

Nursing Diagnoses

The patient receiving a mast cell stabilizer may have the following nursing diagnoses related to drug therapy:

- Acute Pain related to local effects, headache, or GI effects
- Risk for Injury related to CNS effects
- Deficient Knowledge regarding drug therapy

Implementation With Rationale

- Review administration procedures with the patient periodically; *proper use of the delivery device is important in maintaining the effectiveness of this drug.*
- Caution the patient not to discontinue use abruptly; cromolyn and nedocromil should be tapered slowly if discontinuation is necessary *to prevent rebound adverse effects.*
- Caution the patient to continue taking this drug, even during symptom-free periods, *to ensure therapeutic levels of the drug.*
- Administer oral drug 30 minutes before meals and at bedtime *to promote continual drug levels and relief of asthma.*
- Initiate safety precautions if dizziness and fatigue are problems with nedocromil therapy *to prevent patient injury.*
- Advise the patient not to wear soft contact lenses; if cromolyn eye drops (used for allergic reactions) are used *lenses can be stained or warped.*
- Provide thorough patient teaching, including the drug name and prescribed dosage, measures to help avoid adverse effects, warning signs that may indicate problems, and the need for periodic monitoring and evaluation, *to enhance patient knowledge about drug therapy and to promote compliance.*
- Offer support and encouragement *to help the patient cope with the disease and the drug regimen.*

Evaluation

- Monitor patient response to the drug (improved breathing, relief of signs of allergic disorders).
- Monitor for adverse effects (drowsiness, dizziness, headache, GI upset, local irritation).
- Evaluate the effectiveness of the teaching plan (patient can name drug, dosage, adverse effects to watch for, specific measures to avoid adverse effects, measures to take to increase the effectiveness of the drug).
- Monitor the effectiveness of other measures to ease breathing.

WEB LINKS

Health care providers and patients may want to consult the following Internet sources:

http://copd.20m.com Information on living with COPD, aimed at patients and families.

http://www.newtechpub.com/health.html Information on support groups, treatment programs, resources, and research involving COPD and asthma.

http://www.lungusa.org/index.html Information on lung diseases, community support groups, getting involved, treatment, research, and definitions.

Points to Remember

- Pulmonary obstructive diseases include asthma, emphysema, and chronic obstructive pulmonary disease (COPD), which cause obstruction of the major airways, and respiratory distress syndrome (RDS), which causes obstruction at the alveolar level.
- Drugs used to treat asthma and COPD include drugs to block inflammation and drugs to dilate bronchi.
- The xanthine derivatives have a direct effect on the smooth muscle of the respiratory tract, both in the bronchi and in the blood vessels.
- The adverse effects of the xanthines are directly related to the theophylline concentration in the blood and can progress to coma and death.
- Sympathomimetics are drugs that mimic the effects of the sympathetic nervous system; they are used for dilation of the bronchi and to increase the rate and depth of respiration.
- Anticholinergics can be used as bronchodilators because of their effect on the vagus nerve, resulting in a relaxation of smooth muscle in the bronchi, which leads to bronchodilation.
- Steroids are used to decrease the inflammatory response in the airway. Inhaling the steroid tends to decrease the numerous systemic effects that are associated with steroid use.
- Leukotriene receptor antagonists block or antagonize receptors for the production of leukotrienes D_4 and E_4, thus blocking many of the signs and symptoms of asthma.
- Lung surfactants are instilled into the respiratory system of premature infants who do not have enough surfactant to ensure alveolar expansion.
- The mast cell stabilizers are antiasthmatic drugs that block mediators of inflammation and help to decrease swelling and blockage in the airways.

CHECK YOUR UNDERSTANDING

Answers to the questions in this chapter may be found in the Answer Key in the back of the book.

Multiple Choice

Select the best answer to the following.

1. Treatment of obstructive pulmonary disorders is aimed at
   a. opening the conducting airways through muscular bronchodilation or by decreasing the effects of inflammation on the lining of the airway.
   b. blocking the autonomic reflexes that alter respirations.
   c. blocking the effects of the immune and inflammatory systems.
   d. altering the respiratory membrane to increase flow of oxygen and carbon dioxide.

2. The xanthines
   a. block the sympathetic nervous system.
   b. stimulate the sympathetic nervous system.
   c. directly affect the smooth muscles of the respiratory tract.
   d. act in the CNS to cause bronchodilation.

3. Your patient has been maintained on theophylline for many years and has recently taken up smoking. The theophylline levels in this patient would be expected to
   a. rise, because nicotine prevents the breakdown of theophylline.
   b. stay the same, because smoking has no effect on theophylline.
   c. fall, because the nicotine stimulates liver metabolism of theophylline.
   d. rapidly reach toxic levels.

4. A person with hypertension and known heart disease has frequent bronchospasms and asthma attacks that are most responsive to sympathomimetic drugs. This patient might be best treated with
   a. an inhaled sympathomimetic, to decrease systemic effects.
   b. a xanthine.
   c. no sympathomimetics because they would be contraindicated.
   d. an anticholinergic.

5. A patient with many adverse reactions to drugs is tried on an inhaled steroid for treatment of bronchospasm. For the first 3 days, the patient does not notice any improvement. You should
   a. switch the patient to a xanthine.
   b. encourage the patient to continue the drug for 2 to 3 weeks; if no response is noted by then, try another inhaled steroid.
   c. switch the patient to a sympathomimetic.
   d. try the patient on surfactant.

6. Leukotriene receptor antagonists act to block production of a component of SRSA. They are most beneficial in treating
   a. seasonal rhinitis.
   b. pneumonia.
   c. COPD.
   d. asthma.

7. Respiratory distress syndrome occurs in
   a. babies with frequent colds.
   b. babies with genetic allergies.
   c. premature babies and those with low birth weight.
   d. babies stressed during the pregnancy.

8. Lung surfactants used therapeutically are
   a. injected into a developed muscle.
   b. instilled via a nasogastric tube.
   c. injected into the umbilical artery.
   d. instilled into an endotracheal tube properly placed in the baby's lungs.

Multiple Response

Select all that apply

1. Clients who are using inhalers require careful teaching about which of the following?
   a. Avoiding food 1 hour before and 2 hours after dosing
   b. Storage of the drug
   c. Administration techniques to promote therapeutic effects and avoid adverse effects
   d. Lying flat for as long as 2 hours after dosing
   e. Timing of administration
   f. The difference between rescue treatment and prophylaxis

2. A child with repeated asthma attacks may be treated with which of the following drugs?
   a. A leukotriene receptor antagonist
   b. A beta-blocker
   c. An inhaled corticosteroid
   d. An inhaled beta agonist
   e. A surfactant
   f. A mast cell stabilizer

True or False

Indicate whether the following statements are true (T) or false (F).

______ 1. Pulmonary obstructive diseases include asthma, emphysema, chronic obstructive pulmonary disease (COPD), respiratory distress syndrome, and seasonal rhinitis.

______ 2. Drugs used to treat asthma and COPD include agents that block inflammation and dilate bronchi.

______ 3. The xanthine derivatives have a direct effect on the smooth muscle of the respiratory tract.

______ 4. The adverse effects of the xanthines are directly related to the theophylline levels and are fairly insignificant.

______ 5. Sympathomimetics block the effects of the sympathetic nervous system and are used to dilate the bronchi.

______ 6. Anticholinergics can be used as bronchodilators because of their effect on the sympathetic nervous system receptor sites.

______ 7. Steroids are used to decrease the inflammatory response in the airway.

______ 8. Leukotriene receptor antagonists block or antagonize receptors for the production of leukotriene D_4 and E_4, thus blocking many of the signs and symptoms of asthma.

Word Scramble

Unscramble the following letters to form words related to lower respiratory tract diseases and therapies.

1. opehhlelni ______________________________
2. rotbullea ______________________________
3. reeeppininh ______________________________
4. trollmeesa ______________________________
5. trappruimio ______________________________

6. bedsudeion ______________________

7. firstluzkaa ______________________

8. tuzoline ______________________

9. tracbeant ______________________

10. cortapant ______________________

Bibliography and References

Drug facts and comparisons. (2006). St. Louis: Facts and Comparisons.

Gilman, A., Hardman, J. G., & Limbird, L. E. (Eds.). (2006). *Goodman and Gilman's the pharmacological basis of therapeutics* (11th ed.). New York: McGraw-Hill.

Karch, A. M. (2006). *2007 Lippincott's nursing drug guide.* Philadelphia: Lippincott Williams & Wilkins.

Porth, C. M. (2005). *Pathophysiology: Concepts of altered health states* (7th ed.). Philadelphia: Lippincott Williams & Wilkins.

Professional's guide to patient drug facts. (2006). St. Louis: Facts and Comparisons.

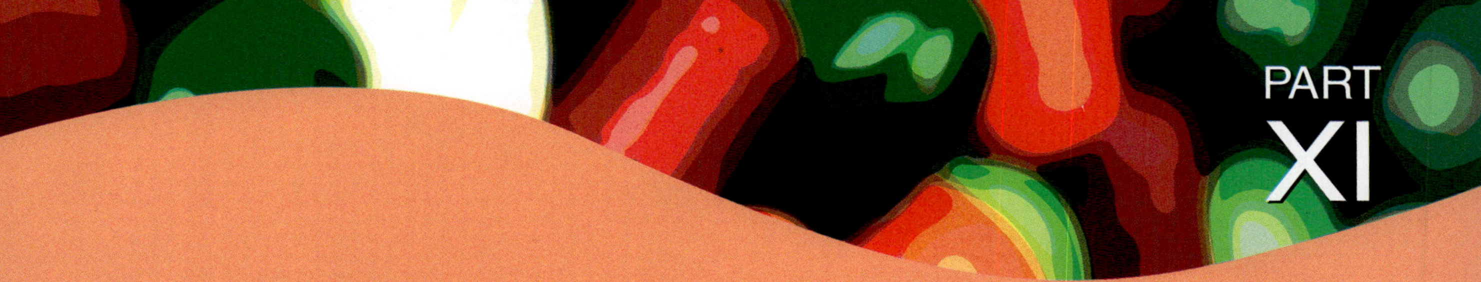

PART XI

Drugs Acting on the Gastrointestinal System

CHAPTER 56

Introduction to the Gastrointestinal System

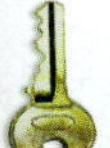

KEY TERMS

bile
chyme
gallstones
gastrin
histamine-2 receptors
hydrochloric acid
local gastrointestinal reflexes
nerve plexus
pancreatic enzymes
peristalsis
saliva
segmentation
swallowing
vomiting

LEARNING OBJECTIVES

Upon completion of this chapter, you will be able to:

1. Label the parts of the gastrointestinal (GI) tract on a diagram and describe secretions, absorption, digestion, and type of motility that occurs in each part.
2. Discuss the nervous control of the GI tract, including influences of the autonomic nervous system on GI activity.
3. List three of the local GI reflexes and describe the clinical application of each.
4. Describe the vomiting reflex and three factors that can stimulate the reflex.
5. Outline the steps involved in swallowing and describe two factors that can influence this reflex.

The gastrointestinal (GI) system is the only system in the body that is open to the external environment. The GI system is composed of one continuous tube that begins at the mouth; progresses through the esophagus, stomach, and small and large intestines; and ends at the anus. The pancreas, liver, and gallbladder are accessory organs that support the functions of the GI system (Figure 56.1). The GI system has four major activities:

- *Secretion*—of enzymes, acid, bicarbonate, and mucus
- *Absorption*—of water and almost all of the essential nutrients needed by the body
- *Digestion*—of food into usable and absorbable components
- *Motility*—movement of food and secretions through the system (what is not used is excreted in the form of feces)

The GI system is responsible for only a very small part of waste excretion. The kidneys and lungs are responsible for excreting most of the waste products of normal metabolism.

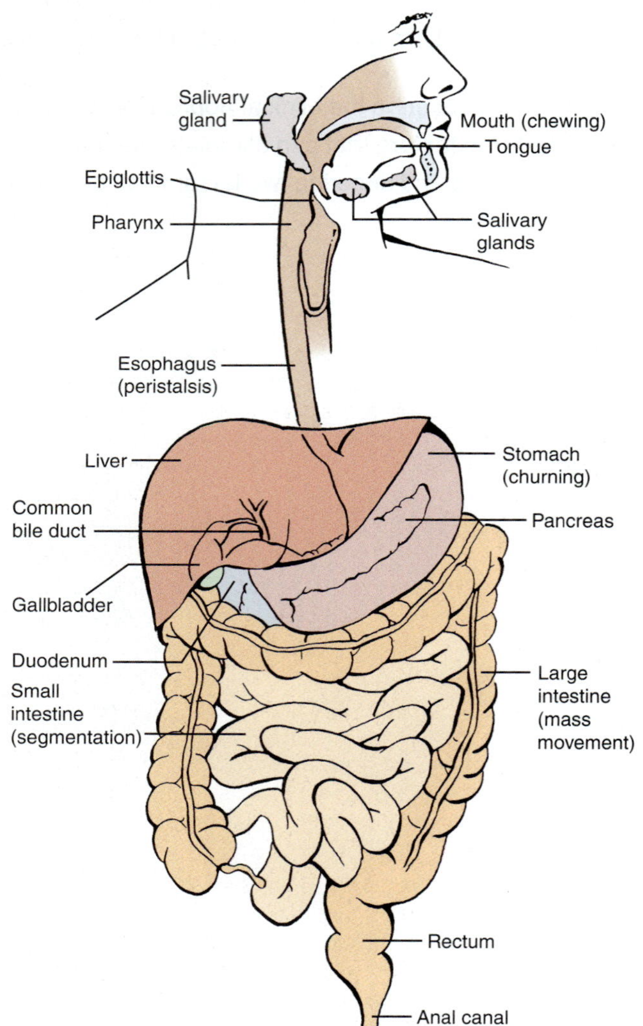

FIGURE 56.1 The gastrointestinal tract.

Composition of the Gastrointestinal Tract

The tube that comprises the GI tract is continuous with the external environment, opening at the mouth and again at the anus. Because of this, the GI tract contains many foreign agents and bacteria that are not found in the rest of the body. The peritoneum lines the abdominal wall and also the viscera, with a small "free space" between the two layers. It helps keep the GI tract in place and prevents a buildup of friction with movement. The greater and lesser omenta hang from the stomach over the lower GI tract and are full of lymph nodes, lymphocytes, monocytes, and other components of the mononuclear phagocyte system. This barrier provides rapid protection for the rest of the body if any of the bacteria or other foreign agents in the GI tract should be absorbed into the body (see Figure 56.1).

The GI tube is composed of four layers: the mucosa, the muscularis mucosa, the **nerve plexus**, and the adventitia.

- The mucosal layer provides the inner lining of the GI tract. It can be seen in the mouth and is fairly consistent throughout the tube. It is important to remember when assessing a patient that if the mouth is very dry or full of lesions, that is a reflection of the state of the entire GI tract and may indicate that the patient has difficulty digesting or absorbing nutrients. This layer has an epithelial component and a connective tissue component.
- The muscularis mucosa layer is made up of muscles. Most of the GI tract has two muscle layers. One layer runs circularly around the tube, helping keep the tube open and squeezing the tube to aid digestion and motility. The other layer runs horizontally, which helps propel the gastrointestinal contents down the tract. The stomach has a third layer of muscle, which runs obliquely and gives the stomach the ability to move contents in a churning motion.
- The nerve plexus has two layers of nerves, one submucosal layer and one myenteric layer. These nerves give the GI tract local control of movement, secretions, and digestion. The nerves respond to local stimuli and act on the contents of the GI tract accordingly. The GI tract is also innervated by the sympathetic and parasympathetic nervous systems. These systems can slow down or speed up the activity in the GI tract but cannot initiate local activity. The sympathetic system is stimulated during times of stress (e.g., "fight or flight" response) when digestion is not a priority. To slow the GI tract, the sympathetic system decreases muscle tone, secretions, and contractions, and increases sphincter tone. By shutting down the GI activity, the body saves energy for other activities. In contrast, the parasympathetic system ("rest and digest" response) stimulates the GI tract, increasing muscle tone, secretions, and contractions and decreasing sphincter tone, allowing easy movement.

- The adventitia, the outer layer of the GI tract, serves as a supportive layer and helps the tube maintain its shape and stay in position (Figure 56.2).

Gastrointestinal Activities

The GI tract has four functions: secretion, digestion, absorption, and motility. These functions are discussed in detail in the following sections.

Secretion

The GI tract secretes various compounds to aid the movement of the food bolus through the GI tube, to protect the inner layer of the GI tract from injury, and to facilitate the digestion and absorption of nutrients (see Figure 56.1). Secretions begin in the mouth. **Saliva**, which contains water and digestive enzymes, is secreted from the salivary glands to begin the digestive process and to facilitate swallowing by making the bolus slippery. Mucus is also produced in the mouth to protect the epithelial lining and to aid swallowing. The esophagus produces mucus to protect the inner lining of the GI tract and to further facilitate the movement of the bolus down the tube.

The stomach produces acid and digestive enzymes. In addition, it generates a large amount of mucus to protect the stomach lining from the acid and the enzymes. In the stomach, secretion begins with what is called the cephalic phase of digestion. The sight, smell, or taste of food stimulates the stomach to begin secreting before any food reaches the stomach. Once the bolus of food arrives at the stomach, **gastrin** is secreted. Gastrin stimulates the stomach muscles to contract, the parietal cells to release **hydrochloric acid**, and the chief cells to release pepsin. Parasympathetic stimulation also leads to acid release. Gastrin and the parasympathetic system stimulate **histamine-2 receptors** near the parietal cells, causing the cells to release hydrochloric acid into the lumen of the stomach. Proteins, calcium, alcohol, and caffeine in the stomach increase gastrin secretion. High levels of acid decrease the secretion of gastrin. Other digestive enzymes are released appropriately, in response to proteins and carbohydrates, to begin digestion. Peptic ulcers can develop when there is a decrease in the protective mucosal layer or an increase in acid production.

As the now-acidic bolus leaves the stomach and enters the small intestine, secretin is released, which stimulates the pancreas to secrete large amounts of sodium bicarbonate (to neutralize the acid bolus), the **pancreatic enzymes** chymotrypsin and trypsin (to break down proteins to smaller amino acids), other lipases (to break down fat), and amylases (to break down sugars). These enzymes are delivered to the GI tract through the common duct, which is shared with the gallbladder.

If fat is present in the bolus, the gallbladder contracts and releases **bile** into the small intestine. Bile contains a detergent-like substance that breaks apart fat molecules so that they can be processed and absorbed. The bile in the gallbladder is produced by the liver during normal metabolism. Once delivered to the gallbladder for storage, it is concentrated; water is removed by the walls of the gallbladder. Some people are prone to develop **gallstones** in the gallbladder when the concentrated bile crystallizes. These stones can move down the duct and cause severe pain or even blockage of the bile duct. See Box 56.1 for information on drugs used to dissolve gallstones.

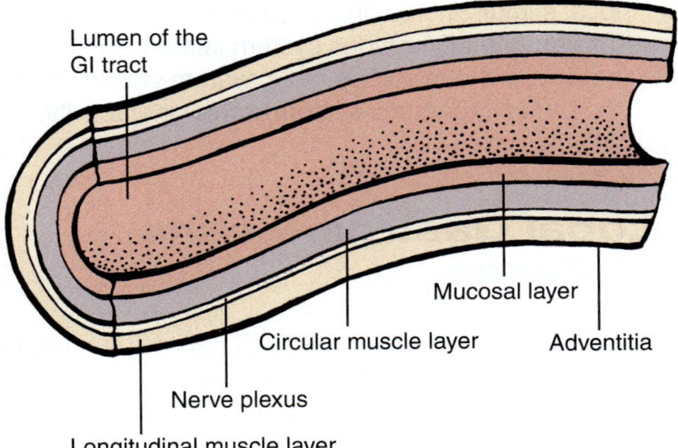

FIGURE 56.2 Layers of the gastrointestinal tract.

BOX 56.1 Gallstone Solubilizers

Surgery is usually the treatment of choice for the removal of gallstones. Severe pain, nausea, and vomiting usually accompany an acute gallbladder attack, and removal is desirable. Some patients are not candidates for surgery because of other underlying medical conditions, and these patients might benefit from the use of gallstone solubilizers to dissolve certain gallstones. Available drugs are

- Chenodiol (*Chenix*), which was the first such drug developed and is now available only as an orphan drug. Because this agent causes serious diarrhea and sometimes hepatitis and even colon cancer, its use must be weighed carefully against the dangers of the obstructed gallbladder.
- Ursodiol (*Actigall*), another oral gallstone solubilizer, which is not associated with severe adverse effects but may require months of therapy to achieve an outcome. It is best used when the gallstones are small and not obstructing. The drug is given at a dose of 8–10 mg/kg/day PO in two or three divided doses. Up to 50% of the patients who do respond to this drug have a recurrence of stones within 5 years.
- Mono-octanoin (*Moctanin*), which is a semisynthetic glycerol that must be delivered by a continuous perfusion pump through a catheter inserted into the common bile duct. Treatment with mono-octanoin must continue for 7 to 21 days. This drug is reserved for postcholecystectomy patients who still have gallstones in the biliary tract.

In response to the presence of food, the small and large intestines may secrete various endocrine hormones, including growth hormone, aldosterone, and glucagon. They also secrete large amounts of mucus to facilitate the movement of the bolus through the rest of the GI tract.

Digestion

Digestion is the process of breaking food into usable, absorbable nutrients. Digestion begins in the mouth, with the enzymes in the saliva starting the process of breaking down sugars and proteins. The stomach continues the digestion process with muscular churning, breaking down some foodstuffs while mixing them thoroughly with the hydrochloric acid and enzymes. The acid and enzymes further break down sugars and proteins into building blocks and separate vitamins, electrolytes, minerals, and other nutrients from ingested food for absorption. The beginning of the small intestine introduces bile to the food bolus, which is now called **chyme**. Bile breaks down fat molecules for processing and absorption into the bloodstream. Digestion is finished at this point, and absorption of the nutrients begins.

Absorption

Absorption is the active process of removing water, nutrients, and other elements from the GI tract and delivering them to the bloodstream for use by the body. The portal system drains all of the lower GI tract, where absorption occurs, and delivers what is absorbed into the venous system directly to the liver. The liver filters, clears, and further processes most of what is absorbed before it is delivered to the body (see Figure 56.1). Some absorption occurs in the lower end of the stomach (e.g., water, alcohol). The small intestine absorbs about 8500 mL/day, including nutrients, drugs, and anything that is taken into the GI tract, as well as any secretions. The small intestine mucosal layer is specially designed to facilitate this absorption, with long villi on the epithelial layer providing a vast surface area for absorption. The large intestine absorbs approximately 350 mL/day, mostly sodium and water.

Motility

The GI tract depends on an inherent motility to keep things moving through the system. The nerve plexus maintains a basic electrical rhythm (BER), much like the pacemaker rhythm in the heart. The cells within the plexus are somewhat unstable and leak electrolytes, leading to the regular firing of an action potential. This rhythm maintains the tone of the GI tract muscles and can be affected by local or autonomic stimuli to increase or decrease the rate of firing.

The basic movement seen in the esophagus is **peristalsis**, a constant wave of contraction that moves from the top to the bottom of the esophagus. The act of **swallowing**, a response to a food bolus in the back of the throat, stimulates the peristaltic movement that directs the food bolus into the stomach. The stomach uses its three muscle layers to produce a churning action. This action mixes the digestive enzymes and acid with the food to increase digestion. A contraction of the lower end of the stomach sends the chyme into the small intestine.

The small intestine uses a process of **segmentation** with an occasional peristaltic wave to clear the segment. Segmentation involves contraction of one segment of small intestine while the next segment is relaxed. The contracted segment then relaxes, and the relaxed segment contracts. This action exposes the chyme to a vast surface area to increase the absorption. The small intestine maintains a BER of 11 contractions per minute.

The large intestine uses a process of mass movement with an occasional peristaltic wave. When the beginning segment of the large intestine is stimulated, it contracts and sends a massive peristaltic movement throughout the entire large intestine. The end result of the mass movement is usually excretion of waste products. Rectal distention after mass movement stimulates a defecation reflex that causes relaxation of the external and internal sphincters. Control of the external sphincter is a learned behavior. The receptors in the external sphincter adapt relatively quickly, and will stretch and require more and more distention to stimulate the reflex if the reflex is ignored.

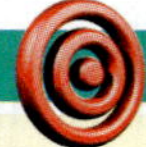

FOCUS POINTS

- The GI system begins at the mouth and ends at the anus; a long tube extends between them and comprises the esophagus, the stomach, the small intestine, and the large intestine. Essential functions are digestion and absorption of nutrients.
- The system secretes enzymes, acid, bicarbonate, and mucus to facilitate the digestion and absorption of nutrients.
- The small intestine is the organ where most absorption occurs. The veins of the small intestine carry the absorbed products to the liver for filtering, cleaning, and biotransformation.
- The nerve plexus controls the GI system by maintaining electrical rhythm and responding to local stimuli (increasing or decreasing activity). The autonomic nervous system influences GI activity, with the sympathetic system slowing and the parasympathetic system increasing activity.

Local Gastrointestinal Reflexes

Stimulation of local nerves within the GI tract causes increased or decreased movement within the system, maintaining homeostasis. Loss of reflexes or stimulation can result in constipation and the lack of movement of the bolus along the GI tract, or diarrhea with increased motility and excretion. The longer a fecal bolus remains in the large intestine, the more sodium and water is absorbed from it and the harder and less mobile it can become. There are many **local gastrointestinal reflexes**, and some knowledge of how they operate makes it easier to understand what happens when the reflexes are blocked or overstimulated and how therapeutic measures are often used to cause reflex activity.

- *Gastroenteric reflex:* Stimulation of the stomach by stretching, the presence of food, or cephalic stimulation causes an increase in activity in the small intestine. It is thought that this prepares the small intestine for the coming chyme.
- *Gastrocolic reflex:* Stimulation of the stomach also causes increased activity in the colon, again preparing to empty any contents to provide space for the new chyme.
- *Duodenal–colic reflex:* The presence of food or stretch in the duodenum stimulates colon activity and mass movement, again to empty the colon for the new chyme.

It is important to remember the gastroenteric, gastrocolic, and duodenal reflexes when helping patients to maintain GI movement. Taking advantage of stomach stimulation (e.g., having the patient drink prune juice or hot water or eat bran) and providing the opportunity of time and privacy for a bowel movement encourages normal reflexes to keep things in control.

Other local GI reflexes include the following:

- *Ileogastric reflex:* The introduction of chyme or stretch to the large intestine slows stomach activity, as well as the introduction of chyme into the small and large intestine, allowing time for absorption. In part, this reflex explains why patients who are constipated often have no appetite: The continued stretch on the ileum that comes with constipation continues to slow stomach activity and makes the introduction of new food into the stomach undesirable.
- *Intestinal–intestinal reflex:* Excessive irritation to one section of the small intestine causes a cessation of activity above that section, to prevent further irritation, and an increase in activity below that section, which leads to a flushing of the irritant. This reflex is active in "Montezuma's revenge" (traveler's diarrhea): Local irritation of the intestine causes increased secretions and movement below that section, resulting in watery diarrhea and a cessation of movement above that section. Loss of appetite or even nausea may occur. An extreme reaction to this reflex can be seen after abdominal surgery, when the handling of the intestines causes intense irritation and the reflex can cause the entire intestinal system to cease activity, leading to a paralytic ileus.
- *Peritoneointestinal reflex:* Irritation of the peritoneum as a result of inflammation or injury leads to a cessation of GI activity, preventing continued movement of the GI tract and thus further irritation of the peritoneum.
- *Renointestinal reflex:* Irritation or swelling of the renal capsule causes a cessation of movement in the GI tract, again to prevent further irritation to the capsule.
- *Vesicointestinal reflex:* Irritation or overstretching of the bladder can cause a reflex cessation of movement in the GI tract, again to prevent further irritation to the bladder from the GI movement. Many patients with cystitis or overstretched bladders from occupational constraints or neurological problems complain of constipation, which can be attributable to this reflex.
- *Somatointestinal reflex:* Taut stretching of the skin and muscles over the abdomen irritates the nerve plexus and causes a slowing or cessation of GI activity to prevent further irritation. During the era when tight girdles were commonly worn, this reflex was often seen among women, and constipation was a serious problem for many women who wore such constraining garments. Tight-fitting clothing (e.g., jeans) can have the same effect. Patients who complain of chronic constipation may be suffering from overactivity of the somatointestinal reflex.

Central Reflexes

Two centrally mediated reflexes—swallowing and vomiting—are very important to the functioning of the GI tract.

The swallowing reflex is stimulated whenever a food bolus stimulates pressure receptors in the back of the throat and pharynx. These receptors send impulses to the medulla, which stimulates a series of nerves that cause the following actions: the soft palate elevates and seals off the nasal cavity; respirations cease in order to protect the lungs; the larynx rises and the glottis closes to seal off the airway; and the pharyngeal constrictor muscles contract and force the food bolus into the top of the esophagus, where pairs of muscles contract in turn to move the bolus down the esophagus into the stomach. This reflex is complex, involving more than 25 pairs of muscles.

This reflex can be facilitated in a number of ways if swallowing (food or medication) is a problem. Icing the tongue by sucking on a *Popsicle* or an ice cube blocks external nerve impulses and allows this more basic reflex to respond. Icing the sternal notch or the back of the neck, although not as appealing, has also proved effective in stimulating the swallowing reflex. In addition, keeping the head straight (not turned to one side) allows the muscle pairs to work together and helps the process. Providing stimulation of the receptors in the mouth through temperature variations and textured foods helps initiate the reflex. Patients who do not produce their own saliva can be given artificial saliva to increase digestion and to lubricate the food bolus, which also help the swallowing reflex.

The **vomiting** reflex is another basic reflex that is centrally mediated and important in protecting the system from unwanted irritants. The vomiting reflex is stimulated by two centers in the medulla. The more primitive center is called the emetic zone. When stimulated, it initiates a projectile vomiting. This type of intense reaction is seen in young children and whenever increased pressure in the brain or brain damage allows the more primitive center to override the more mature chemoreceptor trigger zone (CTZ). The CTZ is stimulated in several ways:

- Tactile stimulation of the back of the throat, a reflex to get rid of something that is too big or too irritating to be swallowed
- Excessive stomach distention
- Increasing intracranial pressure by direct stimulation
- Stimulation of the vestibular receptors in the inner ear (a reaction often seen with dizziness after wild rides in amusement parks)
- Stimulation of stretch receptors in the uterus and bladder (a possible explanation for vomiting in early pregnancy and before delivery)
- Intense pain fiber stimulation
- Direct stimulation by various chemicals, including fumes, certain drugs, and debris from cellular death (a reason for vomiting after chemotherapy or radiation therapy that results in cell death).

Once the CTZ is stimulated, a series of reflexes occurs. Salivation increases, and there is a large increase in the production of mucus in the upper GI tract, which is accompanied by a decrease in gastric acid production. This action protects the lining of the GI tract from potential damage by the acidic stomach contents. (Nauseated patients who start swallowing repeatedly or complain about secretions in their throat are in the process of preparing for vomiting.) The sympathetic system is stimulated, with a resultant increase in sweating, increased heart rate, deeper respirations, and nausea. This prepares the body for fight or flight and the insult of vomiting. The esophagus then relaxes and becomes distended, and the gastric sphincter relaxes. The patient takes one deep respiration; the glottis closes and the palate rises, trapping the air in the lungs and sealing off entry to the lungs. The abdominal and thoracic muscles contract, increasing intra-abdominal pressure. The stomach then relaxes and the lower section of the stomach contracts in waves, approximately six times per minute. With nothing in the stomach, this movement is known as retching, and it can be quite tiring and uncomfortable. This action causes a backward peristalsis and movement of stomach contents up the esophagus and out the mouth. The body thus rids itself of offending irritants.

The vomiting reflex is complex and protective, but it can be undesirable in certain clinical situations, when the stimulant is not something that can be vomited or when the various components of the vomiting reflex could be detrimental to a patient's health status.

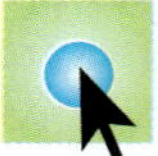

WEB LINK

To explore a virtual GI system, consult the following Internet source:
http://www.InnerBody.com

Points to Remember

- The gastrointestinal (GI) system is composed of one long tube that starts at the mouth; includes the esophagus, the stomach, the small intestine, and the large intestine; and ends at the anus. The GI system is responsible for digestion and absorption of nutrients.
- Secretion of digestive enzymes, acid, bicarbonate, and mucus facilitates the digestion and absorption of nutrients.
- The GI system is controlled by a nerve plexus, which maintains a basic electrical rhythm and responds to local stimuli to increase or decrease activity. The autonomic system can influence the activity of the GI tract, with the sympathetic system slowing and the parasympathetic system increasing activity. Initiation of activity depends on local reflexes.
- A series of local reflexes within the GI tract helps maintain homeostasis within the system. Overstimulation of any of these reflexes can result in constipation (underactivity) or diarrhea (overactivity).
- Swallowing is a centrally mediated reflex that is important in delivering food to the GI tract for processing. It is controlled by the medulla and involves a complex series of timed reflexes.
- Vomiting is controlled by the chemoreceptor trigger zone (CTZ) in the medulla or by the emetic zone in immature or injured brains. The CTZ is stimulated by several different processes and initiates a complex series of responses that first prepare the system for vomiting and then cause a strong backward peristalsis to rid the stomach of its contents.

CHECK YOUR UNDERSTANDING

Answers to the questions in this chapter may be found in the Answer Key in the back of the book.

Multiple Choice

Select the best response to the following.

1. Constipation
   a. results from increased peristaltic activity in the intestinal tract.
   b. occurs only if one does not have a bowel movement at least once a day.
   c. leads to decreased salt and water absorption from the large intestine.
   d. symptoms can be artificially induced by increasing the volume of the large intestine.

2. The pancreas
   a. is only an endocrine gland.
   b. secretes enzymes in response to an increased plasma glucose concentration.
   c. neutralizes the hydrochloric acid secreted by the stomach.
   d. produces bile.

3. Gastrin
   a. stimulates acid secretion in the stomach.
   b. secretion is blocked by the products of protein digestion in the stomach.
   c. secretion is stimulated by acid in the duodenum.
   d. is responsible for the chemical or gastric phase of intestinal secretion.

4. The activities of the GI tract, movement and secretion, are controlled by
   a. the sympathetic nervous system.
   b. the parasympathetic nervous system.
   c. local nerve reflexes initiated in the nerve plexus layer of the GI tract.
   d. the medulla.

5. The presence of fat in the duodenum causes
   a. acid indigestion.
   b. decreased acid production.
   c. increased gastrin release.
   d. contraction of the gallbladder.

6. The basic type of movement that occurs in the small intestine is
   a. peristalsis.
   b. mass movement.
   c. churning.
   d. segmentation.

7. Most of the nutrients absorbed from the GI tract pass immediately into the portal venous system and are processed by the liver. This is possible because almost all absorption occurs through
   a. the lower section of the stomach.
   b. the top section of the large intestine.
   c. the small intestine.
   d. the ileum.

Multiple Response

Select all that apply.

1. The chemoreceptor trigger zone in the brain is activated by which of the following?
   a. Stretch of the uterus
   b. Stretch of the bladder
   c. Decreased GI activity
   d. Radiation
   e. Cell death
   f. Extreme pain

2. Acid production in the stomach is stimulated by which of the following?
   a. Protein in the stomach
   b. Calcium products in the stomach
   c. High levels of acid in the stomach
   d. Alcohol in the stomach
   e. Low levels of acid in the stomach
   f. Histamine-2 stimulation

3. Pancreatic digestive enzymes help in the breakdown of which of the following?
   a. Gastric acid
   b. Fats
   c. Proteins
   d. Sugars
   e. Bile
   f. Lipids

Matching

Match the following words with the appropriate definition.

1. ______________________ bile
2. ______________________ chyme
3. ______________________ gallstones
4. ______________________ gastrin
5. ______________________ histamine-2 receptors

6. ______________________ hydrochloric acid
7. ______________________ nerve plexus
8. ______________________ pancreatic enzymes
9. ______________________ peristalsis
10. ______________________ segmentation

A. Acid released in response to gastrin
B. Sites near the parietal cells of the stomach that cause the release of hydrochloric acid into the stomach.
C. Contents of the stomach
D. Pancreatin and pancrelipase
E. Network of nerve fibers running through the wall of the GI tract
F. Fluid stored in the gallbladder
G. Crystallization of cholesterol in the gallbladder
H. Secreted by the stomach to stimulate the release of hydrochloric acid
I. GI movement characterized by contraction of one segment of small intestine while the next segment is relaxed
J. GI movement characterized by a progressive wave of muscle contraction

Fill in the Blanks

1. The GI system is composed of one long tube and is responsible for ______________________ and ______________________ of nutrients.

2. Secretion of digestive enzymes, ______________________, bicarbonate, and ______________________ facilitates the digestion and absorption of nutrients.

3. The GI system is controlled by a(n) ______________________, which maintains a basic electrical rhythm and responds to local stimuli to increase or decrease activity.

4. The autonomic system can influence the activity of the GI tract; the ______________________ system slows it and the ______________________ system increases activity.

5. Initiation of activity in the GI tract depends on ______________________.

6. Overstimulation of any of the GI reflexes can result in ______________________ (underactivity) or ______________________ (overactivity).

7. Swallowing is a centrally mediated reflex that is important in delivering food to the GI tract for processing. It is controlled by the ______________________.

8. Vomiting is controlled by the ______________________ in the medulla or by the emetic zone in immature or injured brains.

Bibliography and References

Ganong, W. (2003). *Review of medical physiology* (20th ed.). Norwalk, CT: Appleton & Lange.

Gilman, A., Hardman, J. G., & Limbird, L. E. (Eds.). (2006). *Goodman and Gilman's the pharmacological basis of therapeutics* (11th ed.). New York: McGraw-Hill.

Guyton, A. & Hall, J. (2002). *Textbook of medical physiology*. Philadelphia: W. B. Saunders.

Porth, C. M. (2005). *Pathophysiology: Concepts of altered health states* (7th ed.). Philadelphia: Lippincott Williams & Wilkins.

CHAPTER

57

Drugs Affecting Gastrointestinal Secretions

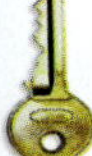

KEY TERMS

acid rebound

antipeptic agents

histamine-2 (H_2) antagonist

peptic ulcer

prostaglandin

proton pump inhibitor

LEARNING OBJECTIVES

Upon completion of this chapter, you will be able to:

1. Describe the current theories on the pathophysiological process responsible for the signs and symptoms of peptic ulcer disease.
2. Describe the therapeutic actions, indications, pharmacokinetics, contraindications, most common adverse reactions, and important drug–drug interactions associated with histamine-2 antagonists, antacids, proton pump inhibitors, antipeptic agents, prostaglandins used to affect gastrointestinal (GI) secretions, and digestive enzymes.
3. Discuss the drugs used to affect GI secretions across the lifespan.
4. Compare and contrast the prototype drugs cimetidine, sodium bicarbonate, omeprazole, and pancrelipase with other agents in their class and with other classes of drugs used to affect GI secretions.
5. Outline the nursing considerations, including important teaching points, for patients receiving drugs used to affect GI secretions.

HISTAMINE-2 ANTAGONISTS

P cimetidine
famotidine
nizatidine
ranitidine

ANTACIDS

aluminum salts
calcium salts
magaldrate
magnesium salts
P sodium bicarbonate

PROTON PUMP INHIBITORS

esomeprazole
lansoprazole
P omeprazole
pantoprazole
rabeprazole

ANTIPEPTIC AGENT

sucralfate

PROSTAGLANDIN

misoprostol

DIGESTIVE ENZYMES

P pancrelipase
saliva substitute

Gastrointestinal (GI) disorders are among the most common complaints seen in clinical practice. Many products are available for the self-treatment of upset stomach, heartburn, and sour stomach. The underlying causes of these disorders can range from dietary excess, stress, hiatal hernia, esophageal reflux, and adverse drug effects to the more serious peptic ulcer disease.

Drugs that affect GI secretions can decrease GI secretory activity, block the action of GI secretions, form protective coverings on the GI lining to prevent erosion from GI secretions, or replace missing GI enzymes that the GI tract or ancillary glands and organs can no longer produce (Figure 57.1). These drugs are used with all age groups (see Box 57.1).

Peptic Ulcers

Erosions in the lining of the stomach and adjacent areas of the GI tract are called **peptic ulcers**. Ulcer patients present with a predictable description of gnawing, burning pain, often occurring a few hours after meals. Many of the drugs that are used to affect GI secretions are designed to prevent, treat, or aid in the healing of these ulcers. The actual cause of chronic peptic ulcers is not completely understood. For many years it was believed that ulcers were caused by excessive acid production, and treatment was aimed at neutralizing acid or blocking the parasympathetic system to decrease normal GI activity and secretions. Further research led many to believe that, because acid production was often nor-

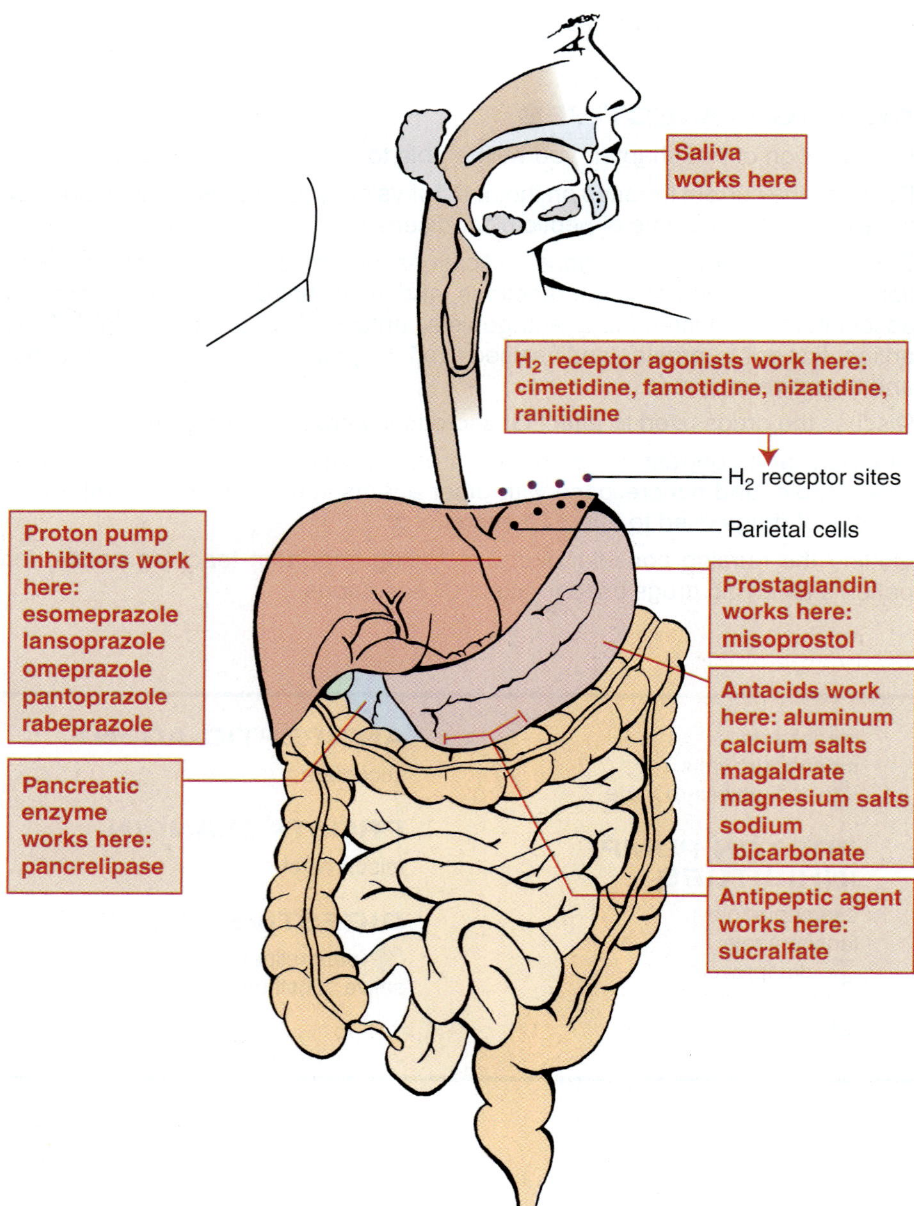

FIGURE 57.1 Sites of action of drugs affecting gastrointestinal secretions.

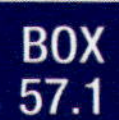
BOX 57.1

DRUG THERAPY ACROSS THE LIFESPAN

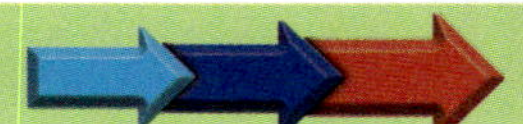

Agents That Affect Gastrointestinal Secretions

CHILDREN

Antacids may be used in children who complain of upset stomach or who are receiving therapy known to increase acid production; 5–15 mL q1–3h is usually an effective dose.

The proton pump inhibitors, although not specifically indicated for use in children, have been very successfully used to decrease ulcer formation related to stress or drug therapy. Dosage should be determined by the age and weight of the child. Famotidine has been approved for use in children if a histamine-2 antagonist is needed. Lansoprazole has established pediatric dosages if a proton pump inhibitor is most appropriate.

Special caution should be used with any of these agents to prevent electrolyte disturbances or any interference with nutrition, which could be especially detrimental to children.

ADULTS

Adults should be cautioned not to overuse these agents and to check with their health care provider if gastrointestinal discomfort continues after repeated use of any of these drugs. Patients should be monitored for any electrolyte disturbances or interference with the absorption or action of other drugs. If antacids are used, they should be spaced 1–2 h before or after the use of other drugs. In 2005, some studies were published that linked prolonged use of these agents with an increased incidence of colitis and other gastrointestinal infections. Until further studies are done, patients should be advised to limit the use of these agents.

The safety of these drugs during pregnancy and lactation has not been established. Misoprostol is an abortifacient and should never be used during pregnancy. Women of childbearing age who use this drug should be advised to use barrier-type contraceptives. Use of these agents should be reserved for those situations in which the benefit to the mother outweighs the potential risk to the fetus. The drugs may enter breast milk and also may alter electrolyte levels or gastric secretions in the neonate. It is advised that caution be used if one of these drugs is prescribed during lactation.

OLDER ADULTS

Older adults frequently are prescribed one or more of these drugs. Older adults are more likely to develop adverse effects associated with the use of these drugs, including sedation, confusion, dizziness, urinary retention, and cardiovascular effects. Safety measures may be needed if these effects occur and interfere with the patient's mobility and balance.

Older adults are also more likely to have renal and/or hepatic impairment related to underlying medical conditions, which could interfere with the metabolism and excretion of these drugs. The dosage for older adults should be started at a lower level than recommended for younger adults. Patients should be monitored very closely, and dosage adjustment should be made based on patient response.

These patients also need to be alerted to the potential for toxic effects when using over-the-counter (OTC) preparations that may contain the same ingredients as many of these agents. They should be advised to check with their health care provider before beginning any OTC drug regimen.

Proton pump inhibitors may be the best choice for treating gastroesophageal reflux disease in older patients because of fewer adverse effects and better therapeutic response with these drugs.

mal in ulcer patients, ulcers were caused by a defect in the mucous lining that coats the inner lumen of the stomach to protect it from acid and digestive enzymes. Treatment was aimed at improving the balance between the acid produced and the mucous layer that protects the stomach lining. Currently it is believed that chronic ulcers may also be the result of bacterial infection by *Helicobacter pylori* bacteria. Combination antibiotics have been found to be quite effective in treating patients with chronic ulcers.

Acute ulcers, or "stress ulcers," are often seen in situations that involve acute stress, such as trauma, burns, or prolonged illness. The activity of the sympathetic nervous system during stress decreases blood flow to the GI tract, leading to weakening of the mucosal layer of the stomach and erosion by acid in the stomach. Many of the drugs available for treating various peptic ulcers act to alter acid-producing activities of the stomach. Five types of drugs are used in the treatment of ulcers:

- **Histamine-2 (H_2) antagonists**, which block the release of hydrochloric acid in response to gastrin
- Antacids, which interact with acids at the chemical level to neutralize them
- **Proton pump inhibitors**, which suppress the secretion of hydrochloric acid into the lumen of the stomach
- **Antipeptic agents**, which coat any injured area in the stomach to prevent further injury from acid
- **Prostaglandins**, which inhibit the secretion of gastrin and increase the secretion of the mucous lining of the stomach, providing a buffer

Recent research studies have begun questioning the effects that lowering acid levels might have on the homeostasis of the GI system (see Box 57.2).

Digestive Enzyme Dysfunction

Some patients require a supplement to the production of digestive enzymes. Patients with strokes, salivary gland disorders, or extreme surgery of the head and neck may not be able to produce saliva. Saliva is important in beginning the digestion of sugars and proteins and is essential in initiating the swallowing reflex. Artificial saliva may be necessary for these patients. Patients with common duct problems,

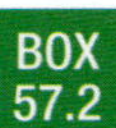

BOX 57.2 FOCUS ON THE **EVIDENCE**

Drugs That Decrease Acid Cause More Diarrhea

In December 2005, the *Journal of the American Medical Association* published a study that followed patients taking proton pump inhibitors (*Nexium, Prevacid, Protonix,* and others) over a period of 10 years. The report showed that patients using these drugs had *Clostridium difficile* infections leading to diarrhea at three times the rate of patients not using these drugs. There was also a reported two-time increase in these infections in patients using histamine-2 (H_2) antagonists (*Tagamet, Pepcid, Axid,* and others). *C. difficile* is a significant cause of diarrhea in the community. Other studies have reported similar findings. Drugs that lower acid levels are changing the normal environment of the gastrointestinal (GI) tract, perhaps allowing bacteria to thrive that would normally be destroyed by the acid. Most of these acid-lowering drugs are available in over-the-counter (OTC) preparations and may be used in excessive doses for prolonged periods of time without the health care provider's knowledge. This information should alert health care providers and patients to the need for caution in using these drugs. If a patient is complaining about diarrhea, the health care provider should specifically ask about the use of acid-lowering products (sometimes patients do not even think of these products as drugs because they can buy them without a prescription). During health care teaching sessions, it is important to remind people to read the labels of OTC drugs carefully and to follow instructions. If a patient feels the need to take one of these products for a prolonged period of time, he or she should be advised to obtain a medical evaluation since the symptoms being treated with these drugs could have an underlying medical cause that should be evaluated.

When evaluating the data from the study, the researchers also noted a similar increase in these GI infections in patients using nonsteroidal anti-inflammatory drugs (ibuprofen, ketoprofen, and others) for a prolonged period of time. The researchers suggested that further study be done on that group of patients to verify the finding.

It is important to keep current with long-term studies on drugs and to remember that changing a normal function or environment in the body will change the balance of homeostasis in the body and could potentially cause other problems.

See Dial, S., Delaney, J. A., Barkun, A. N., and Suissa, S. (2005). Use of gastric acid suppressive agents and the risk of community acquired *Clostridium difficile* associated diarrhea. *JAMA,* 294, 2898–2995.

pancreatic disease, or cystic fibrosis may not be able to produce or secrete pancreatic enzymes. These enzymes may need to be administered to allow normal digestion and absorption of nutrients.

FOCUS POINTS

- Agents used to decrease the acid content of the stomach include H_2 antagonists, which block the release of acid in response to gastrin or parasympathetic release; antacids, which chemically react with the acid to neutralize it; and proton pump inhibitors, which block the last step of acid production to prevent release.
- Acid rebound occurs when the stomach produces more gastrin and more acid in response to lowered acid levels in the stomach. Balancing the reduction of the stomach acid without increasing acid production is a clinical challenge.
- Among the most common complaints addressed in clinical practice are GI symptoms.
- Increased acid production, decrease in the protective mucous lining of the stomach, infection with *Helicobacter pylori* bacteria, or a combination of these are the likely causes of peptic ulcers.
- H_2 antagonists block the release of acid in response to gastrin or parasympathetic release; antacids neutralize stomach acid; and proton pump inhibitors prevent the release of stomach acid.
- To maintain nutrition, replacement digestive enzymes are needed by patients who do not have them because of genetic deficiencies, illness, or medical treatments. Products available for these patient include saliva substitute and pancreatic enzymes.

Histamine-2 Antagonists

The H_2 antagonists selectively block H_2 receptors. These receptors are located on the parietal cells; blocking them prevents gastrin, which causes local release of histamine and stimulation of these receptors, from stimulating the production of hydrochloric acid. This action also decreases pepsin production by the chief cells. Four H_2 antagonists are available (Table 57.1):

- Cimetidine (*Tagamet, Tagamet HB*) was the first drug in this class to be developed. It has been associated with antiadrenergic effects, including gynecomastia and galactorrhea. It is metabolized mainly in the liver and can slow the metabolism of many other drugs that use the same metabolizing enzyme system. It is excreted in urine and is known to cross the placenta and enter breast milk. It should be used with caution during pregnancy, and another method of feeding the baby should be used during lactation. It is available in oral and parenteral forms.
- Ranitidine (*Zantac*), which is longer acting and more potent than cimetidine, is not associated with the antiadrenergic adverse effects or the marked slowing of metabolism in the liver. It is available in oral and parenteral forms. It is also excreted in urine. It crosses the placenta

Table 57.1 DRUGS IN FOCUS

Histamine-2 Antagonists

Drug Name	Usual Dosage	Usual Indications
P cimetidine (*Tagamet, Tagamet HB*)	300 mg PO q.i.d. at meals and at bedtime *or* 800 mg PO at bedtime; 300 mg IV or IM q6–8h or 200 mg PO for heartburn; reduce dosage with geriatric patients or renal impairment Pediatric (1–16 yr): 0.5–1 mg/kg/day PO or 0.25 mg/kg IV q12h	Treatment of duodenal ulcer, benign gastric ulcer, pathological hypersecretory syndrome, gastroesophageal reflux disease (GERD); prophylaxis of stress ulcers; relief of symptoms of heartburn, acid indigestion, sour stomach **Special considerations:** Not for children <16 y old
famotidine (*Pepcid, Pepcid AC*)	20–40 mg PO or IV at bedtime *or* 20 mg PO b.i.d.; 10 mg PO for prevention or relief of heartburn; reduce dosage in renal-impaired or geriatric patients	Treatment of duodenal ulcer, benign gastric ulcer, pathological hypersecretory syndrome, GERD; relief of symptoms of heartburn, acid indigestion, sour stomach
nizatidine (*Axid*)	150–300 mg PO at bedtime *or* 150 mg PO b.i.d., 75 mg PO 30 min before food to prevent heartburn; reduce dosage in renal-impaired or geriatric patients	Treatment of duodenal ulcer, benign gastric ulcer, pathological hypersecretory syndrome, GERD; relief of symptoms of heartburn, acid indigestion, sour stomach in adults **Special considerations:** Not recommended for use in children
ranitidine (*Zantac*)	150 mg daily to b.i.d. PO IM or IV; 75 mg PO as needed for heartburn; reduce dosage in renal impaired or geriatric patients	Treatment of duodenal ulcer, benign gastric ulcer, pathological hypersecretory syndrome, GERD; relief of symptoms of heartburn, acid indigestion, sour stomach in adults **Special considerations:** Not recommended for use in children

and enters breast milk; caution should be used during pregnancy and lactation.

- Famotidine (*Pepcid, Pepcid AC*) is similar to ranitidine in terms of its actions and adverse effects, but it is much more potent than either cimetidine or ranitidine. It can be given orally or intravenously. It is metabolized in the liver and excreted in urine. Famotidine crosses the placenta and enters breast milk; it should be used with caution during pregnancy and lactation. Famotidine is approved for use in children ages 1 to 16 years old.
- Nizatidine (*Axid*), the newest drug in this class, is similar to ranitidine in its effectiveness and adverse effects. It differs from the other three drugs in that it is eliminated by the kidneys, with no first-pass metabolism in the liver. It is the drug of choice for patients with liver dysfunction and for those who are taking other drugs whose metabolism is slowed by the hepatic activity of the other three H_2 antagonists. It is available only in an oral form. It too crosses the placenta and enters the breast milk.

Therapeutic Actions and Indications

H_2 antagonists selectively block histamine-2 receptor sites. This blocking leads to a reduction in gastric acid secretion and reduction in overall pepsin production (see Figure 57.1). H_2 receptor sites are also found in the heart, and high levels of these drugs can produce cardiac arrhythmias.

These drugs are used in the following conditions:

- Short-term treatment of active duodenal ulcer or benign gastric ulcer (reduction in the overall acid level can promote healing and decrease discomfort) (see Critical Thinking Scenario 57-1)
- Treatment of pathological hypersecretory conditions such as Zollinger–Ellison syndrome (blocking the overproduction of hydrochloric acid that is associated with these conditions)
- Prophylaxis of stress-induced ulcers and acute upper GI bleeding in critical patients (blocking the production of acid protects the stomach lining, which is at risk because of decreased mucus production associated with extreme stress)
- Treatment of erosive gastroesophageal reflux (decreasing the acid being regurgitated into the esophagus will promote healing and decrease pain)
- Relief of symptoms of heartburn, acid indigestion, and sour stomach (over-the-counter preparations)

Pharmacokinetics

H_2 antagonists are readily absorbed after oral administration. They cross the placenta and enter breast milk. They are metabolized in the liver and excreted in urine. Nizatidine is the only drug of this class that is not metabolized in the liver, but is directly eliminated by the kidneys.

CRITICAL THINKING SCENARIO 57-1

Histamine-2 Antagonists

The Situation

W.T., a 48-year-old traveling salesman, had experienced increasing epigastric discomfort during a 7-month period. When he finally sought medical care, the diagnosis was a duodenal ulcer. He began taking magaldrate (*Riopan*) for relief of his immediate discomfort, as well as cimetidine (*Tagamet*), 300 mg q.i.d. W.T. was referred to the nurse for patient teaching and given an appointment for a follow-up visit in 3 weeks.

Critical Thinking

Think about the physiology of duodenal ulcers and the various factors that can contribute to aggravating the problem. What patient teaching points should be covered with this patient regarding diet, stress factors, and use of alcohol and tobacco?

What adverse effects of the drugs should this patient be aware of?

What lifestyle changes may be necessary to ensure ulcer healing, and how can W.T. be assisted in making these changes fit into the demands of his job?

Discussion

Further examination indicated that W.T. is a healthy man except for the ulcer. Because he is basically healthy and does not seek medical care unless very uncomfortable (7 months of pain), he may find it difficult to comply with his drug therapy and any suggested lifestyle changes.

W.T. needs patient education, which for purposes of building trust, should preferably be with the same nurse. The instruction should include information on duodenal ulcer disease; ways to decrease acid production (such as avoiding cigarettes, acid-stimulating foods, alcohol, and caffeine); and ways to improve the protective mucous layer of the stomach by decreasing stress and anxiety-causing situations. Cimetidine can cause dizziness and drowsiness, which could be a major problem if W.T. needs to drive to meet his clients. Because of this adverse effect, another histamine-2 inhibitor may be preferable. Dizziness and drowsiness are more often associated with cimetidine than with some of the newer histamine-2 inhibitors. This effect should be discussed with W.T. If driving is an important part of W.T.'s job demands, he may want to explore other means of dealing with his ulcer pain and healing.

In addition, spacing of the cimetidine and antacid doses should be stressed. Cimetidine should be taken 1 hour before or 2 hours after any antacids because they can interfere with the absorption of cimetidine and the patient may not receive a therapeutic dose. W.T. should be encouraged to avoid over-the-counter medications and self-medication because several of these products contain ingredients that could aggravate his ulcer or interfere with the effectiveness of the drugs that have been prescribed. W.T. should be encouraged to return for regular medical evaluation of his drug therapy and his underlying condition.

Finally, W.T. should feel that he has some control over his situation. Because he does not routinely seek medical care, he may be more comfortable with a medical regimen that he has participated in planning. Allow him to suggest ways to decrease stress, ways to cut down on smoking or the use of alcohol without interfering with the demands of his job, and the best times to take the drugs in his schedule. He will learn in time which foods and situations irritate his condition. However, research has not shown that bland or restrictive diets are particularly effective in decreasing ulcer pain or spread, and they may actually increase patient anxiety. W.T. should be encouraged to jot down the situations or times of day that seem to cause him the most problems. This information can help to provide a guide for adjusting lifestyle and/or dietary patterns to aid ulcer healing and prevent further development of ulcers.

Nursing Care Guide For W.T.: Histamine-2 Antagonists

Assessment: History And Examination

Assess W.T.'s health history for allergies to any of these drugs, renal or hepatic failure, and other drugs being taken, such as antimetabolites, alkylating agents, oral anticoagulants, phenytoin, beta-blockers, alcohol, quinidine, lidocaine, theophylline, benzodiazepines, nifedipine, tricyclic antidepressants (TCAs), and carbamazepine.

Focus the physical examination on the following areas:

Neurological: orientation, affect

Skin: color, lesions

CV: pulse, cardiac auscultation

GI: liver evaluation

Laboratory tests: CBC, liver, renal function tests

Histamine-2 Antagonists *(continued)*

Nursing Diagnoses

Acute Pain related to GI or CNS effects

Disturbed Sensory Perception (Kinesthetic, Auditory) related to CNS effects

Decreased Cardiac Output related to cardiac effects

Deficient Knowledge regarding drug therapy

Implementation

Administer with meals and at bedtime.

Provide comfort and safety measures: analgesics, access to bathroom, safety precautions.

Arrange for decreased dose in renal/hepatic disease.

Provide support and reassurance to deal with drug effects and lifestyle changes.

Provide patient teaching regarding drug name, dosage, adverse effects, precautions, and warnings to report.

Evaluation

Evaluate drug effects: relief of GI symptoms, ulcer healing, prevention of ulcer progression.

Monitor for adverse effects: dizziness, confusion, gynecomastia, arrhythmias, GI alterations.

Monitor for drug–drug interactions as listed.

Evaluate effectiveness of patient teaching program.

Evaluate effectiveness of comfort and safety measures.

PATIENT TEACHING FOR W.T.

- ☐ The drug that has been prescribed for you, cimetidine, is called a histamine-2 antagonist. A histamine-2 antagonist decreases the amount of acid that is produced in the stomach. It is used to treat conditions that are aggravated by excess acid.
- ☐ Some of the following adverse effects may occur with this drug:
  - *Diarrhea:* Have ready access to bathroom facilities. This usually becomes less severe over time.
  - *Dizziness, feeling faint on arising, headache:* These usually lessen as your body adjusts to the drug. Change positions slowly. If you fell drowsy, avoid driving or dangerous activities.
  - Report any of the following to your health care provider: *sore throat, unusual bleeding or bruising, confusion, muscle or joint pain, heart palpitations.*
- ☐ Avoid taking any over-the-counter medication without first checking with your health care provider. Several of these medications can interfere with the effectiveness of this drug.
- ☐ If an antacid has been ordered for you, take it exactly as prescribed.
- ☐ Tell any physician, nurse, or other health care provider involved in your care that you are taking this drug.
- ☐ If you are taking any other medications, do not vary the drug schedules. Consult with your primary health care provider if anything should happen to change any of these drugs or your scheduled doses.
- ☐ It is important to have regular medical follow-up while you are taking this drug to evaluate your response to the drug and any possible underlying problems.
- ☐ Keep this drug, and all other medications, out of the reach of children.

Contraindications and Cautions

The H_2 antagonists should not be used with known allergy to any drugs of this class. Caution should be used during pregnancy or lactation and with hepatic or renal dysfunction *that could interfere with drug metabolism and excretion.* (Hepatic dysfunction is not as much of a problem with nizatidine.) Care should also be taken if prolonged or continual use of these drugs is necessary *because they may be masking serious underlying conditions.*

Adverse Effects

The adverse effects most commonly associated with H_2 antagonists include the following: GI effects of diarrhea or constipation; CNS effects of dizziness, headache, somnolence, confusion, or even hallucinations (thought to be related to possible H_2 receptor effects in the CNS); cardiac arrhythmias and hypotension (related to H_2 cardiac receptor blocking; more commonly seen with intravenous or intramuscular administration or with prolonged use); and gynecomastia (more common with long-term use of cimetidine) and impotence.

Clinically Important Drug–Drug Interactions

The three H_2 antagonists that are metabolized in the liver (cimetidine, famotidine, and ranitidine) can slow the metabolism of the following drugs, leading to increased serum levels and possible toxic reactions: warfarin anticoagulants, phenytoin, beta-adrenergic blockers, alcohol, quinidine, lidocaine, theophylline, chloroquine, benzodiazepines, nifedipine, pentoxifylline, tricyclic antidepressants, procainamide, and carbamazepine. It is a good idea to review a patient's other medications carefully any time an H_2 antagonist is prescribed or a patient reports taking an over-the-counter form.

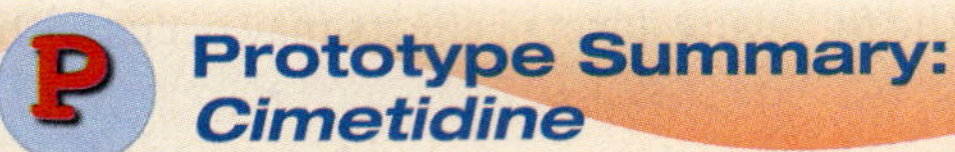

Prototype Summary: Cimetidine

Indications: Short-term treatment of active duodenal or benign gastric ulcers; treatment of pathological hypersecretory conditions; prophylaxis of stress-induced ulcers; treatment of erosive gastroesophageal reflux; relief of symptoms of heartburn and acid indigestion

Actions: Inhibits the actions of histamine at H_2 receptor sites of the stomach, inhibiting gastric acid secretion and reducing total pepsin output

Pharmacokinetics:

Route	Onset	Peak	Duration
Oral	Varies	1–1.5 h	4–5 h
IM, IV	Rapid	1–1.5 h	4–5 h

$T_{1/2}$: 2 hours; metabolized in the liver and excreted in urine

Adverse effects: Dizziness, confusion, headache, somnolence, cardiac arrhythmias, cardiac arrest, diarrhea, impotence, gynecomastia, rash

Nursing Considerations for Patients Receiving Histamine-2 Antagonists

Assessment: History and Examination

Screen for the following conditions, *which could be cautions or contraindications to use of the drug:* history of allergy to any H_2 antagonists; impaired renal or hepatic function; pregnancy or lactation; and a detailed description of the GI problem, including length of time of the disorder and medical evaluation.

Include screening for skin lesions; orientation and affect; baseline pulse and blood pressure, electrocardiogram (if intravenous use is needed); liver and abdominal examination; and liver and renal function tests.

Nursing Diagnoses

The patient who is receiving any H_2 antagonist may have the following nursing diagnoses related to drug therapy:

- Acute Pain related to CNS and GI effects
- Disturbed Sensory Perception (Kinesthetic, Auditory) related to CNS effects
- Decreased Cardiac Output related to cardiac arrhythmias
- Deficient Knowledge regarding drug therapy

Implementation With Rationale

- Administer oral drug with or before meals and at bedtime (exact timing varies with product) *to ensure therapeutic levels when the drug is most needed.*
- Arrange for decreased dosage in cases of hepatic or renal dysfunction *to prevent serious toxicity.*
- Monitor patient continually if giving intravenous doses *to allow early detection of potentially serious adverse effects, including cardiac arrhythmias.*
- Assess patient carefully for any potential drug–drug interactions if giving in combination with other drugs *because of the drug effects on liver enzyme systems.*
- Provide comfort and safety measures, including analgesics, ready access to bathroom facilities, assistance with ambulation, and periodic orientation if GI or CNS effects occur, *to ensure patient safety and improve patient tolerance of the drug and drug effects.*
- Arrange for regular follow-up *to evaluate drug effects and the underlying problem.*
- Provide thorough patient teaching, including drug name, prescribed dosage, measures for avoidance of adverse effects, and warning signs that may indicate possible problems. Instruct patients about the need for periodic monitoring and evaluation *to enhance patient knowledge about drug therapy and to promote compliance.*
- Offer support and encouragement *to help patients cope with the disease and the drug regimen.*

Evaluation

- Monitor patient response to the drug (relief of GI symptoms, ulcer healing, prevention of progression of ulcer).
- Monitor for adverse effects (dizziness, confusion, hallucinations, GI alterations, cardiac arrhythmias, hypotension, gynecomastia).
- Evaluate effectiveness of teaching plan (patient can name drug, dosage, adverse effects to watch for, and specific measures to avoid adverse effects).
- Monitor effectiveness of comfort measures and compliance with regimen.

Antacids

The antacids are a group of inorganic chemicals that have long been used to neutralize stomach acid. Antacids are available over the counter, and many patients use them to self-treat a variety of GI symptoms. All antacids have adverse effects, and there is no perfect antacid.

Administering an antacid frequently causes **acid rebound**. Neutralizing the stomach contents to an alkaline level stimulates gastrin production to cause an increase in acid production and return the stomach to its normal acidic state. In many cases, the acid rebound causes an increase in symptoms, which results in an increased intake of the antacid. This leads to more acid production, and a cycle develops. When more and more antacid is used, the risk for systemic effects rises.

The choice of an antacid depends on adverse effect and absorption factors. Available agents are the following (Table 57.2):

- Sodium bicarbonate (*Bell-Ans*), the oldest drug in this group, is readily available in many preparations, including baking soda. This drug is widely distributed when absorbed, crossing the placenta and entering breast milk. It should be used with caution during pregnancy and lactation because of the potential for adverse effects on the fetus or neonate. It is excreted in urine and can cause serious electrolyte imbalance in people with renal impairment.
- Calcium carbonate (*Oystercal, Tums,* and others), the next antacid to be developed, is actually precipitated chalk. The main drawbacks to this agent are constipation and acid rebound. It can be absorbed systemically and cause calcium imbalance. When absorbed, it is metabolized in the liver and excreted in urine and feces. Known to cross the placenta and enter breast milk, this drug should be used with caution during pregnancy and lactation.
- Magnesium salts (*Milk of Magnesia* and others) are very effective in buffering acid in the stomach but have been known to cause diarrhea. Although these agents are not generally absorbed systemically, absorbed magnesium can lead to nerve damage and even coma. Because they are minimally absorbed systemically, this may be a drug of choice if an antacid is needed during pregnancy or lactation.
- Aluminum salts (*Amphojel* and others) do not cause acid rebound but are not very effective in neutralizing acid. They are bound in feces for excretion. They have been related to severe constipation. Aluminum binds dietary phosphates and causes hypophosphatemia, which can then cause calcium imbalance throughout the system. For that reason, this drug should be used with caution during pregnancy and should be avoided during lactation because of the potential for adverse effects on the fetus and neonate.
- Magaldrate (*Lowsium, Riopan*), an aluminum and magnesium salt combination, minimizes the GI effects of constipation and diarrhea by combining these two salts but may cause a rebound hyperacidity and alkalosis. Magaldrate is not generally absorbed systemically. This drug should be used with caution during pregnancy and lactation because the potential for effects on the fetus or neonate is unclear.

Many of these antacids are available in combination forms to take advantage of the acid-neutralizing effect and block adverse effects. For example, a combination of calcium and aluminum salts (*Maalox*) buffers acid and produces neither constipation nor diarrhea.

Antacids can greatly affect the absorption of drugs from the GI tract. Most drugs are prepared for an acidic environment, and an alkaline environment can prevent them from being broken down for absorption or can actually neutralize them so that they cannot be absorbed. Patients taking antacids should be advised to separate them from any other medications by 1 to 2 hours.

Table 57.2 DRUGS IN FOCUS

Antacids

Drug Name	Usual Dosage	Usual Indications
aluminum salts (*AlternaGEL*)	Adult: 500–1500 mg three to six times per day between meals and at bedtime Pediatric: 50–150 mg/kg PO q24h in divided doses q4–6h	Symptomatic relief of gastrointestinal (GI) hyperacidity; treatment of hyperphosphatemia; prevention of formation of phosphate urinary stones
calcium salts (*Oystercal, Tums*)	0.5–2 g PO as needed as an antacid	Symptomatic relief of GI hyperacidity, treatment of calcium deficiency, prevention of hypocalcemia
magaldrate (*Iosopan, Riopan*)	480–1080 mg PO 1 and 3 h after meals and at bedtime	Symptomatic relief of GI hyperacidity in adults
magnesium salts (*Milk of Magnesia,* others)	280–1500 mg PO q.i.d., dose based on salt used Pediatric: one-half of the adult dose	Symptomatic relief of GI hyperacidity; prophylaxis of stress ulcers; relief of constipation
P sodium bicarbonate (*Bell/Ans*)	Adult: 300–2000 mg PO daily to q.i.d.	Symptomatic relief of GI hyperacidity, minimization of uric acid crystalluria, adjunctive treatment in severe diarrhea

Therapeutic Actions and Indications

Antacids neutralize stomach acid by direct chemical reaction (see Figure 57.1). They are recommended for the symptomatic relief of upset stomach associated with hyperacidity, as well as the hyperacidity associated with peptic ulcer, gastritis, peptic esophagitis, gastric hyperacidity, and hiatal hernia.

Contraindications and Cautions

The antacids are contraindicated in the presence of any known allergy to antacid products. Caution should be used in the following instances: any condition that can be exacerbated by electrolyte or acid–base imbalance; any electrolyte imbalance; GI obstruction, *which could cause systemic absorption;* allergy to any component of the drug; renal dysfunction, *which could lead to electrolyte disturbance if any absorbed antacid is not neutralized properly;* and pregnancy and lactation *because of the potential for adverse effects on the fetus or neonate.*

Adverse Effects

The adverse effects associated with these drugs relate to their effects on acid–base levels and electrolytes. Rebound acidity, in which the stomach produces more acid in response to the alkaline environment, is common. Alkalosis with resultant metabolic changes (nausea, vomiting, neuromuscular changes, headache, irritability, muscle twitching, and even coma) may occur. The use of calcium salts may lead to hypercalcemia and milk-alkali syndrome (seen as alkalosis, renal calcium deposits, or severe electrolyte disorders). Constipation or diarrhea may result, depending on the antacid being used. Hypophosphatemia can occur with the use of aluminum salts. Finally, fluid retention and congestive heart failure can occur with sodium bicarbonate because of its high sodium content.

Drug–Drug Interactions

Antacids affect the absorption of many other drugs. For example they may decrease the absorption of tetracyclines, phenothiazines, and ketoconazole, which is why they should be taken 2 hours before or 2 hours after other medications are taken. If the pH of urine is affected by large doses of antacids, levels of drugs, such as quinidine, may increase and levels of salicylates may decrease.

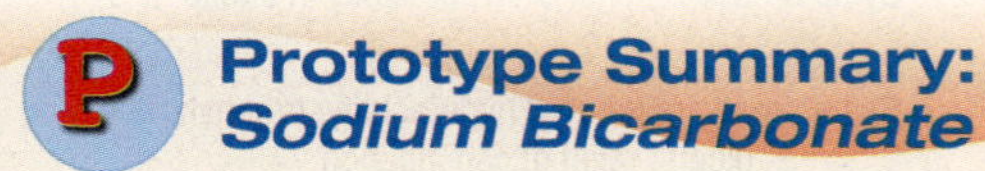

Prototype Summary: Sodium Bicarbonate

Indications: Symptomatic relief of upset stomach from hyperacidity; prophylaxis for GI bleeding and stress ulcers; adjunctive treatment of severe diarrhea; also used for treatment of metabolic acidosis, certain drug intoxications, to minimize uric acid crystallization

Actions: Neutralizes or reduces gastric acidity, resulting in an increase in gastric pH, which inhibits the proteolytic activity of pepsin

Pharmacokinetics:

Route	Onset	Peak	Duration
Oral	Rapid	30 min	1–3 h

$T_{1/2}$: Unknown; excreted unchanged in urine

Adverse effects: Gastric rupture, systemic alkalosis (headache, nausea, irritability, weakness, tetany, confusion), hypokalemia, gastric acid rebound

Nursing Considerations for Patients Receiving Antacids

Assessment: History and Examination

Screen for the following conditions, *which could be cautions or contraindications to use of the drug:* any history of allergy to antacids; renal dysfunction *that might interfere with the drug's metabolism and excretion;* electrolyte disturbances *that could be exacerbated by the effects of the drug;* and pregnancy or lactation, *which would require caution.*

Include screening for baseline data *to assess the effectiveness of the drug and the occurrence of any adverse effects associated with drug therapy.* Assess the following: abdominal sounds, *to ensure GI motility;* mucous membrane status, *to evaluate potential problems with absorption;* and serum electrolytes and renal function tests.

Nursing Diagnoses

The patient receiving antacids may have the following nursing diagnoses related to drug therapy:

- Diarrhea related to GI effects
- Risk for Constipation related to GI effects
- Imbalanced Nutrition: Less Than Body Requirements, related to GI effects
- Risk for Imbalanced Fluid Volume related to systemic effects
- Deficient Knowledge regarding drug therapy

Implementation With Rationale

- Administer the drug apart from any other oral medications (1 hour before or 2 hours after) *to ensure adequate absorption of the other medications.*
- Have patients chew tablets thoroughly and follow with water *to ensure therapeutic levels reach the stomach to decrease acid.*
- Periodically monitor serum electrolytes *to evaluate drug effects.*
- Assess patients for any signs of acid–base or electrolyte imbalance *to arrange for appropriate interventions.*
- Provide thorough patient teaching, including drug name, prescribed dosage, measures for avoidance of adverse effects, and warning signs that may indicate possible problems. Instruct patients about the need for periodic monitoring and evaluation *to enhance patient knowledge about drug therapy and to promote compliance.*
- Offer support and encouragement *to help patients cope with the disease and the drug regimen.*

Evaluation

- Monitor patient response to the drug (relief of GI symptoms caused by hyperacidity).
- Monitor for adverse effects (GI effects, serum electrolytes, and acid–base levels).
- Evaluate effectiveness of teaching plan (patient can give the drug and dosage, as well as describe adverse effects to watch for, specific measures to avoid adverse effects, and measures to take to increase the effectiveness of the drug).
- Monitor effectiveness of comfort measures and compliance with regimen.

Proton Pump Inhibitors

The gastric acid pump or proton pump inhibitors suppress gastric acid secretion by specifically inhibiting the hydrogen–potassium adenosine triphosphatase (H^+,K^+-ATPase) enzyme system on the secretory surface of the gastric parietal cells. This action blocks the final step of acid production, lowering the acid levels in the stomach. Five proton pump inhibitors are currently available (Table 57.3):

- Omeprazole (*Prilosec*) is a faster-acting and more quickly excreted drug. It is used in combination therapy to treat ulcers caused by *H. pylori* bacteria. Omeprazole is also recommended for the relief of symptoms of heartburn and is available over the counter (OTC) for that purpose.
- Esomeprazole (*Nexium*) is a longer-acting drug; it is not broken down as fast in the liver, compared with the parent drug omeprazole. It is indicated for the treatment of gastroesophageal reflux disease (GERD), severe erosive esophagitis, and pathological hypersecretory conditions.

Table 57.3 DRUGS IN FOCUS

Proton Pump Inhibitors

Drug Name	Usual Dosage	Usual Indications
esomeprazole (*Nexium*)	Acute: 20–40 mg/day PO for 4–8 wk; 20–40 mg/day PO for maintenance	Gastroesophageal reflux disease (GERD), severe erosive esophagitis, duodenal ulcers, pathological hypersecretory conditions
lansoprazole (*Prevacid*)	15–30 mg/day PO based on condition and response; 30 mg IV over 30 min for up to 7 days Pediatric: 1–11 yr (≤30 kg)—15 mg/kg/day PO; 1–11 yr (>30 kg)—30 mg/kg/day PO; 12–17 yr—15–30 mg/day PO	Treatment of gastric ulcer, GERD, pathological hypersecretory syndromes; maintenance therapy for healing duodenal ulcers and esophagitis; in combination therapy for the eradication of *Helicobacter pylori* infection
P omeprazole (*Prilosec*)	20–40 mg/day PO for 4–8 wk based on condition and response	Treatment of gastric ulcers, GERD, pathological hypersecretory syndromes; maintenance therapy for healing duodenal ulcers and esophagitis; in combination therapy for the eradication of *H. pylori* infection; heartburn
pantoprazole (*Protonix*)	40 mg PO daily to b.i.d. *or* 40 mg/day IV for 7–10 days	Treatment of GERD in adults
rabeprazole (*Aciphex*)	20–60 mg/day PO based on condition and response	Healing and maintenance of GERD, duodenal ulcers, pathological hypersecretory conditions; in combination therapy for the eradication of *H. pylori* infection

- Lansoprazole (*Prevacid*) is available in a delayed-release form and an IV preparation for use in the treatment of gastric ulcers, GERD, and pathological hypersecretory syndromes; as part of maintenance therapy for healing duodenal ulcers and esophagitis; and in combination therapy for the eradication of *H. pylori* infection. Lansoprazole is approved for use in children.

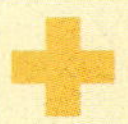

FOCUS ON **PATIENT SAFETY**

With many patients taking NSAIDs over a long term for a variety of conditions, including arthritis and cancers, the incidence of GI ulceration and bleeding could increase. In late 2003, a drug pack called *Prevacid NapraPAC* was marketed to help prevent the GI ulceration associated with NSAID use before it occurs. This drug pack comes in weekly blister packages with 14 naproxen (an NSAID) tablets and 7 lansoprazole capsules. The patient takes one capsule and one tablet each morning with a full glass of water and one tablet in the evening. This combination is approved to decrease the risk of gastric ulcers associated with long-term use of the NSAID naproxen for treatment of arthritis. Many health care providers will prescribe a proton pump inhibitor when prescribing long-term NSAID use to protect the patient from gastric erosion. Providing the patient with a convenient, weekly packet of medication might improve compliance with the drug regimen.

- Pantoprazole (*Protonix*) is used for the treatment of GERD, peptic ulcer, and Zollinger–Ellison syndrome. This drug is also available in a parenteral form for short-term use when the oral form cannot be tolerated.
- Rabeprazole (*Aciphex*) is available only in a delayed-release form and is used to heal and maintain GERD, for the healing of duodenal ulcers, and for the treatment of pathological hypersecretory conditions.

Therapeutic Actions and Indications

Proton pump inhibitors act at specific secretory surface receptors to prevent the final step of acid production and thereby decrease the level of acid in the stomach (see Figure 57.1). They are recommended for the short-term treatment of active duodenal ulcers, GERD, erosive esophagitis, and benign active gastric ulcer; for the long-term treatment of pathological hypersecretory conditions; as maintenance therapy for healing of erosive esophagitis and ulcers; and in combination with amoxicillin and clarithromycin for the treatment of *H. pylori* infection.

Pharmacokinetics

These drugs are acid labile and are rapidly absorbed from the GI tract. They undergo extensive metabolism in the liver and are excreted in urine. There are no adequate studies of these drugs during pregnancy and lactation. Caution should be used, however, because of the potential for adverse effects on the fetus or neonate. The safety and efficacy of these drugs has not been established for patients younger than 18 years of age.

Contraindications and Cautions

These drugs are contraindicated in the presence of known allergy to either the drug or the drug components. Caution should be used in pregnant or lactating women.

Adverse Effects

The adverse effects associated with these drugs are related to their effects on the H^+,K^+-ATPase pump on the parietal and other cells. CNS effects of dizziness and headache are commonly seen; asthenia (loss of strength), vertigo, insomnia, apathy, and dream abnormalities may also be observed. GI effects can include diarrhea, abdominal pain, nausea, vomiting, dry mouth, and tongue atrophy. Upper respiratory tract symptoms, including cough, stuffy nose, hoarseness, and epistaxis, are frequently seen. Other, less common adverse effects include rash, alopecia, pruritus, dry skin, back pain, and fever. In preclinical studies, long-term effects of proton pump inhibitors included the development of gastric cancer.

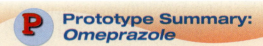

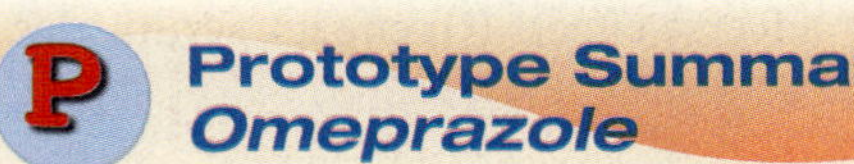

Indications: Short-term treatment of active duodenal ulcer or active benign gastric ulcer; treatment of heartburn or symptoms of gastroesophageal reflux; treatment of pathological hypersecretory syndromes; eradication of *H. pylori* infection as part of combination therapy

Actions: Specifically inhibits the hydrogen–potassium adenosine triphosphatase enzyme system on the secretory surface of the gastric parietal cells, blocking the final step in acid production and decreasing gastric acid levels

Pharmacokinetics:

Route	Onset	Peak	Duration
Oral	Varies	0.5–3.5 h	Varies

$T_{1/2}$: 30–60 min; metabolized in the liver and excreted in urine and bile

Adverse effects: Headache, dizziness, vertigo, insomnia, rash, diarrhea, abdominal pain, nausea, vomiting, upper respiratory infection symptoms, cough

Nursing Considerations for Patients Receiving Proton Pump Inhibitors

Assessment: History and Examination

Screen for any history of allergy to a proton pump inhibitor, pregnancy, or lactation, *which could be cautions or contraindications to use of the drug.*

Include screening *to establish baseline data for assessing the effectiveness of the drug and the occurrence of any adverse effects associated with drug therapy.* Assess skin color and lesions, as well as reflexes, affect, and orientation. In addition, perform an abdominal and respiratory examination.

Nursing Diagnoses

The patient receiving proton pump inhibitors may have the following nursing diagnoses related to drug therapy:

- Diarrhea related to GI effects
- Risk for Constipation related to GI effects
- Imbalanced Nutrition: Less Than Body Requirements, related to GI effects
- Disturbed Sensory Perception (Kinesthetic, Auditory) related to CNS effects
- Deficient Knowledge regarding drug therapy

Implementation With Rationale

- Administer drug before meals; ensure that the patient does not open, chew, or crush capsules; they should be swallowed whole *to ensure therapeutic effectiveness of the drug.*
- Provide appropriate safety and comfort measures if CNS effects occur *to prevent patient injury.*
- Arrange for medical follow-up if symptoms are not resolved after 4 to 8 weeks of therapy *because serious underlying conditions could be causing the symptoms.*
- Provide thorough patient teaching, including drug name, prescribed dosage, measures for avoidance of adverse effects, and warning signs that may indicate possible problems. Instruct patients about the need for periodic monitoring and evaluation *to enhance patient knowledge about drug therapy and to promote compliance.*
- Offer support and encouragement *to help patients cope with the disease and the drug regimen.*

Evaluation

- Monitor patient response to the drug (relief of GI symptoms caused by hyperacidity; healing of erosive GI lesions).
- Monitor for adverse effects (GI effects, CNS changes, dermatological effects, respiratory effects).
- Evaluate effectiveness of teaching plan (patient can name the drug and dosage and describe adverse effects to watch for, specific measures to avoid adverse effects, and measures to take to increase the effectiveness of the drug).
- Monitor effectiveness of comfort and safety measures and compliance with regimen.

Antipeptic Agent

The antipeptic agent sucralfate (*Carafate*) is given to protect eroded ulcer sites in the GI tract from further damage by acid and digestive enzymes (Table 57.4).

Therapeutic Actions and Indications

Sucralfate forms an ulcer-adherent complex at duodenal ulcer sites, protecting the sites against acid, pepsin, and bile salts. This action prevents further breakdown of the area and promotes ulcer healing. The drug also inhibits pepsin activity in gastric juices, preventing further breakdown of proteins in the stomach, including the protein wall of the stomach (see Figure 57.1).

Sucralfate is recommended for the short-term treatment of duodenal ulcers. It is used at a reduced dose for maintenance of duodenal ulcers after healing. In addition, this agent is

Table 57.4 DRUGS IN FOCUS

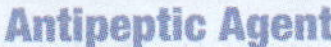

Antipeptic Agent

Drug Name	Usual Dosage	Usual Indications
sucralfate (*Carafate*)	1 g PO b.i.d to q.i.d.	Short-term treatment of duodenal ulcers; maintenance of duodenal ulcers after healing in adults; treatment of oral and esophageal ulcers due to radiation or chemotherapy

undergoing investigation for the treatment of gastric ulcers; gastric damage induced by nonsteroidal anti-inflammatory drugs (NSAIDs); prevention of stress ulcers in acutely ill individuals; and the treatment of oral and esophageal ulcers due to radiation, chemotherapy, or sclerotherapy.

Pharmacokinetics

Sucralfate is rapidly absorbed, metabolized in the liver, and excreted in feces. It crosses the placenta and may enter breast milk. Because of the potential adverse effects on the fetus or neonate, this drug should not be used during pregnancy or lactation unless the benefit to the mother clearly outweighs the potential adverse effects.

Contraindications and Cautions

Sucralfate should not be given to any person with known allergy to the drug or any of its components. It should not be given to individuals with renal failure or undergoing dialysis *because a buildup of aluminum may occur if it is used with aluminum-containing products.* Caution should be used in patients who are pregnant or lactating.

Adverse Effects

The adverse effects associated with sucralfate are primarily related to its GI effects. Constipation is the most frequently seen adverse effect. Diarrhea, nausea, indigestion, gastric discomfort, and dry mouth may also occur. Other adverse effects that have been reported with this drug include dizziness, sleepiness, vertigo, skin rash, and back pain.

Clinically Important Drug–Drug Interactions

If aluminum salts are combined with sucralfate, there is a risk of high aluminum levels and aluminum toxicity. Extreme care should be taken if this combination is used.

In addition, if phenytoin, fluoroquinolone antibiotics (e.g., ciprofloxacin, norfloxacin), or penicillamine is combined with sucralfate, decreased serum levels and drug effectiveness may result. In such combinations, the individual agents should be administered separately, with at least 2 hours between drugs.

Nursing Considerations for Patients Receiving an Antipeptic Agent

Assessment: History and Examination

Screen for the following conditions, *which could be cautions or contraindications to use of the drug:* any history of allergy to sucralfate, renal dysfunction or dialysis, and pregnancy or lactation.

Include screening *to establish baseline data for assessing the effectiveness of the drug and the occurrence of any adverse effects associated with drug therapy.* Assess the following: skin color and lesions; reflexes, affect, and orientation; abdominal examination; and mucous membranes.

Nursing Diagnoses

The patient receiving sucralfate may have the following nursing diagnoses related to drug therapy:

- Diarrhea related to GI effects
- Risk for Constipation related to GI effects
- Imbalanced Nutrition: Less Than Body Requirements, related to GI effects
- Disturbed Sensory Perception (Kinesthetic) related to CNS effects
- Deficient Knowledge regarding drug therapy

Implementation With Rationale

- Administer drug on an empty stomach, 1 hour before or 2 hours after meals and at bedtime, *to ensure therapeutic effectiveness of the drug.*
- Monitor patient for GI pain, *and arrange to administer antacids to relieve pain if needed.*
- Administer antacids between doses of sucralfate, not within 30 minutes of a sucralfate dose, *because sucralfate can interfere with absorption of oral agents.*
- Provide comfort and safety measures if CNS effects occur *to prevent patient injury.*
- Provide frequent mouth care; sugarless lozenges to suck; bowel training as needed; and small, frequent meals *if GI effects are uncomfortable.*
- Provide thorough patient teaching, including drug name, prescribed dosage, measures for avoidance of adverse effects, and warning signs that may indicate possible problems. Instruct patients about the need for periodic monitoring and evaluation to enhance patient knowledge *about drug therapy and to promote compliance.*
- Offer support and encouragement *to help patients cope with the disease and the drug regimen.*

Evaluation

- Monitor patient response to the drug (relief of GI symptoms caused by hyperacidity; healing of erosive GI lesions).
- Monitor for adverse effects (GI effects, CNS changes, dermatologic effects).

- Evaluate effectiveness of teaching plan (patient can name drug and dosage and describe adverse effects to watch for, specific measures to avoid adverse effects, and measures to take to increase the effectiveness of the drug).
- Monitor effectiveness of comfort and safety measures and compliance with regimen.

Prostaglandin

The synthetic prostaglandin E_1 analog, misoprostol (*Cytotec*), is used to protect the lining of the stomach in situations that might lead to serious GI complications (Table 57.5).

Therapeutic Actions and Indications

Prostaglandin E_1 inhibits gastric acid secretion and increases bicarbonate and mucous production in the stomach, thus protecting the stomach lining (see Figure 57.1). Misoprostol is used to prevent NSAID-induced gastric ulcers in patients who are at high risk for complications from a gastric ulcer (e.g., elderly or debilitated patients, patients with a past history of ulcer). It has also been found to be effective for treatment of duodenal ulcers in patients who are not responsive to H_2 antagonists, and it is being investigated for that purpose. This drug is also used with mifepristone as an abortifacient.

Pharmacokinetics

Misoprostol is rapidly absorbed from the GI tract, metabolized in the liver, and excreted in urine. Caution should be used in the presence of hepatic or renal impairment, *which could interfere with the effective metabolism and excretion of the drug.* Misoprostol crosses the placenta and enters breast milk. *It has been associated with fetal deaths in animal studies* and should be given to women of childbearing age only after a negative pregnancy test and with warnings to use a barrier form of contraceptive while taking this drug. If this drug is needed during lactation, another method of feeding the baby should be used.

Contraindications and Cautions

This drug is contraindicated during pregnancy *because it is an abortifacient.* Women of childbearing age should be advised to have a negative serum pregnancy test within 2 weeks of beginning treatment, and they should begin the drug on the second or third day of their next menstrual cycle. In addition, they should be instructed to use barrier contraceptives during therapy. Caution should be used during lactation and with any known allergy to prostaglandins.

Adverse Effects

The adverse effects associated with this drug are primarily related to its GI effects—nausea, diarrhea, abdominal pain, flatulence, vomiting, dyspepsia, and constipation. Genitourinary effects, which are related to the actions of prostaglandins on the uterus, include miscarriages, excessive bleeding, spotting, cramping, hypermenorrhea, dysmenorrhea, and other menstrual disorders. Women taking this drug should be notified, both in writing and verbally, of these potential effects of this drug.

Nursing Considerations for Patients Receiving Prostaglandin

Assessment: History and Examination

Screen for the following *contraindications to the use of the drug:* any history of allergy to misoprostol, and pregnancy or lactation.

Include screening *to establish baseline data for assessing the effectiveness of the drug and the occurrence of any adverse effects associated with drug therapy.* Assess abdominal examination, pregnancy test, and normal menstrual activity.

Nursing Diagnoses

The patient receiving misoprostol may have the following nursing diagnoses related to drug therapy:

- Diarrhea related to GI effects
- Risk for Constipation related to GI effects

Table 57.5 DRUGS IN FOCUS

Prostaglandin

Drug Name	Usual Dosage	Usual Indications
misoprostol (*Cytotec*)	200 mcg PO q.i.d.; reduce dosage with renal impairment	Prevention of NSAID-induced ulcers in adults at high risk for development of these gastric ulcers

- Imbalanced Nutrition: Less Than Body Requirements, related to GI effects
- Sexual Dysfunction related to genitourinary effects
- Deficient Knowledge regarding drug therapy

Implementation With Rationale

- Administer to patients at high risk for NSAID-induced ulcers during the full course of NSAID therapy *to prevent the development of gastric ulcers.* Administer four times a day—with meals and at bedtime.
- Arrange for a serum pregnancy test within 2 weeks before beginning treatment; begin therapy on the second or third day of the menstrual period *to ensure that women of childbearing age are not pregnant and to prevent abortifacient effects associated with this drug.*
- Provide patient with both written and oral information regarding the associated risks of pregnancy *to ensure that the patient understands the risks involved;* advise the use of barrier contraceptives during therapy *to ensure prevention of pregnancy.*
- Assess nutritional status if GI effects are severe *in order to arrange for appropriate measures to relieve discomfort and ensure nutrition.*
- Provide thorough patient teaching, including drug name, prescribed dosage, measures for avoidance of adverse effects, and warning signs that may indicate possible problems. Instruct patients about the need for periodic monitoring and evaluation *to enhance patient knowledge about drug therapy and to promote compliance.*
- Offer support and encouragement *to help patients cope with the disease and the drug regimen.*

Evaluation

- Monitor patient response to the drug (prevention of GI ulcers related to NSAIDs).
- Monitor for adverse effects (GI, genitourinary).
- Evaluate effectiveness of teaching plan (patient can name drug and dosage and describe adverse effects to watch for, specific measures to avoid adverse effects, and measures to take to increase the effectiveness of the drug).
- Monitor effectiveness of comfort and safety measures and compliance with the regimen.

Digestive Enzymes

Some patients—those who have suffered strokes, salivary gland disorders, or extreme surgery of the head and neck, and those with cystic fibrosis or pancreatic dysfunction—may require a supplement to the production of digestive enzymes. Two digestive enzymes are available for replacement in conditions that result in lower than normal levels of these enzymes (Table 57.6):

- Saliva substitute (*MouthKote, Salivart*) helps in conditions that result in dry mouth—stroke, radiation therapy, chemotherapy, and other illnesses. This drug is not generally absorbed systemically.
- Pancrelipase (*Creon, Pancrease*) is used in conditions that result in a lack of pancrelipase to aid the digestion and absorption of fats, proteins, and carbohydrates in conditions that result in a lack of this enzyme. This drug is thought to be processed through normal metabolic systems in the body. Little is known about its pharmacokinetics.

Therapeutic Actions and Indications

Saliva substitute contains electrolytes and carboxymethylcellulose to act as a thickening agent in dry mouth conditions. This makes the food bolus easier to swallow and begins the early digestion process. The pancreatic enzymes are replacement enzymes that help the digestion and absorption of fats, proteins, and carbohydrates (see Figure 57.1). They

Table 57.6 DRUGS IN FOCUS

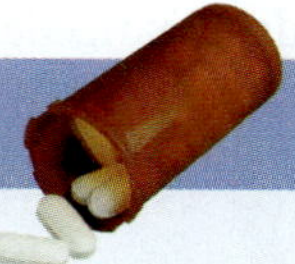

Digestive Enzymes

Drug Name	Usual Dosage	Usual Indications
(P) pancrelipase (*Creon, Pancrease*)	Adult: 4,000–48,000 units PO with each meal and snacks Pediatric: 6 mo–1 yr—2000 units PO per meal; 1–6 yr—4000–8000 units PO with meals, 4000 units with snacks; 7–12 yr—4,000–12,000 units PO with each meal and snack	An aid for digestion and absorption of fats, proteins, and carbohydrates in conditions that result in a lack of this enzyme
saliva substitute (*MouthKote, Salivart*)	Spray or apply to oral mucosa	An aid in conditions resulting in dry mouth—stroke, radiation therapy, chemotherapy, and other illnesses

are used as replacement therapy in patients with cystic fibrosis, chronic pancreatitis, ductal obstruction, pancreatic insufficiency, steatorrhea, or malabsorption syndrome and after pancreatectomy or gastrectomy.

Contraindications and Cautions

Saliva substitute is contraindicated in the presence of known allergy to parabens or any component of the drug. It should be used cautiously in patients with congestive heart failure, hypertension, or renal failure *because there may be an abnormal absorption of electrolytes, including sodium, leading to increased cardiovascular load.* Pancreatic enzymes should not be used with known allergy to the product or to pork products. In addition, they should be used cautiously in pregnancy and lactation.

Adverse Effects

The adverse effects most commonly seen with saliva substitute involve complications from abnormal electrolyte absorption, such as increased levels of magnesium, sodium, or potassium. The adverse effects that most often occur with pancreatic enzymes are related to GI irritation and include nausea, abdominal cramps, and diarrhea.

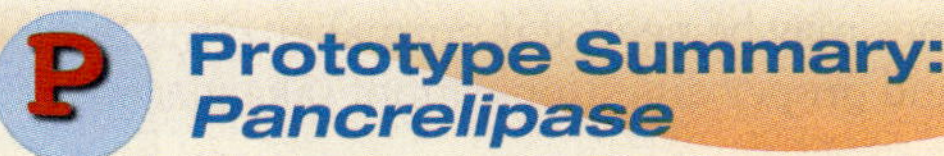

Prototype Summary: Pancrelipase

Indications: Replacement therapy in patients with deficient exocrine pancreatic secretions

Actions: Replaces pancreatic enzymes to aid in the digestion and absorption of fats, proteins, and carbohydrates

Pharmacokinetics: Generally not absorbed systemically

$T_{1/2}$: Generally not absorbed systemically

Adverse effects: Nausea, abdominal cramps, diarrhea, hyperuricosuria

Nursing Considerations for Patients Receiving Digestive Enzymes

Assessment: History and Examination

Screen for the following conditions, *which could be cautions or contraindications to use of the drug:* any history of allergy to any of the drugs or to pork products (pancreatic enzymes); pregnancy or lactation; congestive heart failure or hypertension (saliva substitute).

Include screening *for establishment of baseline data for assessing the effectiveness of the drug and the occurrence of any adverse effects associated with drug therapy.* Assess the following: abdominal examination, mucous membranes, blood pressure, cardiac evaluation, and pancreatic enzyme levels (pancreatic enzymes).

Nursing Diagnoses

The patient receiving digestive enzymes may have the following nursing diagnoses related to drug therapy:

- Diarrhea related to GI effects
- Imbalanced Nutrition: Less Than Body Requirements, related to GI effects
- Deficient Knowledge regarding drug therapy

Implementation With Rationale

- Have patient swish a saliva substitute around the mouth as needed for dry mouth and throat, *to coat the mouth and ensure therapeutic effectiveness of the drug.*
- Monitor swallowing *because it may be impaired and additional therapy may be needed.*
- Administer pancreatic enzymes with meals and snacks so that enzyme is available when it is needed. Avoid spilling powder on the skin *because it may be irritating.* Do not crush the capsule or allow the patient to chew it; it must be swallowed whole *to ensure full therapeutic effects.*
- Assess nutritional status if there are GI effects *in order to arrange for appropriate measures to relieve discomfort and ensure nutrition.*
- Provide thorough patient teaching, including drug name, prescribed dosage, measures for avoidance of adverse effects, and warning signs that may indicate possible problems. Instruct patients about the need for periodic monitoring and evaluation *to enhance patient knowledge about drug therapy and to promote compliance.*
- Offer support and encouragement *to help patients cope with the disease and the drug regimen.*

Evaluation

- Monitor patient response to the drug (e.g., relief of dry mouth and throat; digestion of fats, proteins, and carbohydrates).
- Monitor for adverse effects (e.g., electrolyte imbalance, GI effects).

- Evaluate effectiveness of teaching plan (patient can name the drug and dosage and describe adverse effects to watch for, specific measures to avoid adverse effects, and measures to take to increase the effectiveness of the drug).
- Monitor effectiveness of comfort/safety measures and compliance with regimen.

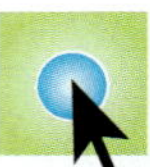

WEB LINKS

Health care providers and patients may want to consult the following Internet sources:

http://www.emedicine.com/EMERG/topic820.htm Information on the anatomy and physiology of the GI tract, pathophysiology of various gastrointestinal ulcer disorders, treatments, and research.

http://www.familydoctor.org/handouts/271.html Information for patients and families about ulcers, including treatments and causes of ulcers and *H. pylori* infection.

http://www.gerd.com Information on gastroesophageal reflux disorders.

http://www.cdc.gov Information about *H. pylori* research and treatment.

http://www.med.unc.edu/medicine/fgidc/bkgrnd.htm Educational materials on a variety of GI disorders.

Points to Remember

- GI complaints are some of the most common symptoms seen in clinical practice.
- Peptic ulcers may result from increased acid production, decrease in the protective mucous lining of the stomach, infection with *Helicobacter pylori* bacteria, or a combination of these.
- Agents used to decrease the acid content of the stomach include H_2 antagonists, which block the release of acid in response to gastrin or parasympathetic release; antacids, which chemically react with the acid to neutralize it; and proton pump inhibitors, which block the last step of acid production to prevent release.
- Acid rebound occurs when the stomach produces more gastrin and more acid in response to lowered acid levels in the stomach. Balancing the reduction of the stomach acid without increasing acid production is a clinical challenge.
- The antipeptic agent sucralfate forms a protective coating over the eroded stomach lining to protect it from acid and digestive enzymes and to aid healing.
- The prostaglandin misoprostol blocks gastric acid secretion while increasing the production of bicarbonate and mucous lining in the stomach.
- Digestive enzymes such as substitute saliva and pancreatic enzymes may be needed if normal enzyme levels are very low and proper digestion cannot take place.

CHECK YOUR UNDERSTANDING

Answers to the questions in this chapter may be found in the Answer Key in the back of the book.

Multiple Choice

Select the best response to the following.

1. Histamine-2 antagonists act to
   a. block the release of gastrin.
   b. selectively block histamine receptors, reducing swelling and inflammation.
   c. selectively block H_2 receptor sites, leading to a reduction in gastric acid secretion and reduction in overall pepsin production.
   d. are effective only with long-term use.

2. H_2 receptors are found throughout the body, including
   a. in the nasal passages, upper airways, and stomach.
   b. in the CNS and upper airways.
   c. in the respiratory tract and the heart.
   d. in the heart, CNS, and stomach.

3. The H_2 receptor blocker of choice for a patient with known liver dysfunction would be
   a. cimetidine.
   b. famotidine.
   c. nizatidine.
   d. ranitidine.

4. A patient receiving intravenous cimetidine (*Tagamet*) for an acute ulcer problem needs to be monitored for
   a. GI upset.
   b. gynecomastia.
   c. cardiac arrhythmias.
   d. constipation.

5. Acid rebound is a condition that occurs when
   a. lowering gastric acid to an alkaline level stimulates the release of gastric acid.
   b. raising gastric acid levels causes heartburn.
   c. combining protein, calcium, and smoking greatly elevates gastric acid levels.
   d. eating citrus fruit neutralizes gastric acid.

6. A nurse taking care of a patient who is receiving a proton pump inhibitor should teach the patient
   a. to take the drug after every meal.
   b. to chew or crush tablets to increase their absorption.
   c. to swallow tablets or capsules whole.
   d. to stop taking the drug after 3 weeks of therapy.

7. Misoprostol (*Cytotec*) is a prostaglandin that is used to
   a. prevent uterine contractions.
   b. prevent NSAID-related gastric ulcers in patients at high risk.
   c. decrease hyperacidity with meals.
   d. relieve the burning associated with hiatal hernia at night.

8. A nurse caring for a patient receiving pancreatic enzymes as replacement therapy should be assessing the patient for
   a. hypertension.
   b. cardiac arrhythmias.
   c. excessive weight gain.
   d. signs of GI irritation.

Multiple Response

Select all that apply.

1. Patients who use antacids frequently can be expected to experience which of the following adverse effects?
   a. Systemic alkalosis
   b. Electrolyte imbalances
   c. Hyperkalemia
   d. Metabolic acidosis
   e. Constipation or diarrhea
   f. Muscle weakness

2. Saliva substitute (*Moi-Stir*) may be useful in which of the following circumstances?
   a. Cancer radiation therapy
   b. Stroke
   c. Parkinson's disease
   d. Brain injury
   e. Situational anxiety
   f. Hypertension

Web Exercise

You are doing a rotation on medicine and working on a gastrointestinal (GI) unit. You are asked to prepare an inservice for the staff covering various GI diseases, treatments, and research and nursing implications involved in the care of patients with these disorders. Because this program will determine 20% of your course grade, you want to be current and thorough. Go to the Internet to prepare the teaching session.

Matching

Match the following drugs with the appropriate class of drugs used to affect GI secretions. (Some classes may be used more than once.)

1. ____________________ misoprostol
2. ____________________ lansoprazole
3. ____________________ sucralfate
4. ____________________ cimetidine
5. ____________________ saliva
6. ____________________ aluminum
7. ____________________ sodium bicarbonate
8. ____________________ pancrelipase
9. ____________________ omeprazole
10. ____________________ famotidine

A. Histamine (H_2) antagonists
B. Antacids
C. Proton pump inhibitors
D. Antipeptic agent
E. Prostaglandin
F. Digestive enzymes

Bibliography and References

Drug facts and comparisons. (2006). St. Louis: Facts and Comparisons.

Gilman, A., Hardman, J. G., & Limbird, L. E. (Eds.). (2006). *Goodman and Gilman's the pharmacological basis of therapeutics* (11th ed.). New York: McGraw-Hill.

Karch, A. M. (2006). *2007 Lippincott's nursing drug guide.* Philadelphia: Lippincott Williams & Wilkins.

Porth, C. M. (2005). *Pathophysiology: Concepts of altered health states* (7th ed.). Philadelphia: Lippincott Williams & Wilkins.

Professional's guide to patient drug facts. (2006). St. Louis: Facts and Comparisons.

CHAPTER
58

Laxative and Antidiarrheal Agents

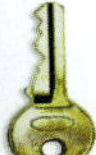

KEY TERMS

antidiarrheal drug
bulk stimulant
cathartic dependence
chemical stimulant
constipation
diarrhea
lubricant

LEARNING OBJECTIVES

Upon completion of this chapter, you will be able to:

1. Describe the underlying processes in diarrhea and constipation and correlate this with the types of drugs used to treat these conditions.
2. Describe the therapeutic actions, indications, pharmacokinetics, contraindications, most common adverse reactions, and important drug–drug interactions associated with chemical stimulant laxatives, bulk laxatives, lubricant laxatives, gastrointestinal stimulants, and antidiarrheal drugs.
3. Discuss the use of laxatives and antidiarrheal agents across the lifespan.
4. Compare and contrast the prototype drugs castor oil, magnesium citrate, mineral oil, metoclopramide, and loperamide with other agents in their class and with other classes of laxatives and antidiarrheals.
5. Outline the nursing considerations, including important teaching points, for patients receiving laxatives and antidiarrheal agents.

LAXATIVES

Chemical Stimulants

bisacodyl
cascara
P castor oil
senna

Bulk Laxatives

lactulose
P magnesium citrate
magnesium hydroxide
magnesium sulfate
polycarbophil
polyethylene glycol-electrolyte solution
psyllium

Lubricants

docusate
glycerin
P mineral oil

GASTROINTESTINAL STIMULANTS

dexpanthenol
P metoclopramide

ANTIDIARRHEAL DRUGS

bismuth subsalicylate
P loperamide
opium derivatives

Drugs used to affect the motor activity of the gastrointestinal (GI) tract can do so in several different ways. They can be used to speed up or improve the movement of intestinal contents along the GI tract when movement becomes too slow or sluggish to allow for proper absorption of nutrients and excretion of wastes, as in **constipation**. Drugs are also used to increase the tone of the GI tract and to stimulate motility throughout the system. They can also be used to decrease movement along the GI tract when rapid movement decreases the time for absorption of nutrients, leading to a loss of water and nutrients and the discomfort of **diarrhea** (Figure 58.1). All of these drugs are used with people of all ages (Box 58.1).

Laxatives

Laxative, or cathartic, drugs are used in several ways to speed the passage of the intestinal contents through the GI tract. Laxatives may be either **chemical stimulants**, which chemically irritate the lining of the GI tract; **bulk stimulants** (also called mechanical stimulants), which cause the fecal matter to increase in bulk; or **lubricants**, which help the intestinal contents move more smoothly (Box 58.2 and Table 58.1).

Chemical Stimulants

Drugs that act as chemical stimulants directly stimulate the nerve plexus in the intestinal wall, causing increased movement and the stimulation of local reflexes. Such laxatives include the following agents:

- Cascara (generic), a reliable agent that leads to intestinal evacuation, may have a slow, steady effect or may cause severe cramping and rapid evacuation of the contents of the large intestine.
- Senna (*Senokot*), another reliable drug with effects similar to cascara, is found in many over-the-counter (OTC) preparations.
- Castor oil (*Neoloid*), an old standby, is used when a thorough evacuation of the intestine is desirable. This agent

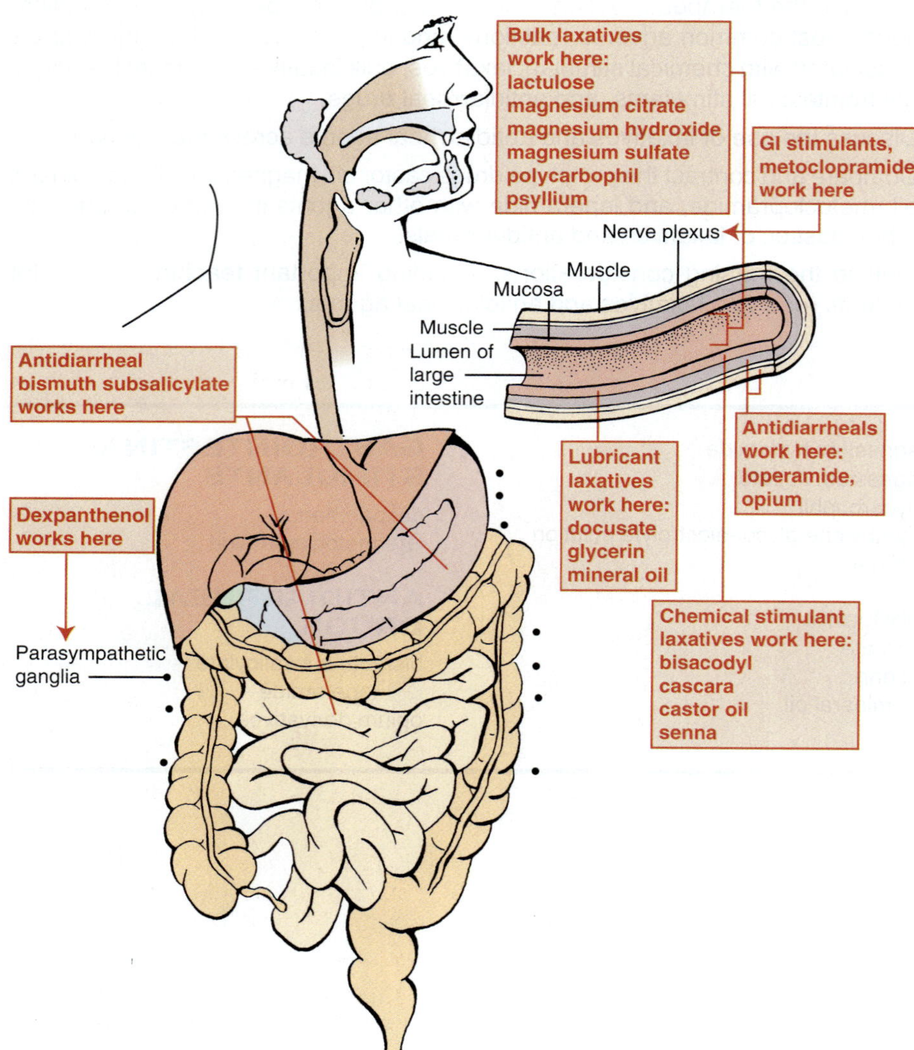

FIGURE 58.1 Sites of action of drugs affecting gastrointestinal motility.

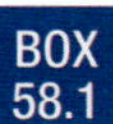

BOX 58.1 DRUG THERAPY ACROSS THE LIFESPAN

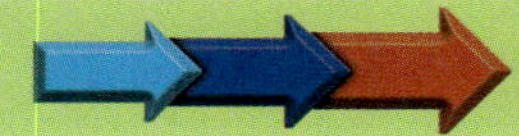

Laxatives and Antidiarrheal Agents

CHILDREN

Laxatives should not be used in children routinely. Proper diet including roughage, plenty of fluids, and exercise should be tried first if a child has a tendency to become constipated. If a laxative is needed, glycerin suppositories are the best choice for infants and young children. Stool softeners can be used in older children; harsh stimulants should be avoided. Children with encopresis, however, are often given senna preparations or mineral oil to help them evacuate the massive stool.

Children receiving these agents should use them for only a short period and should be evaluated for potential underlying medical or nutritional problems if they are not able to return to normal function.

Loperamide may be the antidiarrheal of choice in children >2 years of age if such a drug is needed. Special precautions need to be taken to monitor for electrolyte and fluid disturbances and supportive measures taken as needed.

ADULTS

Adults who use laxatives need to be cautioned not to become dependent. Proper diet, exercise, and adequate intake of fluids should keep the gastrointestinal tract functioning normally. If an antidiarrheal is needed, adults should be carefully instructed in the proper dosing of the drug and monitoring of their total use to avoid excessive dosage.

The safety for the use of these drugs during pregnancy and lactation has not been established. Use should be reserved for those situations in which the benefit to the mother outweighs the potential risk to the fetus. A mild stool softener is often used after delivery. The drugs may enter breast milk and also may affect gastrointestinal activity in the neonate. It is advised that caution be used if one of these drugs is prescribed during lactation.

OLDER ADULTS

Older adults are more likely to develop adverse effects associated with the use of these drugs, including sedation, confusion, dizziness, electrolyte disturbances, fluid imbalance, and cardiovascular effects. Safety measures may be needed if these effects occur and interfere with the patient's mobility and balance.

Older patients also may be taking other drugs that are associated with constipation and may need help to prevent severe problems from developing.

Older adults are more likely to have renal and/or hepatic impairment related to underlying medical conditions, which could interfere with the metabolism and excretion of these drugs. The dosage for older adults should be started at a lower level than recommended for younger adults. The patient should be monitored very closely and dosage adjustment should be made based on patient response.

These patients also need to be alerted to the potential for toxic effects when using over-the-counter (OTC) preparations and should be advised to check with their health care provider before beginning any OTC drug regimen.

A psyllium product is the agent of choice with older adults because there is less risk of adverse reactions. The patient needs to be cautioned to drink plenty of fluid after taking one of these agents, to prevent problems that can occur if the drug starts to pull in fluid while still in the esophagus.

The older adult should be encouraged to drink plenty of fluids, to exercise every day, and to get plenty of roughage in the diet. Many older adults have established routines, such as drinking warm water or prune juice at the same time each morning, that are disrupted with illness or hospitalization. These patients should be encouraged and helped to try to maintain their usual protocol as much as possible.

begins working at the beginning of the small intestine and increases motility throughout the rest of the GI tract. Because castor oil blocks absorption of fats (including fat-soluble vitamins) and may lead to constipation from GI tract exhaustion when there is no stimulus to movement, its frequent use is not desirable.

- Bisacodyl (*Dulcolax*), chemically related to phenolphthalein (the acid-base chemical indicator), is often the drug of choice to empty the bowel before some surgeries or diagnostic tests, such as barium enema. It may be administered orally or rectally.

BOX 58.2 Kinds of Laxatives

Chemical Stimulants

bisacodyl, cascara, castor oil, senna

Bulk Stimulants

lactulose, magnesium citrate, magnesium hydroxide, magnesium sulfate, polycarbophil, psyllium

Lubricants

docusate, glycerin, mineral oil

Bulk Stimulants

Bulk stimulants are rapid-acting, aggressive laxatives that increase the motility of the GI tract by increasing the fluid in the intestinal contents, which enlarges bulk, stimulates local stretch receptors, and activates local activity. Available bulk stimulants include the following agents:

- Magnesium sulfate (*Epsom Salts*), a very potent laxative, is used when total evacuation of the GI tract is needed rapidly, as in cases of GI poisoning. This agent acts by exerting a hypertonic pull against the mucosal wall, drawing fluid into the intestinal contents.
- Magnesium citrate (*Citrate of Magnesia*), found in a citrus-flavored base, is often used to stimulate bowel evacuation before many GI tests and examinations.
- Magnesium hydroxide (*Milk of Magnesia*) is used to stimulate bulk and is a milder and slower-acting laxative. It also works by a saline pull, bringing fluids into the lumen of the GI tract.

Table 58.1 DRUGS IN FOCUS

Laxatives

Drug Name	Usual Dosage	Usual Indications
Chemical Stimulants		
bisacodyl (*Dulcolax*)	10–15 mg PO or 2.5 g in water via enema	Bowel preparation; prevention of constipation and straining after gastrointestinal (GI) surgery, myocardial infarction (MI), obstetrical delivery; short-term treatment of constipation
cascara (*generic*)	325–650 mg PO	Short-term treatment of constipation; evacuation of the large intestine for diagnostic examination
P castor oil (*Neoloid*)	15–30 mL PO	Emptying of the GI tract for diagnostic testing; short-term treatment of constipation
senna (*Senokot*)	One to eight tablets per day at bedtime or 10–25 mL syrup	Short-term treatment of constipation; treatment of encopresis
Bulk Laxatives		
lactulose (*Chronulac*)	15–30 mL PO	Short-term treatment of constipation; especially useful in patients with cardiovascular disorders
P magnesium citrate (*Citrate of Magnesia*)	One glassful; ½ glass for pediatric patients	Bowel evacuation before GI diagnostic tests and examinations
magnesium hydroxide (*Milk of Magnesia*)	15–30 mL PO	Short-term treatment of constipation; prevention of straining after GI surgery, delivery, MI
magnesium sulfate (*Epsom Salts*)	10–25 mg PO	Treatment of GI poisoning; rapid evacuation of the GI tract
polycarbophil (*FiberCon*)	1 g PO, one to four times per day as needed; do not exceed 6 g/day for adults or 3 g/day for children	Mild laxative; short-term treatment of constipation
polyethylene glycol-electrolyte solution (*GoLYTELY*, others)	4 L of oral solution at a rate of 240 mL every 10 min	Bowel cleansing prior to GI examination
psyllium (*Metamucil*)	1 tsp or packet in cold water, one to three times per day; ½ packet for children	Mild laxative; short-term treatment of constipation
Lubricants		
docusate (*Colace*)	50–240 mg PO	Prevention of straining in postoperative, post-MI, and post-partum patients
glycerin (*Sani-Supp*)	4 mL liquid suppository	Short-term treatment of constipation
P mineral oil (*Agoral Plain*)	5–45 mL PO	Short-term treatment of constipation

- Lactulose (*Chronulac*) is the alternative choice for patients with cardiovascular problems. This saltless osmotic laxative pulls fluid out of the venous system and into the lumen of the small intestine.
- Polycarbophil (*FiberCon*) is a natural substance that forms a gelatin-like bulk out of the intestinal contents. This agent stimulates local activity. It is considered milder and less irritating than many other bulk stimulants. Patients must use caution and take polycarbophil with plenty of water. If only a little water is used, it may absorb enough fluid in the esophagus to swell into a gelatin-like mass that can obstruct the esophagus and cause severe problems.
- Psyllium (*Metamucil*), another gelatin-like bulk stimulant, is similar to polycarbophil in action and effect.
- Polyethylene glycol-electrolyte solution (*GoLYTELY*) is a bulk laxative used when a thorough bowel evacuation is needed. This is often used prior to colonoscopy, sigmoidoscopy, or other diagnostic procedures.

Lubricating Laxatives

Sometimes it is desirable to make defecation easier without stimulating the movement of the GI tract; this is done using lubricants. Patients with hemorrhoids and those who have recently had rectal surgery may need lubrication of the stool. Some patients who could be harmed by straining might also benefit from this type of laxative. The type of laxative recommended depends on the condition of the patient, the speed of relief needed, and the possible implication of various adverse effects. Lubricating laxatives include the following:

- Docusate (*Colace*) has a detergent action on the surface of the intestinal bolus, increasing the admixture of fat and water and making a softer stool. This drug is frequently used as prophylaxis for patients who should not strain (such as after surgery, myocardial infarction, or obstetrical delivery).
- Glycerin (*Sani-Supp*) is a hyperosmolar laxative that is used in suppository form to gently evacuate the rectum without systemic effects higher in the GI tract.
- Mineral oil (*Agoral Plain*) is the oldest of these laxatives. It is not absorbed and forms a slippery coat on the contents of the intestinal tract. When the intestinal bolus is coated with mineral oil, less water is absorbed out of the bolus and the bolus is less likely to become hard or impacted. Frequent use of mineral oil can interfere with absorption of the fat-soluble vitamins A, D, E, and K. In addition, leakage and staining may be a problem when mineral oil is used and the stool cannot be retained by the external sphincter.

Therapeutic Actions and Indications

Laxatives work in three ways:

- by direct chemical stimulation of the GI tract
- by production of bulk or increased fluid in the lumen of the GI tract, leading to stimulation of local nerve receptors
- by lubrication of the intestinal bolus to promote passage through the GI tract (see Figure 58.1).

Laxatives are indicated for the short-term relief of constipation; to prevent straining when it is clinically undesirable (such as after surgery, myocardial infarction, or obstetrical delivery); to evacuate the bowel for diagnostic procedures; to remove ingested poisons from the lower GI tract; and as an adjunct in anthelmintic therapy when it is desirable to flush helminths from the GI tract. Measures, such as proper diet and exercise, and taking advantage of the actions of the intestinal reflexes, have eliminated the need for laxatives in many situations; therefore, these agents are used less frequently than they once were in clinical practice.

Most laxatives are available in OTC preparations, and they are often abused by people who then become dependent on them for stimulation of GI movement. Such individuals may develop chronic intestinal disorders as a result.

Pharmacokinetics

Most of these agents are only minimally absorbed and exert their therapeutic effect directly in the GI tract. Changes in absorption, water balance, and electrolytes resulting from GI changes can have adverse effects on patients with underlying medical conditions that are affected by volume and electrolyte changes. Use with caution during pregnancy and lactation because of the lack of studies regarding the effects of these drugs. Castor oil should not be used during pregnancy because its irritant effect has been associated with induction of premature labor. Magnesium laxatives can cause diarrhea in the neonate.

Contraindications and Cautions

Laxatives are contraindicated in acute abdominal disorders, including appendicitis, diverticulitis, and ulcerative colitis, *when increased motility could lead to rupture or further exacerbation of the inflammation.* Laxatives should be used with great caution during pregnancy and lactation. In some cases, stimulation of the GI tract can precipitate labor, and many of these agents cross the placenta and are excreted in breast milk.

Adverse Effects

The adverse effects most commonly associated with laxatives are GI effects such as diarrhea, abdominal cramping, and nausea. CNS effects, including dizziness, headache, and weakness, are not uncommon and may relate to loss of fluid and electrolyte imbalances that may accompany laxative use. Sweating, palpitations, flushing, and even fainting have been reported after laxative use. These effects may be related to a sympathetic stress reaction to intense neurostimulation of the GI tract or to the loss of fluid and electrolyte imbalance.

A very common adverse effect that is seen with frequent laxative use or laxative abuse is **cathartic dependence**. This reaction occurs when patients use laxatives over a long period and the GI tract becomes dependent on the vigorous stimulation of the laxative. Without this stimulation, the GI tract does not move for a period of time (i.e., several days), which could lead to constipation and drying of the stool and ultimately to impaction.

Clinically Important Drug–Drug Interactions

Because laxatives increase the motility of the GI tract and some interfere with the timing or process of absorption, it is advisable not to take laxatives with other prescribed medications. The administration of laxatives and other medications should be separated by at least 30 minutes.

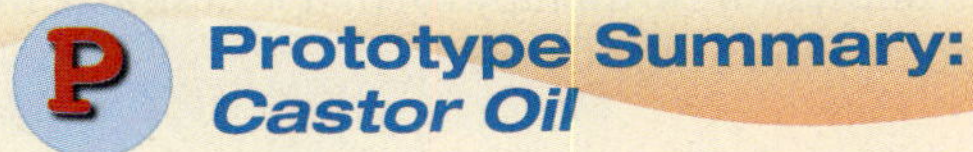

Indications: To evacuate the bowel for diagnostic procedures; to remove ingested poisons from the lower GI tract; an adjunct in anthelmintic therapy when it is desirable to flush helminths from the GI tract

Actions: Directly stimulates the nerve plexus in the intestinal wall, causing increased movement and the stimulation of local reflexes

Pharmacokinetics: Not absorbed systemically

$T_{1/2}$: Not absorbed systemically

Adverse effects: Diarrhea, abdominal cramps, perianal irritation, dizziness, cathartic dependence

Prototype Summary: *Magnesium Citrate*

Indications: Short-term relief of constipation; to prevent straining when it is clinically undesirable; to evacuate the bowel for diagnostic procedures; to remove ingested poisons from the lower GI tract; an adjunct in anthelmintic therapy when it is desirable to flush helminths from the GI tract

Actions: Increases the motility of the GI tract by increasing the fluid in the intestinal contents, which enlarges bulk, stimulates local stretch receptors, and activates local activity

Pharmacokinetics: Not absorbed systemically

$T_{1/2}$: Not absorbed systemically

Adverse effects: Diarrhea, abdominal cramps, bloating, perianal irritation, dizziness

Prototype Summary: *Mineral Oil*

Indications: Short-term relief of constipation; to prevent straining when it is clinically undesirable; to remove ingested poisons from the lower GI tract; an adjunct in anthelmintic therapy when it is desirable to flush helminths from the GI tract

Actions: Forms a slippery coat on the contents of the intestinal tract; less water is absorbed out of the bolus and the bolus is less likely to become hard or impacted

Pharmacokinetics: Not absorbed systemically

$T_{1/2}$: Not absorbed systemically

Adverse effects: Diarrhea; abdominal cramps; bloating; perianal irritation; dizziness; interference with absorption of the fat-soluble vitamins A, D, E, and K; leakage of stool and staining

Nursing Considerations for Patients Receiving Laxatives

Assessment: History and Examination

Screen for the following conditions, *which could be cautions or contraindications to use of the drug:* history of allergy to laxative, fecal impaction, or intestinal obstruction; acute abdominal pain, nausea, or vomiting; and pregnancy or lactation.

Include screening for skin lesions; orientation and affect; baseline pulse rate; abdominal examination, including bowel sounds; and serum electrolyte levels.

Nursing Diagnoses

The patient receiving any laxative may have the following nursing diagnoses related to drug therapy:

- Acute Pain related to CNS and GI effects
- Diarrhea related to drug effects
- Deficient Knowledge regarding drug therapy

Implementation With Rationale

- Administer only as a temporary measure *to prevent development of cathartic dependence.*
- Arrange for appropriate dietary measures, exercise, and environmental controls *to encourage return of normal bowel function.*
- Administer with a full glass of water, and caution the patient not to chew tablets *to ensure that laxative reaches the GI tract to allow for therapeutic effects.* Encourage fluid intake throughout the day as appropriate *to maintain fluid balance and improve GI movement.*
- Do not administer in the presence of acute abdominal pain, nausea, or vomiting, *which might indicate a serious underlying medical problem that could be exacerbated by laxative use.*
- Monitor bowel function *to evaluate drug effectiveness.* If diarrhea or cramping occurs, discontinue the drug *to relieve discomfort and to prevent serious fluid and electrolyte imbalance.*
- Provide comfort and safety measures *to improve patient compliance and to ensure patient safety,*

including ready access to bathroom facilities, assistance with ambulation, and periodic orientation if GI or CNS effects occur.

- Offer support and encouragement *to help patient deal with the discomfort of the condition and drug therapy.*
- Provide thorough patient teaching, including name of drug, dosage prescribed, proper administration, measures to avoid adverse effects, warning signs of problems, and the importance of periodic monitoring and evaluation, *to enhance patient knowledge about drug therapy and promote compliance with the drug regimen.*
- Offer support and encouragement *to help patient deal with the diagnosis and the drug regimen.*

Evaluation

- Monitor patient response to the drug (relief of GI symptoms, absence of straining, evacuation of GI tract).
- Monitor for adverse effects (dizziness, confusion, GI alterations, sweating, electrolyte imbalance, cathartic dependence).
- Evaluate effectiveness of teaching plan (patient can name the drug and dosage as well as describe adverse effects to watch for and specific measures to use to avoid adverse effects).
- Monitor effectiveness of comfort measures and compliance with the regimen

FOCUS POINTS

- Laxative drugs stimulate GI motility and assist excretion.
- Laxatives can be chemical stimulants or lubricants.
- In many cases, implementing diet and exercise strategies and promoting natural intestinal reflexes have decreased the need to use laxatives.
- Chronic use of laxatives can lead to dependence on them and on external stimuli for normal GI function.

Gastrointestinal Stimulants

Some drugs are available for more generalized GI stimulation that results in an overall increase in GI activity and secretions. These drugs stimulate parasympathetic activity or make the GI tissues more sensitive to parasympathetic activity. Such stimulants include the following (Table 58.2):

- Dexpanthenol (*Ilopan*) increases acetylcholine levels and stimulates the parasympathetic system.
- Metoclopramide (*Reglan*) blocks dopamine receptors and makes the GI cells more sensitive to acetylcholine, leading to increased GI activity and rapid movement of food through the upper GI tract.

Therapeutic Actions and Indications

By stimulating parasympathetic activity within the GI tract, these drugs increase GI secretions and motility on a general level throughout the tract (see Figure 58.1). They do not have the local effects of laxatives to increase activity only in the intestines. These drugs are indicated when more rapid movement of GI contents is desirable. Dexpanthenol is indicated in many postoperative situations when intestinal atony or loss of tone could become a problem. Metoclopramide is indicated for relief of symptoms of gastroesophageal reflux disease; for prevention of nausea and vomiting after emetogenic chemotherapy or after surgery; for relief of symptoms of diabetic gastroparesis; and for the promotion of GI movement during small bowel intubation or to promote rapid movement of barium.

Table 58.2 DRUGS IN FOCUS

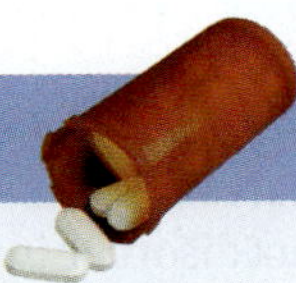

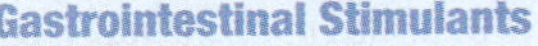
Gastrointestinal Stimulants

Drug Name	Usual Dosage	Usual Indications
dexpanthenol (*Ilopan*)	250–500 mg IM or IV, repeat in 2 h and then q6h as needed	Prevention of intestinal atony in postoperative situations in adults
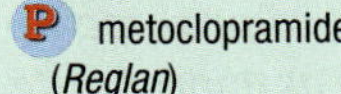 metoclopramide (*Reglan*)	10–20 mg IM, IV, or PO Pediatric: 6–14 yr—2.5–5 mg IV over 1–2 min; <6 yr—0.1 mg/kg IV over 1–2 min	Relief of symptoms of gastroesophageal reflux disease; prevention of nausea and vomiting after emetogenic chemotherapy or postoperatively; relief of symptoms of diabetic gastroparesis; promotion of gastrointestinal movement during small bowel intubation or promotion of rapid movement of barium

Pharmacokinetics

These drugs are rapidly absorbed, metabolized in the liver, and excreted in urine. They cross the placenta and enter breast milk. No adequate studies are available on their effects during pregnancy and lactation, but they should be used only if the benefit to the mother clearly outweighs the potential risk to the fetus or neonate. Metoclopramide is being studied for improvement of lactation in doses of 30 to 45 mg/d. Its effectiveness in improving lactation may be linked to its dopamine-blocking effect, which is often associated with increased prolactin levels.

Contraindications and Cautions

GI stimulants should not be used in patients with a history of allergy to any of these drugs or with any GI obstruction or perforation. They should be used with caution during pregnancy or lactation.

Adverse Effects

The most common adverse effects seen with GI stimulants include nausea, vomiting, diarrhea, intestinal spasm, and cramping. Other adverse effects, such as declining blood pressure and heart rate, weakness, and fatigue, may be related to parasympathetic stimulation.

Clinically Important Drug–Drug Interactions

Metoclopramide has been associated with decreased absorption of digoxin from the GI tract; patients taking this combination should be monitored carefully.

Decreased immunosuppressive effects and increased toxicity of cyclosporine have occurred when these drugs were combined. This combination should be avoided.

Increased sedation can occur if either of these drugs is combined with alcohol or other CNS sedative drugs.

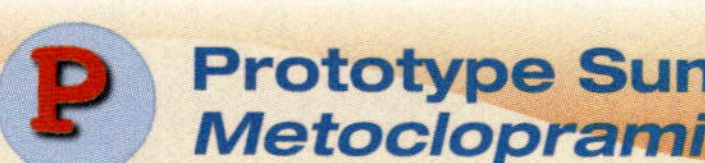

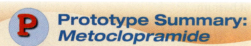

Prototype Summary: Metoclopramide

Indications: Relief of acute and chronic diabetic gastroparesis; short-term treatment of gastroesophageal reflux disorder in adults who cannot tolerate standard therapy; prevention of postoperative nausea and vomiting; facilitation of small bowel intubation; stimulation of gastric emptying; intestinal transit of barium

Actions: Stimulates movement of the upper GI tract without stimulating gastric, pancreatic, or biliary secretions; appears to sensitize tissues to the effects of acetylcholine

Pharmacokinetics:

Route	Onset	Peak	Duration
Oral	30–60 min	60–90 min	1–2 h
IM	10–15 min	60–90 min	1–2 h
IV	1–5 min	60–90 min	1–2 h

$T_{1/2}$: 5–6 hours; metabolized in the liver and excreted in urine

Adverse effects: Restlessness, drowsiness, fatigue, extrapyramidal effects, Parkinson-like reactions, nausea, diarrhea

Nursing Considerations for Patients Receiving Gastrointestinal Stimulants

Assessment: History and Examination

Screen for the following conditions, *which could be cautions or contraindications to the use of the drug:* any history of allergy to these drugs; intestinal obstruction, bleeding, or perforation; and pregnancy or lactation.

Include screening *to establish baseline data for assessing the effectiveness of the drug and the occurrence of any adverse effects associated with drug therapy.* Perform an abdominal evaluation, checking bowel sounds *to ensure GI motility;* assess pulse and blood pressure *to monitor for adverse effects;* and check skin color and lesions *to assess for hypersensitivity reactions.*

Nursing Diagnoses

The patient receiving GI stimulants may have the following nursing diagnoses related to drug therapy:

- Diarrhea related to drug effects
- Acute Pain related to GI effects
- Deficient Knowledge regarding drug therapy

Implementation With Rationale

- Administer at least 15 minutes before each meal and at bedtime *to ensure therapeutic effectiveness.*
- Monitor blood pressure carefully if giving drug intravenously *to detect and consult with the prescriber about treatment for sudden drops in blood pressure.*
- Monitor diabetic patients *in order to arrange for alteration in insulin dose or timing as appropriate.*
- Provide thorough patient teaching, including name of drug, dosage prescribed, proper administration,

measures to avoid adverse effects, warning signs of problems, and the importance of periodic monitoring and evaluation, *to enhance patient knowledge about drug therapy and promote compliance with the drug regimen.*

- Offer support and encouragement *to help the patient deal with the diagnosis and the drug regimen.*

Evaluation

- Monitor patient response to the drug (increased tone and movement of GI tract).
- Monitor for adverse effects (GI effects, parasympathetic activity).
- Evaluate effectiveness of the teaching plan (patient can name the drug and dosage, as well as describe adverse effects to watch for and specific measures to take to avoid adverse effects and increase the effectiveness of the drug).
- Monitor the effectiveness of comfort measures and compliance with the regimen.

Antidiarrheal Drugs

Antidiarrheal drugs that block stimulation of the GI tract are used for symptomatic relief from diarrhea. Available agents include the following (Table 58.3):

- Bismuth subsalicylate (*Pepto-Bismol*) acts locally to coat the lining of the GI tract and soothe any irritation that might be stimulating local reflexes to cause excessive GI activity and diarrhea. This agent has been found to be very helpful in treating traveler's diarrhea (see Critical Thinking Scenario 58-1) and in preventing cramping and distention associated with dietary excess and some viral infections. Bismuth subsalicylate is absorbed from the GI tract, metabolized in the liver, and excreted in urine. It crosses the placenta and should be used in pregnancy only if the benefit to the mother outweighs any potential risk to the fetus. It is not known whether it enters breast milk.
- Loperamide (*Imodium*) has a direct effect on the muscle layers of the GI tract to slow peristalsis and allow increased

BOX 58.3 New Drug for Traveler's Diarrhea

In 2004, rifaximin (*Xifaxan*) was approved by the FDA specifically for treating traveler's diarrhea. A new antibiotic, rifaximin acts locally in the GI tract against noninvasive strains of *Escherichia coli*, the most common cause of traveler's diarrhea. About 80%–90% of the drug is delivered to the intestines without being absorbed through the GI tract.

Rifaximin acts locally in the GI tract to destroy the *E. coli* that causes the signs and symptoms associated with traveler's diarrhea. The drug is taken in 200-mg tablets, three times a day for 3 days once the signs and symptoms of the disorder occur. It should not be used if the patient has bloody diarrhea or if diarrhea persists more than 48 hours or worsens during treatment with the drug. Destroying the causative agent will relieve the GI symptoms of diarrhea, nausea, and anorexia. Prevention remains the best intervention for traveler's diarrhea.

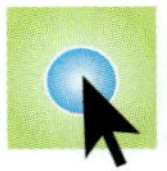

WEB LINKS

Health care providers and patients may want to consult the following Internet sources:

http://www.cdc.gov/travel Information for the traveler about causes, treatments, and prevention of traveler's diarrhea (see also Box 58.3).

http://www.nlm.nih.gov/medlineplus/constipation.html Information on constipation—causes, diagnosis, research, treatment, and prevention across the lifespan.

http://digestive.niddk.nih.gov/diseases/pubs/diarrhea Information on diarrhea—guidelines for prevention and treatment.

Table 58.3 DRUGS IN FOCUS

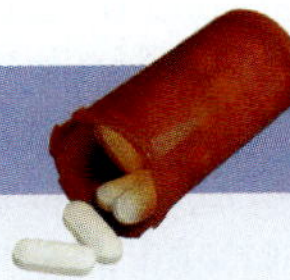

Antidiarrheals

Drug Name	Usual Dosage	Usual Indications
bismuth subsalicylate (*Pepto-Bismol*)	Adult: 524 mg PO q30–60min as needed, up to eight doses per day Pediatric: <3 yr—not recommended; 3–6 yr—⅓ tablet or 5 mL PO; 6–9 yr—⅔ tablet or 10 mL PO; 9–12 yr—one tablet or 15 mL PO	Treatment of traveler's diarrhea; prevention of cramping and distention associated with dietary excess and some viral infections
P loperamide (*Imodium*)	Adult: 4 mg PO, then 2 mg PO after each loose stool Pediatric (2–12 yr—1–2 mg PO t.i.d.; <2 yr—not recommended	Short-term treatment of diarrhea associated with dietary problems, viral infections
opium derivatives (paregoric)	Adult: 5–10 mL PO once to four times daily Pediatric: 0.25–0.5 mL/kg PO once to four times daily as needed	Short-term treatment of cramping and diarrhea

CRITICAL THINKING SCENARIO 58-1

Traveler's Diarrhea

The Situation

P.F. received an all-expenses-paid trip to Mexico to celebrate his graduation from college. He was very excited about getting away for a week of sun and fun and arranged to stay in the same hotel as two college friends who were also celebrating. The three men had a wonderful time visiting the beaches, bars, and nightclubs in the area. On the third day of the trip, P.F. began experiencing nausea, some vomiting, and a low-grade fever. Several hours later he began experiencing intense cramping and diarrhea. For the next 2 days, P.F. felt so ill he was unable to leave his hotel room. The next morning, he arranged for an emergency trip home.

Critical Thinking

What is probably happening to P.F.? *Think about the gastrointestinal reflexes and explain the underlying cause for his signs and symptoms.*

What treatment should be started now?

What could have been done to prevent this problem from occurring?

What possible drug therapy might have been helpful for P.F.?

Discussion

P.F. is probably experiencing the common disorder called traveler's diarrhea. This disorder occurs when pathogens found in the food and water of a foreign environment are ingested. (Because these pathogens are commonly found in the environment, they do not normally cause problems for the people who live in the area.) When the pathogen, usually a strain of *Escherichia coli,* enters a host that is not accustomed to the bacteria, it releases enterotoxins and sets off an intestinal–intestinal reaction in the host.

The intestinal–intestinal reaction results in a reduction of activity above the point of irritation (which causes nausea and in some cases vomiting) and an increase in activity below the point of irritation. The body is trying to flush the invader from the body. A low-grade fever may occur as a reaction to the toxins released by the bacteria. Muscle aches and pains, malaise, and fatigue are often common symptoms. It is important at this stage of the disease to maintain fluid intake to prevent dehydration from occurring.

P.F. may want to return home, but with intense cramping and diarrhea it might not be a good idea. Bismuth subsalicylate (*Pepto-Bismol*), taken four times a day, has been effective in preventing traveler's diarrhea and associated problems. Taken during a course of traveler's diarrhea, it may relieve the stomach upset and nausea and some of the discomfort of the diarrhea. Some patients respond to the prophylactic antibiotics *Bactrim* and *Septra,* combinations of trimethoprim and sulfamethoxazole (TMP-SMZ) that are often prescribed as prophylactic measures for patients who are traveling to areas known to be associated with traveler's diarrhea and for those who are known to be very susceptible to the disorder. Once traveler's diarrhea is diagnosed, rifaximin (*Xifaxan*) can be taken. The 200-mg tablets are taken three times a day. It should not be used if the patient has bloody diarrhea or diarrhea that worsens or persists for more than 48 hours.

The best course of action, however, is prevention. Several measures can be taken to avoid ingestion of the local bacteria: drinking only bottled or mineral water; avoiding fresh fruits and vegetables that may have been washed in the local water, unless they are peeled; avoiding ice cubes in drinks because the ice cubes are made from the local water; avoiding any food that might be undercooked or rare, including shellfish; and even being cautious about using water to brush the teeth or gargle. People who have suffered a bout of traveler's diarrhea are very cautious about exposure to local bacteria when they travel again, often combining prophylactic drug therapy with careful avoidance of local pathogens. P.F. can be reassured that in a few days the diarrhea and associated signs and symptoms should pass and he will regain his strength and energy.

Nursing Care Guide for P.F.: Antidiarrheals

Assessment: History And Examination

Assess the patient's health history for allergies to any of these drugs, acute abdominal pain, concurrent use of aspirin products, methotrexate, valproic acid, corticosteroids, oral tetracyclines, oral antidiabetic agents, or sulfinpyrazone.

Focus the physical examination on the following:

Neurological: orientation, reflexes

Traveler's Diarrhea *(continued)*

GI: abdominal evaluation, bowel sounds
Respiratory: respiratory rate and depth
Laboratory tests: serum electrolyte levels
Other: temperature

Nursing Diagnoses

Acute Pain related to GI, CNS effects
Diarrhea related to GI effects
Deficient Knowledge regarding drug therapy

Implementation

Administer antidiarrheal agent only as a temporary measure.

Provide comfort and safety measures, including assistance, access to bathroom, safety precautions if necessary.

Monitor bowel function.

Provide support and reassurance for coping with drug effects and discomfort.

Provide patient teaching regarding drug name and dosage, adverse effects and precautions, warning signs of serious adverse effects to report.

Evaluation

Evaluate drug effects: relief of GI symptoms.

Monitor for adverse effects: GI alterations, dizziness, confusion, salicylate toxicity.

Monitor for drug–drug interactions as indicated.

Evaluate effectiveness of patient teaching program and comfort and safety measures.

Patient Teaching For P.F.

☐ The drug prescribed for you is called bismuth subsalicylate (*Pepto-Bismol*). This drug is called an antidiarrheal agent. It forms a protective coating over the inner lining of the intestine and soothes the irritated areas.

☐ Take this drug exactly as indicated. Shake the bottle well before using the liquid preparation. If you are using tablets, make sure that you chew them thoroughly; do not swallow them whole.

☐ Common effects of this drug include:

- *Darkening of the stools:* Do not become concerned; this is a normal effect that will go away when you stop taking the drug.
- *Ringing in the ears, rapid respirations:* This is more likely to occur if you are taking other products that contain aspirin, which is also a salicylate.
- Report any of the following conditions to your health care provider: *diarrhea that does not stop within 2 days, ringing in the ears, rapid respirations, fever and/or intense abdominal pain.*

☐ Stay away from any food or beverage that may be contaminated with bacteria. Use bottled water for drinking, as well as for brushing your teeth. Do not wash fruit or vegetables with water from the local supply.

☐ Do not use any other medication that contains aspirin; inadvertent overdose may occur.

☐ Tell any doctor, nurse, or other health care provider involved in your care that you are taking this drug.

☐ Keep this drug and all medications out of the reach of children.

time for absorption of fluid and electrolytes. Loperamide is slowly absorbed, metabolized in the liver, and excreted in urine and feces. It may cross the placenta and enter breast milk. It should be used in pregnancy or lactation only if the benefits clearly outweigh any potential risks to the fetus or neonate.

- Opium derivatives (paregoric) block nerve impulses within the GI tract, stopping peristalsis and diarrhea and associated discomfort. A category C-III controlled substance, opium is readily absorbed, metabolized in the liver, and excreted in urine. It crosses the placenta and enters breast milk and can have adverse effects on the fetus or neonate.

Box 58.4 describes combination antidiarrheal products. See Box 58.5 for a discussion of irritable bowel syndrome and its treatment.

Therapeutic Actions and Indications

Antidiarrheal agents slow the motility of the GI tract through direct action on the lining of the GI tract to inhibit local reflexes (bismuth subsalicylate), through direct action on the muscles of the GI tract to slow activity (loperamide), or through action on CNS centers that cause GI spasm and slowing (opium derivatives). These drugs are indicated for the

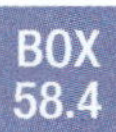

BOX 58.4 Combination Antidiarrheal Products

Two very popular antidiarrheal agents combine atropine with a meperidine-like compound. Meperidine (*Demerol*) has a local effect on the gastrointestinal wall, causing a slowing of intestinal motility. Difenoxin and diphenoxylate are chemically related to meperidine and are used at doses that decrease gastrointestinal activity without having analgesic or respiratory effects. These drugs, which are controlled substances—difenoxin is category C-IV and diphenoxylate is category C-V—are combined with atropine to discourage deliberate use of excessive doses to get the euphoric effects associated with meperidine.

difenoxin with atropine (*Motofen*)	Adult: two tablets PO, then one tablet after each loose stool. Do not exceed eight tablets in 24 h Pediatric: not for use in children <12 yr
diphenoxylate with atropine (*Lomotil, Logen, Lomanate*)	Adult: 5 mg PO q.i.d. Pediatric (2–12 yr): use liquid form only, start with 0.3–0.4 mg/kg/day PO in four divided doses

relief of symptoms of acute and chronic diarrhea, reduction of volume of discharge from ileostomies, and prevention and treatment of traveler's diarrhea (see Figure 58.1).

Pharmacokinetics

In general, the pharmacokinetics of antidiarrheal agents vary depending on the agent (see the descriptions above).

Contraindications and Cautions

Antidiarrheal drugs should not be given to anyone with known allergy to the drug or any of its components. Caution should be used in pregnancy and lactation. Care should also be taken in individuals with any history of GI obstruction, acute abdominal conditions, or diarrhea due to poisonings.

Adverse Effects

The adverse effects associated with antidiarrheal drugs, such as constipation, distention, abdominal discomfort, nausea, vomiting, dry mouth, and even toxic megacolon, are related to their effects on the GI tract. Other adverse effects that have been reported include fatigue, weakness, dizziness, and skin rash.

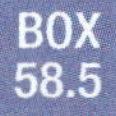

BOX 58.5 Irritable Bowel Syndrome

Irritable bowel syndrome (IBS) is a very common disorder, striking three times as many women as men, and reportedly accounting for half of all referrals to gastrointestinal (GI) specialists. The disorder is characterized by abdominal distress, bouts of diarrhea or constipation, bloating, nausea, flatulence, headache, fatigue, depression, and anxiety. No anatomical cause has been found for this disorder. Underlying causes might be stress related. Patients with this disorder have often suffered for years, not enjoying meals or activities because of their GI pain and discomfort.

Alosetron Returns

Alosetron (*Lotronex*) was the first drug to provide relief to this patient population. This drug, a serotonin 5-HT antagonist, blocks specific serotonin receptors in the enteric nervous system of the GI tract, which leads to decreased perception of abdominal pain and discomfort, decreased GI motility, and increased colon transit time. In late 2000, alosetron was pulled from the market after less than a year of availability. Reports of ischemic colitis, mesenteric colitis, and even death in patients who were using the drug led to this decision. In July 2002, after hearing lots of testimony and reading many petitions from patients, the FDA agreed to approve the release of the drug for marketing. This is the first time in the history of the FDA that a drug pulled from the market because of safety concerns has been re-released. Restrictions have been applied to the use of the drug, and patients who use it must read and sign a Patient–Physician Agreement. The use of *Lotronex* should be discontinued immediately if the patient develops constipation or symptoms of ischemic colitis. It is approved for women with IBS with diarrhea being the predominant complaint.

Tegaserod

Tegaserod (*Zelnorm*), a 5-HT$_4$ modulator, was then approved for the treatment of women with IBS; this slightly different serotonin receptor site is thought to help regulate the normal intestinal reflexes while relieving abdominal pain and discomfort. It is also approved for the treatment of chronic idiopathic constipation for patients older than 65 years of age.

Hyoscyamine

Hyoscyamine (*Anaspaz*), an anticholinergic agent that was found to decrease GI spasm, was approved in 2001 as an adjunctive therapy for the treatment of IBS.

Support and symptomatic relief remain the mainstays of treating this disorder. Stress management and a consistent relationship with a health care provider may help to relieve some of the problems associated with this common, although not entirely understood, disorder.

Drug–Drug Interactions

Drug interactions vary depending on the antidiarrheal agent. Consult individual drug package insert for specific interactions.

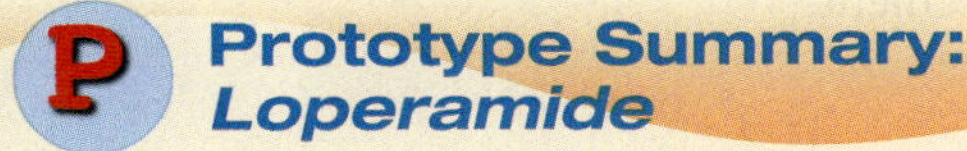

Prototype Summary: Loperamide

Indications: Control and symptomatic relief of acute, nonspecific diarrhea and chronic diarrhea associated with irritable bowel syndrome; reduction of volume of discharge from ileostomies

Actions: Inhibits intestinal peristalsis through direct effects on the longitudinal and circular muscles of the intestinal wall, slowing motility and movement of water and electrolytes

Pharmacokinetics:

Route	Onset	Peak
Oral (capsule)	Varies	5 h

$T_{1/2}$: 10.8 hours; metabolized in the liver and excreted in urine and feces

Adverse effects: Abdominal pain, distention, or discomfort; dry mouth; nausea; constipation; dizziness; tiredness; drowsiness

Nursing Considerations for Patients Receiving Antidiarrheals

Assessment: History and Examination

Screen for the following conditions, *which could be cautions or contraindications to the use of the drug:* any history of allergy to these drugs; acute abdominal conditions; poisoning; and pregnancy or lactation.

Include screening *to establish baseline data for assessing the effectiveness of the drug and the occurrence of any adverse effects associated with drug therapy.* Assess skin color and lesions; abdominal examination; and orientation and affect.

Nursing Diagnoses

The patient receiving antidiarrheal drugs may have the following nursing diagnoses related to drug therapy:

- Constipation related to GI slowing
- Acute Pain related to GI effects
- Disturbed Sensory Perception (Kinesthetic, Gustatory) related to CNS effects
- Deficient Knowledge regarding drug therapy

Implementation With Rationale

- Monitor response carefully. If no response is seen within 48 hours, *the diarrhea could be related to an underlying medical condition.* Arrange to discontinue the drug and arrange for medical evaluation *to allow for diagnosis of underlying medical conditions.*
- Provide appropriate safety and comfort measures if CNS effects occur *to prevent patient injury.*
- Administer drug after each unformed stool *to ensure therapeutic effectiveness.* Keep track of exact amount given *to ensure that dosage does not exceed recommended daily maximum dose.*
- Provide thorough patient teaching, including name of drug, dosage prescribed, proper administration, measures to avoid adverse effects, warning signs of problems, and the importance of periodic monitoring and evaluation *to enhance patient knowledge about drug therapy and promote compliance with the drug regimen.*
- Offer support and encouragement *to help the patient deal with the diagnosis and the drug regimen.*

Evaluation

- Monitor patient response to the drug (relief of diarrhea).
- Monitor for adverse effects (GI effects, CNS changes, dermatologic effects).
- Evaluate effectiveness of teaching plan (patient can name the drug and dosage, as well as describe adverse effects to watch for, specific measures to use to avoid adverse effects, and measures to take to increase the effectiveness of the drug).
- Monitor effectiveness of comfort and safety measures and compliance with the regimen.

Points to Remember

- Laxatives are drugs used to stimulate movement along the GI tract and to aid excretion. They may be used to prevent or treat constipation.
- Laxatives can be chemical stimulants, which directly irritate the local nerve plexus; bulk stimulants, which increase the size of the food bolus and stimulate stretch receptors in the wall of the intestine; or lubricants,

which facilitate movement of the bolus through the intestines.

- Use of proper diet and exercise, as well as taking advantage of the actions of the intestinal reflexes, has eliminated the need for laxatives in many situations.
- Cathartic dependence can occur with the chronic use of laxatives, leading to a need for external stimuli for normal functioning of the GI tract.
- GI stimulants act to increase parasympathetic stimulation in the GI tract and to increase tone and general movement throughout the GI system.
- Antidiarrheal drugs are used to soothe irritation to the intestinal wall; block GI muscle activity to decrease movement; or affect CNS activity to cause GI spasm and stop movement.

CHECK YOUR UNDERSTANDING

Answers to the questions in this chapter may be found in the Answer Key in the back of the book.

Multiple Choice

Select the best response to the following.

1. Laxatives are drugs that are used to
   a. increase the quantity of wastes excreted.
   b. speed the passage of the intestinal contents through the GI tract.
   c. increase digestion of intestinal contents.
   d. increase the water content of the intestinal contents.

2. A laxative of choice when mild stimulation is needed to prevent straining would be
   a. senna.
   b. castor oil.
   c. bisacodyl.
   d. magnesium citrate.

3. Cathartic dependence can occur when
   a. patients do not use laxatives and become very constipated.
   b. chronic use of laxatives leads to a reliance on the intense stimulation of laxatives to cause movement.
   c. patients maintain a good diet including roughage.
   d. patients start an exercise program.

4. Drugs that stimulate parasympathetic activity are used to increase GI activity and secretions. This could be therapeutic in the treatment of
   a. duodenal ulcers.
   b. gastric ulcers.
   c. signs and symptoms of gastroesophageal reflux disease.
   d. poisoning, to induce nausea and vomiting.

5. The drug of choice for treating traveler's diarrhea would be
   a. loperamide.
   b. opium.
   c. bisacodyl.
   d. bismuth subsalicylate.

Multiple Response

Select all that apply.

1. A nurse is preparing a teaching plan for a client who has been prescribed a laxative. The teaching plan should include which of the following?
   a. The importance of proper diet and fluid intake
   b. The need to take the drug for several weeks to get the full effect
   c. The importance of exercise
   d. The need to take advantage of natural reflexes by providing privacy and time to allow them to work
   e. The need to limit fluids
   f. The importance of limiting the duration of laxative use

2. A nurse might expect an order for mineral oil for which of the following patients?
   a. A debilitated patient low on nutrients
   b. A patient with hemorrhoids
   c. A patient with recent rectal surgery
   d. A child with encopresis
   e. A postpartum woman
   f. A patient with Crohn's disease

3. When explaining the actions of laxatives to a client, the nurse would state that they can work by
   a. acting as chemical stimulants.
   b. acting as lubricants of the intestinal bolus.
   c. acting to increase bulk of the intestinal bolus and stimulate movement.
   d. stimulating CNS centers in the medulla to cause GI movement.
   e. blocking the parasympathetic nervous system.
   f. causing central nervous system depression.

Word Scramble

Unscramble the following letters to form the names of frequently used laxatives or antidiarrheal agents.

1. saccara ________________
2. epromledia ________________
3. sadlycoib ________________
4. slyumipl ________________
5. annse ________________
6. romimcatpelode ________________
7. umoip ________________
8. ocatsude ________________

True or False

Indicate whether the following statements are true (T) or false (F).

_____ 1. Laxatives are used to stop movement along the GI tract.

_____ 2. Laxatives are used to prevent or treat constipation.

_____ 3. Chemical stimulants directly irritate the local nerve plexus of the GI tract.

_____ 4. Bulk stimulants decrease the size of the food bolus and stimulate stretch receptors in the intestinal wall.

_____ 5. For many patients, eating a proper diet, exercising, and taking advantage of the actions of the intestinal reflexes has eliminated the need for laxatives.

_____ 6. Cathartic dependence can occur with the occasional use of laxatives, leading to a need for external stimuli for normal functioning of the GI tract.

_____ 7. GI stimulants act to increase sympathetic stimulation in the GI tract.

_____ 8. Antidiarrheal drugs are used to soothe irritation to the intestinal wall, block GI muscle activity to decrease movement, or affect central nervous system activity to cause GI spasm and stop movement.

Bibliography and References

Drug facts and comparisons. (2006). St. Louis: Facts and Comparisons.

Gilman, A., Hardman, J. G., & Limbird, L. E. (Eds.). (2006). *Goodman and Gilman's the pharmacological basis of therapeutics* (11th ed.). New York: McGraw-Hill.

Karch, A. M. (2006). *2007 Lippincott's nursing drug guide.* Philadelphia: Lippincott Williams & Wilkins.

The medical letter on drugs and therapeutics. (2006). New Rochelle, NY: Medical Letter.

Porth, C. M. (2005). *Pathophysiology: Concepts of altered health states* (7th ed.). Philadelphia: Lippincott Williams & Wilkins.

CHAPTER 59

Emetic and Antiemetic Agents

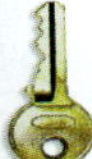

KEY TERMS

antiemetic

emetic

intractable hiccough

phenothiazine

photosensitivity

vestibular

LEARNING OBJECTIVES

Upon completion of this chapter, you will be able to:

1. Outline the vomiting reflex, including factors that stimulate it and how measures used to block it work.
2. Describe the therapeutic actions, indications, pharmacokinetics, contraindications, most common adverse reactions, and important drug–drug interactions associated with phenothiazine and nonphenothiazine antiemetics, anticholinergic/antihistamine antiemetics, 5-HT_3 receptor blockers, substance P/neurokinin 1 receptor antagonists, and miscellaneous antiemetics agents.
3. Discuss the use of antiemetics across the lifespan.
4. Compare and contrast the prototype drugs prochlorperazine, metoclopramide, meclizine, ondansetron, and aprepitant with other agents in their class and with other classes of antiemetics.
5. Outline the nursing considerations, including important teaching points, for patients receiving antiemetics.

ANTIEMETIC AGENTS

Phenothiazines

chlorpromazine

perphenazine

P prochlorperazine

promethazine

thiethylperazine

Nonphenothiazine

P metoclopramide

Anticholinergics/Antihistamines

buclizine

cyclizine

P meclizine

5-HT_3 Receptor Blockers

dolasetron

granisetron

P ondansetron

palonosetron

Substance P/Neurokinin 1 Receptor Antagonist

P aprepitant

Miscellaneous

dronabinol

hydroxyzine

trimethobenzamide

One of the most common and most uncomfortable complaints encountered in clinical practice is that of nausea and vomiting. Vomiting is a complex reflex reaction to various stimuli (see Chapter 56). In some cases of overdose or poisoning, it may be desirable to induce vomiting to rapidly rid the body of a toxin. This can be accomplished by physical stimuli, often to the back of the throat. In some cases, gastric lavage is used to wash out the contents of the stomach. **Emetics**, which cause vomiting, no longer are recommended for at-home poison control (Box 59.1).

In many clinical conditions, the reflex reaction of vomiting is not beneficial in ridding the body of any toxins but is uncomfortable and even clinically hazardous to the patient's condition. In such cases, an **antiemetic** is used to decrease or prevent nausea and vomiting. Antiemetic agents can be centrally acting or locally acting, and they have varying degrees of effectiveness. These drugs are used with all age groups (Box 59.2).

Antiemetic Agents

Drugs used in managing nausea and vomiting are called antiemetics. All of them work by reducing the hyperactivity of the vomiting reflex in one of two ways: locally, to decrease the local response to stimuli that are being sent to the medulla to induce vomiting, or centrally, to directly block the chemoreceptor trigger zone (CTZ) or suppress the vomiting center. The locally acting antiemetics may be antacids, local anesthetics, adsorbents, protective drugs that coat the GI mucosa, or drugs that prevent distention and stretch stimulation of the GI tract. These agents are often reserved for use in mild nausea. Many of these drugs are discussed in Chapter 58.

Centrally acting antiemetics can be classified in several groups: phenothiazines, nonphenothiazines, serotonin (5-HT_3) receptor blockers, substance P/neurokinin 1 receptor antagonist, anticholinergics/antihistamines, and a miscellaneous group (see Tables 59.1 and 59.2).

Phenothiazines

The two most commonly used **phenothiazines** are prochlorperazine (*Compazine*) (see Critical Thinking Scenario 59.1) and promethazine (*Phenergan*), both of which have rapid onset and limited adverse effects. Other drugs in this group include chlorpromazine (*Thorazine*), perphenazine (*Trilafon*), and thiethylperazine (*Torecan*). Chapter 22 discusses the phenothiazines in greater detail.

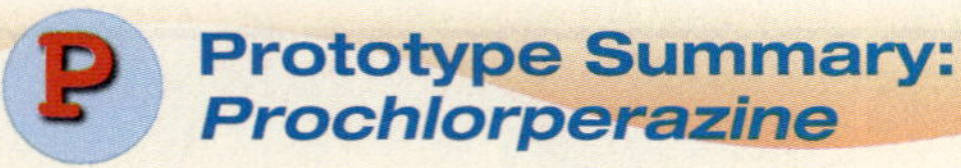

Prototype Summary: Prochlorperazine

Indications: Control of severe nausea and vomiting

Actions: Mechanism of action not understood; depresses various areas of the CNS

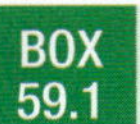

BOX 59.1 FOCUS ON THE EVIDENCE

Ipecac Syrup No Longer Recommended

In the summer of 2003, the U.S. Food and Drug Administration released the results of efficacy and toxicity studies done with the emetic drug syrup of ipecac and ruled that the drug was not effective for its intended use.

In November 2003, the American Academy of Pediatrics (AAP) revised its long-standing recommendation that parents be advised to keep and use ipecac for ingestion of toxic substances. Study findings showed that ipecac did not fully empty the stomach, that inducing vomiting in many cases was more toxic than what was ingested, and that the poison that was ingested needed to be carefully evaluated before the proper treatment was recommended.

History

Until November 2003, syrup of ipecac was the standard emetic agent in use in the United States. It was purchased in prepackaged 1-ounce containers without a prescription to have on hand in case of emergency. Parents were encouraged to keep one of these prepackaged doses at home, just in case it was needed. Ipecac syrup was thought to irritate the GI mucosa locally, which stimulated the chemoreceptor trigger zone (CTZ) in the brain to induce vomiting within 20 minutes. Parents were cautioned not to use ipecac syrup in the following situations: when caustic alkali or corrosive mineral acids were ingested because the potential for serious damage to the upper GI tract and airways overrode any benefit; when a volatile petroleum distillate such as kerosene was swallowed because the risk of aspiration into the lungs, with a resultant fulminant and untreatable pneumonia, was serious; when a patient was comatose or semicomatose or showed signs of convulsing, again because the risk of aspiration was too great; or when a rapid-acting and specific antidote to the poison was available and that treatment would be the most appropriate.

New Guidelines

The new guidelines set forth by the AAP for anticipatory counseling for prenatal and well-infant visits include:

- Keep potential poisons out of sight and out of reach.
- Always return any child-proof caps to the locked position after they are used.
- Never transfer a substance to a different container; it is important to have the information on the original container in case of emergency.
- Safely dispose of all unused or no-longer-needed medication.
- Never refer to medications as candy or a treat.
- Post the telephone number of the poison control center near the phone. If a local poison control center is not available, post 1-800-222-1222.

The AAP recommends that parents be advised to dispose of any ipecac that they may have at home. The organization stresses the importance of prevention and calling an authority if accidental ingestion occurs. Additional information on the AAP policy and position, ipecac study and results, and teaching guidelines and brochures are available at http://aappolicy.org.

BOX 59.2 DRUG THERAPY ACROSS THE LIFESPAN

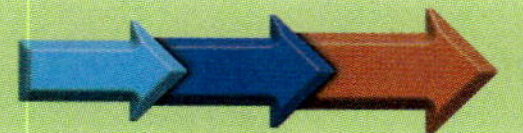

Antiemetic Agents

CHILDREN

Parents should be taught to call their health care provider or a local poison control center if their children ingest potentially toxic substances. The professionals will advise them of the best treatment in each individual case.

Antiemetics should be used with caution in children who are at higher risk for adverse effects, including central nervous system (CNS) effects, as well as fluid and electrolyte disturbances.

Prochlorphenazine is often a drug of choice with children, and it has established oral, rectal, and parenteral doses. Promethazine often has fewer adverse effects, but it should not be used with children who have liver impairment, Reye's syndrome, or sleep apnea. The serotonin 5-HT_3 agents have been very successfully used in children younger than 2 years of age. Care should be used when determining dosage and timing of dosage. Dronabinol does not have established guidelines for children, but if it is used, the child should be constantly supervised, and dosage should be calculated very carefully based on age and weight.

ADULTS

Antiemetics are often used after surgery or chemotherapy, and precautions should be used to ensure that CNS effects do not interfere with mobility or other activities.

The safety of these drugs during pregnancy and lactation has not been established. Use should be reserved for those situations in which the benefit to the mother outweighs the potential risk to the fetus. The drugs may enter breast milk and also may cause fluid imbalance that could interfere with milk production. It is advised that caution be used if one of these drugs is prescribed during lactation.

OLDER ADULTS

Older adults are more likely to develop adverse effects associated with the use of these drugs including sedation, confusion, dizziness, fluid imbalance, and cardiovascular effects. Safety measures may be needed if these effects occur and interfere with the patient's mobility and balance.

Older adults are also more likely to have renal and/or hepatic impairment related to underlying medical conditions, which could interfere with the metabolism and excretion of these drugs. The dosage for older adults should be started at a lower level than recommended for young adults. The patient should be monitored very closely, and dosage adjustment should be made based on patient response.

If dronabinol is used with older patients, special safety precautions should be in place, because the older patient is more likely to experience CNS effects and related problems when using this drug.

Pharmacokinetics:

Route	Onset	Peak	Duration
Oral	30–40 min	Unknown	3–4 h
PR	60–90 min	Unknown	3–4 h
IM	10–20 min	10–30 min	3–4 h
IV	Immediate	10–30 min	3–4 h

$T_{1/2}$: Unknown; metabolized in the liver and excreted in urine

Adverse effects: Drowsiness, dystonia, photophobia, blurred vision, urine discolored pink to red-brown

Nonphenothiazine

The only nonphenothiazine currently available for use as an antiemetic is metoclopramide (*Reglan*), which acts to reduce the responsiveness of the nerve cells in the CTZ to circulating chemicals that induce vomiting. Chapter 58 discusses metoclopramide, which is commonly used to treat gastroparesis, in greater detail.

Anticholinergics/Antihistamines

The anticholinergics/antihistamines used to prevent or treat nausea and vomiting include buclizine (*Bucladin*), cyclizine (*Marezine*), and meclizine (*Antivert*). These drugs are anticholinergics that act as antihistamines and block the trans-

Table 59.1 Focus on Antiemetic Agents

Type	Names
Phenothiazines	chlorpromazine, perphenazine, prochlorperazine, promethazine, thiethylperazine
Nonphenothiazine	metoclopropamide
Anticholinergics/Antihistamines	buclizine, cyclizine, meclizine, antihistamines
5-HT_3 receptor blockers	dolasetron, granisetron, ondansetron, palonosetron
Substance P/neurokinin 1 receptor inhibitor	aprepitant
Miscellaneous	dronabinol, hydroxyzine, trimethobenzamide

Table 59.2 DRUGS IN FOCUS

Antiemetic Agents

Drug Name	Usual Dosage	Usual Indications
Phenothiazines		
chlorpromazine (*Thorazine*)	Adult: 10–25 mg PO q4–6h *or* 50–100 mg PR or 25 mg IM Pediatric: 0.5 mg/kg PO q4–6h; 1.1 mg/kg PR q6–8h or 0.5 mg/kg IM q6–8h	Treatment of nausea and vomiting, including that specifically associated with anesthesia; severe vomiting; intractable hiccoughs
perphenazine (*Trilafon*)	8–16 mg/day PO in divided doses; 5–10 mg IM for rapid control; 5 mg IV in divided doses, slowly	Treatment of severe nausea and vomiting; intractable hiccoughs in patients >12 yr
P prochlorperazine (*Compazine*)	Adult: 5–10 mg PO t.i.d. to q.i.d.; 25 mg PR b.i.d.; 5–10 mg IM q3–4h, up to 40 mg/day; 5–10 mg IM 1–2 h before anesthesia or during or after anesthesia, may repeat in 30 min Pediatric: 9.1–13.2 kg—2.5 mg PO or PR daily to b.i.d., do not exceed 7.5 mg/day; 13.6–17.7 kg—2.5 mg PO or PR b.i.d. to t.i.d., do not exceed 10 mg/day; 18.2–38.6 kg—2.5 mg PO or PR t.i.d. to 5 mg b.i.d., do not exceed 15 mg/day, *or* 0.132 mg/kg IM as a single dose	Treatment of severe nausea and vomiting, including that specifically associated with anesthesia
promethazine (*Phenergan*)	Adult: 25 mg PO or PR, repeat doses of 12.5–25 mg q4–6h as needed; 12.5–25 mg IM or IV q4–6h Pediatric: 1 mg/kg PO q4–6h as needed	Prevention and control of nausea and vomiting associated with anesthesia and surgery
thiethylperazine (*Torecan*)	10–30 mg/day PO in divided doses; 2 mL IM, one to three times per day	Relief of nausea and vomiting in adults
Nonphenothiazine		
P metoclopramide (*Reglan*)	10–20 mg IM at the end of surgery; 2 mg/kg IV over not less than 15 min given 30 min before chemotherapy, then q2h for two doses, then q3h for three doses	Treatment of nausea and vomiting, especially related to chemical stimulation of the chemoreceptor trigger zone in adults
Anticholinergics/Antihistamines		
buclizine (*Bucladin*)	50 mg PO, up to 150 mg/day has been used	Treatment of nausea and vomiting associated with motion sickness in adults
cyclizine (*Marezine*)	Adult: 50 mg PO 30 min before exposure to motion, then q4–6h as needed Pediatric: (6–12 yr): 25 mg PO up to three times per day	Treatment of nausea and vomiting associated with motion sickness
P meclizine (*Antivert*)	25–50 mg PO 1 h before travel, may repeat q24h during trip	Treatment of nausea and vomiting associated with motion sickness in patients >12 yr
5-HT$_3$ Receptor Blockers		
dolasetron (*Anzemet*)	Adult: 100 mg PO within 1 h of procedure; 12.5 mg IV for postoperative vomiting; 1.8 mg/kg IV or 100 mg IV injection before chemotherapy Pediatric (2–16 yr): 1.8 mg/kg PO 1 h before chemotherapy, diluted in apple or apple-grape juice; 1.8 mg/kg IV 30 min before chemotherapy; 1.2 mg/kg IV for postoperative vomiting	Treatment of nausea and vomiting associated with emetogenic chemotherapy; prevention of postoperative nausea and vomiting
granisetron (*Kytril*)	Adult and pediatric (>2 yr): 10 mcg/kg IV over 5 min starting within 30 min of chemotherapy; *or* 1 mg PO b.i.d. beginning up to 1 h before chemotherapy and giving the second dose 12 h after, use only on days of chemotherapy	Treatment of nausea and vomiting associated with emetogenic chemotherapy
P ondansetron (*Zofran*)	Adult: 8 mg PO t.i.d. or 24 mg PO 30 min before chemotherapy; three 0.15-mg/kg doses IV over 15 min beginning before chemotherapy or one 32-mg dose infused over 30 min, given 30 min before chemotherapy; 4 mg IV or 4 mg IM *or* 16 mg PO 1 h before surgery to prevent postoperative vomiting Pediatric (4–12 yr): 4 mg PO t.i.d.; use same IV dose as adults	Treatment of severe nausea and vomiting associated with emetogenic chemotherapy, radiation therapy, postoperative situations
palonosetron (*Aloxi*)	0.25 mg IV as a single dose over 30 sec given 30 min before the start of chemotherapy; do not repeat dose for 7 days	Treatment of acute and delayed vomiting associated with highly emetogenic chemotherapy
Substance P/Neurokinin 1 Receptor Antagonist		
P aprepitant (*Emend*)	125 mg PO 1 h before chemotherapy (day 1); then 80 mg PO in the morning, days 2 and 3, with dexamethasone 12 mg PO day 1 and 8 mg PO days 2–4, and 32 mg ondansetron IV on day 1 only	Prevention of acute and delayed nausea and vomiting associated with highly emetogenic cancer chemotherapy

Table 59.2 DRUGS IN FOCUS *(Continued)*

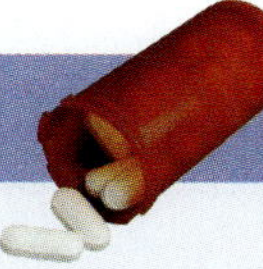

Antiemetic Agents

Drug Name	Usual Dosage	Usual Indications
Miscellaneous Drugs		
dronabinol (*Marinol*)	5 mg/m² PO 1–3 h before chemotherapy, repeat q2–4h as needed for a total of four to six doses per day	Management of nausea and vomiting associated with cancer chemotherapy in adults
hydroxyzine (*Vistaril*)	Adult: 25–100 mg IM Pediatric: 1.1 mg/kg IM	Treatment of prepartum, postpartum, and postoperative nausea and vomiting
trimethobenzamide (*Tigan*)	Adult: 250 mg PO t.i.d. to q.i.d.; 200 mg PR t.i.d. to q.i.d.; 200 mg IM t.i.d. to q.i.d. Pediatric (≥30 lb): 100–200 mg PO or PR t.i.d. to q.i.d. Pediatric (<30 lb): 100 mg PR t.i.d. to q.i.d.	Treatment of nausea and vomiting (not sedating)

mission of impulses to the CTZ. Chapter 33 discusses the anticholinergics in greater detail.

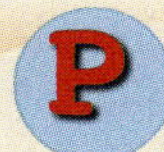

Prototype Summary: Metoclopramide

Indications: Prevention of nausea and vomiting associated with emetogenic cancer chemotherapy; prevention of postoperative nausea and vomiting

Actions: Slows GI activity; sedating

Pharmacokinetics:

Route	Onset	Peak	Duration
Oral	30–60 min	60–90 min	1–2 h
IM	10–15 min	60–90 min	1–2 h
IV	1–3 min	60–90 min	1–2 h

$T_{1/2}$: 5–6 hours; metabolized in the liver and excreted in urine

Adverse effects: Drowsiness, fatigue, restlessness, extrapyramidal symptoms, diarrhea

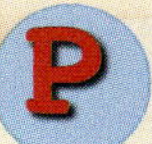

Prototype Summary: Meclizine

Indications: Prevention and treatment of nausea and vomiting, motion sickness

Actions: Blocks cholinergic receptors in the vomiting center, anticholinergic

Pharmacokinetics:

Route	Onset	Peak	Duration
Oral	1 hr	1–2 h	12–24 h

$T_{1/2}$: 6 hours; metabolism unknown; excreted in urine and feces

Adverse effects: Drowsiness, confusion, dry mouth, anorexia, urinary frequency

5-HT$_3$ Receptor Blockers

The 5-HT$_3$ receptor blockers block those receptors associated with nausea and vomiting in the CTZ and locally. These drugs include dolasetron (*Anzemet*), granisetron (*Kytril*), ondansetron (*Zofran*), and palonosetron (*Aloxi*). They are rapidly absorbed, metabolized in the liver, and excreted in urine and feces. Because they are known to cross the placenta and enter breast milk, use during pregnancy and lactation should be limited to situations in which the benefit to the mother outweighs the potential risk to the fetus or neonate. These drugs have proven especially helpful in treating the nausea and vomiting associated with antineoplastic chemotherapy and postoperative nausea and vomiting.

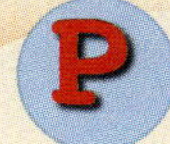

Prototype Summary: Ondansetron

Indications: Control of severe nausea and vomiting associated with emetogenic cancer chemotherapy, radiation therapy; treatment of postoperative nausea and vomiting

Actions: Blocks specific receptor sites associated with nausea and vomiting, peripherally and in the CTZ

Pharmacokinetics:

Route	Onset	Peak	Duration
Oral	30–60 min	60–90 min	1.7–2.2 h
IV	Immediate	60–90 min	Duration of infusion

CRITICAL THINKING SCENARIO 59-1

Handling Postoperative Nausea and Vomiting

The Situation

A.J. is a 16-year-old boy who has undergone reconstructive knee surgery after a football injury. After the surgery, A.J. complains of nausea and vomits three times in 2 hours. A.J. becomes increasingly agitated. Rectal prochlorperazine (*Compazine*) is ordered to relieve the nausea, to be followed by an oral order when tolerated. The prochlorperazine is somewhat helpful in relieving the nausea, but A.J. expresses a desire to try cannabis, which he has read is good for the relief of nausea.

Critical Thinking

What are the important nursing implications in this case?

What other measures could be taken to relieve A.J.'s nausea?

What explanation could be given to the request for cannabis?

Discussion

It is often impossible to pinpoint an exact cause of a patient's nausea and vomiting in a hospital setting. For example, the underlying cause may be related to the pain, a reaction to the pain medication being given, or a response to what A.J. described as the "awful hospital smell." A combination of factors should be considered when dealing with nausea and vomiting. A.J., as a teenager, may become increasingly agitated by the discomfort and possible embarrassment of vomiting. The administration of rectal prochlorperazine may "take the edge off" the nausea. A.J. will have to be reminded that the drug he is being given may make him dizzy, weak, or drowsy and that he should ask for assistance if he needs to move.

Once the nausea and vomiting diminish somewhat, it will be possible to try other interventions to help stop the vomiting reflex. One such intervention is removing the offending odor that A.J. described, if possible, because doing so may relieve a chemical stimulus to the chemoreceptor trigger zone (CTZ). Administration of pain medication, as prescribed, may relieve the CTZ stimulus that comes with intense pain. Other interventions include providing a serene, quiet environment and encouraging A.J. to take slow, deep breaths, which stimulate the parasympathetic system (vagus nerve) and partially override the sympathetic activity stimulated by the CTZ to activate vomiting. For many patients, mouth care, ice chips, or small sips of water may also help to relieve the discomfort and ease the sensation of nausea.

After A.J. has relaxed a bit and his nausea has abated, the use of cannabis for treating nausea can be discussed. This may be a good opportunity to explain the many effects of cannabis to A.J. The drug does relieve nausea and vomiting, especially in patients undergoing chemotherapy. It also decreases activity in the respiratory tract, affects the development of sperm in males, and alters thinking patterns and brain chemistry. The U. S. Food and Drug Administration has approved the use of the active ingredient in cannabis, delta-9-tetrahydrocannabinol, in an oral form (dronabinol [*Marinol*]) for the relief of nausea and vomiting in cancer patients who have not responded to other therapies and for the treatment of anorexia associated with acquired immunodeficiency syndrome (AIDS). It is not approved for use in the postoperative setting.

Nursing Care Guide for A.J.: Antiemetics

Assessment: History And Examination

Assess A.J.'s health history for allergies to any antiemetic, coma, CNS depression, severe hypotension, liver dysfunction, bone marrow depression, epilepsy, and concurrent use of alcohol, anticholinergic drugs, barbiturate anesthetics, and guanethidine.

Focus the physical examination on the following areas:

Neurological: orientation, affect

Skin: color, lesions

CV: pulse, blood pressure, orthostatic blood pressure

GI: abdominal and liver evaluation

Laboratory tests: hematological, CBC, liver function tests

Nursing Diagnoses

Acute Pain related to GI, skin, CNS effects

Risk for Injury related to CNS, CV effects

Deficient Knowledge regarding drug therapy

Implementation

Administer antiemetics only as a temporary measure.

Provide comfort and safety measures including assistance with mobility, access to bathroom, safety precautions, mouth care, and ice chips.

Handling Postoperative Nausea and Vomiting *(continued)*

Monitor A.J. for dehydration and provide remedial measures as needed.

Provide support and reassurance for coping with drug effects and discomfort.

Provide patient teaching regarding drug name, dosage, adverse effects, precautions, warning to report.

Evaluation

Evaluate drug effects, e.g., relief of nausea and vomiting.

Monitor for adverse effects, including GI alterations, orthostatic hypotension, dizziness, confusion, sensitivity to sunlight, and dehydration.

Monitor for drug–drug interactions as appropriate.

Evaluate effectiveness of patient teaching program and comfort and safety measures.

Patient Teaching For A.J.

☐ The drug that has been prescribed for you is called prochlorperazine, or *Compazine.* It belongs to a class of drugs called antiemetics. An antiemetic helps prevent nausea and vomiting and the discomfort they cause.

☐ Common effects of this drug include:

- *Dizziness, weakness:* Change positions slowly. If you feel drowsy, avoid driving or dangerous activities (such as the use of heavy machinery or tasks requiring coordination).
- *Sensitivity to the sun:* Avoid exposure to the sun and ultraviolet light, because serious reactions may occur. If exposure cannot be prevented, use sunscreen and protective clothing to cover the skin.
- *Dehydration:* Avoid excessive heat exposure and try to drink fluids as much as possible because you will have an increased risk for heat stroke.
- Report any of the following conditions to your health care provider: *fever, rash, yellowing of the eyes or skin, dark urine, pale stools, easy bruising, rash, and vision changes.*

☐ Avoid over-the-counter medications. If you feel that you need one, check with your health care provider first.

☐ Tell any doctor, nurse, or other health care provider that you are taking this drug.

☐ Keep this drug and all medications out of the reach of children.

$T_{1/2}$: 3.5–6 hours; metabolized in the liver and excreted in urine

Adverse effects: Headache, dizziness, drowsiness, myalgia, urinary retention, constipation, pain at injection site

Substance P/Neurokinin 1 Receptor Antagonist

The first drug in the newest class of drugs for treating nausea and vomiting is the substance P/neurokinin 1 receptor antagonist aprepitant (*Emend*). This drug acts directly in the CNS to block receptors associated with nausea and vomiting with little to no effect on serotonin, dopamine, or corticosteroid receptors. It is approved for use in treating the nausea and vomiting associated with highly emetogenic antineoplastic chemotherapy, including cisplatin therapy. It is given orally, in combination with dexamethasone. Aprepitant is metabolized in the liver and excreted in urine and feces. This drug is known to cross the placenta and to enter breast milk and should not be used during pregnancy or lactation.

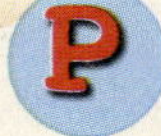

Prototype Summary: Aprepitant

Indications: In combination with other agents for prevention of acute and delayed nausea and vomiting associated with severely emetogenic cancer chemotherapy

Actions: Selectively blocks human substance P/neurokinin 1 (NK1) receptors in the CNS, blocking the nausea and vomiting caused by highly emetogenic chemotherapeutic agents

Pharmacokinetics:

Route	Onset	Peak
Oral	Rapid	4 h

$T_{1/2}$: 9–13 hours; metabolized in the liver and excreted in urine and feces

Adverse effects: Anorexia, fatigue, constipation, diarrhea, liver enzyme elevations, dehydration

Miscellaneous Agents

Miscellaneous agents used as antiemetics include dronabinol (*Marinol*), which contains the active ingredient of cannabis (marijuana); hydroxyzine (*Vistaril*), which may suppress cortical areas of the CNS; and trimethobenzamide (*Tigan*), which is similar to the antihistamines but is not as sedating. Trimethobenzamide is often a drug of choice in this group because it is not associated with as much sedation and CNS suppression as other agents. It is available in oral, parenteral, and suppository forms, and is rapidly absorbed, metabolized in the liver, and excreted in urine. It crosses the placenta and enters breast milk, and use should be reserved for situations in which the benefit to the mother outweighs any potential risk to the fetus or neonate.

Hydroxyzine is used for nausea and vomiting before or after obstetrical delivery or surgery. It is rapidly absorbed, metabolized in the liver, and excreted in urine. It has not been associated with fetal problems during pregnancy and is not thought to enter breast milk; however, as with all drugs, caution should be used during pregnancy and lactation.

Dronabinol is approved for use in managing the nausea and vomiting associated with cancer chemotherapy in cases that have not responded to other treatment. Its exact mechanism of action is not understood. This drug, a category C-III controlled substance, must be used under close supervision because of the possibility of altered mental status. It is readily absorbed and metabolized in the liver, with excretion through the bile and in urine.

Therapeutic Actions and Indications

As stated earlier, the locally active antiemetics are used to relieve mild nausea. The centrally acting antiemetics change the responsiveness or stimulation of the CTZ in the medulla (Figure 59.1). The phenothiazines are recommended for the

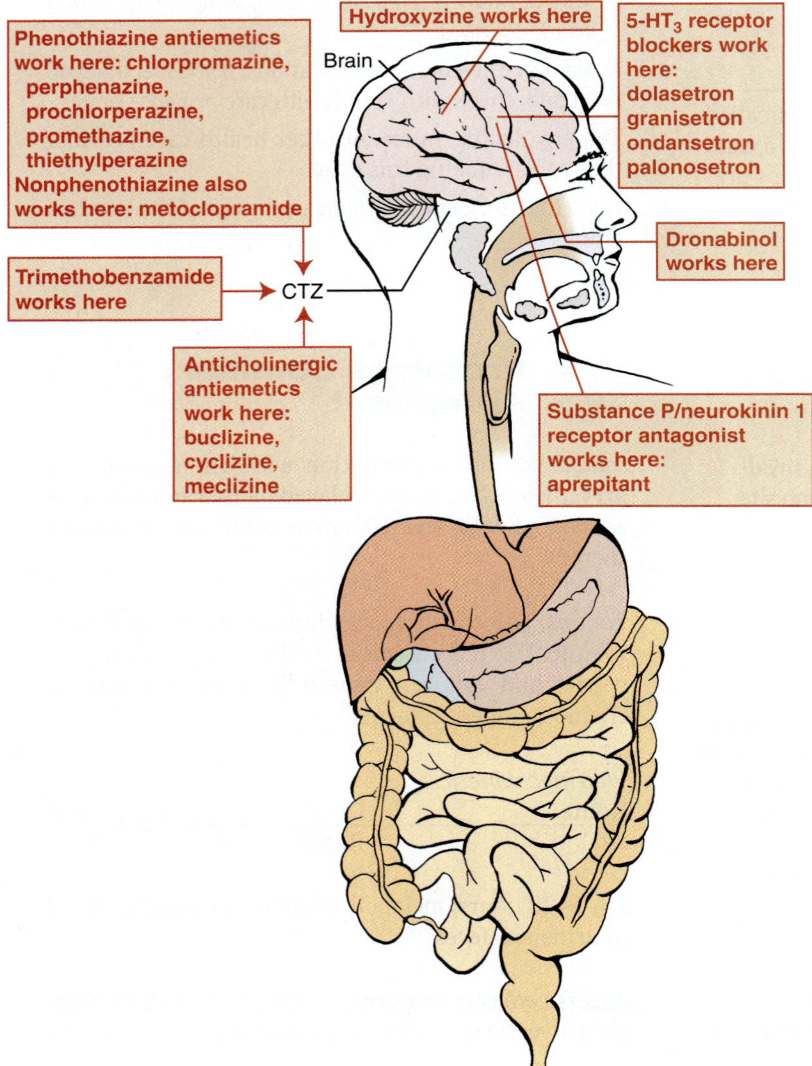

FIGURE 59.1 Sites of action of emetics/antiemetics. CTZ, chemoreceptor trigger zone.

treatment of nausea and vomiting, including that specifically associated with anesthesia; severe vomiting; **intractable hiccoughs**, which occur with repetitive stimulation of the diaphragm and lead to persistent diaphragm spasm; and nausea and vomiting. The anticholinergics that act as antihistamines are recommended for the nausea and vomiting associated with motion sickness or **vestibular** (inner ear) problems. Some of these agents are available over the counter in a reduced dose for prevention or self-treatment of motion sickness. The 5-HT_3 receptor blockers and substance P/neurokinin 1 receptor antagonist are specific for the treatment of nausea and vomiting associated with emetogenic chemotherapy. These are relatively new drugs, and the drug of choice depends on personal preference and experience.

Contraindications and Cautions

In general, antiemetics should not be used in patients with coma or severe CNS depression, or in those who have experienced brain damage or injury *because of the risk of further CNS depression.* Other contraindications include severe hypotension or hypertension and severe liver dysfunction, *which might interfere with the metabolism of the drug.* Caution should be used in individuals with renal dysfunction, active peptic ulcer, or pregnancy and lactation.

Adverse Effects

Adverse effects associated with antiemetics are linked to their interference with normal CNS stimulation or response. Drowsiness, dizziness, weakness, tremor, and headache are common adverse effects. As previously stated, some of the antiemetics are thought to have fewer CNS effects. Other, not uncommon adverse effects include hypotension, hypertension, and cardiac arrhythmias. When the phenothiazines and antihistamines are used as antiemetics, autonomic effects such as dry mouth, nasal congestion, anorexia, pallor, sweating, and urinary retention often occur. **Photosensitivity** (increased sensitivity to the sun and ultraviolet light) is a common adverse reaction with many of the antiemetics. Patients should be advised to use sunscreens and protective garments if exposure cannot be avoided.

Clinically Important Drug–Drug Interactions

Additive CNS depression can be seen with any of the antiemetics if they are combined with other CNS depressants, including alcohol. Patients should be advised to avoid this combination and any over-the-counter preparation unless they check with their health care provider. Other drug–drug interactions are specific to each drug (refer to a nursing drug guide).

Nursing Considerations for Patients Receiving an Antiemetic

Assessment: History and Examination

Screen for the following conditions, *which could be cautions or contraindications to the use of the drug:* history of allergy to antiemetic; impaired renal or hepatic function; pregnancy or lactation; coma or semiconscious state, CNS depression; hypotension or hypertension; active peptic ulcer; and CNS injury.

Include screening for orientation, affect, and reflexes: baseline pulse and blood pressure; skin lesions and color; liver and abdominal examination; and liver and renal function tests.

Nursing Diagnoses

The patient receiving an antiemetic may have the following nursing diagnoses related to drug therapy:

- Acute Pain related to CNS, skin, and GI effects
- Risk for Injury related to CNS effects
- Decreased Cardiac Output related to cardiac effects
- Deficient Knowledge regarding drug therapy

Implementation With Rationale

- Assess the patient carefully for any potential drug–drug interactions if giving antiemetics in combination with other drugs *to avert potentially serious drug–drug interactions.*
- Provide comfort and safety measures, including mouth care, ready access to bathroom facilities, assistance with ambulation and periodic orientation, ice chips to suck, protection from sun exposure, and remedial measures to treat dehydration if it occurs, *to protect patient from injury and to increase patient comfort.*
- Provide support and encouragement, as well as other measures (quiet environment, carbonated drinks, deep breathing), *to help the patient cope with the discomfort of nausea and vomiting and drug effects.*
- Provide thorough patient teaching, including name of drug, dosage prescribed, proper administration, measures to avoid adverse effects, warning signs of problems, the importance of periodic monitoring and evaluation, and the need to avoid overdose and poisoning, *to enhance patient knowledge about drug therapy and promote compliance with the drug regimen.*

Evaluation

- Monitor patient response to the drug (relief of nausea and vomiting).
- Monitor for adverse effects (dizziness, confusion, GI alterations, cardiac arrhythmias, hypotension, gynecomastia).
- Evaluate effectiveness of teaching plan (patient can name the drug and dosage as well as describe adverse effects to watch for and specific measures to avoid these adverse effects).
- Monitor effectiveness of comfort measures and compliance with the regimen.

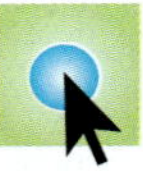

WEB LINKS

Health care providers and patients may want to consult the following Internet sources:

http://www.anzemet.com Information on nausea and vomiting associated with cancer chemotherapy.

http://www.nlm.nih.gov/medlineplus/nauseaandvomiting.html Information on nausea and vomiting, including causes, research, and alternative therapies.

http://quickcare.org/gast/nausea.html Information on causes and treatments for nausea and vomiting.

http://www.mgh.org/poison/index.html Information for patients and health care workers on home treatment of various poisons.

Points to Remember

- Antiemetics are used to manage nausea and vomiting in situations in which these actions are not beneficial and could actually cause harm to the patient.
- Antiemetics act by depressing the hyperactive vomiting reflex, either locally or through alteration of CNS actions.
- The choice of an antiemetic depends on the cause of the nausea and vomiting and the expected actions of the drug.
- Most antiemetics cause some CNS depression with resultant dizziness, drowsiness, and weakness. Care must be taken to protect the patient and advise him or her to avoid dangerous situations.
- Photosensitivity is another common adverse effect with antiemetics. Patients should be protected from exposure to the sun and ultraviolet light. Sunscreens and protective clothing are essential if exposure cannot be prevented.

CHECK YOUR UNDERSTANDING

Answers to the questions in this chapter may be found in the Answer Key in the back of the book.

Multiple Choice

Select the best answer to the following.

1. Prochlorperazine (*Compazine*) would be the antiemetic of choice for
   a. nausea and vomiting after anesthesia.
   b. nausea and vomiting associated with cancer chemotherapy.
   c. motion sickness.
   d. intractable hiccoughs.

2. Most antiemetics work with the CNS to decrease the activity of
   a. the medulla.
   b. the CTZ.
   c. the respiratory center.
   d. the sympathetic nervous system.

3. Photosensitivity is a common adverse effect associated with the use of antiemetic agents. Patients should be cautioned
   a. to avoid having their picture taken.
   b. to cover the head at extremes of temperature.
   c. to take extra precautions to avoid heat stroke.
   d. to wear protective clothing and use a sunscreen if exposed to the sun or ultraviolet light.

4. The 5-HT_3 receptor blockers, including ondansetron (*Zofran*) and granisetron (*Kytril*), are particularly effective in decreasing the nausea and vomiting associated with
   a. vestibular problems.
   b. emetogenic cancer chemotherapy.
   c. pregnancy.
   d. severe pain.

5. Prochlorperazine (*Compazine*) may be the drug of choice for
   a. nausea associated with cisplatin use.
   b. nausea associated with cancer chemotherapy.
   c. nausea associated with food poisoning.
   d. vomiting associated with antineoplastic chemotherapy.

6. A parent calls with concerns that a 2-year-old child ate a bottle of baby aspirin. The nurse would advise the parent

a. to administer ipecac immediately.
b. to induce vomiting by inserting a finger against the back of the child's throat.
c. to force fluids and bring the child in for evaluation.
d. to feed the child charcoal.

Multiple Response

Select all that apply.

1. Nursing interventions for the client receiving an antiemetic drug would include which of the following?
   a. Frequent mouth care and ice chips to suck
   b. Bowel program to deal with constipation
   c. Protection from falls or injury
   d. Fluids to guard against dehydration
   e. Protection from sun exposure
   f. Quiet environment and temperature control

2. Palonosetron (*Aloxi*) would be a drug of choice for a client with which of the following problems?
   a. Nausea and vomiting associated with cancer chemotherapy
   b. A prolonged Q-T interval
   c. Delayed nausea and vomiting associated with antineoplastic chemotherapy
   d. Difficulty swallowing
   e. Hypokalemia
   f. Hypomagnesemia

Web Exercise

You and your neighbor are having a discussion about the use of syrup of ipecac to induce vomiting in children. You are trying to explain the latest guidelines that have been developed regarding this practice. Your neighbor insists that she and her mother and her grandmother have always used ipecac and keep it in the house. Go on-line to find the studies that were done and prepare an informed teaching plan to explain the reasoning for this guideline as well as the guidelines that should be followed in case of accidental ingestion of possible toxins. A good starting place would be:

http://aappolicy.aappublications.org/cgi/content/abstract/pediatrics;112/5/1182

Fill in the Blanks

1. Emetic drugs are used to induce ____________________ in cases of poisoning or drug overdose.

2. ____________________, once the standard emetic in use, is no longer recommended.

3. ____________________ are used to manage nausea and vomiting in situations in which they are not beneficial and could actually cause harm to the patient.

4. Antiemetics act by depressing the ____________________, either locally or through alteration of central nervous system actions.

5. Vomiting is a complex reflex mediated through the ____________________ located in the ____________________.

6. The chemoreceptor trigger zone (CTZ) can be stimulated by ____________________, ____________________, ____________________ or several other mechanisms.

7. Most antiemetics cause some ____________________, with resultant dizziness, drowsiness, and weakness.

8. ____________________ is another common adverse effect with antiemetics. Patients should be protected from exposure to the sun and ultraviolet light.

Bibliography and References

American Association of Pediatrics Committee on Injury, Violence, and Poison Prevention. (2003). Poison treatment in the home. *Pediatrics, 112*(5), 1182–1185.

Drug facts and comparisons. (2006). St. Louis: Facts and Comparisons.

Gilman, A., Hardman, J. G., & Limbird, L. E. (Eds.). (2006). *Goodman and Gilman's the pharmacological basis of therapeutics* (11th ed.). New York: McGraw-Hill.

Karch, A. M. (2006). *2007 Lippincott's nursing drug guide.* Philadelphia: Lippincott Williams & Wilkins.

The medical letter on drugs and therapeutics. (2006). New Rochelle, NY: Medical Letter.

Porth, C. M. (2005). *Pathophysiology: Concepts of altered health states* (7th ed.). Philadelphia: Lippincott Williams & Wilkins.

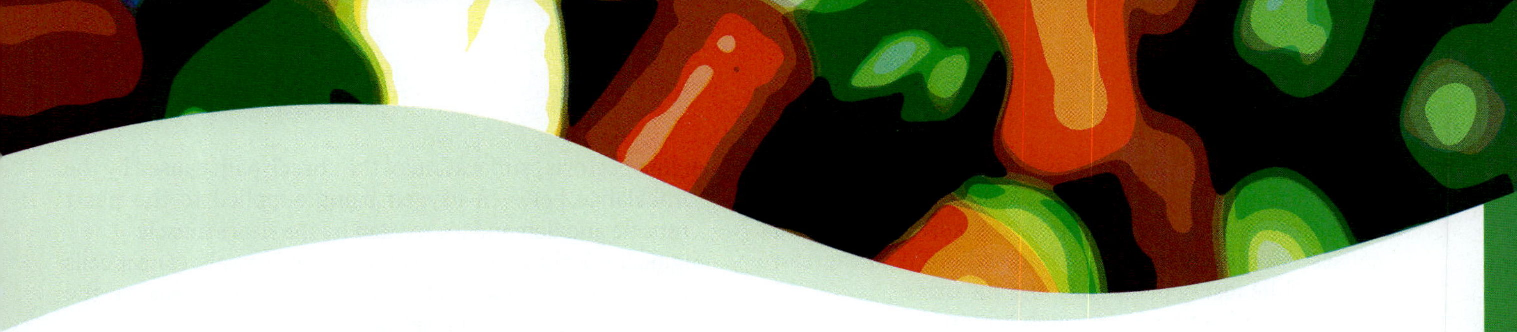

Glossary

A

A fibers large-diameter nerve fibers that carry peripheral impulses associated with touch and temperature to the spinal cord

abortifacients drugs used to stimulate uterine contractions and promote evacuation of the uterus to cause abortion or to empty the uterus after fetal death

absence seizure type of generalized seizure that is characterized by sudden, temporary loss of consciousness, sometimes with staring or blinking for 3 to 5 seconds; formerly known as a petit mal seizure

absorption what happens to a drug from the time it enters the body until it enters the circulating fluid; intravenous administration causes the drug to directly enter the circulating blood, bypassing the many complications of absorption from other routes

ACE inhibitor drug that blocks the enzyme responsible for converting angiotensin I to angiotensin II in the lungs; this blocking prevents the vasoconstriction and aldosterone release related to angiotensin II

acetylcholine receptor site area on the muscle cell membrane where acetylcholine (ACh) reacts with a specific receptor site to cause stimulation of the muscle in response to nerve activity

acetylcholinesterase enzyme responsible for the immediate breakdown of acetylcholine when released from the nerve ending; prevents overstimulation of cholinergic receptor sites

acid rebound reflex response of the stomach to lower-than-normal acid levels; when acid levels are lowered through the use of antacids, gastrin production and secretion are increased to return the stomach to its normal acidity

acidification the process of increasing the acid level; used to treat bladder infections, making the bladder an undesirable place for bacteria

acquired immunodeficiency syndrome (AIDS) collection of opportunistic infections and cancers that occurs when the immune system is severely depressed by a decrease in the number of functioning helper T cells; caused by infection with human immunodeficiency virus (HIV)

acromegaly thickening of bony surfaces in response to excess growth hormone after the epiphyseal plates have closed

actin thin filament that makes up a sarcomere or muscle unit

action potential sudden change in electrical charge of a nerve cell membrane; the electrical signal by which neurons send information

active immunity the formation of antibodies secondary to exposure to a specific antigen; leads to the formation of plasma cells, antibodies, and memory cells to immediately produce antibodies if exposed to that antigen in the future; imparts lifelong immunity

active transport the movement of substances across a cell membrane against the concentration gradient; this process requires the use of energy

A-delta and C fibers small-diameter nerve fibers that carry peripheral impulses associated with pain to the spinal cord

adrenal cortex outer layer of the adrenal gland; produces glucocorticoids and mineralocorticoids in response to adrenocorticotropic hormone (ACTH) stimulation; also responds to sympathetic stimulation

adrenal medulla inner layer of the adrenal gland; a sympathetic ganglion, it releases norepinephrine and epinephrine into circulation in response to sympathetic stimulation

adrenergic agonist a drug that stimulates the adrenergic receptors of the sympathetic nervous system, either directly (by reacting with receptor sites) or indirectly (by increasing norepinephrine levels)

adrenergic receptor receptor sites on effectors that respond to norepinephrine

adrenergic receptor site specificity a drug's affinity for only adrenergic receptor sites; certain drugs may have specific affinity for only alpha- or only beta-adrenergic receptor sites

adverse effects drug effects that are not the desired therapeutic effects; may be unpleasant or even dangerous

aerobic bacteria that depend on oxygen for survival

affect feeling that a person experiences when he or she responds emotionally to the environment

afferent neurons or groups of neurons that bring information to the central nervous system; sensory nerve

agonist a drug that acts like or increases the effects of a specific neurotransmitter or hormone

AIDS-related complex (ARC) collection of less serious opportunistic infections with HIV infection; the decrease in the number of helper T cells is less severe than in fully developed AIDS

aldosterone hormone produced by the adrenal gland that causes the distal tubule to retain sodium, and therefore water, while losing potassium into the urine

alkalosis state of not having enough acid to maintain normal homeostatic processes; seen with loop diuretics, which cause loss of bicarbonate in the urine

alopecia hair loss; a common adverse effect of many antineoplastic drugs, which are more effective against rapidly multiplying cells such as those of hair follicles

alpha-agonist specifically stimulating to the alpha-receptors within the sympathetic nervous system, causing body responses seen when the alpha-receptors are stimulated

alpha-receptors adrenergic receptors that are found in smooth muscles

$alpha_1$-selective adrenergic blocking agents drugs that block the postsynaptic $alpha_1$-receptor sites, causing a decrease in vascular tone and a vasodilation that leads to a fall in blood pressure; these drugs do not block the presynaptic $alpha_2$-receptor sites, and therefore the reflex tachycardia that accompanies a fall in blood pressure does not occur

alternative therapy including herbs and other "natural" products as found in ancient records, these products are not controlled or tested by the U.S. Food and Drug Administration, and because of this, the advertising surrounding these products is not as restricted or as accurate as it would be with classic drugs

alveoli the respiratory sac, the smallest unit of the lungs where gas exchange occurs

Alzheimer's disease degenerative disease of the cortex with loss of acetylcholine-producing cells and cholinergic receptors; characterized by progressive dementia

amebiasis amebic dysentery, which is caused by intestinal invasion of the trophozoite stage of the protozoan *Entamoeba histolytica*

amnesia loss of memory of an event or procedure

anabolic steroids androgens developed with more anabolic or protein-building effects than androgenic effects

anaerobic bacteria that survive without oxygen, which are often seen when blood flow is cut off to an area of the body

analgesia loss of pain sensation

analgesic compounds with pain-blocking properties, capable of producing analgesia

anaplasia loss of organization and structure; property of cancer cells

androgenic effects effects associated with development of male sexual characteristics and secondary characteristics (e.g., deepening of voice, hair distribution, genital development, acne)

androgens male sex hormones, primarily testosterone; produced in the testes and adrenal glands

anemia a decrease in the number of red blood cells (RBCs), leading to an inability to effectively deliver oxygen to the tissues

angina pectoris "suffocation of the chest"; pain caused by the imbalance between oxygen being supplied to the heart muscle and demand for oxygen by the heart muscle

angiogenesis the generation of new blood vessels; cancer cells release an enzyme that will cause angiogenesis or the growth of new blood vessels to feed the cancer cells

angiotensin II receptors specific receptors found in blood vessels and in the adrenal gland that react with angiotensin II to cause vasoconstriction and release of aldosterone

***Anopheles* mosquito** type of mosquito that is essential to the life cycle of *Plasmodium;* injects the protozoa into humans for further maturation

anterior pituitary lobe of the pituitary gland that produces stimulating hormones, as well as growth hormone, prolactin, and melanocyte-stimulating hormone

antiarrhythmics drugs that affect the action potential of cardiac cells and are used to treat arrhythmias and return normal rate and rhythm

antibiotic chemical that is able to inhibit the growth of specific bacteria or cause the death of susceptible bacteria

antibodies immunoglobulins; produced by B cell plasma cells in response to a specific protein; react with that protein to cause its destruction directly or through activation of the inflammatory response

anticholinergic drug that opposes the effects of acetylcholine at acetylcholine receptor sites

anticoagulants drugs that block or inhibit any step of the coagulation process, preventing or slowing clot formation

antidiarrheal drug drug that blocks the stimulation of the gastrointestinal (GI) tract, leading to decreased activity and increased time for absorption of needed nutrients and water

antidiuretic hormone (ADH) hormone produced by the hypothalamus and stored in the posterior pituitary gland; important in maintaining fluid balance; causes the distal tubules and collecting ducts of the kidney to become permeable to water, leading to an antidiuretic effect and fluid retention

antiemetic agent that blocks the hyperactive response of the chemoreceptor trigger zone (CTZ) to various stimuli, the response that produces nonbeneficial nausea and vomiting

antiepileptic drug used to treat the abnormal and excessive energy bursts in the brain that are characteristic of epilepsy

antigen foreign protein

antihistamines drugs that block the release or action of histamine, a chemical released during inflammation that increases secretions and narrows airways

anti-inflammatory blocking the effects of the inflammatory response

antineoplastic agent drug used to combat cancer or the growth of neoplasms

antipeptic drug that coats any injured area in the stomach to prevent further injury from acid or pepsin

antipsychotic drug used to treat disorders involving thought processes; dopamine receptor blocker that helps affected people organize their thoughts and respond appropriately to stimuli

antipyretic blocking fever, often by direct effects on the thermoregulatory center in the hypothalamus or by blockade of prostaglandin mediators

antispasmodics agents that block muscle spasm associated with irritation or neurological stimulation

antitoxins immune sera that contains antibodies to specific toxins produced by invaders; may prevent the toxin from adhering to body tissues and causing disease

antitussives drugs that block the cough reflex

anxiety unpleasant feeling of tension, fear, or nervousness in response to an environmental stimulus, whether real or imaginary

anxiolytic drug used to depress the central nervous system (CNS); prevents the signs and symptoms of anxiety

apothecary system a very old system of measure that was specifically developed for use by apothecaries or pharmacists; it uses the minim as the basic unit of liquid measure and the grain as the basic unit of solid measure.

arachidonic acid released from injured cells to stimulate the inflammatory response through activation of various chemical substances

arrhythmia a disruption in cardiac rate or rhythm

arteries vessels that take blood away from the heart; muscular, resistance vessels

assessment information gathering regarding the current status of a particular patient, including evaluation of past history and physical examination; provides a baseline of information and clues to effectiveness of therapy

asthma disorder characterized by recurrent episodes of bronchospasm (i.e., bronchial muscle spasm leading to narrowed or obstructed airways)

atheroma plaque in the endothelial lining of arteries; contains fats, blood cells, lipids, inflammatory agents, platelets; leads to narrowing of the lumen of the artery, stiffening of the artery, and loss of distensibility and responsiveness

atherosclerosis narrowing of the arteries caused by buildup of atheromas, swelling, and accumulation of platelets; leads to a loss of elasticity and responsiveness to normal stimuli

atrium top chamber of the heart, receives blood from veins

attention-deficit disorder behavioral syndrome characterized by an inability to concentrate for longer than a few minutes and excessive activity

auricle appendage on the atria of the heart, holds blood to be pumped out with atrial contraction

autoimmune disease a disorder that occurs when the body responds to specific self-antigens to produce antibodies or cell-mediated responses against its own cells

automaticity property of heart cells to generate an action potential without an external stimulus

autonomic nervous system portion of the central and peripheral nervous systems that, with the endocrine system, functions to maintain internal homeostasis

autonomy loss of the normal controls and reactions that inhibit growth and spreading; property of cancer cells

axon long projection from a neuron that carries information from one nerve to another nerve or effector

azoles a group of drugs used to treat fungal infections

B

B cells lymphocytes programmed to recognize specific proteins; when activated, these cells cause the production of antibodies to react with that protein

bactericidal substance that causes the death of bacteria, usually by interfering with cell membrane stability or with proteins or enzymes necessary to maintain the cellular integrity of the bacteria

bacteriostatic substance that prevents the replication of bacteria, usually by interfering with proteins or enzyme systems necessary for reproduction of the bacteria

balanced anesthesia use of several different types of drugs to achieve the quickest, most effective anesthesia with the fewest adverse effects

barbiturate former mainstay drug used for the treatment of anxiety and for sedation and sleep induction; associated with potentially severe adverse effects and many drug–drug interactions, which makes it less desirable than some of the newer agents

baroreceptor pressure receptor; located in the arch of the aorta and in the carotid artery; responds to changes in pressure and influences the medulla to stimulate the sympathetic system to increase or decrease blood pressure

basal ganglia lower area of the brain associated with coordination of unconscious muscle movements that involve movement and position

belladonna a plant that contains atropine as an alkaloid; used to dilate the pupils as a fashion statement in the past; used in herbal medicine much as atropine is used today

benign prostatic hyperplasia (BPH) enlargement of the prostate gland, associated with age and inflammation; also called benign prostatic hypertrophy

benzodiazepine drug that acts in the limbic system and the reticular activating system to make gamma-aminobutyric acid (GABA), an inhibitory neurotransmitter, more effective, causing interference with neuron firing; depresses CNS to block the signs and symptoms of anxiety and may cause sedation and hypnosis (extreme sedation with further CNS depression and sleep) in higher doses

beta-adrenergic blocking agents drugs that, at therapeutic levels, selectively block the beta-receptors of the sympathetic nervous system

beta-agonist specifically stimulating to the beta-receptors within the sympathetic nervous system, causing body responses seen when the beta-receptors are stimulated

beta-receptors adrenergic receptors that are found in the heart, lungs, and vascular smooth muscle

$beta_1$-selective adrenergic blocking agents drugs that, at therapeutic levels, specifically block the $beta_1$-receptors in the sympathetic nervous system, while not blocking the $beta_2$-receptors and resultant effects on the respiratory system

bile fluid stored in the gallbladder that contains cholesterol and bile salts; essential for the proper breakdown and absorption of fats

bile acids cholesterol-containing acids found in the bile that act like detergents to break up fats in the small intestine

biogenic amine one of the neurotransmitters norepinephrine, serotonin, or dopamine; it is thought that a deficiency of these substances in key areas of the brain results in depression

biological weapons so-called germ warfare; the use of bacteria, viruses, and parasites on a large scale to incapacitate or destroy a population

biotransformation the alteration of a drug by the body into new chemicals that are less active, less toxic, and more easily excreted by the body; this action usually occurs in the liver

bisphosphonates drugs used to block bone resorption and lower serum calcium levels in several conditions

blood dyscrasia bone marrow depression caused by drug effects on the rapidly multiplying cells of the bone marrow; lower-than-normal levels of blood components can be seen

bone marrow suppression inhibition of the blood-forming components of the bone marrow; a common adverse effect of many antineoplastic drugs, which are more effective against rapidly multiplying cells, such as those in bone marrow; also seen in anemia, thrombocytopenia, and leukopenia

bradycardia slower than normal heart rate (usually <60 beats/min)

bradykinesia difficulty in performing intentional movements and extreme slowness and sluggishness; characteristic of Parkinson's disease

brand name name given to a drug by the pharmaceutical company that developed it; also called trade name

bronchial tree the conducting airways leading into the alveoli; they branch smaller and smaller, appearing much like a tree

bronchodilation relaxation of the muscles in the bronchi, resulting in a widening of the bronchi; an effect of sympathetic stimulation

bronchodilator medication used to facilitate respirations by dilating the airways; helpful in symptomatic relief or prevention of bronchial asthma and bronchospasm associated with chronic obstructive pulmonary disease

bulk stimulant agent that increases in bulk, frequently by osmotic pull of fluid into the feces; the increased bulk stretches the GI wall, causing stimulation and increased GI movement

C

calcitonin hormone produced by the parafollicular cells of the thyroid; counteracts the effects of parathyroid hormone to maintain calcium levels

calor heat, one of the four cardinal signs of inflammation; caused by activation of the inflammatory response

Candida fungus that is normally found on mucous membranes; can cause yeast infections or thrush of the GI tract and vagina in immunosuppressed patients

capacitance system the venous system; distensible, flexible veins that are capable of holding large amounts of blood

capillary small vessel made up of loosely connected endothelial cells that connect arteries to veins

carbonic anhydrase a catalyst that speeds up the chemical reaction combining water and carbon dioxide, which react to form carbonic acid and which immediately dissociate to form sodium bicarbonate

carcinoma tumor that originates in epithelial cells

cardiac cycle a period of cardiac muscle relaxation (diastole) followed by a period of contraction (systole) in the heart

cardiac output the amount of blood the heart can pump per beat; influenced by the coordination of cardiac muscle contraction, heart rate, and blood return to the heart

Cardiac Arrhythmia Suppression Test (CAST) a large research study run by the National Heart and Lung Institute that found that long-term treatment of arrhythmias may have a questionable effect on mortality, and in some cases actually lead to increased cardiac death; basis for the current indication for antiarrhythmics (short-term use to treat life-threatening ventricular arrhythmias)

cardiomegaly enlargement of the heart, seen with chronic hypertension, valvular disease, and congestive heart failure

cardiomyopathy a disease of the heart muscle that leads to an enlarged heart and eventually to complete heart muscle failure and death

cardiovascular center area of the medulla at which stimulation will activate the sympathetic nervous system to increase blood pressure, heart rate, and so forth

cathartic dependence overuse of laxatives that can lead to the need for strong stimuli to initiate movement in the intestines; local reflexes become resistant to normal stimuli after prolonged use of harsher stimulants, leading to further laxative use

cell membrane lipoprotein structure that separates the interior of a cell from the external environment; regulates what can enter and leave a cell

cell cycle life cycle of a cell, which includes the phases G_0, G_1, S, G_2, and M; during the M phase, the cell divides into two identical daughter cells

cerebellum lower portion of the brain associated with coordination of muscle movements, including voluntary motion, as well as extrapyramidal control of unconscious muscle movements

cestode tapeworm with a head and segmented body parts that is capable of growing to several yards in the human intestine

chemical name name that reflects the chemical structure of a drug

chemical stimulant agent that stimulates the normal GI reflexes by chemically irritating the lining of the GI wall, leading to increased activity in the GI tract

chemotaxis property of drawing neutrophils to an area

chemotherapeutic agents synthetic chemicals used to interfere with the functioning of foreign cell populations; this term is frequently used to refer to the drug therapy of neoplasms, but it also refers to drug therapy affecting any foreign cell

Cheyne–Stokes respiration abnormal pattern of breathing characterized by apneic periods followed by periods of tachypnea; may reflect delayed blood flow through the brain

cholesterol necessary component of human cells that is produced and processed in the liver, then stored in the bile until stimulus causes the gallbladder to contract and send the bile into the duodenum via the common bile duct; a fat that is essential for the formation of steroid hormones and cell membranes; it is produced in cells and taken in by dietary sources

cholinergic responding to acetylcholine; refers to receptor sites stimulated by acetylcholine, as well as neurons that release acetylcholine

cholinergic receptor receptor sites on effectors that respond to acetylcholine

chronic obstructive pulmonary disease (COPD) chronic condition that occurs over time; often the result of chronic bronchitis or repeated and severe asthma attacks; leads to destruction of the respiratory defense mechanisms and physical structure

chrysotherapy treatment with gold salts; gold is taken up by macrophages, which then inhibit phagocytosis; it is reserved for use in patients who are unresponsive to conventional therapy and can be very toxic

chylomicron carrier for lipids in the bloodstream, consisting of proteins, lipids, cholesterol, and so forth

chyme contents of the stomach containing ingested food and secreted enzymes, water, and mucus

cilia microscopic, hair-like projections of the epithelial cell membrane lining the upper respiratory tract, which are constantly moving and directing the mucus and any trapped substance toward the throat

cinchonism syndrome of quinine toxicity characterized by nausea, vomiting, tinnitus, and vertigo

Clark's Rule a method of determining the correct drug dose for a child based on the known adult dose (assumes that the adult dose is based on a 150-lb person); it states

$$\text{child's dose} = \frac{\text{weight of child (lb)}}{150\text{ lb}} \times \text{average adult dose}$$

clotting factors substances formed in the liver, many requiring vitamin K, that react in a cascading sequence to cause the formation of thrombin from prothrombin; thrombin then breaks down fibrin threads from fibrinogen to form a clot

coagulation the process of blood's changing from a fluid state to a solid state to plug injuries to the vascular system

common cold viral infection of the upper respiratory tract that initiates the release of histamine and prostaglandins and causes an inflammatory response

complement series of cascading proteins that react with the antigen–antibody complex to destroy the protein or stimulate an inflammatory reaction

conductivity property of heart cells to rapidly conduct an action potential of electrical impulse

congestive heart failure (CHF) a condition in which the heart muscle fails to adequately pump blood around the cardiovascular system, leading to a backup or congestion of blood in the system

constipation slower-than-normal evacuation of the large intestine, which can result in increased water absorption from the feces and can lead to impaction

conversion finding the equivalent values between two systems of measure

convulsion tonic–clonic muscular reaction to excessive electrical energy arising from nerve cells in the brain

coronary artery disease (CAD) characterized by progressive narrowing of coronary arteries, leading to a decreased delivery of oxygen to cardiac muscle cells; leading killer of adults in the Western world

corpus luteum remains of follicle that releases mature ovum at ovulation; becomes an endocrine gland producing estrogen and progesterone

corpus striatum part of the brain that reacts with the substantia nigra to maintain a balance of suppression and stimulation

corticosteroids steroid hormones produced by the adrenal cortex; include androgens, glucocorticoids, and mineralocorticoids

cost comparison a comparison of the relative cost of the same drug provided by different manufacturers to determine the costs to the consumer

cough reflex response to irritation in the respiratory membrane, results in expelling of forced air through the mouth

countercurrent mechanism process used by medullary nephrons to concentrate or dilute the urine in response to body stimuli to maintain fluid and electrolyte balance

cretinism lack of thyroid hormone in an infant; if untreated, leads to mental retardation

critical concentration the concentration a drug must reach in the tissues that respond to the particular drug to cause the desired effect

culture sample of the bacteria (e.g., from sputum, cell scrapings, urine) to be grown in a laboratory to determine the species of bacteria that is causing an infection

cycloplegia inability of the lens in the eye to accommodate to near vision, causing blurring and inability to see near objects

cystic fibrosis a hereditary disease that results in the accumulation of copious amounts of very thick secretions in the lungs, which will eventually lead to obstruction of the airways and destruction of the lung tissue

cystitis inflammation of the bladder, caused by infection or irritation

cytomegalovirus (CMV) DNA virus that accounts for many respiratory, ophthalmic, and liver infections

cytoplasm interior of a cell; contains organelles for producing proteins, energy, and so on

D

decongestants drugs that decrease the blood flow to the upper respiratory tract and decrease the overproduction of secretions

dendrite short projection on a neuron that transmits information

depolarization opening of the sodium channels in a nerve membrane to allow the influx of positive sodium ions, reversing the membrane charge from negative to positive

depolarizing neuromuscular junction (NMJ) blocker stimulation of a muscle cell, causing it to contract, with no allowance for repolarization and restimulation of the muscle; characterized by contraction and then paralysis

depression affective disorder in which a person experiences sadness that is much more severe and long-lasting than is warranted by the event that seems to have precipitated it, with a more intense mood; the condition may not even be traceable to a specific event or stressor

dermatological reactions skin reactions commonly seen as adverse effects of drugs; can range from simple rash to potentially fatal exfoliative dermatitis

diabetes insipidus lack of ADH, which results in the production of copious amounts of glucose-free urine

diabetes mellitus a metabolic disorder characterized by high blood glucose levels and altered metabolism of proteins and fats; associated with thickening of the basement membrane, leading to numerous complications

diarrhea more-frequent-than-normal bowel movements, often characterized as fluid-like and watery because not enough time for absorption is allowed during the passage of food through the intestines

diastole resting phase of the heart; blood is returned to the heart during this phase

diffusion movement of solutes from an area of high concentration to an area of low concentration across a concentration gradient

distribution movement of a drug to body tissues; the places where a drug may be distributed depend on the drug's solubility, perfusion of the area, cardiac output, and binding of the drug to plasma proteins

diurnal rhythm response of the hypothalamus and then the pituitary and adrenals to wakefulness and sleeping; normally, the hypothalamus begins secretion of corticotropin-releasing factor (CRF) in the evening, peaking at about midnight; adrenocortical peak response is between 6 and 9 AM; levels fall during the day until evening, when the low level is picked up by the hypothalamus and CRF secretion begins again

dolor pain, one of the four cardinal signs of inflammation; caused by activation of the inflammatory response

dopaminergic drug that increases the effects of dopamine at receptor sites

drug allergy formation of antibodies to a drug or drug protein; causes an immune response when the person is next exposed to that drug

drugs chemicals that are introduced into the body to bring about some sort of change

dwarfism small stature, resulting from lack of growth hormone in children

dyspnea discomfort with respirations, often with a feeling of anxiety and inability to breathe, seen with left-sided CHF

dysrhythmia a disruption in cardiac rate or rhythm, also called an arrhythmia

dysuria painful urination

E

edema movement of fluid into the interstitial spaces; occurs when the balance between osmotic pull (from plasma proteins) and hydrostatic push (from blood pressure) is upset

effector cell stimulated by a nerve; may be a muscle, a gland, or another nerve

efferent neurons or groups of neurons that carry information from the central nervous system to an effector; motor neurons

electrocardiogram (ECG) an electrical tracing reflecting the conduction of an electrical impulse through the heart muscle; does not reflect mechanical activity

emetic agent used to induce vomiting to rid the stomach of toxins or drugs

endocytosis engulfing substances and moving them into a cell by extending the cell membrane around the substance; pinocytosis and phagocytosis are two kinds of endocytosis

engram short-term memory made up of a reverberating electrical circuit of action potentials

epilepsy collection of various syndromes, all of which are characterized by seizures

ergosterol steroid-type protein found in the cell membrane of fungi; similar in configuration to adrenal hormones and testosterone

ergot derivative drug that causes a vascular constriction in the brain and the periphery; relieves or prevents migraine headaches but is associated with many adverse effects

erythrocytes RBCs, responsible for carrying oxygen to the tissues and removing carbon dioxide; have no nucleus and live approximately 120 days

erythropoiesis process of RBC production and life cycle; formed by megaloblastic cells in the bone marrow, using iron, folic acid, carbohydrates, vitamin B_{12}, and amino acids; they circulate in the vascular system for about 120 days, then are lysed and recycled

erythropoietin glycoprotein produced by the kidneys, released in response to decreased blood flow or oxygen tension in the kidney; controls the rate of RBC production in the bone marrow

essential hypertension sustained blood pressure above normal limits with no discernible underlying cause

estrogen hormone produced by the ovary, placenta, and adrenal gland; stimulates development of female characteristics and prepares the body for pregnancy

evaluation part of the nursing process; determining the effects of the interventions that were instituted for the patient and leading to further assessment and implementation

excretion removal of a drug from the body; primarily occurs in the kidneys but can occur through the skin, lungs, bile, or feces

exocytosis removal of substances from a cell by pushing them through the cell membrane

expectorants drugs that increase productive cough to clear the airways

extrapyramidal tract cells from the cortex and subcortical areas, including the basal ganglia and the cerebellum, which coordinate unconsciously controlled muscle activity; allows the body to make automatic adjustments in posture or position and balance

extrinsic pathway cascade of clotting factors in blood that has escaped the vascular system to form a clot on the outside of the injured vessel

F

fertility drugs drugs used to stimulate ovulation and pregnancy in women with functioning ovaries who are having trouble conceiving

fibrillation rapid, irregular stimulation of the cardiac muscle resulting in lack of pumping activity

filtration passage of fluid and small components of the blood through the glomerulus into the nephron tubule

first-pass effect a phenomenon in which drugs given orally are carried directly to the liver after absorption, where they may be largely inactivated by liver enzymes before they can enter the general circulation; oral drugs frequently are given in higher doses than drugs given by other routes because of this early breakdown

flatworms platyhelminths, including the cestodes or tapeworms; a worm that can live in the human intestine or can invade other human tissues (flukes)

fluid rebound reflex reaction of the body to the loss of fluid or sodium; the hypothalamus causes the release of ADH, which retains water, and stress related to fluid loss combines with decreased blood flow to the kidneys to activate the renin–angiotensin system, leading to further water and sodium retention

focal seizure seizure that involves one area of the brain and does not spread throughout the entire brain; also known as a partial seizure

follicle storage site of each ovum in the ovary; allows the ovum to grow and develop, produces estrogen and progesterone

follicles structural unit of the thyroid gland; cells arranged in a circle

Food and Drug Administration (FDA) federal agency responsible for the regulation and enforcement of drug evaluation and distribution policies

forebrain upper level of the brain; consists of the two cerebral hemispheres, where thinking and coordination of sensory and motor activity occur

Fried's Rule a method of determining a pediatric drug dose for a child younger than 1 year of age; based on the child's age and the usual adult dose (assumes that an adult dose would be appropriate for a 12.5-year-old child); it states

$$\text{dose (for child} < 1\text{ yr)} = \frac{\text{infant's age (mo)}}{150\text{ mo}} \times \text{average adult dose}$$

fungus a cellular organism with a hard cell wall that contains chitin and many polysaccharides, as well as a cell membrane that contains ergosterols

G

ganglion (ganglia) a closely packed group of nerve cell bodies

gastrin secreted by the stomach in response to many stimuli; stimulates the release of hydrochloric acid from the parietal cells and pepsin from the chief cells; causes histamine release at histamine-2 receptors to effect the release of acid

gate control theory theory that states that the transmission of a nerve impulse can be modulated at various points along its path by descending fibers from the brain that close the "gate" and block transmission of pain information and by A fibers that are able to block transmission in the dorsal horn by closing the gate for transmission for the A-delta and C fibers

general anesthetic drug that induces a loss of consciousness, amnesia, analgesia, and loss of reflexes to allow performance of painful surgical procedures

generalized seizure seizure that begins in one area of the brain and rapidly spreads throughout both hemispheres

generic drugs drugs sold by their chemical name; not brand (or trade) name products

generic name the original designation that a drug is given when the drug company that developed it applies for the approval process

genetic engineering process of altering DNA, usually of bacteria, to produce a chemical to be used as a drug

giardiasis protozoal intestinal infection that causes severe diarrhea and epigastric distress; may lead to serious malnutrition

gigantism response to excess levels of growth hormone before the epiphyseal plates close; heights of 7 to 8 feet are not uncommon

glomerulus the tuft of blood vessel between the afferent and efferent arterioles in the nephron; the fenestrated membrane of the glomerulus allows filtration of fluid from the blood into the nephron tubule

glucocorticoids steroid hormones released from the adrenal cortex; they increase blood glucose levels, fat deposits, and protein breakdown for energy

glycogen storage form of glucose; can be broken down for rapid glucose level increases during times of stress

glycogenolysis breakdown of stored glucose to increase the blood glucose levels

glycosuria presence of glucose in the urine

glycosylated hemoglobin a blood glucose marker that provides a 3-month average of blood glucose levels

gram-negative bacteria that accept a negative stain and are frequently associated with infections of the genitourinary or GI tract

gram-positive bacteria that take a positive stain and are frequently associated with infections of the respiratory tract and soft tissues

grand mal seizure *see tonic–clonic seizure*

H

Hageman factor first factor activated when a blood vessel or cell is injured; starts the cascading reaction of the clotting factors, activates the conversion of plasminogen to plasmin to dissolve clots, and activates the kinin system responsible for activation of the inflammatory response

half-life the time it takes for the amount of drug in the body to decrease to one-half of the peak level it previously achieved

heart blocks blocks to conduction of an impulse through the cardiac conduction system; can occur at the atrioventricular node, interrupting conduction from the atria into the ventricles, or in the bundle branches within the ventricles, preventing the normal conduction of the impulse

helminth worm that can cause disease by invading the human body

helper T cell human lymphocyte that helps initiate immune reactions in response to tissue invasion

hemodynamics the study of the forces moving blood throughout the cardiovascular system

hemoptysis blood-tinged sputum, seen in left-sided CHF when blood backs up into the lungs and fluid leaks out into the lung tissue

hemorrhagic disorders disorders characterized by a lack of clot-forming substances, leading to states of excessive bleeding

hemostatic drugs drugs that stop blood loss, usually by blocking the plasminogen mechanism and preventing clot dissolution

herpes DNA virus that accounts for many diseases, including shingles, cold sores, genital herpes, and encephalitis

high-ceiling diuretics powerful diuretics that work in the loop of Henle to inhibit the reabsorption of sodium and chloride, leading to a sodium-rich diuresis

high-density lipoprotein (HDL) loosely packed chylomicron containing fats, able to absorb fats and fat remnants in the periphery; thought to have a protective effect, decreasing the development of CAD

hindbrain most primitive area of the brain, the brainstem; consists of the pons and medulla, which control basic, vital functions and arousal, and the cerebellum, which controls motor functions that regulate balance

hirsutism hair distribution associated with male secondary sex characteristics (e.g., increased hair on trunk, arms, legs, face)

histamine-2 (H_2) antagonist drug that blocks the H_2 receptor sites; used to decrease acid production in the stomach (H_2 sites are stimulated to cause the release of acid in response to gastrin or parasympathetic stimulation)

histamine-2 (H_2) receptors sites near the parietal cells of the stomach which, when stimulated, cause the release of hydrochloric acid into the lumen of the stomach; also found near cardiac cells

histocompatibility antigens proteins found on the surface of the cell membrane, which are determined by genetic code; provide cellular identity as self-cell

HMG-CoA reductase enzyme that regulates the last step in cellular cholesterol synthesis

hormones chemical messengers working within the endocrine system to communicate within the body

human immunodeficiency virus (HIV) retrovirus that attacks helper T cells, leading to a decrease in immune function and AIDS or ARC

hydrochloric acid acid released by the parietal cells of the stomach in response to gastrin release or parasympathetic stimulation; makes the stomach contents more acidic to aid digestion and breakdown of food products

hyperaldosteronism excessive output of aldosterone from the adrenal gland, leading to increased sodium and water retention and loss of potassium

hyperglycemia elevated blood glucose levels (>110 mg/dL) leading to multiple signs and symptoms and abnormal metabolic pathways

hyperlipidemia increased levels of lipids in the serum, associated with increased risk of CAD development

hyperparathyroidism excessive parathormone

hypersensitivity excessive responsiveness to either the primary or the secondary effects of a drug; may be caused by a pathological or individual condition

hyperthyroidism excessive levels of thyroid hormone

hypertonia state of excessive muscle response and activity

hypnosis extreme sedation resulting in CNS depression and sleep

hypnotic drug used to depress the CNS; causes sleep

hypocalcemia calcium deficiency

hypoglycemia lower than normal blood sugar (<40 mg/dL); often results from imbalance between insulin or oral agents and patient's eating, activity, and stress

hypogonadism underdevelopment of the gonads (testes in the male)

hypokalemia low potassium in the blood, which often occurs after diuretic use; characterized by weakness, muscle cramps, trembling, nausea, vomiting, diarrhea, and cardiac arrhythmias

hypoparathyroidism rare condition of absence of parathormone; may be seen after thyroidectomy
hypopituitarism lack of adequate function of the pituitary; reflected in many endocrine disorders
hypotension sustained blood pressure that is lower than that required to adequately perfuse all of the body's tissues
hypothalamic–pituitary axis interconnection of the hypothalamus and pituitary to regulate the levels of certain endocrine hormones through a complex series of negative feedback systems
hypothalamus "master gland" of the neuroendocrine system; regulates both nervous and endocrine responses to internal and external stimuli
hypothyroidism lack of sufficient thyroid hormone to maintain metabolism

I

immune stimulant drug used to energize the immune system when it is exhausted from fighting prolonged invasion or needs help fighting a specific pathogen or cancer cell
immune suppressant drug used to block or suppress the actions of the T cells and antibody production; used to prevent transplant rejection and to treat autoimmune diseases
immune sera preformed antibodies found in immune globulin from animals or humans who have had a specific disease and developed antibodies to it
immunization the process of stimulating active immunity by exposing the body to weakened or less toxic proteins associated with specific disease-causing organisms; the goal is to stimulate immunity without causing the full course of a disease
induction time from the beginning of anesthesia until achievement of surgical anesthesia
influenza A RNA virus that invades tissues of the respiratory tract, causing the signs and symptoms of the common cold or "flu"
inhibin estrogen-like substance produced by seminiferous tubules during sperm production; acts as a negative feedback stimulus to decrease release of follicle-stimulating hormone (FSH)
insulin hormone produced by the beta cells in the pancreas; stimulates insulin receptor sites to move glucose into the cells; promotes storage of fat and glucose in the body
interferon tissue hormone that is released in response to viral invasion; blocks viral replication
interleukins chemicals released by white blood cells (WBCs) to communicate with other WBCs and to support the inflammatory and immune reactions
Internet the world-wide digital information system accessed through computer systems
interneuron neuron in the CNS that communicates with other neurons, not with muscles or glands
interstitial or Leydig cells part of the testes that produce testosterone in response to stimulation by luteinizing hormone (LH)
interstitial cystitis chronic inflammation of the interstitial connective tissue of the bladder; may extend into deeper tissue
intervention action undertaken to meet a patient's needs, such as administration of drugs, comfort measures, or patient teaching
intractable hiccough repetitive stimulation of the diaphragm that leads to hiccough, a diaphragmatic spasm that persists over time
intrinsic pathway cascade of clotting factors leading to the formation of a clot within an injured vessel
iodine important dietary element used by the thyroid gland to produce thyroid hormone
iron deficiency anemia low RBC count with low iron available because of high demand, poor diet, or poor absorption; treated with iron replacement

K

ketosis breakdown of fats for energy, resulting in an increase in ketones to be excreted from the body
kinin system system activated by Hageman factor as part of the inflammatory response; includes bradykinin

L

larynx the vocal chords and the epiglottis, which close during swallowing to protect the lower respiratory tract from any foreign particles
leishmaniasis skin, mucous membrane, or visceral infection caused by a protozoan passed to humans by the bites of sand flies
leukocytes WBCs; can be neutrophils, basophils, or eosinophils
leukotriene receptor antagonists drugs that selectively and competitively block or antagonize receptors for the production of leukotrienes D_4 and E_4, components of slow-reacting substance of anaphylaxis (SRSA)
levothyroxine a synthetic salt of thyroxine (T_4), a thyroid hormone, the most frequently used replacement hormone for treating thyroid disease
limbic system area in the midbrain that is rich in epinephrine, norepinephrine, and serotonin and seems to control emotions
liothyronine (T3) the most potent thyroid hormone, with a short half-life of 12 hours
lipoprotein structure composed of proteins and lipids; bipolar arrangement of the lipids monitors substances passing in and out of the cell
local gastrointestinal reflex reflex response to various stimuli that allows the GI tract local control of its secretions and movements based on the contents or activity of the whole GI system
local anesthetic powerful nerve blocker that prevents depolarization of nerve membranes, blocking the transmission of pain stimuli and, in some cases, motor activity
low-density lipoprotein (LDL) tightly packed fats that are thought to contribute to the development of CAD when

remnants left over from the LDL are processed in the arterial lining

lower respiratory tract the smallest bronchi and the alveoli that make up the lungs; the area where gas exchange takes place

lubricant agent that increases the viscosity of the feces, making it difficult to absorb water from the bolus and easing movement of the bolus through the intestines

lymphocytes white blood cells with large, varied nuclei; can be T cells or B cells

lysosomes encapsulated digestive enzymes found within a cell; they digest old or damaged areas of the cell and are responsible for destroying the cell when the membrane ruptures and the cell dies

M

macrophages mature leukocytes that are capable of phagocytizing an antigen (foreign protein); also called monocytes or mononuclear phagocytes

major tranquilizer former name of antipsychotic drugs; no longer used because it implies that its primary effect is sedation, which is no longer thought to be the desired therapeutic action

malaria protozoal infection with *Plasmodium*, characterized by cyclic fever and chills as the parasite is released from ruptured red blood cells; causes serious liver, CNS, heart, and lung damage

malignant hyperthermia reaction to some NMJ drugs in susceptible individuals; characterized by extreme muscle rigidity, severe hyperpyrexia, acidosis, and in some cases death

mania state of hyperexcitability; one phase of bipolar disorders, which alternate between periods of severe depression and mania

mast cell stabilizer drug that works at the cellular level to inhibit the release of histamine (released from mast cells in response to inflammation or irritation) and the release of slow-reacting SRSA

megaloblastic anemia anemia caused by lack of vitamin B_{12} and/or folic acid, in which RBCs are fewer in number and have a weak stroma and a short lifespan; treated by replacement of folic acid and vitamin B_{12}

menopause depletion of the female ova; results in lack of estrogen and progesterone

menstrual cycle cycling of female sex hormones in interaction with the hypothalamus and anterior pituitary feedback systems

metabolism rate at which the cells burn energy

metastasis ability to enter the circulatory or lymphatic system and travel to other areas of the body that are conducive to growth and survival; property of cancer cells

metric system the most widely used system of measure, based on the decimal system; all units in the system are determined as multiples of ten

midbrain the middle area of the brain; it consists of the hypothalamus and thalamus and includes the limbic system

migraine headache headache characterized by severe, unilateral, pulsating head pain associated with systemic effects, including GI upset and sensitization to light and sound; related to a hyperperfusion of the brain from arterial dilation

mineralocorticoids steroid hormones released by the adrenal cortex; they cause sodium and water retention and potassium excretion

miosis constriction of the pupil; relieves intraocular pressure in some types of glaucoma

mitochondria rod-shaped organelles; they produce adenosine triphosphate (ATP) for energy within the cell

monoamine oxidase (MAO) enzyme that breaks down norepinephrine to make it inactive

monoamine oxidase inhibitor (MAOI) drug that prevents the enzyme monoamine oxidase from breaking down norepinephrine (NE), leading to increased NE levels in the synaptic cleft; relieves depression and also causes sympathomimetic effects

monoclonal antibodies specific antibodies produced by a single clone of B cells to react with a very specific antigen

mucolytics drugs that increase or liquefy respiratory secretions to aid the clearing of the airways

muscarinic receptors cholinergic receptors that also respond to stimulation by muscarine

myasthenia gravis autoimmune disease characterized by antibodies to cholinergic receptor sites, leading to destruction of the receptor sites and decreased response at the neuromuscular junction; it is progressive and debilitating, leading to paralysis

mycosis disease caused by a fungus

mydriasis relaxation of the muscles around the pupil, leading to pupil dilation

myelocytes leukocyte-producing cells in the bone marrow that can develop into neutrophils, basophils, eosinophils, monocytes, or macrophages

myocardial infarction end result of vessel blockage in the heart; leads to ischemia and then necrosis of the area cut off from the blood supply; it can heal, with the dead cells replaced by scar tissue

myocardium the muscle of the heart

myosin thick filament with projections that makes up a sarcomere or muscle unit

myxedema severe lack of thyroid hormone in adults

N

narcolepsy mental disorder characterized by daytime sleepiness and periods of sudden loss of wakefulness

narcotic agonists–antagonists drugs that react at some opioid receptor sites to stimulate their activity and at other opioid receptor sites to block activity

narcotic agonists drugs that react at opioid receptor sites to stimulate the effects of the receptors

narcotic antagonists drugs that block the opioid receptor sites; used to counteract the effects of narcotics or to treat an overdose of narcotics

narcotics drugs, originally derived from opium, that react with specific opioid receptors throughout the body

negative feedback system control system in which increasing levels of a hormone lead to decreased levels of releasing and stimulating hormones, leading to decreased hormone levels, which stimulates the release of releasing and stimulating hormones; allows tight control of the endocrine system

nematode a roundworm such as the commonly encountered pinworm, whipworm, threadworm, *Ascaris*, or hookworm

neoplasm new or cancerous growth; occurs when abnormal cells have the opportunity to multiply and grow

nephron functional unit of the kidney, composed of Bowman's capsule, the proximal and distal convoluted tubules, and the collecting duct

nerve gas irreversible acetylcholinesterase inhibitor used in warfare to cause paralysis and death by prolonged muscle contraction and parasympathetic crisis

nerve plexus network of nerve fibers running through the wall of the GI tract that allows local reflexes and control

neuroendocrine system the combination of the nervous and endocrine systems, which work closely together to maintain regulatory control and homeostasis in the body

neuroleptic a drug with many associated neurological adverse effects that is used to treat disorders that involve thought processes (e.g., schizophrenia)

neuron structural unit of the nervous system

neurotransmitter chemical produced by a nerve and released when the nerve is stimulated; reacts with a specific receptor site to cause a reaction

nicotinic receptors cholinergic receptors that also respond to stimulation by nicotine

nitrates drugs used to cause direct relaxation of smooth muscle, leading to vasodilation and decreased venous return to the heart with decreased resistance to blood flow; this rapidly decreases oxygen demand in the heart and can restore the balance between blood delivered and blood needed in the heart muscle of patients with angina

nocturia getting up to void at night, reflecting increased renal perfusion with fluid shifts in the supine position when a person has gravity-dependent edema related to CHF; other medical conditions, including urinary tract infection, increase the need to get up and void

nondepolarizing neuromuscular junction (NMJ) blocker no stimulation or depolarization of the muscle cell; prevents depolarization and stimulation by blocking the effects of acetylcholine

nonsteroidal anti-inflammatory drugs (NSAIDs) drugs that block prostaglandin synthesis and act as anti-inflammatory, antipyretic, and analgesic agents

nucleosides drugs that inhibit cell protein synthesis by HIV, leading to viral death

nucleus the part of a cell that contains the DNA and genetic material; regulates cellular protein production and cellular properties

nursing the art of nurturing and administering to the sick combined with the scientific application of chemistry, anatomy, physiology, biology, nutrition, psychology, and pharmacology to the particular clinical situation

nursing diagnosis statement of an actual or potential problem, based on the assessment of a particular clinical situation, which directs needed nursing interventions

nursing process the problem-solving process used to provide efficient nursing care; it involves gathering information, formulating a nursing diagnosis statement, carrying out interventions, and evaluating the process

O

off-label uses uses of a drug that are not part of the stated therapeutic indications for which the drug was approved by the FDA

oncotic pressure the pulling pressure of the plasma proteins, responsible for returning fluid to the vascular system at the capillary level

opioid receptors receptor sites on nerves that react with endorphins and enkephalins, which are receptive to narcotic drugs

organelles distinct structures found within the cell cytoplasm

orphan drugs drugs that have been discovered but are not available for use by those who could benefit from them, usually because they are not financially profitable

orthopnea difficulty breathing when lying down, often referred to by the number of pillows required to allow a person to breath comfortably

osmosis movement of water from an area of low solute concentration to an area of high solute concentration in an attempt to equalize the concentrations

osmotic pull drawing force of large molecules on water, pulling it into a tubule or capillary; essential for maintaining normal fluid balance within the body; used to draw out excess fluid into the vascular system or the renal tubule

OTC drugs see *over-the-counter (OTC) drugs*

ova eggs; the female gamete; contain half of the information needed in a human nucleus

ovaries female sexual glands that store ova and produce estrogen and progesterone

over-the-counter (OTC) drugs drugs that are available without a prescription for self-treatment of a variety of complaints

oxytocics drugs that act like the hypothalamic hormone oxytocin; they stimulate uterine contraction and contraction of the lacteal glands in the breast, promoting milk ejection

P

Paget's disease a genetically linked disorder of overactive osteoclasts that are eventually replaced by enlarged and softened bony structures

pancreatic enzymes digestive enzymes secreted by the exocrine pancreas, including pancreatin and pancrelipase, which are needed for the proper digestion of fats, proteins, and carbohydrates

paralysis lack of muscle function

parasympathetic nervous system "rest and digest" response mediator that contains CNS cells from the cranium or sacral area of the spinal cord, long preganglionic axons, ganglia near or within the effector tissue, and short postganglionic axons that react with cholinergic receptors

parasympatholytic lysing or preventing parasympathetic effects

parasympathomimetic mimicking the effects of the parasympathetic nervous system bradycardia, hypotension, pupil constriction, increased GI secretions and activity, increased bladder tone, relaxation of sphincters, bronchoconstriction

parathormone hormone produced by the parathyroid glands; responsible for maintaining calcium levels in conjunction with calcitonin

Parkinson's disease debilitating disease, characterized by progressive loss of coordination and function, which results from the degeneration of dopamine-producing cells in the substantia nigra

partial seizures also called focal seizures; seizures involving one area of the brain that do not spread throughout the entire organ

passive diffusion movement of substances across a semipermeable membrane with the concentration gradient; this process does not require energy

passive immunity the injection of preformed antibodies into a host at high risk for exposure to a specific disease; immunity is limited by the amount of circulating antibody

penile erectile dysfunction condition in which the corpus cavernosum does not fill with blood to allow for penile erection; can be related to aging or to neurological or vascular conditions

peptic ulcer erosion of the lining of stomach or duodenum; results from imbalance between acid produced and the mucous protection of the GI lining, or possibly from infection by *Helicobacter pylori* bacteria

peripheral resistance force that resists the flow of blood through the vessels, mostly determined by the arterioles, which contract to increase resistance; important in determining overall blood pressure

peristalsis type of GI movement that moves a food bolus forward; characterized by a progressive wave of muscle contraction

pernicious anemia megaloblastic anemia characterized by lack of vitamin B_{12} secondary to low production of intrinsic factor by gastric cells; vitamin B_{12} must be replaced by intramuscular injection or nasal spray because it cannot be absorbed through the GI tract

petit mal seizure see *absence seizure*

phagocytes neutrophils that are able to engulf and digest foreign material

phagocytosis the process of engulfing and digesting foreign material

pharmacodynamics the science that deals with the interactions between the chemical components of living systems and the foreign chemicals, including drugs, that enter living organisms; the way a drug affects a body

pharmacogenomics the study of genetically determined variations in the response to drugs

pharmacokinetics the way the body deals with a drug, including absorption, distribution, biotransformation, and excretion

pharmacology the study of the biological effects of chemicals

pharmacotherapeutics clinical pharmacology, the branch of pharmacology that deals with drugs; chemicals that are used in medicine for the treatment, prevention, and diagnosis of disease in humans

phase I study a pilot study of a potential drug done with a small number of selected, healthy human volunteers

phase II study a clinical study of a drug by selected physicians using actual patients who have the disorder the drug is designed to treat; patients must provide informed consent

phase III study use of a drug on a wide scale in the clinical setting with patients who have the disease the drug is thought to treat

phase IV study continual evaluation of a drug after it has been released for marketing

phenothiazine antianxiety drug that blocks the responsiveness of the CTZ to stimuli, leading to a decrease in nausea and vomiting

pheochromocytoma a tumor of the chromaffin cells of the adrenal medulla that periodically releases large amounts of norepinephrine and epinephrine into the system with resultant severe hypertension and tachycardia

photosensitivity hypersensitive reaction to the sun or ultraviolet light, seen as an adverse reaction to various drugs; can lead to severe skin rash and lesions as well as damage to the eye

pinworm nematode that causes a common helminthic infection in humans; lives in the intestine and causes anal and possible vaginal irritation and itching

pituitary gland gland found in the sella turcica of the brain; produces hormones, endorphins, and enkephalins and stores two hypothalamic hormones

placebo effect documented effect of the mind on drug therapy; if a person perceives that a drug will be effective, the drug is much more likely to actually be effective

plasma the liquid part of the blood; consists mostly of water and plasma proteins, glucose, and electrolytes

plasma esterase enzyme found in plasma that immediately breaks down ester-type local anesthetics

plasminogen natural clot-dissolving system; converted to plasmin (also called fibrinolysin) by many substances to dissolve clots that have formed and to maintain the patency of injured vessels

Plasmodium a protozoan that causes malaria in humans; its life cycle includes the *Anopheles* mosquito, which injects protozoa into humans

platelet aggregation property of platelets to adhere to an injured surface and then attract other platelets, which clump together or aggregate at the area, plugging up an injury to the vascular system

platyhelminth flatworm or fluke such as the tapeworm

***Pneumocystis carinii* pneumonia (PCP)** opportunistic infection that occurs when the immune system is depressed; a frequent cause of pneumonia in patients with AIDS and in those who are receiving immunosuppressive therapy

pneumonia inflammation of the lungs that can be caused by bacterial or viral invasion of the tissue or by aspiration of foreign substances

poisoning overdose of a drug that causes damage to multiple body systems and the potential for fatal reactions

polydipsia increased thirst; seen in diabetes when loss of fluid and increased tonicity of the blood lead the hypothalamic thirst center to make the patient feel thirsty

polyphagia increased hunger; sign of diabetes when cells cannot use glucose for energy and feel that they are starving, causing hunger

positively inotropic causing an increased force of contraction

posterior pituitary lobe of the pituitary that receives ADH and oxytocin via neuraxons from the hypothalamus and stores them to be released when stimulated by the hypothalamus

postmenopausal osteoporosis dropping levels of estrogen allow calcium to be pulled out of the bone, resulting in a weakened and honeycombed bone structure

preclinical trial initial trial of a chemical thought to have therapeutic potential; uses laboratory animals, not human subjects

premature atrial contraction (PAC) caused by an ectopic focus in the atria that stimulates an atrial response

premature ventricular contraction (PVC) caused by an ectopic focus in the ventricles that stimulates the cells and causes an early contraction

Prinzmetal's angina drop in blood flow through the coronary arteries caused by a vasospasm in the artery, not by atherosclerosis

proarrhythmic tending to cause arrhythmias; many of the drugs used to treat arrhythmias have been found to generate arrhythmias

progesterone hormone produced by the ovary, placenta, and adrenal gland; promotes maintenance of pregnancy

progestin female sex hormone; important in maintaining a pregnancy and supporting many secondary sex characteristics

prophylaxis treatment to prevent an infection before it occurs, as in the use of antibiotics to prevent bacterial endocarditis or antiprotozoals to prevent malaria

prostaglandin any one of numerous tissue hormones that have local effects on various systems and organs of the body, including vasoconstriction, vasodilation, increased or decreased GI activity, and increased or decreased pancreatic enzyme release

prostate gland gland located around the male urethra; responsible for producing an acidic fluid that maintains sperm and lubricates the urinary tract

protease inhibitors drugs that block the activity of the enzyme protease in HIV; protease is essential for the maturation of infectious virus, and its absence leads to the formation of an immature and noninfective HIV particle

proton pump inhibitor drug that blocks the H^+, K^+-ATPase enzyme system on the secretory surface of the gastric parietal cells, thus interfering with the final step of acid production and lowering acid levels in the stomach

protozoan a single-celled organism that passes through several stages in its life cycle, including at least one phase as a human parasite; found in areas of poor sanitation and hygiene and crowded living conditions

puberty point at which the hypothalamus starts releasing gonadotropin-releasing factor (GnRF) to stimulate the release of FSH and LH and begin sexual development

pulmonary edema severe left-sided CHF with backup of blood into the lungs, leading to loss of fluid into the lung tissue

pulse pressure the systolic blood pressure minus the diastolic blood pressure; reflects the filling pressure of the coronary arteries

pyelonephritis inflammation of the pelves of the kidney, frequently caused by backward flow problems or by bacteria ascending the ureter

pyramidal tract fibers within the CNS that control precise, intentional movement

pyrogen substance that resets the thermoregulatory center in the hypothalamus to elevate the body temperature, thus speeding metabolism; some pyrogens are released by active neutrophils as part of the inflammatory response

R

ratio and proportion an equation in which the ratio containing two known equivalent amounts is on one side of the equation and the ratio containing the amount desired to convert and its unknown equivalent is on the other side

reabsorption the movement of substances from the renal tubule back into the vascular system

rebound congestion occurs when the nasal passages become congested as the effect of a decongestant drug wears off; patients tend to use more drug to decrease the congestion and a vicious circle of congestion, drug, and congestion develops, leading to abuse of the decongestant; also called rhinitis medicamentosa

receptor sites sites on cell membranes that react with specific other chemicals to cause an effect; a drug may be effective because it reacts with a specific receptor site on particular cells in the body

recombinant DNA technology use of bacteria to produce chemicals normally produced by human cells

releasing hormones or factors chemicals released by the hypothalamus into the anterior pituitary to stimulate the release of anterior pituitary hormones

renin–angiotensin system compensatory process that leads to increased blood pressure and blood volume to ensure perfusion of the kidneys; important in the day-to-day regulation of blood pressure

repolarization return of a membrane to a resting state, with more sodium ions outside the membrane and a relatively negative charge inside the membrane

resistance ability of bacteria over time to adapt to an antibiotic and produce cells that are no longer affected by a particular drug

resistance system the arteries; the muscles of the arteries provide resistance to the flow of blood, leading to control of blood pressure

respiration the act of breathing

respiratory distress syndrome (RDS) disorder found in premature neonates whose lungs have not had time to mature and who are lacking sufficient surfactant to maintain open airways to allow for respiration

respiratory membrane area through which gas exchange must be made; made up of the capillary endothelium, the capillary basement membrane, the interstitial space, the alveolar basement membrane, the alveolar endothelium, and the surfactant layer

reticulocyte red blood cell (RBC) that has lost its nucleus and entered circulation just recently, not yet fully matured

reverse transcriptase inhibitors drugs that block the transfer of both RNA- and DNA-dependent DNA polymerase activities; prevents the transfer of information that allows the virus to replicate and survive

rhinitis medicamentosa reflex reaction to vasoconstriction caused by decongestants; a rebound vasodilation that often leads to prolonged overuse of decongestants; also called rebound congestion

ribosomes membranous structures that are the sites of protein production within a cell

risk factors factors that have been identified to increase the risk of the development of a disease; for CAD, risk factors include genetic predisposition, gender, age, high-fat diet, sedentary lifestyle, gout, hypertension, diabetes, and estrogen deficiency

roundworm worm such as *Ascaris* that causes a common helminthic infection in humans; can cause intestinal obstruction as the adult worms clog the intestinal lumen or severe pneumonia when the larvae migrate to the lungs and form a pulmonary infiltrate

rubor redness, one of the four cardinal signs of inflammation; caused by activation of the inflammatory response

S

salicylates salicylic acid compounds, used as anti-inflammatory, antipyretic, and analgesic agents; they block the prostaglandin system

saliva fluid produced by the salivary glands in the mouth in response to tactile stimuli and cerebral stimulation; contains enzymes to begin digestion as well as water and mucus to make the food bolus slippery and easier to swallow

sarcoma tumor that originates in the mesenchyme and is made up of embryonic connective tissue cells

sarcomere functional unit of a muscle cell, composed of actin and myosin molecules arranged in layers to give the unit a striped or striated appearance

schistosomiasis infection with a blood fluke that is carried by a snail; it poses a common problem in tropical countries, where the snail is the intermediary in the life cycle of the worm; larvae burrow into the skin in fresh water and migrate throughout the human body, causing a rash and then symptoms of diarrhea and liver and brain inflammation

schizophrenia the most common type of psychosis; characteristics include hallucinations, paranoia, delusions, speech abnormalities, and affective problems

Schwann cell insulating cell found on nerve axons; allows "leaping" electrical conduction to speed the transmission of information and prevent tiring of the neuron

seasonal rhinitis inflammation of the nasal cavity, commonly called hay fever; caused by reaction to a specific antigen

secretion the active movement of substances from the blood into the renal tubule

sedation loss of awareness of and reaction to environmental stimuli

sedative drug that depresses the CNS; produces a loss of awareness of and reaction to the environment

segmentation GI movement characterized by contraction of one segment of small intestine while the next segment is relaxed; the contracted segment then relaxes, and the relaxed segment contracts; exposes the chyme to a vast surface area to increase absorption

seizure sudden discharge of excessive electrical energy from nerve cells in the brain

selective serotonin reuptake inhibitor (SSRI) drug that specifically blocks the reuptake of serotonin and increases its concentration in the synaptic cleft; relieves depression and is not associated with anticholinergic or sympathomimetic adverse effects

selective toxicity property of a chemotherapeutic agent that affects only systems found in foreign cells, without affecting healthy human cells (e.g., specific antibiotics can affect certain proteins or enzyme systems used by bacteria but not by human cells)

self-care tendency for patients to self-diagnose and determine their own treatment needs

seminiferous tubules part of the testes that produce sperm in response to stimulation by FSH

sensitivity testing evaluation of bacteria obtained in a culture to determine to which antibiotics the organisms are sensitive to and which agent would be appropriate for treatment of a particular infection

serum sickness reaction of a host to injected antibodies or foreign sera; host cells make antibodies to the foreign proteins, and a massive immune reaction can occur

shock severe hypotension that can lead to accumulation of waste products and cell death

sinoatrial (SA) node the normal pacemaker of the heart; composed of primitive cells that constantly generate an action potential

sinuses air-filled passages through the skull that open into the nasal passage

sinusitis inflammation of the epithelial lining of the sinus cavities

sliding filament theory theory explaining muscle contraction as a reaction of actin and myosin molecules when they are freed to react by the inactivation of troponin after calcium is allowed to enter the cell during depolarization

sneeze reflex response to irritation in the nasal passages; results in expelling of forced air through the nose

soma cell body of a neuron; contains the nucleus, cytoplasm, and various granules

spasticity sustained muscle contractions

spectrum range of bacteria against which an antibiotic is effective (e.g., broad-spectrum antibiotics are effective against a wide range of bacteria)

sperm male gamete; contains half of the information needed for a human cell nucleus

spinothalamic tract nerve pathway from the spine to the thalamus along which pain impulses are carried to the brain

Starling's law of the heart addresses the contractile properties of the heart: the more the muscle is stretched, the stronger it will react, until it is stretched to a point at which it will not react at all

status epilepticus state in which seizures rapidly recur; most severe form of generalized seizure

stomatitis inflammation of the mucous membranes related to drug effects; can lead to alterations in nutrition and dental problems

street drugs nonprescription drugs with no known therapeutic use; used to enhance mood or increase pleasure

stroke volume the amount of blood pumped out of the ventricle with each beat; important in determining blood pressure

substantia nigra a part of the brain rich in dopamine and dopamine receptors; site of degenerating neurons in Parkinson's disease

sulfonylureas oral antidiabetic agents used to stimulate the pancreas to release more insulin

superinfections infections caused by the destruction of bacteria of the normal flora by certain drugs, which allows other bacteria to enter the body and cause infection; may occur during the course of antibiotic therapy

surfactant lipoprotein that reduces surface tension in the alveoli, allowing them to stay open to allow gas exchange

swallowing complex reflex response to a bolus in the back of the throat; allows passage of the bolus into the esophagus and movement of ingested contents into the GI tract

sympathetic nervous system "fight or flight" response mediator; composed of CNS cells from the thoracic or lumbar areas, short preganglionic axons, ganglia near the spinal cord, and long postganglionic axons that react with adrenergic receptors

sympatholytic a drug that lyses, or blocks, the effects of the sympathetic nervous system

sympathomimetic mimicking of the sympathetic nervous system (SNS) with the signs and symptoms seen when the SNS is stimulated

sympathomimetics drugs that mimic the effects of the sympathetic nervous system

synapse junction between a nerve and an effector; consists of the presynaptic nerve ending, a space called the synaptic cleft, and the postsynaptic cell

syncytium intertwining network of muscle fibers that make up the atria and the ventricles of the heart; allows for a coordinated pumping contraction

synergistic drugs that work together to increase drug effectiveness

systole contracting phase of the heart, during which blood is pumped out of the heart

T

T cells lymphocytes programmed in the thymus gland to recognize self-cells; may be effector T cells, helper T cells, or suppressor T cells

tachycardia faster than normal heart rate (usually >100 beats/min)

tachypnea rapid and shallow respirations, seen with left-sided CHF

teratogenic having adverse effects on the fetus

testes male sexual gland that produces sperm and testosterone

testosterone male sex hormone; produced by the interstitial or Leydig cells of the testes

thiazide type of diuretic acting in the renal tubule to block the chloride pump, which prevents reabsorption of sodium and chloride, leading to a loss of sodium and water in the urine

thioamides drugs used to prevent the formation of thyroid hormone in the thyroid cells, lowering thyroid hormone levels

threadworm pervasive nematode that can send larvae into the lungs, liver, and CNS; can cause severe pneumonia or liver abscess

thromboembolic disorders disorders characterized by the formation of clots or thrombi on injured blood vessels with potential breaking of the clot to form emboli that can travel to smaller vessels, where they become lodged and occlude the vessel

thrombolytic drugs drugs that lyse, or break down, a clot that has formed; these drugs activate the plasminogen mechanism to dissolve fibrin threads

thyroxine (T_4) a thyroid hormone that is converted to triiodothyronine (T_3) in the tissues; it has a half-life of 1 week

tinea fungus called ringworm that causes such infections as athlete's foot, jock itch, and others

tocolytics drugs used to relax the gravid uterus to prolong pregnancy

tonic–clonic seizure type of generalized seizure that is characterized by serious clonic–tonic muscular reactions and loss of consciousness, with exhaustion and little memory of the event on awakening; formerly known as a grand mal seizure

trachea the main conducting airway leading into the lungs

trichinosis disease that results from ingestion of encysted roundworm larvae in undercooked pork; larvae migrate throughout the body to invade muscles, nerves, and other tissues; can cause pneumonia, heart failure, and encephalitis

trichomoniasis infestation with a protozoan that causes vaginitis in women but no signs or symptoms in men

tricyclic antidepressant (TCA) drug that blocks the reuptake of norepinephrine and serotonin; relieves depression and has anticholinergic and sedative effects

triptan selective serotonin receptor blocker that causes a vascular constriction of cranial vessels; used to treat acute migraine attacks

trophozoite a developing stage of a parasite, which uses the host for essential nutrients needed for growth

troponin chemical in heart muscle that prevents the reaction between actin and myosin, leading to muscle relaxation; it is inactivated by calcium during muscle stimulation to allow actin and myosin to react, causing muscle contraction

trypanosomiasis African sleeping sickness, which is caused by a protozoan that inflames the CNS and is spread to humans by the bite of the tsetse fly; also, Chagas' disease, which causes a serious cardiomyopathy after the bite of the house fly

tumor swelling, one of the four cardinal signs of inflammation; caused by activation of the inflammatory response

tyramine an amine found in food that causes vasoconstriction and raises blood pressure; ingesting foods high in tyramine while taking an MAOI poses the risk of a severe hypertensive crisis

U

unconsciousness loss of awareness of one's surroundings

upper respiratory tract the conducting airways, composed of the nose, mouth, pharynx, larynx, trachea, and upper bronchial tree

urgency the feeling that one needs to void immediately; associated with infection and inflammation in the urinary tract

urinary frequency the need to void often; usually seen in response to irritation of the bladder, age, and inflammation

uterus the womb; site of growth and development of the embryo and fetus

V

vaccine immunization containing weakened or altered protein antigens to stimulate a specific antibody formation against a specific disease; refers to a product used to stimulate active immunity

veins vessels that return blood to the heart; distensible tubes

ventilation the exchange of gases at the alveolar level across the respiratory membrane

ventricle bottom chamber of the heart, which contracts to pump blood out of the heart

vestibular referring to the apparatus of the inner ear that controls balance and sense of motion; stimulus to this area can cause motion sickness

virus particle of DNA or RNA surrounded by a protein coat that survives by invading a cell to alter its functioning

volatile liquid liquid that is unstable at room temperature and releases vapors; used as an inhaled general anesthetic, usually in the form of a halogenated hydrocarbon

vomiting complex reflex mediated through the medulla after stimulation of the CTZ; protective reflex to remove possibly toxic substances from the stomach

W

whipworm worm that attaches itself to the intestinal mucosa and sucks blood; may cause severe anemia and disintegration of the intestinal mucosa

X

xanthines naturally occurring substances, including caffeine and theophylline, that have a direct effect on the smooth muscle of the respiratory tract, both in the bronchi and in the blood vessels

Y

Young's rule a method for determining pediatric drug dosage based on the child's age and the usual adult dose; it states

$$\text{dose (child 1–12 yr)} = \frac{\text{child's age (yr)}}{\text{child's age (yr)} + 12} \times \text{average adult dose}$$

Answer Key

Chapter 1

Multiple Choice

1. b 2. d 3. c 4. c 5. a 6. d 7. b 8. c

Multiple Response

1. c, d, e, f
2. a, c, d, f

Matching

1. G 2. F 3. A 4. H 5. E 6. I 7. C 8. J 9. B 10. D

Chapter 2

Multiple Choice

1. c 2. b 3. d 4. b 5. c 6. a 7. a

Multiple Response

1. c, g
2. a, d, e, f
3. b, e, f

Word Scramble

1. biotransformation
2. distribution
3. placebo
4. excretion
5. pharmacokinetics
6. receptor site
7. half-life
8. pharmacotherapeutics

Fill in the Blanks

1. pharmacodynamics
2. pharmacokinetics
3. chemotherapeutic agents
4. critical concentration
5. absorption, biotransformation, distribution, excretion
6. first-pass effect
7. enzyme induction
8. half-life

Chapter 3

Multiple Choice

1. c 2. d 3. b 4. d 5. b 6. c

Multiple Response

1. a, b, f
2. a, b, c, d, e, f
3. a, b, e, f
4. b, c, d, e

Matching

1. e 2. c 3. a 4. f 5. b 6. d

Fill in the Blanks

1. gentamicin
2. hypoglycemia
3. chloroquine
4. ototoxicity
5. blood dyscrasia
6. dizziness, drowsiness, confusion

Chapter 4

Multiple Choice

1. c 2. a 3. c 4. a 5. d 6. c 7. a

Multiple Response

1. a, b, c
2. b, c, d
3. a, b, d, e

Complete the List

1. Correct drug and patient
2. Correct storage of the drug
3. Correct and most effective route
4. Correct dosage
5. Correct preparation
6. Correct timing
7. Correct recording of administration

Fill in the Blanks

1. assessment
2. evaluation
3. Nursing diagnoses
4. over-the-counter drugs or herbal therapies
5. dose
6. avoid driving a car or operating dangerous machinery

Chapter 5

Multiple Choice

1. b 2. c 3. d 4. d 5. b 6. b 7. d 8. b

Matching

1. E 2. A 3. F 4. C 5. D 6. B

Complete the Problems

1. a. 0.1 g b. 1.5 kg c. 100 mL d. 0.5 L
2. a. 9 g b. 15 mg c. 2 mL d. 2 L
3. a. 1 tsp b. 2 tbsp
4. a. 77 kg b. 7 lb
5. 11.25 mL
6. 15 mg
7. 0.65 mL
8. 0.58 (0.6) mL
9. 1.6 mL
10. 1.9 mL

Chapter 6

Multiple Choice

1. c 2. b 3. a 4. c 5. b 6. c

Multiple Response

1. c, e, f
2. b, d, e

Matching

1. c 2. d 3. a 4. e 5. a 6. e 7. a 8. c 9. b 10. b

Definitions

1. self-care: a tendency for patients to self-diagnose and determine their own treatment needs
2. Internet: a worldwide digital information system accessed through computer systems
3. OTC drugs: drugs that are available without a prescription for self-treatment of a variety of complaints
4. alternative therapies: includes herbs and other "natural" products as found in ancient records; these products are not controlled by the Food and Drug Administration (FDA) and, because of this, the advertising surrounding these products is not as restricted or accurate as it would be with classic drugs
5. off-label uses: when drugs are used for therapeutic indications other than those for which they were approved by the FDA
6. cost comparisons: a comparison of the relative cost of the same drug provided by different manufacturers to determine the cost to the consumer

Chapter 7

Multiple Choice

1. d 2. a 3. b 4. c 5. b 6. c 7. c

Multiple Response

1. b, c, e, f
2. b, d, e
3. a, d, f

Matching

1. E 2. D 3. B 4. C 5. A

Word Scramble

1. diffusion
2. endocytosis
3. pinocytosis
4. phagocytosis
5. osmosis
6. mitosis
7. passive transport
8. active transport

Chapter 8

Multiple Choice

1. c 2. c 3. a 4. c 5. b 6. c 7. d

Multiple Response

1. a, b, c
2. a, c, d

Definitions

1. culture: sample of bacteria (from sputum, cell scraping, urine, etc.) to grow in a laboratory to determine the species of bacteria that is causing an illness
2. prophylaxis: treatment to prevent an infection before it occurs, as in the use of antibiotics to prevent diseases such as bacterial endocarditis or antiprotozoals to prevent malaria
3. resistance: ability of bacteria over time to adapt to an antibiotic and produce cells that are no longer affected by the drug
4. selective toxicity: property of antibiotics that allows them to affect certain proteins or enzyme systems used by bacteria but not by human cells, sparing the human cells from the destructive effects of the antibiotics
5. sensitivity testing: evaluation of bacteria obtained in a culture to determine to what antibiotics the organisms are sensitive and which agent would be appropriate for treatment of a particular infection
6. spectrum: range of bacteria against which an antibiotic is effective (eg, broad-spectrum antibiotics are effective against a wide range of bacteria)

Matching

1. c 2. a 3. b 4. e 5. f 6. d

Chapter 9

Multiple Choice

1. d 2. c 3. b 4. a 5. d 6. c 7. b 8. c 9. c 10. b

Multiple Response

1. b, d, f
2. a, b, c, f

True or False

1. T 2. F 3. F 4. T 5. F 6. T 7. F 8. T

Web Exercise

Log on to http://www.cdc.gov. Select Health and Related Topics. Select Diseases and Conditions. Using the alphabet list at the top of the page, click on T. Select tuberculosis. On the left-hand side of the page you have several options that will help you prepare a teaching plan. Click on Fact Sheet for general information on tuberculosis; Education and Training Materials will give you specific guidelines and information for making up your teaching plan.

Matching

1. G 2. F 3. I 4. A 5. B 6. J 7. C 8. D 9. E 10. C 11. A 12. H

Chapter 10

Multiple Choice

1. c 2. b 3. c 4. d 5. c 6. b 7. a 8. b

Multiple Response

1. a, d, e, f
2. a, e, f

Matching

1. C 2. D 3. B 4. A 5. A

Fill in the Blanks

1. zanamivir
2. ribavirin
3. amantadine
4. foscarnet
5. valacyclovir
6. acyclovir
7. zidovudine
8. penciclovir

Chapter 11

Multiple Choice

1. b 2. c 3. d 4. c 5. b 6. c 7. b 8. c

Multiple Response

1. a, d, f
2. a, c, f

Web Exercise

Log on to http://www.athletesfoot.com to get all types of information about the fungus that causes athlete's foot. Click on information for prevention, such as Sweaty Feet or Tennis Shoe. Click on Treatment and you will be connected to many products with explanations of how they work. Use this information to prepare your teaching plan.

Fill in the Blanks

1. hard, ergosterol
2. mycosis
3. hepatic, renal
4. Candida
5. tinea
6. systemically
7. wounds
8. burning, irritation, pain

Chapter 12

Multiple Choice

1. d 2. b 3. d 4. b 5. c 6. d 7. c 8. a 9. c

Multiple Response

1. c, d, f

Web Exercise

Log on to http://www.cdc.gov. Select Traveler's Health from the selections on the right side of the page. Select the destination your friend is traveling to. Click on Vaccines, Diseases, and other categories to prepare a teaching outline for your friend, including vaccines needed, things to avoid, and precautions that should be taken.

Matching

1. A 2. B 3. A 4. C 5. A 6. D 7. A 8. D

Chapter 13

Multiple Choice

1. b 2. a 3. c 4. d 5. a 6. b 7. a

Multiple Response

1. a, c, f

Definitions

1. cestode: tapeworm with a head and segmented body parts that is capable of growing to several yards in the human intestine
2. nematode: roundworm such as the commonly encountered pinworm, whipworm, threadworm, *Ascaris,* or hookworm
3. pinworm: nematode that causes a common helminthic infection in humans; lives in the intestine and causes anal and possible vaginal irritation and itching
4. round worm: worm such as *Ascarix* that causes a common helminthic infection in humans; can cause intestinal obstruction because the adult worms clog the intestinal lumen or severe pneumonia when the larvae migrate to the lungs and form a pulmonary infiltrate
5. schistosomiasis: infection with blood fluke that is carried by a snail, poses a common problem in tropical countries, where the snail is the intermediary in the life cycle of the worm; larvae burrow into the skin in fresh water and migrate throughout the human body, causing a rash and then symptoms of diarrhea and liver and brain inflammation
6. trichinosis: disease that results from ingestion of encysted roundworm larvae in undercooked pork; larvae migrate throughout the body to invade muscle and nervous tissue; can cause pneumonia, heart failure, and encephalitis.
7. thread worm: worm that attaches itself to the intestinal mucosa and sucks blood; may cause severe anemia and disintegration of the intestinal mucosa
8. whip worm: worm that attaches itself to the intestinal mucosa and sucks blood; may cause severe anemia and disintegration of the intestinal mucosa

Learning Activity

Patient Teaching Checklist

Mebendazole

An anthelmintic acts to destroy certain helminths or worms that have invaded your body. You must take the full course of the drug that has been prescribed for you to ensure that you have cleared all of the worms, in all phases of their life cycle, from your body. Your drug has been prescribed to treat pinworms.

Your drug can be taken with meals or with a light snack to decrease any stomach upset that you may experience.

Common effects of the drug include:

- Nausea, vomiting, loss of appetite—Take the drug with meals and eat small, frequent meals.
- Dizziness, drowsiness—If this happens, avoid driving a car or operating dangerous machinery; change positions slowly to avoid falling or injury.

Report any of the following to your health care provider: fever, chills, rash, headache, weakness, tremors.

It is very important to take the complete prescription that has been ordered for you.

Never use this drug to self-treat any other infection or give it to any other person.

Tell any doctor, nurse, or other health care provider that you are taking this drug.

Keep this drug, and all medication, out of the reach of children.

Follow these guidelines to help to prevent reinfection with the worms or the spread of this infection to any other family members:

- Wash hands vigorously with soap after using toilet facilities.
- Shower in the morning to wash away any ova deposited in the anal area during the night.
- Change and launder undergarments, bed linens and pajamas every day.
- Disinfect toilets and toilet seats daily and bathroom and bedroom floors periodically.

Chapter 14

Multiple Choice

1. c 2. d 3. a 4. c 5. b 6. b 7. b 8. c

Multiple Response

1. a, b, c, e, f
2. a, b, d

Matching

1. D 2. G 3. C 4. E 5. F 6. A 7. H 8. B

Word Scramble

1. vinblastine
2. carmustine
3. carboplatin
4. cisplatin
5. tamoxifen
6. bleomycin
7. dacarbazine
8. etoposide

Chapter 15

Multiple Choice

1. d 2. b 3. a 4. b 5. d 6. b 7. d 8. a

Multiple Response

1. a, b, c
2. a, b, d

True or False

1. T 2. F 3. T 4. F 5. F 6. F 7. F 8. T 9. F 10. T

Definitions

1. interleukin: chemical released by WBCs to communicate with other WBCs and to support the inflammatory and immune reactions
2. rubor: redness, one of the four cardinal signs of inflammation; caused by activation of the inflammatory response
3. pyrogen: substance that resets the thermoregulatory center in the hypothalamus to elevate body temperature, thus speeding metabolism; some pyrogens are released by active neutrophils as part of the inflammatory response

4. antibody: an immune globulin; produced by B cell plasma cells in response to specific protein; reacts with that protein to cause its destruction directly or through activation of the inflammatory response
5. chemotaxis: property of drawing neutrophils to an area
6. dolor: pain, one of the four cardinal signs of inflammation; caused by activation of the inflammatory response
7. neutrophil: white blood cell that is the first responder to an inflammatory reaction, phagocytizes invading pathogens, injured cells
8. antigen: foreign protein

Chapter 16

Multiple Choice

1. d 2. c 3. d 4. b 5. d 6. a 7. c 8. c

Multiple Response

1. a, b, c, f
2. c, e, f

Web Exercise

Information sheet will vary with each individual accessing the site.

Matching

1. D 2. G 3. E 4. C 5. B 6. F 7. A

Chapter 17

Multiple Choice

1. d 2. c 3. d 4. a 5. d 6. c

Multiple Response

1. a, b, d
2. a, c, d

Definitions

1. autoimmune: having antibodies to self-cells or self-proteins; leads to chronic inflammatory disease and cell destruction
2. interferon: protein released by cells in response to viral invasion, prevents viral replication in other cells
3. interleukin: "between white cells"; substance released by active white cells to communicate with other white cells and support the inflammatory and immune reaction
4. monoclonal antibodies: specific antibodies produced by a single clone of B cells to react with a specific antigen
5. immune suppressant: drugs used to block or suppress the actions of the T cells and antibody production; used to prevent transplant rejection and treat autoimmune disease

Fill in the Blanks

1. monoclonal antibodies
2. basiliximab, daclizumab, muromonab CD3
3. Crohn's
4. respiratory syncytial virus
5. trastuzumab
6. rituximab
7. omalizumab
8. alemtuzumab

Chapter 18

Multiple Choice

1. b 2. a 3. d 4. b 5. d 6. b 7. a

Multiple Response

1. a, b, c, f
2. c, e, f
3. b, c

Web Exercise

Go to http://www.aap.org/family/parents/vaccine.htm. This contains the guidelines and frequently asked questions about vaccinations from the American Academy of Pediatrics.

Information can be downloaded and printed out for the parent.

True or False

1. F 2. T 3. T 4. T 5. T 6. T 7. F 8. F

Chapter 19

Multiple Choice

1. b 2. b 3. c 4. a 5. b 6. c 7. a 8. b

Multiple Response

1. a, b, c
2. a, c, f

Matching

1. G 2. C 3. B 4. J 5. I 6. H 7. A 8. F 9. E 10. D

Definitions

1. neuron: structural unit of the nervous system
2. neurotransmitter: chemical produced by a nerve and released when a nerve is stimulated; reacts with a specific receptor site to cause an action
3. limbic system: area of the brain above the hypothalamus, high in norepinephrine levels; thought to be the site of emotions in the human brain
4. Schwann cell: insulating cell found on nerve axons; allows "leaping" electrical conduction to speed the transmission of information and prevent tiring of the nerve
5. myelination: property of a nerve axon that has Schwann's cells
6. soma: cell body of a neuron; contains the nucleus, cytoplasm and various granules
7. synapse: junction between a nerve and an effector; consists of the presynaptic nerve ending, a space called the synaptic cleft, and the postsynaptic cell
8. repolarization: return of a membrane to a resting state, with more sodium ions outside the membrane and a relatively negative charge inside the membrane

Chapter 20

Multiple Choice

1. d 2. a 3. a 4. c 5. c 6. d 7. a 8. c

Multiple Response

1. a, b, c, e
2. a, b, c, f

Fill in the Blanks

1. anxiety
2. motivator
3. sedatives
4. hypnotics
5. tension, fear
6. sedation
7. depress
8. benzodiazepines

Matching

1. C 2. E 3. A 4. B 5. G 6. H 7. D 8. F 9. J 10. I

Chapter 21

Multiple Choice

1. c 2. c 3. d 4. b 5. d 6. b 7. d 8. c

Multiple Response

1. a, c, d
2. a, c, d

Word Scramble

1. bupropion
2. fluoxetine
3. clomipramine
4. venlafaxine
5. phenelzine

6. paroxetine
7. imipramine

Fill in the Blanks

1. norepinephrine, dopamine, serotonin
2. breakdown, synaptic cleft
3. reuptake
4. norepinephrine, serotonin
5. tyramine
6. PMDD (premenstrual dysphoric disorder)
7. bupropion
8. anticholinergic

Chapter 22

Multiple Choice

1. c 2. c 3. a 4. c 5. b 6. a 7. d 8. d

Multiple Response

1. a, b, c, d
2. a, b, d

Matching

1. F 2. C 3. B 4. G 5. D 6. A 7. E

Web Exercise

Go to http://www.mhsource.com. Select Disorders from the pull down menu under Resources. Read the Ask the Expert information under Seasonal Affective Disorder to learn about treatment options—herbal and alternative therapies and light therapy, including insurance backing of the purchase of lights.

Chapter 23

Multiple Choice

1. c 2. d 3. b 4. a 5. a 6. c 7. a 8. b

Multiple Response

1. b, e
2. b, c, d

Fill in the Blanks

1. epilepsy
2. seizure
3. convulsion
4. antiepileptics
5. grand mal seizure
6. absence seizure
7. myoclonic seizures
8. febrile seizures
9. status epilepticus
10. focal

Web Exercise

Each student will prepare a teaching plan based on information found at http://www.aesnet.org.

Chapter 24

Multiple Choice

1. d 2. c 3. c 4. a 5. b 6. c 7. b 8. b

Multiple Response

1. a, b, c
2. a, c, f

Word Scramble

1. levodopa
2. procyclidine
3. pergolide
4. biperiden
5. amantadine
6. ropinirole
7. benztropine
8. bromocriptine

Web Exercise

Go to http://www.ninds.nih.gov.

From the Disorders Quick Links, pull-down menu, select Parkinson's. Choose topics from the information page that would be of interest to this family—research, surgery, support groups, and so on.

Chapter 25

Multiple Choice

1. c 2. d 3. d 4. c 5. d 6. c 7. c

Multiple Response

1. a, b, d, f
2. a, c, d, e, f

Matching

1. C 2. E 3. H 4. F 5. A 6. B 7. G 8. D

True or False

1. F 2. T 3. F 4. F 5. T 6. F 7. T 8. F 9. T 10. F

Chapter 26

Multiple Choice

1. b 2. c 3. c 4. c 5. b 6. d 7. b 8. c

Multiple Response

1. b, c, d, e
2. a, c, f

Matching

1. G 2. F 3. D 4. I 5. C 6. B 7. H 8. E 9. A

Definitions

1. A fibers: large-diameter nerve fibers that carry peripheral impulses associated with touch and temperature to the spinal cord
2. A-delta and C fibers: small-diameter nerve fibers that carry peripheral impulses associated with pain to the spinal cord
3. gate-control theory: theory that the transmission of nerve impulses can be modulated at several points along its path by the closing and opening of "gates"
4. migraine headache: headache characterized by severe, unilateral, pulsating head pain and associated with systemic effects, including GI upset, light and sound sensitization
5. narcotics: drugs originally derived from opium that react with specific opioid receptors in the body
6. narcotic agonist: drugs that act at opioid receptors to simulate the effects of the receptors
7. narcotic agonist-antagonists: drugs that act at some opioid receptors to stimulate activity and at other opioid receptors to block activity
8. narcotic antagonists: drugs that block opioid receptors, used to counteract the effects of narcotics and to treat narcotic overdose
9. opioid receptors: receptor sites on nerves that react with enkephalins and endorphins and that are receptive to narcotic drugs
10. triptan: selective serotonin receptor blocker that causes a vascular constriction of cranial vessels, used to treat acute migraine attacks

Chapter 27

Multiple Choice

1. b 2. c 3. b 4. c 5. a

Multiple Response

1. a, b, d, f
2. a, b, d, e
3. a, b, c, f

Fill in the Blanks

1. pain relief, analgesia, amnesia, unconsciousness
2. loss of sensation, death
3. induction of anesthesia
4. balanced anesthesia
5. depolarization of the nerve membrane
6. central nervous system depression

7. sensation, mobility, the ability to communicate
8. skin breakdown, self-injury, biting oneself

Web Exercise

Logging on to http://www.anesthesiologyonline.com will give you access to appropriate teaching protocols. Prepare a comparison of the types and actions for the patient to review with you.

Chapter 28

Multiple Choice

1. a 2. b 3. c 4. b 5. c 6. b 7. a

Multiple Response

1. a, b, c

Matching

1. A 2. C 3. D 4. F 5. E 6. B

Web exercise

Answer will vary with individual search.

Chapter 29

Multiple Choice

1. c 2. b 3. d 4. c 5. d 6. b 7. d 8. a

Multiple Response

1. a, b, f
2. a, b, d

Matching

1. K 2. C 3. F 4. B 5. I 6. G 7. H 8. A 9. J
10. E 11. L 12. D

Chapter 30

Multiple Choice

1. c 2. b 3. c 4. d 5. c 6. a

Multiple Response

1. b, c, e, f
2. c, e, f

Word Scramble

1. ephedrine
2. clonidine
3. dopamine
4. ritodrine
5. dobutamine
6. norepinephrine
7. metaraminol
8. phenylephrine
9. epinephrine
10. isoproterenol

Definitions

1. adrenergic agonist: a drug that stimulates the adrenergic receptors of the sympathetic nervous system, either directly, by reacting with the receptor site, or indirectly by increasing norepinephrine levels
2. alpha-agonist: specifically stimulating the alpha receptors within the sympathetic nervous system, causing body responses seen when the alpha receptors are stimulated
3. beta-agonist: specifically stimulating the beta receptors within the sympathetic nervous system, causing body responses seen when the beta receptors are stimulated
4. glycogenolysis: breakdown of stored glucose to increase the blood glucose levels
5. sympathomimetic: a drug that mimics the effects of the sympathetic nervous system

Chapter 31

Multiple Choice

1. d 2. c 3. a 4. b 5. a 6. c 7. d 8. c

Multiple Response

1. a, b, d, f
2. a, b, d, f

Web Exercise

Individual response will vary with what the student decides to explore.

True or False

1. F 2. T 3. F 4. T 5. T 6. F 7. T 8. T

Chapter 32

Multiple Choice

1. b 2. c 3. a 4. c 5. b 6. d 7. b 8. c

Multiple Response

1. a, b, d
2. a, b, d

Matching

1. D 2. E 3. A, C 4. B 5. B 6. A, C 7. D 8. E

Fill in the Blanks

1. acetylcholine
2. parasympathomimetic
3. direct-acting
4. indirect-acting
5. Alzheimer's disease
6. myasthenia gravis
7. nausea, vomiting, diarrhea, increased salivation
8. bradycardia, hypotension, heart block

Chapter 33

Multiple Choice

1. a 2. c 3. c 4. d

Multiple Response

1. a, b, c
2. a, e, f

Fill in the Blanks

1. acetylcholine
2. parasympatholytic
3. increase, decrease
4. sweating
5. cyclopegia
6. mydriatic
7. atropine
8. dry mouth, difficulty swallowing

Web Exercise

Going to www.cdc.gov and finding the latest info on bioterrorism will lead to information on treating and preventing nerve gas paralysis. A teaching guide can be developed using this information.

Chapter 34

Multiple Choice

1. d 2. b 3. a 4. c 5. d 6. d 7. c

Multiple Response

1. a, b, e, f
2. a, b, d
3. c, e, f

Matching

1. D 2. H 3. F 4. A 5. G 6. C 7. E 8. B

Word Scramble

1. pituitary gland
2. diurnal rhythm
3. releasing factors
4. insulin
5. hypothalamus
6. negative feedback

7. hormones
8. posterior pituitary
9. pancreas
10. hypothalamic-pituitary axis

Chapter 35

Multiple Choice

1. a 2. c 3. d 4. b 5. c 6. c 7. d 8. b

Multiple Response

1. d, e, f
2. c, e

Web Exercise

Entering the search word "Turner's Syndrome" will link to many organizations and medical sites that will provide the information needed for the project.

Matching

1. C 2. E 3. G 4. A 5. D 6. H 7. B 8. F

Chapter 36

Multiple Choice

1. b 2. c 3. d 4. a 5. a 6. d 7. a 8. c

Multiple Response

1. a, b, c, f
2. a, b, d, f

Word Scramble

1. prednisone
2. triamcinolone
3. betamethasone
4. hydrocortisone
5. budesonide
6. flunisolide
7. cortisone
8. dexamethasone

True or False

1. F 2. F 3. F 4. T 5. T 6. F 7. F 8. T 9. T 10. T

Chapter 37

Multiple Choice

1. b 2. c 3. c 4. b 5. d 6. b 7. c 8. b

Multiple Response

1. a, c, d
2. b, c, d

Matching

1. E 2. A 3. F 4. B 5. J 6. C 7. H 8. D 9. G 10. I

Word Scramble

1. calcitonin
2. thyroxine
3. cretinism
4. bisphosphonates
5. parathormone
6. iodine
7. osteoporosis
8. hyperthyroidism
9. myxedema
10. liothyronine

Chapter 38

Multiple Choice

1. c 2. c 3. a 4. b 5. b 6. d 7. c 8. a

Multiple Response

1. a, b, c, e, f
2. a, b, d, f

Web Exercise

Go to http://www.diabetes.org, the American Diabetes Association website. Click on "Type 2 Diabetes" to get information on the disease. Click "Medical Information" to get information on specific drugs that J.L. might be taking. Click "Meal Planning" to get nutrition information as well as recipes that J.L. or his wife might like to review. If they seem interested in support groups, enter their zip code to find local ADA chapters and pertinent support. Print out anything that would be useful in preparing a teaching program for the patient.

Fill in the Blanks

1. diabetes mellitus
2. insulin, glucagons, somatostatin
3. glycogen, lipids, proteins
4. glycosuria
5. polyphagia
6. Polydipsia
7. ketosis
8. diet, exercise
9. sulfonylureas
10. metformin

Chapter 39

Multiple Choice

1. a 2. b 3. b 4. c 5. b 6. c 7. d 8. a

Multiple Response

1. a, b, c, f
2. a, c, d, e

Web Exercise

Go to http://www.InnerBody.com and select sexual development. Prepare posters, handouts, easy explanations of the process.

True or False

1. F 2. T 3. T 4. F 5. T 6. F 7. F 8. T

Chapter 40

Multiple Choice

1. b 2. c 3. a 4. b 5. b 6. c 7. c

Multiple Response

1. b, c, e, f
2. a, b, c, e, f
3. a, b, d, e

Word Scramble

1. toremifene
2. estradiol
3. estrone
4. raloxifene
5. dienestrol
6. estropipate
7. diethylstilbestrol
8. chlorotrianisene

Fill in the Blanks

1. oxytocics
2. tocolytics
3. osteoporosis, hot flashes, coronary artery disease
4. thrombi, emboli
5. Raloxifene
6. injection
7. fertility drugs
8. abortifacients

Chapter 41

Multiple Choice

1. a 2. d 3. c 4. b 5. c 6. a 7. c 8. d

Multiple Response

1. a, b, d
2. b, d, e, f

True or False
1. T 2. F 3. T 4. T 5. F 6. F 7. T 8. T 9. F 10. F

Fill in the Blanks
1. Androgenic
2. Anabolic
3. Testosterone
4. anemias
5. Erectile penile dysfunction
6. prostaglandin, injected
7. Sildenafil
8. sexual stimulation

Chapter 42

Multiple Choice
1. c 2. c 3. d 4. c 5. a 6. b 7. a 8. c 9. c

Multiple Response
1. a, b, c, e, f
2. a, b, c, f

Definition
1. troponin: chemical in muscle that prevents actin and myosin from reacting, leading to muscle relaxation; inactivated by calcium during muscle stimulation to allow actin and myosin to react, causing muscle contraction
2. actin: thin filament that makes up a sarcomere or muscle unit
3. myosin: thick filament that makes up a sarcomere or muscle unit
4. arrhythmia: a disruption in cardiac rate or rhythm
5. Starling's Law of the Heart: addresses the contractile properties of the heart; the more the muscle is stretched, the stronger it will react until stretched to a point at which it will not react at all
6. fibrillation: rapid, irregular stimulation of the cardiac muscle resulting in lack of pumping activity
7. capillary: small vessel made up of loosely connected endothelial cells that connect arteries to veins
8. resistance system: the arteries; the muscles of the arteries provide resistance to the flow of blood, leading to control of blood pressure

Matching
1. H 2. C 3. F 4. E 5. D 6. L 7. J 8. A 9. K
10. G 11. I 12. B

Chapter 43

Multiple Choice
1. b 2. b 3. d 4. d 5. c 6. b 7. c 8. d

Multiple Response
1. a, b, c, e
2. a, b, d, e

Matching
1. B 2. A 3. E 4. B 5. D 6. D 7. A 8. B 9. C 10. D
11. A 12. C

True or False
1. F 2. T 3. F 4. F 5. T 6. F 7. T 8. T 9. F 10. T

Chapter 44

Multiple Choice
1. b 2. c 3. a 4. c 5. d 6. b 7. c 8. b

Multiple Response
1. a, b, c
2. a, c, d, e

Web Exercise
Go to the American Heart Association home page at http://www.americanheart.org. Select "Your Heart." Now select "Diseases and Conditions." Then select "Congestive Heart Failure." Print out pertinent information that might be useful for J.D. Return to the home page and enter your zip code, then print out information on support groups and help in your specific area.

Word Scramble
1. dyspnea
2. milrinone
3. nocturia
4. orthopnea
5. tachypnea
6. congestive heart failure
7. digoxin
8. hemoptysis
9. cardiomyopathy
10. immune fab

Chapter 45

Multiple Choice
1. d 2. c 3. c 4. b 5. d 6. a 7. c 8. d

Multiple Response
1. a, c, d, f
2. a, b, c, e, f

Fill in the Blanks
1. tachycardia, bradycardia
2. cardiac output
3. action potential
4. CAST study
5. automaticity
6. Beta receptor
7. digoxin
8. lidocaine

Word Scramble
1. amiodarone
2. esmolol
3. bretylium
4. verapamil
5. procainamide
6. propranolol
7. flecainide
8. digoxin

Chapter 46

Multiple Choice
1. a 2. b 3. d 4. b 5. d 6. b

Multiple Response
1. a, b, d, e, f
2. a, b, c, f
3. a, b, d, e,
4. c, e, f

Matching
1. C 2. F 3. E 4. G 5. A 6. B 7. D 8. H

True or False
1. F 2. T 3. F 4. T 5. F 6. F 7. T 8. T

Chapter 47

Multiple Choice
1. b 2. b 3. c 4. d 5. b 6. c 7. c 8. d

Multiple Response
1. a, b, f
2. a, b, e, f

Web Exercise

Go to the American Heart Association home page at http://www.americanheart.org. Click on "Warning signs," then "Risk Assessment" for a survey of risk factors. Return to the home page. Click on "Diseases and Conditions," then "Cholesterol" for the diet and drug guidelines. Print out useful information.

Word Scramble

1. cholesterol
2. clofibrate
3. niacin
4. hyperlipidemia
5. colestipol
6. atorvastatin
7. gemfibrozil
8. bile acids
9. lipoprotein
10. lovastatin

Chapter 48

Multiple Choice

1. c 2. b 3. c 4. d 5. b 6. c

Multiple Response

1. a, b, c
2. b, c, d
3. a, b, c, f
4. a, b, c, e, f

True or False

1. T 2. F 3. T 4. F 5. T 6. F 7. T 8. F 9. F 10. T

Web Exercise

Go to www.ptinr.com. Select Patient-Consumer information. Select Patient Education. Click on "Using Warfarin Safely at Home." Select and print out any useful information.

Chapter 49

Multiple Choice

1. c 2. b 3. a 4. c 5. d 6. c 7. c 8. d

Multiple Response

1. b, c, e, f
2. a, c, d

Word Scramble

1. erythrocytes
2. plasma
3. megaloblastic
4. pernicious
5. epoetin
6. folic acid
7. anemia
8. erythropoiesis
9. reticulocyte
10. deficiency

True or False

1. T 2. F 3. F 4. T 5. T 6. T 7. F 8. T

Chapter 50

Multiple Choice

1. a 2. d 3. a 4. c 5. c 6. d 7. b

Multiple Response

1. a, b, c, e, f
2. a, c, d, e, f
3. a. c, f

Word Scramble

1. glomerulus
2. filtration
3. secretion
4. aldosterone
5. reabsorption
6. tubule
7. renin
8. prostate

Fill in the Blanks

1. 25%
2. nephron, Bowman's capsule, loop of Henle, collecting duct
3. glomerular filtration, tubular secretion, tubular reabsorption
4. aldosterone
5. concentration, dilution
6. aldosterone
7. Vitamin D
8. renin

Chapter 51

Multiple Choice

1. b 2. c 3. b 4. c 5. d 6. a 7. d 8. c

Multiple Response

1. a, b, d, f
2. a, c, d, f

Definitions

1. edema: movement of fluid into the interstitial spaces; occurs when the balance between osmotic pull and hydrostatic push is upset
2. fluid rebound: reflex reaction of the body to the loss of fluid or sodium; hypothalamus causes the release of ADH, which leads to the retention of water and stress related to the fluid loss combines with decreased blood flow to the kidneys to activate the renin-angiotensin-aldosterone system, leading to further sodium and water retention
3. thiazide: type of diuretic acting in the renal tubule to block the chloride pump, which prevents reabsorption of sodium and chloride, leading to a loss of sodium and water in the urine
4. hypokalemia: low potassium in the blood; often occurs with diuretic use; characterized by weakness, muscle cramps, trembling, nausea, vomiting, diarrhea, and cardiac arrhythmias
5. high-ceiling diuretics: powerful diuretics that work in the loop of Henle to inhibit the reabsorption of sodium and chloride, leading to a sodium-rich diuresis
6. alkalosis: state of not having enough acid to maintain normal homeostatic processes; seen with loop diuretics, which cause the loss of bicarbonate in the urine
7. hyperaldosteronism: excessive output of aldosterone from the adrenal gland, leading to an increased sodium and water retention and loss of potassium
8. osmotic pull: drawing force of large molecules on water; pulling it into the tubule or capillary; essential for maintaining normal fluid balance within the body; used to draw excessive fluid into the vascular system or the renal tubule

Matching

1. A 2. E 3. C 4. B 5. B 6. A 7. D 8. B 9. D 10. C

Chapter 52

Multiple Choice

1. d 2. b 3. d 4. b 5. a 6. a 7. b 8. c

Multiple Response

1. a, b, d, e
2. a, b, d, f

Web Exercise

You could start by going to www.pslgroup.com/ENLARGPROST.htm.

On the home page, click on "Enlarged Prostate Information" then click on "Prostate Gland" to get information on the gland and problems that can occur. Print out the information that looks most useful for the clients. You could also click on "Treatments" to get helpful information. Returning to the home page you can also seek out additional information on PSA levels, the TUNA approach, and others.

True or False

1. T 2. F 3. F 4. T 5. F 6. T 7. F 8. T

Chapter 53

Multiple Choice

1. c 2. a 3. c 4. d 5. c 6. d 7. b

Multiple Response

1. a, b, c
2. a, b, d, e, f
3. a, b, c, e, f

Matching

1. K 2. D 3. B 4. J 5. E 6. A 7. C 8. G 9. L
10. F 11. I 12. H

Web Exercise

A good place to start is to go to www.niaid.nih/gov/factsheets/cold.htm. This will give you most of the basic information you will need to prepare a teaching program for your interested clients.

Chapter 54

Multiple Choice

1. d 2. c 3. d 4. b 5. a 6. c 7. d

Multiple Response

1. a, b, c, e
2. a, c, d, e
3. a, b, d, e, f

Web Exercise

Go to www.nlm.nih.gov/medlineplus/healthtopics.html. Select "A," then "Allergy." Print out pertinent pages to prepare a teaching program for R.W.

Word Scramble

1. clemastine
2. dextromethorphan
3. ephedrine
4. tetrahydrozoline
5. pseudoephedrine
6. budesonide
7. fluticasone
8. astemizole

Chapter 55

Multiple Choice

1. a 2. c 3. c 4. a 5. b 6. d 7. c 8. c

Multiple Response

1. b, c, e, f
2. a, c, d

True or False

1. F 2. T 3. T 4. F 5. F 6. F 7. T

Word Scramble

1. theophylline
2. albuterol
3. epinephrine
4. salmeterol
5. ipratropium
6. budesonide
7. zafirlukast
8. zileuton
9. beractant
10. poractant

Chapter 56

Multiple Choice

1. d 2. c 3. a 4. c 5. d 6. d 7. c

Multiple Response

1. a, b, c, e, f
2. a, b, d, e, f
3. b, c, d, f

Matching

1. F 2. C 3. G 4. H 5. B 6. A 7. E 8. D 9. J 10. I

Fill in the Blanks

1. digestion, absorption
2. acid, mucous
3. nerve plexus
4. sympathetic, parasympathetic
5. local reflexes
6. constipation, diarrhea
7. medulla
8. chemoreceptor trigger zone (CTZ)

Chapter 57

Multiple Choice

1. c 2. d 3. c 4. c 5. a 6. c 7. b 8. c

Multiple Response

1. a, b, c, e, f
2. a, b, d

Web Exercise

Go to www.nlm.nih.gov/medlineplus/healthtopics.html. Select "D," then "Digestive Diseases." Choose several different complaints and using the information presented for each one, prepare a teaching session including the following: causes, lifestyle changes, disease occurrence, treatment, medical follow-up.

Matching

1. E 2. C 3. D 4. A 5. F 6. B 7. B 8. F 9. C 10. A

Chapter 58

Multiple Choice

1. b 2. c 3. b 4. c 5. d

Multiple Response

1. a, c, d, f
2. b, c, d
3. a, b, c

Word Scramble

1. cascara
2. loperamide
3. bisacodyl
4. psyllium
5. senna
6. metoclopramide
7. opium
8. docusate

True or False

1. F 2. T 3. T 4. F 5. T 6. F 7. F 8. T

Chapter 59

Multiple Choice

1. a 2. b 3. d 4. b 5. c 6. c

Multiple Response

1. a, c, d, e, f
2. a, c, d

Web Exercise

Go to http://aappolicy.aappublications.org/cgi/content/abstract/pediatrics;112/5/1182.

Prepare an educational program for your neighbor that could be used with new parents, based on the information provided at this site.

Fill in the Blanks

1. vomiting
2. Ipecac syrup
3. Antiemetics
4. vomiting reflex
5. CTZ, medulla
6. pain, chemicals, uterine stretch
7. CNS depression
8. Photosensitivity

APPENDIX A

Parenteral Agents

Parenteral preparations are fluids that are given either intravenously (IV) or through a central line.

Therapeutic Actions and Indications

Parenteral agents are used for the following purposes: to provide replacement fluids, sugars, electrolytes, and nutrients to patients who are unable to take them in orally; to provide ready access for administration of drugs in an emergency situation; to provide rehydration; and to restore electrolyte balance. The composition of the IV fluids needed for a patient depends on the patient's fluid and electrolyte status.

Parenteral nutrition (PN) is the administration of essential proteins, amino acids, carbohydrates, vitamins, minerals, trace elements, lipids, and fluids. PN is used to improve or stabilize the nutritional status of cachectic or debilitated patients who cannot take in or absorb oral nutrition to the extent required to maintain their nutritional status. The exact composition of the PN solution is determined after a nutritional assessment and must take into account the patient's current health status, age, and metabolic needs.

Contraindications and Cautions

PN is contraindicated in anyone with known allergies to any component of the solution. (Multiple combination products are available, so a suitable solution may be found.) PN should be used with caution in patients with unstable cardiovascular status, because of the change in fluid volume that may occur and the resultant increased workload on the heart. These preparations also should be used with caution in patients with unstable fluid and electrolyte status, who could react adversely to sudden changes in fluids and electrolytes.

Adverse Effects

Adverse effects associated with the use of PN include IV irritation, extravasation of the fluid into the tissues, infection of the insertion site, fluid volume overload, vascular problems related to fluid shifts, and potential electrolyte imbalance related to dilution of the blood. PN also is associated with mechanical problems related to insertion of the line, such as pneumothorax, infections, or air emboli; emboli related to protein or lipid aggregation; infections related to nutrient-rich solution and invasive administration; metabolic imbalances related to the composition of the solution; gallstone development (especially in children); and nausea (especially related to the administration of lipids).

Clinically Important Drug–Drug Interactions

Some IV drugs can be diluted only with particular IV solutions to avoid precipitation or inactivation of the drug. A drug guide should be checked before diluting any IV drug in solution.

Nursing Considerations

Assessment: History and Examination

Obtain a nutritional assessment. Screen for any medical conditions and drugs being taken.

Evaluate insertion site; skin hydration; orientation and affect; height and weight; pulse, blood pressure, and respirations; and blood chemistries, complete blood count with differential, and glucose levels.

Nursing Diagnoses

The patient receiving a parenteral agent may have the following nursing diagnoses related to drug therapy:

- Acute Pain related to administration of the fluid
- Risk for Infection related to invasive delivery system

- Risk for Imbalanced Nutrition related to fluid composition
- Deficient Knowledge regarding drug therapy

Implementation

- Assess patient's general physical condition before beginning test *to decrease the potential for adverse effects.*
- Monitor IV insertion site or central line regularly; consult with prescriber *to discontinue site of infusion and treat any infection or extravasation as soon as it occurs.*
- Follow these administration guidelines *to provide the most therapeutic use of PN with the fewest adverse effects:*

  Refrigerate PN solutions until ready to use.
  Check contents before hanging to ensure that no precipitates are present.
  Do not hang bag for longer than 24 hours.
  Suggest the use of on-line filters to decrease bacterial invasion and infusion of aggregate as appropriate.
- Discontinue PN only after an alternative source of nutrition has been established *to ensure continued nutrition for the patient; taper slowly to avoid severe reactions.*
- Provide comfort measures *to help the patient tolerate drug effects* (e.g., provide proper skin care as needed, analgesics, hot soaks to extravasation sites).
- Include information about the solution being used in a test (e.g., what to expect, adverse effects that may occur, follow-up tests that may be needed) *to enhance patient knowledge about drug therapy and promote compliance with the drug regimen.*

Evaluation

- Monitor patient response to the drug (stabilization of nutritional state, fluid and electrolyte balance, laboratory values).
- Monitor for adverse effects (local irritation, infection, fluid and electrolyte imbalance).
- Evaluate effectiveness of teaching plan (patient can name adverse effects to watch for, specific measures to avoid adverse effects; patient understands importance of follow-up that will be needed).
- Monitor effectiveness of comfort measures and compliance with regimen.

Table A Parenterals

Solution	Caloric Content (cal/L)	Osmolarity (mOsm/L)	Usual Indications
In Solutions			
Dextrose Solutions			
2.5% (25 g/L)	85	126	Provide calories and fluid
5% (50 g/L)	170	253	Provide calories and fluid, keep vein open for administration of IV drugs; frequent choice for dilution of IV drugs
10% (100 g/L)	340	505	Hypertonic solution used after admixture with other fluids; provide calories and fluid
20% (200 g/L)	680	1010	Hypertonic solution used after admixture with other fluids; provide calories and fluid
25% (250 g/L)	850	1330	Hypertonic solution used after admixture with other fluids; provide calories and fluid; treatment of acute hypoglycemic episodes in infants to restore glucose levels and suppress symptoms; sclerosing agent for varicose veins
30% (300 g/L)	1020	1515	Hypertonic solution used after admixture with other fluids; provide calories and fluid
40% (400 g/L)	1360	2020	Hypertonic solution used after admixture with other fluids; provide calories and fluid
50% (500 g/L)	1700	2525	Hypertonic solution used after admixture with other fluids; provide calories and fluid; treatment of hyperinsulinemia; sclerosing agent for varicose veins
60% (600 g/L)	2040	3030	Hypertonic solution used after admixture with other fluids; provide calories and fluid
70% (700 g/L)	2380	3535	Hypertonic solution used after admixture with other fluids; provide calories and fluid

Solution	Sodium Content (mEq/L)	Chloride Content (mEq/L)	Osmolarity (mOsm/L)	Usual Indications
Saline Solutions				
0.45% (½ normal saline)	77	77	155	Hydrating solution; may be used to evaluate kidney function; treatment of hyperosmolar diabetes
0.9% (normal saline)	154	154	310	Replacement of fluid, sodium, and chloride; flushing lines and catheters; dilution of IV medications; priming of dialysis machines; neonate blood transfusions

Table A Parenterals (Continued)

Solution	Sodium Content (mEq/L)	Chloride Content (mEq/L)	Osmolarity (mOsm/L)	Usual Indications
3%	513	513	1030	Hypertonic solution to treat sodium and chloride depletion; emergency treatment of water intoxication or severe salt depletion
5%	855	855	1710	Hypertonic solution to treat sodium and chloride depletion; emergency treatment of water intoxication or severe salt depletion

Commonly Used Combination Fluids*

Solution	Na Content (mEq/L)	K Content (mEq/L)	Cl Content (mEq/L)	Ca Content (mEq/L)	Mg Content (mEq/L)	Lactate (mEq/L)	Acetate (mEq/L)	Osmolarity (mOsm/L)
Plasma-Lyte-R	140	10	103	5	3	8	47	312
Ringer's Injection	147	4	156	4	—	—	—	310
Lactated Ringer's	130	4	109	3	—	28	—	273
Normosol-R	140	5	96	—	3	—	27	295

Typical Central Parenteral Nutrition Solution*—1 Liter

(Actual concentration of solution and components of any particular solution will be determined by the assessment of the patient's current status and nutritional needs.)

Component	Purpose	Dosage	Special Considerations
10% Amino acids	Provides 50 g protein for growth and healing	500 mL	Monitor BP, cardiac output, blood chemistries, urine to determine effect of intravascular protein pull.
50% Dextrose	Provides 850 calories for energy	500 mL	Monitor blood sugar; evaluate injection site for any sign of infection, irritation.
20% Fat emulsion	Provides 500 fat calories, ready energy	250 mL	Monitor for any sign of emboli (e.g., shortness of breath, chest pain, deep leg pain, neurological changes). Carefully monitor patients for any sign of increased vascular workload, especially very young and geriatric patients.
Sodium chloride	Provides sodium and chloride needed for various chemical reactions within the body	40 mEq	Monitor cardiac rhythm, serum electrolytes.
Calcium gluconate	Provides essential calcium for muscle contraction, blood clotting, numerous chemical reactions	4.8 mEq	Monitor cardiac rhythm, muscle strength, serum electrolytes.
Magnesium sulfate	Provides magnesium for various chemical reactions within the body	8 mEq	Monitor BP, deep tendon reflexes, and serum electrolytes.
Potassium phosphate	Provides needed potassium for nerve functioning, muscle contractions, etc.	9 mM	Monitor P, including rhythm, muscle function, and serum electrolytes.
Multivitamins	Provide a combination of essential vitamins to maintain cell integrity, promote healing	10 mL	Monitor for signs of vitamin deficiency or toxicity.
Trace elements	Provide small amounts of elements essential for numerous chemical reactions in the body and maintenance of cell integrity and healing		Periodically monitor blood chemistries to determine adequacy of replacement.
Zinc		3 mg	
Copper		1.2 mg	
Manganese		0.3 mg	
Chromium		12 mcg	
Selenium		20 mcg	
Total nonprotein calories: 1350			
Total volume of solution: 1250 mL			
Dextrose concentration: 25%			
Amino acid concentration: 5%			
Osmolarity: 1900 mOsm/L			

(*continued*)

Table A Parenterals *(Continued)*

Typical Peripheral Parenteral Nutrition Solution*—1 Liter

(Actual concentration of solution and components of any particular solution will be determined by the assessment of the patient's current status and nutritional needs. Solutions used for peripheral therapy are usually less concentrated and less irritating to the vessel.)

Component	Purpose	Dosage	Special Considerations
8.5% Amino acids	Provides 41 g protein for growth and healing	500 mL	Monitor BP, cardiac output, blood chemistries, urine to determine effect of intravascular protein pull.
20% Dextrose	Provides 340 calories for energy	500 mL	Monitor blood sugar; evaluate injection site for any sign of infection, irritation.
20% Fat emulsion	Provides 500 fat calories, ready energy	250 mL	Monitor for any sign of emboli (e.g., shortness of breath, chest pain, deep leg pain, neurological changes). Carefully monitor patients for any sign of increased vascular workload, especially very young and geriatric patients.
Sodium chloride	Provides sodium and chloride needed for various chemical reactions within the body	40 mEq	Monitor cardiac rhythm, serum electrolytes.
Calcium gluconate	Provides essential calcium for muscle contraction, blood clotting, numerous chemical reactions	4.8 mEq	Monitor cardiac rhythm, muscle strength, serum electrolytes.
Magnesium sulfate	Provides magnesium for various chemical reactions within the body	8 mEq	Monitor BP, deep tendon reflexes, and serum electrolytes.
Potassium phosphate	Provides needed potassium for nerve functioning, muscle contractions, etc.	9 mMoles	Monitor P, including rhythm, muscle function, and serum electrolytes.
Multivitamins	Provide a combination of essential vitamins to maintain cell integrity, promote healing, etc.	10 mL	Monitor for signs of vitamin deficiency or toxicity.
Trace elements	Provide small amounts of elements essential for numerous chemical reactions in the body and maintenance of cell integrity and healing.		Periodically monitor blood chemistries to determine adequacy of replacement.
Zinc		3 mg	
Copper		1.2 mg	
Manganese		0.3 mg	
Chromium		12 mcg	
Selenium		20 mcg	
Total nonprotein calories: 840			
Total volume of solution: 1250 mL			
Dextrose concentration: 10%			
Amino acid concentration: 4.25%			
Osmolarity: 900 mOsm/L			

* Note: Multiple combination preparations are available commercially. Each preparation varies in the concentration of one or more components and should be checked carefully before hanging.

APPENDIX B

Topical Agents

Topical agents are intended for surface use only and are not meant for ingestion or injection. They may be toxic if absorbed into the system, but they have several useful purposes when applied to the surface of the skin or mucous membranes. Some forms of drugs are prepared to be absorbed through the skin for systemic effects. These drugs may be prepared as transdermal patches (e.g., nitroglycerin, estrogens, nicotine), which are designed to provide a slow release of the drug from the vehicle. Drugs prepared for this type of administration are discussed with the specific drug in the text and are not addressed in this appendix.

Therapeutic Actions and Indications

Topical agents are used to treat a variety of disorders in a localized area. Table B describes the usual uses for the many different types of topical agents. Because these drugs are designed for topical application, they are minimally absorbed systemically and, if used properly, should have minimal systemic effects.

Contraindications and Cautions

The use of topical agents is contraindicated in cases of allergy to the drugs and in the presence of open wounds or abrasions, which could lead to the systemic absorption of the drugs. Caution should be used during pregnancy if there is any possibility that the agent might be absorbed. Caution should also be used in the presence of any known allergy to the vehicles of preparation (creams, lotions).

Adverse Effects

Because these drugs are not intended to be absorbed systemically, the adverse effects usually associated with topical agents are local effects, including local irritation, stinging, burning, or dermatitis. Toxic effects are associated with inadvertent systemic absorption.

Nursing Considerations

Assessment: History and Examination

Screen for the presence of any known allergy to the drug, which would be a contraindication to its use.

Include screening for baseline status before beginning therapy and for any potential adverse effects. Assess the following: condition of area to be treated.

Nursing Diagnoses

The patient receiving a topical agent may have the following nursing diagnoses related to drug therapy:

- Risk for Injury related to toxic effects associated with absorption
- Acute Pain related to local effects of the drug
- Deficient Knowledge regarding drug therapy

Implementation

- Ensure proper administration of drug *to provide best therapeutic effect and least adverse effects as follows*:

  Apply sparingly. Some preparations come with applicators, some should be applied while wearing protective gloves, and others are dropped onto the site with no direct contact. Consult information regarding the individual drug being used for specific procedures.

  Do not use with open wounds or broken skin, *which could lead to systemic absorption and toxic effects*.

  Avoid contact with the eyes, *which could be injured by the drug*.

  Do not use with occlusive dressings, *which could increase the risk of systemic absorption*.

- Monitor area being treated *to evaluate drug effects on the condition being treated*.

- Provide comfort measures *to help the patient tolerate drug effects* (e.g., analgesia as needed for local pain, itching).
- Provide patient teaching *to enhance patient knowledge about drug therapy and promote compliance with the drug regimen*:

  Teach the patient the proper administration technique for the topical agent ordered.

  Caution the patient that transient stinging or burning may occur.

  Instruct the patient to report severe irritation, allergic reaction, or worsening of the condition being treated.

Evaluation

- Monitor patient response to the drug (improvement in condition being treated).
- Monitor for adverse effects (local stinging or inflammation).
- Evaluate effectiveness of teaching plan (patient can name drug, dosage, adverse effects to watch for, specific measures to avoid adverse effects; patient understands importance of continued follow-up).
- Monitor effectiveness of comfort measures and compliance with regimen.

Table B Topical Agents

Drug	Brand Name	Dosage	Usual Indication/Special Considerations
Emollients			
boric acid ointment	*Borofax*	Apply as needed	Relieves burns, itching, irritation
dexpanthenol	*Panthoderm*	Apply daily to b.i.d.	Relieves itching and aids in healing for mild skin irritations
lanolin		Ointment base, applied generously	Allergy to sheep or sheep products—use caution; base for many ointments
urea	*Aquacare* *Carmol* *Gordon's Urea* *Nutraplus* *Ureacin*	Apply two to four times per day to area affected	Rub in completely. Used to restore nails—cover with plastic wrap; keep dry and remove in 3, 7, or 14 days.
vitamins A & D	*generic*	Apply locally with gentle massage b.i.d. to q.i.d.	Relieves minor burns, chafing, skin irritations Consult health care provider if not improved within 7 days.
zinc oxide	*Borofax Skin Protectant*	Apply as needed	Relieves burns, abrasion, diaper rash
Growth Factor			
becaplermin	*Regranax*	Apply to diabetic foot ulcers b.i.d. to q.i.d.	Increases the incidence of healing of diabetic foot ulcers as adjunctive therapy; must have an adequate blood supply
Lotions and Solutions			
Burow's solution aluminum acetate	*Bluboro Powder* *Boropak Powder* *Domeboro Powder* *Pedi-Boro Soak Paks*	Dissolve one packet in a pint of water; apply q15–30min for 4–8 h	Astringent wet dressing for relief of inflammatory conditions, insect bites, athlete's foot, bruise, sores; do not use occlusive dressing.
calamine lotion	*generic*	Apply to affected area t.i.d. to q.i.d.	Relieves itching, pain of poison ivy, poison sumac and oak, insect bites, and minor skin irritations
hamamelis water	*Witch Hazel* *A-E-R*	Apply locally up to six times per day	Relieves itching and irritation of vaginal infection, hemorrhoids, postepisiotomy discomfort, posthemorrhoidectomy care
Antiseptics			
benzalkonium chloride	*Benza* *Zephiran* *Bacto-Shield*	Mix in solution as needed; spray for preoperative	Thoroughly rinse detergents and soaps from skin before use; add anti-rust tablets for instruments stored in solution; dilute solution as indicated for use.
chlorhexidine gluconate	*Dyna-Hex* *Exidine* *Hibistat* *Hibiclens*	Scrub or rinse; leave on for 15 sec; for surgical scrub—3 min	Use for surgical scrub, preoperative skin preparation, wound cleansing; preoperative bathing and showering
hexachlorphene	*pHisoHex* *Septisol*	Apply as wash	Surgical wash, scrub; do not use with burns or on mucous membranes; rinse thoroughly.

Table B Topical Agents *(Continued)*

Drug	Brand Name	Dosage	Usual Indication/Special Considerations
iodine	*generic*	Wash affected area	Highly toxic; avoid occlusive dressings; stains skin and clothing. Iodine allergy is common.
povidone-iodine	*ACU-dyne* *Betadine* *Betagen* *Iodex* *Operand*	Apply as needed	Treated areas may be bandaged. HIV is inactivated in this solution; causes less irritation than iodine; less toxic
sodium hypochlorite	*Dakin's*	Apply as antiseptic	Caution—chemical burns can occur.
thimersol	*Aeroaid* *Mersol*	Apply daily to b.i.d.	Contains mercury compound; used preoperatively and as first aid for abrasions, wounds
Antibiotic			
ciprofloxacin/ dexamethasone	*Ciprodex*	Apply drops to ears or outer ear canal	Treatment of acute otitis media with tympanostomy tubes; acute otitis externa.
mupirocin	*Bactroban*	Apply small amount to affected area t.i.d.	Used to treat impetigo caused by *Staphylococcus aureus*, *Streptococcus*, *S. pathogens*; may be covered with a gauze pad; monitor for signs of superinfection, reevaluate if no clinical response in 3–5 days.
Antivirals			
acyclovir	*Zovirax*	Apply ½-inch ribbon to affected area six times per day for 7 days	Treatment of herpes simplex cold sores and fever blisters (cream); initial herpes simplex virus genital infections (ointment)
docosanal	*Abreva*	Apply daily to b.i.d.	Used for treatment of oral and facial herpes simplex cold sores and fever blisters. Caution patient not to overuse.
imiquimod	*Aldara*	Apply thin layer to warts and rub in three times per week at bedtime for 16 wk	For treatment of genital warts and perianal warts; remove with soap and water after 6–10 h.
penciclovir	*Denavir*	Apply thin layer to affected area q2h while awake for 4 days	Treatment of cold sores in healthy patients; begin use at first sign of cold sore. Reserve use for herpes labialis on lips and face; avoid mucous membranes.
Antipsoriatics			
anthralin	*Anthra-Derm* *Drithocreme*	Apply daily only to psoriatic lesions	May stain fabrics, skin, hair, fingernails; use protective dressing.
calcipotriene	*Dovonex*	Apply thin layer twice a day	Monitor serum calcium levels with extended use; use only for disorder prescribed; may cause local irritation; is a synthetic vitamin D_3
calcipotriene/ betamethasone	*Taclonex*	Apply once daily for up to 4 wk	Monitor serum calcium levels and check for endocrine imbalance.
Antiseborrheics			
chloroxine	*Capitrol*	Massage into wet scalp; leave lather on for 3 min	May discolor blond, gray, or bleached hair. Do not use on active lesions.
selenium sulfide	*Selsun Blue*	Massage 5–10 mL into scalp; rest 2–3 min, rinse	May damage jewelry, remove before use; discontinue if local irritation occurs.
Antifungals			
butenafine HCl	*Mentax*	Apply to affected area once a day for 4 wk	Treatment of athlete's foot (intradigital pedia), tinea corporis, ringworm, tinea cruris
butoconazole nitrate	*Gynazole 1*	Apply intravaginally as one dose	Treatment of vaginal yeast infections; culture fungus, if no response, reculture. Ensure full course of therapy.
ciclopirox	*Loprox* *Penlac* *Penlac Nail Lacquer*	Apply directly to affected fingernails or toenails	Treatment of onychomycosis of the fingernails and toenails in immunocompromised patients

(continued)

Table B Topical Agents *(Continued)*

Drug	Brand Name	Dosage	Usual Indication/Special Considerations
clotrimazole	*Cruex* *Lotrimin* *Mycelex*	Gently massage into affected area b.i.d.	Cleanse area before applying; use for up to 4 wk. Discontinue if irritation or worsening of condition occurs.
econozole nitrate	*Spectazole*	Apply locally daily to b.i.d.	Treatment of athlete's foot (intradigital pedia), tinea corporis, ringworm, tinea cruris; cleanse area before applying; treat for 2–4 wk; for athlete's foot, change socks and shoes at least once a day.
gentian violet	*generic*	Apply locally b.i.d.	May stain skin and clothing; do not apply to active lesions.
ketoconazole	*Nizoral*	Shampoo daily	Reduction of scaling due to dandruff; burning may occur.
naftitine HCl	*Naftin*	Gently massage into affected area b.i.d.	Avoid occlusive dressings; wash hands thoroughly after application. Do not use longer than 4 wk.
oxiconazole	*Oxistat*	Apply daily to b.i.d.	May be needed for up to 1 mo.
sertaconazole nitrate	*Ertaczo*	Apply to affected areas and surrounding tissue b.i.d. for 4 wk	Treatment of tinea pedis.
terbinafine	*Lamisil*	Apply to area b.i.d. until clinical signs are improved; 1–4 wk	Do not use occlusive dressings; report local irritation; discontinue if local irritation occurs.
tolnaftate	*Aftate* *Genaspor* *Tinactin* *Ting*	Apply small amount b.i.d. for 2–3 wk, 4–6 wk may be needed if skin is very thick	Cleanse skin with soap and water before applying drug, dry thoroughly; wear loose, well-fitting shoes; change socks at least q.i.d.
Pediculocides/ Scabicides			
lindane	*G-Well*	Apply thin layer to entire body; leave on 8–12 h; wash thoroughly; shampoo 1–2 oz into dry hair and leave in place for 4 min	Single application is usually sufficient; reapply after 7 days at signs of live lice. Teach hygiene and prevention; treat all contacts. Assure parents this is a readily communicable disease.
malathion	*Ovide Lotion*	Apply to dry hair and leave on for 8–12 h; repeat in 7–9 days	Avoid use with open lesions. Change bed linens and clothing daily; treat all contacts.
crotamiton	*Eurax*	Thoroughly massage into skin over entire body, repeat in 24 h. Take a cleansing bath or shower 48 h after last application	Change all bed linens and clothing the next day. Contaminated clothing can be dry cleaned or washed in hot water. Shake well before using.
permethrin	*Acticin* *Elimite* *Nix*	Thoroughly massage into all skin areas; wash off after 8–14 h. Shampoo into freshly washed, rinsed, and towel-dried hair, leave on for 10 min, rinse	Single application is usually curative. Notify health care provider if rash, itch becomes worse. Approved for prophylactic use during head lice epidemics
Keratolytics			
podophyllium resin	*Podocon-25* *Podofin*	Applied only by physician	Do not use if wart is inflamed or irritated. Very toxic; minimum amount possible is used to avoid absorption.
podofilox	*Condylox*	Apply q12h for 3 consecutive days	Allow to dry before using area; dispose of used applicator; may cause burning and discomfort
Topical Hemostatics			
absorbable gelatin	*Gelfoam*	Smear or press to cut surface; when bleeding stops, remove excess. Apply sponge and allow to remain in place; will be absorbed	Prepare paste by adding 3–4 mL sterile saline to contents of jar. Apply sponge dry or saturated with saline. Assess for signs of infection. Do not use in presence of infection.
microfibrillar collagen	*Avitene* *Hemopad* *Hemotene*	Use dry. Apply directly to source of bleeding, apply pressure for 3–5 min. Discard leftover product.	Monitor for infection. Remove any excess material once bleeding has stopped.
thrombin	*Thrombinar* *Thrombogen* *Thrombostat*	Prepare in sterile distilled water; mix freely with blood on the surface of the injury	Contraindicated in the presence of any bovine allergies. Watch for severe allergic reactions in sensitive individuals.

Table B Topical Agents (Continued)

Drug	Brand Name	Dosage	Usual Indication/Special Considerations
Pain Relief			
capsaicin	*Capsin* *Dolorac* *Pain-X* *Zostrix*	Do not apply more than three to four times per day	Provides temporary relief from the pain of osteoarthritis, rheumatoid arthritis, neuralgias. Do not bandage tightly. Stop use and seek medical help if condition worsens or persists after 14–28 days.
Burn Preparations			
mafenide	*Sulfamylon*	Apply to a clean, debrided wound, one to two times per day. Cover burns at all times with drug; reapply as needed	Bathe patient in a whirlpool daily to debride wound. Continue debridement with a gloved hand. Cover. Continue until healing occurs. Monitor for infection and toxicity, especially acidosis. May cause severe discomfort requiring premedication before application
nitrofurazone	*Furacin*	Apply directly to burn or place on gauze; reapply daily	Flushing the dressing with sterile water will facilitate removal. Monitor for superinfections and treat appropriately. Rash is common.
silver sulfadiazine	*Silvadene* *SSD Cream* *Thermazene*	Apply daily to b.i.d. to a clean, debrided wound; use $\frac{1}{16}$-inch thickness	Bathe the patient in a whirlpool to aid debridement. Dressings are not necessary but may be used; reapply when necessary. Monitor for fungal infections.
Estrogens			
estradiol hemihydrate	*Vagifem*	Insert one tablet intravaginally daily for 2 wk, then one tablet intravaginally two times per wk	Treatment of atrophic vaginitis. Attempt to taper every 3–6 mo.
Acne Products			
adapalene	*Differin*	Apply a thin film to affected area after washing	Do not use near cuts or open wounds; avoid sun-burned areas; do not combine with other products; limit exposure to the sun. Less drying than most acne products
altretinoin	*Panretin*	1% gel; apply as needed to cover lesion b.i.d.	Treatment of lesions of Kaposi's sarcoma. Inflammation, peeling, redness may occur.
azelaic acid	*Azelex* *Finevin (20%)*	Wash and dry skin; massage thin layer into skin b.i.d.	Wash hands thoroughly after application. Improvement usually seen within 4 wk. Initial irritation usually passes with time.
clindamycin	*Evoclin*	Wash and dry area; massage into area morning and evening	Do not use occlusive dressings; may cause transient burning
metronidazole	*MetroGel* *Noritate*	Apply cream to affected area	Treatment of rosacea
sodium sulfacetamide	*Klaron*	Apply a thin film b.i.d.	Wash affected area with mild soap and water, pat dry. Avoid use in denuded or abraded areas.
tarazotene	*Tazorac*	Apply thin film daily in the evening	Avoid use in pregnancy. Drying, causes photosensitivity. Do not use with products containing alcohol.
tretinoin, 0.025% cream	*Avita*	Apply thin layer daily	Discomfort, peeling, redness, and worsening of acne may occur for first 2–4 wk
tretinoin, 0.05% cream	*Renova*	Apply thin coat in evening	Use for the removal of fine wrinkles.
tretinoin, gel	*Retin-A-micro*	Apply to cover daily, after cleansing	Exacerbation of inflammation may occur at first. Therapeutic effects usually seen in first 2 wk.
Mouth Products			
amlexanox	*Aphthasol* *OraDisc A*	Apply to aphthous ulcers q.i.d. after meals and at bedtime, following oral hygiene; for 10 days	Consult with dentist if ulcers are not healed within 10 days. May cause local pain
Antihistamine			
azelastine HCl	*Astelin*	Two sprays per nostril b.i.d.	Avoid use of alcohol and OTC antihistamines; dizziness and sedation may occur.

(continued)

Table B Topical Agents *(Continued)*

Drug	Brand Name	Dosage	Usual Indication/Special Considerations
Nasal Corticosteroid			
fluticasone	*Flonase* *Flovent Rotadisk*	Adult: 88–440 mcg intranasal b.i.d.; lower dose if also on corticosteroids Pediatric: 500–600 mcg b.i.d. via rotodisk	Preventive treatment for asthma, not a primary treatment. May take several weeks to see effects Pediatric use for children 4–11 yr
Hair Removal			
eflornithine	*Vaniqa*	Apply to unwanted facial hair b.i.d. for up to 24 wk	Approved for use in women only
Skin Substitute			
graftskin lasting	*Alpigraf*	Apply to wound, keep clean, loose cover	Treatment of venous leg ulcers lasting >1 mo; diabetic foot ulcers lasting >3 wk
Topical Corticosteroids			
These drugs enter cells and bind to cytoplasmic receptors, initiating complex reactions that are responsible for the anti-inflammatory, anti-pruritic, and anti-proliferative effects of these drugs. They are used to relieve the inflammation and pruritic manifestations of corticosteroid-sensitive dermatoses and for temporary relief of minor skin irritations and rashes. These agents should always be applied sparingly because of the risk of systemic corticosteroid effects if absorbed systemically. Occlusive dressings and tight coverings should be avoided. Prolonged use should also be avoided because of the risk of systemic effects and local irritation and breakdown. These agents are applied topically two to three times daily.			
alclometasone dipropionate	*Aclovate*	Ointment, cream: 0.05% concentration	Occlusive dressings may be used for the management of refractory lesions of psoriasis and deep-seated dermatoses.
amcinonide	*Cyclocort*	Ointment, cream, lotion: 0.1% concentration	
betamethasone dipropionate	*Diprosone, Maxivate, Teledar*	Ointment, cream, lotion, aerosol: 0.05% concentration	
betamethasone dipropionate, augmented	*Diprolene*	Ointment, cream, lotion: 0.05% concentration	
betamethasone valerate	*Betaderm, Beta-Val, Valisone*	Ointment, cream, lotion: 0.01% concentration	
clobetasol propionate	*Cormax, Temovate* *Clobex*	Ointment, cream: 0.05% concentration Spray 0.05%	
clocortolone pivalate	*Cloderm*	Cream: 0.1% concentration	
desonide	*DesOwen, Tridesiolon*	Ointment, cream: 0.05% concentration	
desoximetasone	*Topicort*	Ointment, cream: 0.25% concentration Gel: 0.05% concentration	
dexamethasone	*Decaspray* *Aeroseb-Dex*	Gel: 0.1% concentration Aerosol: 0.01% concentration Aerosol: 0.04% concentration	
dexamethasone sodium phosphate	*generic*	Cream: 0.1% concentration	
diflorasone diacetate	*Florone, Maxiflor, Psorcon* *Florone E*	Ointment, cream: 0.05% concentration Cream: 0.5% concentration	
fluocinolone acetonide	*Flurosyn, Synalar* *Flurosyn, Synalar, Synemol* *Fluonid, Flurosyn, Synalar*	Ointment: 0.025% concentration Cream: 0.01% concentration Cream: 0.025% concentration Solution: 0.01% concentration	
fluocinonide	*Lidex* *Fluonex, Lidex, Vasoderm* *Lidex, Topsyn Gel* *Vanos*	Ointment: 0.05% concentration Cream: 0.05% concentration Solution, gel: 0.05% concentration Cream: 0.1%	

Table B Topical Agents (Continued)

Drug	Brand Name	Dosage	Usual Indication/Special Considerations
flurandrenolide	*generic*	Ointment, cream: 0.025% concentration Ointment, cream, lotion: 0.05% concentration Tape: 4 mcg/cm^2	
fluticasone propionate	*Cutivate*	Cream: 0.05% concentration Ointment: 0.005% concentration	
halcinonide	*Halog*	Ointment, cream, solution: 0.1% concentration	
halobetasol propionate	*Ultravate*	Ointment, cream: 0.05% concentration	
hydrocortisone	*Cortizone 5, Bactine Hydrocortisone, Cort-Dome, Dermolate, Dermtex HC, HydroTex* *Cortizone 10, Hycort, Tegrin-HC* *Hytone*	Lotion: 0.25% concentration Cream, lotion, ointment, aerosol: 0.5%, 1% concentration Cream, lotion, ointment, solution: 1% concentration	
hydrocortisone acetate	*Cortaid, Lanacort-5* *Corticaine (R$_x$), FoilleCort, Gynecort, Lanacort 5* *Anusol-HC* *Cortaid with Aloe*	Ointment: 0.5% concentration (OTC preparations) Cream: 0.5% concentration (OTC preparations) Cream: 1% concentration Cream: 0.5%, 1% concentration (OTC preparation)	
hydrocortisone buteprate	*generic*	Cream: 0.1% concentration	
hydrocortisone butyrate	*Locoid*	Ointment, cream: 0.1% concentration	
hydrocortisone valerate	*Westcort*	Ointment, cream: 0.2% concentration	
mometasone furoate	*Elocon* *Nasonex* *Asmanex Twisthaler*	Ointment, cream, lotion: 0.1% concentration Nasal spray: 0.2% concentration Solution for inhalation: 220 mcg/actuation	
prednicarbate	*Dermatop*	Cream: 0.1% concentration: preservative free	
triamcinolone acetonide	*Flutex, Kenalog* *Aristocort, Flutex, Kenalog* *Aristocort, Flutex, Kenalog, Triacet, Triderm*	Ointment: 0.025% concentration Ointment: 0.1% concentration and 0.5% concentration Cream: 0.025% concentration and 0.5% concentration Cream: 0.1% concentration Lotion: 0.025% and 0.1% concentration	

APPENDIX C

Ophthalmic Agents

Ophthalmic agents are drugs that are intended for direct administration into the conjunctiva of the eye. These drugs are used to treat glaucoma (miotics constrict the pupil and decrease the resistance to aqueous flow), to aid in the diagnosis of eye problems (mydriatics dilate the pupil for examination of the retina; cycloplegics paralyze the muscles that control the lens to aid refraction); to treat local ophthalmic infections or inflammation; and to provide relief from the signs and symptoms of allergic reactions.

These drugs are not generally absorbed systemically because of their method of administration. They are classified in Pregnancy Category C, and caution should always be used when giving drugs during pregnancy or lactation.

Contraindications and Cautions

These drugs are contraindicated in the presence of allergy to the specific drug or to any component of the product being used. Although they are seldom absorbed systemically, caution should be used in any patient who would have problems with the systemic effects of the drugs if they were absorbed systemically.

Adverse Effects

Adverse effects of these drugs include local irritation, stinging, burning, blurring of vision (prolonged when using ointments), tearing, and headache.

Clinically Important Drug–Drug Interactions

Because of their actions on the eye or because of the components of the drug, many of these drugs cannot be given at the same time but should be spaced 1 to 2 hours apart. Check the specific drug being used for details.

Dosage

The usual dosage for any of these drugs is one to two drops in each eye or in the affected eye two to four times daily, or 0.25 to 0.5 inches of ointment in the affected eye or eyes.

Nursing Considerations

Assessment

Screen for the following: allergy to the specific drug or components of the preparation; underlying medical conditions that would be affected if the drug were absorbed systemically.

Evaluate eye, conjunctival color; note any lesions. A vision examination may be appropriate.

Nursing Diagnoses

The patient receiving an ophthalmic agent may have the following nursing diagnoses related to drug therapy:

- Acute Pain related to administration of the drug
- Risk for Injury related to changes in vision
- Deficient Knowledge regarding drug therapy

Implementation

- Assess patient's general physical condition before beginning test *to decrease the potential for adverse effects.*
- Follow these administration guidelines *to provide the most therapeutic use of the drug with the fewest adverse effects*:

  Solution or drops: Wash hands thoroughly before administering; do not touch dropper to eye or to any other surface. Have patient tilt head backward or lie down, and stare upward. Gently grasp lower eyelid and pull eyelid away from the eyeball; instill drops into pouch formed by eyelid. Release lid slowly; have patient close the eye and look downward. Apply gentle pressure to

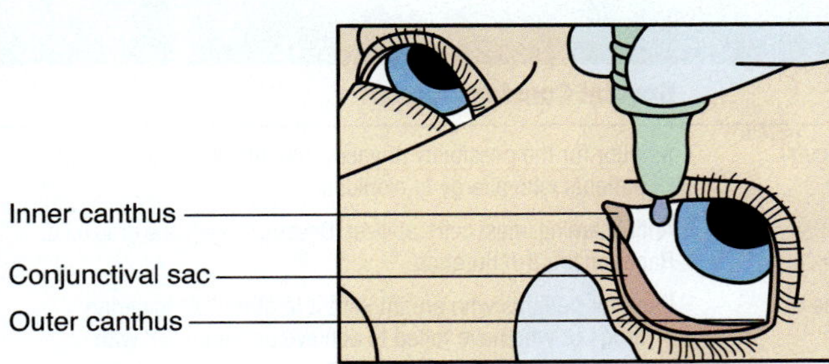

FIGURE C.1 Administration of ophthalmic drops.

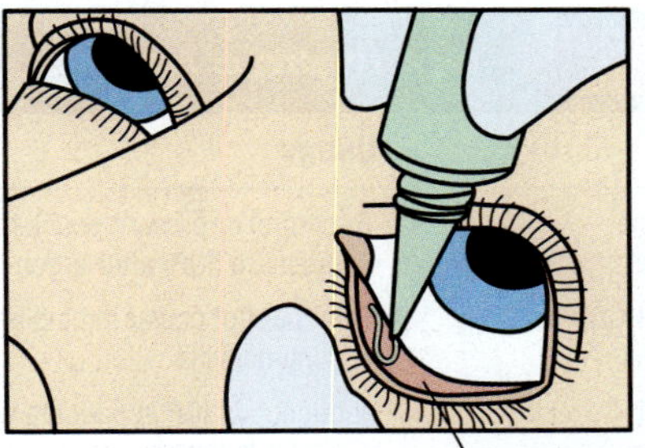

FIGURE C.2 Administration of ophthalmic ointment.

the inside corner of the eye for 3 to 5 minutes to retard drainage. Do not rub eyes; do not rinse eyedropper. Do not use eye drops that have changed color; if more than one type of eye drop is used, wait at least 5 minutes between administrations. Refer to Figure C.1.

Ointment: Wash hands thoroughly before administering; hold tube between hands for several minutes to warm ointment; discard the first centimeter of ointment when opening the tube for the first time. Tilt head backward or have patient lie down and stare upward. Gently pull out lower lid to form pouch; place 0.25 to 0.5 inches of ointment inside the lower lid. Have patient close the eye for 1 to 2 minutes and roll the eyeball in all directions; remove any excess ointment from around the eye. If using more than one kind of ointment, wait at least 10 minutes between administrations. Refer to Figure C.2.

- Provide comfort measures *to help patient tolerate drug effects* (e.g., control light, analgesics as needed).
- Include the following information—in addition to the proper administration technique for the drug—in the teaching program for the patient *to improve compliance and provide safety and comfort measures as necessary:* safety measures may need to be taken if blurring of vision should occur; burning and stinging may occur on administration but should pass quickly; the pupils will dilate with mydriatic agents and the eyes may become very sensitive to light (the use of sunglasses is recommended); any severe eye discomfort, palpitations, nausea, or headache should be reported to the health care provider.

Evaluation

- Monitor patient response to the drug (changes in pupil size, relief of pressure of glaucoma, relief of itching and tearing related to allergic reaction).
- Monitor for adverse effects (local irritation, blurring of vision, headache).
- Evaluate effectiveness of teaching plan (patient can name adverse effects to watch for, specific measures to avoid adverse effects; patient understands importance of follow-up that will be needed).
- Monitor effectiveness of comfort measures and compliance with regimen.

Table C Ophthalmic Agents

Drug	Usage	Special Considerations
apraclonidine (*Lopidine*)	To control or prevent postsurgical elevations of intraocular pressure (IOP) after argon–laser eye surgery	Monitor for the possibility of vasovagal attack; do not give to patients with allergy to clonidine.
azelastine (HCl) (*Optivar*)	Treatment of ocular itching associated with allergic conjunctivitis	Antihistamine, mast cell stabilizer. Dosage (≥3 yr): one drop b.i.d. Rapid onset, 8-h duration
bimatoprost (*Lumigan*)	Reduction of IOP in patients with open-angle glaucoma or ocular hypertension	Used for patients who are intolerant to other IOP-lowering drugs or who have failed to achieve optimum IOP with other IOP-lowering medications
brimonidine tartrate (*Alphagan, Alphagan P*)	Treatment of open-angle glaucoma and ocular hypertension	Selective alpha$_2$-antagonist; minimal effects on cardiovascular and pulmonary systems. Do not use with monoamine oxidase inhibitors. Dosage: one drop t.i.d.
brinzolamide (*Azopt*)	To decrease intraocular pressure in open-angle glaucoma	May be given with other agents. Dosage: one drop t.i.d. Give 10 min apart from any other agents.
bromfenac (*Xilorom*)	Treatment of postoperative inflammation following cataract surgery	One drop in affected eye b.i.d. starting 24 h after surgery for 2 wks
carbachol (*Carbastat, Miostat,Carboptic*)	Direct-acting miotic; for treatment of glaucoma; miosis during surgery	Surgical dose: a one-use-only portion. For glaucoma: one to two drops up to t.i.d. as needed
cyclopentolate (*Ak-Pentolate, Cyclogyl,Pentolair*)	Mydriasis/cycloplegia in diagnostic procedures	Individuals with dark-pigmented irises may require higher doses; compress lacrimal sac for 1–2 min after administration to decrease any systemic absorption.
cyclosporine emulsion (*Restasis*)	Increases tear production in patients with decreased tear production related to inflammation or keratoconjunctivitis sicca	One drop in each eye b.i.d., approx. 12 h apart; remove contact lenses during use.
dapiprazole (*Rev-Eyes*)	Miotic: iatrogenically induced mydriasis produced by adrenergic or parasympathetic agents	Not for use to reduce IOP; do not use if constriction is undesirable. Do not use more than once a week.
diclofenac sodium (*Voltaren Ophthalmic*)	Photophobia: for use in patients undergoing incisional refractive surgery	Apply one drop q.i.d. beginning 24 h after cataract surgery; continue through the first 2 wk after surgery.
dipivefrin (*Propine, AK Pro*)	Control of IOP in chronic open-angle glaucoma	One drop q12h; monitor closely with tonometry.
dorzolamide (*Trusopt*)	Treatment of elevated IOP in open-angle glaucoma or ocular hypertension	A sulfonamide; monitor patients taking parenteral sulfonamides for possible adverse effects.
dorzolamide 2% and timolol 0.5% (*Cosopt*)	To decrease IOP in open-angle glaucoma or ocular hypertension in patients who do not respond to beta-blockers alone	Administer one drop in affected eye b.i.d. Monitor for cardiac failure; if absorbed, may mask symptoms of hypoglycemia or thyrotoxicosis
echothiopate (generic)	Treatment of glaucoma; irreversible cholinesterase inhibitor; long-acting Accommodative esotropia	Given only once a day because of long duration of action; tolerance may develop with prolonged use but usually returns after a rest period.
emedastine (*Emadine*)	Temporary relief of signs and symptoms of allergic conjunctivitis	One drop in affected eye up to q.i.d. Do not wear contact lenses if eyes are red; may cause headache, blurred vision
epinastine (*Elestat*)	Prevention of itching caused by allergic conjunctivitis	One drop in each eye b.i.d. for entire time of exposure Remove contact lenses before use.
fluocinolone (*Retisert*)	Treatment of noninfectious uveitis in posterior segment of eye	One implant every 3 months
fluorometholone (*Flarex, Fluor-Op*)	Topical corticosteroid used for treatment of inflammatory conditions of the eye	Improvement should occur within several days, discontinue if no improvement is seen. Discontinue if swelling of the eye occurs.
fomivirsen sodium (*Vitravene*)	Treatment of retinal cytomegalovirus in AIDS patients who cannot tolerate other agents	Injected into affected eye every other week for two doses, then every 4 wk; do not use if previously treated with cidofivir within past 2–4 wk.
gatifloxacin (*Zymar*)	Treatment of bacterial conjunctivitis caused by susceptible strains	Contacts should not be worn. Can cause blurred vision.

Table C Ophthalmic Agents (*Continued*)

Drug	Usage	Special Considerations
homatropine (*Isopto-Homatropine, Homatropin HBr*)	Long-acting mydriatic and cycloplegic used for refraction and treatment of inflammatory conditions of the uveal tract	Individuals with dark-pigmented irises may require larger doses; 5–10 min is usually required for refraction.
ketotifen (*Zaditor*)	Temporary relief of itching due to allergic conjunctivitis	Remove contact lenses before use—may be replaced 10 min after administration. An antihistamine/mast cell stabilizer
latanoprost (*Xalatan*)	Treatment of open-angle glaucoma or ocular hypertension in patients intolerant or unresponsive to other agents	Remove contact lenses before use and for 15 min after use; allow at least 5 min between this and the use of any other agents; expect blurring of vision
levobetaxolol (*Betaxon*)	Reduction of IOP with chronic open-angle glaucoma, ocular hypertension	One drop b.i.d.; may take up to 2 wk to see results; do not combine with beta-adrenergics.
levobunolol (*AK Beta, Betagan Liquifilm*)	Lowering of IOP with chronic open-angle glaucoma, ocular hypertension	One to two drops b.i.d. Do not combine with beta-blockers.
levofloxin (*Quixin*)	Treatment of bacterial conjunctivitis caused by susceptible bacteria	One to two drops per day in affected eye
lodoxamide (*Alomide*)	Treatment of vernal conjunctivitis and keratitis	Patients should not wear contact lenses while using this drug; discontinue if stinging or burning persists after instillation.
loteprednol etabonate (*Lotemax [0.5%]*) (*Alrex [0.2%]*)	Treatment of steroid-resistant ocular disease Treatment of postoperative inflammation after ocular surgery	One to two drops q.i.d. One to two drops q.i.d. beginning 24 h after surgery and continuing for 2 wk. Shake vigorously before use. Discard after 14 days. Prolonged use may cause nerve or eye damage.
metipranolol (*OptiPranolol*)	Beta-blocker; used in treating chronic open-angle glaucoma and ocular hypertension	Concomitant therapy may be needed; caution patient about possible vision changes.
moxifloxacin (*Vigamox*)	Treatment of bacterial conjunctivitis caused by susceptible strains	Contact lenses should not be worn. Can cause blurred vision.
natamycin (*Natacyn*)	Antibiotic used to treat fungal blepharitis, conjunctivitis, and keratitis; drug of choice for Fusarium sotani keratitis	Shake well before each use; store at room temperature. Failure to improve in 7–10 days suggests a nonsusceptible organism; re-evaluate.
nedocromil (*Alcoril*)	Treatment of itching of allergic conjunctivitis	One to two drops in each eye b.i.d. for entire allergy season
nepafenac (*Nevanac*)	Relief of pain and inflammation after cataract surgery	One drop in affected eye t.i.d., starting 24 h before surgery, day of surgery, next 2 wks. Do not wear contact lenses.
olopatadine hydrochloride (*Patanol*)	Mast cell stabilizer and antihistamine; provides fast onset of relief of itching due to conjunctivitis and has prolonged action	Not for use with contact lenses; headache is a common side effect.
pemirolast potassium (*Alamast*)	Prevention of itchy eyes due to allergic conjunctivitis	One to two drops q.i.d.
pilocarpine (*Adsorbocarpine, Akarpine, Isopto Carpine, Pilocar, Piloptic, Pilostat*)	Chronic and acute glaucoma; treatment of mydriasis caused by drugs; direct-acting mitotic	Can be stored at room temperature for up to 8 wk, then discard. May use 1–2 drops up to six times per day, based on patient response
polydimethylsiloxane (*AdatoSil*)	Treatment of retinal detachments when other therapy is not effective or is inappropriate; primary choice for retinal detachment caused by AIDS-related cytomegalovirus retinitis or viral infection	Monitor for cataracts; must be injected directly into the aqueous humor
rimexolone (*Vexol*)	Corticosteroid; postoperative ocular surgery for the treatment of anterior uveitis	Monitor for signs of steroid absorption.
suprofen (*Profenal*)	NSAID; used to inhibit intraoperative miosis	Local burning may occur; monitor patient for cross-sensitivities to other nonsteroidal anti-inflammatory drugs (NSAIDs).
timolol (*Timoptic-XE*)	Treatment of elevated IOP in ocular hypertension or open-angle glaucoma	One drop in affected eye(s) each day in the morning

(*continued*)

Table C **Ophthalmic Agents** *(Continued)*

Drug	Usage	Special Considerations
travoprost (*Travatan*)	Reduction of intraocular pressure in patients with open-angle glaucoma or ocular hypertension	Reserve for patients who are intolerant of other IOP-lowering medications or who have failed to achieve optimum IOP with other IOP-lowering medications.
trifluridine (*Viroptic*)	Antiviral; used to treat primary keratoconjunctivitis and recurrent epithelial keratitis due to herpes simplex virus types 1 and 2	Transient burning or stinging may occur; reconsider drug choice if improvement is not seen within 7 days. Do not administer longer than 21 days at a time.
tropicamide (*Mydriacyl Opticyl*)	Mydriatic and cyclopegic for refraction	One to two drops, repeat in 5 min. May repeat in 30 min for prolonged effects
unoprostone (*Rescula*)	Treatment of open-angle glaucoma ocular hypertension in patients who do not respond to other agents	One drop b.i.d.; not for use in children or during pregnancy or lactation. Remove contact lenses during use.

APPENDIX D

Vitamins

Vitamins are substances that the body requires for carrying out essential metabolic reactions. The body cannot synthesize enough of these components to meet all of its needs, therefore, they must be obtained from animal and vegetable tissues taken in as food. Vitamins are needed only in small amounts because they function as coenzymes that activate the protein portions of enzymes, which catalyze a great deal of biochemical activity. Vitamins are either water soluble and excreted in the urine, or they are fat soluble and capable of being stored in adipose tissue in the body.

Therapeutic Actions and Indications

Vitamins act as coenzymes to activate a variety of proteins on enzymes that catalyze biochemical activity. They are indicated for the treatment of vitamin deficiencies, as dietary supplements when needed, and as specific therapy related to the activity of the vitamin.

Contraindications and Cautions

These drugs are contraindicated in the presence of any known allergy to the drug or the colorants, additives, or preservatives used in the drug. They are categorized as Pregnancy Category C and are used to maintain adequate vitamin levels during pregnancy and lactation.

Adverse Effects

The adverse effects primarily associated with these drugs are related to gastrointestinal upset and irritation, which is caused by direct gastrointestinal contact with the drugs.

Clinically Important Drug–Drug Interactions

Pyridoxine, vitamin B_6, interferes with the effectiveness of levodopa.

Fat-soluble vitamins may not be absorbed if given concurrently with mineral oil, cholestyramine, or colestipol.

Nursing Considerations

Assessment

Obtain a nutritional assessment. Screen for any medical conditions and drugs being taken and for any known allergies.

Evaluate skin, and mucous membranes; pulse, respirations, and blood pressure. Complete blood count (CBC) and clotting times may need to be evaluated with specific vitamins.

Nursing Diagnoses

The patient receiving vitamins may have the following nursing diagnoses related to drug therapy:

- Acute Pain related to GI discomfort
- Risk for Imbalanced Nutrition related to replacement therapy
- Deficient Knowledge regarding drug therapy

Implementation

- Assess patient's general physical condition before beginning test *to decrease the potential for adverse effects and assure need for the drug.*
- Advise patient to avoid the use of over-the-counter preparations that contain the same vitamins *to prevent inadvertent overdose of the vitamin.*
- Provide comfort measures *to help patient tolerate drug effects* (e.g., take drug with meals to alleviate gastrointestinal distress).
- Include information about the solution being used in a test (e.g., what to expect, adverse effects that may occur,

follow-up tests that may be needed) *to enhance patient knowledge about drug therapy and promote compliance with drug regimen.*

Evaluation

- Monitor patient response to the drug (adequate vitamin intake).
- Monitor for adverse effects (GI upset).
- Evaluate effectiveness of teaching plan (patient can name adverse effects to watch for, specific measures to avoid adverse effects; patient understands importance of follow-up that will be needed).
- Monitor effectiveness of comfort measures and compliance with the regimen.

Table D Vitamins

Vitamin	Solubility Type	Recommended Dietary Allowance	Therapeutic Uses/Special Considerations
A (*Aquasol A, Palmitate-A 5000*)	Fat	1000 mcg (male) 800 mcg (female) 1300 mcg (lactation) 375–700 mcg (pediatric)	Severe deficiency: 500,000 International Units/day for 3 days, then 50,000 International Units/day for 2 wk given IM or PO. Protect IM vial from light. Hypervitaminosis A can occur, including cirrhotic-like liver syndrome with central nervous system effects; gastrointestinal drying, rash, and liver changes. Treat by discontinuing the vitamin and give saline, prednisone, and calcitonin IV. Liver damage may be permanent.
ascorbic acid (*Cecon, Cevi-Bid, Dull C, Vita-C, N'Ice Vitamin C Drops*)	Water	50–60 mg (male) 50–60 mg (female) 70–90 mg (lactation) 70 mg (pregnancy) 30–45 mg (pediatric)	May be given PO, IM, slow IV, or Sub-Q. Treatment of scurvy: 300–1000 mg daily. Enhanced wound healing: 300–500 mg/day for 7–10 days. Burns: 1–2 g/day. Also being studied for treatment of common cold, asthma, coronary artery disease, cancer, and schizophrenia. May be very toxic at high doses.
calcifediol (D_3) (*Calderol*)	Fat		Management of metabolic bone disease or hypocalcemia in patients receiving chronic renal dialysis: 300–350 mcg/wk daily or on alternate days. Discontinue if hypercalcemia occurs.
cholecalciferol (D_3) (*Delta-D*)	Fat	200–400 International Unit (male) 200–400 International Unit (female) 400 International Unit (lactation) 400 International Unit (pregnancy) 300–400 International Unit (pediatric)	Vitamin D deficiency: 400–1000 International Unit/day. May be useful for the treatment of hypocalcemic tetany and hypoparathyroidism
cyanocobalamin (B_{12}) (*Big Shot B_{12}, Crystamine, Crysti 1000, Cyanoject, Cyomin, Rubersol 1000*)	Water	2 mcg (male) 2 mcg (female) 2.6 mcg (lactation) 2.2 mcg (pregnancy) 0.3–1.4 mcg (pediatric)	Deficiency: 25–250 mcg/day. (Note: oral route is not for the treatment of pernicious anemia.) Pernicious anemia: 100 mcg IM each month for life; given with folic acid; nasal route is preferable.
D	Fat	200–400 International Unit (male) 200–400 International Unit (female) 400 International Unit (lactation) 400 International Unit (pregnancy) 300–400 International Unit (pediatric)	Vitamin D deficiency: 400–1000 International Units/day. May be useful for the treatment of hypocalcemic tetany and hypoparathyroidism. Encourage balanced diet and exposure to sunlight. Do not use with mineral oil.
dihydrotachysterol (*DHT, D_2*)(*DHT, Hytakerol*)	Fat		Treatment of postoperative tetany, idiopathic tetany, and hypoparathyroidism. Initial dose: 0.8–2.4 mg/day for several days, then 0.2–1 mg/day to achieve normal serum calcium. May supplement with oral calcium.

Table D Vitamins (*Continued*)

Vitamin	Solubility Type	Recommended Dietary Allowance	Therapeutic Uses/Special Considerations
E (*Aquavil-E, Vita-Plus E Softgels*)	Fat	15 International Unit (male) 12 International Unit (female) 16–18 International Unit (lactation) 15 International Unit (pregnancy) 4–10 International Unit (pediatric)	Used in certain premature infants to reduce the toxic effects of oxygen on the lung and retina; do not give IV; report fatigue, weakness, nausea, or headache.
ergocalciferol (D_2) (*Calciferol, Drisdol Drops*)	Fat	200–400 International Unit (male) 200–400 International Unit (female) 400 International Unit (lactation) 400 International Unit (pregnancy) 300–400 International Unit (pediatric)	Give IM in gastrointestinal, biliary, or liver disease. Refractory rickets: 12,000–500,000 International Unit/day. Hypoparathyroidism: 50,000–2,000,000 International Unit/day. Familial hypophosphatemia: 10,000–80,000 International Unit/day plus 1–2 g phosphorus.
niacin (B_3) (*Niacor, Nicotinic Acid, Nicotinex, SLO-Niacin, Niaspan*)	Water	15–20 mg (male) 13–15 mg (female) 20 mg (lactation) 17 mg (pregnancy) 5–13 mg (pediatric)	Prevention and treatment of pellagra: up to 500 mg/day. Niacin deficiency: up to 100 mg/day. Also used for the treatment of hyperlipidemia if no response to diet and exercise: 1–2 g t.i.d. Do not exceed 6 g/day. Feelings of warmth or flushing may occur with administration but usually pass within 2 h.
nicotinamide (B_3) (*Niacinamide*)	Water	15–20 mg (male) 13–15 mg (female) 20 mg (lactation) 17 mg (pregnancy) 5–13 mg (pediatric)	Prevention and treatment of pellagra: up to 50 mg, 3–10 times per day.
P (*bioflavonoids*) (*Amino Opti-C, Bio-Acerola C, Citro-Flav 2000, Flavons 500, Pan C-500, Peridin C, Quercetin, Span C*)	Water	Unknown	Used to treat bleeding, abortion, poliomyelitis, diabetes, and other conditions. There is little evidence that these uses have any clinical efficacy.
phytonadione (K) (*Mephyton*)	Fat	45–80 mcg (male) 45–65 mcg (female) 65 mcg (lactation) 65 mcg (pregnancy) 5–30 mcg (pediatric)	Hypoprothrombinemia due to anticoagulant use: 2.5–10 mg PO, IM. Hemorrhagic disease of the newborn: 0.5–1 mg IM within 1 h of birth: 1–5 mg IM may be given to the mother before delivery. Hypoprothrombinemia in adult: 2.5–25 mg PO or IM
pyridoxine HCl (B_6) (*Aminoxin, Nestrex*)	Water	1.7–2 mg (male) 1.4–1.6 mg (female) 2.1 mg (lactation) 2.2 mg (pregnancy) 0.3–1.4 mg (pediatric)	Deficiency: 10–20 mg/day PO or IM for 3 wk. Vitamin B_6 deficiency syndrome: up to 600 mg/day for life. Isoniazid poisoning (give an equal amount of pyridoxine): 4 g IV followed by 1 g IM q30min. Reduces the effectiveness of levodopa and leads to serious toxic effects—avoid this combination.
riboflavin	Water	1.4–1.8 mg (male) 1.2–1.3 mg (female) 1.7 –1.8 mg (lactation) 1.6 mg (pregnancy) 0.4–1.2 mg (pediatric)	Treatment of deficiency: 5–15 mg/day. May cause a yellow or orange discoloration to the urine
thiamine HCl (B_1) (*Thiamilate*)	Water	1.2–1.5 mg (male) 1–1.1 mg (female) 1.6 mg (lactation) 1.5 mg (pregnancy) 0.3–1 mg (pediatric)	Treatment of wet beriberi: 10–30 mg IV t.i.d. Treatment of beriberi: 10–20 mg IM t.i.d. for 2 wk with multivitamin containing 5–10 mg/day for 1 mo. Do not mix in alkaline solutions. Used orally as a mosquito repellant, alters body sweat composition. Feeling of warmth and flushing may occur with administration but usually passes within 2 h.

APPENDIX E

Alternative and Complementary Therapies

Many natural substances are used by the public for self-treatment of many complaints. These substances, derived from folklore of various cultures, often have ingredients that have been identified and have known therapeutic activities. Some of these substances have unknown mechanisms of action but over the years have been reliably used to relieve specific symptoms. There is an element of the placebo effect in using some of these substances. The power of believing that something will work and that there is some control over the problem is often very beneficial in achieving relief from pain or suffering. Some of these substances may contain yet unidentified ingredients, which, when discovered, may prove very useful in the modern field of pharmacology. Because these products are not regulated or monitored, there is always a possibility of toxic effects. Some of these products may contain ingredients that interact with prescription drugs. A history of the use of these alternative therapies may explain unexpected reactions to some drugs.

Substance	Reported Use
acidophilus	Oral: prevention or treatment of uncomplicated diarrhea; decreases effectiveness of warfarin
alfalfa	Topical: healing ointment, relief of arthritis pain Oral: arthritis treatment, strength giving
allspice	Topical: anesthetic for teeth and gums; soothes sore joints and muscles Oral: treatment of indigestion, flatulence, diarrhea, fatigue Seizures have been reported with excessive dosage.
aloe leaves	Topical: treatment of burns, healing of wounds Oral: treatment of chronic constipation
androstenedione	Oral spray: anabolic steroid effects to increase muscle mass
angelica	Oral: "cure all" for gynecological problems, headaches, and backaches; increases circulation in the periphery Risk of bleeding if combined with anticoagulants
anise	Oral: relief of dry cough, treatment of flatulence
apple	Oral: control of blood glucose, constipation
arnica gel	Topical: relief of pain from muscle or soft tissue injury
ashwagandha	Oral: enhancement of mental and physical functioning; general tonic; used to protect cells during cancer chemotherapy and radiation therapy Avoid use during pregnancy and lactation.
astragalus	Oral: increases stamina and energy; improves immune function and resistance to disease Do not use with fever or acute infection.
barberry	Oral: antidiarrheal, antipyretic, cough suppressant Risk of spontaneous abortion if taken during pregnancy
bayberry	Topical: to promote wound healing Oral: stimulant, emetic, antidiarrheal

Substance	Reported Use
bee pollen	Oral: treatment of allergies, asthma, impotence, prostatitis; suggested use to decrease cholesterol levels Risk of hyperglycemia; do not use in diabetic patients or with antidiabetic drugs.
betel palm	Oral: mild stimulant, digestive aid Increased risk of hypertension with MAOIs, decreased heart rate with digoxin, beta-blockers
bilberry	Oral: treatment of diabetes; cardiovascular problems; lowers cholesterol and triglycerides; treatment of diabetic retinopathy; treatment of cataracts, night blindness
birch bark	Topical: treatment of infected wounds, cuts Oral: as tea for relief of stomach ache
blackberry	Oral: as tea for generalized healing; treatment of diabetes
black cohosh root	Oral: treatment of PMS, menopausal disorders, rheumatoid arthritis Contains estrogen-like components. Do not use with hormone replacement therapy or hormonal contraceptives; avoid use in pregnancy and lactation; may lower blood pressure with sedatives, antihypertensives
bromelain	Oral: treatment of inflammation, sports injuries, URIs, PMS, and adjunctive therapy in cancer treatments Associated with nausea, vomiting, diarrhea, menstrual disorders
burdock	Oral: treatment of diabetes; atropine-like side effects, uterine stimulant May lower blood sugar with antidiabetics
capsicum	Topical: external analgesic Oral: treatment of bowel disorders, chronic laryngitis, peripheral vascular disease Risk of bleeding with warfarin, aspirin
catnip leaves	Oral: treatment of bronchitis, diarrhea
cat's claw	Oral: treatment of allergies, arthritis; adjunct in the treatment of cancers and AIDS Do not use with pregnancy, lactation, transplant recipients; increased risk of bleeding episodes if taken with oral anticoagulants
cayenne pepper	Topical: treatment of burns, wounds, relief of toothache
celery	Oral: lowers blood glucose, acts as a diuretic; may cause potassium depletion Use caution with diabetics.
chamomile	Topical: treatment of wounds, ulcer, conjunctivitis Oral: treatment of migraines, gastric cramps, relief of anxiety Contains coumarin—closely monitor patients taking anticoagulants. May cause depression; monitor patients on antidepressants. Cross-reaction with ragweed allergies may occur. Do not use during pregnancy or lactation.
chaste-tree berry	Oral: progesterone-like effects; used to treat PMS and menopausal problems, and to stimulate lactation Use caution with hormone replacement therapy and hormonal contraceptives.
chicken soup	Oral: breaks up respiratory secretions, bronchodilator, relieves anxiety
chicory	Oral: treatment of digestive tract problems, gout; stimulates bile secretions
Chinese angelica (dong quai)	Oral: general tonic; treatment of anemias, PMS, menopause, antihypertensive, laxative Use caution with the flu, hemorrhagic diseases. Monitor patients on antihypertensives or vasodilators for toxic effects. Use caution with hormone replacement therapy.
chondroitin	Oral: treatment of osteoarthritis and related disorders Risk of increased bleeding if combined with anticoagulants
chong cao fungi	Oral: antioxidant, promotes stamina, sexual function Avoid use in children.
coleus forskohlii	Oral: treatment of asthma, hypertension, eczema Use caution with antihypertensives or antihistamines; severe additive effects can occur. Avoid use with hypotension or peptic ulcers.
comfrey	Topical: treatment of wounds, cuts, ulcers Oral: gargle for tonsillitis
coriander	Oral: weight loss, lowers blood glucose
creatine monohydrate	Oral: enhancement of athletic performance
dandelion root	Oral: treatment of liver and kidney problems; decreases lactation (after delivery or with weaning); lowers blood glucose Use caution with antidiabetics.
DHEA	Oral: slows aging, improves vigor ("Fountain of Youth"); androgenic side effects
di huang	Oral: treatment of diabetes mellitus
dried root bark of lycium Chinese mill	Oral: lowers cholesterol, lowers blood glucose

(*continued*)

Substance	Reported Use
echinacea (cone flower)	Oral: treatment of colds, flu; stimulates the immune system, attacks viruses; causes immunosuppression May be liver toxic. Do not use longer than 8 wk. Do not give with liver-toxic drugs or immunosuppressants. Avoid use with antifungals; serious liver injury could occur. Avoid use in patients with SLE, tuberculosis, AIDS.
elder bark and flowers	Topical: gargle for tonsillitis, pharyngitis Oral: treatment of fever, chills
ephedra	Oral: increases energy, relieves fatigue May cause serious complications; banned by FDA
ergot	Oral: treatment of migraine headaches, treatment of menstrual problems, hemorrhage
eucalyptus	Topical: treatment of wounds Oral: decreases respiratory secretions, suppresses cough
evening primrose	Oral: treatment of PMS, menopause, rheumatoid arthritis, diabetic neuropathy Do not use with phenothiazines, antidepressants—increases risk of seizures; avoid use in patients with epilepsy, schizophrenia.
false unicorn root	Oral: treatment of menstrual and uterine problems Do not use during pregnancy or lactation.
fennel	Oral: treatment of colic, gout, flatulence; enhances lactation
fenugreek	Oral: lowers cholesterol levels; reduces blood glucose; aids in healing; use caution with antidiabetics, anticoagulants.
feverfew	Oral: treatment of arthritis, fever, migraine Use caution with anticoagulants; may increase bleeding. Avoid use before or immediately after surgery because of bleeding risk.
fish oil	Oral: treatment of coronary diseases, arthritis, colitis, depression, aggression, attention deficit disorder
gamboge	Oral: appetite suppressant, lowers cholesterol, promotes weight loss
garlic	Oral: treatment of colds, diuretic; prevention of coronary artery disease, intestinal antiseptic; lowers blood glucose, anticoagulant Use caution with diabetic patients, oral anticoagulants. Known to affect blood clotting. Do not use with warfarin.
ginger	Oral: treatment of nausea, motion sickness, postoperative nausea (may increase risk of miscarriage) Affects blood clotting. Do not give with anticoagulants.
ginkgo	Oral: vascular dilation; increases blood flow to the brain, improving cognitive function; used in treating Alzheimer's disease; antioxidant Can inhibit blood clotting. Do not give with aspirin or NSAIDs. Can interact with phenytoin, carbamazepine, phenobarbital, TCAs, and MAOIs; use caution with other drugs.
ginkobe	Oral: increases cerebral blood flow, improves concentration and memory
ginseng	Oral: aphrodisiac, mood elevator, tonic; antihypertensive; decreases cholesterol levels; lowers blood glucose; adjunct in cancer chemotherapy and radiation therapy May cause irritability if combined with caffeine. Inhibits clotting. Do not use with anticoagulants, aspirin, NSAIDs. Do not use for longer than 3 mos. May cause headaches, manic episodes if used with phenelzine, MAOIs. Additive effects of estrogens and corticosteroids. May also interfere with cardiac effects of digoxin. Monitor patients closely. Use caution with antidiabetics.
glucosamine	Oral: treatment of osteoarthritis and joint diseases, usually combined with chondroitin
goldenrod leaves	Oral: treatment of renal disease, rheumatism, sore throat, eczema
goldenseal	Oral: lowers blood glucose, aids healing; treatment of bronchitis, colds, flulike symptoms, cystitis. High doses may cause paralysis. Affects blood clotting; do not give with anticoagulants.
gotu kola	Topical: treatment of cellulites, scleroderma, open wounds, pressure sores
grape seed extract	Oral: treatment of allergies, asthma; improves circulation; decreases platelet aggregation Use caution with oral anticoagulants; may increase bleeding
green tea leaf	Oral: antioxidant, used as a preventative for cancer and cardiovascular disease Use caution with oral anticoagulants; may increase bleeding
guayusa	Oral: lowers blood glucose; promotes weight loss
hawthorn	Oral: treatment of angina, arrhythmias, blood pressure problems; decreases cholesterol Use caution with digoxin, ACE inhibitors; may potentiate effects
hop	Oral: sedative; aids healing; alters blood glucose
horehound	Oral: expectorant; treatment of respiratory problems, GI disorders Use caution with antidiabetics, antihypertensives.
horse chestnut seed	Oral: treatment of varicose veins, hemorrhoids Use caution with oral anticoagulants; may increase bleeding
hyssop	Topical: treatment of cold sores, genital herpes, burns, wounds Oral: treatment of coughs, colds, indigestion, and flatulence

Substance	Reported Use
Java plum	Oral: treatment of diabetes mellitus
jojoba	Topical: promotion of hair growth, relief of skin problems Toxic if ingested.
juniper berries	Oral: increases appetite, aids digestion; diuretic; urinary tract disinfectant; lowers blood glucose Use caution with antidiabetics.
kava	Oral: treatment of nervous anxiety, stress, restlessness; tranquilizer Do not use with alprazolam—may cause coma. Do not use with Parkinson's disease or history of stroke. Do not combine with St. John's wort, antianxiety drugs, or alcohol.
kudzu	Oral: reduces cravings for alcohol; being researched for use with alcoholics
lavender	Topical: astringent for minor cuts, burns Oral: treatment of insomnia, restlessness Use caution with CNS depressants.
ledum tincture	Topical: treatment of insect bites, puncture wounds; dissolves some blood clots and bruises
licorice	Oral: prevents thirst, soothes coughs; treats "incurable" chronic fatigue syndrome; treatment of duodenal ulcer Acts like aldosterone. Blocks spironolactone effects. Can lead to digoxin toxicity because of effects of lowering aldosterone. Use extreme caution. Contraindicated with renal or liver disease, hypertension, CAD, pregnancy, lactation. Do not combine with thyroid drugs, antihypertensives, hormonal contraceptives.
ma huang	Oral: treatment of colds, nasal congestion, asthma. Contains ephedrine. Do not use with antihypertensives, diabetes, MAOIs, or digoxin. Serious side effects could occur.
mandrake root	Oral: treatment of fertility problems
marigold leaves and flowers	Oral: relief of muscle tension, increases wound healing
melatonin	Oral: relief of jet lag, treatment of insomnia Use caution with benzodiazepines, antihypertensives.
milk thistle	Oral: treatment of hepatitis, cirrhosis, fatty liver due to alcohol or drugs
milk vetch	Oral: improves resistance to disease; adjunct therapy in cancer chemotherapy and radiation therapy
mistletoe leaves	Oral: promotes weight loss; relief of signs and symptoms of diabetes
momordica charantia (Karela)	Oral: blocks intestinal absorption of glucose; lowers blood glucose; weight loss Use caution with antidiabetics.
nettle	Topical: stimulation of hair growth, treatment for bleeding Oral: treatment of rheumatism, allergic rhinitis; antispasmodic; expectorant Do not use during pregnancy or lactation.
nightshade leaves and roots	Oral: stimulates circulatory system; treatment of eye disorders
octacosanol	Oral: treatment of parkinsonism, enhancement of athletic performance Do not use during pregnancy or lactation; avoid use with carbidopa-levodopa.
parsley seeds and leaves	Oral: treatment of jaundice, asthma, menstrual difficulties, conjunctivitis Risk of serotonin syndrome with SSRIs
passion flowervine	Oral: sedative and hypnotic May increase sedation with other CNS depressants, MAOIs. Avoid alcohol while using this drug.
peppermint leaves	Oral: treatment of nervousness, insomnia, dizziness, cramps, coughs Topical: rubbed on forehead to relieve tension headaches
psyllium	Oral: treatment of constipation; lowers cholesterol Can cause severe gas and stomach pain; may interfere with nutrient absorption. Avoid use with warfarin, digoxin, lithium—absorption of drug may be blocked. Do not combine with laxatives.
raspberry	Oral: healing of minor wounds; control and treatment of diabetes
red clover	Oral: estrogen replacement in menopause; suppression of whooping cough Risk of bleeding with anticoagulants, antiplatelets; avoid use in pregnancy.
rose hips	Oral: laxative, to boost the immune system and prevent illness
rosemary	Topical: relief of rheumatism, sprains, wounds, bruises, eczema Oral: gastric stimulation, relief of flatulence, stimulation of bile release, relief of colic
rue extract	Topical: relief of pain associated with sprains, groin pulls, whiplash
saffron	Oral: treatment of menstrual problems, abortifacient
sage	Oral: lowers blood pressure; lowers blood glucose

(*continued*)

Substance	Reported Use
SAM-e (adomet)	Oral: promotion of general well-being and health Associated with frequent GI complaints and headache
sarsaparilla	Oral: treatment of skin disorders, rheumatism
sassafras	Topical: treatment of local pain, skin eruptions Oral: enhancement of athletic performance, "cure" for syphilis Oil has been toxic to fetus, children, and adults when ingested.
saw palmetto	Oral: treatment of benign prostatic hyperplasia Do not use with estrogen-replacement or hormonal contraceptives—may greatly increase side effects. May decrease iron absorption. Do not combine with finasteride; toxicity could occur.
schisandra	Oral: health tonic, liver protectant; adjunct in cancer chemotherapy and radiation therapy Do not use in pregnancy; causes uterine stimulation
squaw vine	Oral: diuretic, tonic, aid in labor and childbirth, treatment of menstrual problems Associated with hepatic toxicity
St. John's wort	Oral: treatment of depression, PMS symptoms; antiviral Topical: treatment of puncture wounds, insect bites, crushed fingers or toes Avoid tyramine-containing foods; hypertensive crisis is possible. Can increase sensitivity to light; do not combine with drugs that cause photosensitivity. Severe photosensitivity can occur in light-skinned people. Serious drug interactions have been reported with SSRIs, MAOIs, kava, digoxin, theophylline, AIDS antiviral agents, antineoplastics, hormonal contraceptives. Avoid these combinations.
sweet violet flowers	Oral: treatment of respiratory disorders, emetic
tarragon	Oral: weight loss; prevents cancer; lowers blood glucose
tea tree oil	Topical: antifungal, antibacterial; used in the treatment of burns, insect bites; used as a mouth wash
thyme	Topical: liniment, treatment of wounds, gargle Oral: antidiarrheal, relief of bronchitis and laryngitis Can increase sensitivity to light; do not combine with drugs that cause photosensitivity. Do not use with MAOIs or with SSRIs—can cause serious side effects.
turmeric	Oral: antioxidant, anti-inflammatory; used to treat arthritis May cause GI distress. Do not use with known biliary obstruction. May cause increased bleeding with oral anticoagulants
Valerian	Oral: sedative and hypnotic; reduces anxiety, relaxes muscles Can cause severe liver damage. Do not use with barbiturates, alcohol, CNS depressants, or antihistamines; can cause serious sedation
went rice	Oral: cholesterol- and triglyceride-lowering effects Do not use in pregnancy, liver disease, alcoholism, or acute infections.
white willow bark	Oral: treatment of fevers
xuan shen	Oral: lowers blood glucose; slows heart rate; treatment of congestive heart failure. Use caution with antidiabetics.
yohimbe	Oral: treatment of erectile dysfunction Can affect blood pressure; CNS stimulant; has cardiac effects; use caution—manic episodes have been reported in psychiatric patients.

From Karch, A. M. (2006). *2007 Lippincott's nursing drug guide* (pp.1248–1256). Philadelphia: Lippincott Williams & Wilkins.

APPENDIX F

Diagnostic Agents

Some pharmacological agents are used solely to diagnose particular conditions. Diagnostic tests that use these agents include

- In vitro tests, which are done outside the body to measure the presence of particular elements (e.g., proteins, blood glucose, bacteria)
- In vivo tests, which introduce drugs into the body to evaluate specific physiological functions (e.g., cardiac output, intestinal absorption, gastric acid secretion)

Therapeutic Actions and Indications

In vitro tests are often performed as part of the nursing evaluation of a patient, or they may be done at home by the patient as part of a medical regimen. These drugs can include reagents that react with specific enzymes or chemicals, such as glucose, blood, or human chorionic gonadotropin (HCG). Drugs used for in vivo tests may stimulate or suppress normal body reactions, such as a glucose challenge to evaluate insulin release or thyroid suppression tests to evaluate thyroid response. Specific tests of blood, urine, or other bodily fluids are often needed to evaluate the body's response to these drugs and to make a diagnosis. Drugs given as part of in vivo tests are administered under the supervision of medical personnel who are either conducting the test or making the diagnosis. They are usually given only once or used over a short period of time. Their use is part of an overall diagnostic plan to determine the underlying source of a particular problem.

Contraindications and Cautions

The use of any of the in vivo drugs is contraindicated in cases of allergy to the drugs themselves or to the colorants or preservatives used in them. Specific agents may be contraindicated in conditions that could be exacerbated by the stimulation of particular body responses. These drugs should be used cautiously during pregnancy or lactation.

Adverse Effects

The adverse effects seen with diagnostic agents are usually associated with the suppression or stimulation of the response they are being used to test. Because these drugs are given as only part of a test, the adverse effects usually last for a short period and can be tolerated by the patient.

Clinically Important Drug–Drug Interactions

Drug interactions vary with the particular agent that is being used. Consult a drug guide for specific information before giving any diagnostic agent.

Clinically Important Drug–Food Interactions

Because these tests are designed to elicit very specific responses, there is often the possibility that food will interfere with the actions or sensitivity of the test. Consult a drug guide for specific information about drug–food interactions before giving any diagnostic agent.

Nursing Considerations

Assessment: History and Examination

Screen for the following conditions, which could be contraindications to use of the agent: presence of known allergy to any of these drugs or to the colorants or preservatives used in these drugs.

Include screening for baseline status before beginning therapy and for any potential adverse effects. Assess the following: skin and mucous membrane condition; orientation, affect, and reflexes; pulse, blood pressure, and respirations; abdominal examination; bowel sounds; and blood and urine tests required for the particular test being performed.

Nursing Diagnoses

The patient receiving a diagnostic agent may have the following nursing diagnoses related to drug therapy:

- Acute Pain related to effects of the drugs
- Fear related to the test being done and possible test results
- Disturbed Body Image related to testing procedure and related tests that must be done
- Deficient Knowledge regarding drug therapy

Implementation

- Assess patient's general physical condition before beginning test *to decrease the potential for adverse effects.*
- Provide comfort measures *to help patient tolerate drug effects* (e.g., give drug with food to decrease gastrointestinal upset, provide proper skin care as needed, administer analgesics for headache as appropriate, provide privacy for the collection and storage of urine samples).
- Include information about the drug being used in a test (e.g., what to expect, adverse effects that may occur, follow-up tests that may be needed) *to enhance patient knowledge about drug therapy and promote compliance with the drug regimen.*

Evaluation

- Monitor patient response to the drug (adverse reactions, collection of diagnostic information).
- Monitor for adverse effects (neurological effects, gastrointestinal upset, skin reaction, hypoglycemia, constipation).
- Evaluate effectiveness of teaching plan (patient can name adverse effects to watch for, specific measures to avoid adverse effects; patient understands importance of follow-up that will be needed).
- Monitor effectiveness of comfort measures and compliance with the regimen.

Table F Diagnostic Agents

Test Object	Brand Names	Usual Indication	Special Considerations
In Vitro Tests			
acetone	*Acetest* *Chemstrip K* *Ketostix*	Test for ketones in urine, blood, serum, or plasma	Most frequently used to test urine; *Acetest* is the only product that is also used for blood products.
albumin	*Albustix* *Chemstrip Micral*	At-home urine test for the presence of proteins	Advise patients to follow product storage instructions.
urine bacteria	*Microstix-3* *Uricult* *Isocult for Bacteriuria*	Test for urine nitrates, uropathogens, gram-negative bacteria	Most accurate if used with a clean-catch urine sample
bilirubin	*Icotest*	Test for urine bilirubin levels	Most accurate if used with a clean-catch urine sample
blood urea nitrogen	*Azostix*	Estimate of BUN	Used as a reagent strip with whole blood
Candida tests	*Isocult for Candida* *CandidaSure*	Culture paddles or reagent slides for testing vaginal smears	Rapid test for presence of *Candida* with vaginal examination
Chlamydia trachomatis	*Amplicor* *Chlamydiazyme* *MicroTrak for Chlamydia* *Sure Cell Chlamydia* *Clearview Chlamydia*	Kits and slides for testing urogenital, rectal, conjunctival, and nasopharyngeal specimens for the presence of *Chlamydia*	Kits are specific for testing specimens.
cholesterol	*Advanced Care Cholesterol Test*	At-home cholesterol test	Kit includes audio cassette with instructions; patients should be cautioned to seek medical care and advice.
glucose, blood	*Chemstrip bG* *Dextrostrip* *Glucostix* *Glucometer Elite* *Accu-Check Advantage* and others	At-home testing of blood glucose levels	Patients should be taught how to calibrate the machine, proper blood drawing technique, and importance of seeking follow-up medical care.

Table F Diagnostic Agents *(Continued)*

Test Object	Brand Names	Usual Indication	Special Considerations
In Vitro Tests			
glucose, urine	*Clinitest* *Clinistix* *Diastix*	At-home testing of urine glucose levels	Patients should be taught how to read strips, proper storage of products, and importance of seeking follow-up medical care.
gonorrhea	*Biocult-GC* *Gonozyme Diagnostic* *Isocult for Neisseria gonorrhoeae*	Kits and culture paddles for the detection of *Neisseria gonorrhea* on endocervical, rectal, urethral, and oropharyngeal specimens	Test kits containing reagents, preservatives as needed for detection of *Neisseria gonorrhea* during physical examination
mononucleosis	*Mono-Plus* *Mono-Diff* *Mono-Sure* and others	Kits, reagents, and slides for the testing of serum and blood for mononucleosis	Rapid tests for suspected cases of mononucleosis; all necessary reagents and preservatives included in kit
occult blood	*ColoCare* *EZ Detect* *Hemoocult II* and others	Kits and slides for the testing of fecal swabs for the presence of occult blood	Card forms can be used by patients at home in routine screening programs.
ovulation	*Answer* *OvuQuick Self-Test* *First Response Ovulation Predictor* and others	Kits to determine the levels of LH in the urine as a predictor of ovulation	Used at home by patients as part of fertility programs; patients may need instruction.
pregnancy	*Advance, First Response* *Pregnosis* and others	Kits or urine strips to detect the presence of HCG (human chorionic gonadotropin) as a predictor of pregnancy	May be used at home; patients may need instruction and should be advised to seek follow-up medical care.
rheumatoid factor	*Rheumatex* *Rheumaton*	Slide tests for the presence of rheumatoid factor in blood, serum, or synovial fluid	An aid in the diagnosis of autoimmune diseases
sickle cell	*Sickledex*	Kit for the testing of blood for the presence of hemoglobin S	Diagnostic for sickle cell anemia
streptococci	*Sure Cell Streptococci* *Culturette 10 Minute Group A Strep ID* *Bactigen Strep B* and others	Kits, slides, and culture paddles for the identification of streptococcal infection in blood, serum, urine, throat, and cerebrospinal fluid	Early detection of streptococcal infection to facilitate beginning of treatment before culture and sensitivity results are known
In Vivo Tests			
aminohippurate	*PAH* *Aminohippurate Sodium*	Estimation of renal plasma flow and to measure the functional capacity of the renal secretory mechanism	Injected as a 20% aqueous solution; requires careful urine collection
arbutamine	*GenESA*	Diagnosis of CAD in patients who cannot exercise adequately	Causes stress to evaluate body response; must be given with its own delivery device
arginine	*R-Gene 10*	Diagnostic aid to assess pituitary reserve of growth hormone	IV infusion, followed by blood tests to monitor response
benzylpenicilloyl-polylysine	*Pre-Pen*	Skin test to evaluate sensitivity to penicillin and safety of administering penicillin in potentially sensitive individuals	Intradermal or scratch test is used; positive reaction is usually seen within 10–15 min
gonadorelin	*Factrel*	Evaluation of gonadotropic capacity of the pituitary gland	Given IV or Sub-Q; monitor closely for potential hypersensitivity reactions.
histamine phosphate	*Histamine-Phosphate*	Sub-Q—to evaluate ability of gastric mucosa to produce HCl IV—diagnosis of pheochromocytoma	May cause severe symptoms, including shock, cardiovascular collapse, even death; monitor patient closely.
indocyanine green	*Cardio-Green*	Determining cardiac output, hepatic function, and liver blood flow; also used for ophthalmic angiography	Use caution with known allergy to dyes.
inulin	*Inulin injection*	Measurement of glomerular filtration rate	Requires blood tests and urine collection
methacholine chloride	*Provocholine*	Diagnosis of bronchial airway hypersensitivity in patients without documented asthma	Inhaled with pulmonary function test immediately; may cause hypotension, chest pain, or GI upset
pentagastrin	*Peptavlon*	Evaluation of gastric acid secretory function	Given Sub-Q; may cause abdominal pain, flushing, nausea, vomiting, diarrhea, tachycardia

(*continued*)

Table F Diagnostic Agents *(Continued)*

Test Object	Brand Names	Usual Indication	Special Considerations
In Vivo Tests			
secretin	*Secretin-Ferring Powder*	Diagnosis of pancreatic exocrine disease Diagnosis of gastrinoma	Requires a 12–15-h fast; passing of a radiopaque tube for pancreatic function or repeated blood samples for gastrinoma diagnosis
sermorelin	*Geref*	Evaluation of pituitary ability to secrete growth hormone	Single IV injection; follow-up blood tests will be needed to determine response
sincalide	*Kinevac*	Stimulation of gallbladder contractions, pancreatic secretion to evaluate for stones, enzyme activity	Gallbladder—given IV over 30–60 sec; pancreatic function—given IV over 60 min
sodium iodide	*Sodium Iodide I[123]*	Diagnosis of thyroid function or morphology	Handle with care; oral capsules are radioactive, dispose of properly; thyroid can be evaluated for radiation content within 6 h of dose
thyrotropin alpha	*Thyrogen*	Differentiation of thyroid function to estimate thyroid reserve	Given IM every 24 h for two doses; follow with radioactive iodine and thyroid scan
tolbutamide	*Orinase Diagnostic*	Diagnosis of pancreatic islet cell adenoma	Given IV after 3 days of high-carbohydrate diet; prepare to support patient if severe hypoglycemia occurs.

APPENDIX G

Canadian Drug Information

Presented here is a list of Canadian brand names for frequently used drugs. The brand name appears in italics with the corresponding generic name listed in parentheses.

A

Abenol (acetaminophen)
Acet-Amp (theophylline)
Acilac (lactulose)
Acti 12 (hydroxocobalamin)
Actiprofen (ibuprofen)
Albert Glyburide (glyburide)
Alcomicin (gentamicin)
Allerdryl (diphenhydramine)
Alti-Acyclovir (acyclovir)
Alti-Diltiazem (diltiazem)
Alti-Doxepin (doxepin)
Alti-Ibuprofen (ibuprofen)
Alti-Ipratropium (ipratropium)
Alti-Minocycline (minocycline)
Alti-MPA (medroxyprogesterone)
Alti-Nadolol (nadolol)
Alti-Piroxicam (piroxicam)
Alti-Ranitidine (ranitidine)
Alti-Sulfasalazine (sulfasalazine)
Alti-Trazadone (trazodone)
Alti-Triazolam (triazolam)
Alti-Valproic (valproic acid)
Ampicin (ampicillin)
Anapolon 50 (oxymetholone)
Anexate (flumazenil)
Anturan (sulfinpyrazone)
Apo-Acetazolamide (acetazolamide)
Apo-Allopurinol (allopurinol)
Apo-Alpraz (alprazolam)
Apo-Amoxi (amoxicillin)
Apo-Ampi (ampicillin)
Apo-Asa (aspirin)
Apo-Atenol (atenolol)
Apo-Baclofen (baclofen)
Apo-Beclomethasone (beclomethasone)
Apo-Benztropine (benztropine)
Apo-Bromocriptine (bromocriptine)
Apo-Cal (calcium carbonate)
Apo-Capto (captopril)
Apo-Carbamazepine (carbamazepine)
Apo-Ceclor (cefaclor)
Apo-Cephalex (cephalexin)
Apo-Chlorodiazepoxide (chlordiazepoxide)
Apo-Chlorpropamide (chlorpropamide)
Apo-Chlorthalidone (chlorthalidone)
Apo-Cimetidine (cimetidine)
Apo-Clomipramine (clomipramine)
Apo-Clonazepam (clonazepam)
Apo-Clonidine (clonidine)
Apo-Clorazepate (clorazepate)
Apo-Cyclobenzaprine (cyclobenzaprine)
Apo-Desipramine (desipramine)
Apo-Diazepam (diazepam)
Apo-Diflunisal (diflunisal)
Apo-Diltiaz (diltiazem)
Apo-Dimenhydrinate (dimenhydrinate)
Apo-Dipyridamole (dipyridamole)
Apo-Doxepin (doxepin)
Apo-Doxy (doxycycline)
Apo-Erythro (erythromycin)
Apo-Erythro ES (erythromycin)
Apo-Erythro-S (erythromycin)
Apo-Famotidine (famotidine)
Apo-Ferrous Gluconate (ferrous gluconate)
Apo-Ferrous Sulfate (ferrous sulfate)
Apo-Fluoxetine (fluoxetine)
Apo-Fluphenazine (fluphenazine)
Apo-Flurbiprofen (flurbiprofen)
Apo-Fluvoxamine (fluvoxamine)
Apo-Furosemide (furosemide)
Apo-Gemfibrozil (gemfibrozil)
Apo-Haloperidol (haloperidol)

Apo-Hydralazine (hydralazine)
Apo-Hydro (hydrochlorothiazide)
Apo-Hydroxyzine (hydroxyzine)
Apo-Ibuprofen (ibuprofen)
Apo-Imipramine (imipramine)
Apo-Indomethacin (indomethacin)
Apo-Ipravent (ipratropium)
Apo-ISDN (isosorbide dinitrate)
Apo-K (potassium chloride)
Apo-Lisinopril (lisinopril)
Apo-Loperamide (loperamide)
Apo-Lorazepam (lorazepam)
Apo-Lovastatin (lovastatin)
Apo-Mefenamic (mefenamic acid)
Apo-Megestrol (megestrol)
Apo-Meprobamate (meprobamate)
Apo-Metoclop (metoclopramide)
Apo-Metoprolol (metoprolol)
Apo-Metronidazole (metronidazole)
Apo-Nadolol (nadolol)
Apo-Napro-Na (naproxen)
Apo-Naproxen (naproxen)
Apo-Nifed (nifedipine)
Apo-Nitrofurantoin (nitrofurantoin)
Apo-Nizatidine (nizatidine)
Apo-Oxazepam (oxazepam)
Apo-Oxybutynin (oxybutynin)
Apo-Perphenazine (perphenazine)
Apo-Pindol (pindolol)
Apo-Piroxicam (piroxicam)
Apo-Prazo (prazosin)
Apo-Prednisone (prednisone)
Apo-Primidone (primidone)
Apo-Procainamide (procainamide)
Apo-Propranolol (propranolol)
Apo-Quinidine (quinidine)
Apo-Sotalol (sotalol)
Apo-Sucralfate (sucralfate)
Apo-Sulfinpyrazone (sulfinpyrazone)
Apo-Sulin (sulindac)
Apo-Tamox (tamoxifen)
Apo-Temazepam (temazepam)
Apo-Tetra (tetracycline)
Apo-Timol (timolol)
Apo-Tolbutamide (tolbutamide)
Apo-Trazadone (trazodone)
Apo-Triazo (triazolam)
Apo-Trifluoperazine (trifluoperazine)
Apo-Trihex (trihexyphenidyl)
Apo-Trimip (trimipramine)
Apo-Zidovudine (zidovudine)
Aquacort (hydrocortisone)
Atasol (acetaminophen)
Avirax (acyclovir)
Avlosulfan (dapsone)
Ayercillin (penicillin G procaine)

B

Baciguent (bacitracin)
Balminin DM (dextromethorphan)
Barbilixir (phenobarbital)
Barbita (phenobarbital)
Beclodisk (beclomethasone)
Beclovent Rotocaps (beclomethasone)
Bentylol (dicyclomine)
Benuryl (probenecid)
Betabloc (metoprolol)
Betacort (betamethasone)
Betaderm (betamethasone)
Betnesol (betamethasone)
Betnovate (betamethasone)
Bretylate (bretylium)
Burinex (bumetanide)
Busodium (butabarbital)
Butalan (butabarbital)

C

Calcite 500 (calcium carbonate)
Caltine (calcitonin, salmon)
Candistatin (nystatin)
Canesten Vaginal (clotrimazole)
Carbolith (lithium)
Cedocard SR (isosorbide dinitrate)
Celestoderm (betamethasone)
C.E.S. (estrogens, conjugated)
Charcolate (charcoal)
Chlorpromanyl (chlorpromazine)
Chlor-Tripolon (chlorpheniramine)
Cibalith-S (lithium)
Ciloxin (ciprofloxacin)
Clinda-Derm (clindamycin)
Clonapam (clonazepam)
Clotrimaderm (clotrimazole)
Combantrin (pyrantel)
Congest (estrogens, conjugated)
Creon (pancrelipase)
Crysticillin-AS (penicillin G procaine)
Cyclomen (danazol)

D

Dalacin C (clindamycin)
Dehydral (methenamine)
Deproic (valproic acid)
Dermovate (clobetasol)
Diarr-Eze (loperamide)
Diazemuls (diazepam)
Dihydroergotamine Sandoz (dihydroergotamine)
Diodoquin (iodoquinol)
Diomycin (erythromycin)
Dionephrine (phenylephrine)
Dipridacot (dipyridamole)
Dixarit (clonidine)
Dopamet (methyldopa)

Doxycin (doxycycline)
Doxytec (doxycycline)
Duralith (lithium)
Duretic (methyclothiazide)

E

Eltor (pseudoephedrine)
Endantadine (amantadine)
Entocort (budesonide)
Entrophen (aspirin)
Epimorph (morphine)
Epival (valproic acid)
Ergomar (ergotamine)
Erybid (erythromycin)
Erythrocin (erythromycin)
Erythrocin I.V. (erythromycin)
Erythromid (erythromycin)
Estromed (estrogens, esterified)
Etibi (ethambutol)
Euflex (flutamide)
Euglucon (glyburide)

F

Falapen (penicillin G potassium)
Ferodan (ferrous salts)
Fero-Grad (ferrous salts)
Fertinorm HP (urofollitropin)
Fluor-A-Day (sodium fluoride)
Fluotic (sodium fluoride)
Formulex (dicyclomine)
Froben (flurbiprofen)
Froben-SR (flurabiprofen)
Furoside (furosemide)

G

Gen-Atenolol (atenolol)
Gen-Baclofen (baclofen)
Gen-Captopril (captopril)
Gen-Cimetidine (cimetidine)
Gen-Clomipramine (clomipramine)
Gen-Clonazepam (clonazepam)
Gen-Diltiazem (diltiazem)
Gen-Fibro (gemfibrozil)
Gen-Glybe (glyburide)
Gen-Medroxy (medroxyprogesterone)
Gen-Minocycline (minocycline)
Gen-Nifedipine (nifedipine)
Gravol (dimenhydrinate)

H

Haldol LA (haloperidol)
Hepalean (heparin)
Hepalean-Lok (heparin)
Heparin Leo (heparin)
Hip-Rex (methenamine)
Humulin U (insulin)
Hycort (hydrocortisone)
Hydromorph Contin (hydromorphone)

I

Iletin PZI (insulin)
Immunine VH (factor IX)
Impril (imipramine)
Indocid P.D.A. (indomethacin)
Indotec (indomethacin)
Infufer (iron dextran)
Isotamine (isoniazid)
Isotrex (isotretinoin)

K

Kabolin (nandrolone)
K-Exit (sodium polystyrene)
Kidrolase (asparaginase)
Koffex (dextromethorphan)

L

Lactulax (lactulose)
Lanvis (thioguanine)
Largactil (chlorpromazine)
Laxilose (lactulose)
Lopresor (metoprolol)
LoSec (omeprazole)
Loxapac (loxapine)
Lyderm Cream (fluocinonide)

M

Mandelamine (methenamine)
Maxeran (metoclopramide)
Megace OS (megestrol)
Megacillin (penicillin G benzathine)
Meprolone (methylprednisolone)
Mesasal (mesalamine)
M-Eslon (morphine)
MetroCream (metronidazole)
Micozole (miconazole)
Minims (atropine)
Minims Sodium Chloride (sodium chloride)
Minox (minoxidil)
Minoxigaine (minoxidil)
Mireze (nedocromil)
Modecate Deconate (fluphenazine)
Moditen Enanthate (fluphenazine)
Monazole 7 (miconazole)
Monitan (acebutolol)
Multipax (hydroxyzine)
Mycifradin (neomycin)
Mycil (chlorphenesin)
Myclo (clotrimazole)
Myrosemide (furosemide)

N

Nadopen-V (penicillin V)
Nadostine (nystatin)

Nalcrom (cromolyn)
Natulan (procarbazine)
Naxen (naproxen)
Neo-Tric (metronidazole)
NidaGel (metronidazole)
Norlutate (norethindrone)
Norventyl (nortriptyline)
Norzine (thiethylperazine)
Novahistex DM (dextromethorphan)
Novahistine DM (dextromethorphan)
Novamoxin (amoxicillin)
Novasen (aspirin)
Novo-Alprozol (alprazolam)
Novo-Ampicillin (ampicillin)
Novo-Atenol (atenolol)
Novo-AZT (zidovudine)
Novo-Baclofen (baclofen)
Novo-Butamide (tolbutamide)
Novo-Captopril (captopril)
Novo-Carbamaz (carbamazepine)
Novo-Cefadroxil (cefadroxil)
Novo-Cholamine (cholestyramine)
Novo-Cholamine Light (cholestyramine)
Novo-Cimetine (cimetidine)
Novo-Clonidine (clonidine)
Novo-Clopamine (clomipramine)
Novo-Clopate (clorazepate)
Novo-Cycloprine (cyclobenzaprine)
Novo-Desipramine (desipramine)
Novo-Difenac (diclofenac)
Novo-Diflunisal (diflunisal)
Novo-Digoxin (digoxin)
Novo-Diltiazem (diltiazem)
Novo-Doxepin (doxepin)
Novo-Doxylin (doxycycline)
Novo-Famotidine (famotidine)
Novo-Fluoxetine (fluoxetine)
Novo-Flurbiprofen (flurbiprofen)
Novo-Flutamide (flutamide)
Novo-Furan (nitrofurantoin)
Novo-Gemfibrozil (gemfibrozil)
Novo-Hydrazide (hydrochlorothiazide)
Novo-Hydroxyzin (hydroxyzine)
Novo-Hylazin (hydralazine)
Novo-Ipramide (ipratropium)
Novo-Lexin (cephalexin)
Novolin ge (insulin)
Novolin ge lente (insulin)
Novolin ge Toronto (insulin)
Novolin ge ultralente (insulin)
Novo-Loperamide (loperamide)
Novo-Lorazem (lorazepam)
Novo-Maprotiline (maprotiline)
Novo-Medopa (methyldopa)
Novo-Medrone (medroxyprogesterone)
Novomepro (meprobamate)
Novo-Metoprol (metoprolol)
Novo-Mexiletine (mexiletine)
Novo-Minocycline (minocycline)
Novo-Nadolol (nadolol)
Novo-Naprox (naproxen)
Novo-Nidazol (metronidazole)
Novo-Nifedin (nifedipine)
Novo-Oxybutynin (oxybutynin)
Novo-Pen G (penicillin G)
Novo-Pen VK (penicillin V)
Novo-Pentobarb (pentobarbital)
Novoperidol (haloperidol)
Novo-Pindol (pindolol)
Novo-Pirocam (piroxicam)
Novo-Poxide (chlordiazepoxide)
Novo-Pramine (imipramine)
Novo-Pranol (propranolol)
Novo-Prazin (prazosin)
Novo-Prednisolone (prednisolone)
Novo-Prednisone (prednisone)
Novo-Profen (ibuprofen)
Novo-Propoxyn (propoxyphene)
Novo-Pyrazone (sulfinpyrazone)
Novo-Ranidine (ranitidine)
Novo-Rythro (erythromycin)
Novo-Salmol (albuterol)
Novo-Secobarb (secobarbital)
Novo-Sotalol (sotalol)
Novosoxazole (sulfisoxazole)
Novo-Spiroton (spironolactone)
Novo-Sucralfate (sucralfate)
Novo-Sundac (sulindac)
Novo-Tamoxifen (tamoxifen)
Novo-Temazepam (temazepam)
Novotetra (tetracycline)
Novo-Tolmetin (tolmetin)
Novo-Triolam (triazolam)
Novo-Tripramine (trimipramine)
Novo-Triptyn (amitriptyline)
Novoxapam (oxazepam)
Nu-Alpraz (alprazolam)
Nu-Amoxi (amoxicillin)
Nu-Ampi (ampicillin)
Nu-Capto (captopril)
Nu-Cephalex (cephalexin)
Nu-Cimet (cimetidine)
Nu-Clonidine (clonidine)
Nu-Cloxi (cloxacillin)
Nu-Diclo (diclofenac)
Nu-Diflunisal (diflunisal)
Nu-Diltiaz (diltiazem)
Nu-Doxycycline (doxycycline)
Nu-Erythromycin-S (erythromycin)
Nu-Hydral (hydralazine)
Nu-Ketoprofen (ketoprofen)
Nu-Loraz (lorazepam)

Nu-Medopa (methyldopa)
Nu-Metoclopramide (metoclopramide)
Nu-Metop (metoprolol)
Nu-Pindol (pindolol)
Nu-Pirox (piroxicam)
Nu-Prazo (prazosin)
Nu-Ranit (ranitidine)
Nu-Tetra (tetracycline)
Nu-Trazodone (trazodone)

O

Octostim (desmopressin)
Ocu-Phrin (phenylephrine)
Opium TCT (opium)
Oracort (triamcinolone)
Orafen (ketoprofen)
Orfenace (orphenadrine)

P

Palafer (ferrous fumarate)
Parvolex (acetylcysteine)
PCE (erythromycin)
PDF (sodium fluoride)
Pedi-Dent (sodium fluoride)
Penbritin (ampicillin)
Pentacarinat (pentamidine)
Pentids (penicillin G)
Peptol (cimetidine)
Phenazine (perphenazine)
Phenazo (phenazopyridine)
Phenytex (phenytoin)
PMS-ASA (aspirin)
PMS Bethanecol Chloride (bethanechol)
PMS-Ceclor (cefaclor)
PMS-Cephalexin (cephalexin)
PMS-Chloral Hydrate (chloral hydrate)
PMS-Desipramine (desipramine)
PMS-Egozinc (zinc)
PMS-Fluoxetine (fluoxetine)
PMS-Fluphenazine (fluphenazine)
PMS-Hydromorphone (hydromorphone)
PMS-Isoniazid (isoniazid)
PMS-Lithium Carbonate (lithium)
PMS-Loxapine (loxapine)
PMS-Mefenamic Acid (mefenamic acid)
PMS-Methylphenidate (methylphenidate)
PMS-Metronidazole (metronidazole)
PMS-Neostigmine Methylsulfate (neostigmine)
PMS-Nortriptyline (nortriptyline)
PMS-Nystatin (nystatin)
PMS-Prochlorperazine (prochlorperazine)
PMS-Procyclidine (procyclidine)
PMS-Promethazine (promethazine)
PMS-Propranolol (propranolol)
PMS-Pyrazinamide (pyrazinamide)
Ponstan (mefenamic acid)
Prandase (acarbose)
Pressyn (vasopressin)
Prevex B (betamethasone)
Primene (amino acids)
Procan SR (procainamide)
Procyclid (procyclidine)
Procytox (cyclophosphamide)
Progestilin (progesterone)
Propaderm (beclomethasone)
Propanthel (propantheline)
Propyl-Thyracil (propylthiouracil)
Purinol (allopurinol)

Q

Quinate (quinidine)
Quintasa (mesalamine)

R

Reactine (cetirizine)
Renedil (felodipine)
Revimine (dopamine)
Rhinalar (flunisolide)
Rhinocort Tubuhaler (budesonide)
Rhodacine (indomethacin)
Rhodis (ketoprofen)
Rhodis EC (ketoprofen)
Rhodis SR (ketoprofen)
Rho-Fluphenazine Deconate (fluphenazine)
Rholosone (betamethasone)
Rhoprosone (betamethasone)
Rhotral (acebutolol)
Rhotrimine (trimipramine)
Rhovail (ketoprofen)
Riphenidate (methylprednisolone)
Rivotril (clonazepam)
Rofact (rifampin)
Rogitine (phentolamine)
Roychlor (potassium chloride)
Rylosol (sotalol)
Rythmodan (disopyramide)

S

Salazopyrin (sulfasalazine)
Salbutamol (albuterol)
Saline from Otrivin (sodium chloride)
Salinex (sodium chloride)
Salofalk (mesalamine)
Sarisol #2 (butabarbital)
S.A.S. (sulfasalazine)
Sotacar (sotalol)
Stemitil (prochlorperazine)
Stemitil Suppositories (prochlorperazine)
StieVA-A (tretinoin)
Sulcrate (sucralfate)
Supeudol (oxycodone)
Synacthen Depot (cosyntropin)
Synflex (naproxen)

T

Tamofen (tamoxifen)
Tamone (tamoxifen)
Tanta Orciprenaline (metaproterenol)
Taro-Sone (betamethasone)
Tebrazid (pyrazinamide)
Teejel (choline salicylate)
Tenolin (atenolol)
Texacort (hydrocortisone)
Topsyn Gel (fluocinonide)
Travel Tabs (dimenhydrinate)
Triadapin (doxepin)
Trichlorex (trichlormethiazide)
Trikacide (metronidazole)
Triptil (protriptyline)

U

Ultradol (etodolac)
Urasal (methenamine)
Urozide (hydrochlorothiazide)
Ursofalk (ursodiol)

V

Vamin 18 (amino acids)
Velbe (vinblastine)
Ventodisk (albuterol)
Vivol (diazepam)
Voltaren Ophtha (diclofenac)
Voltaren Rapide (diclofenac)

W

Warfilone (warfarin)
Winpred (prednisone)

X

Xanax-TS (alprazolam)

Y

Yodoquinal (iodoquinol)

Z

Zoladex L.A. (goserelin)
Zonalon (doxepin)

APPENDIX H

Canadian Regulations

Table H Narcotic, Controlled Drugs, Benzodiazepines, and Other Targeted Substances

This table summarizes the requirements for prescribing, dispensing, and record-keeping for narcotics, controlled drugs, benzodiazepines, and other targeted substances. This information is not intended to present a comprehensive review; the reader is therefore encouraged to seek additional and confirmatory information (e.g., Controlled Drugs and Substances Act, Narcotic Control Regulations, parts G and J of the Food and Drug Regulations, Benzodiazepines, and Other Targeted Substances Regulations).

Classification and Description	Legal Requirements
Narcotic Drugs*	
• 1 narcotic (e.g., cocaine, codeine, hydromorphone, morphine) • 1 narcotic + 1 active non-narcotic ingredient (e.g., *Empracet-30, Novahistex DH, Tylenol No. 4*) • All narcotics for parenteral use (e.g., fentanyl, pethidine) • All products containing diamorphine (hospitals only), hydrocodone, oxycodone, methadone, or pentazocine • Dextropropoxyphene, propoxyphene (straight) (e.g., *Darvon-N, 642*)	• Written prescription required. • Verbal prescriptions not permitted. • Refills not permitted. • Written prescription may be prescribed to be dispensed in divided portions (part-fills). • For part-fills, copies of prescriptions should be made in reference to the original prescription. Indicate on the original prescription the new prescription number, the date of the part-fill, the quantity dispensed, and the pharmacist's initials. • Transfers not permitted. • Record and retain all documents pertaining to all transactions in a manner that permits an audit. • Sales reports required except for dextropropoxyphene, propoxyphene. • Report any loss or theft of narcotic drugs within 10 days to the Office of Controlled Substances at the address indicated on the forms.
Narcotic Preparations*	
• Verbal prescription narcotics: 1 narcotic + 2 or more active non-narcotic ingredients in a recognized therapeutic dose (e.g., *Fiorinal with Codeine, Robitussin AC, 692, 282, 292, Tylenol No. 2* and *No. 3*) • Exempted codeine compounds: contain codeine up to 8 mg/solid dosage form or 20 mg/30 mL liquid + 2 or more active non-narcotic ingredients (e.g., *Atasol-8, Robitussin with Codeine*)	• Written or verbal prescriptions permitted. • Refills not permitted. • Written or verbal prescriptions may be prescribed to be dispensed in divided portions (part-fills). • For part-fills, copies of prescriptions should be made in reference to the original prescription. Indicate on the original prescription the new prescription number, the date of the part-fill, the quantity dispensed, and the pharmacist's initials. • Transfers not permitted. • Exempted codeine compounds when dispensed pursuant to a prescription follow the same regulations as for verbal prescription narcotics. • Record and retain all documents pertaining to all transactions for a period of at least 2 yr, in a manner that permits an audit. • Sales reports not required. • Report any loss or theft of narcotic drugs within 10 days to the Office of Controlled Substances at the address indicated on the forms.
Controlled Drugs*	
• Part I For example, amphetamines (*Dexedrine*) methylphenidate (*Ritalin*) pentobarbital (*Nembutal*) secobarbital (*Seconal, Tuinal*) preparations: 1 controlled drug + 1 or more active noncontrolled drug(s) (*Cafergot-PB*)	• Written or verbal prescriptions permitted. • Refills not permitted for verbal prescriptions. • Refills permitted for written prescriptions if the prescriber has indicated in writing the number of refills and dates for, or intervals between, refills. • Written or verbal prescriptions may be prescribed to be dispensed in divided portions (part-fills). • For refills and part-fills, copies of prescriptions should be made in reference to the original prescription. Indicate on the original prescription the new prescription number, the date of the repeat or part-fill, the quantity dispensed, and the pharmacist's initials.

(continued)

Table H Narcotic, Controlled Drugs, Benzodiazepines, and Other Targeted Substances *(Continued)*

Classification and Description	Legal Requirements
Controlled Drugs* ***(continued)***	
	• Transfers not permitted. • Record and retain all documents pertaining to all transactions for a period of at least 2 yr, in a manner that permits an audit. • Sales reports required except for controlled drug preparations. • Report any loss or theft of controlled drugs within 10 days to the Office of Controlled Substances at the address indicated on the forms.
• Part II For example, barbiturates (amobarbital, phenobarbital) butorphanol (*Stadol NS*) diethylpropion (*Tenuate*) nalbuphine (*Nubain*) phentermine (*Lonamin*) preparations: 1 controlled drug + 1 or more active noncontrolled ingredient(s) (*Fiorinal, Neo-Pause, Tecnal*)	• Written or verbal prescriptions permitted. • Refills permitted for written or verbal prescriptions if the prescriber has authorized in writing or verbally (at the time of issuance) the number of refills and dates for, or intervals between, refills. • Written or verbal prescriptions may be prescribed to be dispensed in divided portions (part-fills). • For refills and part-fills, copies of prescriptions should be made in reference to the original prescription. Indicate on the original prescription the new prescription number, the date of the repeat or part-fill, the quantity dispensed, and the pharmacist's initials.
• Part III For example, anabolic steroids (methyltestosterone, nandrolone decanoate)	• Transfers not permitted. • Record and retain all documents pertaining to all transactions for a period of at least 2 yr, in a manner that permits an audit. • Sales reports not required. • Report the loss or theft of controlled drugs within 10 days to the Office of Controlled Substances at the address indicated on the forms.
Benzodiazepines and Other Targeted Substances	
For example, alprazolam (*Xanax*) bromazepam (*Lectopam*) chlordiazepoxide (*Librium*) clobazam (*Frisium*) ethchlorvynol lorazepam (*Ativan*) mazindol meprobamate oxazepam (*Serax*)	• Written and verbal prescriptions permitted. • Refills for written or verbal prescriptions permitted if indicated by prescriber. • Part-fills permitted as per prescriber's instructions. • For refills or part-fills of prescriptions, record the following information: date of the repeat or part-fill, prescription number, quantity dispensed, and the pharmacist's initials. • Transfer of prescriptions permitted except a prescription that has been already transferred. • Record and retain all documents pertaining to all transactions for a period of at least 2 yr, in a manner that permits an audit. • Sales reports not required. • Report any loss or theft of benzodiazepines and other targeted substances within 10 days to the Office of Controlled Substances at the address indicated on the forms.

*The products noted are examples only.

Adapted with permission from the Canadian Pharmacists Association. (2004). *Compendium of pharmaceuticals and specialties* (p. A1). Ottawa, Canada: Author.

Reviewed 2004 by the Office of Controlled Substances, Health Canada.

Adverse Reactions: Reporting and Surveillance

The following is a description of the Canadian Adverse Drug Reaction Monitoring Program (CADRMP). This information is not intended to present a comprehensive review.

Reviewed 2004 by the Marketed Health Products Directorate, Health Canada (L. Loorand-Stiver).

Suspected adverse reaction reporting: Although health products are carefully tested to ensure safety and efficacy before licensing, inherent limitations of premarketing clinical trials including limited sample size, short duration of study, and controlled conditions prevent the identification of some rarely occurring adverse reactions (ARs). Therefore, until a health product is used by the general population, the effects of confounders such as comorbidities (e.g., renal or hepatic dysfunction), extremes of age, pregnancy, or the influence of concomitant drugs and therapies may only then be identified.

Reporting of suspected ARs by health professionals and consumers to Health Canada's CADRMP is a valuable source of information for the safety and efficacy of marketed health products. The identification of many rare and/or serious ARs have been based on a compilation of information submitted in suspected AR reports. It is the collection, evaluation, and investigation of these reports that contribute to changes in product safety information, and ultimately improved patient care. For more information on the CADRMP, contact the appropriate Regional AR Centre for your province as indicated on page 1045.

What to report? ARs to Canadian marketed health products including prescription, nonprescription, biological (including blood products as well as therapeutic and diagnostic vaccines), natural health, and radiopharmaceutical products are collected by the CADRMP. The Food and Drugs Act Regulations define an adverse "drug" reaction as a "noxious and unintended response to a drug which occurs at doses normally used or tested for the diagnosis, treatment, or prevention of a disease or the modification of an organic function." This includes *any* undesirable patient effect suspected to be associated with drug use. Unintended response, abuse, overdose, interaction (including drug–drug and drug–food interactions), and unusual lack of therapeutic efficacy are considered to be reportable ARs. AR reports are, for the most part, only *suspected* associations. A temporal or possible association is sufficient for a report to be made. Reporting of an AR does not imply a definitive causal link.

All suspected ARs should be reported, especially those that are:

- **Unexpected,** regardless of their severity (i.e., not consistent with the product information or labelling), or
- **Serious,** whether expected or not. The Canadian Regulations pertaining to reporting ARs for marketed drug products define a serious adverse drug reaction as "a noxious and unintended response to a drug, that occurs at any dose and that requires in-patient hospitalization or prolongation of existing hospitalization, causes congenital malformation, results in persistent or significant disability or incapacity, is life-threatening or results in death"; or
- **Reactions to recently marketed health products** (on the market for less than five years) regardless of their nature or severity.

How to report? To report a suspected AR for health products (pharmaceuticals, biologics [including blood products, therapeutic and diagnostic vaccines], natural health products, or radiopharmaceuticals) marketed in Canada, health professionals or consumers (preferably in conjunction with their health professional) should complete a copy of the reporting form provided in this section. This form may also be obtained from www.hc-sc.gc.ca/hpfb-dgpsa/tpd-dpt/adverse_e.pdf, your Regional AR Centre, or the National AR Centre (see contact information on page 1045).

Health professionals may also report ARs to the market authorization holder (i.e., manufacturer) and should indicate on the AR report sent to Health Canada if a case was also reported to the product(s)' manufacturer.

The success of the program depends on the quality and accuracy of the information submitted by the reporter.

For further information, visit www.hc-sc.gc.ca/hpfb-dgpsa/tpd-dpt/index_adverse_e.html. Readers may find the fact sheet entitled "How Adverse Reaction Information on Health Products is Used" of particular interest. It is available at www.hc-sc.gc.ca/hpfb-dgpsa/tpd-dpt/fact_adr_e.html.

Electronic subscription to the Canadian Adverse Drug Reaction Newsletter and drug advisories is now available: You may now join the Health_Prod_Info mailing list to subscribe electronically to this Newsletter and to receive notices of health professional advisories. Go to www.hc-sc.gc.ca/hpfb-dgpsa/tpd-dpt/subscribe_e.html.

Regional AR Centres

To facilitate the receipt of drug safety information, health professionals and consumers may use the following toll-free numbers to report ARs. Calls will be automatically routed to the appropriate regional or national AR centre.
Telephone: 1-866-234-2345
Fax: 1-866-678-6789

British Columbia
British Columbia Region AR Centre
c/o BC Drug and Poison Information Centre
1081 Burrard St.
Vancouver BC V6Z 1Y6
Tel.: (604) 806-8625
Fax: (604) 806-8262
Email: adr@dpic.ca

Saskatchewan
Saskatchewan Regional AR Centre
c/o Saskatchewan Drug Information Service
College of Pharmacy and Nutrition
University of Saskatchewan
110 Science Place
Saskatoon SK S7N 5C9
Tel.: (306) 966-6329
Fax: (306) 966-2286
Email: Sask.AR@usask.ca

Ontario
Ontario Regional AR Centre
c/o LonDIS Drug Information Centre
London Health Sciences Centre
339 Windermere Road
London ON N6A 5A5
Tel.: (519) 663-8801
Fax: (519) 663-2968
Email: adr@lhsc.on.ca

Quebec
Quebec Regional AR Centre
Drug Information Centre
Hôpital du Sacré-Coeur de Montréal
5400, boul. Gouin ouest
Montréal QC H4J 1C5
Tel.: (514) 338-2961
Fax: (514) 338-3670
Email: pharmacovigilance.hsc@ssss.gouv.qc.ca

Atlantic
Atlantic Regional AR Centre For New Brunswick, Nova Scotia, Prince Edward Island, Newfoundland and Labrador
c/o Queen Elizabeth II Health Sciences Centre
Drug Information Centre
1796 Summer St., Rm. 2421
Halifax NS B3H 3A7
Tel.: (902) 473-7171
Fax: (902) 473-8612
Email: adr@cdha.nshealth.ca

All other provinces and territories
National AR Centre
Marketed Health Products Safety and Effectiveness Information Division
Marketed Health Products Directorate
Tunney's Pasture
Address locator: 0701C Ottawa ON K1A 0K9
Tel.: (613) 957-0337
Fax: (613) 957-0335
Email: cadrmp@hc-sc.gc.ca

Adapted with permission from the Canadian Pharmacists Association. (2004). *Compendium of pharmaceuticals and specialties* (p. A7). Ottawa, Canada: Author.

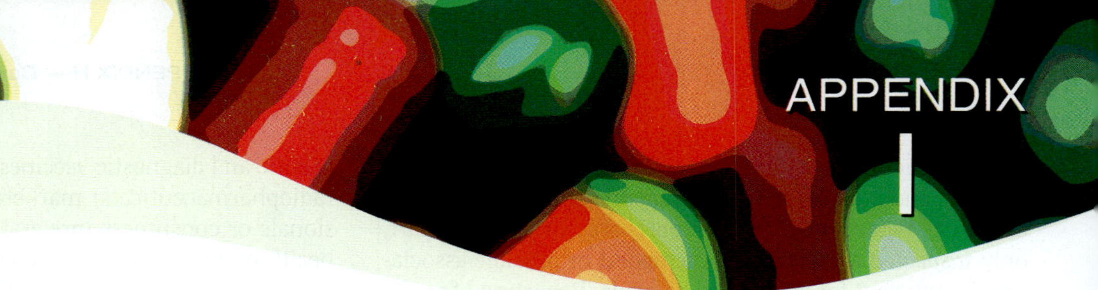

Canadian National Advisory Committee on Immunization (NACI) Recommended Immunization Schedule for Infants, Children, and Youth March 16, 2005

This is an update of the NACI Recommended Routine Immunization Schedule for Infants and Children published in the *Canadian Immunization Guide, 6th Edition* (2002). Publicly funded immunization programs may vary by province and territory. For more information on specific vaccines and on the NACI recommended immunization schedules for children who did not commence their immunization in early infancy, please consult the *Canadian Immunization Guide, 6th Edition* (2002) (http://www.phac-aspc.gc.ca/publicat/cig-gci/index.html) and the vaccine manufacturer's package insert.

Age at vaccination	DTaP-IPV	Hib	MMR	Var	Hep B	Pneu-C	Men-C	dTap	Flu
Birth					Infancy 3 doses				
2 months	○	✳			★	◈	◗		
4 months	○	✳				◈	◗		
6 months	○	✳				◈	◗ or		6–23 months
12 months			■	❖		◈ 12–15 months	◗ if not yet given		◆ 1–2 doses
18 months	○	✳	■ or		or				
4–6 years	○		■						
14–16 years					Pre-teen/teen 2–3 doses if not yet given		◗ if not yet given	🌢	

○	**DTaP-IPV**	Diphtheria, Tetanus, acellular Pertussis, and inactivated Polio virus vaccine
✳	**Hib**	Haemophilus Influenzae type b conjugate vaccine
■	**MMR**	Measles, mumps and rubella vaccine
❖	**Var**	Varicella vaccine
★	**Hep B**	Hepatitis B vaccine
◈	**Pneu-C**	Pneumococcal conjugate vaccine
◗	**Men-C**	Meningococcal C conjugate vaccine
🌢	**dTap**	Diphtheria, Tetanus, acellular Pertussis vaccine (adult formulation)
♦	**Flu**	Influenza Vaccine

Notes

○ **Diphtheria, tetanus, acellular pertussis, and inactivated polio virus vaccine (DTaP-IPV):** DTaP-IPV vaccine is the preferred vaccine for all doses in the vaccination series, including completion of the series in children who have received one dose of DPT (whole cell) vaccine (e.g., recent immigrants).

✳ ***Haemophilus influenzae*** **type b conjugate vaccine (Hib):** Hib schedule shown is for the Haemophilus b capsular polysaccharide (PRP), conjugated to tetanus toxoid (*Act-HIB*) or the Haemophilus b oligosaccharide conjugate (HbOC) (*HibTITER*) vaccines.

■ **Measles, mumps, and rubella vaccine (MMR):** A second dose of MMR is recommended, at least 1 month after the first dose for the purpose of better measles protection. For convenience, options include giving it with the next scheduled vaccination at 18 months of age or at school entry (4–6 years) (depending on the provincial/territorial policy), or at any intervening age that is practical. The need for a second dose of mumps and rubella vaccine is not established but may benefit (given for convenience as MMR). The second dose of MMR should be given at the same visit as DTaP-IPV (± Hib) to ensure high uptake rates.

❖ **Varicella vaccine (Var):** Children aged 12 months to 12 years should receive one dose of varicella vaccine. Individuals 13 years of age or older should receive two doses at least 28 days apart.

◆ **Influenza vaccine (Flu):** Previously unvaccinated children in the 6 to 23-month age group require two doses with an interval of at least 4 weeks. The second dose is not required if the child has received one or more doses of influenza vaccine during the previous immunization season.

★ **Hepatitis B vaccine (Hep B):** Hepatitis B vaccine can be routinely given to infants or preadolescents, depending on the provincial/territorial policy. For infants born to chronic carrier mothers, the first dose should be given at birth (with hepatitis B immunoglobulin); otherwise, the first dose can be given at 2 months of age to fit more conveniently with other routine infant immunization visits. The second dose should be administered at least 1 month after the first dose, and the third at least 2 months after the second dose, but again may fit more conveniently into the 4- and 6-month immunization visits. A two-dose schedule for adolescents is an option.

◈ **Pneumococcal conjugate vaccine—7-valent (Pneu-C):** Recommended schedule, number of doses, and subsequent use of 23-valent polysaccharide pneumococcal vaccine depend on the age of the child when vaccination is begun.

◗ **Meningococcal C conjugate vaccine (Men-C):** Recommended schedule and number of doses of meningococcal vaccine depend on the age of the child. If the provincial/territorial policy is to give Men-C after 12 months of age, one dose is sufficient.

🌢 **Diphtheria, tetanus, acellular pertussis vaccine—adult/adolescent formulation (dTap):** A combined adsorbed "adult-type" preparation for use in people 7 years of age or older contains less diphtheria toxoid and pertussis antigens than preparations given to younger children and is less likely to cause reactions in older people.

Index

Note: Page numbers followed by f indicate figures; those followed by t indicate tables; and those followed by b indicate boxed text.

B

C

E

F

G

H

M

N

O

P

S

T